Evolve®

W9-CDA-750

YOU'VE JUST PURCHASED

MORE THAN A TEXTBOOK!

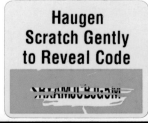

Evolve Student Resources for *Ulrich & Canale's Nursing care planning guides, 8th Edition*, include the following:

- **Online Care Planner**
  Build, edit, and print a customized care plan by choosing from more than 30 nursing diagnoses from the 8th edition of *Ulrich & Canale's Nursing Care Planning Guides*. Select each set of Diagnoses, Outcomes, and Interventions you wish to include in the care plan.

- **Additional Care Plans** ☺▶
  Choose from 14 nursing care plans and disorder care plans for further study and guidance.

- **Animations/Videos**
  Review 67 detailed pathophysiology animations and 36 skills videos.

Activate the complete learning experience that comes with each textbook purchase by registering at

http://evolve.elsevier.com/Haugen/careplanning/

Haugen
Scratch Gently to Reveal Code

REGISTER TODAY!

ELSEVIER

You can now purchase Elsevier products on Evolve!
Go to evolve.elsevier.com/shop to search and browse for products.

2018v1.0

Ulrich & Canale's

NURSING CARE PLANNING GUIDES

Prioritization, Delegation, and Clinical Reasoning

8th Edition

Nancy Haugen, PhD, RN
Associate Professor and Associate Dean
Prelicensure and Undergraduate Programs
School of Nursing
Samuel Merritt University
Oakland, California

Sandra J. Galura, PhD, RN, CCRP
Assistant Professor
College of Nursing
University of Central Florida
Orlando, Florida

ELSEVIER

ULRICH AND CANALE'S NURSING CARE PLANNING GUIDES:
PRIORITIZATION, DELEGATION, AND CLINICAL REASONING,
EIGHTH EDITION

ISBN: 978-0-323-59542-1

Copyright © 2020, by Elsevier Inc. All rights reserved.
Previous editions copyrighted 2011, 2005, 2001, 1998, 1994, 1990, 1986

All rights reserved. No part of this publication may be reproduced or transmitted in any form or by any means, electronic or mechanical, including photocopying, recording, or any information storage and retrieval system, without permission in writing from the publisher. Details on how to seek permission, further information about the Publisher's permissions policies and our arrangements with organizations such as the Copyright Clearance Center and the Copyright Licensing Agency, can be found at our website: www.elsevier.com/permissions.

This book and the individual contributions contained in it are protected under copyright by the Publisher (other than as may be noted herein).

T. Heather Herdman/Shigemi Kamitsuru (Eds.), NANDA International, Inc. Nursing Diagnoses: Definitions and Classification 2018-2020, Eleventh Edition © 2017 NANDA International, ISBN 978-1-62623-929-6. Used by arrangement with the Thieme Group, Stuttgart/New York.

Notices

Knowledge and best practice in this field are constantly changing. As new research and experience broaden our understanding, changes in research methods, professional practices, or medical treatment may become necessary.

Practitioners and researchers must always rely on their own experience and knowledge in evaluating and using any information, methods, compounds, or experiments described herein. In using such information or methods they should be mindful of their own safety and the safety of others, including parties for whom they have a professional responsibility.

With respect to any drug or pharmaceutical products identified, readers are advised to check the most current information provided (i) on procedures featured or (ii) by the manufacturer of each product to be administered, to verify the recommended dose or formula, the method and duration of administration, and contraindications. It is the responsibility of practitioners, relying on their own experience and knowledge of their patients, to make diagnoses, to determine dosages and the best treatment for each individual patient, and to take all appropriate safety precautions.

To the fullest extent of the law, neither the Publisher nor the authors, contributors, or editors assume any liability for any injury and/or damage to persons or property as a matter of products liability, negligence or otherwise, or from any use or operation of any methods, products, instructions, or ideas contained in the material herein.

ISBN: 978-0-323-59542-1

Executive Content Strategists: Kellie White/Lee Henderson
Content Development Manager: Lisa Newton
Publishing Services Manager: Jameel Shereen
Project Manager: Nadhiya Sekar
Design Direction: Patrick Ferguson

Printed in the United States
Last digit is the print number: 9 8 7 6 5 4 3 2 1

ELSEVIER

3251 Riverport Lane
St. Louis, Missouri 63043

Working together
to grow libraries in
developing countries

www.elsevier.com • www.bookaid.org

To my husband David and my children Jeffery and Sara
Thank you for your love and support. You are my pride and joy!
—Nancy Haugen

To my son Jacob, husband Mike, and all of my past and current students who
continue to challenge me to be the very best at whatever role I assume!
—Sandra J. Galura

About the Authors

Nancy Haugen, PhD, RN, has more than 35 years of experience in nursing and nursing education. She has clinical experience in medical-surgical nursing, obstetrics, critical care, and post anesthesia care and nursing research. She has also worked in health care facilities as the Director of Education, Infection Control, and Employee Health. Dr. Haugen's academic experience includes teaching in associate degree, generic baccalaureate degree, and accelerated baccalaureate degree programs. Her areas of teaching include medical-surgical nursing, health assessment, pharmacology, and pathophysiology. Dr. Haugen is currently an Associate Professor and Associate Dean, Prelicensure and Undergraduate Programs in the School of Nursing at Samuel Merritt University, in Oakland, California. She received her ASN and BSN from Southern Adventist University, her MN from Louisiana State University, and her PhD from the University of Florida. She is a member of Sigma Theta Tau International, Nu XI chapter.

Sandra J. Galura, PhD, RN, CCRP, has more than 30 years of clinical and leadership experience in critical care, post anesthesia nursing practice, and nursing research. She is currently an Assistant Professor in the College of Nursing at the University of Central Florida in Orlando, Florida. Dr. Galura's academic experience includes teaching in associate degree, baccalaureate, and master's degree nursing programs. Her current areas of teaching include nursing leadership and management. She received her BSN from Troy University in Troy, Alabama, and her MSN and PhD from the University of Central Florida in Orlando, Florida. She is active both locally and nationally in professional organizations including the American Society of PeriAnesthesia Nurses (ASPAN) where she has served as a member of multiple committees at the local, state, and national level. She is a member of Sigma Theta Tau International, Theta Epsilon chapter.

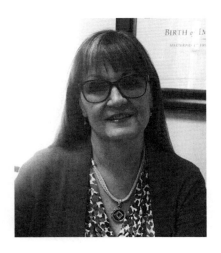

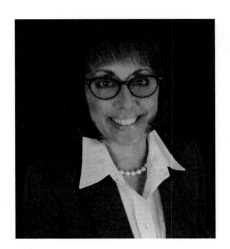

Reviewers

Mary Pinto Englert, DNP, NP-C, CNE
Nursing Faculty
College of Health Professions
Western Governors University
Salt Lake City, Utah

Michelle L. Finch, PhD, RN, CPN
Assistant Professor
Nursing
Middle Tennessee State University
Murfreesboro, Tennessee

Christina D. Keller, MSN, RN, CHSE
Instructor, Clinical Simulation Center
School of Nursing
Radford University
Radford, Virginia

Melissa A. Layne, MSN, RN
Capito Department of Nursing
Bert Bradford Department of Health Sciences
University of Charleston
Charleston, West Virginia

Rosemary Macy, PhD, RN, CNE, CHSE
Associate Professor
Nursing
Boise State University
Boise, Idaho

Nancy Noble, MSN, RN, CNE
Associate Professor
Nursing
Marian University
Fond Du Lac, Wisconsin

Charles D. "Chad" Rogers, MSN, APRN, FNP-C
Associate Professor of Nursing
Nursing
Morehead State University
Morehead, Kentucky

Preface

Ulrich and Canale's Nursing Care Planning Guides provide a comprehensive guide for the planning of nursing care for adults with common and chronic medical-surgical conditions. The care plans provided include information that is applicable to clients receiving nursing care in acute care, community, extended care, and home care settings. The book includes the most recent NANDA International (NANDA-I)–approved nursing diagnoses, Nursing Outcomes Classification (NOC), and Nursing Interventions Classification (NIC) labels.

Each of the care plans in the book provide a description of the medical condition or surgery and identifies the relevant nursing diagnoses and collaborative diagnoses. For each diagnosis there is a specific etiology statement, a desired outcome, NIC and NOC, and a comprehensive list of nursing actions. This edition provides comprehensive etiology statements, comprehensive coverage of potential complications (collaborative diagnoses), and thorough client teaching. The content represents standards of nursing care and can be used as a guide for students and practitioners in planning individualized client-centered care.

Chapter 1 discusses prioritization, management, and delegation of nursing care. It can be used as a guide on how to prioritize, manage, and delegate nursing care and how to modify and individualize nursing care plans. Included in the chapter is a step-by-step approach to delegating nursing actions to both patient care assistants and licensed practical or vocational nurses. Guidelines are provided for modifying and individualizing nursing care using a case-study approach to demonstrate the components of the nursing process used to provide individualized client-centered care.

Chapter 2 focuses on nurse-sensitive indicators that reflect the structure (supply and skill level of nursing staff), processes (assessment, intervention), and outcomes (patient outcomes) of nursing care. Nurse-sensitive indicators provide a reliable means to support and evaluate nursing care quality in the hospital setting. Hospitals use data provided by measures of nurse-sensitive indicators to evaluate, improve, and demonstrate nursing care quality. Improving nursing care quality improves patient outcomes while reducing costs associated with patient care. The nurse-sensitive indicators examined in this chapter include falls, hospital-acquired pressure ulcers (HAPU), and hospital acquired conditions (HACs) including catheter-associated urinary tract infections (CAUTI), central-line associated bloodstream infections (CLABSI), and ventilator acquired pneumonia (VAP).

Chapter 3 presents frequently used nursing diagnoses. Importantly, this unit includes the rationale for nursing actions that provides the nursing student and practitioner with a strong understanding of how each intervention helps to achieve a positive, client-centered outcome. Information accompanying each nursing diagnosis in this unit includes: NANDA-I–definition, related factors or risk factors, defining characteristics, desired outcomes, documentation criteria, and suggested NIC interventions and NOC outcomes. Information provided in this chapter can facilitate the planning of care for a client with a medical-surgical condition not addressed in this text.

Chapter 4 focuses on care of the client having surgery. The chapter includes standardized care plans on procedural sedation and preoperative and postoperative nursing care.

Chapters 5 through 15 include care plans that provide information regarding conditions and/or treatment modalities. These chapters are divided according to body systems. Care plans within each chapter deal with conditions often seen in health care settings. The care plans in Chapter 15 cover treatment modalities for specific neoplastic disorders.

Chapter 16 focuses on care of the elderly client. It includes the nursing diagnoses that reflect the biopsychosocial changes that commonly occur with the aging process and can be intensified with the stress of illness. The information is applicable to care of the elderly in all health care settings and can be used independently or in combination with care plans appropriate to the client's concurrent medical condition(s) and/or surgical situation.

Chapter 17 focuses on care at the end of life. The information applies clients in acute and community care settings. Nursing diagnoses included in the care plans are those common to all persons facing death and should be used in conjunction with care plans pertinent to the client's specific medical diagnoses.

Each of the standardized care plans in this book can be used to plan care for a client with a medical condition not covered in this text. The content in each care plan is organized in a traditional nursing care plan format that can readily be adapted to other plan-of-care formats used by health care providers (e.g., critical pathways, clinical practice guidelines, nursing protocols). Each care plan is organized as follows:

INTRODUCTION

The reader is provided with an overview of the condition including a basic definition and pathophysiological mechanisms involved and/or a description of the surgical procedure and/or selected treatment modality. This overview is not a substitute for the information provided in medical-surgical nursing texts or other references, but rather provides a quick review or a beginning point for additional research.

OUTCOME/DISCHARGE CRITERIA

When client care is provided, the nurse should focus on the outcomes required to support return to optimal health. This section includes outcome criteria that serve as a guide for determining the client's readiness for discharge from the specific health care setting. Recognizing that client education is a vital aspect of health care, the authors use client outcomes as the basis for detailed teaching included at the end of each care plan.

NURSING AND COLLABORATIVE DIAGNOSES

The nursing and collaborative diagnoses for each plan of care describe actual or potential health problems a client with a particular condition may experience. Nursing diagnoses were selected from those approved by NANDA-I through 2020 and are indicated with the **NDx** symbol. Nursing diagnoses that are not unique to a particular condition but may be relevant for a client (e.g., spiritual distress) have not consistently been included but should be considered when individualizing each care plan. Collaborative diagnoses have been included to incorporate potential client alterations for which there are no established nursing diagnostic labels. Pathophysiological and psychosocial factors are provided for the majority of nursing and collaborative diagnoses. As with other portions of the standardized care plans, these etiologies are to be individualized for each client. In most instances, the authors did not include etiologies for the nursing diagnosis labels that deal directly with client teaching (i.e., deficient knowledge, ineffective health maintenance, ineffective health management) because of the numerous individual variables that may affect a client's ability to learn, maintain health, and manage his/her treatment regimen.

In order to provide consistency in the care plans, the nursing and collaborative diagnoses statements have usually been listed in the same order. Within each care plan, an effort has been made to prioritize the diagnoses; however, individual patient circumstances may necessitate reprioritization. Priorities will need to be established by the student and practitioner based on the individual client's current needs.

CLINICAL MANIFESTATIONS

The clinical manifestations for the nursing and collaborative diagnosis provide assessment criteria for the client. Clinical manifestations are differentiated between subjective and objective manifestations and supporting data is provided for selection and prioritization of the appropriate nursing diagnosis.

DESIRED OUTCOMES

The desired outcomes for all diagnoses include evaluation criteria to evaluate effectiveness of care provided. The student and practitioner should modify goals and specific outcome criteria as needed to reflect what is realistic to maintain client-centered care. Target dates for the desired outcomes are not included as these are determined in collaboration with the patient and based on the client's current status.

SUGGESTED NIC AND NOC LABELS

Suggested Nursing Interventions Classification (NIC) and the Nursing Outcomes Classification (NOC) are listed for the nursing diagnoses in each care plan. These classification systems are included to demonstrate how they are linked to nursing diagnoses and to increase awareness and use of standardized outcome criteria and for determining nursing interventions in the care planning process.

NURSING ASSESSMENT, NURSING ACTIONS, AND SELECTED PURPOSES/RATIONALES

These columns contain nursing actions/interventions that can assist the client to achieve desired outcomes. The actions include detailed assessments based on clinical manifestations associated with each diagnostic label as identified in the literature and/or as defined by NANDA-I. These assessments can be used to determine if the nursing or collaborative diagnosis is an actual problem or if the client is at risk for developing it. The nursing interventions are specific and realistic yet broad enough to allow for regional and multidisciplinary variations in standards of care. Rationales have been included to clarify actions that may not be fundamental nursing knowledge.

CLIENT TEACHING/CONTINUED CARE

Although client teaching is included throughout the care plans, the majority of the teaching is found in the actions for the nursing diagnoses of deficient knowledge, ineffective health maintenance, ineffective health management, and/or ineffective family health management. Included client teaching uses terminology that most clients can understand.

ONLINE RESOURCES

The eighth edition's companion ⊖volve website provides even more planning and study resources. The *Online Care Planner* offers access to all of the nursing diagnoses care plans printed in the edition in electronic format, allowing users to build care plans for specific conditions by selecting and customizing nursing diagnoses. All care plans can then be saved to another location and printed. Additional in-depth care plans are provided on the ⓔvolve website. A comprehensive list of all care plans, both print and electronic, is located inside the front cover of this book. In addition, the companion website now also features more than 100 narrated, 3-D, pathophysiology-based animations that correspond to disorders content in the text.

The value of a systematic approach to individualized client-centered care is measured by its effect on the quality of care provided to the client. While overall care of a client is coordinated, and planned by registered nurses, many interventions are delegated to licensed and unlicensed members of the health care delivery team. Within each care plan, actions that can be delegated to licensed practical nurse/licensed vocational nurse (LPN/LVN) or nursing assistive personnel are indicated with a(*) at the bottom of each page. Although actions may be indicated as delegatable, students and practitioners should consult their individual state's Nurse Practice Act as well as organizational policies when deciding whether to delegate nursing interventions.

The authors hope that the eighth edition of this book will assist with the integration of the numerous aspects of client-centered care, facilitate critical thinking and implementation of the nursing process, and provide both the student and the practitioner with a guide for planning and implementing high-quality client care.

ACKNOWLEDGMENTS

The authors of the eighth edition of *Ulrich & Canale's Nursing Care Planning Guides* would like to acknowledge the work by reviewers of this text. Updating and revising a book of this scope is no small undertaking; however, it cannot be done without external feedback. We would also like to acknowledge all the nurses who continue to develop and revise, the NANDA-I diagnoses. Their work provides all nurses with tools by which they can improve client-centered care.

Contents

*For a full, detailed care plan on this topic, go to http://evolve/elsevier.com/Haugen/careplanning/

Prioritization, Delegation, and Critical Thinking in Client Management

The management and provision of nursing care is an exciting, challenging, and rewarding experience. Nurses practice in a variety of care settings as critical members of an interdisciplinary health care team. The delivery of nursing care is accomplished with registered nurses (RNs), licensed vocational nurses (LVNs)/licensed practical nurses (LPNs), and unlicensed assistive personnel. The RN is responsible for management of client care and includes clinical decision making and proper delegation of client care to other members of the care delivery team. While each member of the team plays an important role in the care of the client, it is the RN's responsibility to determine which nursing interventions are to be safely assigned and/or delegated to specific team members.

PRIORITIZATION

The nurse is responsible for prioritizing and individualizing a client's plan of care. Prioritization is defined as " deciding which needs or problems require immediate action and which ones could tolerate a delay in response until a later time because they are not urgent". (L Silvestri and A Silvestri, 2017, p. 67). The RN must use all steps in the nursing process and collaborate with the client to individualize care. Interventions should be client-centered and prioritized to achieve optimum client outcomes. However, planning care that is prioritized, client-centered, and comprehensive can be challenging owing to lack of time and adequate resources.

Alfaro-LeFevre (2017, p. 170) provides steps for setting nursing priorities. All priority setting should be determined through the lens of maintaining patient and care giver safety. The first level priority setting is to maintain airway, breathing, and circulation. Additional priority setting includes identification and treatment of abnormal vital signs and life-threatening lab values. Second level client priorities include issues related to mental health changes, untreated medical problems, pain, and urinary elimination problems. Lastly, the nurse should address any health challenges that do not fall into the other categories.

An additional level of priority setting includes Maslow's hierarchy of needs, which spans the continuum from the most crucial needs necessary for survival to self-actualization. Physiologic needs necessary for the continued function of the human body often require the greatest attention when client care is being prioritized. However, attention to safety needs, such as the prevention of accidents and adverse client outcomes, must be considered a high priority as long as the client's physiologic needs have been stabilized.

DELEGATION

Both the National Council of State Boards of Nursing (NCSBN) and the American Nurses Association (ANA) define delegation as "the process for a nurse to direct another person to perform nursing tasks and activities" (ANA and NCSBN, 2017, p. 1). Nurses responsible for delegation must be aware of many variables aside from the client's condition. To safely and appropriately delegate nursing care, the nurse must have an understanding of the appropriate state's Nurse Practice Act, which identifies which tasks may be delegated, when the tasks may be delegated, and to whom the tasks may be delegated.

The first step in the delegation process is assessment of the client. In addition, to delegate safely, the nurse must assess the qualifications of each member of the health care delivery team. Once the nurse determines the client's condition and the tasks to be delegated, he or she then identifies the team member to whom the task will be delegated based on an understanding of the member's qualifications and skills. Once the tasks to be delegated have been determined, the nurse must communicate the actions to the team member, including what to do, when to do it, and to whom it should be done. These individuals should also be informed of the circumstances under which they should ask for assistance. Clear communication in the transfer of information is critical, so that each person has a complete understanding of the delegated task as well as of the conditions that require the assistance of an RN. The Five Rights of Delegation (ANA and NCSBN, 2017) summarize the process and include the following:

1. The right task
2. Under the right circumstance
3. To the right person
4. With the right directions and communication
5. Under the right supervision and evaluation

Although the RN is responsible for the safe delegation of nursing tasks to the appropriate team members, responsibility and accountability for the safe completion of interventions are not delegated and remain the ultimate responsibility of the RN. The nurse must monitor the implementation of the task and determine whether the task was completed appropriately and in a timely manner. After the completion of delegated tasks, the nurse must evaluate both the delegation process and the client outcomes. Questions that should be answered in evaluating this process include the following:

Was the task delegated to the appropriate individual?

Did that individual perform the task correctly and in a timely manner?

Was the expected client outcome achieved?

Was the client satisfied with the care received?

Was the communication between the nurse and the team member appropriate to accomplish the required intervention?

What if anything did not go as planned, and what could have prevented this from occurring?

The algorithm in Fig. 1.1 may serve to assist the nurse in the delegation process.

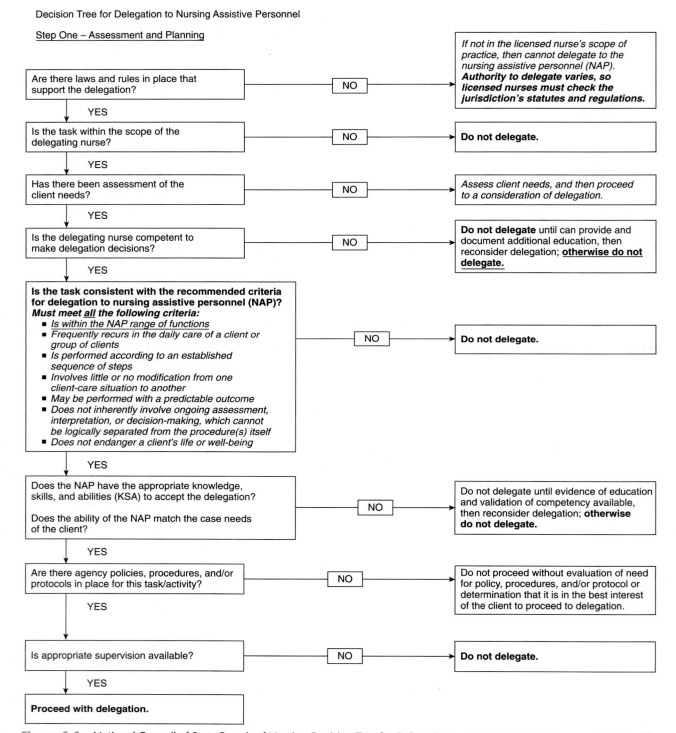

Figure 1-1   National Council of State Boards of Nursing Decision Tree for Delegation to Nursing Assistive Personnel.   From the American Nurses Association and the National Council of State Boards of Nursing: *Joint statement on delegation* [2005]. https://www.nursingworld.org/practice-policy/nursing-excellence/official-position-statements/id/joint-statement-on-delegation-by-ANA-and-NCSBN/. Accessed March 16, 2017.

Step Two – Communication

Communication must be a two-way process.

The nurse:	The NAP:	Documentation:

▪ Assesses the assistant's understanding
  ○ How the task is to be accomplished
  ○ When and what information is to be reported, including:
    ✓ Expected observations to report and record
    ✓ Specific client concerns that would require prompt reporting
▪ Individualizes for the NAP and client situation
▪ Addresses any unique client requirements and characteristics, and clear expectations of:
  ○ Assesses the assistant's understanding of expectations, providing clarification if needed
  ○ Communicates his or her willingness and availability to guide and support assistant
  ○ Assures appropriate accountability by verifying that the receiving person accepts the delegation and accompanying responsibility
	▪ **Asks questions regarding the delegation and seeks clarification of expectations if needed**
	▪ Informs the nurse if the assistant has not done a task/function/activity before, or has only done infrequently
	▪ Asks for additional training or supervision
	▪ Affirms understanding of expectations
	▪ Determines the communication method between the nurse and the NAP
	▪ Determines the communication and plan of action in emergency situations
		Timely, complete, and accurate documentation of provided care:
		▪ Facilitates communication with other members of the health care team
		▪ Records the nursing care provided

Step Three – Surveillance and Supervision

The purpose of surveillance and monitoring is related to nurse's responsibility for client care within the context of a client population. The nurse supervises the delegation by monitoring the performance of the task or function and assures compliance with standards of practice, policies, and procedures. Frequency, level, and nature of monitoring vary with needs of client and experience of assistant.

The nurse considers the:	The nurse determines:	The nurse is responsible for:

▪ Client's health care status and stability of condition
▪ Predictability of responses and risks
▪ Setting where care occurs
▪ Availability of resources and support infrastructure
▪ <u>Complexity of the task being performed</u>
	▪ The frequency of onsite supervision and assessment based on:
	  ○ Needs of the client
	  ○ Complexity of the delegated function/task/activity
	  ○ Proximity of nurse's location
		▪ Timely intervening and follow-up on problems and concerns. Examples of the need for intervening include:
		  ○ Alertness to subtle signs and symptoms (which allows nurse and assistant to be proactive before a client's condition deteriorates significantly)
		  ○ Awareness of assistant's difficulties in completing delegated activities
		  ○ Providing adequate follow-up to problems and/or changing situations is critical aspect of delegation

Step Four – Evaluation and Feedback

Evaluation is often the forgotten step in delegation.

In considering the effectiveness of delegation, the nurse addresses the following question:

▪ Was the delegation successful?
  ○ Was the task/function/activity performed correctly?
  ○ Was the client's desired and/or expected outcome achieved?
  ○ Was the outcome optimal, satisfactory, or unsatisfactory?
  ○ Was communication timely and effective?
  ○ What went well? What was challenging?
  ○ Were there any problems or concerns? If so, how were they addressed?
▪ Is there a better way to meet the client need?
▪ Is there a need to adjust the overall plan of care, or should this approach be continued?
▪ Were there any "learning moment" for the assistant and/or the nurse?
▪ Was appropriate feedback provided to the assistant regarding the performance of the delegation?
▪ Was the assistant acknowledged for accomplishing the task/activity/function?

Figure 1-1, cont'd

CRITICAL THINKING

To deliver client-centered, prioritized, individualized, and safe nursing care, the professional nurse must be able to think critically by analyzing information. This information is obtained from multiple sources to determine the best plan of action that will safely and effectively meet the client's basic physiologic needs. Critical thinking is composed of attitudes, knowledge, and skills.

The attitude of inquiry enables the professional nurse to recognize the existence of a client problem and to seek out both assessment and collaborative data that describe the encountered problem. Knowledge enables the professional nurse to weigh the accuracy of different kinds of evidence as the client's plan of care is altered to address prioritized problems. Finally, skill enables the professional nurse to apply both inquiry and knowledge in the delivery of safe client-centered care.

The nursing process (assess, diagnose, plan, implement, evaluate) provides a framework by which the professional nurse can connect clinical events and data obtained from a variety of sources with the appropriate interventions to safely manage and evaluate client care.

This book is intended to facilitate the care planning process with adults with common and recurring medical-surgical conditions. Within each care plan specific interventions are identified that may be delegated to members of the nursing care team. Within each care plan are nursing and collaborative diagnoses with etiologic factors, desired outcomes with measurable behavioral criteria, and independent and dependent nursing actions and delegable actions with selected purposes or rationales. Safe, comprehensive care can be planned in a minimal amount of time using this book.

CREATING AN INDIVIDUALIZED, PRIORITIZED PLAN OF CARE

To be most effective, the standardized nursing care plan must be adapted in collaboration with the client to meet his or her individual needs. A process for planning individualized, prioritized client care follows:

1. Read the nurse's admission assessment/history information and the medication administration record of the assigned client.
2. Review the history, current lab, and diagnostic test results; nurses' notes for the last 48 hrs; progress notes of health care providers (e.g., physician, dietitian, physical and occupational therapists, pain management specialist, social worker, discharge planner), and current consultation reports.
3. Interview the client and complete an assessment using the tool provided by your nursing school or health care facility. Discuss with clients what they would like to be the focused outcome of their care.
4. Read about the client's medical diagnosis and appropriate nursing care in a current medical-surgical nursing text.
5. Select the appropriate standardized care plan or plans from this text and read the introductory information at the beginning of each care plan.
6. Select the nursing and collaborative diagnoses that are appropriate for your client and supported by assessment findings; choose the etiologic factors that are relevant and modify them as appropriate.
7. Modify the collaboratively identified and desired outcomes so that they are measurable and realistic for your client; establish appropriate target dates.
8. Select and prioritize the nursing actions that are relevant to the client's immediate care needs; add to or modify the actions required to meet these needs; include specific medications and treatments as well as client preferences and other actions that will facilitate achievement of the desired client outcomes.
9. Determine whether the client is stable and to which team member nursing interventions may be delegated.
10. Communicate delegable actions to the appropriately qualified individual.
11. Evaluate the delegation process, the quality of the delegated task, and client outcomes.

The following situation serves to illustrate how these standardized nursing care plans can be used by the student and the practitioner in planning individualized client care.

Mary G. is a 30-year-old woman hospitalized following a spinal cord injury suffered in a motor vehicle collision (MVC). She has been bedridden for the past 3 weeks due to a thoracic spine injury at the T-10 level. It resulted in paraplegia. The client has improving upper body strength, movement of the upper extremities, and diminished respiratory capacity and endurance. She has two children between the ages of 3 and 6 years. Both Mary and her husband have been trying to prepare the children for Mary's physical disability. They have no other family members living nearby.

1. **Read the nurse's admission assessment/history information and the medication administration record of the assigned client.**

    It is determined that Mary is a 30-year-old married woman. Her religious preference is Protestant. Her diagnosis is spinal cord transection at T-10. She is receiving morphine sulfate, 15 mg every 8 hrs (q 8 h); Dialose, 100 mg/day; and milk of magnesia, 30 mL orally (PO) every evening.

2. **Review the history, current diagnostic test results, nurses' notes for the last 48 hrs, progress notes of health care providers (e.g., physician, dietitian, physical and occupational therapists, pain management specialist, social worker, discharge planner), and consultation reports.**

    From the history it is determined that Mary had an MVC 3 weeks ago. She is experiencing back pain related to nerve root irritation at the site of her spinal cord injury. She has been bedridden since the time of her accident. The physician's progress notes indicate that Mary's paraplegia is permanent, and the goal of care is to optimize her current physiologic state and keep her comfortable.

    Diagnostic test results reveal that Mary's red blood cell (RBC) count, hemoglobin (Hgb), hematocrit (Hct), and serum protein levels are decreased.

    The nurses' notes reveal that Mary needs assistance with all activities. She is able to feed herself but is consuming only 10% of her meals. She had a bowel movement this morning following digital stimulation. Mary has an indwelling urinary catheter, and her intake and output are balanced. She has been crying frequently and states that neither she nor her husband are coping well with her disability.

3. **Interview the client and complete an assessment using the tool provided by your nursing school or health care facility.**

    The interview and physical assessment reveal that Mary has persistent reddened areas on her left hip and coccyx; diminished breath sounds in both lung bases, shallow respirations of 24 breaths per minute; crackles (rales) in both lungs; and a cough that is productive of yellow, foul-smelling sputum. She has normal bowel sounds and states that she usually has a bowel movement every other day following digital stimulation. Mary is alert, oriented, and able to move her upper extremities. She has no movement in her lower extremities but is able to transfer herself with assistance to a wheelchair. She complains of pain in her back.

4. **Read about the client's diagnosis and nursing care in a current medical-surgical nursing text.**

   Review **Spinal Cord Injury** and **Impaired Physical Mobility. NDx**

5. **Select the appropriate standardized care plan or plans from this text and read the introductory information at the beginning of the care plans.**

   The physician has sstated that Mary's primary treatment plan is focused on optimizing her current physical condition and controlling her pain, and Mary agrees with that plan. The appropriate care plans for Mary are **Spinal Cord Injury** and **Impaired Physical Mobility.**

6. **Select and prioritize the nursing and collaborative diagnoses that are appropriate for your client. Choose the etiologic factors that are relevant and modify them as appropriate.**

   It is determined that there are numerous diagnoses and etiologic factors from the care plan on **Spinal Cord Injury.**

Examples of some of the nursing diagnoses within this care plan are as follows (the etiologic factors have been modified to reflect Mary's situation):

a. **Ineffective Breathing Pattern NDx related to**
   1. The depressant effect of narcotic (opioid) analgesics loss of abdominal and intercostal muscle function (innervation of these muscles at the thoracic level)
b. **Ineffective Airway Clearance NDx related to:**
   1. Decreased mobility, decreased effectiveness of cough resulting from diminished lung/chest wall expansion, depressant effect of narcotic (opioid) analgesics
c. **Acute/Chronic Pain NDx**: back-, rib-, and pelvic-related nerve root irritation at the site of spinal cord injury metastases
d. **Ineffective Coping NDx** related to ongoing grieving associated with spinal cord injury and its effect on body function

7. **Determine which nursing interventions may be delegated to the appropriately qualified individual within the nursing care team.**

   The process for individualization of etiologies and delegation of nursing actions is demonstrated using the nursing diagnosis of **Risk for Constipation NDx** as a prototype.

STANDARDIZED

Risk for chronic functional constipation NDx related to: **(Etiologies from the care plan on Impaired Physical Mobility NDx)**

a. Diminished defecation reflex associated with:
   1. Suppression of urge to defecate because of lack of privacy and reluctance to use bedpan
   2. Decreased gravity filling of lower rectum resulting from horizontal positioning

b. Weakened abdominal muscles associated with generalized loss of muscle tone resulting from prolonged immobility and lack of innervation
c. Decreased gastrointestinal motility associated with decreased activity and the increased sympathetic nervous system activity that occurs with anxiety

INDIVIDUALIZED

Risk for chronic functional constipation NDx related to:

a. Diminished defecation reflex associated with:
   1. Lack of awareness of stool in rectum associated with sensory loss below the level of injury
   2. Decreased gravity filling of lower rectum resulting from horizontal positioning
   3. Loss of central nervous system control over defecation reflex
b. Loss of autonomic nervous system function below the level of injury (T-10) during a period of spinal shock

c. Decreased activity

8. **Modify the desired outcomes so that they are measurable and realistic for your client. Establish appropriate target dates.**

The process for individualization of a desired outcome is demonstrated using the nursing diagnosis of **Risk for chronic functional constipation NDx** as a prototype.

STANDARDIZED

(Outcome from the care plan on Immobility)
The client will not experience constipation as evidenced by:
a. Usual frequency of bowel movements
b. Passage of soft, formed stool
c. Absence of abdominal distention and pain, feeling of rectal fullness or pressure, and straining during defecation

INDIVIDUALIZED

Mary will not experience constipation as evidenced by:
a. Passing soft, formed stool at least every other day
b. Absence of abdominal distention and abdominal pain

NDx = NANDA Diagnosis   **D** = Delegatable Action   ● = UAP   ✦ = LVN/LPN   ⊖▶ = Go to ℮volve for animation

9. **Select the nursing actions that are relevant to the client's care. Add to or modify the actions to meet the needs of your client. Include specific medications and treatments as well as client preferences and other actions that will facilitate the achievement of the desired client outcomes.**

The process for individualization of nursing actions is demonstrated below using the nursing diagnosis of risk for chronic functional constipation NDx as a prototype.

STANDARDIZED

(Actions from impaired physical mobility NDx)
a. Assess for signs and symptoms of constipation (e.g., decrease in frequency of bowel movements; passage of hard, formed stools; anorexia; abdominal distention and pain; feeling of fullness or pressure in rectum; straining during defecation).
b. Assess bowel sounds. Report a pattern of decreasing bowel sounds.
c. Implement measures to prevent constipation:
   1. Encourage client to defecate whenever the urge is felt.

   2. Place client in high Fowler's position for bowel movements unless contraindicated.
   3. Encourage client to relax, provide privacy, and have call signal within reach during attempts to defecate. (Measures to promote relaxation enable client to relax the levator ani muscle and external anal sphincter, which facilitates evacuation of stool.)
   4. Encourage client to establish a regular time for defecation, preferably within an hour after a meal.
   5. Instruct client to increase intake of foods high in fiber (e.g., bran, whole-grain breads and cereals, fresh fruits and vegetables) unless contraindicated.
   6. Instruct client to maintain a minimum fluid intake of 2500 mL/day unless contraindicated.

   7. Encourage client to drink hot liquids upon arising in the morning in order to stimulate peristalsis.
   8. Encourage client to perform isometric abdominal strengthening exercises unless contraindicated.
   9. If client is taking analgesics for pain management, encourage the use of nonnarcotic rather than narcotic (opioid) analgesics when appropriate.
   10. Increase activity as allowed.

   11. Administer laxatives or cathartics and/or enemas if ordered.
d. Consult physician about checking for an impaction and digitally removing stool if client has not had a bowel movement in 3 days, if client is passing liquid stool, or if other signs and symptoms of constipation are present.
e. Consult appropriate health care provider if signs and symptoms of constipation persist and appear to be an ongoing problem.

INDIVIDUALIZED

a. Assess Mary every shift for signs and symptoms of constipation (e.g., no bowel movement for 3 days; passage of hard, formed stools; increased anorexia; abdominal distention).

b. Assess bowel sounds. Report a pattern of decreasing bowel sounds.
c. Implement measures to prevent Mary's constipation:
   1. Encourage Mary to use regular rectal stimulation to have a regular bowel movement.
   2. Place Mary on bedpan in high Fowler's position for bowel movements.
   3. Turn on soft music, provide privacy, and have call signal within reach during attempts to defecate.

   4. Encourage Mary to attempt digital rectal stimulation about 30 minutes after breakfast.
   5. Offer bran cereal and fresh fruit for breakfast; encourage Mary to select foods high in fiber for lunch and dinner.
   6. Encourage Mary to increase her fluid intake; offer 200 mL of apple juice, orange juice, or water every hour while she is awake.
   7. Offer hot tea or hot water with lemon with breakfast.
   8. Omit; not appropriate for a client with spinal cord injury.
   9. Omit; Mary currently requires the narcotic analgesic for effective pain management.

   10. Increase passive and active range-of-motion (ROM) exercises as indicated.
   11. Administer milk of magnesia, 30 mL PO, each evening, and Dialose, 100 mg PO, each morning.
d. Consult physician about checking for an impaction and digitally removing stool if Mary has not had a bowel movement for 4 days and other signs and symptoms of constipation are present.
e. Consult appropriate health care provider if signs and symptoms of constipation occur and this appears to be an ongoing problem.

SAMPLE INDIVIDUALIZED CARE PLAN

Individualized Care Plan for Mary for the Nursing Diagnosis of Risk for Constipation NDx

DATA

Mary states had a bowel movement this morning.

Normal bowel sounds.

Physician's orders: milk of magnesia, 30 mL PO each evening; Dialose, 100 mg PO, every morning.

Bedridden for 3 weeks.

Consuming only 10% of meals.

Mary states she usually has a bowel movement every other day (QOD) about 30 minutes after breakfast.

Activity: bed rest. Mary requires assistance with all activities.

Receiving morphine sulfate every 2 hrs.

NURSING DIAGNOSIS

Risk for chronic functional constipation NDx related to:

a. Diminished defecation reflex associated with decreased nervous system responses in spinal cord injury state and decreased gravity filling of lower rectum resulting from horizontal positioning

b. Decreased ability to respond to urge to defecate associated with weakened abdominal muscles and impaired physical mobility

c. Decreased gastrointestinal motility associated with decreased activity, use of morphine sulfate, and increased sympathetic nervous system activity that occurs with anxiety and pain

d. Decreased intake of fluids and foods high in fiber

DESIRED OUTCOME

Mary will not experience constipation as evidenced by:

a. Passing a soft, formed stool at least QOD

b. Absence of abdominal distention

NURSING ACTIONS

a. Assess Mary every shift for signs and symptoms of constipation (e.g., no bowel movement for 3 days; passage of hard, formed stool; increased anorexia; abdominal distention; abdominal pain.

b. Assess bowel sounds. Report a pattern of decreasing bowel sounds.

c. Implement measures to prevent Mary's constipation. **D** ● ◆

  1. Place Mary on bedpan in high Fowler's position for bowel movements. **D** ● ◆
  2. Turn on soft music, provide privacy, and have call signal within reach during attempts to defecate. **D** ● ◆
  3. Encourage Mary to attempt to digital rectal stimulation about 30 minutes after breakfast. **D** ◆
  4. Offer bran cereal and fresh fruit for breakfast; encourage Mary to select foods high in fiber for lunch and dinner. **D** ◆
  5. Encourage Mary to increase her fluid intake; offer 200 mL of apple juice, orange juice, or water every hour while she is awake. **D** ◆
  6. Offer hot tea with breakfast. **D** ◆
  7. Administer milk of magnesia, 30 mL PO, each evening; give Dialose, 100 mg PO, each morning. **D** ◆

d. Consult physician about checking for an impaction and digitally removing stool if Mary has not had a bowel movement for 4 days and other signs and symptoms of constipation are present.

e. Consult appropriate health care provider if signs and symptoms of constipation occur and given the clients condition, constipation could be an ongoing problem.

See spinal cord injury care plan for additional nursing diagnosis.

NDx = NANDA Diagnosis   **D** = Delegatable Action   ● = UAP   ◆ = LVN/LPN   ⊜▶ = Go to ⊜volve for animation

Nurse-Sensitive Indicators

FALLS

Patient falls and falls with injury are nurse-sensitive indicators that represent both the processes and outcomes associated with quality nursing care. The National Quality Forum (NQF) defines a fall as an unplanned descent to the floor (or extension of the floor, e.g., trash can or other equipment) with or without injury to the patient. The Agency for Healthcare Research and Quality (2017) estimates that in the United States, up to 1 million hospitalized patients and approximately half of the 1.6 million nursing home residents fall each year. In addition, more than one-third of falls occurring in hospitals result in injury, including serious injury (e.g., head trauma, fractures). Falls are associated with increased length of stay, higher rates of discharge to extended care facilities, and greater health care utilization. The Centers for Medicare and Medicaid services (CMS) have identified falls as an event that is preventable and one that should never occur. As a result, falls are listed as a hospital-acquired condition (HAC) for which reimbursement is limited. In addition, the CMS does not reimburse hospitals for additional costs associated with patient falls.

There are multiple categories of risk factors associated with falls including age, gender, alterations in mobility or the use of assistive devices, medications (e.g., polypharmacy, medications for sedation, pain), alternations in mental status, medical diagnoses, and alterations in continence. Different clients may have different combinations of risk factors that change over time during hospitalization. Although client risk for falls may vary, with some being at higher risk, by virtue of illness, all patients should be considered at risk for falls.

To better understand falls in terms of contributing risk factors, researchers have classified falls into three key categories—anticipated physiologic falls, unanticipated physiologic falls, and accidental falls. Most in-hospital falls are classified as anticipated physiologic, occurring in clients identified as having risk factors for falls that can be identified in advance such as altered mental status, abnormal gait, frequent toileting, or high-risk medications. Unanticipated physiologic falls occur in clients normally of low fall risk but occur due to an event, the timing of which could not be predicted, such as a stroke, syncopal episode, or seizure. Accidental falls occur in otherwise low-risk clients, due to an environmental hazard. Some researchers have further suggested categorizing falls as either preventable or nonpreventable.

Given the patient safety challenges presented by falls, hospitals are charged with treating not only the problem that prompted admission to the hospital but keeping the patient safe, which requires balancing fall prevention with other care priorities. Successful fall prevention requires an interdisciplinary approach with some standardized interventions that include both environmental measures and clinical interventions that are individualized to each client's specific risk profile. Many health care facilities adopt standardized fall intervention "bundles" which represent the latest available evidence related to fall prevention interventions. Nurses and nurse leaders within health care organizations are tasked with and accountable for monitoring the outcome of nursing interventions aimed at fall prevention, which includes the number of falls and the number of falls with various levels of injury.

This care plan focuses on care of the adult client at risk for falls and hospitalized in an acute care setting. Given the need to balance patient safety with other care priorities, this care plan should be used in conjunction with the plan of care developed for the primary admitting diagnosis of the client. Much of this information is applicable to clients receiving follow-up care in an extended care facility or home setting.

OUTCOME/DISCHARGE CRITERIA

The client will:
1. Remain free from injury
2. Return to baseline mobility
3. Demonstrate understanding of risk factors for falls and risk reduction strategies.

Nursing Diagnosis   RISK FOR FALLS NDx

Definition: Susceptible to increased susceptibility to falling, which may cause physical harm and compromise health.

CLINICAL MANIFESTATIONS

Subjective	Objective
Expressed concern for safety during ambulation; stated history of previous falls	Unsteadiness when ambulating; use of ambulation aids; visual field deficits; confusion; orthostatic hypotension; medication therapy (e.g., antihypertensives, diuretics, hypnotics, antianxiety agents, narcotics, antidepressants); anemias, arthritis

RISK FACTORS

- Age ≥65 yr
- History of falls
- Environmental
  - Cluttered environment
  - Insufficient lighting
  - Unfamiliar setting
  - Use of restraints
- Physiologic
  - Alterations in blood glucose levels
  - Decrease in lower extremity strength (deconditioning)
- Gait difficulty
- Impaired mobility
- Incontinence/urinary urgency
- Sleeplessness
- Associated conditions
  - Acute illness
  - Alterations in cognitive function
  - Anemia
  - Arthritis
  - Hearing impairment
  - Impaired balance
- Impaired vision
- Lower limb prosthetics
- Neuropathy
- Orthostatic hypotension
- Pharmaceutic agents
- Postoperative recovery period
- Use of assistive devices
- Vascular disease

DESIRED OUTCOMES

The client will remain free from falls and injury associated with falls.

DOCUMENTATION

- Standardized fall risk assessment score
- Universal fall precaution interventions
- Mobility/ambulation; use of assistive devices
- Restraints

NURSING OUTCOMES CLASSIFICATION (NOC)

Falls prevention behavior; falls occurrence; risk detection; knowledge: personal safety

NURSING INTERVENTIONS CLASSIFICATION (NIC)

Environmental management: safety; fall prevention

NURSING ASSESSMENT

Assess client's risk for falls using standardized assessment tool (e.g., Morse Falls Scale, on admission, transfer from one care unit to another, and/or following a significant change in patient condition). Assessment should include evaluation of:
- History of falls
- Mobility problems/use of assistive devices
- Mental status
- Continence

Consult organizational policy and/or standard operating procedures for assessment frequency.

Assess client's gait, balance, and mobility skills.

Evaluate client's medications to determine whether they place the client at increased risk for falls.

RATIONALE

Determining the client's risk for falls allows implementation of standardized and individualized preventive measures. Risk factors and a client's overall risk may vary during hospitalization and should be assessed at the appropriate intervals, as defined by organizational policy and/or standard operating procedures.

Determining the client's baseline status allows for the implementation of the appropriate preventive measures.

Some medications may cause excessive drowsiness, altered mental states, or physiologic changes, such as orthostatic hypotension, that can increase the risk of falls in clients. Early identification of such medications allows for implementation of appropriate preventive measures.

THERAPEUTIC INTERVENTIONS

RATIONALE

Independent Actions

Implement scheduled rounding protocols (e.g., 5 P's - pain, personal needs, position, placement, prevent falls) according to organizational policy and/or standard operating procedure **D** ● ✦.

Hourly rounding is an excellent proactive strategy to ensure client's needs are met, potentially reducing the risk for falls.

Continued...

THERAPEUTIC INTERVENTIONS	RATIONALE

Implement measures to prevent falls: **D** ● ✦

- Orient client to surroundings (e.g., room; nurse call system).
- Instruct client to call for assistance with movement as appropriate.
- Place articles within easy reach of the client.
- Reduce clutter in client's immediate environment.
- Assist unsteady client with ambulation.
- Have client wear safe footwear when ambulating (e.g., nonskid shoes/slippers).
- Have client wear prescription glasses as appropriate.
- Ensure adequate lighting in client's room.
- Encourage client to use ambulation aids and glasses.
- Keep bed in lowest position.
- Keep bed wheels in locked position
- Use side rails of appropriate height and length.
- Keep floor surfaces clean and dry.
- Implement appropriate alerts identifying clients at high risk for falls (e.g., room signage; wrist identification bands [ID])
- Apply bed sensor pad/bed alarms.
- Apply wheelchair lap belt/safety belt as appropriate.
- Monitor client's ability to transfer to and from a bed, wheelchair, and toilet. **D** ● ✦
- Use proper technique when transferring a patient to and from a bed, wheelchair, and toilet.
- Involve family to aid with activities of daily living and prevention of falls. **D** ● ✦

Physical hazards in the client's immediate environment increase the risk for accidental injury. Falls are usually a result of both intrinsic (e.g., illness, drug therapy) and extrinsic, or environmental, factors. Extrinsic factors are much easier to modify and eliminate. Many organizations implement fall prevention "bundles" that are based on the most recent scientific evidence and are independent nursing actions. Consult organizational policy and standard operating procedures for fall prevention bundles.

Older adults are more likely to fall in the bedroom and the bathroom, with most falls occurring when transferring from beds, chairs, and toilets.

In the acute care environment, frequent observation of clients at risk for falls is necessary to reduce the risk for falls.

Dependent/Collaborative Actions

Collaborate with multidisciplinary team members to monitor and minimize side effects of medications that increase the risk of falls.

Implement the use of restraints as ordered.

Consult physical therapy for strengthening, exercises, gait training, and help with balance to increase mobility.

Notify physician of client falls.

Intrinsic factors increasing the risk of falls may be modified or eliminated if identified and discussed with the appropriate health care provider.

Avoid the use of restraints if at all possible. If restraints must be used, choose the least restrictive device and follow institutional policy for the monitoring and documentation of the client's condition.

Collaboration with other disciplines is an important part of a client's plan of care. Additional resources provided during the hospital stay, as well as in preparation for discharge, can assist the client in gaining the strength, mobility, and endurance to reduce the risk for falls.

Notifying the appropriate health care provider allows for modification of the treatment plan.

Nursing Diagnosis ## DEFICIENT KNOWLEDGE NDx

Definition: Absence of cognitive information related to a specific topic, or its acquisition.

CLINICAL MANIFESTATIONS

Subjective	Objective
Verbal self-report acknowledging lack of understanding of fall risk.	Inaccurate follow-through of instructions; insufficient knowledge

RISK FACTORS

- Alteration in cognitive function
- Insufficient interest in learning
- Insufficient information

DESIRED OUTCOMES

The client will:
- Identify ways to reduce the risk for falls
- Remain free of falls and/or injury from falls

NDx = NANDA Diagnosis   **D** = Delegatable Action   ● = UAP   ✦ = LVN/LPN   ⊖▶ = Go to ⊖volve for animation

NOC OUTCOMES	NIC INTERVENTIONS
Knowledge: personal safety	Teaching: individual; learning: readiness enhancement; learning: facilitation

NURSING ASSESSMENT	RATIONALE
Assess for client's understanding of fall risk upon admission to the hospital.	*Client engagement in his or her health care could lead to safe hospital stays. Many clients may not be aware of their risk for falls and prevention interventions.*
Assess client's ability and readiness to learn.	*Learning is more effective when the client is motivated and understands the importance of what is to be learned. Readiness to learn changes based on situations and physical and emotional challenges.*
Assess client's understanding of teaching.	*It is important for the nurse to ensure client's understanding of teaching. Further education using different instructional modalities may be necessary.*

THERAPEUTIC INTERVENTIONS	RATIONALE

Independent Actions

- Instruct client, family, and visitors regarding factors that contribute to the risk for falls in the hospital setting.
- Effects of medications
- Changes in mobility
- Deconditioning—weakness resulting from prolonged periods of bed rest
- Age
- Comorbid conditions
- Instruct and reinforce institutional fall prevention interventions that will be implemented during hospital stay—including standard interventions and interventions tailored to client's clinical condition.

Clients without alterations in mobility may not be aware of factors that may increase their risk for fall while hospitalized. Family and visitors should be included.

Instructing clients, including visitors and family members, regarding fall prevention interventions can potentially increase client engagement and adherence. Instructions may need to be reinforced frequently

ADDITIONAL NURSING DIAGNOSES

IMPAIRED PHYSICAL MOBILITY NDx
Related to:
- Physical deconditioning
- Disuse
- Reluctance to initiate movement

RISK FOR INJURY NDx
Related to:
- Physical deconditioning
- Extremes of age
- Impaired primary defense mechanisms
- Alterations in cognitive/psychomotor functioning

⊖▶ HOSPTAL ACQUIRED PRESSURE ULCERS/INJURIES

Another nurse-sensitive indicator associated with processes and outcomes related to quality nursing care is pressure ulcers (e.g., bed sores, decubitus ulcers, pressure sores). Pressure ulcers are one of the biggest challenges health care organizations face on a day-to-day basis. Pressure ulcers interfere with a client's functional recovery and may be complicated by pain and infection, contributing to longer hospital stays. Each year, more than 2.5 million people in the United States develop pressure ulcers, which bring pain, increased risk for serious infection, and increased health care utilization and costs. Approximately 60,000 patients die each year as a direct result of a pressure ulcer. In the United States, pressure ulcers costs $9.1 to $11.6 billion per year, with individual patient costs ranging from $20,900 to $151,700 per pressure ulcer. As of 2008, the CMS no longer pays for additional costs associated with hospital-acquired pressure ulcers, a potentially preventable condition.

In 2016, national definitions for pressure ulcers where redefined by the National Pressure Ulcer Advisory Panel. The updated definition changes terminology from pressure ulcer to pressure injury defined as localized damage to the skin and underlying soft tissue usually over a bony prominence or related to a medical or other device. The injury can present as intact skin, or an open ulcer and may be painful. The injury occurs as a result of intense and/or prolonged pressure or pressure in combination with shear and/or friction. The tolerance of soft tissue for pressure and shear may also be affected by the microclimate, which is defined as the climate between the support surface and the client and influenced by temperature, humidity, airflow, nutrition, comorbidities, and the condition of the soft tissue. Pressure injuries are classified based on stages. The current classification includes: stage 1: nonblanchable erythema of intact skin; stage 2: partial-thickness skin loss with exposed dermis; stage 3: Full-thickness skin loss; stage 4: full-thickness skin loss and tissue loss; unstageable: obscured full-thickness skin and tissue loss; and deep tissue: persistent non-blanchable deep red, maroon, or purple discoloration. Additional pressure injury definitions include pressure injuries related to medical devices and mucosal membrane pressure injuries. Clients at high risk for the development of pressure injuries include the elderly and the critically ill. Critically ill patients are at higher risk due to the use of mechanical/medical devices (e.g., nasal cannula tubing, braces, splints, respiratory masks), hemodynamic instability, and the use of vasoactive drugs which may compromise blood flow to the tissues.

Prevention of pressure injuries is a patient safety priority and requires an interdisciplinary approach to care involving physicians, dieticians, physical therapists, nurses (often including wound ostomy certified nurses), patients, and their family members. As with falls, prevention and treatment of pressure injury involve implementation of evidence-based intervention using a "bundle" of standardized interventions. Key elements of a pressure injury prevention bundle include comprehensive assessment, standardized pressure ulcer risk assessment, and

care planning and implementation to address areas of risk. Detailed strategies outlined by the National Pressure Ulcer Advisory Panel include risk assessment (starting point), skin care (protection and monitoring), nutrition (prevention of under-nutrition), position and mobilization (immobility significantly contributes to pressure injuries), and monitoring training and leadership support related to process improvement initiatives. Nurses and nurse leaders within health care organizations are tasked with and accountable for monitoring the outcome of nursing interventions aimed at the prevention of pressure injury, which includes the prevalence of stage 3 or stage 4 pressure injury acquired after admission to a health care facility.

This care plan focuses on care of the adult client at risk for hospital-acquired pressure ulcers/injury and hospitalized in an acute care setting. Given the need to balance patient safety with other care priorities, this care plan should be used in conjunction with the plan of care developed for the primary admitting diagnosis of the client. Much of this information is applicable to clients receiving follow-up care in an extended care facility or home setting.

Nursing Diagnosis RISK FOR PRESSURE ULCER NDx

Definition: Susceptible to localized injury to the skin and/or underlying tissue usually over a bony prominence as a result of pressure, or pressure in combination with shear (NPUAP), 2007.

CLINICAL MANIFESTATIONS

Subjective	Objective
Verbal self-report of localized pain in affected skin/tissue area.	Localized damage to the skin and soft underlying tissue usually over a bony prominence; stage 1: intact skin with localized area of nonblanchable erythema, changes in sensation, temperature, or firmness; stage 2: partial-thickness loss of skin with exposed dermis; stage 3: full-thickness loss of skin with visible exposed adipose (fat); stage 4: full-thickness loss of skin and tissue loss with exposed fascia, muscle, or bone; deep tissue pressure injury: persistent nonblanchable deep red, maroon, or purple discoloration; unstageable pressure injury: obscured full-thickness skin and tissue loss; mucosal membrane injury.

RISK FACTORS

- Decrease in mobility/immobility
- Extended period of immobility on a hard surface (e.g., surgery)
- Inadequate nutrition
- Incontinence
- Shearing/friction forces (e.g., client rubbing feet across sheets); force of gravity added to friction (e.g., same agitate client with head of bed elevated)
- Microclimate with high humidity (e.g., linen with insufficient moisture wicking property)
- Diabetes
- Circulatory impairment
- Smoking

DESIRED OUTCOMES

The client will remain free from pressure injury as evidenced by intact skin and mucous membranes.

DOCUMENTATION

- Standardized risk assessment score (e.g., Braden Scale)
- Skin care
- Nutrition
- Positioning/mobilization
- Skin/mucous membrane changes
- Photo documentation of wounds

NDx = NANDA Diagnosis   **D** = Delegatable Action   ● = UAP   ✦ = LVN/LPN   ⊖▶ = Go to ⊖volve for animation

NOC OUTCOMES

Risk control: pressure injury; immobility consequences: physiologic

NIC INTERVENTIONS

Positioning; intraoperative; pressure ulcer prevention; pressure ulcer care; skin surveillance; skin care: topical treatment

NURSING ASSESSMENT

Assess client's risk for using standardized/structured risk assessment tool (e.g., Braden Scale) on admission (at minimum within 8 hours from admission). Risk assessment should be repeated at regular intervals and with change in condition. Frequency of assessments based on acuity levels:
- Acute care: every shift
- Long-term care: weekly for 4 weeks, then quarterly
- Home care: at every nurse visit.

Assess client for additional risk factors:
- Fragile skin
- Existing pressure injury of any stage, including those ulcers that are healed or closed
- Impaired blood flow (poor perfusion) to the extremities.
- Pain in areas exposed to pressure
- Poor nutritional status
- Evaluate the client's ability to eat independently
- Increased skin moisture.
- Inspect skin upon admission and at least daily.
- Inspect skin at least daily for signs of pressure injury (e.g., nonblanchable erythema, ulcerations, color, firmness)
- Inspect skin for excessive moisture/dryness
- Inspect mucous membranes for areas of discoloration or breakdown
- Inspect skin for rashes and abrasions
- In dark pigmented clients, look for changes in skin tone, skin temperature, and tissue consistency compared with adjacent skin.

Assess bony prominences (e.g., sacrum, coccyx, buttocks, heels, ischium, trochanters, elbows, and beneath medical devices (e.g., NG tubes, nasal cannula/oxygen masks).

Assess for sources of pressure and friction (e.g., prolonged pressure of objects against skin, rubbing of sheets against skin).

Assess for presence of pain using standardized pain assessment scale.

RATIONALE

Determining the client's risk for pressure injury allows implementation of standardized and individualized preventive measures based upon areas of risk. Risk factors and a client's overall risk may vary during hospitalization and should be assessed at the appropriate intervals as defined by organizational policy and/or standard operating procedures.

Preexisting skin wounds/prior pressure injuries must be documented accordingly on admission so as to not adversely impact hospital reimbursement. Additional risk factors should be considered in addition to standardized risk score when developing the plan of care.

Inspection of skin upon admission and identification of preexisting wounds is critical to the classification of a wound as hospital acquired, which impacts reimbursement of associated costs. Early identification of signs of pressure injury and/or signs of microclimate (e.g. dryness/excessive moisture) that can contribute to injury allows for prompt modification of the treatment plan.

Pressure exerted over bony prominences reduces blood flow to the tissues, resulting in hypoxia, increasing risk for the development of a pressure injury.
Identification of sources of pressure, shear, and friction allows for modification of the treatment plan.

Pain is associated with pressure injury. Assessment of pain provides for modification of the treatment plan.

THERAPEUTIC INTERVENTIONS

Independent Actions
Implement pressure injury prevention measures:
Skin care D ● ✦
- Keep skin clean and dry, removing excessive moisture from perspiration, wound drainage, and/or incontinence.
- Cleanse skin promptly following episodes of incontinence, use pH-balanced skin cleanser, and avoid use of hot water.
- Consider use of a breathable incontinence pad.

RATIONALE

Presence of skin damage from moisture may increase the risk for pressure ulceration/injury. Use of a breathable incontinence pad may be helpful when using microclimate management surfaces.

Continued...

THERAPEUTIC INTERVENTIONS	RATIONALE
• Moisturize dry, unbroken skin.	*Use a skin moisturizer to hydrate dry skin to reduce the risk of damage. Consult organizational policies and standard operating procedures and/or skin care bundles for evidence-based interventions.*
• Apply protective barriers, such as creams or moisture absorbing pads, to remove excess moisture as appropriate.	*Presence of skin damage from moisture may increase the risk for pressure ulceration/injury. Consult organizational policies and standard operating procedures and/or skin care bundles for evidence-based interventions.*
• Do not massage or vigorously rub skin at risk of pressure ulcers.	*Friction massage can cause mild destruction or provoke inflammatory reactions, particularly in frail older adults.*
• Do not apply heating devices (e.g., hot water bottles, heating pads) directly on skin.	*Heat increases the metabolic rate, induces sweating, and decreases the tolerance of skin/tissue for pressure.*

Repositioning D ● ✦

- Reposition all individuals at risk for development of pressure injuries.
- Avoid positioning on an area of erythema whenever possible.
- Frequency of repositioning based upon:
  - Support surface
  - Tolerance of skin for pressure
  - Individual preferences
- Reposition the client in a manner that relieves pressure or redistributes pressure avoiding shear/friction forces.

Repositioning serves to reduce the duration and magnitude of pressure over vulnerable areas of the body and contribute to comfort, hygiene, dignity, and functional ability.

Erythema indicates the body/skin area has not recovered from previous pressure loading and requires further rest.

Regular repositioning may not be possible for all clients based upon medical condition—alternate strategies may need to be considered (e.g., high-specification mattress).

When repositioning, it is important to assess whether pressure is actually relieved or redistributed. Lift—do not drag—the client when repositioning. Use a hand to determine if sacrum is off the bed.

- Avoid repositioning on bony prominences with preexisting areas of erythema.

Erythema is an indication of the early signs of pressure injury. Further compromise to blood supply may occur, thereby worsening damage.

- Repositioning individuals in bed:
  - Use the 30-degree, tilted side-lying position (alternate right side, back, left side) or the prone position if tolerated
  - Avoid head of bed elevation that places pressure and shear on the coccyx and sacrum
  - Ensure heels are free of the surfaces of the bed—use heel suspension devices (e.g., pillow elevating heels off bed)
  - Maintain knee in slight flexion (e.g. 5–10 degrees)

  - Repositioning seated individuals (e.g., wheelchair)
  - Adjust footrests and armrests to maintain proper posture and pressure distribution
  - Provide adequate sit tilt to prevent sliding forward.

Elevating HOB greater than 30 degrees has potential to increase pressure, shear, and friction, increasing the risk for tissue damage.

Individuals should be positioned and supported to prevent sliding down in bed and creating shearing forces.

Heels should be free of all pressure. Suspension devices should be removed frequently to assess for skin breakdown.

Hyperextension of the knee may cause obstruction of the popliteal vein.

The ischia bear intense pressure when a client is seated in a wheelchair. Positioning should minimize pressure and shear exerted on soft tissues.

Positioning Devices D ● ✦

- Apply elbow and heel protectors as appropriate.

Protection of bony prominence areas prone to shear friction may prevent tissue injury.

- Use devices on bed that protect individual (e.g., natural sheepskin).
- Do not use ring- or donut-shaped devices.

Natural sheep skin, not synthetic sheep skin, may assist in preventing pressure ulcers.

Edges of ring- or donut-shaped devices crease areas of high pressure that may damage skin/tissue.

Keep bed linens clean and wrinkle free D ● ✦

- Consider using silk-like fabrics to reduce friction/shear.

Mobilization D ● ✦

- Increase activity as tolerated developing a plan for progressive sitting.

Clients on bed rest should progress to sitting and ambulation as rapidly as tolerated to help offset deconditioning seen in clients on bed rest.

NDx = NANDA Diagnosis   **D** = Delegatable Action   ● = UAP   ✦ = LVN/LPN   ●▶ = Go to ℮volve for animation

Continued...

THERAPEUTIC INTERVENTIONS	RATIONALE

Medical Devices
- Remove medical devices as soon as feasibly possible.
- Keep skin clean and dry under medical devices.
- Do not reposition client directly on the medical device unless it is unavoidable.
- Rotate or reposition medical device when possible (e.g., ET tube).

Adults with medical devices should be considered at risk for pressure injury and appropriate prevention measures should be implemented.

Nutrition
- Provide and encourage adequate daily fluid intake as appropriate to client's underlying condition.

Implement measures to decrease pain associated with pressure injury.
- Organize care to ensure coordination with pain medication administration.
- Encourage client to request a "time-out" during any treatment procedures that may cause pain.
- Reduce pressure ulcer pain by keeping wound bed covered, moist, and using a nonadherent dressing.
- Use a lift or transfer sheet to minimize friction and/or shear when repositioning.
- If an ulcer is present, reposition off ulcer whenever possible.

Adequate hydration is essential to transport of essential nutrients critical to sustain the health state of the client.

Pain is often associated with pressure injury and should be addressed accordingly with multimodal interventions.

Dependent/Collaborative Actions
Implement measures to prevent pressure injury:

Consult Dietician/Nutrition
- Screen nutritional status for the client at risk or with a pressure ulcer.
- In collaboration with interprofessional team, develop and individualized nutritional plan based on the individual's nutritional needs. The following needs should be addressed in the plan:
  - Energy/caloric intake appropriate to client's condition using appropriate fortified foods and/or high-calorie, high-protein oral nutritional supplements.
  - For inadequate oral intake, consideration of enteral or parenteral nutritional strategies.
  - Hydration/daily fluid intake
  - Vitamins and minerals.

A qualified member of the health care team should perform a comprehensive nutrition assessment in patients at risk for pressure injury. An appropriate diet is necessary to sustain normal body functions and promote tissue healing. The focus of the assessment should be on energy intake, unintended weight change, and the impact of stress. In addition, the client's individual caloric, protein, and/or fluid requirements.

Consult wound care advanced practice nurse (APN)/ physician for appropriate support surface
- Collaborate with members of the health care team to select the support surface that best meets the needs of the client and is based on:
- Level of immobility
- Need for microclimate control
- Size and weight of individual
- Risk for development of new pressure injuries
- Number, severity, and location of pressure injuries.

- Use a high-specification reactive foam mattress for all individuals assessed for being at risk.

Support surfaces are specialized devices for pressure redistribution designed for managing tissue load, microclimate, and/or other therapeutic functions. The type of support surface selected should be compatible to the care setting, be used according to manufacturer's recommendations, and be used with compatible bed lines and other positioning devices. Note: organizations may have decision algorithms to drive selection of support surfaces. Review organizational policies and/or standard operating procedures for evidence-based practices.

Support surfaces/mattresses are designed to either reduce pressure or sequentially alter the parts of the body that bear load to reduce the time of pressure on any given part of the body.

- For seated support surfaces, select cushion with consideration for body size, effects of posture and deformity on pressure distribution, and mobility and lifestyle needs.
- Cushion cover should be breathable and fit loosely on the top surface of the cushion.

Pressure redistribution surfaces should be used in clients sitting in a chair whose mobility is reduced.

A tight cover will adversely impact cushion performance.

Continued...

THERAPEUTIC INTERVENTIONS	RATIONALE

Consult wound care APN/physician for the use of prophylactic dressings.
- Consider application of a polyurethane foam dressing to a bony prominence (e.g., heels/elbows/sacrum).
- Selection of dressing for prophylactic or existing wounds should be based on ability of dressing to manage microclimate (e.g., moisture), ease of application/removal; ability to regularly assess skin; anatomic location to be applied; and the correct size.
- Consider type of medical device in use as applicable.

Implement measures to manage existing pressure injuries

Consult wound care APN/physician for wound management
- Wound care cleansing as ordered by physician or APN.

Prophylactic dressings placed in anatomic areas prone to friction and shear (e.g., heels, elbows, sacrum) can reduce the risk of injury. Prophylactic dressings differ in qualities, therefore the selected dressings must be appropriate to clinical use and the individual. Note, application of a prophylactic dressing may be considered an independent nursing action—consult organizational policies and/or standard operating procedures.

Cleansing of the wound is the first step in preparing the pressure injury to heal by removing surface debris. Wound cleansing is most often completed by APNs using evidence-based treatment protocols developed collaboratively by members of the health care team. Cleansing allows for better visualization and assessment of a wound.

- Wound care debridement as ordered by a physician or APN.

Debridement is performed only when there is evidence of adequate perfusion to the tissue. Debridement of devitalized tissue within the wound bed and/or edges of pressure ulcer when appropriate to the client's condition. Wound debridement is completed by a physician or APN.

- Biophysical agents for use in wound healing as ordered by physician or APN:
  - Negative pressure wound therapy
  - Whirlpool
  - Pulsatile lavage
  - Hyperbaric oxygen therapy.
- Administer pain medications (opioids/nonopioids) as ordered for acute pain associated with pressure injury and/or cleansing/débriding procedures.
- Consult appropriate pain resources for management of chronic pain associated with pressure injury.

Listed adjunct therapies promote healing by providing a form of biophysical energy. Indications for therapy vary depending upon status of the pressure injury.

Acute pain associated with pressure injury should be evaluated and treated according to client's pain goals.

Nursing Diagnosis ## DEFICIENT KNOWLEDGE NDx

Definition: Absence of cognitive information related to a specific topic, or its acquisition.

CLINICAL MANIFESTATIONS

Subjective	**Objective**
Verbal self-report acknowledging lack of understanding of strategies to reduce risk for pressure injury.	Inaccurate follow-through of instructions; insufficient knowledge

RISK FACTORS
- Alteration in cognitive function
- Insufficient interest in learning
- Insufficient information

DESIRED OUTCOMES
The client will:
- Identify ways to reduce the risk for pressure injury
- Remain free of pressure injury

NOC OUTCOMES
Knowledge: treatment regimen

NIC INTERVENTIONS
Teaching: individual; learning: readiness enhancement; learning: facilitation

NDx = NANDA Diagnosis　**D** = Delegatable Action　● = UAP　◆ = LVN/LPN　　⊖▶ = Go to ⊖volve　for animation

NURSING ASSESSMENT	RATIONALE
Assess for client's understanding of pressure injury prevention upon admission to the hospital.	*Client engagement in his or her health care could lead to safe hospital stays. Many clients may not be aware of their risk for pressure injury and prevention interventions.*
Assess client's ability and readiness to learn.	*Learning is more effective when the client is motivated and understands the importance of what is to be learned. Readiness to learn changes based on situations and physical and emotional challenges.*
Assess client's understanding of teaching.	*It is important for the nurse to ensure client's understanding of teaching. Further education using different instructional modalities may be necessary.*

THERAPEUTIC INTERVENTIONS	RATIONALE

Independent Actions

Instruct client and family on individual risk for pressure injury, including signs and symptoms of skin breakdown.	*Clients, including family members, should be instructed on the client's individual risk factors for pressure injury and signs and symptoms of skin breakdown that should be promptly reported to a health care provider.*
Instruct client and family on preventative skin care: • Keep skin clean and dry. • Cleanse skin promptly following incontinent episode. • Do not massage or vigorously rub skin prone to breakdown. • Protect skin from excessive moisture using prescribed barrier products. • Apply skin moisturizer to hydrate skin. • Application of prophylactic dressings to bony prominence areas.	*Clients, including family members, should be instructed on the appropriate interventions to keep skin dry and intact, reducing the risk for breakdown.*
Instruct client and family on repositioning techniques: • Reposition at least every 2 hours. • Avoid shearing/friction (e.g., do not drag) during repositioning (e.g., use assist devices such as overhead trapeze, mechanical lift). • Avoid postures that increase pressure (e.g., 90 degrees side-lying; semi-recumbent position). • Avoid repositioning on areas or erythema. • Avoid repositioning on medical devices. • "Pressure relief lifts" (e.g. alleviating pressure/lifting off areas of pressure at intervals). • Elevate/pad heels/bony prominences.	*Clients and family should be instructed on appropriate repositioning techniques, with special attention on how to reduce friction and shear when moving. Instruction should also include ensuring that pressure is truly alleviated with change in position.*
Instruct client and family on the proper use of support surfaces and positioning devices.	*Support surface and positioning devices must be used in accordance with manufacturers recommendations to prevent unintended injury.*
Encourage caloric and fluid intake conducive to client's clinical condition/comorbid conditions.	*Appropriate caloric and fluid intake is necessary to ensure maintenance of skin integrity and/or appropriate healing.*
Instruct client and family on the importance of increasing activity as rapidly as tolerated conducive to the client's clinical condition/comorbid conditions.	*Increasing activity as quickly as tolerated reduces the risk of pressure injury by reducing pressure load on areas at risk for skin breakdown.*

ADDITIONAL NURSING DIAGNOSES

ACUTE PAIN NDx

Related to
• Alterations in skin integrity
• Pressure load on erythematic areas of the skin

RISK FOR INFECTION NDx

Related to
• Bacteria present on skin surfaces that invade wounds when primary defense provided by intact skin is lost.
• Unfavorable microclimate (temperature of skin combined with humidity or skin surface moisture) that promotes bacterial growth.

HEALTH CARE–ASSOCIATED INFECTIONS

Health care–associated infections (HAIs), or infections acquired while receiving health care for another condition, can occur in a variety of health care settings, including hospitals, ambulatory surgery centers, and long-term care facilities. It is estimated that on any given day, approximately 1 in 25 hospitalized patients has at least one HAI. HAIs are often considered preventable and present a major threat to patient safety.

HAIs, caused by bacteria, fungi, viruses, and other pathogens, are a significant cause of death and emotional, financial, and additional medical consequences. Factors known to increase the risk of HAIs include the presence of catheters, surgical procedures, injections, improper cleaning and disinfecting of hospital settings/equipment, communicable diseases passed between patients and health care workers, and overuse/improper use of antibiotics. Common infections acquired in hospital settings include urinary tract infections, central line–associated bloodstream infections (CLASBIs), pneumonia, surgical site infections, methicillin-resistant *Staphylococcus aureus* (MRSA) infections, and *Clostridium difficile* infections.

At the national level the 2018 National Patient Safety Goals as issued by the Joint Commission on Accreditation of Healthcare Organizations include "reducing the risk of health care–associated infections" as one of 15 goals addressing current concerns related to patient safety. HAIs, identified as nursing sensitive and associated with the quality of nursing care, include catheter-associated urinary tract infections (CAUTIs), CLABSIs, and ventilator-associated pneumonia (VAP).

As with other nurse-sensitive indicators, the approach to prevention of these HAIs rests on implementation of evidence-based "bundles" based on the most current evidence supporting interventions. Nurses and nurse leaders within health care organizations are tasked with and accountable for monitoring the outcome of nursing interventions aimed at the prevention of HAIs which include rates of each type of HAIs (CAUTI, CLABSI, VAP). Effective in 2015, hospitals risked a reduction in reimbursement from Medicare and Medicaid for how they performed in meeting HAI outcome measures.

This care plan focuses on care of the adult client at risk for HAIs (including CAUTI, CLABSI, and VAP), identified as nurse sensitive, and in an acute care setting. Given the need to balance patient safety with other care priorities, this care plan should be used in conjunction with the plan of care developed for the primary admitting diagnosis of the client. Much of this information is applicable to clients receiving follow-up care in an extended care facility or home setting.

Nursing Diagnosis | ## RISK FOR INFECTION NDx

Definition: Susceptible to invasion and multiplication of pathogenic organisms, which may compromise health.

CLINICAL MANIFESTATIONS

Subjective	**Objective**
CAUTI	**CAUTI**
Verbal self-report of pain in the bladder, groin, lower abdomen, or pelvic area; verbal self-report of fatigue	Fever and/or chills not related to infection at another site; foul-smelling urine; cloudy, dark, and/or blood urine; laboratory evidence of elevated WBCs, RBCs, and/or bacteria in urinalysis
	CLABSI
CLABSI	Fever and/or chills not related to infection at another site; redness at or near the catheter insertion site; drainage from skin around the catheter; laboratory evidence of a recognized pathogen from one or more blood cultures drawn on separate occasions and catheter tip cultures and catheter site exudate if present.
Verbal self-report of pain or tenderness along path of catheter or insertion site	
	VAP
VAP	Fever; purulent, increased, or change in pulmonary secretions; positive tracheal cultures; abnormal breath sounds (e.g., rales/rhonchi, crackles); tachypnea/dyspnea; hypoxia
N/A	

RISK FACTORS

CAUTI
- Meatal, rectal, or vaginal organism colonization
- Contaminated hands of health care personnel during insertion or manipulation of the collection system.
- Break in the urine closed drainage system

- Contamination of the urine collection system.
- Prolonged/inappropriate catheterization
- Older age
- Impaired immunity
- Comorbid conditions (e.g., diabetes, renal dysfunction)

CLABSI
- Contaminated hands of health care personnel during insertion, manipulation during changing of the line dressing, or during administration of medication through the line.
- Prolonged time in place.

NDx = NANDA Diagnosis **D** = Delegatable Action ● = UAP ✦ = LVN/LPN ⊖▶ = Go to ⊝volve for animation

VAP
- Mechanical ventilation/presence of an endotracheal tube >48 hours (aspiration/leakage of secretions above the cuff of an endotracheal tube
- Ventilator circuit (e.g., collection of condensation in circuitry)

- Contaminated hands of health care personnel
- Loss of gag reflex/cough reflex associated with decreased level of consciousness and/or sedation.
- Patient positioning (e.g., higher in supine patients)

- Presence of a nasogastric or orogastric tube (increased risk for reflux and aspiration)
- Comorbid conditions (e.g., immunosuppression, chronic obstructive pulmonary disease [COPD], adult respiratory distress syndrome [ARDS])

DESIRED OUTCOMES

The client will remain free from infection as evidenced by:
CAUTI
- Absence of WBCs, RBCs, and/or bacteria in urine
- Normal or baseline urine color

CLABSI
- Absence of cultured pathogens from blood, catheter tip, or site samples

VAP
- Normal or baseline chest x-ray
- Normal or baseline respiratory rate
- Normal or baseline oxygen saturation (arterial blood gases as indicated)
- Absence of purulent, excessive secretions

DOCUMENTATION

CAUTI
- Catheter insertion date/time
- Perineal/catheter maintenance care

CLABSI
- Central line insertion date/time
- Dressing change date/time

VAP
- Intubation date/time
- Oral care
- Insertion depth of ET tube (ET cm marking at lip)*
- ET cuff pressure*

NOC OUTCOMES

Risk control: infectious process; infection severity

NIC INTERVENTIONS

CAUTI—Infection control; infection protection; urinary catheterization; tube care: urinary
CLABSI—Infection control; infection protection; central venous access device management
VAP—Infection control; infection protection; aspiration prevention; mechanical ventilation management—pneumonia prevention

NURSING ASSESSMENT

Assess for systemic and localized signs and symptoms of infection.
Systemic
- Fever
- Fatigue
- Headache
- Nausea

Localized
CAUTI
- Foul-smelling urine
- Cloudy, dark, and/or blood urine

CLABSI
- Pain at insertion site
- Exudate at insertion site
- Redness/swelling at insertion site.

VAP
- Purulent, increased, or change in pulmonary secretions
- Abnormal breath sounds
- Dyspnea, tachypnea

RATIONALE

Identification of signs and symptoms of infection, both systemic and localized to the site, allows for prompt intervention.

---

*Documentation may be responsibility of respiratory therapy

Continued...

NURSING ASSESSMENT	RATIONALE
Assess laboratory values/cultures for values indicating infection: • Absolute granulocyte count • WBC • Differential • Cultures (e.g., blood, sputum, urine, site, catheter tip as applicable)	*Serum lab results indicative of infection include abnormal values in WBC and differential cell counts. National guidelines define collection methods and interpretation of findings specific to infection sites to be classified as hospital acquired/associated. Refer to organizational policies and standard operating procedures for processes to follow when collecting site specific culture for infection determination. Collection of cultures from devices such as catheter tips requires following detailed steps to prevent untoward contamination.*
Assess applicable radiographic results for evidence of infection (e.g., chest x-ray)	*Supporting evidence for diagnosis of VAP is presence of a new infiltrate on chest radiograph.*

THERAPEUTIC INTERVENTIONS	RATIONALE
Independent Actions Follow appropriate hand hygiene practices • Before touching a client • Before a procedure • After a procedure or exposure to body fluid • After touching a client • After touching a client's surroundings	*Hand hygiene must be followed by all health care professionals when providing care and should be based upon CDC/World Health Organization guidelines.*
Implement infection prevention measures during insertion, maintenance care, and removal of devices as appropriate **CAUTI** Insertion: • Adhere to aseptic technique during insertion using sterile equipment—performing hand hygiene prior to insertion. • Cleanse meatus with appropriate antiseptic solution.	*Organizations implement written guidelines and care bundles that are evidence based and based on national clinical practice recommendations by leading infection prevention organizations (e.g., Society for Healthcare Epidemiology of America [SHEA]; Association for Professionals in Infection Control and Epidemiology [APIC]), as best practices to reduce the risk of infections. To ensure quality care, nurses must be aware of and adhere to organizational policy and standard operating procedures specific to devices with increased risk for infection.*
• Use smallest catheter as possible consistent with proper drainage. Maintenance:	*Use of the smallest appropriate catheter reduces the risk of urethral trauma, which may provide an avenue for infection.*
• Properly secure indwelling catheters after insertion.	*Prevents movement and urethral traction/trauma, which may provide an avenue for infection.*
• Maintain sterile, continuously closed drainage system.	*Prevents contamination and reduces the risk for infection. If leaks or breaks in the drainage system occur, replace catheter and collection system using aseptic technique.*
• Maintain unobstructed urine flow, keeping the drainage bag below the level of the bladder and tubing free from kinks.	*Allows for free drainage of urine, preventing backflow of urine into the bladder which increases the risk for infection.*
• Perform routine hygiene, cleaning the metal area with soap and water. **CLABSI** Insertion:	*Current guidelines state cleansing with antiseptic solutions is unnecessary. Refer to organizational policy and standard operating procedures for frequency of routine hygiene.*
• Ensure adherence to aseptic technique performing hand hygiene prior to procedure. • Maximum sterile barrier precautions should be observed at bedside (e.g., sterile gown, gloves, caps, client drapes).	*Central line insertions, often done at the bedside, are often accomplished with the use of a procedural checklist to ensure adherence to aseptic technique and safety procedures. Although insertion is a function of the physician, all providers assisting should be empowered to stop the procedure if aseptic technique is not maintained or safety procedures are not being followed.*
• Skin preparation with alcoholic chlorhexidine Maintenance:	*Reduces skin microbes. Skin prep must be allowed to dry before puncture.*
• ICU clients should be bathed with a broad-spectrum topical antimicrobial agent (e.g., chlorhexidine) daily.	*Daily bathing with a broad-spectrum topical antimicrobial agent (e.g., chlorhexidine) may reduce HAIs.*
• Disinfect catheter hubs, needless connectors, and injection ports before accessing catheters. • Vigorously scrub with friction for no less than 5 seconds.	*Before accessing central venous access catheters for infusions, ports should be vigorously scrubbed with an alcoholic chlorhexidine preparation. Refer to organizational policy and/or standard operating procedures.*

Continued...

THERAPEUTIC INTERVENTIONS	RATIONALE
• Change central venous access catheter dressings, performing site care with a chlorhexidine- based antiseptic every 5–7 days or immediately if dressing is soiled, loose, or damp.	*Refer to organizational policy/standard operating procedures for dressing change frequency. Chlorhexidine, an antimicrobial topical solution, has been effective in preventing CLABSIs-many commercial dressing change kits include a chlorhexidine-impregnated dressing.*
VAP Maintenance: • Minimize pooling of secretions above the endotracheal tube cuff • Suctioning the oropharynx as needed	*The majority of interventions focused on the prevention of VAP are implemented during maintenance while the client is intubated and mechanically ventilated. Keeping the oropharynx free of subglottic secretions reduces the risk of aspiration of secretions and the development of pneumonia. Some endotracheal tubes may have subglottic drainage ports and be used in clients expected to be ventilated for more than 48–72 hours.*
• Perform oral care with chlorhexidine • Consider brushing teeth	*Oral care with chlorhexidine had demonstrated a decrease in VAP rates in clinical research studies. Refer to organizational policies and standard operating procedures for frequency of oral care.*
• Endotracheal suctioning should be performed only when assessment findings indicate (e.g., rhonchi) using aseptic technique.	*Endotracheal suctioning should be performed only as needed, using sterile technique to avoid cross-contamination. Instilling of saline prior to suctioning is no longer a recommended practice.*
• Maintain and improve physical conditioning by providing early exercise and mobilization.	*Interventions that promote early mobility in ventilated patients increase the rate of return to independent function/extubation and reduce the risk of VAP.*
Ensure appropriately trained personnel are involved in the insertion, maintenance, and removal of indwelling devices (e.g., urinary catheters, central venous access catheters).	*Delegation practices vary by institution. Nurses must be aware of unlicensed assistive personnel who are appropriately trained in the insertion (e.g., urinary catheters) and/or maintenance (e.g., perineal care, chlorhexidine bathing, central line dressing changes) of indwelling devices prone to infection. Review organizational policy and standard operating procedures before delegating care.*

Dependent/Collaborative Actions

THERAPEUTIC INTERVENTIONS	RATIONALE
Collaborate with other health care providers in implementing evidence-based care bundles for the appropriate use, insertion, and maintenance of indwelling devices: • Urinary catheters • Central venous access catheters. • Endotracheal tubes/intubation.	*To reduce the risk for hospital-acquired infections, many organizations have established evidence-based written guidelines/care bundles for the appropriate use, insertion, and maintenance of urinary catheters, central venous access devices, and endotracheal tubes/intubation. In addition, many organizations have implemented nurse driven protocols for the removal of these same devices. Nurses must be aware of these guidelines and collaborate with other members of the health care team to ensure adherence.*
Collaborative with other members of the health care team to ensure indwelling devices (e.g., urinary catheters, central venous access catheters, endotracheal tubes) are removed as soon as no longer necessary.	*Indwelling devices (e.g., urinary catheters/central venous access catheters) should be removed as soon as no longer necessary, to reduce the risk for infection. Many organizations implement electronic reminders and/or continued use documentation requirements in the electronic health record to ensure continued use of these devices is justified.*
Collaborate with other members of the health care team for specific interventions to reduce **VAP**: • Minimize sedation in intubated/mechanically ventilated clients • Interrupt sedation (sedation vacation) once a day in clients without contraindications) • Conduct spontaneous breathing trials	*Goal of interventions is to reduce intubation time and progress client towards extubation, reducing the risk for infection.*
• Administer prophylactic probiotics as ordered by physician or advance practice provider (ARNP, PA).	*Some research evidence has reported reduction of VAP rates with use of probiotics.*

Continued...

THERAPEUTIC INTERVENTIONS	RATIONALE
If signs and symptoms of infection are observed, consult physician or advanced practice provider (e.g. ARNP; PA).	*Allows for modification of the treatment plan.*
● Obtain blood, urine, site, and/or device-specific cultures as ordered in accordance with hospital policy/standard operating procedures for collection methods.	*Organizational policies and/or standard operating procedures must be followed when obtaining cultures, specimens with potential to confirm an infection, classify the infection as hospital acquired, and guide medical treatment. Not following appropriate collection methods may result in cross-contamination, prescribing of inappropriate antibiotic therapy, and inappropriate classification of the infection as hospital acquired.*
● Administered ordered antibiotics and antifungals as ordered and guided by results of cultures and serum lab values.	

Nursing Diagnosis DEFICIENT KNOWLEDGE NDx

Definition: Absence of cognitive information related to a specific topic, or its acquisition.

CLINICAL MANIFESTATIONS

Subjective	Objective
Verbal self-report acknowledging lack of understanding of strategies to reduce risk for pressure injury.	Inaccurate follow-through of instructions; insufficient knowledge

RISK FACTORS
- Alteration in cognitive function
- Insufficient interest in learning
- Insufficient information

DESIRED OUTCOMES

The client will:
- Identify ways to reduce the risk for infection
- Remain free of hospital associated infection

NOC OUTCOMES

Knowledge: treatment regimen

NIC INTERVENTIONS

Teaching: disease process; learning readiness enhancement; learning facilitation

NURSING ASSESSMENT	RATIONALE
Assess for client's understanding of the risk for acquiring infections upon admission to the hospital.	*Client engagement in his or her health care could lead to safe hospital stays. Many clients may not be aware of their risk for acquiring infections in the hospital and prevention interventions.*
Assess client's ability and readiness to learn.	*Learning is more effective when the client is motivated and understands the importance of what is to be learned. Readiness to learn changes based on situations and physical and emotional challenges.*
Assess client's understanding of teaching.	*It is important for the nurse to ensure client's understanding of teaching. Further education using different instructional modalities may be necessary.*

THERAPEUTIC INTERVENTIONS	RATIONALE

Independent Actions

Instruct client and family on proper handwashing/use of alcohol-based foam.

- Instruct client and family to monitor health care provider adherence to handwashing when entering the client's room.
- Instruct client and family members on when and how best to perform handwashing.
- Hand hygiene should be performed before preparing or eating food; before touching eyes, nose, or mouth; after using the restroom; after blowing nose, coughing, or sneezing; after touching hospital surfaces (e.g., bed rails, bedside tables, phone).
- Hand hygiene can be performed using alcohol-based hand sanitizer or with soap and water.

Encourage client and family to "speak up" about hand hygiene practices, instructing them it is OK to ask health care providers if they have cleaned their hands.

Instruct client and family on individual risk for acquiring an infection, including signs and symptoms of infection.

Hand hygiene is the first line of defense against infection. Clients and family members can contribute to reducing the risk for infection by participating in hand hygiene.

Best practices for hand hygiene include the use of either soap and water or alcohol-based hand sanitizer. Sanitizing with alcohol-based sanitizers involves covering hands with alcohol-based hand sanitizer, rubbing hands together for approximately 20 seconds, covering all surfaces until hands feel dry. Soap and water hand hygiene involves application of soap, rubbing hands together for approximately 15 seconds, rinsing under warm water, and drying with a paper towel.

Engaging clients in their care helps to hold all members of the health care team accountable for preventing infection.

Clients and family members should be instructed on the client's individual risk factors for infection and signs and symptoms that should be promptly reported to a health care provider.

3

Selected Nursing Diagnoses, Interventions, Rationales, and Documentation

---

Nursing Diagnosis **ACTIVITY INTOLERANCE** NDx

Definition: Insufficient physiological or psychological energy to endure or complete required or desired daily activities.

CLINICAL MANIFESTATIONS

Subjective	**Objective**
Verbal self-report of fatigue or weakness	Abnormal heart rate or blood pressure response to activity; exertional discomfort or dyspnea; electrocardiographic changes reflecting dysrhythmias or ischemia; unable to speak with physical activity

RISK FACTORS

- Bedrest or immobility
- Physical deconditioning
- Sedentary lifestyle
- Imbalance between oxygen supply/demand

DESIRED OUTCOMES

The client will demonstrate an increased tolerance for activity as evidenced by:
a. Verbalization of feeling less fatigued and weak
b. Ability to perform activities of daily living without exertional dyspnea, chest pain, diaphoresis, dizziness, and significant changes in vital signs

DOCUMENTATION

- Activity level
- Statements of weakness and fatigue
- Exertional dyspnea, chest pain, diaphoresis, or dizziness
- Vital signs before, during, and after activity
- Therapeutic interventions
- Client teaching

NURSING OUTCOMES CLASSIFICATION (NOC) OUTCOMES

Activity tolerance; discomfort level; endurance; fatigue level; psychomotor energy; self-care status; self-care: activities of daily living; vital signs; energy conservation

NURSING INTERVENTION CLASSIFICATION (NIC) INTERVENTIONS

Activity therapy; energy management; oxygen therapy; nutrition management; sleep enhancement; cardiac care; cardiac rehabilitation; teaching regarding prescribed activity

NURSING ASSESSMENT	**RATIONALE**
Assess for signs and symptoms of activity intolerance: • Statements of fatigue or weakness • Exertional dyspnea, chest pain, diaphoresis, or dizziness • Abnormal heart rate response to activity (e.g., increase in rate of 20 beats/min above resting rate, rate not returning to preactivity level within 3 minutes after stopping activity, change from regular to irregular rate) • A significant change (e.g. 15–20 mmHg) in blood pressure with activity.	*Early recognition of signs and symptoms of activity intolerance allows for prompt intervention.*
Assess complete blood cell count (CBC) and report abnormal values.	*Anemia results in decreased oxygen-carrying capacity of the blood.*

THERAPEUTIC INTERVENTIONS	RATIONALE

Independent Actions

Implement measures to promote rest and/or conserve energy (e.g., maintain prescribed activity restrictions, minimize environmental activity and noise, provide uninterrupted rest periods, assist with care, and limit the number of visitors). **D** ● ✦

Cells use oxygen and fat, protein, and carbohydrate to produce the energy needed for all body activities. Rest and activities that conserve energy result in a lower metabolic rate, which preserves nutrients and oxygen for necessary activities.

Discourage smoking and excessive intake of beverages high in caffeine such as coffee, tea, and colas.

Both nicotine and excessive caffeine intake can increase cardiac workload and myocardial oxygen utilization, thereby decreasing the amount of oxygen necessary for energy production.

Implement measures to improve respiratory status (e.g., encourage use of incentive spirometer; elevate head of bed; assist with turning, coughing, and deep breathing) if ineffective breathing pattern, ineffective airway clearance, or impaired gas exchange is contributing to client's activity intolerance. **D** ✦

Altered respiratory function can lead to inadequate tissue oxygenation, which results in less efficient energy production and a reduced ability to tolerate activity. Improving respiratory status increases the amount of oxygen available for energy production. It also eases the work of breathing, which reduces energy expenditure.

Instruct client to report a decreased tolerance for activity and to stop any activity that causes chest pain, shortness of breath, dizziness, or extreme fatigue or weakness.

These symptoms indicate that insufficient oxygen is reaching the tissues and that activity has been increased beyond a therapeutic level.

Dependent/Collaborative Actions

Implement measures to increase cardiac output (e.g., administer positive inotropic agents, vasodilators, or antidysrhythmics as ordered; elevate the head of the bed) if decreased cardiac output is contributing to the client's activity intolerance.

Sufficient cardiac output is necessary to maintain an adequate blood flow and oxygen supply to the tissues. Adequate tissue oxygenation promotes more efficient energy production, which subsequently improves client's activity tolerance.

Implement measures to reduce fever if present (e.g., administer tepid sponge bath, administer antipyretics as ordered). **D** ✦

An elevated temperature increases the metabolic rate with subsequent depletion of available energy and a decrease in the ability to tolerate activity.

Maintain oxygen therapy as ordered.

An oxygen deficiency results in anaerobic metabolism, which is less efficient than the aerobic mechanism of energy supply. Supplemental oxygen helps to alleviate hypoxia and restore the more efficient aerobic metabolism, thereby improving energy levels and activity tolerance.

Implement measures to maintain an adequate nutritional status (e.g., provide a diet high in essential nutrients, provide dietary supplements as indicated, and administer vitamins and minerals as ordered).

Metabolism is the process by which nutrients are transformed into energy. If nutrition is inadequate, energy production is decreased, which subsequently reduces one's ability to tolerate activity.

Implement measures to treat anemia if present (e.g., administer prescribed iron, folic acid, and/or vitamin B12; administer packed red blood cells as ordered).

Anemia reduces the oxygen-carrying capacity of the blood. Resolution of anemia increases oxygen availability to the cells, which increases the efficiency of energy production and subsequently improves activity tolerance.

Increase client's activity gradually as allowed and tolerated. **D** ● ✦

A gradual increase in activity helps prevent a sudden increase in cardiac workload and myocardial oxygen consumption and the subsequent imbalance between oxygen supply and demand. Progressive activity also helps strengthen the myocardium, which enhances cardiac output and improves activity tolerance.

Consult physician if signs and symptoms of activity intolerance persist.

Notifying the physician allows for modification of the treatment plan.

Nursing Diagnosis # INEFFECTIVE AIRWAY CLEARANCE NDx

Definition: Inability to clear secretions or obstructions from the respiratory tract to maintain a clear airway.

CLINICAL MANIFESTATIONS

Subjective	Objective
Verbal self-report of shortness of breath	Dyspnea, orthopnea; diminished breath sounds; adventitious breath sounds (e.g., crackles, rhonchi, wheezes); cough, ineffective or absent sputum production; difficulty vocalizing; wide-eyed; restlessness; changes in respiratory rate and rhythm; cyanosis

RISK FACTORS

- **Environmental:** Smoking; smoke inhalation; second-hand smoke; air quality/pollutants
- **Obstructed airway:** Airway spasm; retained secretions; excessive mucus; presence of artificial airway; foreign body in airway; secretions in the bronchi; exudates in the alveoli
- **Physiologic:** Neuromuscular dysfunction; hyperplasia of the bronchial walls; chronic obstructive pulmonary disease; infection; asthma; allergic/reactive airways

DESIRED OUTCOMES

The client will maintain clear, open airways as evidenced by:
a. Normal breath sounds
b. Normal rate and depth of respirations
c. Absence of dyspnea

DOCUMENTATION

- Breath sounds
- Rate, depth, and ease of respirations
- Characteristics of cough
- Description of sputum
- Therapeutic interventions
- Client teaching

NOC OUTCOMES

Risk control: aspiration; mechanical ventilation response: respiratory status: airway patency; respiratory status: ventilation

NIC INTERVENTIONS

Respiratory monitoring; airway management; airway suctioning; chest physiotherapy; cough enhancement

NURSING ASSESSMENT

Assess for signs and symptoms of ineffective airway clearance:
- Abnormal breath sounds
- Rapid, shallow respirations
- Dyspnea
- Nonproductive cough

RATIONALE

Early recognition of signs and symptoms of ineffective airway clearance allows for prompt intervention.

THERAPEUTIC INTERVENTIONS

Independent Actions
Implement measures to decrease pain if present:
- Splint chest or abdominal incisions with pillow when coughing and deep breathing. **D** ✦

Instruct and assist client to change position, deep breathe, and cough or "huff" every 1 to 2 hrs. **D** ✦

RATIONALE

Pain often interferes with a client's willingness to move, cough, and deep breathe. Pain reduction enables the client to increase activity and cough and deep breathe more effectively, all of which promote effective airway clearance.

Repositioning helps mobilize secretions. Deep breathing helps clear the airways by loosening secretions and promoting a more effective cough. Coughing or "huffing" (i.e., a forced expiration technique) accelerates airflow through the airways, which helps mobilize and clear mucus and foreign matter from the respiratory tract.

Continued...

THERAPEUTIC INTERVENTIONS	RATIONALE
Discourage smoking.	*Irritants present in smoke increase mucus production, impair ciliary function, and can cause inflammation and damage to the bronchial walls. This results in narrowed airways and stasis of pulmonary secretions.*
Perform oral suctioning if needed. **D** ✦	*Suctioning removes secretions from the large airways. It also stimulates coughing, which helps clear airways of mucus and foreign matter.*

Dependent/Collaborative Actions

Implement measures to decrease pain: • Administer prescribed analgesics before planned activity. **D** ✦	*Pain often interferes with a client's willingness to move, cough, and deep breathe. Pain reduction enables the client to increase activity and cough and deep breathe more effectively, all of which promote effective airway clearance.*
Increase activity as allowed and tolerated. **D** ● ✦	*Activity helps to mobilize secretions and promotes deeper breathing. Deep breathing can help loosen secretions and enhance the effectiveness of coughing.*
Implement measures to thin secretions and maintain adequate moisture of the respiratory mucous membranes: • Maintain a fluid intake of 2500 mL/day, if tolerated • Humidify inspired air **D** ✦	*Adequate hydration and humidified inspired air help thin secretions, which facilitates the mobilization and expectoration of secretions. These actions also reduce dryness of the respiratory mucous membrane, which helps enhance mucociliary clearance.*
Assist with the administration of mucolytics (e.g., acetylcysteine) and diluting or hydrating agents (e.g., water, saline) via nebulizer as ordered.	*Mucolytics and diluents or hydrating agents are mucokinetic substances that reduce the viscosity of mucus, thus making it easier for the client to mobilize and clear secretions from the respiratory tract.*
Administer expectorants if ordered (e.g., guaifenesin, dornase alfa). **D** ✦	*Expectorants reduce the viscosity of sputum, making it easier to be removed by coughing or suctioning.*

Administer the following medications if ordered:
• Bronchodilators
  • Methylxanthines (e.g., theophylline, aminophylline, oxtriphylline)
  • Sympathomimetic (adrenergic) agents (e.g., albuterol, terbutaline, metaproterenol, salmeterol)
  • Anticholinergic agents (e.g., ipratropium)
• Corticosteroids
  • Prednisone
  • Methylprednisolone
  • Beclomethasone
  • Flunisolide
  • Triamcinolone
  • Budesonide
• Leukotriene modifiers
  • Montelukast
  • Zafirlukast ✦
	These medications increase the patency of the airways and enhance bronchial airflow. Methylxanthines and sympathomimetics produce bronchodilation by relaxing the bronchial smooth muscle. Anticholinergic agents block cholinergic reflex constriction of the bronchioles and decrease mucus production. Corticosteroids and leukotriene modifiers reduce inflammation in the airways, which results in decreased bronchial hyperactivity and constriction and mucus production.

Administer central nervous system depressants judiciously.	*Central nervous system depressants depress the cough reflex, which can result in stasis of secretions.*
Assist with or perform postural drainage therapy if ordered.	*Postural drainage therapy techniques (e.g., vibration, percussion, postural drainage) use the forces of motion and gravity to mobilize secretions from the periphery of the lungs to the larger central airways where they can be removed by coughing or suctioning.*
Consult the appropriate health care provider (e.g., physician, respiratory therapist) if signs and symptoms of ineffective airway clearance persist.	*Notifying the appropriate health care provider allows for modification of the treatment plan.*

Nursing Diagnosis ANXIETY NDx

Definition: Vague, uneasy feeling of discomfort or dread accompanied by an autonomic response (the source is often nonspecific or unknown to the individual); a feeling of apprehension caused by anticipation of danger. It is an alerting sign that warns of impending danger and enables the individual to take measures to deal with that threat.

CLINICAL MANIFESTATIONS

Subjective	Objective
Behavioral: Verbal self-report of concerns due to change in life events	**Behavioral:** Diminished productivity; scanning and vigilance; poor eye contact; restlessness; glancing about; extraneous movement (e.g., foot shuffling, hand/arm movements); insomnia; fidgeting
Affective: Verbal self-report of painful and persistent increased helplessness; uncertainty; increased wariness; feelings of inadequacy	**Affective:** Regretful; irritability, anguish; scared; jittery; overexcited; rattled; focus on self; fearful; distressed; worried, apprehensive; anxious
Physiologic: Verbal self-report of dry mouth; nausea, fatigue	**Physiologic:** Voice quivering; trembling/hand tremors; shakiness; urinary urgency; increased pulse; pupil dilation; increased reflexes; abdominal pain; sleep disturbance; tingling in extremities; cardiovascular excitation; increased perspiration; facial tension; anorexia; heart pounding; diarrhea; weakness; facial flushing; superficial vasoconstriction; twitching; faintness; respiratory difficulties; increased blood pressure
Cognitive: Verbal self-report of fear of unspecified consequences; awareness of physiological symptoms	**Cognitive:** Blocking of thought; confusion; preoccupation; forgetfulness; rumination; impaired attention; decreased perceptual field; tendency to blame others; difficulty concentrating; diminished ability to problem solve; diminished ability to learn

RISK FACTORS

- Exposure to toxins
- Threat to or change in role status
- Unconscious conflict about essential values/goals of life
- Familial association/hereditary
- Unmet needs
- Interpersonal transmission/contagion
- Situational/maturational crises
- Threat of death
- Threat to or change in health status
- Threat to or change in interaction patterns
- Threat to or change in role function
- Threat to self-concept
- Threat to or change in environment
- Stress
- Threat to or change in economic status
- Substance abuse

DESIRED OUTCOMES

The client will experience a reduction in anxiety as evidenced by:
a. Verbalization of feeling less anxious
b. Usual sleep pattern
c. Relaxed facial expression and body movements
d. Stable vital signs
e. Usual perceptual ability and interaction with others

DOCUMENTATION

- Verbalization of feeling anxious
- Sleep pattern
- Facial expression and body movement
- Vital signs
- Focus on self
- Client's perception of precipitating factors
- Therapeutic interventions
- Client/family teaching

NOC OUTCOMES

Anxiety level; anxiety self-control; concentration; coping; hyperactivity level

NIC INTERVENTIONS

Anxiety reduction; calming technique; emotional support; presence

---

NDx = NANDA Diagnosis   **D** = Delegatable Action   ● = UAP   ✦ = LVN/LPN   ⊖▶ = Go to ⊖volve for animation

NURSING ASSESSMENT	**RATIONALE**
Assess for signs and symptoms of anxiety: • Verbalization of feeling anxious • Insomnia • Tenseness • Shakiness • Restlessness • Diaphoresis • Tachycardia • Elevated blood pressure • Self-focused behaviors	*Early recognition of signs and symptoms of anxiety allows for prompt intervention.*

THERAPEUTIC INTERVENTIONS	**RATIONALE**

Independent Actions

Encourage verbalization of feelings and concerns and assist client to identify specific stressors that may be causing anxiety. Provide feedback.	*Verbalization of feelings and concerns helps the client identify factors that are causing anxiety. Providing feedback helps the client clarify and validate feelings and concerns, and identify techniques that can reduce anxiety.*
Orient client to environment, equipment, and routines. **D ✦ ●**	*Familiarity with the environment and usual routines reduces the client's anxiety about the unknown, provides a sense of security, and increases his/her sense of control, all of which help decrease anxiety.*
All care providers should properly introduce themselves and identify their role. If possible, maintain consistency in staff assigned to his/her care.	*Introduction to staff familiarizes the client with those individuals who will be working with him/her, which provides the client with a feeling of stability, which reduces the anxiety that typically occurs with change.*
Assure client that staff members are nearby. Respond to call signal as soon as possible.	*Close contact and a prompt response to requests provide a sense of security and facilitates the development of trust, thus reducing the client's anxiety.*
All care providers should maintain a calm, supportive, confident manner when interacting with the client. **D ✦ ●**	*A sense of calmness and confidence conveys to the client that someone is in control of the situation, which helps reduce anxiety.*
Reinforce physician's explanations and clarify misconceptions the client has about the diagnostic tests, disease condition, treatment plan, surgical procedure, and/or prognosis.	*Factual information and an awareness of what to expect help decrease the anxiety that arises from uncertainty.*
Implement measures to reduce respiratory distress if present: • Elevate the head of the bed • Encourage the client to breathe deeply and more slowly	*Improvement of respiratory status helps relieve anxiety associated with the feeling of not being able to breathe.*
Implement measures to reduce pain if present: • Instruct and assist with relaxation techniques.	*Pain can create or increase anxiety because it is often perceived as a threat to well-being. Pain also causes sympathetic nervous system stimulation with subsequent feelings of tenseness and increased anxiety.*
Provide a calm, restful environment. **D ✦ ●**	*A calm, restful environment facilitates relaxation and promotes a sense of security, which reduces anxiety.*
When appropriate, assist the client to meet spiritual needs (e.g., arrange for a visit from the clergy).	*Spiritual support is a source of comfort and security for many people and can help reduce the client's anxiety.*
Encourage significant others to project a caring, concerned attitude without obvious anxiousness.	*Anxiety is easily transferable from one person to another. If significant others convey empathy, provide reassurance, and do not appear anxious, they can help reduce the client's anxiety.*
Include significant others in orientation and teaching sessions and encourage their continued support of the client.	*Significant others can help reduce the client's anxiety by reinforcing information that he/she has difficulty understanding or recalling. In addition, the presence of significant others often provides the client with a sense of support and security, which helps to reduce anxiety.*
Provide information based on current needs of client at a level he/she can understand. Encourage the client to ask questions and to seek clarification of information provided.	*Providing the client with information that he/she is not ready to process or cannot understand tends to increase anxiety. Making the client feel comfortable enough to ask questions or clarify information helps to reduce anxiety.*

THERAPEUTIC INTERVENTIONS	RATIONALE
Include significant others in orientation and teaching sessions and encourage their continued support of the client.	*Significant others can help reduce the client's anxiety by reinforcing information that he/she has difficulty understanding or recalling. In addition, the presence of significant others often provides the client with a sense of support and security, which helps reduce anxiety.*

Dependent/Collaborative Actions

Administer oxygen therapy as ordered. **D** ✦	*Improvement of respiratory status helps relieve anxiety associated with the feeling of not being able to breathe.*
Administer prescribed analgesics if pain is present. **D** ✦	*Pain can create or increase anxiety because it is often perceived as a threat to well-being. Pain also causes sympathetic nervous system stimulation with subsequent feelings of tenseness and increased anxiety.*
Administer prescribed antianxiety agents if indicated. **D** ✦	*Medications are sometimes prescribed to help reduce the client's anxiety. Benzodiazepines (e.g., lorazepam, diazepam, alprazolam, chlordiazepoxide) are the drugs of choice for management of short-term anxiety. These drugs augment the inhibitory effect of gamma-aminobutyric acid (GABA) on cell membrane responses to excitatory neurotransmitters.*
Initiate a social service referral and/or assist client to identify and contact appropriate community resources if indicated.	*Concerns about factors such as finances, follow-up medical care, and home maintenance can be a source of great anxiety. Facilitating contact with the appropriate resources can help reduce the client's anxiety and provide ongoing support.*
Consult appropriate health care provider (e.g., psychiatric nurse practitioner, psychologist, psychiatrist, physician) if above actions fail to control anxiety.	*Notifying the appropriate health care provider allows for modification of the treatment plan.*

Nursing Diagnosis **RISK FOR ASPIRATION** NDx

Definition: Susceptible to entry of gastrointestinal secretions, oropharyngeal secretions, solids, or fluids to the tracheobronchial passages, which may compromise health.

CLINICAL MANIFESTATIONS

Subjective	**Objective**
Verbal self-report of shortness of breath, difficulty swallowing	Rhonchi; dull percussion note over affected lung area; cough; tachypnea; tachycardia; presence of tube feeding in tracheal aspirate; dyspnea, cough, excessive drooling

RISK FACTORS

- Reduced level of consciousness
- Depressed cough and gag reflexes
- Presence of tracheostomy or endotracheal tube
- Incompetent lower esophageal sphincter

- Gastrointestinal tubes
- Tube feedings
- Medication administration
- Situations hindering elevation of upper body
- Increased intragastric pressure

- Increased gastric residual
- Decreased gastrointestinal motility
- Delayed gastric emptying
- Impaired swallowing
- Facial, oral, neck surgery or trauma
- Wired jaws

DESIRED OUTCOMES

The client will not aspirate secretions or foods/fluids as evidenced by:
a. Clear breath sounds
b. Resonant percussion note over lungs
c. Absence of cough, tachypnea, and dyspnea

DOCUMENTATION

- Breath sounds
- Percussion note over lungs
- Respiratory rate and effort
- Presence of cough
- Pulse rate
- Color of tracheal aspirate
- Therapeutic interventions
- Client/family teaching

NDx = NANDA Diagnosis   **D** = Delegatable Action   ● = UAP   ✦ = LVN/LPN   ⊖▶ = Go to ⊖volve for animation

NOC OUTCOMES

Risk control: aspiration; body positioning; gastrointestinal function; nausea and vomiting control; respiratory status; swallowing status

NIC INTERVENTIONS

Aspiration precautions; respiratory monitoring; swallowing therapy; airway suctioning

NURSING ASSESSMENT	RATIONALE
Assess for and report signs and symptoms of aspiration of secretions or foods/fluids: • Rhonchi • Dull percussion note over affected lung area • Cough • Tachypnea • Dyspnea • Tachycardia • Presence of tube feeding in tracheal aspirate	*Early recognition of signs and symptoms of aspiration allows for prompt intervention.*
Assist with diagnostic studies to determine if aspiration is occurring during swallowing (e.g., videofluoroscopy).	*Aspiration of foods/fluids during swallowing process is evident on studies such as video fluoroscopy. Knowing when aspiration occurs during the swallowing process aids in the development of an individualized plan of care to prevent further aspiration.*
Monitor chest radiograph results. Report findings of pulmonary infiltrate.	*Evidence of pulmonary infiltrate on chest radiograph results can indicate that aspiration has occurred.*

THERAPEUTIC INTERVENTIONS	RATIONALE
Independent Actions Implement measures to prevent aspiration if client has a depressed or absent gag reflex, severe dysphagia, and/or decreased level of consciousness: • Withhold oral foods/fluids. **D** ✦	*The risk for aspiration is high when mechanisms to protect the client's airway (e.g., gag reflex, swallowing reflex) are impaired or the client has a decreased level of consciousness.* *Withholding oral foods/fluids eliminates the possibility of aspiration of same.*
• Place client in a side-lying position unless contraindicated. **D** ● ✦	*Placing the client in a side-lying position allows oral secretions to accumulate in the mouth where they can be expectorated or removed by suctioning rather than flow into the pharynx where they can enter the larynx and be aspirated.*
• Perform oral hygiene and/or oropharyngeal suctioning as often as needed to remove excess secretions. **D** ✦	*Removing excess secretions from the mouth and pharynx prevents them from entering the larynx and being aspirated.*
Implement measures to prevent vomiting (e.g., eliminate noxious sights and odors). **D** ✦	*When the client vomits, gastric contents move up the esophagus, through the pharynx, and into the mouth. While vomitus is in the pharynx, it can spill into the larynx resulting in aspiration.*
If client is receiving tube feedings, check tube placement before each feeding or on a routine basis if tube feeding is continuous. **D** ✦	*Verification of feeding tube placement ensures that the tube feeding solution goes into the alimentary tract rather than the lungs.*
Implement measures to prevent aspiration when client is eating and drinking:	*When the client is eating and drinking, there is a high risk for aspiration before the swallowing reflex is triggered (i.e., the larynx and pharynx are at rest and the airway is open at this time), during swallowing if the larynx does not close completely, and after swallowing when the larynx opens again.*
• Place client in high Fowler's position unless contraindicated. **D** ● ✦	*This position uses gravity to facilitate movement of foods/fluids through the pharynx into the esophagus where the risk for aspiration is greatly reduced.*
• Instruct client to avoid laughing or talking when swallowing.	*Normally, when the swallowing reflex is triggered, the folds of the larynx that form its three valves contract so that aspiration does not occur as foods/fluids pass from the back of the mouth through the pharynx. When the client talks and laughs, air is forced through the trachea and the larynx opens. Instructing the client to avoid talking and laughing when swallowing reduces the risk of the airway being open when food/fluid is in the pharynx.*

THERAPEUTIC INTERVENTIONS	RATIONALE
• Encourage client to concentrate on eating and drinking and allow ample time for meals and snacks.	*If the client becomes distracted and/or is rushed during meals or snacks, swallowing and breathing attempts can become uncoordinated. This results in the larynx being open when the food/fluid is in the pharynx, which greatly increases the risk for aspiration.*
• Instruct client to dry swallow, cough twice, or clear his or her throat after swallowing if indicated.	*If the client has a swallowing impairment such as decreased pharyngeal peristalsis, food/fluid can remain in the pharyngeal recesses after the swallowing reflex has occurred. Dry swallowing, coughing, or clearing the throat helps ensure that the pharynx is clear after swallowing, which reduces the risk for aspiration.*
• Instruct and assist the client to perform oral hygiene after meals.	*Good oral hygiene after meals results in removal of remaining food particles that could enter the larynx and be aspirated into the lungs.*

Dependent/Collaborative Actions

Administer antiemetics as ordered. **D** ✦	*When the client vomits, gastric contents move up the esophagus, through the pharynx, and into the mouth. While vomitus is in the pharynx, it can spill into the larynx resulting in aspiration.*
Implement measures to reduce the risk of regurgitation (i.e., maintain gastric decompression as ordered, provide small meals rather than large ones, evaluate patient clinical tolerance of tube feedings if gastric residual >200–250 mL), maintain client in high Fowler's position for at least 30 minutes after meals and tube feedings, administer upper gastrointestinal stimulants as ordered. **D** ✦	*As gastric secretions or foods/fluids accumulate in the stomach, upward pressure is placed on the lower esophageal sphincter (LES). If the pressure increases significantly and/or the client has an incompetent LES, regurgitation can occur. Contents that move up through the esophagus into the pharynx can spill into the larynx, resulting in aspiration.*
Perform actions to improve swallowing if indicated (e.g., select foods/fluids appropriate to client's swallowing ability, reinforce exercises to strengthen and develop muscles used in swallowing).	*Improving the ability to swallow helps ensure that foods/fluids do not enter the larynx when the client is eating or drinking.*

Nursing Diagnosis # INEFFECTIVE BREATHING PATTERN NDx

Definition: Inspiration and/or expiration that does not provide adequate ventilation.

CLINICAL MANIFESTATIONS

Subjective	**Objective**
Verbal self-report of shortness of breath	Dyspnea; orthopnea; respiratory rate (adults [ages ≥14 years], <11 or >24 breaths/min; infants, <25 or >60 breaths/min; ages 1–4 years, <20 or >30 breaths/min; ages 5–14 years, <14 or >25 breaths/min); depth of breathing (tidal volume: adults, 500 mL at rest; infants, 6–8 mL/kg); decreased inspiratory/expiratory pressure; decreased minute ventilation; decreased vital capacity; nasal flaring; use of accessory muscles to breathe; assumption of three-point position; altered chest excursion; pursed-lip breathing; prolonged expiration phases; increased anterior-posterior chest diameter; decreased pulse oximetry readings

RISK FACTORS

- Hyperventilation
- Respiratory muscle fatigue
- Pain
- Perception/cognitive impairment
- Anxiety
- Decreased energy/fatigue
- Neuromuscular dysfunction
- Musculoskeletal impairment
- Chest wall deformity
- Obesity
- Spinal cord injury
- Body position that inhibits lung expansion
- Neurologic immaturity

NDx = NANDA Diagnosis   **D** = Delegatable Action   ● = UAP   ✦ = LVN/LPN   ⊖▶ = Go to ℮volve for animation

DESIRED OUTCOMES

The client will maintain an effective breathing pattern as evidenced by:
a. Normal rate and depth of respirations
b. Symmetric chest excursion
c. Absence of dyspnea

DOCUMENTATION

- Rate, depth, and ease of respirations
- Chest excursion
- Oximetry results
- Therapeutic interventions
- Client teaching

NOC OUTCOMES

Respiratory status: airway patency; respiratory status: ventilation; respiratory status: gas exchange; vital signs

NIC INTERVENTIONS

Respiratory monitoring; ventilation assistance; anxiety reduction

NURSING ASSESSMENT

Assess for signs and symptoms of an ineffective breathing pattern (e.g., shallow respirations, tachypnea, limited chest excursion, dyspnea, use of accessory muscles when breathing).

Monitor for and report a significant decrease in oximetry results.

RATIONALE

Early recognition of signs and symptoms of an ineffective breathing pattern allows for prompt intervention.

Oximetry is a noninvasive method of measuring arterial oxygen saturation. The results assist in evaluating respiratory status.

THERAPEUTIC INTERVENTIONS

Independent Actions

Implement measures to reduce chest or abdominal pain if present (e.g., splint incision with pillow during coughing and deep breathing). **D** ✦

Implement measures to decrease fear and anxiety (e.g., assure client that breathing deeply will not dislodge tubes or cause incision to break open, interact with client in a confident manner).

Implement measures to increase strength and activity tolerance if client is weak and fatigued (e.g., provide uninterrupted rest periods, maintain optimal nutrition). **D** ✦

Place client in a semi- to high-Fowler's position unless contraindicated. Position with pillows to prevent slumping. **D** ● ✦

If client must remain flat in bed, assist with position change at least every 2 hrs. **D** ● ✦

Instruct client to deep breathe or use incentive spirometer every 1 to 2 hrs. **D** ✦

Instruct client in and assist with diaphragmatic and pursed-lip breathing techniques if appropriate. NOTE: Diaphragmatic breathing is most often indicated for clients who have had thoracic surgery or clients who have chronic airflow limitation (e.g., emphysema) or neuromuscular conditions that cause fixation or weakening of the diaphragm.

Instruct client to breathe slowly if hyperventilating.

RATIONALE

A client with chest or upper abdominal pain often guards respiratory efforts and breathes shallowly in an attempt to prevent additional discomfort.

Fear and anxiety may cause a client to breathe shallowly or to hyperventilate. Decreasing fear and anxiety allows the client to focus on breathing more slowly and taking deeper breaths.

An increase in strength and activity tolerance enables the client to breathe more deeply and participate in activities to improve breathing pattern.

A semi- to high-Fowler's position allows for maximal diaphragmatic excursion and lung expansion. Prevention of slumping is essential because slumping causes the abdominal contents to be pushed up against the diaphragm and restricts lung expansion.

Compression of the thorax and subsequent limited chest wall and lung expansion occur when the client lies in one position. Frequent repositioning promotes maximal chest wall and lung expansion.

Deep breathing and use of an incentive spirometer promote maximal inhalation and lung expansion. Deep inhalation also stimulates surfactant production, which lowers alveolar surface tension and subsequently increases lung compliance and ease of inflation.

Diaphragmatic breathing promotes greater movement of the diaphragm and decreases the use of accessory muscles for inspiration. Use of this technique eases the work of breathing and ultimately promotes an increased efficiency of alveolar ventilation. Pursed-lip breathing causes a mild resistance to exhalation, which creates positive pressure in the airways. This pressure helps prevent airway collapse and subsequently promotes more complete alveolar emptying.

Hyperventilation is an ineffective breathing pattern that can eventually lead to respiratory alkalosis. The client can often slow breathing rate if he/she concentrates on doing so.

THERAPEUTIC INTERVENTIONS	RATIONALE
Dependent/Collaborative Actions	
Administer prescribed analgesics before planned activity. **D** ✦	*Pain reduction enables the client to breathe more deeply.*
Assist with positive airway pressure techniques (e.g., continuous positive airway pressure [CPAP], bilevel positive airway pressure [BiPAP], flutter/positive expiratory pressure [PEP] device) if ordered.	*Positive airway pressure techniques increase intrapulmonary (i.e., alveolar) pressure, which helps reexpand collapsed alveoli and prevent further alveolar collapse.*
Instruct client in and assist with segmental or localized breathing exercises if appropriate (may be indicated for clients with painful respiratory conditions or clients who have had thoracic or abdominal surgery).	*Segmental or localized breathing exercises improve expansion of apical and/or basal areas of the lung by having the client focus on selectively expanding these areas of the chest.*
Increase activity as allowed and tolerated. **D** ✦	*During activity, especially ambulation, the client usually takes deeper breaths, thus increasing lung expansion.*
Administer central nervous system depressants judiciously. Hold medication and consult physician if respiratory rate is less than 12/min.	*Central nervous system depressants cause depression of the respiratory center in the brainstem, which can result in a decreased rate and depth of respiration.*
Consult appropriate health care provider (e.g., physician, respiratory therapist) if ineffective breathing pattern continues.	*Notifying the appropriate health care provider allows for modification of treatment plan.*

Nursing Diagnosis **DECREASED CARDIAC OUTPUT** NDx

Definition: Inadequate blood pumped by the heart to meet the metabolic demands of the body.

CLINICAL MANIFESTATIONS

Subjective	Objective
Behavioral/Emotional: Verbal self-report of anxiety; restlessness	**Altered Heart Rate/Rhythm:** Dysrhythmias; palpitations; electrocardiogram (ECG) changes
	Altered Preload: Jugular vein distention (JVD); fatigue; edema; murmurs; increased/decreased central venous pressure (CVP); increased/decreased pulmonary artery wedge pressure (PAWP); weight gain
	Altered Afterload: Cold/clammy skin; shortness of breath/dyspnea; oliguria; prolonged capillary refill; decreased peripheral pulses; variations in blood pressure (BP) readings; increased/decreased systemic vascular resistance (SVR); increased/decreased pulmonary vascular resistance (PVR); skin color changes
	Altered Contractility: Crackles; cough; orthopnea/paroxysmal nocturnal dyspnea; cardiac output (CO) <4, L/min; cardiac index <2.5 L/min; decreased ejection fraction, stroke volume index (SVI), left ventricular stroke work index (LVSWI); S₃ or S₄ sounds

RISK FACTORS

- Altered heart rate/rhythm
- Altered stroke volume
- Altered preload
- Altered afterload
- Altered contractility

DESIRED OUTCOMES

The client will maintain adequate CO as evidenced by:
a. BP within normal range for client
b. Apical pulse regular and 60 to 100 beats/min
c. Absence of gallop rhythms
d. Absence of fatigue and weakness
e. Unlabored respirations at 12 to 20 breaths/min
f. Clear, audible breath sounds
g. Usual mental status

DOCUMENTATION

- Vital signs
- Heart sounds
- Activity tolerance
- Breath sounds
- Ease of respirations
- Mental status
- Peripheral pulses
- Capillary refill time
- Skin color and temperature
- Urine output
- Presence of edema
- Presence of JVD
- Hemodynamic measurements (e.g., CO, pulmonary artery pressure [PAP], pulmonary capillary wedge pressure [PCWP], CVP)
- Therapeutic interventions
- Client teaching
- Dysrhythmias

NOC OUTCOMES

Cardiac pump effectiveness; cardiopulmonary status; circulation status; fluid overload severity; tissue perfusion: abdominal organs, cardiac, cellular, cerebral, and peripheral; vital signs

NIC INTERVENTIONS

Cardiac care: acute; invasive hemodynamic monitoring; hemodynamic regulation; cardiac precautions; dysrhythmia management; oxygen therapy; hypovolemia management; hypervolemia management; electrolyte management: hypomagnesemia; electrolyte management: hyperkalemia; cardiac care: rehabilitative

NURSING ASSESSMENT

Assess for and report signs and symptoms of decreased CO:
- Variations in BP (may be increased because of compensatory vasoconstriction; may be decreased when compensatory mechanisms and pump fail)
- Tachycardia
- Presence of gallop rhythm
- Fatigue and weakness
- Dyspnea, tachypnea
- Crackles (rales)
- Restlessness, change in mental status
- Dizziness, syncope
- Diminished or absent peripheral pulses
- Cool extremities
- Pallor or cyanosis of skin
- Capillary refill time greater than 2 to 3 seconds
- Oliguria
- Edema
- JVD
- Hemodynamic abnormalities such as decreased CO and increased PAP, PCWP, and CVP

Monitor ECG readings and report significant abnormalities.

Monitor chest radiograph results. Report findings of cardiomegaly, pulmonary vascular congestion, pleural effusion, or pulmonary edema.

RATIONALE

Early recognition of signs and symptoms of decreased CO allows for prompt intervention.

ECG readings provide data regarding functioning of the heart's electrical conduction system. Altered generation or transmission of electrical impulses often causes an abnormal heart rate or rhythm that can lead to decreased CO.

Chest radiograph films provide data regarding the size of the heart, volume of blood in the pulmonary vessels, and fluid accumulation in the pleural space, pulmonary interstitium, and alveoli. Cardiomegaly often results in decreased CO, whereas pulmonary vascular congestion, pleural effusion, and pulmonary edema are often a result of decreased CO.

NURSING ASSESSMENT	RATIONALE
Monitor serum electrolytes, cardiac enzymes, troponin, and brain natriuretic peptide (BNP) levels.	*Alterations in serum electrolytes such as potassium and magnesium can precipitate cardiac dysrhythmias that may significantly alter CO/tissue perfusion. Serum troponin level alterations can indicate myocardial tissue damage, while serum BNP levels can indicate congestive heart failure. The presence of either situation can influence optimum CO.*

THERAPEUTIC INTERVENTIONS	RATIONALE

Independent Actions

Implement measures to reduce cardiac workload:	*Cardiac workload is the effort the heart expends to pump blood. The work of the heart is determined largely by the volume of blood distending the ventricles at the end of diastole (preload) and the amount of tension the ventricle must pump against to eject blood (afterload). Decreasing cardiac workload reduces the work that the compromised heart must perform in order to pump an adequate amount of blood. This results in increased CO.*
• Place client in a semi- to high-Fowler's position. **D** ● ✦	*Elevation of client's upper body reduces cardiac workload by decreasing venous return from the periphery and subsequently reducing preload.*
• Instruct client to avoid activities that create a Valsalva response (e.g., straining to have a bowel movement, holding breath while moving up in bed).	*When a client exhales after the Valsalva maneuver, the intrathoracic pressure falls, causing a sudden increase in venous return and a subsequent increase in preload and cardiac workload. The rebound increase in heart rate and BP that occurs after the Valsalva maneuver also causes an increase in cardiac workload.*
• Perform actions to promote physical and emotional rest (e.g., maintain a calm, quiet environment; limit the number of visitors; maintain activity restrictions). **D** ✦	*Physical rest reduces cardiac workload by lowering the body's energy requirements and subsequent need for oxygen. Promoting emotional rest reduces cardiac workload by preventing the increase in heart rate and BP that accompanies stress-induced sympathetic nervous system stimulation.*
• Perform actions to promote adequate tissue oxygenation (e.g., encourage deep breathing exercises and use of incentive spirometer). **D** ✦	*When tissue oxygenation is adequate, the heart does not need to work as hard to supply oxygen to the tissues; thus more oxygen is available for myocardial use.*
• Discourage smoking.	*Nicotine stimulates catecholamine output, which increases heart rate and causes vasoconstriction and subsequently increases cardiac workload. Smoking also reduces oxygen availability because hemoglobin has a greater affinity for the carbon monoxide in smoke than for oxygen. This increases cardiac workload as the heart tries to compensate for the reduced oxygen levels.*
• Discourage excessive intake of beverages high in caffeine such as coffee, tea, and colas	*Excessive caffeine can increase cardiac workload because caffeine is a myocardial stimulant and can increase the rate and force of myocardial contractions.*
• Provide small meals rather than large ones.	*Large meals can increase cardiac workload because they require a greater increase in blood supply to the gastrointestinal tract to aid digestion.*

Dependent/Collaborative Actions

Implement measures to prevent hypovolemia (e.g., maintain a minimal fluid intake of 1000 mL/day unless ordered otherwise, consult physician before giving diuretics if excessive weight loss has occurred or client develops postural hypotension, administer blood and/or colloid or crystalloid solutions as ordered).	*Hypovolemia reduces venous return to the heart, which subsequently decreases the amount of blood in the ventricles at the end of diastole (preload). This results in a decrease in stroke volume and CO.*
Maintain oxygen therapy as ordered. **D** ✦	*When tissue oxygenation is adequate, the heart does not need to work as hard to supply oxygen to the tissues; thus more oxygen is available for myocardial use.*
Perform actions to prevent or treat fluid volume excess (e.g., maintain prescribed fluid and dietary sodium restrictions, administer diuretics as ordered).	*Preventing or treating excess fluid volume reduces vascular volume, which decreases preload and afterload and subsequently reduces cardiac workload.*

Continued...

THERAPEUTIC INTERVENTIONS	RATIONALE
Increase activity gradually as allowed and tolerated. **D** ●	*A gradual increase in activity prevents a sudden increase in cardiac workload. A graded activity program also helps strengthen and tone the myocardium, which ultimately increases CO.*
Administer the following medications if ordered:	
• Positive inotropic agents (e.g., digitalis preparations, dobutamine, dopamine, inamrinone, milrinone)	*Positive inotropic agents increase CO by improving myocardial contractility.*
• Nitrates (e.g., nitroglycerin, isosorbide dinitrate)	*Nitrates decrease cardiac workload and myocardial oxygen demands by relaxing peripheral veins and, to a lesser extent, arterioles. This reduces venous return to the heart (preload) and peripheral vascular resistance (afterload). Nitrates also dilate nonsclerosed coronary arteries, which improves coronary blood flow and myocardial oxygen supply.*
• Direct-acting vasodilators (e.g., sodium nitroprusside, hydralazine) or centrally acting or alpha-adrenergic inhibitors (e.g., clonidine, prazosin, doxazosin)	*Vasodilators reduce cardiac workload by dilating the arterioles and subsequently decreasing peripheral vascular resistance (afterload). Certain vasodilators also dilate the veins, which decreases venous return and lowers diastolic ventricular filling pressure (preload).*
• Angiotensin-converting enzyme (ACE) inhibitors (e.g., captopril, enalapril, lisinopril, benazepril, fosinopril, quinapril) or angiotensin II receptor antagonists (e.g., losartan, valsartan)	*ACE inhibitors/angiotensin II receptor antagonists block the formation/effect of angiotensin II (a potent vasoconstrictor), which subsequently also causes a decrease in aldosterone output. The reduction in angiotensin II and aldosterone results in a decrease in total peripheral vascular resistance and reduced sodium and water retention, which leads to decreased cardiac workload.*
• Beta-adrenergic blocking agents (e.g., propranolol, metoprolol, atenolol, nadolol, sotalol)	*Beta-adrenergic blockers reduce cardiac workload by blocking sympathetic nervous system stimulation of beta-receptors in the heart.*
• Anticholinergic agents (e.g., atropine)	*CO is dependent on stroke volume and heart rate. Anticholinergics increase the heart rate (i.e., have a positive chronotropic effect) and are used to increase CO in clients with bradydysrhythmias.*
• Antidysrhythmics (e.g., flecainide, lidocaine, disopyramide, procainamide, amiodarone, esmolol, sotalol, adenosine)	*Antidysrhythmics improve CO by correcting automaticity and/or conduction abnormalities in the heart. By slowing the heart rate and/or decreasing irregularity of the heart rate, the diastolic filling time is prolonged, resulting in an increased preload and stroke volume.*
• Calcium channel blocking agents (e.g., nifedipine, verapamil, diltiazem, nicardipine, amlodipine)	*Calcium channel blockers dilate the coronary arteries, thus improving coronary blood flow and myocardial oxygen supply. They also reduce cardiac workload by dilating peripheral arteries and subsequently reducing afterload. Certain calcium channel blockers (e.g., diltiazem, verapamil) also have an antidysrhythmic effect, which subsequently increases CO by helping restore normal heart rate and rhythm.*
Consult physician if signs and symptoms of decreased CO persist or worsen.	*Notifying the physician allows for modification of treatment plan.*

Nursing Diagnosis **READINESS FOR ENHANCED COMFORT** NDx

For a full, detailed care plan on this topic, go to http://evolve.elsevier.com/Haugen/careplanning/.

Nursing Diagnosis **ACUTE CONFUSION** NDx

Definition: Reversible disturbances of consciousness, attention, cognition, and perception that develop over a short period of time, and which lasts less than 3 months.

CLINICAL MANIFESTATIONS

Subjective	Objective
Verbal self-report of visual, auditory hallucinations	Exaggerated emotional responses; fluctuations in level of consciousness/cognition; alterations in normal sleep/wake cycle; increased agitation/restlessness; altered perceptive ability (inappropriate responses); lack of ability to initiate or follow through with goal-directed or purposeful behavior

RISK FACTORS

- Medication reaction/drug-to-drug interaction
- Substance abuse
- Delirium
- Metabolic imbalances
- Chronic illness exacerbation
- Elderly
- Dementia
- Hypoxemia
- Pain
- Sleep deprivation
- Infection

DESIRED OUTCOMES

The client will regain usual reality orientation and level of consciousness as evidenced by:
a. Ability to participate independently in activities of daily living
b. Decrease in agitation/restlessness
c. Improvement in sleep/wake cycles
d. Appropriate responses to environmental stimuli

DOCUMENTATION

- Level of consciousness/orientation
- Electrolyte values
- Oxygenation
- Vital signs
- Safety risk
- Restraint use

NOC OUTCOMES

Cognitive orientation; neurologic status: consciousness; fatigue level; anxiety level; agitation level; sleep; electrolyte and acid-base balance; respiratory status: gas exchange; blood glucose level

NIC INTERVENTIONS

Delirium management; electrolyte monitoring; electrolyte management; acid-base management; oxygen therapy; peripheral sensation management

NURSING ASSESSMENT

	RATIONALE
Assess for signs and symptoms of acute confusion (e.g., changes in level of consciousness, changes in baseline behavior, increased agitation, hallucinations, and impaired perceptive ability).	*Early recognition of signs and symptoms of acute confusion allows for prompt intervention.*
Assess vital signs for evidence of poor perfusion (e.g., hypotension, tachycardia, tachypnea).	*Poor perfusion to vital organs such as the brain, which can be exacerbated by hypotension or extreme tachycardia, can alter normal cognitive states, leading to confusion.*
Monitor serum glucose levels, drug levels for abnormalities. Monitor pulse oximetry for hypoxemia.	*Altered metabolic parameters (e.g., hypoglycemia and hypoxia) can contribute to confusion and as a priority must be ruled out as potential causes of confusion. Failure to rule out possible metabolic causes of confusion can lead to serious adverse patient outcomes.*
Assess for contributing factors (e.g., substance abuse/withdrawal, episodes of high fever, exposure to toxic substances, drug-to-drug interactions, chronic illness exacerbations, sleep alterations, diet/nutritional alterations, infection).	*Because of the reversible nature of acute confusion, contributing factors should be identified and corrected to return the patient to his/her normal state of cognition.*

THERAPEUTIC INTERVENTIONS

	RATIONALE
Independent Actions Implement measures to maintain a safe patient care environment (e.g., supervision/sitter, family member assistance, side rails). **D ✦** *Note: the use of restraints should be limited because this may worsen the situation by increasing agitation.*	*A confused patient is at risk for injury. Measures must be implemented that protect the patient from injury. Restraints must be used with extreme caution (e.g., behavior that is indicative of violence) because use may increase the risk of patient injury.*

NDx = NANDA Diagnosis **D** = Delegatable Action ● = UAP ✦ = LVN/LPN ⊜▶ = Go to ⊜volve for animation

Continued...

THERAPEUTIC INTERVENTIONS	RATIONALE
Implement measures that assist with client orientation (e.g., clock/calendar within visual field of the client). **D** ● ✦	*The use of orientation aids will assist the patient in establishing an awareness of self and the environment.*
Establish routines as much as possible when providing care and be as consistent as possible in following the routine. **D** ● ✦	*A consistent routine aids in task completion and helps reduce confusion. A consistent, stable environment reduces confusion and frustration.*
Implement measures that reduce sensory overload to the patient: **D** ● ✦	*Reducing sensory overload by limiting environmental noise and stimulation will help prevent the patient from becoming more confused.*
• Cluster nursing care to provide adequate rest periods.	
• Maintain a calm environment, eliminating any unnecessary noise.	
• Provide undisturbed periods of rest.	
Implement measures that foster an awareness of self and environment: **D** ● ✦	*Fostering a sense of self and environment will aid in regaining/maintaining usual reality orientation.*
• Address patient by name.	
• Mention the date, time, and place frequently during the day.	
Provide simple instructions allowing patient adequate time to respond, communicate, and make decisions. **D** ● ✦	*These actions help to decrease confusion, reduce frustration, and promote task completion.*
Encourage family members to share stories, discuss familiar people and events, and assist with orientation. **D** ✦	*Sharing familiar events promotes a sense of continuity and creates a sense of overall security and comfort in a confused patient.*

Dependent/Collaborative Actions

Administer short-acting sleep aids as ordered to facilitate undisturbed periods of rest. **D** ✦	*Undisturbed rest periods will help restore cognitive orientation in acutely confused patients without metabolic alterations.*
Administer psychotropics cautiously to control restlessness, hallucinations, and agitation. **D** ✦	*Medication to reduce restlessness, hallucinations, and agitation can help calm a confused patient. It is most important that metabolic alterations are ruled out as the cause of the confusion/agitation and restlessness before medication administration.*
Notify physician of continued or intensifying confusion, concerning drug-to-drug interactions, signs and symptoms of infection, and abnormal laboratory results.	*Notifying the appropriate health care provider allows for modification of the treatment plan.*

Nursing Diagnosis   **CONSTIPATION** NDx

Definition: Decrease in normal frequency of defecation accompanied by difficult or incomplete passage of stool and/or passage of excessively hard, dry stool.

CLINICAL MANIFESTATIONS

Subjective	Objective
Verbal self-report of straining with defecation; pain with defecation; increased abdominal pressure; feeling of rectal fullness or pressure; inability to pass stool; headache; indigestion; verbalization of abdominal pain and tenderness, and nausea	Change in bowel pattern; bright red blood with stool; presence of soft, pastelike stool in rectum; distended abdomen; dark, black, or tarry stool; percussed abdominal dullness; decreased volume of stool; decreased frequency; dry, hard, formed stool; palpable rectal mass; abdominal pain; anorexia; change in abdominal growling (borborygmi); atypical presentation in older adults (e.g., change in mental status, urinary incontinence; unexplained falls, elevated body temperature); severe flatus; hypoactive or hyperactive bowel sounds; palpable abdominal mass; abdominal tenderness with or palpable muscle resistance; nausea and/or vomiting; oozing liquid stool

RISK FACTORS

- **Functional:** Recent environmental changes; habitual denying/ignoring of urge to defecate; insufficient physical activity; irregular defecation habits; inadequate toileting (e.g., timeliness, positioning for defecation, privacy); abdominal muscle weakness
- **Psychologic:** Depression; emotional stress; mental confusion; decreased mobility/immobility
- **Pharmacologic:** Anticonvulsants; antilipemic agents; laxative overdose; calcium carbonate; aluminum-containing antacids; nonsteroidal antiinflammatory agents; opiates; anticholinergics; diuretics; iron salts; phenothiazines; sedatives; sympathomimetics; bismuth salts; antidepressants; calcium channel blockers
- **Mechanical:** Rectal abscess or ulcer; pregnancy; rectal anal fissures; tumors; megacolon (Hirschsprung's disease); electrolyte imbalance; rectal prolapse; prostate enlargement; neurologic impairment; rectal anal stricture; rectocele; postsurgical obstruction; hemorrhoids; obesity
- **Physiologic:** Poor eating habits; decreased motility of gastrointestinal tract; inadequate dentition or oral hygiene; insufficient fiber intake; insufficient fluid intake; change in usual foods and eating pattern; dehydration

DESIRED OUTCOMES

The client will maintain usual bowel elimination pattern as evidenced by:
a. Usual frequency of bowel movements
b. Passage of soft, formed stool
c. Absence of abdominal distention and pain, feeling of rectal fullness or pressure, and straining during defecation

DOCUMENTATION

- Occurrence of last bowel movement
- Characteristics of stool
- Abdominal distention or report of pain
- Reports of fullness or pressure in rectum
- Reports of straining at stool
- Bowel sounds
- Therapeutic interventions
- Client teaching

NOC OUTCOMES

Bowel elimination; gastrointestinal function; hydration; nausea and vomiting severity; symptom control

NIC INTERVENTIONS

Constipation/impaction management

NURSING ASSESSMENT	RATIONALE
Ascertain client's usual bowel elimination habits.	*Knowledge of the client's usual bowel elimination habits is essential in determining whether constipation is present, because the frequency of defecation varies among individuals.*
Assess for signs and symptoms of constipation: • Decrease in frequency of bowel movements • Passage of hard, formed stools • Anorexia • Abdominal distention and pain • Feeling of fullness or pressure in rectum • Straining during defecation	*Early recognition of signs and symptoms of constipation allows for prompt intervention.*
Assess bowel sounds. Report a pattern of decreasing bowel sounds.	*Bowel sounds are produced by peristaltic activity. A pattern of decreasing bowel sounds indicates a decrease in bowel motility, which can lead to and be present with constipation.*

THERAPEUTIC INTERVENTIONS	RATIONALE

Independent Actions

| Encourage client to defecate whenever the urge is felt. **D** ● ✦ | *If the client feels the urge to defecate but suppresses it by contracting the external anal sphincter, the defecation reflex will subside after a few minutes and not recur for several hours or until additional feces enter the rectum. Repeated inhibition of the defecation reflex results in progressive weakening of the reflex. In addition, when the defecation reflex is inhibited, feces remain in the colon longer and water continues to be absorbed from the feces, making the stool drier, harder, and subsequently more difficult to evacuate.* |

Continued...

THERAPEUTIC INTERVENTIONS	RATIONALE
Assist client to toilet or bedside commode or place in high-Fowler's position on bedpan for bowel movements unless contraindicated. **D** ● ✦	*A sitting position aids in the expulsion of stool by taking advantage of gravity. This position also enhances the client's ability to perform the Valsalva maneuver, which increases intra-abdominal pressure and forces the fecal contents downward and into the rectum where the defecation reflex is then elicited.*
Encourage client to relax, provide privacy, and have call signal within reach during attempts to defecate. **D** ✦	*If the client is able to relax during attempts to defecate, he/she will be able to relax the levator ani muscle and external anal sphincter, thus facilitating the passage of stool.*
Encourage client to establish a regular time for defecation, preferably within an hour after a meal. **D** ✦	*Attempting to have a bowel movement within an hour after a meal, particularly breakfast, takes advantage of mass peristalsis, which occurs only a few times a day and is strongest after meals. Mass peristalsis is stimulated by the gastrocolic reflex, which is initiated by the presence of foods/fluids in the stomach and duodenum.*
Instruct client to increase intake of foods high in fiber (e.g., bran, whole grain breads and cereals, fresh fruits and vegetables) unless contraindicated.	*Foods high in fiber provide bulk to the fecal mass and keep the stool soft because of the ability of fiber to absorb water. The increased bulkiness (i.e., mass) of the stools stimulates peristalsis, which promotes more rapid movement of stool through the colon. Also, the shorter the time that feces remain in the intestine, the less water is absorbed from it, which helps prevent the formation of hard, dry stools that are difficult to expel.*
Encourage client to drink hot liquids (e.g., coffee, tea) upon arising in the morning. **D** ✦	*Ingestion of hot fluids can stimulate peristalsis.*
Encourage client to increase activity as tolerated/as condition allows. **D** ✦	*Increase in activity increases bowel motility, decreasing risk for constipation.*

Dependent/Collaborative Actions

Instruct client to maintain a minimal fluid intake of 2500 mL/day unless contraindicated.	*Inadequate fluid intake reduces the water content of feces, which results in hard, dry stool that is difficult to evacuate.*
Increase activity as allowed and tolerated. **D** ● ✦	*Ambulation stimulates peristalsis, which promotes the passage of stool through the intestines.*
When appropriate, encourage the use of nonnarcotic rather than opioid analgesics for pain management.	*Narcotic analgesics slow peristalsis, which delays transit of intestinal contents. This delay also results in increased absorption of fluid from the fecal mass with the subsequent formation of hard, dry stool.*
Administer laxatives or cathartics (e.g., stool softeners, bulk-forming agents, irritants/stimulants, lubricants, saline/osmotic agents) as ordered. **D** ✦	*Laxatives/cathartics act in a variety of ways to soften the stool, increase stool bulk, stimulate bowel motility, and/or lubricate the fecal mass and thereby promote the evacuation of stool.*
Administer cleansing and/or oil retention enemas if ordered. **D** ● ✦	*A cleansing enema stimulates peristalsis and evacuation of stool by distending the colon with a large volume of solution and/or by irritating the colonic mucosa. An oil retention enema facilitates the passage of stool by softening the fecal mass and lubricating the rectum and anal canal.*
Consult physician about checking for an impaction and digitally removing stool if the client has not had a bowel movement in 3 days, if he/she is passing liquid stool, or if other signs and symptoms of constipation are present.	*An impaction prohibits the normal passage of feces. Digital removal of an impacted fecal mass may be necessary before normal passage of stool can occur.*
Consult appropriate health care provider if diarrhea persists.	*Notifying the appropriate health care provider allows for modification of the treatment plan.*

Nursing Diagnosis CONTAMINATION NDx/

Definition:
* Exposure to environmental contaminants in doses sufficient to cause adverse health effects.

CLINICAL MANIFESTATIONS

Subjective	Objective
Verbal report of exposure to potentially toxic agents	*Note*: Health effects will depend upon the type of contaminant and may include all body systems. Principal routes of exposure include inhalation, absorption, ingestion, and injection. Types of contaminants include incapacitating agents, chemical agents (organophosphates), nerve agents (sarin), cyanide agents, vesicant/blister agents (nitrogen mustards), pulmonary/choking agents (chlorine), riot control agents (pepper spray/tear gas). Objective assessment data will reflect the offending agent and route of absorption.
Pesticides/Chemicals/Biologicals: Verbal self-report of a "stomachache"; cramping; blurred vision; joint and muscle aches; difficulty breathing; flu symptoms; verbalization of nausea; hallucinations	Cardiac dysrhythmias; hypertension/hypotension; diarrhea; nausea; muscle weakness; confusion; seizures; decreased level of consciousness; cough; labored breathing; cyanosis; skin lesions (e.g., rash, pustules, scabs)
Radiation: Verbal self-report of nausea; visual changes; difficulty breathing; verbalization of weakness; fatigue; skin irritation; abdominal pain	Symptoms of radiation sickness (i.e., weakness, hair loss, changes in blood chemistries, hemorrhage, diminished organ function); paresthesias; confusion; lethargy; changes in level of consciousness; skin irritation; itching; blistering; burns; erythema; ulcerations
Waste: Verbal self-report of nausea; abdominal cramps	Anorexia; diarrhea; weight loss; jaundice; weakness; fever
Pollution: Verbal self-report of difficulty breathing; chest pain; headaches; shortness of breath	Reddened conjunctiva; tearing; wheezing; pulmonary congestion; nasal congestion

RISK FACTORS
* **External:** Chemical contamination of food and/or water; bioterrorism; disasters; insufficient or absent use of decontamination protocol; inappropriate or no use of protective clothing; living in poverty; poor sanitation; climate conditions
* **Internal:** Gestational age during exposure; developmental stage; gender; nutritional factors; the presence of preexisting disease

DESIRED OUTCOMES

The client will experience minimal health alterations.

DOCUMENTATION

* Therapeutic interventions
* Decontamination protocol
* Isolation precautions

NOC OUTCOMES

Respiratory status: gas exchange; physical injury severity; anxiety level; fear level; community disaster readiness

NIC INTERVENTIONS

Triage: disaster; infection control; anxiety reduction; crisis intervention; environmental risk protection; bioterrorism preparedness

NURSING ASSESSMENT	RATIONALE
Assess vital signs, including temperature, noting signs and symptoms of inhalation, absorption, ingestion, or injection of environmental contaminants by performing frequent, prioritized multisystem assessment.	*Early recognition of signs and symptoms of contamination allows for prompt intervention.*
• Monitor airway and respiratory status (e.g., rate and depth of breathing, adventitious breath sounds, pulse oximetry).	*Effects of contaminants can be delayed 2 to 24 hrs. Rapid onset of pulmonary symptoms indicates a poor prognosis. Early detection allows for aggressive treatment of symptoms.*

Continued...

NURSING ASSESSMENT	RATIONALE
• Monitor cardiac rhythm.	*Cardiac monitoring should be implemented for any patients exhibiting irregularity (i.e., symptomatic bradycardia, symptomatic tachycardia) to allow for prompt intervention.*
• Assess neuromuscular status.	*Variable routes of exposure to nerve agents may result in symptoms that may not appear for 30 minutes to 18 hrs. Vaporized nerve agents are most toxic, with symptoms appearing within seconds. Diagnosis and treatment are based on observations of signs and symptoms.*
• Assess integumentary system.	*Contaminants absorbed through the skin or eyes produce immediate symptoms. Prompt assessment allows for early implementation of interventions.*
• Monitor serum chemistry and complete blood cell count (CBC) results, reporting abnormalities.	*Monitoring lab values allows for the assessment of hematologic and multisystem consequences of exposure to contaminants.*

THERAPEUTIC INTERVENTIONS	RATIONALE

Independent Actions
Actual exposure:

Provide protective clothing for all health care providers caring for the exposed client (e.g., disposable scrubs, waterproof shoe covers, gowns with seams taped, hat, mask, goggles, double gloves taped at the wrist). **D** ● ✦	*Health care providers must protect themselves from contamination and control further spread.*

Institute decontamination protocols:

• Remove and isolate clothing for decontamination. Clothing exposed to radiation must be sealed in an airtight container and labeled appropriately.	*Prompt removal of contaminated clothing prevents further exposure of skin to contaminants, prevents further absorption of contaminants, and facilitates effective decontamination. Removing clothing can reduce contamination 80% to 90%.*
• Wash intact skin or damaged skin with soap and water. **D** ● ✦	*Washing exposed skin reduces the amount of contaminants absorbed.*
• Irrigate exposed/injured eyes copiously with water. **D** ✦	*Irrigation of eyes reduces the amount of contaminants absorbed.*
• Implement appropriate isolation precautions (e.g., universal, airborne, droplet, and contact isolation). **D** ✦	*Appropriate isolation precautions will assist in reducing the further spread of contaminants and protect health care providers caring for the exposed client.*
Explain decontamination protocols and the need for isolation to patient and family to help alleviate anxiety.	*Providing factual information to the patient and family concerning treatment will help in reducing anxiety associated with fear.*
Encourage patient to verbalize feelings, perceptions, and fears. **D** ✦	*Verbalization of fears or concerns can assist the health care practitioner in identifying knowledge deficits amenable to education while alleviating apprehension on the part of the client.*

Dependent/Collaborative Actions

Establish intravenous access for the administration of medications. **D** ✦	*Many of the drugs used to treat environmental contamination are administered intravenously requiring establishment of access.*
Administer oxygen, bronchodilators, corticosteroids for pulmonary symptoms. **D** ✦	*The use of supplemental oxygen will improve the client's arterial oxygen level, which may become compromised with the development of pulmonary edema. Bronchodilators and corticosteroids will assist with treating inflammatory changes occurring with pulmonary pathology, improving oxygenation and ventilation.*
Wash exposed skin with 0.5% sodium hypochlorite solution for 10 minutes. **D** ✦	*Use of this solution is helpful with gross contamination of the skin, rendering offending contaminants harmless.*
Administer activated charcoal as quickly as possible for gastrointestinal decontamination. **D** ✦	*Activated charcoal should be administered as soon as possible because it absorbs almost all commonly ingested drugs and chemicals except iron, lithium, ethanol, and potassium. Emesis and gastric lavage should be avoided.*

THERAPEUTIC INTERVENTIONS	RATIONALE
Administer drugs for treatment of nerve agent poisoning (e.g., atropine, pralidoxime, and diazepam). **D** ✦	*Atropine administration is indicated for clients exhibiting muscarinic cholinergic excess (e.g., drying of bronchial secretions and decreasing adverse effects including salivation, lacrimation, urination, defecation, and emesis). Pralidoxime administration is indicated for all patients requiring atropine and in those with or at risk for nicotinic cholinergic (e.g., decreased atropine requirements) and treatment of muscle fasciculations and weakness (e.g., nicotinic signs of poisoning). Diazepam or other benzodiazepines are indicated in patients with signs of severe toxicity or seizures.*
Administer drugs for the treatment of cyanide poisoning (e.g., intranasal amyl nitrate, sodium nitrite, sodium thiosulfate). **D** ✦	*Amyl nitrite is administered as an inhalant, followed by sodium nitrite and sodium thiosulfate, which are given intravenously. The nitrites are given to convert hemoglobin in the red blood cell to methemoglobin, which attracts the cyanide away from the cytochrome oxidase and allows the cell to continue the process of aerobic metabolism. Thiosulfate is given to facilitate detoxification of cyanide by the body's own cyanide clearance system.*
Administer antibiotics for secondary bacterial infections. **D** ✦	*Clients exhibiting signs and symptoms of infection (e.g., fever, chills, sweating, increased white blood cell count, pus in open wounds) require the administration of antibiotics to help the body and normal defenses overcome infections.*

Risk for Exposure

Conduct surveillance for environmental contamination. Notify agencies authorized to protect the environment of contaminants in the area.	*Assessment of the client's community and immediate environment can assist with the identification of contaminants that could threaten individual and community health status.*
Assist individuals to modify the environment to minimize risk or assist in relocating to a safer environment.	*Nurses can assist individuals and communities in incorporating environmentally responsible ways in dealing with activities of daily living.*
Collaborate with other agencies to schedule mass casualty and disaster readiness drills.	*In the event a disaster that predisposes a community to contaminants becomes a reality, local health care providers and the community at large must be prepared to respond appropriately.*

Nursing Diagnosis ## INEFFECTIVE COPING NDx

For a full, detailed care plan on this topic, go to http://evolve.elsevier.com/Haugen/careplanning/.

Nursing Diagnosis ## READINESS FOR ENHANCED DECISION-MAKING NDx

For a full, detailed care plan on this topic, go to http://evolve.elsevier.com/Haugen/careplanning/.

Nursing Diagnosis ## DIARRHEA NDx

Definition: Passage of loose, unformed stools.

CLINICAL MANIFESTATIONS

Subjective	Objective
Verbal self-report of urgency, abdominal pain and cramping	Hyperactive bowel sounds; at least three loose liquid stools per day

---

NDx = NANDA Diagnosis   **D** = Delegatable Action   ● = UAP   ✦ = LVN/LPN   ⊝▶ = Go to ⊝volve for animation

RISK FACTORS

- **Situational:** Alcohol abuse; toxins; laxative abuse; radiation; tube feedings; adverse effects of medications; contaminants; travel

- **Psychosocial:** High stress levels and anxiety

- **Physiologic:** Inflammation; malabsorption; infectious processes; irritation; parasites

DESIRED OUTCOMES

The client will have fewer bowel movements and more formed stool.

DOCUMENTATION

- Frequency of defecation
- Characteristics of stool
- Complaints of abdominal cramping
- Bowel sounds
- Therapeutic interventions
- Client teaching

NOC OUTCOMES

Bowel continence; bowel elimination; fluid balance; symptom severity; gastrointestinal function

NIC INTERVENTIONS

Diarrhea management

NURSING ASSESSMENT	RATIONALE
Ascertain client's usual bowel elimination habits.	*Knowledge of the client's usual bowel elimination habits helps determine the severity of the diarrhea.*
Assess for and report signs and symptoms of diarrhea (e.g., frequent loose stools; urgency; abdominal cramping; hyperactive bowel sounds).	*Early recognition of signs and symptoms of diarrhea allows for prompt intervention.*
Assess for factors that may be causing diarrhea (e.g., antimicrobial agents, laxative use, tube feedings, gastrointestinal disorder, change in dietary intake, intestinal infection).	*Knowing the cause of the diarrhea is a critical component in identifying the appropriate treatment.*

THERAPEUTIC INTERVENTIONS	RATIONALE

Independent Actions

As diet advances, gradually progress from fluids to small meals. **D** ● ✦	*Gradual introduction of small amounts of fluid and then food helps prevent a sudden increase in peristalsis and diarrhea.*
Instruct the client to avoid the following foods/fluids:	
• Those known to aggravate diarrhea such as spicy foods, alcohol, coffee, and fatty foods	*These substances are thought to increase intestinal motility and may also cause excessive mucus secretion, which increases the liquidity of the intestinal contents.*
• Those that are extremely hot or cold	*Extremes in temperature of ingested foods/fluids often stimulate peristalsis.*
• Those high in lactose such as milk and milk products	*Diarrhea may temporarily deplete the gastrointestinal enzyme lactase, which is essential for the hydrolysis and subsequent absorption of lactose. The nonabsorbed lactose has an osmotic effect and draws water into the colon, which results in more liquid stool. The lactose also serves as a base for bacterial fermentation in the colon. The lactic and fatty acids produced by this fermentation process irritate the colon, with a subsequent increase in bowel motility and diarrhea.*
• Those foods high in fiber such as whole-grain cereals, raw fruits, and vegetables	*Fiber increases bulk of the stool because of its ability to absorb water. The increased mass (i.e., bulk) of the stools stimulates peristalsis. Limiting fiber intake decreases the water content of the stool, which results in drier, firmer, and less bulky stools. The decrease in bulk (i.e., mass) results in less stimulation of peristalsis, and the dryness of the stools slows intestinal transit time.*
• Those foods made with synthetic, nonabsorbable sugars (e.g., sorbitol) that are found in many dietetic foods	*Synthetic, nonabsorbable sugars are not well absorbed from the gastrointestinal tract and tend to draw water into the intestine by osmosis. This excess water in the intestine increases fluidity and volume of stool.*

THERAPEUTIC INTERVENTIONS	RATIONALE

Implement measures to reduce fear and anxiety:
- Provide client teaching.
- All care providers are to interact with the client in a calm manner.

Encourage the client to rest. **D** ✦

Parasympathetic activity may dominate in some stressful situations and cause increased gastrointestinal motility and diarrhea.

Physical activity stimulates peristalsis.

Dependent/Collaborative Actions

Limit oral intake to clear liquids and replacement solutions as ordered. **D** ✦
- Pedialyte
- Resol
- Rehydrate
- Administer prescribed antianxiety agents. **D** ✦

Peristalsis is stimulated by the presence of foods/fluids in the stomach and duodenum. Restricting oral intake to clear liquids and/or replacement solutions during the acute phase of diarrhea not only allows the bowel to rest but also helps prevent malnutrition and fluid and electrolyte imbalances.

If the client is receiving tube feeding, administer the solution at room temperature. Consult physician about reducing the rate of administration and/or the concentration of the tube feeding solution if diarrhea occurs. **D** ✦

Tube feeding can increase peristalsis if the solution is given while cold or if large amounts are given too quickly. Full-strength tube feeding solution has relatively high osmolality, which subsequently draws water into the intestine and causes an osmotic diarrhea. Reducing the concentration of the feeding solution lessens the risk for osmotic diarrhea.

Consult physician regarding measures to remove fecal impaction if present (e.g., digital removal of stool, oil retention enema).

When a fecal impaction is present, the secretory activity of the bowel increases in an attempt to lubricate and promote evaluation of the impacted feces. The liquid portion of the feces above the mass then leaks around the impaction, resulting in a continuous oozing of diarrheal stool.

Administer the following antidiarrheal agents if ordered: **D** ✦
- Opioids (e.g., paregoric) or synthetic opioids (e.g., loperamide, diphenoxylate hydrochloride)

Opioids and synthetic opioids decrease gastrointestinal motility, which delays the passage of intestinal contents and subsequently allows more time for water to be reabsorbed from the feces. This results in fewer bowel movements and more formed stool.

- Bulk-forming agents (e.g., methylcellulose, psyllium hydrophilic mucilloid, polycarbophil)

Bulk-forming agents absorb water in the bowel, resulting in a more formed stool.

- Adsorbents/protectants (e.g., attapulgite [Kaopectate], bismuth subsalicylate [Pepto-Bismol])

Adsorbents/protectants act locally to coat the walls of the gastrointestinal tract and absorb toxins that are stimulating gut motility and/or secretions.

Consult appropriate health care provider if diarrhea persists.

Notifying the appropriate health care provider allows for modification of the treatment plan.

Nursing Diagnosis # DEFICIENT FLUID VOLUME NDx

Definition: Decreased intravascular, interstitial, and/or intracellular fluid. This refers to dehydration, water loss alone without change in sodium.

CLINICAL MANIFESTATIONS

Subjective	Objective
Verbal self-report of thirst; weakness	Decreased urine output; increased urine concentration; sudden weight loss (except in third spacing); decreased venous filling; increased body temperature; decreased pulse volume/pressure; change in mental status; elevated hematocrit (Hct); decreased skin/tongue turgor; dry skin/mucous membranes; increased pulse rate; decreased blood pressure (BP)

RISK FACTORS
- Active fluid volume loss
- Failure of regulatory mechanisms

DESIRED OUTCOMES

The client will not experience a deficient fluid volume as evidenced by:
a. Normal skin turgor
b. Moist mucous membrane
c. Stable weight
d. BP and pulse within normal range for client and stable with position change
e. Capillary refill time less than 2 to 3 seconds
f. Usual mental status
g. Blood urea nitrogen (BUN) and Hct within normal range
h. Balanced intake and output

DOCUMENTATION
- Vital signs
- Condition of skin and mucous membranes
- Weight
- Capillary refill time
- Appearance of neck veins when client is supine
- Mental status
- Intake and output
- Presence of nausea, vomiting, or other contributing factors
- Intravenous fluid therapy
- Client teaching

NOC OUTCOMES

Fluid balance; hydration; kidney function; vital signs; risk control

NIC INTERVENTIONS

Fluid management; fluid monitoring; fluid resuscitation; hypovolemia management; intravenous therapy

NURSING ASSESSMENT	**RATIONALE**
Assess for signs and symptoms of deficient fluid volume: • Decreased skin turgor • Dry mucous membranes, thirst • Weight loss of 2% or greater over a short period • Postural hypotension and/or low BP • Weak, rapid pulse • Capillary refill time greater than 2 to 3 seconds • Neck veins flat when client is supine • Change in mental status • Decreased urine output	*Early recognition of signs and symptoms of deficient fluid volume allow for prompt intervention.*
Assess BUN/Hct for abnormal elevations.	*Net fluid volume deficits result in decreased renal blood flow, decreased glomerular filtration, acute tubular necrosis, and resulting elevated blood urea nitrogen (BUN) levels. Hypovolemia results in hemoconcentration resulting in elevated hematocrit (Hct) levels.*

THERAPEUTIC INTERVENTIONS	**RATIONALE**
Independent Actions Implement measures to reduce nausea and vomiting if present: • Instruct client to ingest food/fluid slowly. • Eliminate noxious sights and odors.	*Nausea often causes the client to have decreased fluid volume intake. Persistent vomiting results in excessive loss of fluid.*
Implement measures to control diarrhea if present: • Discourage intake of spicy foods and foods high in fiber or lactose.	*Persistent or severe diarrhea results in excessive loss of gastrointestinal fluid.*
Implement measures to reduce fever if present: **D ● ✦** • Sponge bath client with tepid water. • Remove excessive clothing or bedcovers.	*Fever may be accompanied by diaphoresis, which can result in excessive loss of fluid.*
Carefully measure drainage: **D ✦** • Nasogastric • Wound • Urine	*Accurate intake/output records must be maintained to ensure fluid loss is replaced appropriately.*
Maintain a fluid intake of at least 2500 mL/day unless contraindicated. **D ✦**	*Adequate fluid intake needs to be provided in order to ensure adequate hydration.*

THERAPEUTIC INTERVENTIONS	RATIONALE
Dependent/Collaborative Actions	
Administer antiemetics as ordered. **D** ✦	*Nausea often causes the client to have decreased fluid volume intake. Persistent vomiting results in excessive loss of fluid.*
Administer antidiarrheal agents as ordered. **D** ✦	*Persistent or severe diarrhea results in excessive loss of gastrointestinal fluid.*
Administer antipyretics as ordered. **D** ✦	*Fever may be accompanied by diaphoresis, which can result in excessive loss of fluid*
Administer and maintain intravenous replacement fluids as ordered. **D** ✦	*Replacing fluid volume that is lost helps prevent/treat deficient fluid volume.*
Consult physician if signs and symptoms of deficient fluid volume persist or worsen.	*Notifying the physician allows for modification of the treatment plan.*

Nursing Diagnosis ## EXCESS FLUID VOLUME NDx

Definition: Surplus intake and/or retention of fluid.

CLINICAL MANIFESTATIONS

Subjective	**Objective**
Verbal self-report of shortness of breath	Jugular venous distention; decreased hemoglobin and hematocrit (Hct); weight gain over short period; dyspnea; intake exceeds output; pleural effusion; orthopnea; S_3 heart sound; pulmonary congestion; change in respiratory pattern; change in mental status; blood pressure (BP) changes; pulmonary artery pressure changes; oliguria; specific gravity changes; azotemia; altered electrolytes; restlessness; anxiety; abnormal breath sounds (crackles); edema, may progress to anasarca; increased central venous pressure (CVP); positive hepatojugular reflex

RISK FACTORS
- Compromised regulatory mechanism
- Excess fluid intake
- Excess sodium intake

DESIRED OUTCOMES

The client will not experience excess fluid volume as evidenced by:
a. Stable weight
b. BP within normal range
c. Absence of S_3 heart sound
d. Normal pulse volume
e. Balanced intake and output
f. Usual mental status
g. Normal breath sounds
h. Blood urea nitrogen (BUN) and Hct within normal limits
i. Absence of dyspnea, orthopnea, peripheral edema, and distended neck veins
j. CVP within normal range

DOCUMENTATION
- BP
- Weight
- Heart sounds
- Pulse volume
- Intake and output
- Mental status
- Breath sounds, ease of respirations
- Presence of edema and neck vein distention
- CVP readings
- Therapeutic interventions
- Client teaching

NOC OUTCOMES

Cardiopulmonary status; fluid balance; fluid overload severity; kidney function; respiratory status; vital signs; weight: body mass

NIC INTERVENTIONS

Fluid management; fluid monitoring; hypervolemia management

NURSING ASSESSMENT	RATIONALE
Assess for signs and symptoms of excess fluid volume: • Weight gain of 2% or greater in a short period • Elevated BP (Note: BP may not be elevated if fluid has shifted out of the vascular space) • Presence of an S₃ heart sound • Bounding pulse • Intake greater than output • Change in mental status • Crackles (rales), diminished or absent breath sounds • Dyspnea, orthopnea • Peripheral edema • Distended neck veins • Elevated CVP	*Early recognition of signs and symptoms of excess fluid volume allows for prompt intervention.*
Monitor chest radiograph results. Report findings of pulmonary vascular congestion, pleural effusion, or pulmonary edema.	*Chest radiograph films provide data about pulmonary vascular status and fluid accumulation in the pleural space, pulmonary interstitium, and alveoli.*
Monitor BUN, Hct, and electrolytes for abnormalities.	*Fluid volume excess results in a decreased Hct because of hemodilution and a decreased BUN. Electrolyte values will be altered in the presence of excess fluid volume.*

THERAPEUTIC INTERVENTIONS	RATIONALE

Independent Actions

Encourage client to rest periodically in a recumbent position if tolerated. **D** ✦	*Lying flat promotes venous return, which leads to increased cardiac output and renal blood flow. This increases the glomerular filtration rate and promotes diuresis.*

Dependent/Collaborative Actions

Maintain fluid restrictions as ordered. **D** ✦	*Fluid restriction helps to reduce total body water and prevent the accumulation of excess fluid.*
Restrict sodium intake as ordered. **D** ✦	*Excess fluid volume is an isotonic retention of both sodium and water. Restricting sodium intake will result in less sodium and subsequently less water being reabsorbed by the kidneys.*
If client is receiving intravenous fluids that contain a sizeable amount of sodium (e.g., 0.9% normal saline, lactated Ringer's), consult physician about a change in the solution or rate of infusion.	*Excess fluid volume can result from overzealous or prolonged intravenous administration of sodium-containing fluids, particularly ones that contain sizable amounts of sodium.*
If client is receiving numerous and/or large-volume intravenous medications, consult pharmacist about ways to prevent excessive fluid administration. Stop primary infusion during administration of intravenous medications, dilute medications in the minimum amount of solution.	*Limiting the amount of intravenous solution infused at any one time and maximizing the concentration of intravenous medications help prevent an additional fluid burden in the person who has or is at risk for fluid volume overload.*
Administer diuretics as ordered. **D** ✦	*Most diuretics inhibit sodium reabsorption in the renal tubules. This results in decreased water reabsorption and subsequent excretion of excess fluid.*
Consult physician if signs and symptoms of excess fluid volume persist or worsen.	*Notifying the physician allows for modification of the treatment plan.*

Nursing Diagnosis | **IMPAIRED GAS EXCHANGE** NDx

Definition: Excess or deficit in oxygenation and/or carbon dioxide elimination at the alveolar-capillary membrane.

CLINICAL MANIFESTATIONS

Subjective	**Objective**
Verbal self-report of visual disturbances; headache upon awakening	Decreased CO_2; tachycardia; hypercapnia; restlessness; somnolence; irritability; hypoxia; confusion; dyspnea; abnormal arterial blood gases; cyanosis (in neonates only); abnormal skin color (pale, dusky); hypoxemia; abnormal rate, rhythm, depth of breathing; diaphoresis; nasal flaring; low partial pressure of oxygen (O_2) in arterial blood (PaO_2); low pulse oximetry

RISK FACTORS
* Ventilation/perfusion imbalance
* Alveolar-capillary membrane changes

DESIRED OUTCOMES

The client will experience adequate gas (O_2/CO_2) exchange as evidenced by:
a. Usual mental status
b. Unlabored respirations at 12 to 20 breaths/min
c. Oximetry results within normal range
d. Arterial blood gas (ABG) values within normal range
e. Normal breath sounds
f. Normal rate and depth of respirations
g. Absence of dyspnea

DOCUMENTATION

* Respiratory rate
* Difficulty breathing
* Mental status
* Oximetry results
* Route and rate of O_2 administration
* Therapeutic interventions
* Client teaching

NOC OUTCOMES

Respiratory status: ventilation; gas exchange; activity tolerance; airway patency; tissue perfusion: pulmonary; vital signs

NIC INTERVENTIONS

Respiratory monitoring; oxygen therapy; airway management; chest physiotherapy; cough enhancement; acid-base management

NURSING ASSESSMENT	**RATIONALE**
Assess for and report signs and symptoms of impaired gas (O_2/CO_2) exchange: • Restlessness, irritability • Confusion, somnolence • Tachypnea, dyspnea • Decreased PaO_2 and/or increased partial pressure of CO_2 in arterial blood ($PaCO_2$)	*Early recognition of signs and symptoms of impaired gas exchange allows for prompt intervention.*
Monitor for and report a significant decrease in oximetry results.	*Oximetry is a noninvasive method of measuring arterial O_2 saturation. The results assist in evaluating respiratory status.*

THERAPEUTIC INTERVENTIONS	**RATIONALE**
Independent Actions Place client in a semi- to high-Fowler's position unless contraindicated. Position with pillows to prevent slumping. If client is experiencing dyspnea or orthopnea, position overbed table so he/she can lean on it if desired. **D** ● ✦	*These positions allow for increased diaphragmatic excursion and maximum lung expansion, which promotes optimal alveolar ventilation and O_2/CO_2 exchange.*

Continued...

THERAPEUTIC INTERVENTIONS	RATIONALE
Instruct client to change position, deep breathe, and cough or "huff" every 1 to 2 hrs.	*Frequent repositioning helps mobilize secretions and aids lung expansion. Deep breathing helps loosen secretions and promotes a more effective cough. It also promotes maximum lung expansion and stimulates surfactant production. Coughing or "huffing" (a forced expiration technique) mobilizes secretions and facilitates removal of these secretions from the respiratory tract. These actions promote optimal alveolar ventilation and O_2/CO_2 exchange.*
Reinforce correct use of incentive spirometer every 1 to 2 hrs. **D** ✦	*Incentive spirometer use promotes slow, deep inhalation, which improves lung expansion and helps clear airways by loosening secretions and promoting a more effective cough. These actions enhance alveolar ventilation and the exchange of O_2/CO_2.*
Implement measures to reduce chest or abdominal pain if present (e.g., splint incision with pillow during coughing and deep breathing). **D** ● ✦	*A client with chest or abdominal pain often guards respiratory efforts and breathes shallowly in an attempt to prevent additional discomfort. Pain reduction enables the client to breathe more deeply, which enhances alveolar ventilation and O_2/CO_2 exchange.*
Implement measures to decrease fear and anxiety (e.g., assure client that breathing deeply will not dislodge tubes or cause incision to break open, interact with client in a confident manner). **D** ● ✦	*Fear and anxiety may cause a client to breathe shallowly or to hyperventilate. Decreasing fear and anxiety allows the client to focus on breathing more slowly and taking deeper breaths, which subsequently enhances alveolar ventilation and the exchange of O_2/CO_2.*
Instruct client in, and assist with, diaphragmatic breathing and pursed-lip breathing techniques if appropriate. NOTE: Diaphragmatic breathing is most often indicated for clients who have had thoracic surgery or clients who have chronic airflow limitation (e.g., emphysema) or neuromuscular conditions that cause fixation or weakening of the diaphragm.	*Diaphragmatic breathing promotes greater movement of the diaphragm and decreases the use of the accessory muscles for inspiration. Use of this technique eases the work of breathing and ultimately promotes an increased efficiency of alveolar ventilation. Pursed-lip breathing causes a mild resistance to exhalation, which creates positive pressure in the airways. This pressure helps prevent airway collapse and subsequently promotes more complete alveolar emptying.*
Discourage smoking. **D** ✦	*Smoking impairs gas exchange because it:*
	• *Reduces effective airway clearance by increasing mucus production and impairing ciliary function.*
	• *Decreases O_2 availability as hemoglobin binds with the carbon monoxide in smoke rather than with O_2.*
	• *Causes damage to the bronchial and alveolar walls.*
	• *Causes vasoconstriction and subsequently reduces pulmonary blood flow.*

Dependent/Collaborative Actions

Implement measures to facilitate removal of pulmonary secretions (e.g., suction, postural drainage, percussion, vibration) if ordered.	*Excessive secretions and/or client's inability to clear secretions from the respiratory tract lead to stasis of secretions, which can impair O_2/CO_2 exchange. Suction and chest physiotherapy techniques may be necessary to facilitate removal of pulmonary secretions and thereby promote adequate gas exchange.*
Assist with positive airway pressure techniques (e.g., continuous positive airway pressure [CPAP], bilevel positive airway pressure [BiPAP], flutter/positive expiratory pressure [PEP] device) if ordered.	*Positive airway pressure techniques increase intrapulmonary (alveolar) pressure, which helps reexpand collapsed alveoli and prevent further alveolar collapse so that gas exchange can take place.*
Maintain O_2 therapy as ordered. **D** ● ✦	*Supplemental O_2 increases the concentration of O_2 in the alveoli, which increases the diffusion of O_2 across the alveolar-capillary membrane.*
Maintain activity restrictions as ordered. Increase activity gradually as allowed and tolerated. **D** ● ✦	*Restricting activity lowers the body's O_2 requirements and thus increases the amount of O_2 available for gas exchange. A gradual increase in activity conserves energy and thereby lessens O_2 utilization, yet promotes mobilization.*

THERAPEUTIC INTERVENTIONS	RATIONALE
Administer medications that may be ordered to improve client's respiratory status (e.g., bronchodilators, analgesics, antibiotics, corticosteroids, anticoagulants, diuretics). **D** ✦	*Medication therapy is an integral part of treating many respiratory conditions that impair alveolar gas exchange (e.g., bronchodilators improve bronchial airflow and subsequently increase O_2/CO_2 exchange; analgesics can reduce pain and promote deeper breathing and increased activity; antibiotics help resolve certain respiratory infections; corticosteroids reduce inflammation in the lungs and improve bronchial airflow; anticoagulants treat thromboemboli of the pulmonary vessels and subsequently improve pulmonary perfusion; diuretics reduce fluid accumulation in the pulmonary interstitium and alveoli, which subsequently improves gas exchange).*
Administer central nervous system depressants judiciously. Hold medication and consult physician if respiratory rate is less than 12 breaths/min.	*Central nervous system depressants cause depression of the respiratory center and cough reflex. This can result in hypoventilation and stasis of secretions with subsequent impaired gas exchange.*
Consult appropriate health care provider (e.g., physician, respiratory therapist) if signs and symptoms of impaired gas exchange persist or worsen.	*Notifying the appropriate health care provider allows for modification of treatment plan.*

Nursing Diagnosis ## RISK FOR UNSTABLE BLOOD GLUCOSE LEVEL NDx

Definition: Susceptible to variation in serum levels of glucose from the normal range, which may compromise health.

CLINICAL MANIFESTATIONS

Subjective	Objective
Hypoglycemia: Verbal self-report of hunger; lightheadedness and weakness	**Hypoglycemia:** Confusion; difficulty speaking; shakiness; sweating; below-normal blood glucose levels
Hyperglycemia: Verbal self-report of frequent hunger; blurred vision; weight loss; dry mouth	**Hyperglycemia:** Frequent urination; elevated blood glucose levels

RISK FACTORS

- Type I and II diabetes, prediabetes, poor diet and nutrition
- Obesity
- Sedentary lifestyle
- Family history of diabetes
- Giving birth to a baby weighing >9 lb
- High-density lipoprotein (HDL) cholesterol <35 mg/dL
- High triglyceride levels
- High blood pressure
- Age >45 years
- History of gestational diabetes
- Ethnic background of Hispanic, black, Native American, and Asian
- Metabolic syndrome
- Deficient knowledge of diabetes management

DESIRED OUTCOMES

The client will not experience unstable glucose levels as evidenced by:
a. Serum fasting serum glucose levels of 70 to 110 mg/dL
b. 2-hrs postprandial serum glucose readings of:
  - 0 to 50 years <140 mg/dL
  - 50 to 60 years <150 mg/dL
  - ≥60 years <160 mg/dL
c. Glycosylated hemoglobin levels (hemoglobin A_{1c}) <7%
d. Demonstrated ability to accurately monitor blood glucose
e. Demonstrated ability to accurately administer insulin
f. Identification of self-care measures if blood glucose is too high or too low

DOCUMENTATION

- Blood glucose levels
- Diet and nutrition
- Therapeutic interventions
- Client and family teaching

NOC OUTCOMES	NIC INTERVENTIONS
Healthy diet; stable blood glucose levels; diabetes self-management; medication adherence; health-promoting behaviors	Hyperglycemia management; hypoglycemia management

NURSING ASSESSMENT	RATIONALE
Assess for and report signs and symptoms of variations in blood glucose levels: • Anxiety • Confusion • Irritability • Lethargy or behavior changes • Drowsiness or fatigue • Polydipsia • Nausea • Vomiting • Dry mouth • Blurred vision • Cold, clammy skin • Shakiness • Nervousness • Fainting	*Early recognition of signs and symptoms of abnormal blood glucose levels allows for prompt intervention.*
Obtain blood glucose levels and hemoglobin A_{1c} levels and report abnormalities.	*Blood glucose levels and hemoglobin A_{1c} levels indicate the effectiveness of monitoring and treatment.*
Assess self-management skills related to blood glucose levels.	*Assessment determines need for education and support in self-management of blood glucose levels.*
Monitor hemoglobin A_{1c} levels.	*Provides the health care team with a 2- to 3-month overview of how well the client has controlled glucose levels. These data are helpful in discharge planning.*
Evaluate client's medication regimen for medications that can alter blood glucose levels.	*Some medication can cause hyperglycemia or hypoglycemia.*

THERAPEUTIC INTERVENTIONS	RATIONALE

Independent Actions

Monitor intake and output. **D** ● ✦	*Individuals at risk for blood glucose alterations are at a significant risk for dehydration.*
Client and family teaching and discharge planning on control of blood glucose level through:	*Education has been shown to improve control of blood glucose levels and client self-monitoring, and client sense of control over disease.*
• Diet	*Adherence to a diabetic diet can be used to help regulate blood glucose levels.*
• Exercise	*A regular exercise routine has been shown to control blood glucose levels and decrease the amount of adipose tissue.*
• Medication administration	*Improves client's sense of control over the disease process and maintenance of blood glucose levels*
• Self-monitoring of blood glucose	*Reduces incidences of hyperglycemia or hypoglycemic episodes and reduces complications of disease*
• Recognition and treatment of signs and symptoms of hyperglycemia and hypoglycemia	*Allows for prompt intervention and decreases large variations in blood glucose levels*
• Smoking cessation	*Smoking has been associated with worsening glucose control and insulin resistance.*

Dependent/Collaborative Actions

Monitor blood glucose levels at meals and at bedtime. More frequent monitoring of blood glucose levels (e.g., every 4–6 hrs) is required when client is to have nothing by mouth (NPO). Refer to facility policy for frequency. **D** ● ✦	*Frequent blood glucose testing is important for maintenance of appropriate blood glucose levels. When the client is NPO, this is important to prevent significant declines in blood glucose levels.*

THERAPEUTIC INTERVENTIONS	RATIONALE
Monitor blood glucose levels every hour in a client who is receiving continuous intravenous insulin. **D** ✦	*Blood glucose levels change quickly and may require immediate intervention.*
Administer oral hypoglycemics and insulin as needed. NOTE: Always check blood glucose levels before insulin administration. **D** ✦	*Timely administration of insulin assists in maintaining appropriate blood glucose levels and prevents progression to diabetes ketoacidosis.*
Administer 1/2 cup of fruit juice for hypoglycemia if client is able to take fluids. Administer 50% dextrose in water (D50W) or intramuscular glucagon if client is unable to take oral carbohydrates. NOTE: Review hospital policy for variations.	*Early treatment of hypoglycemia can prevent more severe hypoglycemia. D50W is an alternative to oral carbohydrates when the patient is unable to take fluids.*
Refer client for dietary counseling and diabetic education.	*Dietary counseling and diabetic education are interventions that can increase client knowledge of the disease process. Knowledge of disease process can facilitate adherence to treatment plans.*
Refer client and family to community resources.	*Provides for continuum of care.*

Nursing Diagnosis   GRIEVING NDx

Definition: A normal, complex process that includes emotional, physical, spiritual, social, and intellectual responses and behaviors by which individuals, families, and communities incorporate an actual, anticipated, or perceived loss into their daily lives.

CLINICAL MANIFESTATIONS

Subjective	Objective
Verbal self-report of sorrow, guilt, pain; changes in dream patterns	Changes inactivity level; anger; blame, detachment; disorganization; difficulty in expressing the loss; denial of loss; changes in sleep patterns

RISK FACTORS

- Loss of an object (e.g., people, possessions, job status, home, ideals, parts and processes of the body)

DESIRED OUTCOMES

The client will demonstrate beginning progression through the grieving process as evidenced by:
a. Verbalization of feelings about the loss
b. Usual sleep pattern
c. Participation in treatment plan and self-care activities
d. Use of available support systems

DOCUMENTATION

- Verbalization of feelings about the loss
- Participation in activities
- Eating pattern
- Sleep pattern
- Interaction with others
- Measures used to adapt to loss
- Client/family teaching

NOC OUTCOMES

Grief resolution

NIC INTERVENTIONS

Grief work facilitation; emotional support; support system enhancement

NURSING ASSESSMENT	RATIONALE
Assess for signs and symptoms of grieving: • Expression of distress about the loss • Change in eating habits • Inability to concentrate • Insomnia • Anger • Sadness • Withdrawal from significant others • Denial of loss	*Assessment of signs and symptoms of grieving helps the nurse determine the phase of grieving the client is experiencing. This knowledge aids in the development of effective strategies that can assist the client to progress through the phases of grieving.*
Assess for factors that may hinder and facilitate client's acknowledgment of the loss.	*In order for grief work to begin, the client needs to acknowledge the loss. An awareness of factors that may hinder and facilitate this acknowledgment assists in the development of effective strategies to accomplish this goal.*

THERAPEUTIC INTERVENTIONS	RATIONALE

Independent Actions

Assist client to acknowledge the loss (e.g., encourage conversation about the loss including how or why it occurred and its impact on his/her future).	*The client needs to acknowledge the loss in order for grief work to begin.*
Discuss the grieving process and assist client to accept the phases of grieving as an expected response to an actual and/or anticipated loss.	*An awareness of the feelings and behaviors commonly associated with each phase of the grieving process assists the client to accept his/her responses to the loss.*
Allow time for client to progress through the phases of grieving phases vary among theorists but progress from shock and alarm to acceptance.	*Grieving is a process that occurs in phases or stages that progress over time. Some phases may not be experienced by the client, and some may overlap or recur. The amount of time necessary to reach resolution of grief is very individual, may take months to years, and must be allowed to occur in order to reduce the risk for dysfunctional grieving.*
Provide an atmosphere of care and concern (e.g., provide privacy, be available and nonjudgmental, display empathy and respect). **D** ● ✦	*A supportive, nonthreatening environment provides the basis for a constructive, therapeutic relationship between the client and nurse. This allows the client to express feelings of grief and work toward its resolution.*
Implement measures to promote trust (e.g., answer questions honestly, provide requested information). **D** ● ✦	*A feeling of trust in the caregiver promotes the development of a therapeutic relationship in which the client can feel free to verbalize feelings. This facilitates the progression of grief work.*
Encourage the verbal expression of anger and sadness about the loss experienced. Recognize displacement of anger and assist client to see the actual cause of angry feelings and resentment. Establish limits on abusive behavior if demonstrated. **D** ● ✦	*The verbal expression of feelings of anger and sadness facilitates movement toward resolution of grief. Displacement of angry feelings needs to be acknowledged so that grieving can progress but should not be allowed to interfere with the therapeutic process.*
Encourage client to express feelings in whatever ways are comfortable (e.g., writing, drawing, conversation). **D** ● ✦	*Expression of feelings helps the client integrate both positive and negative aspects of the loss and move toward its acceptance.*
Assist client to use techniques that have helped him/her cope in previous situations of loss.	*Techniques that have previously facilitated the client's adjustment to situations of loss are often effective when used to help him/her cope with the current loss.*
Support behaviors suggesting successful grief work (e.g., verbalizing feelings about loss, focusing on ways to adapt to loss, learning needed skills, developing or renewing relationships).	*Positive feedback about behaviors that suggest successful grief work reinforces those behaviors and promotes positive adaptation to loss.*
Explain the phases of the grieving process to significant others. Encourage their support and understanding.	*When significant others are knowledgeable about the phases of the grieving process, they are more likely to understand and accept the client's behavior and assist him/her to move toward resolution of grief.*

THERAPEUTIC INTERVENTIONS	RATIONALE
Facilitate communication between the client and significant others. Be aware that they may be in different phases of the grieving process.	*Effective communication between the client and significant others enhances the client's ability to express feelings and successfully move through the phases of grieving.*

Dependent/Collaborative Actions

Provide information about counseling services and support groups that might assist client in working through grief.	*Counseling and support groups can assist the client in working through grief by:* • *Providing insight into his/her responses to the loss* • *Decreasing the feelings of aloneness and isolation that frequently accompany a loss* • *Helping identify methods or skills that can be used to help cope with the loss*
When appropriate, assist client to meet spiritual needs (e.g., arrange for a visit from clergy).	*Spiritual support can be a source of strength and solace to the client and can facilitate resolution of grief.*
Consult appropriate health care provider (e.g., psychiatric nurse practitioner, grief counselor, physician) if signs of dysfunctional grieving (e.g., persistent denial of losses, excessive anger or sadness, emotional lability) occur.	*Notifying the appropriate health care provider allows for modification of the treatment plan.*

Nursing Diagnosis | ## RISK-PRONE HEALTH BEHAVIOR NDx

For a full, detailed care plan on this topic, go to http://evolve.elsevier.com/Haugen/careplanning/.

Nursing Diagnosis | ## RISK FOR INFECTION NDx

Definition: Susceptible to invasion and multiplication of pathogenic organisms, which may compromise health.

CLINICAL MANIFESTATIONS*

Subjective	Objective
Verbal self-report of chills; loss of energy; loss of appetite; reports of pain, frequency, urgency, or burning with urination	Elevated temperature; increased heart rate; abnormal breath sounds; productive cough of purulent, green, or rust-colored sputum Cloudy urine Increase WBC count in urinalysis; presence of bacteria Heat, swelling, and/or unusual drainage in an area Increase WBC count for significant change in differential

RISK FACTORS

- Inadequate primary defenses (broken skin, traumatized tissue, decrease in ciliary action, stasis of body fluids, change in pH of secretions, altered peristalsis)
- Inadequate secondary defenses (e.g., decreased hemoglobin, leukopenia, suppressed inflammatory response)
- Immunosuppression
- Inadequate acquired immunity
- Trauma
- Tissue destruction and increased environmental exposure
- Chronic disease
- Malnutrition
- Invasive medical procedures
- Pharmaceutic agents (e.g., immunosuppressants)
- Rupture of amniotic membranes
- Insufficient knowledge to avoid exposure to pathogens

---

*Clinical manifestations vary depending on the site of infection.

DESIRED OUTCOMES

The client will remain free of infection as evidenced by:
a. Absence of fever and chills
b. Pulse rate within normal limits
c. Usual mental status
d. Normal breath sounds
e. Cough productive of clear mucus only
f. Voiding clear urine without reports of frequency, urgency, and burning
g. Absence of heat, pain, redness, swelling, and unusual drainage in any area
h. White blood cell (WBC) and differential counts within normal range for client
i. Negative results of cultured specimens

DOCUMENTATION

- Temperature
- Pulse rate
- Presence of chills
- Mental status
- Breath sounds
- Characteristics of urine, sputum, and wound drainage
- Evidence of inflammation in any area
- Evidence of unusual drainage from any area
- Therapeutic interventions
- Client/family teaching

NOC OUTCOMES

Infection severity

NIC INTERVENTIONS

Infection control; infection protection; incision site care; tube care; wound care; nutrition management

NURSING ASSESSMENT

Assess for and report signs and symptoms of infection NOTE: Be aware that some signs and symptoms vary depending on the site of infection, the causative agent, and the age and immune status of the client:
- Elevated temperature
- Chills
- Increased pulse rate
- Malaise, lethargy, acute confusion
- Loss of appetite
- Abnormal breath sounds
- Productive cough of purulent, green, or rust-colored sputum
- Cloudy urine
- Reports of frequency, urgency, or burning when urinating
- Urinalysis showing a WBC count greater than 5, positive leukocyte esterase or nitrites, or presence of bacteria
- Heat, pain, redness, swelling, or unusual drainage in any area
- Elevated WBC count and/or significant change in differential

Obtain specimens (e.g., urine, wound drainage, vaginal drainage, sputum, blood) for culture as ordered. Report positive results.

RATIONALE

Early recognition of signs and symptoms of infection allows for prompt intervention.

Cultures are done to identify the specific organism(s) causing the infection. Culture results provide information that helps determine the most effective treatment.

THERAPEUTIC INTERVENTIONS

Independent Actions

Maintain a fluid intake of at least 2500 mL/day unless contraindicated. **D** ✦

Use good hand hygiene and encourage client to do the same. **D** ● ✦

RATIONALE

Adequate hydration helps prevent infection by:
- *Helping maintain adequate blood flow and nutrient supply to the tissues.*
- *Promoting urine formation and subsequent voiding, which flushes pathogens from the bladder and urethra.*
- *Thinning respiratory secretions so that they can more easily be removed by coughing or suctioning (respiratory secretions provide a good medium for growth and colonization of microorganisms).*

Good hand hygiene removes transient flora, which reduces the risk of transmission of pathogens. Use of products such as an antibacterial soap, a chlorhexidine solution, or an alcohol-based hand rub agent can actually inhibit the growth of or kill microorganisms, which further reduces infection risk.

THERAPEUTIC INTERVENTIONS	RATIONALE
Adhere to the appropriate precautions established to prevent transmission of infection to the client (e.g., standard precautions, transmission-based precautions on other clients, neutropenic precautions). **D** ● ✦	*Adhering to the appropriate precautions that have been established to help prevent the transmission of microorganisms reduces the client's risk of infection.*
Use sterile technique during invasive procedures (e.g., urinary catheterizations, venous and arterial punctures, injections, tracheal suctioning, wound care and dressing changes). **D** ✦	*Use of sterile technique reduces the possibility of introducing pathogens into the body.*
Anchor catheters/tubings (e.g., urinary, intravenous, wound drainage) securely. **D** ✦	*Catheters/tubings that are not securely anchored have some degree of in-and-out movement. This movement increases the risk of infection because it allows for the introduction of pathogens into the body. It can also cause tissue trauma, which can result in colonization of microorganisms.*
Change equipment, tubings, and solutions used for treatments, such as intravenous infusions, respiratory care, irrigations, and enteral feedings according to hospital policy.	*The longer that equipment, tubings, and solutions are in use, the greater the chance of colonization of microorganisms, which can then be introduced into the body.*
Maintain a closed system for drains (e.g., wounds, chest tubes, urinary catheters) and intravenous infusions whenever possible.	*Each time a drainage or infusion system is opened, pathogens from the environment have an opportunity to enter the body. Maintaining a closed system decreases this risk, which reduces the possibility of infection.*
Change peripheral intravenous line sites according to hospital policy. **D** ✦	*Peripheral intravenous line sites are changed routinely to reduce persistent irritation of one area of a vein wall and the resultant colonization of microorganisms at that site.*
Protect client from others with infections. **D** ● ✦	*Protecting the client from others with infections reduces his/her risk of exposure to pathogens.*
Implement measures to maintain healthy, intact skin (e.g., keep skin lubricated, clean, and dry; instruct or assist client to turn every 2 hrs; keep bed linens dry and wrinkle-free). **D** ● ✦	*Healthy, intact skin reduces the risk for infection by:* • *Providing a physical barrier against the introduction of pathogens into the body.* • *Removing many of the microorganisms on the surface of the skin by means of the constant shedding of the epidermis.* • *Inhibiting the growth of some bacteria on the surface of the skin sebum contains fatty acids, which create a slightly acidic environment that inhibits the growth of some bacteria.*
Implement measures to reduce stress (e.g., reduce fear, anxiety, and pain; help client identify and use effective coping mechanisms). **D** ✦	*Stress causes an increased secretion of cortisol. Cortisol interferes with some immune responses, which subsequently increases the client's susceptibility to infection.*
Maintain an optimal nutritional status.	*Adequate nutrition is needed to maintain normal function of the immune system.*
Instruct and assist client to perform good perineal care routinely and after each bowel movement. **D** ✦	*The perineal area contains a large number of organisms. Routine cleansing of the area reduces the risk of colonization of organisms and subsequent perineal, urinary tract, and/or vaginal infection.*
Instruct and assist client to perform good oral hygiene as often as needed. **D** ✦	*Frequent oral hygiene helps prevent infection by removing most of the food, debris, and many of the microorganisms that are present in the mouth. It also helps maintain the integrity of the oral mucosa, which provides a physical and chemical barrier to pathogens.*
Implement measures to prevent urinary retention (e.g., instruct client to urinate when the urge is felt, promote relaxation during voiding attempts).	*A client experiencing urinary retention is at increased risk for urinary tract infection because:* • *The urine that accumulates in the bladder creates an environment conducive to the growth and colonization of microorganisms.* • *Voiding does not occur so microorganisms are not flushed from the mucous lining of the urethra; these microorganisms can colonize and ascend into the bladder.*
Implement measures to prevent stasis of respiratory secretions (e.g., assist client to turn, cough, and deep breathe; increase activity as allowed and tolerated; perform tracheal suctioning if indicated). **D** ✦	*Respiratory secretions provide a good medium for growth of microorganisms. By preventing stasis, there is less chance of colonization of the microorganisms and a decreased risk for development of respiratory tract infection.*

Continued...

THERAPEUTIC INTERVENTIONS	RATIONALE
Instruct client to receive immunizations (e.g., influenza vaccine, pneumococcal vaccine) if appropriate.	*Immunizations are often recommended to reduce the possibility of some infections in high-risk clients (e.g., those clients who are immunosuppressed, elderly, or have a chronic disease).*

Dependent/Collaborative Actions

Administer vitamins and minerals as ordered. **D** ✦	*Adequate nutrition is needed to maintain normal function of the immune system.*
Provide appropriate wound care (e.g., use dressing materials that maintain a moist wound surface, assist with debridement of necrotic tissue, use dressing materials that absorb excess exudate, protect granulating tissue from trauma and contamination, maintain patency of wound drains). **D** ✦	*Proper wound care facilitates wound healing and reduces the number of pathogens that enter or are present in the wound, which reduces the risk of the wound becoming infected.*
Administer bethanechol as ordered. **D** ✦	*Relaxes the bladder sphincter muscles and stimulates urination.*
Consult appropriate health care provider regarding initiation of antimicrobial therapy if indicated. Question orders that do not seem appropriate (e.g., prolonged use of antimicrobials, excessively high dose of an antimicrobial, unnecessary use of broad-spectrum or multiple antimicrobials).	*Most antimicrobials disrupt cell wall synthesis, which halts the growth of, or kills, microorganisms. This can effectively reduce the client's risk for infection. Antimicrobial orders that seem inappropriate should be questioned because they can result in the elimination of normal flora and/or the development of drug-resistant microorganisms, which actually increase the client's risk for infection.*

Nursing Diagnosis **IMPAIRED PHYSICAL MOBILITY** NDx

Definition: Limitation in independent, purposeful movement of the body or of one or more extremities.

CLINICAL MANIFESTATIONS

Subjective	Objective
Verbal self-report of pain; discomfort; fatigue	Decreased reaction time; difficulty moving; engages in substitution for movement; supporting the affected limb; exceptional dyspnea; contractures; limited ability to perform gross and fine motor skills; limited range of motion (ROM); intentional movement-induced tremor; postural instability; uncoordinated movements

RISK FACTORS

- Sedentary lifestyle
- Limited cardiovascular endurance
- Joint stiffness or contracture
- Pain and/or discomfort
- Depression and/or anxiety

- Neuromuscular impairment
- Prescribed movement restrictions
- Decreased muscle strength and/or mass
- Activity intolerance

- Cognitive impairment
- Lack of knowledge regarding the value of physical activity
- Loss of bone mass
- Sensoriperceptual impairments

DESIRED OUTCOMES

The client will improve mobility as evidenced by:
a. Increased physical activity
b. Movement of affected limb or limbs
c. Participation in activities of daily living (ADLs)
d. Demonstration of appropriate use of assistive devices to improve movement

DOCUMENTATION

- ADLs
- Muscle strength
- Distance ambulated
- Passive or active ROM
- Therapeutic interventions
- Client/family teaching

NOC OUTCOMES	NIC INTERVENTIONS
Activity tolerance; cardiovascular status; fall prevention behavior; endurance; joint movement	Positioning; ambulation; pain relief; active and/or passive ROM

NURSING ASSESSMENT	RATIONALE
Assess client's movement ability and activity tolerance. Use a tool such as the Assessment Tool for Safe Patient Handling and Movement or the Functional Independence Measures (FIM).	*Assessment of mobility is used to best determine how to facilitate movement. Assessment of activity tolerance provides a baseline for patient strength and endurance with movement.*
Assess for cause of immobility.	*It is important to determine if the cause of immobility is physical or psychologic, and to plan interventions to improve mobility.*
Assess circulation, motion, and feeling in digits.	*Circulation may be compromised by edema of extremities, which can lead to tissue necrosis and/or contractures.*
Assess skin integrity.	*Routine examination of the skin provides for early detection and intervention of pressure sores. Pressure sores develop quickly in patients who are immobile.*
Assess emotional response to immobility.	*Determine client's acceptance of temporary or permanent limitations. This impacts implementation of therapeutic interventions.*
Assess need for assistive devices.	*Determine client's needs for assistive devices as well as proper use of wheelchairs, walkers, canes, etc., to reduce incidence of falls.*

THERAPEUTIC INTERVENTIONS	RATIONALE

Independent Actions

Encourage and implement strength training activities: • Active and/or passive ROM • Ambulation • Use of trapeze for pull-ups • ADLs **D** ● ✦	*Inactivity contributes to muscle weakening. Contractures can develop as early as 8 hrs of immobility. These activities maintain and increase the client's strength and ability to move.*
Use assistive devices to help client with movement: • Crutches • Gait belt • Walker **D** ● ✦	*Assistive devices help the caregivers decrease the potential for falls and/or injuries.*
Cluster treatments and care activities to allow for uninterrupted periods of rest. **D** ● ✦	*Increases client's tolerance and strength for activities.*
Encourage patient with positive reinforcement during activities. **D** ● ✦	*A positive approach to activities supports the client's accomplishment, engagement in new activities, and improves self-esteem.*
Implement falls protocol.	*Client safety is a priority.*
Maintain the bed in low position and keep side rails up. **D** ● ✦	*Reduces prolonged pressure on tissues, decreasing potential for tissue ischemia and pressure sores.*
For bedridden patients, turn and reposition every 2 hrs. **D** ● ✦	*Turning clients allows for appropriate circulation to tissues.*
Position client with appropriate devices (e.g., wedges, pillows, kinetic bed, air bed, gel mattress). **D** ● ✦	*Reduces prolonged pressure on tissues, decreasing potential for tissue ischemia and pressure sores.*
Use sequential compression devices or antiembolic stockings. **D** ● ✦	*Improves venous circulation and helps to prevent thrombophlebitis in lower extremities.*
Implement measures to maintain healthy, intact skin (e.g., keep skin lubricated, clean, and dry; instruct or assist client to turn every 2 hrs; keep bed linens dry and wrinkle-free). **D** ● ✦	*Healthy, intact skin reduces the risk of pressure sores and infection.*
Maintain an optimal nutritional status. Increase protein intake.	*Adequate nutrition is needed to maintain adequate energy level.*
Increase fluid intake to 2000 to 3000 mL/day unless contraindicated.	*Increased fluid maintains adequate hydration and helps prevent constipation and hardening of the stool.*
Encourage coughing and deep breathing exercises and use of incentive spirometry.	*Prevents buildup of secretions and promotes lung expansion.*
Initiate bowel program.	*Prolonged immobility can lead to constipation.*
Assist client with acceptance of immobility.	*Helps patient accept limitations and focus on a new quality of life.*

NDx = NANDA Diagnosis   **D** = Delegatable Action   ● = UAP   ✦ = LVN/LPN   ⊕▶ = Go to ⊖volve for animation

Continued...

THERAPEUTIC INTERVENTIONS	RATIONALE

Dependent/Collaborative Actions

Consult appropriate health care provider: dietitian, physician, and occupational therapist.

These individuals provide specific activities and exercise programs to improve strength and mobility.

Administer pain medications before activities. **D** ✦

Reduces muscle stiffness and tension, allowing the client to participate in activities.

Nursing Diagnosis # IMBALANCED NUTRITION: LESS THAN BODY REQUIREMENTS NDx

Definition: Intake of nutrients insufficient to meet metabolic needs.

CLINICAL MANIFESTATIONS

Subjective	Objective
Verbal of lack of appetite; fatigue; irritability; poor self-esteem; verbalization of sore mucous membranes	Loss of weight with adequate food intake; body weight 20% or more under ideal weight; sore, inflamed buccal cavity; capillary fragility; pale conjunctiva and mucous membranes; poor muscle tone; excessive hair loss; amenorrhea; decreased blood urea nitrogen (BUN) and elevated creatinine levels; decreased albumin and prealbumin levels; decreased hematocrit (Hct), decreased hemoglobin (Hgb), and decreased white blood cells

RISK FACTORS

- Inability to ingest or digest food or absorb nutrients because of biologic, psychologic, or economic factors

DESIRED OUTCOMES

The client will maintain an adequate nutritional status as evidenced by:
a. Weight within normal range for the client
b. Normal BUN and serum albumin, prealbumin, Hct, Hgb, and lymphocyte levels
c. Usual strength and activity tolerance
d. Healthy oral mucous membrane

DOCUMENTATION

- Weight
- Activity tolerance
- Condition of oral mucous membrane
- Type of diet and amount consumed
- Therapeutic interventions
- Client/family teaching

NOC OUTCOMES

Appetite; body image; bowel elimination; compliance behavior: prescribed diet; hydration; weight maintenance behavior

NIC INTERVENTIONS

Nutritional monitoring; nutritional counseling; nutritional management; nutrition therapy; weight gain assistance; weight management

NURSING ASSESSMENT	RATIONALE

Assess for and report signs and symptoms of malnutrition:
- Weight significantly below client's usual weight or below normal for client's age, height, and body frame
- Increased BUN and low serum albumin, prealbumin, Hct, Hgb, and lymphocyte levels
- Weakness and fatigue
- Sore, inflamed oral mucous membrane
- Pale conjunctiva

Early recognition of signs and symptoms of malnutrition allows for prompt intervention.

Monitor percentage of meals and snacks client consumes. Report a pattern or inadequate intake.

An awareness of the amount of foods/fluids the client consumes alerts the nurse to deficits in nutritional intake. Reporting an inadequate intake allows for prompt intervention.

NURSING ASSESSMENT	**RATIONALE**
Perform or assist with anthropometric measurements such as skinfold thickness, body circumferences (e.g., hip, waist, mid-upper arm), and bioelectrical impedance analysis if indicated. Report results that are lower than normal.	*Anthropometric measurements provide information about the amount of muscle mass, body fat, and protein reserves the client has. These assessments assist in evaluating the client's nutritional status.*

THERAPEUTIC INTERVENTIONS	**RATIONALE**

Independent Actions

Implement measures to prevent vomiting if indicated (e.g., eliminate noxious sites and odors). **D** ● ✦	*Vomiting results in actual loss of nutrients.*
Implement measures to control diarrhea if present (e.g., discourage intake of spicy foods and foods high in fiber or lactose). **D** ● ✦	*Increased intestinal motility that occurs with or causes diarrhea results in a decreased absorption of nutrients in the bowel. In addition, diarrhea causes an actual loss of nutrients.*
Implement measures to improve oral intake:	*Decreases client's appetite and oral intake.*
• Perform actions to reduce nausea, pain, fear, and anxiety if present. **D** ● ✦	
• Perform actions to relieve gastrointestinal distention if present (e.g., encourage and assist client with frequent ambulation) unless contraindicated. **D** ● ✦	*Distention of the gastrointestinal tract, especially the stomach and duodenum, can result in stimulation of the satiety center and subsequent inhibition of the feeding center in the hypothalamus. This effect, along with the discomfort that occurs with distention, decreases appetite.*
• Increase activity as allowed and tolerated. **D** ● ✦	*Activity usually promotes a general feeling of well-being, which can result in improved appetite.*
• Maintain a clean environment and a relaxed, pleasant atmosphere. **D** ● ✦	*Noxious sites and odors can inhibit the feeding center in the hypothalamus. Maintaining a clean environment helps prevent this from occurring. In addition, maintaining a relaxed, pleasant atmosphere can help reduce the client's stress and promote a feeling of well-being which tends to improve appetite and oral intake.*
• Encourage a rest period before meals if indicated. **D** ● ✦	*The physical activity of eating requires some expenditure of energy. Fatigue can reduce the client's desire and ability to eat.*
• Provide oral hygiene before meals. **D** ● ✦	*Oral hygiene moistens the oral mucous membrane, which may make it easier to chew and swallow. It also freshens the mouth and removes unpleasant tastes. This can improve the taste of foods/fluids, which helps stimulate appetite and increase oral intake.*
• Serve foods/fluids that are appealing to the client and adhere to personal and cultural (e.g., religious, ethnic) preferences whenever possible. **D** ● ✦	*Foods/fluids that appeal to the client's senses, especially sight and smell, and are in accordance with personal and cultural preferences are most likely to stimulate appetite and promote interest in eating.*
• Serve frequent, small meals rather than large ones if client is weak, fatigues easily, and/or has a poor appetite. **D** ● ✦	*Providing small rather than large meals can enable a client who is weak or fatigues easily to finish a meal. Also, a client who has a poor appetite is often more willing to attempt to eat smaller meals because they seem less overwhelming than larger ones. If smaller meals are served, the number of meals per day should be increased to help ensure adequate nutrition.*
• Encourage significant others to bring in client's favorite foods unless contraindicated and eat with him/her if client desires.	*A client's favorite foods/fluids tend to stimulate his/her appetite more than institutional foods/fluids. The presence of significant others during meals helps create a familiar social environment that can stimulate appetite and improve oral intake.*
• If client is experiencing dyspnea, place him/her in a high-Fowler's position and provide supplemental oxygen therapy during meals if indicated.	*Because a person cannot swallow and breathe at the same time, relief of dyspnea increases the likelihood of maintaining a good oral intake. In addition, relieving dyspnea decreases the client's anxiety about and preoccupation with breathing efforts and increases the ability to focus on eating and drinking.*
• Perform actions to compensate for taste alterations if present (e.g., add extra sweeteners to foods unless contraindicated, encourage client to experiment with different flavorings and seasonings, provide alternative sources of protein if meats such as beef or pork taste bitter or rancid).	*Enhancing the taste of foods/fluids and providing nutritious alternatives to those that taste unpleasant to the client help to stimulate appetite and improve oral intake.*

Continued...

THERAPEUTIC INTERVENTIONS	RATIONALE
• Allow adequate time for meals; reheat foods/fluids if necessary. **D** ● ✦	*A client who feels rushed during meals tends to become anxious, loses his/her appetite, and stops eating. Appetite is also suppressed if foods/fluids normally served hot or warm become cold and do not appeal to the client.*
• Limit fluid intake with meals unless the fluid has a high nutritional value. **D** ● ✦	*When the stomach becomes distended, its volume receptors stimulate the satiety center in the hypothalamus, and the client reduces his/her oral intake. Drinking liquids with meals distends the stomach and may cause satiety before an adequate amount of food is consumed.*
Ensure that meals are well balanced and high in essential nutrients.	*The client must consume a diet that is well balanced and high in essential nutrients in order to meet his/her nutritional needs. Dietary supplements are often needed to help accomplish this.*
Allow the client to assist in the selection of foods/fluids that meet nutritional needs. **D** ● ✦	*The client who is actively involved in menu planning is more likely to adhere to the diet plan. In addition, the involvement increases his/her sense of control, which promotes a feeling of well-being and can lead to an increased oral intake.*

Dependent/Collaborative Actions

Administer medications that may be ordered to improve client's nutritional status (e.g., antiemetics, antidiarrheals, gastrointestinal stimulants, and vitamins and minerals). **D** ✦	*Medications may relieve vomiting, diarrhea, and distention of the gastric tract, which decreases the discomfort that occurs with each of these signs and symptoms. Vitamins and minerals are needed to maintain metabolic functioning. If the client's dietary intake does not provide adequate amounts of them, oral and/or parenteral supplements may be necessary.*
Obtain a dietary consult if necessary.	*A dietitian is best able to evaluate whether the foods/fluids selected will meet the client's nutritional needs.*
Perform a calorie count if ordered. Report information to the dietitian and physician.	*A calorie count provides information about the caloric and nutritional value of the foods/fluids the client consumes. The information obtained helps the dietitian and physician determine whether an alternative method of nutritional support is needed.*
Consult the physician about an alternative method of providing nutrition (e.g., parenteral nutrition, tube feeding) if the client does not consume enough food or fluids to meet nutritional needs.	*If the client's oral intake is inadequate, an alternative method of providing nutrients needs to be implemented.*

Nursing Diagnosis **IMPAIRED ORAL MUCOUS MEMBRANE INTEGRITY** NDx

Definition: Injury to the lips, soft tissue, buccal cavity, and/or oropharynx.

CLINICAL MANIFESTATIONS

Subjective	Objective
Self-report of sensitive tongue; bad taste in the mouth; oral pain/discomfort; self-report of difficulty eating or swallowing; self-report of diminished or absent taste	Purulent drainage or exudates; gingival recession, pockets deeper than 4 mm; enlarged tonsils beyond what is developmentally appropriate; smooth, atrophic geographic tongue; mucosal denudation; presence of pathogens; difficult speech; gingival or mucosal pallor; xerostomia (dry mouth); vesicles, nodules, or papules; white patches/plaques, spongy patches, or white curdlike exudate; oral lesions or ulcers; halitosis; edema; hyperemia; desquamation; coated tongue; stomatitis; bleeding; macroplasia; gingival hyperplasia; fissures, cheilitis; red or bluish masses (e.g., hemangiomas)

RISK FACTORS

- Chemotherapy
- Chemical (e.g., alcohol, tobacco, acidic foods, drugs, regular use of inhalers or other noxious agents)
- Depression
- Immunosuppression
- Aging-related loss of connective, adipose, or bone tissue
- Barriers to professional care
- Cleft lip or palate
- Medication side effects

- Lack of or decreased salivation
- Trauma
- Pathologic conditions: oral cavity (e.g., radiation to head or neck)
- Nothing by mouth (NPO) for more than 24 hrs
- Mouth breathing
- Malnutrition or vitamin deficiency
- Dehydration
- Infection
- Ineffective oral hygiene

- Mechanical (e.g., ill-fitting dentures, braces, tubes [endotracheal/nasogastric], surgery in oral cavity)
- Decreased platelets
- Immunocompromised
- Radiation therapy
- Barriers to oral self-care
- Diminished hormone levels (women)
- Stress
- Loss of supportive structures

DESIRED OUTCOMES

The client will maintain a healthy oral cavity as evidenced by:
a. Absence of inflammation and discomfort
b. Pink, moist, intact mucosa

DOCUMENTATION

- Client reports of oral dryness and/or discomfort
- Condition of oral mucous membranes
- Therapeutic interventions
- Client teaching

NOC OUTCOMES

Oral health; tissue integrity: skin and mucous membranes; hydration; nutritional status

NIC INTERVENTIONS

Oral health maintenance; oral health restoration; oral health promotion

NURSING ASSESSMENT	RATIONALE
Assess for and report signs and symptoms of impaired oral mucous membrane (e.g., reports of oral dryness and discomfort, coated tongue, inflamed and/or ulcerated oral mucosa).	*Early recognition of signs and symptoms of impaired oral mucous membrane allows for prompt intervention.*
Culture oral lesions as ordered. Report positive results.	*A positive culture reveals the organisms present in a lesion, which provides direction for the treatment plan.*

THERAPEUTIC INTERVENTIONS	RATIONALE

Independent Actions

Assist client to perform oral hygiene as often as needed (e.g., after meals and at bedtime, at least every 2 hrs if NPO). **D** ● ✦	*Good oral hygiene helps maintain health of the oral mucous membrane by removing food particles and debris that harbor or promote the growth of pathogenic organisms that can cause inflammation and infection. Brushing the teeth also stimulates circulation to the gums.*
Assist client to perform oral hygiene using a soft bristle toothbrush or sponge-tipped swab and to floss teeth gently. **D** ● ✦	*Use of appropriate oral hygiene devices and techniques helps to effectively remove food particles and debris from client's mouth without causing trauma to the oral mucous membrane.*
Avoid use of mouthwashes containing alcohol and oral care products that contain lemon and glycerin. **D** ● ✦	*Mouthwashes containing alcohol and oral care products containing lemon and glycerin have a drying and irritating effect on the oral mucous membrane. Excessive use of the lemon-glycerin products also increases acidity in the mouth, which results in further irritation of the oral mucosa.*
Encourage client to rinse mouth frequently with water. **D** ● ✦	*Frequent rinsing of the mouth helps alleviate dryness, which reduces the risk for cracking and breakdown of the oral mucosa. Rinsing also helps prevent inflammation and infection in the mouth by removing food particles and debris that can harbor or promote the growth of pathogenic organisms.*
Lubricate client's lips frequently. **D** ● ✦	*Lubricating the client's lips helps keep them moist, which helps prevent drying and cracking of the lips.*
Encourage client to breathe through nose rather than mouth. **D** ✦	*Air inspired through the nose is humidified by the layer of mucus that coats the lining of the nasal cavity. Air inspired through the mouth lacks this moisture and is drying to the oral mucous membrane.*

Continued...

THERAPEUTIC INTERVENTIONS	RATIONALE
Encourage client not to smoke or chew tobacco.	*Smoking dries the oral mucous membrane. Irritation and subsequent inflammation can occur when tobacco is in contact with the oral mucosa.*
Encourage a fluid intake of at least 2500 mL/day unless contraindicated. **D** ● ✦	*Adequate hydration helps keep the oral mucosa moist, which reduces the risk of cracking and breakdown.*
Encourage client to suck on hard candy if allowed. **D** ✦	*Sucking on hard candy stimulates salivation, which helps alleviate dryness of the oral mucosa and the subsequent risk of cracking and breakdown. Saliva also helps maintain oral mucosal health by washing away food particles and debris that harbor or promote the growth of pathogenic organisms and by directly destroying some of the bacteria present in the mouth.*
Assist client to select foods of moderate temperature and those that are soft and bland. **D** ● ✦	*Foods that are extremely hot or cold; hard, crusty, or rough; spicy; and/or acidic may cause thermal, mechanical, or chemical trauma to the oral mucosa.*
Encourage client to maintain an optimal nutritional status.	*Adequate nutrition is needed to maintain the high cellular turnover of the oral mucous membrane. Good nutrition also promotes optimal function of the immune system, which reduces the client's risk of oral cavity infection.*
Inspect client's dentures. Note if they are rough, cracked, or ill-fitting.	*Rough, cracked, or ill-fitting dentures can cause mechanical trauma and subsequent inflammation and breakdown of the oral mucosa. The discomfort in the affected area(s) can result in a decreased oral intake, which further compromises the health of the oral mucosa.*

Dependent/Collaborative Actions

Administer topical anesthetics, oral protective agents, analgesics, and antimicrobials if ordered. **D** ✦	*Topical anesthetics, oral protective agents, and analgesics promote comfort if the oral mucous membrane is inflamed or if breakdown is present. The increased comfort can result in an improved oral intake, which helps maintain health of the oral mucosa. Antimicrobials prevent or treat infection of the oral mucosa.*
Consult appropriate health care provider if dryness, irritation, discomfort, and/or breakdown of the oral cavity persist or worsen. Consult the physician about an alternative treatment plan	*Notifying the appropriate health care provider allows for modification of the treatment plan.*
Consult a dentist if dentures are rough, cracked, or ill-fitting.	*Notifying a dentist to improve fit and condition of dentures will help improve the health of the oral mucosa.*

Nursing Diagnosis   # ACUTE PAIN NDx

Definition: Unpleasant sensory and emotional experience associated with actual or potential tissue damage. or described in terms of such damage (International Association for the Study of Pain); sudden or slow onset of any intensity from mild to severe with an anticipated or predictable end, and with a duration of less than 3 months.

CLINICAL MANIFESTATIONS

Subjective	Objective
Verbal self-report of pain; self-sleep disturbance; self-focus; narrowed focus (altered time perception, impaired thought processes)	Autonomic responses (e.g., facial mask diaphoresis; changes in blood pressure [BP], respiration, pulse rate; pupillary dilatation); expressive behavior (e.g., restlessness, moaning, crying, vigilance, irritability, sighing); changes in appetite and eating; protective gestures; guarding behavior; eyes lack luster, fixed or scattered movement, beaten look, grimace; reduced interaction with people and environment; autonomic change in muscle tone may span from listless to rigid; distraction behavior (e.g., pacing, seeking out other people and/or activities, repetitive activities)

RISK FACTORS
- Injury agents (e.g., biologic, chemical, physical, psychologic)

DESIRED OUTCOMES

The client will experience diminished pain as evidenced by:
a. Verbalization of decrease in or absence of pain
b. Relaxed facial expression and body positioning
c. Increased participation in activities
d. Stable vital signs

DOCUMENTATION

- Verbal description of pain
- Rating of pain intensity
- Facial expression
- Body movement and position
- Vital signs
- Participation in activities
- Factors that precipitate, aggravate, and alleviate pain
- Therapeutic interventions
- Client/family teaching

NOC OUTCOMES

Pain control; comfort status: physical discomfort level; pain level; stress level

NIC INTERVENTIONS

Pain management; environmental management: comfort; analgesic administration

NURSING ASSESSMENT	RATIONALE
Assess for signs and symptoms of pain (e.g., verbalization of pain, grimacing, reluctance to move, restlessness, diaphoresis, increased BP, tachycardia).	*Early recognition of signs and symptoms of pain allows for prompt intervention and improved pain control.*
Assess client's perception of the severity of pain using a pain intensity rating scale.	*An awareness of the severity of pain being experienced helps determine the most appropriate intervention(s) for pain management. Use of a pain intensity rating scale gives the nurse a clearer understanding of the pain being experienced and promotes consistency when communicating with others about the client's pain experience.*
Assess the client's pain pattern (e.g., location, quality, onset, duration, precipitating factors, aggravating factors, alleviating factors).	*Knowledge of the client's pain pattern assists in the identification of effective pain management interventions.*
Ask the client to describe previous pain experiences and methods used to manage pain effectively.	*Many variables affect a client's response to pain (e.g., age, sex, coping style, previous experience with pain, culture, cause of pain). Knowledge of the client's usual response to pain and methods previously used to manage pain effectively enables the nurse to evaluate the client's pain more accurately and facilitates the identification of effective strategies for pain management.*

THERAPEUTIC INTERVENTIONS	RATIONALE
Independent Actions Implement measures to reduce fear and anxiety (e.g., assure client that his/her need for pain relief is understood, plan methods for achieving pain control with client, provide a calm environment).	*Fear and anxiety can decrease the client's threshold and tolerance for pain and thereby heighten the perception of pain. In addition, pain management methods are not as effective if the client is tense and unable to relax.*
Implement measures to promote rest (e.g., minimize environmental activity and noise). **D** ● ✦	*Fatigue can decrease the client's threshold and tolerance for pain and thereby heighten the perception of pain. If the client is well rested, he/she often experiences decreased pain and increased effectiveness of pain management measures.*
Provide or assist with nonpharmacologic methods for pain relief. Examples include: • Relaxation techniques (e.g., progressive relaxation exercises, meditation, guided imagery) • Distraction measures (e.g., listening to music, conversing, watching television, playing cards, reading) • Position change	*Nonpharmacologic pain management includes a variety of interventions. It is believed that most of these are effective because they stimulate closure of the gating mechanism in the spinal cord and subsequently block the transmission of pain impulses. In addition, some interventions are thought to stimulate the release of endogenous analgesics (e.g., endorphins) that inhibit the transmission of pain impulses and/or alter the client's perception of pain. Many of the nonpharmacologic interventions also help decrease pain by promoting relaxation.*

NDx = NANDA Diagnosis **D** = Delegatable Action ● = UAP ✦ = LVN/LPN ⊖▶ = Go to ⊖volve for animation

Continued...

THERAPEUTIC INTERVENTIONS	RATIONALE

Dependent/Collaborative Actions

Administer analgesics before activities and procedures that can cause pain and before pain becomes severe. **D** ✦

The administration of analgesics before a pain-producing event helps minimize the pain that will be experienced. Analgesics are also more effective if given before pain becomes severe because mild to moderate pain is controlled more quickly and effectively than severe pain.

Administer the following medications as ordered: **D** ✦
- Opioid (narcotic) analgesics
- Nonopioid (nonnarcotic) analgesics such as acetaminophen and salicylates and other nonsteroidal antiinflammatory agents (e.g., ketorolac, ibuprofen, naproxen)

- Anesthetic agents (e.g., bupivacaine, etidocaine).

Pharmacologic therapy is an effective method of reducing or relieving pain.

Opioid analgesics act mainly by altering the client's perception of pain and emotional response to the pain experience.

Nonopioid analgesics are thought to interfere with the transmission of pain impulses by inhibiting prostaglandin synthesis.

Anesthetics help control pain by inhibiting the initiation and conduction of pain impulses along the sensory pathways at and near the infusion site.

Provide or assist with nonpharmacologic methods for pain relief such as cutaneous stimulation measures (e.g., pressure, massage, heat and cold applications, transcutaneous electrical nerve stimulation [TENS], acupuncture).

It is believed that most of these are effective because they stimulate closure of the gating mechanism in the spinal cord and subsequently block the transmission of pain impulses.

Consult physician about an order for patient-controlled analgesia (PCA) if indicated.

The use of PCA allows the client to self-administer analgesics within parameters established by the physician. This method facilitates pain management by ensuring prompt administration of the drug when needed, providing more continuous pain relief, and increasing the client's control over the pain.

Consult appropriate health care provider (e.g., physician, pharmacist, pain management specialist) if above measures fail to provide adequate pain relief.

Notifying the appropriate health care provider allows for modification of the treatment plan.

Nursing Diagnosis   # READINESS FOR ENHANCED SELF-CARE NDx

Definition: A pattern of performing activities for oneself to meet health-related goals, which can be strengthened.

Related to:

CLINICAL MANIFESTATIONS

Subjective	Objective
Verbal self-expressed desire to advance independence in maintaining life; enhance independence in maintaining health; enhance independence in maintaining personal development; enhance independence in maintaining well-being; enhance knowledge of strategies for self-care	Not applicable

DESIRED OUTCOMES

The client will have enhanced self-care as evidenced by:
a. Identification and performance of desired self-care activities
b. Expressed desire to improve self-care habits
c. Ability to evaluate effectiveness of self-care habits

DOCUMENTATION

- Client/family teaching

NOC OUTCOMES	NIC INTERVENTIONS
Adherence behavior; health-seeking behavior; health promotion behavior; information processing; decision-making; health promoting behavior; patient engagement behavior; self-care status	Active listening; family integrity promotion; self-care assistance; self-responsibility facilitation; support system enhancement; spiritual growth facilitation; self-care teaching

NURSING ASSESSMENT	RATIONALE
Assess client's current self-care habits.	*Assessment of the client's current self-care activities provides the basis for planning further self-care activities.*
Assess client's confidence in ability to perform more self-care habits.	*It is important to determine whether the client has the confidence to perform new self-care activities. Confidence in one's ability to change behaviors impacts the success in maintaining change.*

THERAPEUTIC INTERVENTIONS	RATIONALE
Independent Actions	
Encourage client in pursuit of enhanced self-care activities.	*Encouragement will support the client to begin and maintain self-care activities.*
Collaborate with the client to set realistic goals.	*Developed goals should include short- and long-term goals. Short-term goals are more achievable and provide the client confidence to reach the long-term goals. Goals should be specific and realistic, with consideration for the patient's ability.*
Provide positive reinforcement when behaviors are met.	*Positive reinforcement promotes a sense of self-efficacy in the client.*
Promote family involvement in developing self-care activities.	*Self-care activities help improve a client's health and decrease the incidence of repeated hospitalizations. The client's family plays a significant role in promoting success of self-care behaviors.*
Implement culturally sensitive interventions.	*Recognize the impact of culture on self-care. A client's cultural background influences self-care activities and adherence to them.*
Provide client with information to enhance self-care behaviors.	*Specific self-care needs are based on the type of disease process and/or symptoms experienced by the client.*
Inform client of community resources available to support and enhance self-care.	*Client should know what community resources are available to enhance self-care behaviors.*
Use a variety of teaching strategies to enhance self-care behaviors.	*Learning is enhanced when a variety of teaching methods are used.*
Evaluate effectiveness of self-care behaviors.	*This helps the client realize the progress made and verifies the client's ability to maintain self-care behaviors and/or identify new behaviors.*
Educate client and family to evaluate the effectiveness of self-care activities.	*This helps the client determine when and/or if progress is being made and improves the client's confidence in his/her ability to improve well-being.*

Nursing Diagnosis ## READINESS FOR ENHANCED SELF-CONCEPT NDx

For a full, detailed care plan on this topic, go to http://evolve.elsevier.com/Haugen/careplanning/.

Nursing Diagnosis ## RISK FOR IMPAIRED SKIN INTEGRITY NDx

Definition: Susceptible to alteration in epidermis and/or dermis, which may compromise health.

CLINICAL MANIFESTATIONS

Subjective	Objective
Verbal self-report of areas of decreased sensation	Pallor, redness, and breakdown of skin covering bony prominences, dependent areas, pruritic areas, perineum, and areas of decreased sensation

NDx = NANDA Diagnosis **D** = Delegatable Action ● = UAP ✦ = LVN/LPN ⊖▶ = Go to ⊖volve for animation

RISK FACTORS

- **External:** Radiation; physical immobilization; hypothermia or hyperthermia; chemical substance; mechanical factors (e.g., shearing forces, pressure, restraint); humidity; excretions and/or secretions; moisture; extremes of age
- **Internal:** Medication; skeletal prominence; immunologic factors; developmental factors; altered sensation; altered pigmentation; altered metabolic state; altered circulation; alterations in skin turgor (changes in elasticity); alterations in nutritional state (e.g., obesity, emaciation); psychogenetic

DESIRED OUTCOMES

The client will maintain skin integrity as evidenced by:
a. Absence of redness and irritation
b. No skin breakdown

DOCUMENTATION

- Appearance of skin
- Therapeutic interventions
- Client/family teaching

NOC OUTCOMES

Tissue integrity: skin and mucous membranes

NIC INTERVENTIONS

Pressure ulcer prevention; skin surveillance; bathing; pressure management; skin care: topical treatments; positioning; bedrest care

NURSING ASSESSMENT

Determine client's risk for skin breakdown using a risk assessment tool (e.g., Norton Scale, Braden Scale, Gosnell Scale).

Inspect the skin especially bony prominences, dependent areas, pruritic areas, perineum, and areas of decreased sensation and/or edema for pallor, redness, and breakdown.

RATIONALE

Prompt identification of the client's risk for skin breakdown leads to earlier implementation of actions to maintain skin integrity. Use of a risk assessment tool aids in the identification of factors that could cause skin breakdown.
Early recognition of signs of impaired skin integrity allows for prompt intervention.

THERAPEUTIC INTERVENTIONS

Independent Actions
Implement measures to prevent prolonged and/or excessive pressure on any area of the skin: **D** ● ✦

- Assist client to turn at least every 2 hrs unless contraindicated.
- Instruct or assist client to shift weight at least every 30 minutes.
- Position client properly using supportive devices such as pillows and pads as needed.
- Keep bed linens wrinkle-free.
- Ensure that external devices such as braces, casts, and restraints are applied properly.
- Ensure that client is not lying on tubings.
- Use pressure-reducing or pressure-relieving devices (e.g., gel or foam cushions, alternating pressure mattress, airfluidized bed) if indicated.

Gently massage around reddened areas at least every 2 hrs. **D** ● ✦

Implement measures to prevent shearing (e.g., keep head of bed as flat as possible, gatch knees slightly when head of bed is elevated 30 degrees or higher, limit length of time client is in semi-Fowler's position to 30-minute intervals). **D** ● ✦

RATIONALE

Prolonged and/or excessive pressure on the skin obstructs capillary blood flow to that area. The resultant hypoxia, impaired flow of nutrients, and accumulation of waste products in the area of obstructed blood flow make that tissue more susceptible to breakdown. Measures that prevent the excessive pressure or ensure that pressure is relieved often enough to avoid obstruction of capillary blood flow help maintain skin integrity.

Massage stimulates circulation to the skin and underlying tissues. The improved blood flow helps maintain skin integrity by increasing the supply of oxygen and nutrients available to the cells and by removing waste products of metabolism. To avoid damaging the capillaries, massage should be gentle rather than deep, and massage over reddened areas should be avoided.
When one tissue layer slides past another in an opposite direction (i.e., shearing), the capillaries in the affected area are kinked, stretched, or severed. This compromises the area's blood supply and increases the risk of tissue breakdown. A client in a semi-Fowler's position is likely to slide down in the bed. When this occurs, his/her skin tends to remain stationary while the underlying tissues and skeletal structures shift position, resulting in shearing.

THERAPEUTIC INTERVENTIONS	**RATIONALE**
Implement measures to reduce friction between the skin and another surface (e.g., apply a protective covering such as a hydrocolloid or transparent membrane dressing to susceptible areas of the skin, apply thin layer of a dry lubricant such as powder or cornstarch to bottom sheet or client's skin, lift and move client carefully using turn sheet and adequate assistance, adequately secure restraints and tubings, pat skin dry rather than rub). **D** ● ✦	*The outermost layers of skin can be damaged when dragged along or rubbed against another surface. Reducing friction helps prevent skin surface irritation and abrasion.*
Keep client's skin clean. **D** ● ✦	*Keeping the skin clean removes many of the surface microorganisms, which, if allowed to accumulate, increase the risk of irritation or infection and subsequent skin breakdown.*
Use a mild soap when bathing client. **D** ● ✦	*Sebum, which is secreted by the skin, helps maintain skin integrity by preventing excess evaporation of moisture, keeping the skin soft and pliable, and destroying some of the bacteria on the skin's surface. Using a mild rather than a harsh, alkaline soap helps ensure that some sebum remains on the skin after bathing.*
Implement measures to keep skin free of excessive moisture: • Thoroughly dry skin after bathing and as often as needed, paying special attention to skinfolds and opposing skin surfaces (e.g., axillae, perineum, beneath breasts). **D** ● ✦ • Keep bed linens dry. **D** ✦ • Protect skin surrounding wound from drainage (e.g., change dressing when damp, apply a drainage collection device if needed). **D** ✦ • If use of absorbent products such as pads or undergarments is necessary, select those that effectively absorb moisture and keep it away from the skin.	*Excessive moisture on the skin or prolonged exposure of the skin to moisture softens the epidermal cells and makes them less resistant to damage. Moisture also harbors microorganisms that can cause irritation or infection, and it increases the possibility of friction between the skin and the surface it is against. Removing excessive moisture and protecting the skin from prolonged contact with moisture reduces the risk of skin irritation and subsequent breakdown.*
Increase activity as allowed and tolerated. **D** ● ✦	*Activity stimulates circulation, which helps maintain skin integrity by increasing the flow of oxygen and nutrients to the skin and underlying tissues. In addition, increasing activity reduces the risk of prolonged pressure occurring on any area as a result of decreased mobility.*
Maintain an optimal nutritional status.	*An inadequate nutritional status results in muscle atrophy, a decrease in the amount of subcutaneous tissue, and skin that is thin and less elastic. Subsequently, the skin and tissue are more vulnerable to injury because they are less able to withstand minor trauma. In addition, a malnourished client is more susceptible to the effects of pressure because there is less padding between the skin and underlying bone.*
Implement measures to prevent drying of the skin: • Encourage a fluid intake of 2500 mL/day unless contraindicated. • Apply a moisturizing lotion and/or emollient to the skin at least once a day. **D** ● ✦	*Dry skin is more prone to cracking and has decreased elasticity, which makes it susceptible to damage.* • *An adequate fluid intake helps ensure that the skin remains well hydrated.* • *Moisturizing lotion and some emollients provide a source of moisture to the skin. Emollients also form a protective barrier on the epidermis, which reduces the evaporation of moisture.*
Protect skin from contact with urine and feces (e.g., perform actions to prevent incontinence and/or diarrhea, keep perineal area clean and dry, apply a protective ointment or cream to perineal area). **D** ● ✦	*Urine and feces are irritants that can cause inflammation and breakdown of the skin. In addition, the moisture in urine and feces softens epidermal cells and increases friction between opposing skin surfaces and between the skin and bed linen.*
If edema is present, handle edematous areas carefully and implement measures to reduce fluid accumulation in dependent areas (e.g., instruct client in and assist with range of motion exercises, elevate affected extremities whenever possible).	*Edematous areas have an increased risk for skin breakdown because the oxygen and nutrient supply to the skin is compromised by the increased distance that exists between the capillaries and the cells. Handling edematous areas carefully and implementing measures to reduce edema decrease the risk for skin breakdown.*

Continued...

THERAPEUTIC INTERVENTIONS	RATIONALE
If the client is experiencing pruritus, implement measures to reduce the itching sensation (e.g., apply cool compress to pruritic area), keep his/her nails trimmed, and apply mittens if necessary. **D** ● ✦	*The client experiencing pruritus is likely to scratch the affected areas, which irritates the skin and can cause excoriation. Implementing measures to reduce the itching sensation helps prevent scratching. Trimming the client's nails and applying mittens if necessary reduce the risk of trauma to the skin if he/she does scratch the pruritic areas.*

Dependent/Collaborative Actions

Administer antihistamines as prescribed. **D** ✦	*Administering antihistamines can decrease itching.*
Notify appropriate health care provider (e.g., physician, enterostomal therapist, wound care specialist) if skin breakdown occurs.	*Notifying the appropriate health care provider allows for modification of treatment plan.*

Nursing Diagnosis # DISTURBED SLEEP PATTERN NDx

Definition: Time-limited awakenings due to external factors.

CLINICAL MANIFESTATIONS

Subjective	Objective
Verbal self-report of difficulty falling asleep, not feeling well rested, and/or dissatisfaction with sleep	Awakening earlier than desired; prolonged awakenings; sleep maintenance insomnia; self-induced impairment of normal pattern; sleep onset greater than 30 minutes; early morning insomnia; increased proportion of stage 1 sleep; less than age-normed total sleep time; three or more nighttime awakenings; decreased proportion of stages 3 and 4 sleep (e.g., hyporesponsiveness, excess sleepiness, decreased motivation); decreased proportion of rapid eye movement (REM) sleep (e.g., REM rebound, hyperactivity, emotional lability, agitation and impulsivity, atypical polysomnographic features); decreased ability to function

RISK FACTORS

- **Psychologic:** Ruminative pre-sleep thoughts; daytime activity pattern; thinking about home; body temperature; temperament; dietary; childhood onset; inadequate sleep hygiene; sustained use of anti-sleep agents; circadian asynchrony; frequently changing sleep-wake schedule; depression; loneliness; frequent travel across time zones; daylight/darkness exposure; grief; anticipation; shift work; delayed or advanced sleep phase syndrome; loss of sleep partner, life change; preoccupation with trying to sleep; periodic gender-related hormonal shifts; biochemical agents; fear; separation from significant others; social schedule inconsistent with chronotype; aging-related sleep shifts; anxiety; medications; fear of insomnia; maladaptive conditioned wakefulness; fatigue; boredom
- **Environmental:** Noise; unfamiliar sleep furnishings; ambient temperature, humidity; lighting; other-generated awakening; excessive stimulation; physical restraint; lack of sleep privacy/control; interruptions for therapeutics, monitoring, lab tests; sleep partner; noxious odors
- **Parental:** Mother's sleep-wake pattern; parent-infant interaction; mother's emotional support
- **Physiologic:** Urinary urgency, incontinence; fever; nausea; stasis of secretions; shortness of breath; position; gastroesophageal reflux

DESIRED OUTCOMES

The client will attain optimal amounts of sleep as evidenced by:
a. Statements of feeling well rested
b. Ability to perform normal daily activities

DOCUMENTATION

- Statements of difficulty falling asleep, interruptions in sleep, and/or not feeling well rested
- Therapeutic interventions
- Client teaching

NOC OUTCOMES	NIC INTERVENTIONS
Rest; sleep; personal well-being	Sleep enhancement; energy management

NURSING ASSESSMENT	RATIONALE
Assess for signs and symptoms of a disturbed sleep pattern (e.g., statements of difficulty falling asleep, sleep interruptions, or not feeling well rested).	*Early recognition of signs and symptoms of a disturbed sleep pattern allows for prompt intervention.*
Determine client's usual sleep habits.	*Knowledge of the client's usual sleep-wake cycle and routines that help induce and maintain sleep helps the nurse plan interventions aimed at preventing a sleep pattern disturbance.*

THERAPEUTIC INTERVENTIONS	RATIONALE

Independent Actions

Discourage long periods of sleep during the day unless signs and symptoms of sleep deprivation exist or daytime sleep is usual for client. **D** ● ✦	*Long periods of sleep during the day are often a change in the client's usual sleep-wake cycle and cause desynchronization of his/her circadian rhythm. This can result in a poorer quality of sleep.*
Implement measures to reduce fear and anxiety (e.g., maintain a calm, confident manner when working with client; assist client to identify specific stressors and ways to cope with them).	*Fear and anxiety stimulate the sympathetic nervous system, which increases alertness and makes it difficult for the client to fall asleep. Sympathetic nervous system stimulation is also believed to shorten the duration of nonrapid eye movement (NREM) and REM sleep, which results in a poorer quality of sleep.*
Encourage participation in relaxing diversional activities during the evening. **D** ● ✦	*Involvement in relaxing activities in the evening helps the client fall asleep more easily.*
Discourage intake of foods/fluids high in caffeine (e.g., chocolate, coffee, tea, colas) in the evening. **D** ● ✦	*Caffeine acts as a central nervous system stimulant and can interfere with relaxation and subsequent sleep induction. Caffeine also acts as a diuretic, which can cause an interruption in sleep if the client awakens in response to the urge to urinate.*
Offer client an evening snack that includes milk unless contraindicated. **D** ● ✦	*Milk contains the amino acid l-tryptophan, which is believed to help induce and maintain sleep.*
Allow client to continue usual sleep practices (e.g., position; time; presleep routines such as reading, watching television, listening to music, and meditating) whenever possible. **D** ● ✦	*Adherence to usual sleep practices promotes mental and physical relaxation that assists the client to maintain his/her usual sleep-wake cycle.*
Reduce environmental distractions (e.g., close door to client's room; use night light rather than overhead light whenever possible; lower volume of paging system; keep staff conversations at a low level and away from client's room; close curtains between clients in a semi-private room or ward; keep beepers and alarms on low volume; provide client with "white noise" such as a fan, soft music, or tape-recorded sounds of the ocean or rain; have sleep mask and earplugs available for client if needed). **D** ● ✦	*Environmental activity, noise, and light can interfere with the client's ability to fall asleep and stay asleep. Reducing stimuli helps prevent a sleep pattern disturbance.*
Encourage client to avoid drinking alcohol in the evening.	*Although alcohol can induce drowsiness, which promotes sleep induction, it is known to interfere with REM sleep. Alcohol also inhibits the release of antidiuretic hormone (ADH), which can cause an interruption in sleep if the client awakens in response to the urge to urinate.*
Encourage client to avoid smoking before bedtime. **D** ● ✦	*Nicotine is a stimulant that can interfere with sleep by making it difficult for the client to relax and fall asleep and to stay asleep.*
Implement measures to reduce interruptions during sleep (e.g., restrict visitors, group care whenever possible) so that client is able to sleep undisturbed for 70- to 100-minute intervals. **D** ✦	*One sleep cycle takes about 70 to 100 minutes to complete. Each time the cycle is interrupted, it begins again with NREM stage 1 sleep so the client loses portions of NREM and/or REM sleep. When the client is deprived of NREM sleep, lethargy and depression occur. Loss of REM sleep results in irritability and anxiety. Reducing the frequency of sleep interruptions helps ensure that the client progresses through all the sleep stages and does not experience a sleep pattern disturbance.*

NDx = NANDA Diagnosis   **D** = Delegatable Action   ● = UAP   ✦ = LVN/LPN   ⊜▶ = Go to ⊜volve for animation

Continued...

THERAPEUTIC INTERVENTIONS	RATIONALE
Dependent/Collaborative Actions	
If possible, administer medications that can interfere with sleep (e.g., steroids, diuretics) early in the day rather than late afternoon or evening. **D** ✦	*Administering these medications as early as possible during the day helps prevent nighttime insomnia and/or frequent awakenings.*
Administer prescribed sedative-hypnotics if indicated. **D** ✦	*Sedative-hypnotics are central nervous system depressants that promote sleep by reducing anxiety, shortening sleep induction, and/or reducing arousal level (wakefulness). These medications should be used for only a short time because they interfere with the length of REM sleep and can actually create a disturbance in the client's sleep-wake cycle.*
Consult appropriate health care provider if signs and symptoms of sleep deprivation (e.g., irritability, lethargy, agitation, inability to concentrate) occur and persist or worsen.	*Notifying the appropriate health care provider allows for modification of treatment plan.*

Nursing Diagnosis   IMPAIRED SWALLOWING NDx

Definition: Abnormal functioning of the swallowing mechanism associated with deficits in oral, pharyngeal, or esophageal structure or function.

CLINICAL MANIFESTATIONS

Subjective	Objective
Esophageal phase impairment: Verbal self-report of heartburn or epigastric pain; unexplained irritability surrounding mealtime; complaints of "something stuck"	**Pharyngeal phase impairment:** Altered head positions; inadequate laryngeal elevation; food refusal; unexplained fevers; delayed swallow; recurrent pulmonary infections; gurgly voice quality; nasal reflux; choking, coughing, or gagging; multiple swallows; abnormality in pharyngeal phase by swallow study **Oral phase impairment:** Lack of tongue action to form bolus; weak suck resulting in inefficient nippling; incomplete lip closure; food pushed out of mouth; slow bolus formation; premature entry of bolus; piecemeal deglutition; lack of chewing; food falls from mouth; nasal reflux; inability to clear oral cavity; long meals with little consumption; coughing, choking, gagging before a swallow; abnormality in oral phase of swallow study; pooling in lateral sulci; sialorrhea or drooling **Esophageal phase impairment:** Acidic-smelling breath; vomitus on pillow; repetitive swallowing or ruminating; regurgitation of gastric contents or wet burps; bruxism; nighttime coughing or awakening; observed evidence of difficulty in swallowing (e.g., stasis of food in oral cavity, coughing or choking); hyperextension of head, arching during or after meals; abnormality in esophageal phase by swallow study; odynophagia; hematemesis; vomiting

RISK FACTORS

- **Congenital deficits:** Upper airway anomalies; failure to thrive or protein-energy malnutrition; conditions with significant hypotonia; respiratory disorders; history of tube feeding; behavioral feeding problems; self-injurious behavior; neuromuscular impairment (e.g., decreased or absent gag reflex, decreased strength or excursion of muscles involved in mastication, perceptual impairment, facial paralysis); mechanical obstruction (e.g., edema, tracheostomy tube, tumor); congenital heart disease; cranial nerve involvement
- **Neurologic problems:** Upper airway anomalies; laryngeal abnormalities; achalasia; gastroesophageal reflux disease; acquired anatomic defects; cerebral palsy; internal traumas; tracheal, laryngeal, esophageal defects; traumatic head injury; developmental delay; external traumas; nasal or nasopharyngeal cavity defects; oral cavity or oropharynx abnormalities; premature infants

DESIRED OUTCOMES

The client will experience an improvement in swallowing as evidenced by:
a. Verbalization of same
b. Absence of food in oral cavity after swallowing
c. Absence of coughing and choking when eating and drinking

DOCUMENTATION

- Verbalization of difficulty swallowing
- Stasis of food in oral cavity
- Coughing or choking when eating or drinking
- Consistency of foods/fluids client is able to swallow without difficulty
- Therapeutic interventions
- Client/family teaching

NOC OUTCOMES

Swallowing status; swallowing status: oral phase; swallowing status: pharyngeal phase

NIC INTERVENTIONS

Swallowing therapy; aspiration precautions; positioning; risk identification

NURSING ASSESSMENT

Assess for signs and symptoms of impaired swallowing (e.g., statements of difficulty swallowing, stasis of food in oral cavity, coughing or choking when eating or drinking).

Assist with studies to evaluate client's swallowing (e.g., video-fluoroscopy) if ordered.

RATIONALE

Early recognition of signs and symptoms of impaired swallowing allows for prompt intervention.

Swallowing is a complex act that consists of voluntary and involuntary neuromotor components. Studies that evaluate the client's ability to swallow help identify the specific physiologic dysfunction, which aids in planning effective interventions.

THERAPEUTIC INTERVENTIONS

Independent Actions

If client has viscous oral secretions, implement measures to liquefy these secretions (e.g., encourage a fluid intake of 2500 mL/day unless contraindicated, administer a papain product before meals as ordered). **D** ● ✦

If client's mouth is dry, implement measures to moisten mouth before meals and snacks (e.g., provide good oral care, stimulate salivation by having client suck on hard candy unless contraindicated, encourage use of a saliva substitute such as Salivart). **D** ● ✦

Instruct and assist client to select foods/fluids that are appropriate for his/her swallowing ability. Some general guidelines include:

- Avoiding foods that tend to fall apart in the mouth (e.g., applesauce, cake, muffins) and those that consist of small food particles (e.g., rice, peas, corn, nuts) if client has impaired tongue control

- Avoiding foods that are sticky (e.g., peanut butter, soft bread, honey)

- Moistening dry foods with gravy or sauces (e.g., catsup, sour cream, salad dressing)
- Selecting thick rather than thin fluids or adding a thickening agent (e.g., "Thick-It," gelatin, baby cereal) if client has a delayed swallowing reflex and/or poor tongue control

Place client in a high-Fowler's position for meals and snacks unless contraindicated. **D** ● ✦

RATIONALE

Thick oral secretions interfere with movement of food in the mouth. Liquefying these secretions makes it easier for a bolus of food to be formed and moved to the back of the mouth. Liquefying the secretions also helps ensure that the bolus formed is moist so that it stays intact and triggers an effective swallowing reflex.

A moist mouth helps lubricate food, which makes it easier to chew, form into a bolus, and manipulate toward the back of the mouth. A formed, moist bolus more effectively triggers the swallowing reflex and moves more easily through the esophagus.

Impaired swallowing can result from structural or neurologic problems. The types of foods/fluids a client can swallow effectively vary depending on the particular swallowing difficulty.

Clients with impaired tongue movement have difficulty keeping foods that tend to fall apart in the mouth or consist of small pieces in a bolus that can be transferred to the back of the mouth. Some small pieces of food may fall to the back of the mouth, but because the food is not in a bolus, it will not trigger a strong swallowing reflex.

Sticky foods are difficult to move through the mouth because they tend to adhere to various structures, especially the hard palate. It is also difficult to form these foods into the distinct bolus needed to trigger the swallowing reflex.

Moist foods are more easily formed into a bolus and moved through the mouth and esophagus.

Thin fluids pass rapidly through the mouth and can pour over the back of the tongue without triggering an effective swallow. Thick fluids remain more cohesive and are able to stimulate the swallowing reflex more effectively.

A high-Fowler's position uses gravity to aid in the flow of foods/fluids through the esophagus.

Continued...

THERAPEUTIC INTERVENTIONS	RATIONALE
If client has difficulty chewing and maneuvering a bolus of food to the back of the mouth, instruct him/her to tilt head down when chewing and forming a bolus, then raise chin slightly when ready to swallow.	*Tilting the head down allows client more time to chew and form a bolus because the food is in the front of the mouth where it does not trigger the swallowing reflex. Raising the chin facilitates movement of the bolus to the back of the mouth so that the swallowing reflex can be triggered. NOTE: Caution client to avoid tilting head back when swallowing since this position increases the risk for aspiration.*
Serve foods/fluids that are hot or cold instead of room temperature. **D** ● ✦	*Foods/fluids that are hot or cold trigger a more effective swallowing reflex because they have a greater stimulatory effect on the sensory receptors in the mouth.*
If client has motor and sensory dysfunction of one side of the mouth or face, instruct and assist him/her to tilt head toward the unaffected side when eating and drinking and to place food in the unaffected side of the mouth.	*When foods/fluids are directed toward the unaffected side of the mouth, the client is able to more effectively chew and use his/her tongue to form a bolus and move it to the back of the mouth. The unaffected side of the mouth also has more tension in the buccal musculature so foods/fluids are more likely to get to the back of the mouth rather than collect between the cheek and the mandible. Sensory receptors on the unaffected side also trigger a stronger swallowing reflex than those on the affected side.*
Encourage client to concentrate on the act of swallowing. Provide verbal cueing as needed.	*The client can achieve a more effective swallow by focusing on chewing and moving foods/fluids to the back of the mouth where the swallowing reflex is triggered.*
Instruct client to avoid putting too much food/fluid in mouth at one time. **D** ● ✦	*Overfilling the mouth makes it difficult for the client to form a distinct bolus and effectively move it to the back of the mouth where it triggers the swallowing reflex.*
Encourage client to perform exercises to strengthen tongue and facial muscles if indicated (e.g., drinking through a straw; opening mouth and moving tongue anteriorly, posteriorly, and laterally; pushing tongue upward against resistance using an object such as a tongue blade, Popsicle, or sucker).	*Strong tongue and facial muscles increase the client's ability to chew food, form a bolus, and direct the bolus to the back of the mouth where it triggers the swallowing reflex.*

Dependent/Collaborative Actions

Consult speech pathologist about methods for dealing with client's specific swallowing impairment.	*Consulting with persons who are knowledgeable about the management of swallowing difficulties aids in the development of an individualized plan of care to improve the client's swallowing.*
Implement measures to reduce oral and pharyngeal discomfort if indicated (e.g., administer topical and/or systemic analgesics as ordered). **D** ✦	*Oral and pharyngeal discomfort can interfere with the client's ability and willingness to adequately chew food and swallow effectively.*
Consult appropriate health care provider (e.g., physician, speech pathologist) if swallowing difficulties persist or worsen.	*Notifying the appropriate health care provider allows for modification of treatment plan.*

Nursing Diagnosis   # IMPAIRED URINARY ELIMINATION* NDx

Definition: Dysfunction in urine elimination
- **Functional urinary incontinence:** Inability of a usually continent person to reach the toilet in time to avoid unintentional loss of urine.
- **Overflow urinary incontinence:** Involuntary loss of urine associated with overdistention of the bladder.
- **Reflex urinary incontinence:** Involuntary loss of urine at somewhat predictable intervals when a specific bladder volume is reached.
- **Stress urinary incontinence:** Sudden leakage of urine with activities that increase intra-abdominal pressure.
- **Urge urinary incontinence:** Involuntary passage of urine occurring soon after a strong sensation or urgency to void.

---

*NANDA International identifies five types of urinary incontinence: functional, overflow, reflex, urge, and stress. A client can experience a combination of types of incontinence, and the actions for various types often are similar. The information presented here focuses on incontinence in general rather than a specific type.

CLINICAL MANIFESTATIONS

Subjective **Functional:** Verbal self-report of need to void **Overflow:** Verbal self-report of voluntary leakage of small volumes of urine; nocturia **Reflex:** Verbal self-report of no sensation to void; sensation of urgency without voluntary inhibition of bladder contraction; sensations associated with full bladder (e.g., restlessness, abdominal discomfort); inability to voluntarily inhibit voiding; loss of urine with activities that place pressure on the bladder **Stress:** Verbal self-report of involuntary leakage of small amounts of urine. **Urge:** Verbal self-report of urinary urgency; involuntary loss of urine with bladder contractions and spasms; inability to reach toilet in time to avoid urine loss	**Objective** **Functional:** Loss of urine before reaching toilet; may be incontinent only in early morning **Overflow:** Bladder distention; high post void residual volume; observed involuntary leakage of small volumes of urine **Reflex:** Inability to voluntarily inhibit voiding; incomplete emptying of bladder with lesions above sacral and pontine micturition center **Stress:** Loss of urine with activities that place pressure on the bladder (i.e., coughing, sneezing, laughing, running) **Urge:** Observed involuntary loss of urine

RISK FACTORS

- **Functional:** Changes in environmental factors; impaired cognition/vision; neuromuscular limitations; psychological factors; weakened supporting pelvic structures
- **Overflow:** Bladder outlet obstruction; fecal impaction; urethral obstruction; detrusor external sphincter dyssynergia; detrusor hypocontractility; severe pelvic prolapse; side effects of medications—anticholinergics, calcium channel blockers, decongestants
- **Reflex:** Tissue damage; neurologic impairment above level of sacral or pontine micturition center
- **Urge:** Alcohol intake; atrophic urethritis/vaginitis; bladder infections; caffeine intake; decreased bladder capacity; fecal impaction; use of diuretics; detrusor hyperactivity with impaired bladder contractility
- **Stress:** Degenerative changes in pelvic muscles; weak pelvic muscles; high intra-abdominal pressure; intrinsic urethral sphincter deficiency

DESIRED OUTCOMES

The client will experience urinary continence.

DOCUMENTATION

- Episodes of urinary incontinence
- Statements of being unable to control urinary elimination
- Therapeutic interventions
- Client teaching

NOC OUTCOMES

Symptom control; urinary continence; urinary elimination; knowledge: disease process

NIC INTERVENTIONS

Urinary incontinence care; prompted voiding; self-care assistance: toileting; urinary habit training; urinary bladder training; pelvic muscle exercise

NURSING ASSESSMENT

Assess for and report urinary incontinence.

Monitor client's pattern of fluid intake and urination (e.g., times and amounts of fluid intake, types of fluids consumed, times and amounts of voluntary and involuntary voiding, reports of sensation of need to void, activities preceding incontinence).

Assist with urodynamic studies (e.g., urethral pressure profile, uroflowmetry, cystometrogram) if ordered.

RATIONALE

Early recognition of signs and symptoms of urinary incontinence allows for prompt intervention.

Knowledge of the client's fluid intake and urination pattern assists in the identification of factors that may be causing urinary incontinence. This information helps the nurse plan individualized interventions that promote urinary continence.

Urodynamic studies may be done to determine the cause(s) of urinary incontinence. The studies provide information about the motor and sensory function of the bladder and urethra.

THERAPEUTIC INTERVENTIONS	RATIONALE

Independent Actions

Offer bedpan or urinal, or assist client to bedside commode or bathroom every 2 to 4 hrs if indicated. **D** ● ✦

Urinary incontinence occurs when the pressure in the bladder becomes greater than the pressure exerted by the urinary sphincters. Emptying the bladder before the pressure becomes too great reduces the risk of incontinence.

Allow client to assume a normal position for voiding (usually sitting for females and standing for males) unless contraindicated. **D** ● ✦

A sitting or standing position uses gravity to facilitate bladder emptying. The more completely the bladder is emptied, the less risk there is of incontinence.

Implement measures to reduce delays in toileting (e.g., have call signal within client's reach and respond promptly to requests for assistance; have bedpan, urinal, or bedside commode readily available to client; provide easy access to bathroom; provide client with easy-to-remove clothing such as pajamas with Velcro closures or an elastic waistband). **D** ● ✦

If client is having difficulty controlling urination, any delay in toileting increases the risk of incontinence. Measures that enable the client to use a bedpan, urinal, bedside commode, or toilet in a timely manner help reduce the risk of incontinence.

Instruct client to perform pelvic floor muscle exercises (e.g., stopping and starting stream during voiding; squeezing buttocks together, then relaxing the muscles) if appropriate.

Pelvic floor muscle exercises help strengthen the pelvic floor muscles and improve the tone of the external urinary sphincter. As this is achieved, the risk for incontinence decreases.

Instruct client to space fluids evenly throughout the day rather than drinking a large quantity at one time.

Drinking a large amount of fluid at one time results in rapid filling of the bladder, which increases pressure in the bladder and the subsequent risk of incontinence.

Limit oral fluid intake in the evening. **D** ● ✦

As the client's bladder fills and pressure in the bladder increases during sleep, he/she is less likely to be aware of and/or able to respond to the urge to urinate. By limiting fluid intake in the evening, bladder filling during the night is decreased, which reduces the risk of incontinence.

Instruct client to avoid drinking alcohol and beverages containing caffeine such as colas, coffee, and tea.

Alcohol and caffeinated beverages increase urine formation because of their mild diuretic effect. With increased urine formation, bladder filling increases, causing a rise in pressure in the bladder, which subsequently increases the risk of incontinence. Alcohol and caffeine also act as chemical irritants to the bladder and contribute to urge incontinence.

Dependent/Collaborative Actions

Administer the following medications if ordered:

- Cholinergic (parasympathomimetic) agents (e.g., bethanechol) **D** ✦

If incontinence results from incomplete bladder emptying, cholinergic (parasympathomimetic) drugs may be prescribed to stimulate contraction of the detrusor muscle (smooth muscle of the bladder). This enhances bladder emptying and reduces the risk of incontinence.

- Anticholinergics (e.g., tolterodine, oxybutynin) **D** ✦

Hyperactivity of the bladder detrusor muscle can cause a sudden increase in pressure in the bladder and result in incontinence, especially if there is decreased bladder outlet resistance. Anticholinergics may be prescribed to reduce bladder detrusor muscle activity and thereby reduce the risk of incontinence.

Consult appropriate health care provider if urinary incontinence persists.

Notifying the appropriate health care provider allows for modification of treatment plan.

Nursing Diagnosis # URINARY RETENTION NDx

Definition: Inability to empty bladder completely.

CLINICAL MANIFESTATIONS

Subjective	Objective
Verbal self-report of sensation of bladder fullness or difficulty urinating	Bladder distention; small, frequent voiding or absence of urine output; dribbling of urine; residual urine; overflow incontinence

RISK FACTORS

- High urethral pressure caused by weak detrusor
- Inhibition of reflex arc
- Strong urinary sphincter
- Blockage of urine

DESIRED OUTCOMES

The client will not experience urinary retention as evidenced by:
a. Voiding at normal intervals
b. No reports of bladder fullness and suprapubic discomfort
c. Absence of bladder distention and dribbling of urine
d. Balanced intake and output

DOCUMENTATION

- Frequency of urination and amount voided each time
- Reports of bladder fullness and/or suprapubic discomfort
- Bladder distention
- Evidence or statements of dribbling of urine
- Patency of urinary catheter if present
- Intake and output
- Therapeutic interventions
- Client teaching

NOC OUTCOMES

Urinary elimination

NIC INTERVENTIONS

Urinary retention care; fluid management; bladder training; intermittent catheterization

NURSING ASSESSMENT	RATIONALE
Assess for signs and symptoms of urinary retention: • Frequent voiding of small amounts (25–60 mL) of urine • Reports of bladder fullness or suprapubic discomfort • Bladder distention • Dribbling of urine • Output less than intake	*Early recognition of signs and symptoms of urinary retention allows for prompt intervention.*
Assist with urodynamic studies (e.g., urethral pressure profile, uroflowmetry, cystometry) if ordered.	*Urodynamic studies may be indicated when neurogenic dysfunction is the suspected cause of urinary retention. The studies provide information about the motor and sensory function of the bladder and urethra.*

THERAPEUTIC INTERVENTIONS	RATIONALE
Independent Actions Instruct client to urinate when the urge is first felt. **D** ● ✦	*If the client feels the urge to urinate but suppresses it by contracting the external urinary sphincter, the urge will subside and not recur until the bladder fills more. If the client repeatedly suppresses the urge to urinate and the bladder fills too much or is chronically distended, the micturition reflex becomes less sensitive and does not effectively stimulate urination when the bladder fills.*
Implement measures to promote relaxation during voiding attempts (e.g., provide privacy, hold a warm blanket against abdomen, encourage client to read). **D** ● ✦	*If the client is relaxed when trying to urinate, he/she is better able to relax the pelvic floor muscles and external urinary sphincter and allow voiding to occur.*
If client is having difficulty voiding, run water, place his/her hands in warm water, and/or pour warm water over perineum unless contraindicated. **D** ✦ ●	*These measures have been found to trigger the micturition reflex and thereby promote voiding. They also promote a sense of relaxation, which facilitates voiding.*
Allow client to assume a normal position for voiding (usually sitting for females and standing for males) unless contraindicated. **D** ● ✦	*A sitting or standing position uses gravity to facilitate bladder emptying. Allowing the client to assume a normal voiding position also promotes relaxation, which facilitates voiding.*
Instruct and assist client to lean upper body forward and/or gently press downward on the lower abdomen when attempting to void unless contraindicated. **D** ● ✦	*Leaning forward or gently pressing downward on the lower abdomen increases pressure on the bladder. This pressure helps create a sensation of bladder fullness, which stimulates the micturition reflex.*

Continued...

THERAPEUTIC INTERVENTIONS	RATIONALE

Dependent/Collaborative Actions

Administer cholinergic (parasympathomimetic) drugs (e.g., bethanechol) if ordered. **D** ✦

Administer prescribed analgesic if client has pain.

If an indwelling urinary catheter is present, implement measures to ensure its patency (e.g., keep tubing free of kinks, keep collection bag below bladder level, irrigate catheter if indicated). **D** ● ✦

Consult appropriate health care provider if signs and symptoms of urinary retention persist.

Cholinergic (parasympathomimetic) drugs promote urination by stimulating contraction of the bladder detrusor muscle.

Pain blocks the client's ability to relax and subsequently relax the pelvic floor muscles and external urinary sphincter and allow voiding to occur.

Maintaining patency of the indwelling catheter prevents urinary retention.

Notifying the appropriate health care provider allows for modification of treatment plan.

4

Nursing Care of the Client Having Surgery

PROCEDURAL SEDATION

In the acute care setting, many clients undergo invasive procedures using sedation. The depth of sedation required for a client to tolerate an invasive procedure exists along a continuum that allows for balancing the client's ability to tolerate a procedure without compromising optimum respiratory and circulatory function. The American Society of Anesthesiologists (2014) defines four levels of sedation:

1. Minimal Sedation (Anxiolysis)—a drug-induced state during which clients responds to verbal commands. Although cognitive function and physical coordination may be impaired, airway reflexes and ventilatory and cardiovascular function are unaffected.

2. Moderate Sedation/Analgesia ("Conscious Sedation")—a drug-induced depression of consciousness during which clients respond purposefully to verbal commands, either alone or accompanied by light tactile stimulation. No interventions are required to maintain a patent airway, and spontaneous ventilation is adequate. Cardiovascular function is usually maintained.

3. Deep Sedation/Analgesia—a drug-induced depression of consciousness during which clients cannot be easily aroused but respond purposefully following repeated or painful stimulation. The ability to maintain independent ventilatory function may be impaired. Clients may require assistance in maintaining a patent airway, and spontaneous ventilation may be inadequate. Cardiovascular function is usually maintained.

4. General Anesthesia—a drug-induced loss of consciousness during which clients are not arousable, even by painful stimulation. The ability to maintain independent ventilatory function is often impaired. Clients often require assistance in maintaining a patent airway, and positive pressure ventilation may be required because of depressed spontaneous ventilation or drug-induced depression of neuromuscular function. Cardiovascular function may be impaired.

Sedatives routinely used to improve the client's tolerance of an invasive procedure include benzodiazepines (e.g., midazolam [Valium], lorazepam [Versed]). Opioids (e.g., morphine, meperidine [Demerol], fentanyl [Sublimaze]) are commonly used in procedural sedation along with sedatives to reduce the incidence and severity of pain associated with procedures.

Currently, acute care settings are charged with ensuring policies and procedures are in place that specify the minimum qualifications for each type of licensed provider (anesthesia/nonanesthesia) permitted to provide procedural sedation. Although deep sedation/analgesia and general anesthesia are routinely provided by licensed anesthesia providers (anesthesiologist, certified registered nurse anesthetist [CRNA]), many state boards of nursing have position statements, declaratory rules, or guidelines allowing the administration of sedation medications by a professional registered nurse with demonstrated competency in both the administration of sedation medications and physiologic monitoring of the client's response.

This care plan focuses on the care of the adult client who is receiving or has received sedation for an invasive procedure. Because of the nature of ongoing assessment, intervention, and evaluation of the client's tolerance to medications and the invasive procedure, delegation rarely occurs. Much of the information is applicable to clients undergoing conscious sedation in an outpatient setting (e.g., physician's office, surgical care center).

OUTCOME/DISCHARGE CRITERIA

The client will:
1. Maintain optimum respiratory function
2. Maintain optimum circulatory function
3. Return of protective reflexes (e.g., gag reflex, cough reflex)
4. Return to baseline cognition
5. Remain free from injury
6. Obtain adequate pain control

Nursing Diagnosis ACTUAL/RISK FOR IMPAIRED RESPIRATORY FUNCTION*

Ineffective breating pattern **NDx**
Definition: Inspiration and/or expiration that does not provide adequate ventilation.
Impaired gas exchange **NDx**
Definition: Excess or deficit in oxygenation and/or carbon dioxide elimination at the alveolar-capillary membrane.

Related to:
Ineffective breathing pattern:
- Procedure-related anxiety
- Procedure-related pain
- Body position that inhibits lung expansion

Impaired gas exchange:
- Depressed ventilation associated with administration of sedatives and/or opioids

CLINICAL MANIFESTATIONS

Subjective	Objective
Verbal self-report of difficulty breathing	Abnormal breathing pattern (e.g., bradypnea, dyspnea, tachypnea); use of accessory muscles to breathe; abnormal pulse oximetry/capnography/arterial blood gas (ABG) values; diaphoresis; irritability; restlessness; tachycardia; cyanosis

RISK FACTORS
- Administration of pharmacologic agents with potential to depress normal respiratory function (opioids, benzodiaze-pines)
- Altered level of consciousness
- Airway obstruction
- Procedure-related positioning
- Procedure-related pain

DESIRED OUTCOMES

The client will maintain effective respiratory function, as evidenced by:
a. Self-report of ability to breathe comfortably
b. Rate, depth, and of respirations within client's base-line range
c. Pulse oximetry, capnography, and/or ABG values within client's baseline range
d. Baseline mental status

NOC OUTCOMES

Respiratory status: airway patency; gas exchange; ventilation; postprocedure recovery

NIC INTERVENTIONS

Airway management; aspiration precautions; oxygen therapy; respiratory monitoring

NURSING ASSESSMENT	RATIONALE
Assess for anxiety.	*Early identification of anxiety, which may alter normal breathing patterns and indicate early respiratory distress, allows for appropriate intervention.*
Assess rate, depth, and effort of respirations every 5–15 minutes or more frequently as client condition warrants during and after the administration of sedation. Report signs and symptoms of ineffective respiratory function: • Tachypnea • Bradypnea • Apnea • Dyspnea • Restlessness • Diaphoresis • Irritability	*Early recognition of signs and symptoms of ineffective respiratory function allows for prompt intervention.*
Assess for signs of airway obstruction.	*Occlusion of the airway by the tongue can occur in an unconscious client. Loss of consciousness in a patient undergoing sedation is an untoward side effect and report to the physician immediately.*

*This diagnostic label includes the following nursing diagnoses: ineffective breathing pattern and impaired gas exchange.

NURSING ASSESSMENT	RATIONALE
Assess continuous pulse oximetry during the procedure and post procedure until client has returned to baseline status. Consider monitoring continuous capnography for deeper levels of sedation.	*Early recognition of low arterial oxygen saturation (SaO₂) values allows for prompt intervention. Pulse oximetry provides an indirect measure of oxygen saturation.* *An early marker of sedation-induced respiratory depression can be obtained using capnography, which measures exhaled carbon dioxide. Capnography monitoring is currently recommended for use during moderate and deep sedation.*
Assess ABG values as indicated.	*Allows for a more direct assessment of a client's oxygenation status, including carbon dioxide level, if warranted by clinical condition.*
Assess level of consciousness.	*To ensure the administered level of sedation does not compromise the client's level of consciousness, risking aspiration.*

THERAPEUTIC INTERVENTIONS	RATIONALE

Independent Actions

Implement measures to decrease fear and anxiety: • Assure client during the procedure.	*Fear and anxiety associated with the procedure may cause the client to breathe shallowly or hyperventilate. Decreasing anxiety may allow client to focus on breathing more slowly and regularly.*
If the procedure allows, position the client to maximize optimum ventilation: • Side-lying position	*A side-lying position will prevent the tongue from falling back and occluding the client's posterior pharynx.*
If the procedure allows, encourage the client to deep breathe periodically during the procedure.	*Periodic deep breathing allows for ventilation of carbon dioxide that may accumulate if the client's ventilations become too shallow.*
Post procedure, encourage the client to deep breathe at intervals to assist with recovery: Stir-up regimen" which consists of five post-procedure activities: 1. Deep breathing 2. Coughing 3. Positioning 4. Mobilization 5. Pain management	*After the conclusion of the procedure and conscious sedation, stimulating the patient to deep breathe at intervals assists in returning the patient to a more conscious state and enhances the elimination of carbon dioxide.*
Monitor for the recurrence of respiratory depression if narcotic/sedative reversal agents were administered.	*Extended monitoring of the client's respiratory status is necessary if reversal agents were administered, because the half-life of administered sedatives/opioids may outlast the effects of reversal agents.*
Monitor the effectiveness of ventilation. • Pulse oximetry • Capnography (as indicated) • ABGs (as indicated)	*Ongoing monitoring of continuous pulse oximetry, capnography, and/or ABGs allows for early identification of respiratory depression and prompt intervention to prevent hypoxemia.*
Implement appropriate safety measures • Keep suction setup available	*Suction should be readily available to clear airway of accumulated secretions, thereby preventing aspiration should the client not be able to do so independently.*

Dependent/Collaborative Actions

Administer supplemental oxygen as ordered. • Monitor the oxygen liter flow • Monitor position of oxygen delivery device • Periodically check oxygen delivery device to ensure prescribed concentration is being delivered.	*Administer supplemental oxygen as needed to keep SaO₂ >95% or within client's normal range. Administer oxygen with caution to clients with chronic obstructive pulmonary disease (COPD), because this action may take away their hypoxic stimulus to breathe.*
Implement measures to reverse apnea: • Ventilate the apneic client with an Ambu bag that delivers a fraction of inspired oxygen (FIO₂) of 100%. • Administer opioid/sedative reversal agents as ordered. • Naloxone (Narcan) • Flumazenil (Romazicon) • Prepare to assist with intubation/mechanical ventilation if apnea is not corrected.	*Apnea is an adverse effect of sedative/narcotic administration. While preparing to administer the appropriate reversal agents, the nurse should assist with proper ventilation of the client until spontaneous respiratory effort returns or the client is intubated.*
Notify the appropriate health care provider of continued signs and symptoms of ineffective respiratory function.	*Notifying the appropriate health care provider allows for modification of the treatment plan.*

Nursing Diagnosis | **RISK FOR INJURY** NDx

Definition: Susceptible to physical damage due to environmental conditions interacting with the individual's adaptive and defensive resources, which may compromise health.

CLINICAL MANIFESTATIONS

Subjective	**Objective**
Verbal self-report of auditory, visual, or sensory hallucinations	Changes in vital signs (e.g. blood pressure (BP), heart rate (HR), and/or respiratory rate (RR))

RISK FACTORS

- Procedural sedation
- Age

DESIRED OUTCOMES

The client will
- Maintain vital signs within normal range
- Remain free of injury

NOC OUTCOMES

Safe health care environment; vital signs

NIC INTERVENTIONS

Interventions: vital sign monitoring; environmental management: safety

NURSING ASSESSMENT	RATIONALE
Assess client's baseline vital signs before start of procedure: Vital signs: blood pressure, heart rate, respiratory rate, temperature, pulse oximetry Cardiac rhythm Pain level Cognitive orientation	*Assessment of client's baseline status provides comparison values by which to evaluate response to procedural sedation.*
Assess safety needs of patient based on level of cognitive and physical functions.	*Early identification of environmental factors that may contribute to injury in the sedated client allows for implementation of the appropriate safety precautions. Ensure appropriate emergency equipment is functioning properly and readily available in procedural area (e.g., oxygen, suction, defibrillator).*

THERAPEUTIC INTERVENTIONS	RATIONALE
Independent Actions Before procedure, ensure the availability of essential equipment for resuscitation: • Oxygen and delivery sources • Suction apparatus • Noninvasive blood pressure device • Electrocardiograph • Pulse oximeter • Opioid and sedative reversal agents • Naloxone (Narcan) • Flumazenil (Romazicon)	*In the event of an adverse reaction to pharmacologic agents used for conscious sedation or an adverse reaction to a procedure, the appropriate emergency equipment must be available and in proper working order.*
Modify environment to minimize hazards and risk of client injury. • Ensure proper positioning of the client during the procedure, to prevent injury: Maintain proper body alignment. Avoid pressure on bony prominences • Ensure the bed is locked and in the lowest possible position and appropriate protective devices are present to secure patient during the procedure: Side rails Safety straps	*If the procedure is done at the bedside, ensure the client's bed is in the locked and lowest possible position that does not interfere with the procedure. Side rails and safety straps may be necessary to secure the client, preventing injury.* *During a procedure requiring conscious sedation, a client's mobility may be limited.* *Maintaining proper body alignment and padding bony prominences will help to protect the client from injury.*

THERAPEUTIC INTERVENTIONS	RATIONALE
During and following the procedure, monitor client's response to procedural sedation: • Vital signs (i.e., BP, HR, RR) monitored every 5–15 minutes, or more frequency as condition warrants, for deviation from normal values for client • Cognitive orientation agents (sedatives/opioids; intravenous (IV) fluids)	*Evaluation of client's response to procedural sedation by comparison with baseline values allows for early identification of abnormal responses, and intervention and prevention of injury.*

Dependent/Collaborative Actions
Monitor the environment for changes in safety status.
• Alterations in cognition (obtunded level of consciousness; increased confusion/disorientation).

Ongoing collaborative monitoring during and immediately following procedural sedation will allow for prompt intervention preventing client harm.

Nursing Diagnosis **ACUTE PAIN** NDx

Definition: Unpleasant sensory and emotional experience associated with actual or potential tissue damage, or described in terms of such damage (International Association for the Study of Pain); sudden or slow onset of any intensity from mild to severe with an anticipated or predictable end, and with a duration of less than 3 months.

CLINICAL MANIFESTATIONS

Subjective	Objective
Verbal self-report of pain/discomfort	Crying; wincing; muscle tension or rigidity; diaphoresis; elevated blood pressure; increased heart rate; increased respiratory rate

RISK FACTORS
• Physical injury agents (e.g. medical/surgical procedure)

DESIRED OUTCOMES

The client will report pain to be relieved or controlled at a satisfactory level.

NOC OUTCOMES	NIC INTERVENTIONS
Pain level	Pain management: acute

NURSING ASSESSMENT	RATIONALE
Using standardized pain assessment scale, assess the client for signs and symptoms of pain frequently during the course of the procedure: • Verbalization of pain • Grimacing • Restlessness • Increased blood pressure • Tachycardia	*Early recognition of signs and symptoms of pain allows for prompt intervention.*

THERAPEUTIC INTERVENTIONS	RATIONALE
Independent Actions Implement measures to reduce fear and anxiety: • Assure client that a nurse will be present during the entire procedure to assess and ensure that adequate sedation and pain relief are provided.	*Fear and anxiety can decrease the client's threshold and tolerance for pain and thereby heighten the perception of pain.*

Continued...

THERAPEUTIC INTERVENTIONS	RATIONALE
Incorporate nonpharmacologic interventions as appropriate: • Position the patient for comfort as the procedure allows: • Pad bony prominences. **D** ✦ • Provide joint support as needed. **D** ✦	*Proper positioning of limbs and support of bony prominences may assist in alleviating pain associated with lying prolonged in one position during a procedure.*
Monitor sedation and respiratory status before administrating opioids.	*Cautiously administer opioids when administered in combination with sedatives to avoid respiratory depression.*
Dependent/Collaborative Actions Administer opioids as ordered.	*Opioids act mainly by altering the client's perception of pain and emotional response to the pain experience. It is important for the nurse to address pain needs because sedation alone will not relieve pain.*
Consult appropriate health care provider if aforementioned measures fail to provide adequate pain relief.	*Notifying the appropriate health care provider allows for modification of the treatment plan.*

Nursing Diagnosis   **RISK FOR ACUTE CONFUSION** NDx

Definition: Susceptible to reversible disturbances of consciousness, attention, cognition, and perception that develop over a short period of time, which may compromise health.

CLINICAL MANIFESTATIONS

Subjective Verbal self-report of hallucinations	**Objective** Fluctuation in consciousness; level of consciousness; increased agitation; increased restlessness; exaggerated emotional responses

RISK FACTORS

• Pain
• Pharmaceutic agent
• Invasive procedure

DESIRED OUTCOMES

The client will not exhibit signs and symptoms of acute confusion, as evidenced by:
a. Orientation to person, place, and time
b. Return to baseline cognition

NOC OUTCOMES	NIC INTERVENTIONS
Cognitive orientation	Delirium management

NURSING ASSESSMENT	RATIONALE
Assess the client for signs and symptoms of acute confusion: • Fluctuations in consciousness • Hallucinations • Increased agitation • Increased restlessness	*Early recognition of signs and symptoms of acute confusion allows for prompt intervention.*
Assess for and report possible physiologic alterations: • Hypoglycemia • Hypoxia • Hypotension • Adverse effects of medications	*Acute confusion is a clinical manifestation of a variety of physiologic alterations. To reduce the risk of injury/untoward outcomes, it is critical that any physiologic alteration is ruled out as a contributing factor. Prompt attention to these physiologic factors may shorten the duration of the confusion.*

THERAPEUTIC INTERVENTIONS	RATIONALE
Independent Actions Reorient the patient as indicated: • Address the client by a familiar name. **D** ✦	*Use of reality orientation can help to improve the cognition of a client.*

THERAPEUTIC INTERVENTIONS	RATIONALE
Communicate clearly and provide simple explanations to the client. **D** ✦	*Simple explanations are more readily understood by a confused client.*
Provide the patient with ongoing information and reassurance as needed. **D** ✦	*Actions may help to reduce the frustration/anxiety that may accompany confusion.*
Maintain a hazard-free environment:	*A confused client is at risk for injury.*
• Keep side rails up. **D** ✦	*Protective measures help to ensure risk reduction. These measures should be continued until return of the client's baseline cognition.*
• Provide constant surveillance. **D** ✦	
Dependent/Collaborative Actions	
Administer medications for anxiety/agitation as ordered.	*Confusion may be treated with medications.*
	The client must be monitored for side effects of these medications.
Use soft physical restraints as needed only if client is at an increased risk for injury and if all other interventions fail to correct confusion.	*A confused client is at risk for injury.*
	Protective measures help to ensure risk reduction. These measures should be continued until return of the client's baseline cognition.

ADDITIONAL CARE PLANS

RISK FOR ASPIRATION
Related to medication administration altering normal level of consciousness

ANXIETY
Related to stressors (unfamiliar environment; procedure)

PREOPERATIVE CARE

The preoperative phase begins when the client decides to have surgery and ends when the client enters the operating room area. Although surgical procedures are performed in a variety of settings (e.g., hospitals, day surgery centers, physicians' offices), basic preoperative client care is similar. The goals of preoperative care are to prepare the client physically and psychologically for the surgery and the postoperative period. Thorough preoperative preparation reduces the client's postoperative fear and anxiety and the risk of postoperative complications. To individualize this care plan, the client's psychological and physiologic status, the surgical setting, the length of time before the surgical procedure, the type of anesthesia to be used, and the planned surgical procedure must be considered.

This care plan focuses on the adult client who is scheduled for a surgical procedure. It should be used in conjunction with each surgical care plan.

PREOPERATIVE GOALS

The client will:
- Share thoughts and feelings about the impending surgery and its anticipated effects
- Verbalize an understanding of the surgical procedure, preoperative care, and postoperative sensations and care
- Demonstrate the ability to perform activities designed to prevent postoperative complications
- Adhere to preoperative instructions as validated in the preoperative care area on the day of surgery.

Nursing Diagnosis **FEAR** NDx/**ANXIETY** NDx

Definition: Fear: Response to perceived threat that is consciously recognized as a danger; **Anxiety:** Vague, uneasy feeling of discomfort or dread accompanied by an autonomic response (the source is often nonspecific or unknown to the individual); a feeling of apprehension caused by anticipation of danger. It is an alerting sign that warns of impending danger and enables the individual to take measures to deal with that threat.

CLINICAL MANIFESTATIONS

Subjective	Objective
Verbal self-report expressing concern due to surgical procedure; scared, rattled, distressed; apprehensive; fearful; sense of impending doom; fear of consequences	Preoccupation; impaired attention; difficulty concentrating; forgetfulness; increased pulse; increased blood pressure; increased respiratory rate, trembling hands/facial tension

NDx = NANDA Diagnosis **D** = Delegatable Action ● = UAP ✦ = LVN/LPN ⊝▶ = Go to ⊝volve for animation

RISK FACTORS

- Unfamiliar setting
- Separation from support system
- Learned response to threat
- Stressors related to surgical procedure and findings
- Threat of death

DESIRED OUTCOMES

The client will experience a reduction in fear and anxiety, as evidenced by:
a. Verbalization of feeling less anxious
b. Usual sleep pattern
c. Relaxed facial expression and body movements
d. Stable vital signs
e. Usual perceptual ability and interactions with others

NOC OUTCOMES

Anxiety level; anxiety self-control; fear level; fear self-control

NIC INTERVENTIONS

Anxiety reduction; calming technique; relaxation therapy

NURSING ASSESSMENT	RATIONALE
Assess client for signs and symptoms of fear and anxiety: • Verbalization of feeling anxious • Insomnia • Tenseness • Shakiness • Restlessness • Diaphoresis • Tachycardia • Elevated blood pressure • Self-focused behaviors	*Early recognition of signs and symptoms of anxiety allows for prompt intervention.*
Gather the following assessment data from the client during the preoperative period: • Level of understanding of planned surgical procedure • Perceptions about the surgery and its anticipated results • Significance of the surgical procedure and hospitalization • Previous surgical and hospital experiences • Availability of adequate support systems • Arrangements made for responsibilities such as job, child care, meal preparation, and home maintenance if needed during the recovery period	*Assessment of the client's baseline knowledge and understanding of the procedure allows for the nurse to formulate individualized preoperative teaching.* *Identification of available support systems assists with the discharge planning process.*

THERAPEUTIC INTERVENTIONS	RATIONALE
Independent Actions Implement measures to reduce fear and anxiety: • Orient client to environment, equipment, and routines. **D ● ✦**	*Familiarity with the environment and routines reduces the client's anxiety about the unknown, provides a sense of security, and increases the client's sense of control, all of which help to reduce anxiety.*
• Introduce client to staff who will be participating in care; if possible, maintain consistency in staff assigned to client's care.	*Introduction of staff familiarizes the client with those individuals who will be working with him/her, which provides a sense of comfort with the environment. Consistency in staff assignment provides the client with a feeling of stability, which reduces anxiety associated with change.*
• Assure client that staff members are nearby; respond to call signal as soon as possible. **D ● ✦**	*Close contact and a prompt response to requests provide a sense of security and facilitate the development of trust, reducing the client's anxiety.*

• Maintain a calm, supportive, confident manner when interacting with client:
  • Provide a calm, restful environment.
  • Instruct client in relaxation techniques and encourage participation in diversional activities.
	A sense of calmness and confidence conveys to the client that someone is in control of the situation, which helps reduce anxiety.

• Encourage verbalization of fear and anxiety; provide feedback: • Assist client to identify specific stressors and ways to cope with them.	*Verbalization of fears, feelings, and concerns helps the client identify factors that are causing anxiety.*

THERAPEUTIC INTERVENTIONS	RATIONALE

• Reinforce physician's explanations and clarify misconceptions the client has about the surgical procedure, including purpose, size and location of incision, and anticipated outcome:
  • Explain all pre-surgical diagnostic tests.
  • Provide information about preoperative routines and anticipated postoperative care.
  • Provide information based on current needs of the client at a level that the client can understand; encourage questions and clarification of information provided.
  • Assure client that blood is screened carefully and that the risk for contracting blood-borne disease is minimal.
	Factual information and an awareness of what to expect help to decrease the anxiety that arises from uncertainty.

• Perform actions to help client maintain a sense of dignity:
  • Provide privacy when appropriate.
  • Avoid unnecessary body exposure during preoperative procedures.
  • Allow client to wear dentures, glasses, wig, etc. into the operating room suite if possible.
	Increasing a client's sense of control regarding his/her body can help the client to maintain a sense of dignity, which can reduce anxiety.

• Orient client to measures implemented to ensure safety in the surgical setting:
  • Instruct client that they will be involved in marking the surgical site—at minimum when there is more than one possible location for the procedure and when performing the procedure in a different location could harm the patient (e.g., aterality [left/right]; spinal procedures)
  • Instruct client that before the start of any invasive medical procedure, a time-out is taken by the operating room staff to confirm the correct client, procedure, and site
  • Instruct client that it is OK to ask questions if there is reason for concern
	National patient safety goal requirements issued by The Joint Commission require the implementation of safety measures designed to reduce surgical errors.
	
	The "Speak Up" Universal Protocol for Preventing Wrong Site, Wrong Procedure, and Wrong Person Surgery published by The Joint Commission outlines processes including preprocedure verification, marking of the surgical and performance of a "time-out" to help prevent errors and patient harm.

• Assure client that pain relief needs will be met postoperatively.	*Fear and anxiety can decrease the client's threshold for pain and heighten a client's perception of pain. Anxiety can be reduced if the client is assured that pain needs will be met after surgery.*
• Encourage significant others to project a caring, concerned attitude without obvious anxiousness. • Include significant others in orientation and teaching sessions and encourage their continued support of client.	*Anxiety is easily transferable from one person to another. If significant others covey empathy, provide reassurance, and do not appear anxious, they can help reduce a client's anxiety. In addition, significant others can help to reduce anxiety by reinforcing information that the client has difficulty understanding or recalling.*

• Enable client to maintain a sense of control by:
  • Including client in planning of preoperative care and allowing choices whenever possible
  • Explaining that the purpose of the written consent form is to indicate voluntary and informed consent and to protect against unsanctioned surgery
  • Discussing the purpose and benefits of an advanced directive for health care and providing assistance as needed to complete the necessary documents
	Enabling the client to make health care decisions can enhance feelings of autonomy and decrease anxiety.

• When appropriate, assist client to meet spiritual needs • Arrange for a visit from clergy.	*Spiritual support is a source of comfort and security for many people and can help reduce a client's anxiety.*

Dependent/Collaborative Actions

Implement measures to reduce fear and anxiety:

• Initiate a social service referral if indicated	*Concerns about factors such as finances, follow-up medical care, and home maintenance can be a source of great anxiety.* *Facilitating contact with the appropriate resources can help reduce the client's anxiety and provide ongoing support.*

Continued...

THERAPEUTIC INTERVENTIONS	RATIONALE
• Administer prescribed antianxiety agents if indicated.	*Medications are sometimes prescribed to help reduce the client's anxiety. Benzodiazepines (e.g., lorazepam, diazepam, alprazolam, chlordiazepoxide) are the drugs of choice for managing short-term anxiety.*
Consult appropriate health care provider (e.g., psychiatric nurse clinician, physician) if aforementioned actions fail to control fear and anxiety.	*Notifying the appropriate health care provider can allow for modification of the treatment plan.*

CLIENT TEACHING

Nursing Diagnosis **DEFICIENT KNOWLEDGE** NDx

Definition: Absence of cognitive information related to a specific topic, or its acquisition.

CLINICAL MANIFESTATIONS

Subjective	Objective
• Verbal self-report of lack of knowledge related to surgical process/procedures.	• Inaccurate follow-through of instruction; inaccurate performance of test; inappropriate behaviors (e.g., hysterical, hostile, agitated, apathetic); insufficient knowledge

RISK FACTORS

- Alteration in cognitive functioning
- Alteration in memory
- Lack of understanding regarding the surgical procedure

NOC OUTCOMES	NIC INTERVENTIONS
Knowledge: diagnostic and therapeutic procedures; treatment procedures; treatment regimen	Health literacy enhancement; teaching: individual; teaching preoperative

NURSING ASSESSMENT	RATIONALE
Assess client's cognitive, psychomotor, and affective abilities or disabilities.	*Identification of client limitations will allow for modification of the teaching plan and determine the need for family caregiver presence during education sessions.*
Assess client's previous experiences with surgery, background, culture, and current level of knowledge related to surgical procedure.	*Identifying the client's baseline knowledge level will allow for the development of the appropriate, patient-centered teaching plan.*
Assess the client's baseline literacy level through formal or informal assessments.	*A client's health literacy level should be assessed before providing instruction so the appropriate teaching plan can be developed.*
	Unless the nurse considers the client's intellectual abilities when developing the teaching plan, teaching will be unsuccessful.
Assess client's learning needs and preferred learning style.	*Identification of specific client learning needs and preferred learning styles allows for development of an individualized teaching plan using methods appropriate for the identified learning style.*

THERAPEUTIC INTERVENTIONS	RATIONALE

Desired Outcomes: The client will demonstrate:
a. An understanding of the surgical procedure, preoperative care, and postoperative sensations and care
b. The ability to perform activities designed to prevent post-operative complications

THERAPEUTIC INTERVENTIONS	**RATIONALE**

Independent Actions

Provide information about usual preoperative routines for the surgery to be performed, such as preoperative testing, including but not limited to blood work, electrocardiogram [ECG], urinalysis, chest radiograph, insertion of urinary catheter and/or nasogastric tube, bowel and skin preparation, and removal of prosthetic devices.

Providing information about procedures enhances knowledge and decreases anxiety because clients have a better understanding of what to expect during a procedure.

Provide information about:

- Scheduled time and estimated length of surgery
- Food and fluid restrictions before surgery
- Preoperative medications and planned anesthesia
- Body position during surgical procedure
- Purpose for and estimated length of stay in preoperative holding area and postanesthesia care unit (PACU)
- Sensations that can occur after surgery such as dryness of mouth, sore throat after endotracheal intubation, and pain at surgical site

Provides client a sense of control and time to ask questions concerning procedure or postoperative experience.

Inform client of the anticipated postoperative care:

- Equipment such as dressings, intravenous lines, drainage tubes, traction devices, antiembolism stockings, and intermittent pneumatic compression device
- Activity limitations and expectations
- Dietary modifications
- Treatments, such as respiratory care, circulatory management, and wound care, and the expected frequency
- Assessments, such as intake and output, lung sounds, vital signs, neurologic checks, and bowel sounds, and the expected frequency
- Medications such as antiemetics, analgesics, and antimicrobials
- Pain management measures such as oral, parenteral, and/or intravenous medications; epidural analgesia; patient controlled analgesia [(PCA)]; positioning; and relaxation techniques

Allows client time to ask questions and to identify areas of concern.

Provide instructions about activities the client will be expected to perform postoperatively, allowing time for return demonstration. These may include:

- Techniques for splinting incision, coughing, and deep breathing techniques
- Correct use of incentive spirometer (IS)
- Active foot and leg exercises
- Correct methods for moving in bed, getting out of bed, early ambulation

Return demonstration provides the nurse a better understanding of clients' skills and where more teaching is necessary.

Allow time for questions and clarification.

Allowing time for questions and clarification allows the nurse to evaluate the effectiveness of teaching and make the appropriate adjustments to the teaching plan.

Reinforce information provided by the anesthesiologist and surgeon about the surgery.

Reinforcing important information allows the nurse to both summarize key concepts and further assess the client's understanding of instructions.

⊖▶ POSTOPERATIVE CARE

The postoperative phase begins when the client is transferred from surgery to a postanesthesia care unit (PACU). and ends with discharge from the hospital. The length of the postoperative phase varies depending on factors such as the client's age and preoperative health status, the type of anesthesia used, the length and type of surgery, and the client's physiologic and psychological responses postoperatively.

This care plan focuses on postoperative care of an adult client who has received general anesthesia and has been transferred from the recovery area to the clinical care unit. Much of the information is applicable to clients having surgery in an outpatient setting (e.g., physician's office, surgical care center) and to those receiving follow-up care in an extended care facility or home setting.

NDx = NANDA Diagnosis   **D** = Delegatable Action   ● = UAP   ✦ = LVN/LPN   ⊖▶ = Go to ⊖volve for animation

This care plan should be used in conjunction with all surgical care plans.

OUTCOME/DISCHARGE CRITERIA

The client will:
1. Tolerate prescribed diet
2. Tolerate expected level of activity
3. Have adequate surgical pain controlled
4. Have clear, audible breath sounds throughout lungs
5. Have evidence of normal wound healing.
6. Have no signs and symptoms of infection or postoperative complications.
7. Identify ways to prevent postoperative infection.
8. Demonstrate ability to perform wound care.
9. State signs and symptoms to report to health care provider.
10. Share thoughts and feelings about the surgery, diagnosis, prognosis, and treatment plan.
11. Develop a plan for adhering to the recommended follow-up care including future appointments with health care provider, dietary modifications, activity level, treatments, and medications prescribed.

Nursing Diagnosis   INEFFECTIVE BREATHING PATTERN NDx

Definition: Inspiration and/or expiration that does not provide adequate ventilation.

CLINICAL MANIFESTATIONS

Subjective	Objective
Verbal self-report of dyspnea/difficulty breathing	Alterations in depth of breathing; altered chest excursion; bradypnea; decreased minute ventilation; use of accessory muscles to breathe, nasal flaring, orthopnea, tachypnea

RISK FACTORS

- Increased rate of respirations associated with fear and anxiety
- Decreased rate and depth of respirations associated with the depressant effect of anesthesia and some medications (e.g., opioid, analgesics, some antiemetics)
- Reluctance to breathe deeply because of pain, fear, anxiety, weakness, and fatigue
- Restricted chest expansion resulting from positioning and elevation of the diaphragm if abdominal distention is present

DESIRED OUTCOMES

The client will maintain an effective breathing pattern, as evidenced by:
a. A normal rate and depth of respirations
b. Absence of dyspnea

NOC OUTCOMES

Respiratory status

NIC INTERVENTIONS

Ventilation assistance

NURSING ASSESSMENT	RATIONALE
Assess for signs and symptoms of an ineffective breathing pattern:	*Early recognition of signs and symptoms of an ineffective breathing pattern allows for prompt intervention.*
• Auscultate breath sounds, noting decreased or absent ventilation/presence of adventitious breath sounds	
• Tachypnea, dyspnea, bradypnea	
• Limited chest excursion	
• Use of accessory muscles when breathing	
⊖▶ Assess/monitor pulse oximetry (SaO_2) and ABGs as indicated.	*Monitoring continuous SaO_2 readings allows for the early detection of hypoxia. Assessment of ABGs allows for a more direct measurement of both the partial pressure of oxygen in arterial blood (PaO_2) and the partial pressure of carbon dioxide in arterial blood ($PaCO_2$), which reflect the adequacy of ventilation.*

THERAPEUTIC INTERVENTIONS	RATIONALE

Independent Actions

Implement measures to improve breathing pattern: **D** ● ✦
- Perform actions to reduce fear and anxiety:
  - Promote a calm, restful environment.
- Perform actions to reduce pain: **D** ✦
  - Reposition client for comfort
  - Instruct client to support incision when moving or coughing.
- Perform actions to reduce the accumulation of gas and fluid in the gastrointestinal tract: **D** ✦
  - Maintain patency of nasogastric, gastric, or intestinal tubes if present.
- Perform actions to increase strength and improve activity tolerance:
  - Implement measures to conserve energy (e.g., organize care to allow for periods of rest; decrease noise).
- Have client deep breathe using incentive spirometry (IS) every 1–2 hrs. **D** ✦
- Instruct client to breathe slowly if hyperventilating.

- Place client in a semi- to high-Fowler's position unless contraindicated. **D** ●
- If client must remain flat in bed, assist with position change at least every 2 hrs. **D** ●

Reducing fear and anxiety helps to prevent shallow and/or rapid breathing.

Reducing pain helps to increase the client's willingness to move and breathe more deeply.

Reducing the accumulation of gas in the gastrointestinal tract decreases pressure on the diaphragm, facilitating more effective ventilation.

Increasing activity tolerance enables the client to breathe more deeply and participate in activities to improve breathing pattern.

Use of an incentive spirometry (IS) promotes maximal inhalation and lung expansion.

Hyperventilation is an ineffective breathing pattern that can lead to respiratory alkalosis. A client can often slow breathing rate by concentrating on doing so.

A semi- to high-Fowler's position allows for maximal diaphragmatic excursion and lung expansion.

Compression of the thorax and subsequent limited chest wall expansion occur when the client lies in one position. Frequent repositioning promotes maximal chest wall and lung expansion.

Dependent/Collaborative Actions

Implement measures to improve breathing pattern:
- Increase activity as allowed and tolerated, ambulating three to four times per day as appropriate. **D** ● ✦
- Assist with positive airway pressure techniques if ordered.
  - Continuous positive airway pressure (CPAP)
  - Bilevel positive airway pressure (BiPAP)
  - Flutter/positive expiratory pressure ([PEP] device)
- Administer central nervous system depressants judiciously.
- Hold medication and consult physician if respiratory rate is less than 12/min.
- Perform actions to reduce pain:
  - Administer analgesics before activities and procedures that can cause pain and before pain becomes severe. **D** ✦
  - Consider nonpharmacologic interventions as appropriate to client condition (e.g., guided imagery, music therapy).

Consult appropriate health care provider if:
- Ineffective breathing pattern continues.
- Client develops signs and symptoms of impaired gas exchange such as restlessness, irritability, confusion, significant decrease in oximetry results, decreased PaO_2, and increased $PaCO_2$ levels.

During activity, especially ambulation, the client usually takes deeper breaths, thus increasing lung expansion.

Positive airway pressure techniques increase intrapulmonary alveolar pressure, which helps to reexpand collapsed alveoli and prevent further alveoli collapse.

Central nervous system depressants cause depression of the respiratory center in the brainstem, which can result in a decreased rate and depth of respiration.

Reducing pain helps to increase the client's willingness to move and breathe more deeply.

Notifying the appropriate health care provider allows for modification of treatment plan.

NDx = NANDA Diagnosis   **D** = Delegatable Action   ● = UAP   ✦ = LVN/LPN   ⊜▶ = Go to ⊜volve for animation

Nursing Diagnosis INEFFECTIVE AIRWAY CLEARANCE NDx

Definition: Inability to clear secretions or obstructions from the respiratory tract to maintain a clear airway.

CLINICAL MANIFESTATIONS

Subjective	Objective
Verbal self-report of dyspnea/difficulty breathing	Dyspnea, orthopnea; diminished breath sounds; adventitious breath sounds (e.g. crackles, rhonchi, wheezes); cough, ineffective or absent sputum production; difficulty vocalizing; wide eyed; restlessness; changes in respiratory rate and rhythm; cyanosis

RISK FACTORS

- Occlusion of the pharynx in the immediate postoperative period associated with relaxation of the tongue, resulting from the effects of anesthesia and some medications (e.g., narcotic [opioid] analgesics)
- Stasis of secretions associated with (1) decreased activity, (2) depressed ciliary function resulting from the effects of anesthesia, and (3) difficulty coughing up secretions resulting from the depressant effects of anesthesia and some medications (e.g., [opioid] analgesics, some antiemetics), pain, weakness, fatigue, and the presence of tenacious secretions can occur as a result of deficient fluid volume
- Increased secretions associated with irritation of the respiratory tract (can result from inhalation anesthetics and endotracheal intubation)

DESIRED OUTCOMES

The client will maintain clear, open airways, as evidenced by:
a. Normal breath sounds
b. Normal rate and depth of respirations
c. Absence of dyspnea

NOC OUTCOMES

Respiratory status: airway patency

NIC INTERVENTIONS

Airway management; cough enhancement; respiratory monitoring;

NURSING ASSESSMENT	RATIONALE
Assess for signs and symptoms of ineffective airway clearance: • Abnormal breath sounds • Rapid, shallow respirations • Dyspnea • Cough	*Early recognition of signs and symptoms of an ineffective airway clearance allows for prompt intervention.*
Assess/monitor pulse oximetry (SaO$_2$) and ABGs as indicated.	*Monitoring continuous SaO$_2$ readings allows for the early detection of hypoxia. Assessment of ABGs allows for a more direct measurement of both PaO$_2$ and PaCO$_2$, which reflect the adequacy of ventilation.*

THERAPEUTIC INTERVENTIONS	RATIONALE

Independent Actions
Implement measures to promote effective airway clearance:

- Position client on side and/or insert an artificial airway if necessary.

  An artificial airway helps prevent obstruction of airway by tongue.

- Perform actions to reduce pain:
- Reposition client for comfort. **D** ✦ ●

  Reducing pain helps to increase the client's willingness to move and breathe more deeply.

- Instruct client to support incision when moving or coughing. **D** ✦

THERAPEUTIC INTERVENTIONS	RATIONALE
• Instruct and assist client to change position at least every 2 hrs while in bed. **D** ● ✦	*Repositioning helps mobilize secretions.*
• Perform actions to promote the removal of secretions:	*Deep breathing can help loosen secretions and enhance the effectiveness of coughing.*
• Instruct and assist client to deep breathe and cough every 1–2 hrs **D** ✦	
• Assist client in using a pillow or rolled blanket as a splint against incision when coughing. **D** ✦	
• Assist with IS. **D** ✦	
• Discourage smoking.	*Irritants in smoke increase mucus production, impair ciliary function, and can cause inflammation and damage to the bronchial walls.*
• Perform suctioning if needed. **D** ✦	*Suctioning removes secretions from the large airways. It also stimulates coughing, which helps to clear airways of mucus and foreign matter.*

Dependent/Collaborative Actions

Implement measures to promote effective airway clearance:	
• Implement measures to thin tenacious secretions and reduce drying of the respiratory mucous membrane:	*Adequate hydration and humidified inspired air help thin secretions, which facilitates the mobilization and expectoration of secretions.*
• Maintain a fluid intake of at least 2500 mL/day unless contraindicated	*These actions also reduce dryness of the respiratory mucous membrane, which helps enhance mucociliary clearance.*
• Humidify inspired air as ordered. **D** ✦	
• Assist with administration of mucolytics and diluent or hydrating agents via nebulizer if ordered:	*Mucolytics and diluents or hydrating agents are mucokinetic substances that reduce the viscosity of mucus, thus making it easier for the client to mobilize and clear secretions from the respiratory tract.*
• Acetylcysteine	
• Water, saline	
• Assist with administration of bronchodilators as appropriate.	*Bronchodilators are substances that dilate airways facilitating air exchange.*
• Increase activity as allowed and tolerated. **D** ● ✦	*Activity helps to mobilize secretions and promotes deeper breathing.*
• Administer central nervous system depressants judiciously.	*Central nervous system depressants depress the cough reflex, which can result in stasis of secretions.*
Consult appropriate health care provider such as a physician or respiratory therapist if:	*Notifying the appropriate health care provider allows for modification of the treatment plan.*
• Signs and symptoms of ineffective airway clearance persist	
• Signs and symptoms of impaired gas exchange are present:	
• Restlessness	
• Irritability	
• Confusion	
• Significant decrease in oximetry results	
• Decreased PaO_2 and increased $PaCO_2$	

Nursing Diagnosis **ACUTE PAIN** NDx

Definition: Unpleasant sensory and emotional experience associated with actual or potential tissue damage, or described in terms of such damage (International Association for the Study of Pain); sudden or slow onset of any intensity from mild to severe with an anticipated or predictable end, and with a duration of less than 3 months.

CLINICAL MANIFESTATIONS

Subjective	**Objective**
Verbal self-report of pain in the cognitively aware patient can be rated using a standardized pain intensity scale (e.g., 0–10)	Facial expression of pain; guarding behavior; inability to take a deep breath (e.g., splinting), guarding, elevated blood pressure, elevated pulse rate, diaphoresis, increase in the rate and depth of breathing

RISK FACTORS

- Tissue trauma and reflex muscle spasms associated with the surgery
- Irritation from drainage tubes
- Stress on surgical area associated with deep breathing, coughing, and/or movement

DESIRED OUTCOMES

The client will experience diminished pain, as evidenced by:
a. Verbalization of a decrease or absence of pain
b. Relaxed facial expression and body positioning
c. Increased participation in activities
d. Stable vital signs

NOC OUTCOMES

Pain control; pain: disruptive effects; pain level

NIC INTERVENTIONS

Pain management: acute; analgesic administration

NURSING ASSESSMENT

Assess for signs and symptoms of acute pain, including non-verbal cues in clients unable to communicate:
- Verbalization of pain
- Grimacing
- Reluctance to move
- Restlessness
- Diaphoresis
- Increased B/P
- Tachycardia

Assess client's perception of the severity of pain using a pain intensity rating scale. Assessment to include:
- Location
- Quality
- Onset
- Duration
- Precipitation factors
- Aggravating factors
- Alleviating factors

RATIONALE

Early recognition of signs and symptoms of pain allows for prompt intervention.

An awareness of the severity of pain being experienced helps to determine the most appropriate interventions for pain management. Use of a pain intensity rating scale gives the nurse a clearer understanding of the pain being experienced and promotes consistency with others about the client's pain experience.

THERAPEUTIC INTERVENTIONS

Independent Actions

Implement measures to reduce pain:
- Perform actions to reduce fear and anxiety about the pain experience:
    - Assure client that the need for pain relief is understood
    - Plan methods for achieving pain control with client.
- Perform actions to promote rest:
    - Minimize environmental activity and noise. **D** ●
- Provide or assist with nonpharmacologic methods for pain relief: **D** ● ✦
    - Massage
    - Position change
    - Progressive relaxation exercises
    - Restful environment
    - Diversional activities such as watching television, reading, or conversing

- Instruct and assist client to support abdominal or chest incision with a pillow or hands when turning, coughing, and deep breathing. **D** ✦
- If an abdominal incision is present, instruct the client to bend knees while coughing and deep breathing. **D** ✦

Monitor pain using a valid and reliable rating tool appropriate for age and ability to communicate.

RATIONALE

Fear and anxiety can decrease the client's threshold and tolerance for pain and thereby heighten the perception of pain. In addition, pain management methods are not as effective if the client is tense and unable to relax.

Promoting rest helps to reduce fatigue and subsequently increase the client's threshold and tolerance for pain.

Nonpharmacologic pain management includes a variety of interventions. It is believed that most of these are effective because they stimulate closure of the gating mechanism in the spinal cord and subsequently block the transmission of pain impulses. In addition, some interventions are thought to stimulate the release of endorphins that inhibit the transmission of nerve impulses and/or alter the client's perception of pain. Many of the nonpharmacologic interventions also help to decrease pain by promoting relaxation.

The action of "splinting" an incision or providing support to the incision when turning, coughing, and deep breathing helps to provide support and reduce tension on the incision.

Bending the knees while coughing and deep breathing helps to reduce tension on abdominal muscles and incisions.

Quantifies pain level for evaluating response to therapy.

Ensures client safety

THERAPEUTIC INTERVENTIONS	RATIONALE
Monitor sedation and respiratory status before administration of opioids and at regular intervals when opioids are administered.	

Dependent/Collaborative Actions

Implement measures to reduce pain:

- Use combination/multimodal analgesics for severe pain **D** ✦

- Opioid analgesics

- Nonopioid analgesics such as acetaminophen and salicylates and other nonsteroidal antiinflammatory agents (NSAIDs)

- Local anesthetics (e.g., bupivacaine, etidocaine)

- Muscle relaxants

- Encourage client to use PCA device as instructed

- Maintain integrity of analgesia delivery system:
  - Epidural
  - Intravenous
  - Subcutaneous
  - Transdermal

- Administer analgesics before activities and procedures that can cause pain and before pain becomes severe. **D** ✦

Consult appropriate health care provider if aforementioned measures fail to provide adequate pain relief:

- Physician

- Pharmacist

- Pain management specialist

Pharmacologic therapy is an effective method of reducing or relieving pain. All medications reduce pain by a variety of pharmacologic effects.

Better understanding of the pain management treatment approach can help to improve control of pain.

Maintaining integrity of the delivery system ensures client receives full benefit of the prescribed medication.

The administration of analgesics before a pain-producing event helps to minimize the pain that will be experienced. Analgesics are also more effective if given before pain becomes severe because mild to moderate pain is controlled more quickly and effectively than severe pain.

Notifying the appropriate health care provider allows for modification of the treatment plan.

Nursing Diagnosis **RISK FOR VENOUS THROMBOEMBOLISM** NDx

Definition: Susceptible to the development of a blood clot in a deep vein, commonly in the thigh, calf, or upper extremity, which can break off and lodge in another vessel, which may compromise health.

CLINICAL MANIFESTATIONS

Subjective	Objective
Verbal self-report of pain or tenderness in an extremity	Increase in circumference of extremity; distention of superficial vessels in extremity; unusual warmth of extremity; positive Homans sign (Note: not always a reliable indicator)

RISK FACTORS

- Venous stasis associated with decreased activity, positioning during and after surgery, increased blood viscosity
- Hypercoagulability associated with increased release of tissue thromboplastin into the blood
- Obesity
- Impaired mobility
- Trauma to vein walls during surgery

DESIRED OUTCOMES

The client will not develop a deep vein thrombus, as evidenced by:

a. Absence of pain, tenderness, swelling, and distended superficial vessels in extremities

b. Usual temperature of extremities

NDx = NANDA Diagnosis   **D** = Delegatable Action   ● = UAP   ✦ = LVN/LPN   ⊙▶ = Go to ⊖volve for animation

NOC OUTCOMES	NIC INTERVENTIONS
Tissue perfusion: peripheral	Embolus precautions; embolus care: peripheral

NURSING ASSESSMENT	RATIONALE
Assess for and report signs and symptoms of a deep vein thrombus: • Pain or tenderness in extremity • Increase in circumference of extremity • Distention of superficial vessels in extremity • Unusual warmth of extremity	*Early recognition of signs and symptoms of venous thromboembolism allows for prompt intervention.*

THERAPEUTIC INTERVENTIONS	RATIONALE

Independent Actions

Implement measures to prevent embolus formation: **D** ✦
* Perform actions to prevent peripheral pooling of blood such as leg exercises:
  * Ankle rotation
  * Alternate dorsiflexion and plantar extension of feet and legs at least 10 times every hour
  * Passive or active range of motion
  * Change position every 2 hrs
  * Encourage early mobilization/ambulate as tolerated

Leg and ankle exercises help promote venous return and reduce the risk of venous thromboembolism.

If signs and symptoms of a deep vein thromboembolism occur: **D** ✦
* Maintain client on bed rest until activity orders received.
* Elevate foot of bed 20 degrees or greater above heart level.
* Discourage positions that compromise blood flow (e.g., pillows under knees, crossing legs, sitting for long periods).

Avoid putting pressure on the posterior knees because this action will compress leg veins, increasing turbulent blood flow, and increase the risk of venous thromboembolism formation. If a thrombus is suspected, elevate the affected extremity and do not massage the area because of the danger of dislodging the thrombus.

Dependent/Collaborative Actions

Implement measures to prevent thrombus formation:
* Apply mechanical devices designed to increase venous return in the immobile patient: **D** ✦
  * Intermittent pneumatic compression device stockings
  * Graduated elastic compression stockings or sleeves
* Maintain a minimum fluid intake of 2500 mL/day (unless contraindicated). **D** ✦
* Administer prophylactic low dose anticoagulants or antiplatelet medications:
  * Low- or adjusted-dose heparin
  * Fondaparinux
  * Warfarin
  * Dextran
  * Low-molecular-weight heparin **D** ✦

These devices decrease venous stasis in the lower extremities and increase venous return through the deep leg veins, which are prone to the formation of a venous thromboembolism. These devices should remain in place until the patient is ambulatory.
Adequate hydration helps to reduce blood viscosity, which may contribute to the formation of a thromboembolism.
Anticoagulants, if indicated, help to suppress the formation of clots.

If signs and symptoms of a venous thromboembolism occur:
* Prepare client for diagnostic studies (e.g., venography, duplex ultrasound, impedance plethysmography, D dimer for pulmonary embolism [PE]).

Additional studies may be indicated to confirm the presence of a thromboembolism so the appropriate interventions can be implemented.

Nursing Diagnosis **RISK FOR IMBALANCED FLUID VOLUME** NDx **AND RISK FOR ELECTROLYTE IMBALANCE** NDx

Definition: Risk for Imbalanced Fluid Volume NDx: Susceptible to a decrease, increase, or rapid shift from one to the other of intravascular, interstitial, and/or intracellular fluid, which may compromise health. This refers to body fluid loss, gain, or both.
Risk for Electrolye Imbalance NDx: Susceptible to changes in serum electrolyte levels, which may compromise health.

CLINICAL MANIFESTATIONS

Subjective	Objective
Decreased fluid volume: verbal self-report of increased thirst; headaches; muscle cramps **Increased fluid volume:** verbal self-report of swelling; nausea, shortness of breath **Electrolyte loss:** verbal self-report of muscle cramps; nausea; palpitations; paresthesia; dizziness	**Decreased fluid volume:** restlessness; weakness; postural hypotension; inability to concentrate; tachycardia; decreased urine output **Increased fluid volume:** adventitious breath sounds, blood pressure changes, oliguria, S_3 heart sound, changes in mental status, distended neck veins **Electrolyte loss:** confusion, altered mental status, muscle twitching/spasms, EKG changes, arrhythmias

RISK FACTORS

- **Decreased fluid volume:** restricted oral fluid intake before, during, and after surgery; blood loss; and loss of fluid associated with vomiting, nasogastric tube drainage, and/or profuse wound drainage
- **Increased fluid volume:** vigorous fluid therapy during and immediately after surgery and an increased secretion of antidiuretic hormone (ADH). Note: ADH is stimulated by trauma, pain, and anesthetic agents.
- **Electrolyte imbalance: hypokalemia, hypochloremia, and metabolic alkalosis:** loss of electrolytes and hydrochloric acid associated with vomiting and nasogastric tube drainage

DESIRED OUTCOMES

1. The client will not experience deficient fluid volume, hypokalemia, hypochloremia, or metabolic alkalosis, as evidenced by:
   a. Clear lung sounds and being free of dyspnea
   b. Absence of an S_3 heart sound
   c. B/P and pulse within normal range for client and stable with position change
   d. Capillary refill time less than 2–3 secs
   e. Normal pulse volume
   f. Urine output greater than 30 mL/h
   g. Usual mental status
   h. Balanced intake and output within 48 hrs after surgery
   i. Return of peristalsis within expected time
   j. Absence of cardiac dysrhythmias, muscle weakness, paresthesias, twitching, spasms, and dizziness
   k. Serum electrolyte and ABGs (as indicated) values within normal range
   l. Normal skin turgor
   m. Moist mucous membranes
   n. Stable weight
2. The client will not experience excess fluid volume, as evidenced by:
   a. Stable weight
   b. Stable B/P
   c. Absence of an S_3 heart sound
   d. Normal pulse volume
   e. Balanced intake and output within 48 hrs after surgery
   f. Usual mental status
   g. Blood urea nitrogen (BUN)/hematocrit (Hct) and serum sodium and osmolality levels within normal range
   h. Absence of dyspnea, orthopnea, edema, and distended neck veins

NOC OUTCOMES

Fluid balance; electrolyte balance

NIC INTERVENTIONS

Electrolyte management; electrolyte monitoring; fluid/electrolyte management; fluid monitoring

NURSING ASSESSMENT	RATIONALE
Assess for and report signs and symptoms of deficient fluid volume: • Decreased skin turgor, dry mucous membranes, thirst • Weight loss of 2% or greater over a short period • Postural hypotension and/or low B/P • Weak, rapid pulse • Capillary refill time greater than 2–3 secs • Neck veins flat when client is supine • Change in mental status • Continued low urine output 48 hrs after surgery with a change in specific gravity • Elevated BUN	*Early recognition of signs and symptoms of imbalanced fluid and electrolytes allows for prompt intervention.* *The specific gravity will usually increase with an actual fluid volume deficit but may be decreased depending on the cause of the deficit*

NDx = NANDA Diagnosis   **D** = Delegatable Action   ● = UAP   ✦ = LVN/LPN   ⊖▶ = Go to ⊖volve for animation

Continued...

NURSING ASSESSMENT	RATIONALE
Assess for and report signs and symptoms of electrolyte imbalance (hypochloremia, hypokalemia, hyponatremia): • Cardiac dysrhythmias • Postural hypotension • Muscle weakness/twitching • Nausea/vomiting • Abdominal cramping/pain	*Identification of physical assessment findings indicative of electrolyte imbalances allows for prompt intervention preventing potential patient harm and delaying recovery.*
Assess for and report signs and symptoms of excess fluid volume: • Weight gain of 2% or greater over a short period • Elevated BP Note: BP may not be elevated if fluid has shifted out of vascular space • Presence of an S_3 heart sound • ECG • Bounding pulse • Intake that continues to be greater than output 48 hrs postoperatively • Change in mental status • Crackles (rales), diminished or absent breath sounds • Low serum sodium level and low osmolality indicate hypoosmolar overhydration. • Decreased BUN and Hct Note: Low HCT could also indicate blood loss • Dyspnea, orthopnea • Edema • Distended neck veins • Chest radiograph results showing pulmonary vascular congestion, pleural effusion, or pulmonary edema	*Assessment findings indicative of fluid volume overload allows for prompt intervention preventing potential patient harm and delaying recovery.*
Assess serum electrolyte levels, hemogram, serum osmolality, and ABG values as indicated.	*Assessing serum electrolyte levels, hemogram, and serum osmolality allows for the early detection of fluid/electrolyte imbalances.* *Assessment of ABG values allows for a more direct measurement of both pH and $PaCO_2$, which may influence electrolyte imbalances.*
Assess results of chest radiograph as indicated.	*Chest radiograph films provide data about pulmonary vascular status and fluid accumulation in the pleural space, pulmonary interstitium, and alveoli.*

THERAPEUTIC INTERVENTIONS	RATIONALE
Independent Actions Implement measures to prevent or treat deficient fluid volume, hypokalemia, hyponatremia, and/hypochloremia, and/or acid/base imbalances: • Perform actions to prevent nausea and vomiting: 　• Encourage client to take deep, slow breaths when nauseated. **D** ✦	*Nausea often causes the client to have decreased fluid volume intake. Persistent vomiting results in excess loss of fluid and electrolytes.*
• If a nasogastric tube is present and needs to be irrigated frequently and/or with large volumes of solution, irrigate it with normal saline rather than water. **D** ✦	*Irrigation of a nasogastric tube with normal saline instead of water helps to prevent excess loss of gastric electrolytes.*
• Perform actions to reduce fever if present: 　• Sponge client with tepid water. **D** ● 　• Remove excessive clothing or bedcovers. **D** ●	*Fever may be accompanied by diaphoresis, which can result in excessive loss of fluid.*
• Carefully measure drainage: **D** ✦ 　• Wound 　• Nasogastric	*Accurate intake/output records must be maintained to ensure fluid loss is replaced appropriately.*

THERAPEUTIC INTERVENTIONS	RATIONALE

• When oral intake is allowed and tolerated, assist client to select foods/fluids high in potassium: **D** ✦
  • Bananas
  • Orange juice
  • Potatoes
  • Raisins
  • Cantaloupe
  • Tomato juice
Implement measures to prevent or treat excess fluid volume:
• Maintain fluid restrictions if ordered. **D** ✦
	Intake of foods/fluids high in potassium helps correct hypokalemia.

Dependent/Collaborative Nursing Actions

Implement measures to prevent or treat deficient fluid volume, hypokalemia, hypochloremia, and metabolic alkalosis: • Perform actions to prevent nausea and vomiting: • Administer antiemetics and gastrointestinal stimulants as ordered. **D** ✦	*Nausea often causes the client to have decreased fluid volume intake. Persistent vomiting results in excess loss of fluid.*
• Perform actions to reduce fever if present: • Administer antipyretics as ordered. **D** ✦	*Fever may be accompanied by diaphoresis, which can result in excessive loss of fluid*
• Administer fluid and electrolyte replacements if ordered.	*Replacing lost fluid/electrolyte volume helps prevent/treat deficient fluid volume.*
• Maintain a fluid intake of at least 2500 mL/day unless contraindicated. **D** ✦	*Provide adequate fluid intake needs to ensure adequate hydration.*
Implement measures to prevent or treat excess fluid volume: • Administer fluid replacement therapy judiciously, especially within first 48 hrs after surgery.	*The stress of surgery along with anesthesia can trigger the secretion of ADH, which can lead to fluid retention/positive fluid balance. The client must be monitored for fluid volume excess until perioperative fluids are mobilized.*
• If client is receiving intravenous fluids that contain sizable amounts of sodium such as 0.9% sodium chloride (NaCl) or lactated Ringer solution, consult physician about a change in the solution or a decrease in the rate of infusion.	*Excess fluid volume can result from overzealous or prolonged intravenous administration of sodium-containing fluids, particularly ones that contain sizable amounts of sodium.*
• If client is receiving numerous and/or large-volume intravenous medications, consult pharmacist about ways to prevent excessive fluid administration: • Stop primary infusion during administration of intravenous medications, dilute medication in the minimum amount of solution.	*Limiting the amount of intravenous solution infused at any one time and maximizing the concentration of intravenous medications help prevent an additional fluid burden in the person who has or is at risk for fluid volume overload.*
• Administer diuretics, if ordered, to increase excretion of water. **D** ✦	*Most diuretics inhibit sodium reabsorption in the renal tubules. This results in decreased water reabsorption and subsequent excretion of excess fluid.*
Consult physician if signs and symptoms of deficient fluid volume, excess fluid volume, and electrolyte imbalances persist or worsen.	*Notifying the physician allows for modification of the treatment plan.*

Nursing Diagnosis **IMBALANCED NUTRITION: LESS THAN BODY REQUIREMENTS NDx**

Definition: Intake of nutrients insufficient to meet metabolic needs.

CLINICAL MANIFESTATIONS

Subjective	Objective
Verbal self-report of abdominal cramping or pain; aversion toward eating; lack of interest in food; altered taste sensation; weakness/fatigue; sore, painful mucous membranes	Inadequate food intake; inability to ingest food; diarrhea; hypoactive or absent bowel sounds; weakness of muscles of mastication; weight significantly below client's usual weight; pale conjunctiva; inflamed mucous membranes

NDx = NANDA Diagnosis **D** = Delegatable Action ● = UAP ✦ = LVN/LPN ⊝▶ = Go to ⊝volve for animation

RISK FACTORS

- Inability to ingest food and/or absorb nutrients, decreased oral intake associated with prescribed dietary modifications, pain, weakness, fatigue, nausea, dislike of prescribed diet, and feeling of fullness. This can occur as a result of abdominal distention
- Inadequate nutritional replacement therapy
- Loss of nutrients associated with vomiting
- Increased nutritional needs associated with the increased metabolic rate that occurs during wound healing

DESIRED OUTCOMES

The client will maintain an adequate nutritional status, as evidenced by:
a. Weight within normal range for client
b. Normal BUN, serum albumin, Hct, and hemoglobin (Hgb) levels and lymphocyte count
c. Usual strength and activity tolerance
d. Healthy oral mucous membrane

NOC OUTCOMES

Nutritional status: biochemical measures; food and fluid intake; nutrient intake

NIC INTERVENTIONS

Nutritional monitoring; nutrition management; nutrition therapy; diet staging

NURSING ASSESSMENT

Assess for and report signs and symptoms of malnutrition:
- Weight significantly below client's usual weight or below normal for client's age, height, and body frame
- Weakness and fatigue
- Sore, inflamed oral mucous membrane
- Pale conjunctiva

Assess for return of bowel function every 2–4 hrs.

Monitor serum albumin, prealbumin, serum total protein, serum ferritin, transferrin, Hgb, Hct, and electrolyte levels as indicated.

When oral intake is allowed, monitor percentage of meals and snacks client consumes. Report pattern of inadequate intake.

RATIONALE

Early recognition of signs and symptoms of malnutrition allows for prompt intervention.

Once the client begins to expel flatus, notify the health care provider so oral intake can be resumed as soon as possible.

Serum albumin level less than 3.5 g/100 mL is considered an indicator of poor nutritional status. Early recognition of abnormal lab values reflective of the client's overall nutritional state allows for prompt intervention.

An awareness of the amount of foods/fluids a client consumes alerts the nurse to deficits in nutritional intake. Reporting inadequate intake allows for prompt intervention.

THERAPEUTIC INTERVENTIONS

Independent Actions

When food or oral fluids are allowed, implement measures to maintain an adequate nutritional status:
- Implement measures to prevent nausea and vomiting: **D** ● ✦
  - Eliminate noxious sights and odors from the environment
  - Encourage the client to take deep, slow breaths when nauseated
  - Instruct client to change positions slowly
  - Apply a cold washcloth to the client's forehead
  - Consider alternative therapies (e.g., aromatherapy; acupressure bands).
- Implement measures to reduce pain:
  - Instruct client to support incision with movement. **D** ✦
- Implement measures to reduce the accumulation of gas and fluid in the gastrointestinal tract and prevent constipation:
  - Encourage frequent position changes **D** ✦
  - Encourage ambulation. **D** ✦
- Encourage a rest period before meals. **D** ✦
- Provide nursing assistance during meals. **D** ●
- Maintain a clean environment and a relaxed, pleasant atmosphere. **D** ●
- Provide oral hygiene before meals. **D** ●

RATIONALE

The presence of nausea can decrease the appetite. Preventing nausea and vomiting can improve the client's appetite.

The presence of pain decreases the appetite.

The subsequent feeling of fullness that accompanies gas accumulation leads to an early feeling of satiety.

To conserve energy for consuming meals, rest periods before eating should be encouraged.

A pleasant environment helps to promote adequate intake.

Good oral hygiene enhances appetite. A moist oral mucosa makes chewing and swallowing easier. Oral hygiene can also remove unpleasant tastes, improving the taste of foods/fluids.

THERAPEUTIC INTERVENTIONS	**RATIONALE**
• Serve frequent, small meals rather than large ones if client is weak, fatigues easily, and/or has a poor appetite. **D** ✦	*Small, frequent meals are better tolerated in clients with a poor appetite.*
• Encourage significant others to bring in client's favorite foods unless contraindicated. **D** ✦	*Food preferences enhance a client's appetite.*
• Allow adequate time for meals; reheat foods/fluids if necessary. **D** ●	*Research has demonstrated that it takes 35 minutes to feed the client who is willing to eat.*
• Limit fluid intake with meals unless the fluid has high nutritional value. **D** ✦	*A high fluid intake with meals promotes a feeling of fullness and early satiety that may decrease actual food intake.*

Dependent/Collaborative Nursing Actions

When food or oral fluids are allowed, implement measures to maintain an adequate nutritional status:

• Administer antiemetics as ordered. **D** ✦	*The presence of nausea can decrease the appetite. Preventing nausea and vomiting can improve the client's appetite.*
• Administer pain medications as ordered. **D** ✦	*The presence of pain decreases the appetite.*
• Increase activity as tolerated and allowed. **D** ●	*Activity promotes gastric emptying, which reduces feeling of gastric fullness; it also usually promotes a sense of well-being, which can improve appetite.*
• Obtain a dietary consult if necessary, to assist client in selecting foods/fluids that meet nutritional needs, are appealing, and adhere to personal and cultural preferences, as well as the prescribed dietary modifications.	*A dietician or nutritional support team can help clients individualize their diet within prescribed dietary restrictions. Providing food in line with client preferences can enhance adherence to prescribed diet.*
• Ensure that meals are well balanced and high in essential nutrients; offer dietary supplements if indicated.	*Dietary supplements have shown a positive relationship with weight gain, reduced mortality, and reduced length of hospitalization.*
• Administer vitamins and minerals if ordered. **D** ✦	*Vitamins and minerals are essential to many metabolic processes in the body.*
• Perform a calorie count if ordered. Report information to dietitian and physician. **D** ✦	*Information gathered from an accurate calorie count is used to determine the adequacy of a client's daily diet or the need for nutritional support.*

Consult physician about an alternative method of providing nutrition if client does not consume enough food or fluids to meet nutritional needs:	*Notifying the physician allows for modification of the treatment plan.*

• Enteral tube feedings
• Parenteral nutrition.

Nursing Diagnosis **NAUSEA** NDx

Definition: A subjective phenomenon of an unpleasant feeling in the back of the throat and stomach, which may or may not result in vomiting.

CLINICAL MANIFESTATIONS

Subjective	**Objective**
Verbal self-report of nausea/aversion toward food; sour taste in the mouth	Gagging; increased salivation; increase in swallowing

RISK FACTORS

- Stimulation of visceral afferent pathways resulting from abdominal distention and/or the irritating effect of some medications on the gastric mucosa
- Stimulation of the cerebral cortex resulting from pain, stress, and/or noxious environmental stimuli
- Stimulation of the chemoreceptor trigger zone resulting from rapid movement and the effect of some medications (e.g., morphine)

DESIRED OUTCOMES

The client will experience relief of nausea and vomiting, as evidenced by:
a. Verbalization of relief of nausea
b. Absence of vomiting

NDx = NANDA Diagnosis   **D** = Delegatable Action   ● = UAP   ✦ = LVN/LPN   ⊖▶ = Go to ℮volve for animation

NOC OUTCOMES	NIC INTERVENTIONS
Nausea and vomiting control; nausea and vomiting severity; nausea and vomiting disruptive effects	Nausea management; vomiting management; environmental management: comfort

NURSING ASSESSMENT	RATIONALE
Assess for nausea and vomiting.	*Early recognition of signs and symptoms of nausea and vomiting allows for prompt intervention.*

THERAPEUTIC INTERVENTIONS	RATIONALE

Independent Actions

Implement measures to prevent nausea and vomiting:
- Perform actions to reduce the accumulation of gas and fluid in the gastrointestinal tract: **D** ✦
  - Frequent position changes
  - Early ambulation
  - Expel flatus when urge felt

As gas accumulates in the intestines, the bowel wall stretches causing feelings of fullness, pain, and cramping that can contribute to nausea.

- Consider alternative therapies for the treatment of nausea:
  - Inhalation of isopropyl alcohol
  - Continuous acupressure with bands or buttons on the wrist

Inhalation of isopropyl alcohol for clients who have undergone general anesthesia has been shown to be somewhat effective for postoperative nausea and vomiting (PONV). Acupressure was demonstrated to be a noninvasive, inexpensive, safe treatment for PONV.

- Perform nonpharmacologic actions to reduce pain:
  - Proper positioning
  - Splinting of incisions

Pain is known to contribute to PONV.

- Eliminate noxious sights and odors from the environment.

Implement distraction techniques when client experiences nausea:
- Slow, deep breaths
- Guided imagery

Noxious stimuli can cause stimulation of the vomiting center.
Distraction techniques can help to draw attention away from nausea. Slow, deep breaths in the immediate postanesthesia period can help to rid the body of inhaled anesthetic agents.

- Instruct client to change positions slowly.

Rapid movement can result in chemoreceptor trigger zone stimulation and subsequent excitation of the vomiting center.

- Provide oral hygiene after each emesis. **D** ●
- When oral intake is allowed:
  - Advance diet slowly usually beginning with clear liquids and progressing to solid food.

Oral care can help remove foul tastes associated with vomiting.
Slow advances in diet allow for gradual adjustment of the digestive tract to the presence of food.

- Avoid serving foods with an overpowering aroma; remove lids from hot foods before entering room.

Sudden, concentrated food odors can stimulate nausea.

- Provide small, frequent meals rather than three (3) large ones.

Nausea can be prevented by ingesting small meals.

- Instruct client to ingest foods and fluids slowly.
- Instruct client to avoid foods/fluids that irritate the gastric mucosa (e.g., spicy foods; caffeine-containing beverages such as coffee, tea, and colas).

Eating slowly can reduce the incidence of nausea.
Foods that irritate the gastric mucosa may lead to the development of nausea.

- Encourage client to consume foods that prevent nausea (e.g., dry, bland foods such as toast/crackers and liquids such as ginger ale).

Foods that are bland and dry are better tolerated by a nauseated client. Ginger root has been demonstrated to be an effective treatment for nausea and vomiting.

- Instruct client to avoid foods high in fat.
- Instruct client to rest after eating with head of bed elevated.

Fat delays gastric emptying and may contribute to nausea.
Resting in a sitting position after eating may help prevent nausea.

Dependent/Collaborative Nursing Actions

Implement measures to prevent nausea and vomiting:
- Administer antiemetics and gastrointestinal stimulants (e.g., metoclopramide) if ordered. **D** ✦

Antiemetic medications can reduce the incidence of nausea. Gastrointestinal stimulants promote peristalsis.

- Administer medications known to cause gastric irritation (e.g., aspirin and aspirin-containing products, corticosteroids, ibuprofen) with or immediately after meals unless contraindicated.

Administering medications known to irritate the stomach with foods helps to reduce the potential for nausea and enhance absorption of the medications.

Consult physician if aforementioned measures fail to control nausea and vomiting.

Notifying the appropriate health care provider allows for modification of the treatment plan.

Nursing Diagnosis RISK FOR DELAYED SURGICAL RECOVERY NDx

Definition: Susceptible to an extension of the number of postoperative days required to initiate and perform activities that maintain life, health, and well-being, which may compromise health.
Related to:
- Type of procedure performed
- Prolonged or extensive surgery
- Persistent nausea/vomiting
- Surgical site infection
- Impaired mobility

CLINICAL MANIFESTATIONS

Subjective	Objective
Verbal self-report of pain exceeding agreed upon pain goal; loss of appetite; nausea	Interrupted healing of surgical area; impaired mobility; required self-care assistance; vomiting

RISK FACTORS

- Extremes of age
- Obesity
- Malnutrition
- Pain
- Comorbidities (e.g., diabetes mellitus)

DESIRED OUTCOMES

The client will meet length of stay goal for admitting diagnosis/procedure.

NOC OUTCOMES

Surgical recovery: immediate postoperative; convalescence

NIC INTERVENTIONS

Nutrition management; pain management: acute; nausea management; vomiting management; exercise therapy: ambulation; wound care

NURSING ASSESSMENT	RATIONALE
Assess pain to include location, onset, duration, frequency, and location.	*Persistent, uncontrolled pain can delay surgical recovery and interfere with the ability to achieve discharge criteria*
• Identify client's knowledge and beliefs about pain, including cultural influences.	
• Identify client's pain goal that allows a state of comfort and appropriate function.	
Assess for the presence of persistent nausea/vomiting including frequency, duration, severity, and precipitating factors.	*Persistent, unrelieved nausea and vomiting can be indicative of surgical complications (e.g., paralytic ileus) which can delay surgical recovery.*
• Assess for the presence of bowel sounds, abdominal distention/pain.	
• Identify factors that contribute to nausea/vomiting	
• Identify treatment past treatment options successful in the management of nausea/vomiting	
Assess client's nutritional status and ability to meet nutritional needs.	*Inadequate nutrition can delay wound healing, resulting in delayed surgical recover and discharge.*
• Identify food preferences	
Assess surgical site for presence of drainage, color, odor, and approximation of wound edges.	*Routine assessment of surgical wound integrity allows for the identification of inadequate wound healing and allows for prompt intervention.*
Assess client's ability to ambulate including level of assistance and the need for ambulation aids.	*The ability to independently and safely ambulate will determine client's discharge potential and the need for further rehabilitation.*

THERAPEUTIC INTERVENTIONS	RATIONALE

Independent Actions

Implement measures to achieve client's pain goals:

- Monitor pain using a valid and reliable rating tool appropriate for age and ability to communicate.
- Ensure client receives prompt analgesic care before pain-inducing activities and/or before the pain becomes severe.
- Incorporate nonpharmaceutic interventions to pain management incorporating patient preference as appropriate (e.g., application of ice; guided imagery; meditation). **D** ●

Implement measures to relieve persistent nausea/vomiting

- Control environmental factors that may contribute to nausea/vomiting (e.g., aversive smells, sound, unpleasant visual stimulation). **D** ●
- Reduce client factors that may precipitate nausea/vomiting (e.g., anxiety, fear, fatigue).
- Incorporate frequent oral hygiene into care to promote comfort. **D** ●
- Consider alternative therapies (e.g., acupressure; aroma-therapy).

Implement measures to improve appetite.

- Provide optimum environment for meal consumption (e.g., clean, well ventilated). **D** ●
- Ensure food is prepared in a manner optimum for consumption.
- Assist patient with eating if needed. **D** ●
- Monitor caloric and dietary intake.

Implement measures to ensure progressive wound healing. **D** ●

- Ensure client and provider observe hand hygiene practices.
- Position patient to prevent tension on wound as appropriate.
- Ensure healthy diet to promote would healing.
- Ensure client does not smoke during postoperative period.

Implement measures to progress independent mobility.

- Provide low-height bed as appropriate. **D** ●

- Provide footwear that promotes safe ambulation. **D** ●
- Encourage client to sit on side of bed (dangle) as tolerated.
- Assist patient with initial ambulation as necessary. **D** ●
- Assist patient to stand and ambulate specified distances. **D** ●
- Encourage patient to be up "ad lib" as appropriate to condition. **D** ●

Dependent/Collaborative Actions

Implement measures to achieve client's pain goals: **D** ●

- Consider administration of analgesics around the clock for the first 24–48 hrs after surgery unless contraindicated by level of sedation or respiratory status.
- Use combination analgesics if pain is severe (e.g., opioids/nonopioids).
- Consider alternative therapies (e.g., guided imagery; meditation).

Ongoing monitoring of pain level allows for evaluation of response to therapy and adjustment of the treatment plan if unable to achieve client's pain goals.

Nonpharmacologic pain relief practices may reduce the need for opioid narcotics and contribute to progressive recovery.

Persistent, unrelieved nausea and/or vomiting interferes with adequate nutritional intake, which can impair wound healing and overall recovery.

Adequate nutritional intake is necessary for optimum wound healing. Enhances client's desire to eat.

Assures that client intake is appropriate to support healing. Healthy diet is necessary to promote wound healing.

Smoking causes vasoconstriction and can interfere with wound healing.

Early ambulation is necessary to prevent muscle atrophy, reduce the risk for falls, improve circulation, reduce edema, and prevent additional surgical complications.

Improves ability for independence and prevents potential for falls or other injury.

Administration of pain medication around the clock during the first 24–48 hrs after surgery when pain is most intense will enhance recovery by facilitating client's ability to comply with postoperative activities (e.g., ambulation, coughing).

THERAPEUTIC INTERVENTIONS	RATIONALE
Implement measures to relieve persistent nausea/vomiting **D** ●	*Unrelieved, persistent nausea/vomiting delays surgical recovery by interfering with adequate nutritional intake and increasing tension on wound (e.g., abdominal), risking dehiscence.*
• Monitor fluid and electrolyte intake, gradually increasing fluids if no vomiting occurs.	
• Administer appropriate antiemetic medications.	
Implement measures to improve appetite.	*Identification of weight loss/inadequate nutritional intake can delay wound healing/discharge. Consultation with dietician allows for appropriate modification of the treatment plan.*
• Monitor trends in weight loss/weight gain.	
• Offer nutrient-dense snacks	
• Obtain referral for dietician for supplemental nutrition as indicated	
Implement measures to ensure progressive wound healing. **D** ●	*Surgical dressings, if applied, should be kept dry and intact—either reinforcing or changing in accordance with physician's orders to ensure an optimum environment for wound healing. Sterile technique, when necessary, must be adhered to in order to prevent infection.*
• Maintain sterile dressing technique when changing dressings/performing wound care as appropriate.	
• Change dressings according to the amount of exudate and drainage.	
• Reinforce dressings as needed.	
Implement measures to progress independent mobility.	*Early, progressive ambulation is an independent function of the nurse. Any barriers to achieving ambulation should be discussed with physical therapy in a timely manner to prevent delayed recovery and/or discharge.*
• Consult physical therapy about ambulation plan as needed.	
Consult physician if signs and symptoms of any of the following occur:	*Notifying the appropriate health care provider allows for modification of the treatment plan.*
• Self-reported, unrelieved pain that exceeds identified goals for comfort and optimum functioning.	
• Self-reported, persistent, unrelieved nausea and vomiting.	
• Inadequate nutritional/caloric intake.	
• Signs/symptoms of wound infection or delayed healing (e.g., swelling, odor, foul discharge/drainage, wound edges that are not approximated).	
• Inability to safety ambulate independently.	

Nursing Diagnosis ## IMPAIRED ORAL MUCOUS MEMBRANE INTEGRITY NDx

Definition: Injury to the lips, soft tissue, buccal cavity, and/or oropharynx.

CLINICAL MANIFESTATIONS

Subjective	Objective
Verbal self-report of difficulty swallowing, oral discomfort, or bad taste in the mouth	Difficult speech; decreased salivation; halitosis; impaired ability to swallow; white patches in mouth; coated tongue

RISK FACTORS

- Deficient fluid volume associated with restricted oral intake and fluid loss
- Decreased salivation associated with food and fluid restrictions and the effect of anesthesia and some medications (e.g., narcotic [opioid] analgesics)
- Inability to perform self–oral care
- Malnutrition

DESIRED OUTCOMES

The client will maintain a moist, intact oral mucous membrane.

NOC OUTCOMES

Oral health

NIC INTERVENTIONS

Oral health maintenance; oral health promotion; oral health restoration

---

NDx = NANDA Diagnosis   **D** = Delegatable Action   ● = UAP   ✦ = LVN/LPN   ●▶ = Go to ⊖volve for animation

NURSING ASSESSMENT	RATIONALE
Assess for dryness of the oral mucosa.	*Early recognition of signs and symptoms of a dry oral mucosa allows for prompt intervention.*

THERAPEUTIC INTERVENTIONS	RATIONALE

Independent Actions

Implement measures to relieve dryness of the oral mucous membrane: **D** ✦

• Instruct and assist client to perform oral hygiene as often as needed.	
• Avoid use of products that contain lemon and glycerin and use of mouthwashes containing alcohol.	*These products have a drying and irritating effect on the oral mucous membrane.*
• Encourage client to rinse mouth frequently with water. **D** ●	*Prevents oral dryness and flushes out unwanted substances and bacteria.*
• Lubricate client's lips frequently. **D** ●	*Frequent lubrication of the lips helps prevent drying and cracking.*
• Encourage client to breathe through nose rather than mouth.	*Breathing through the nose allows for the proper warming and humidification of air, which is bypassed with mouth breathing.*
• Encourage client not to smoke.	*Smoking dries the oral mucosa and has been linked to mucous membrane breakdown and oral cancer.*
• Encourage client to suck on hard candy unless contraindicated.	*Action helps to stimulate salivation, moistening the oral mucosa.*

Dependent/Collaborative Actions

Implement measures to relieve dryness of the oral mucous membrane:

• Maintain intravenous fluid therapy as ordered.	*Intravenous fluid therapy enhances hydration and helps to improve the condition of dry mucous membranes.*
• Increase oral fluid intake as ordered. **D** ● ✦	*Increasing oral fluid intake promotes hydration and stimulates salivation.*
Consult physician if signs and symptoms of parotitis (e.g., pain, tenderness, and swelling at the angle of the jaw; fever) occur.	*Notifying the appropriate health care provider allows for modification of the treatment plan.*

Nursing Diagnosis ## BATHING, DRESSING, FEEDING, AND TOILETING SELF-CARE DEFICIT

Definition: **Bathing Self-Care Deficit NDx:** Inability to independently complete cleansing activities; **Dressing Self-Care Deficit NDx:** Inability to independently put on or remove clothing; **Feeding Self-Care Deficit NDx:** Inability to eat independently; **Toileting Self-Care Deficit NDx:** Inability to independently perform tasks associated with bowel and bladder elimination.

CLINICAL MANIFESTATIONS

Subjective	**Objective**
Verbal self-report of inability to perform basic personal care activities	Inability to access bathroom; inability to wash body; inability to maintain appearance at acceptable level; inability to put on necessary items of clothing

RISK FACTORS

• Impaired physical mobility associated with weakness, fatigue, pain, nausea, depressant effect of some medications, fear of dislodging tubes and compromising surgical wound, and activity restrictions

DESIRED OUTCOMES

The client will perform self-care activities within physical limitations and postoperative activity restrictions.

NOC OUTCOMES	NIC INTERVENTIONS
Self-care assistance: bathing/hygiene; dressing/grooming; feeding; toileting	Self-care assistance: bathing/hygiene; dressing/grooming; feeding; toileting

NURSING ASSESSMENT	RATIONALE
Assess for physical limitations or postoperative restrictions that may interfere with a client's ability to perform self-care: bathing/hygiene; dressing/grooming; feeding; toileting.	*Early recognition of signs and symptoms of physical limitations allows for prompt intervention.*

THERAPEUTIC INTERVENTIONS	RATIONALE

Independent Actions

With client, develop a realistic plan for meeting daily basic personal care activities.

Including the client in developing a plan of care promotes autonomy and helps to establish a sense of control.

Assist the client with activities he/she is unable to perform independently. **D** ● ✦

Implement measures to facilitate the client's ability to perform self-care activities: **D** ● ✦

- Schedule care at a time when client is most likely to be able to participate (e.g., when analgesics are at peak effect, after rest periods, not immediately after meals or treatments).

Pain relief facilitates range of motion, which may increase the client's ability to perform self-care.

- Keep needed objects within easy reach.
- Allow adequate time for accomplishment of self-care activities.
- Perform actions to increase physical mobility.

Obtain assistive devices as necessary.

- Toileting: bedside commode/urinal
- Feeding: adaptive devices (e.g., utensils with small straps; long-handled utensils; large-handled cups)
- Dressing: extension equipment for pulling on clothing as appropriate

Environmental and/or physical factors may interfere with the client's ability to perform self-care activities. The ability to perform self-care activities may be enhanced with adaptation of the client's care environment.

Encourage maximum independence within physical limitations and postoperative activity restrictions. **D** ● ✦

Inform significant others of client's abilities to perform own care. Explain the importance of encouraging and allowing client to maintain an optimal level of independence.

The ability to perform self-care is essential for optimum self-esteem.

Dependent Collaborative Actions

Consult with physician and/or case management to evaluate client for needed support services to assist with activities of daily living bathing, dressing, feeding, toileting.

Inability of client to perform activities of daily living, including feeding, may hamper postoperative recovery. If family is unable to support, home care services or rehabilitation services may be required to ensure appropriate recovery.

Nursing Diagnosis ## URINARY RETENTION NDx

Definition: Inability to empty bladder completely.

CLINICAL MANIFESTATIONS

Subjective	**Objective**
Verbal self-report of inability to urinate; feelings of the need to strain to empty the bladder	Palpable distended bladder; urinary dribbling; absence of urinary output; frequent voiding

RISK FACTORS

- Increased tone of the urinary sphincters associated with sympathetic nervous system stimulation resulting from pain, fear, and anxiety
- Decreased perception of bladder fullness associated with depressant effect of anesthesia and some medications (e.g., opioid analgesics)
- Relaxation of the bladder muscle associated with depressant effect of anesthesia and some medications (e.g., opioid analgesics) and stimulation of the sympathetic nervous system (can result from pain, fear, and anxiety)

DESIRED OUTCOMES

The client will not experience urinary retention, as evidenced by:
a. Voiding at normal intervals
b. No reports of bladder fullness and suprapubic discomfort
c. Absence of bladder distention and dribbling of urine
d. Balanced intake and output within 48 hrs after surgery

NOC OUTCOMES

Urinary continence; urinary elimination

NIC INTERVENTIONS

Urinary catheterization; urinary elimination management

NURSING ASSESSMENT	RATIONALE
Assess for signs and symptoms of urinary retention: • Frequent voiding of small amounts (25–60 mL) of urine • Reports of bladder fullness or suprapubic discomfort • Bladder distention • Dribbling of urine Monitor intake and output.	*Early recognition of signs and symptoms of urinary retention allows for prompt intervention.* *Administration of anesthetic agents impairs normal bladder emptying. Adequate volume replacement is necessary to fill bladder and stimulate micturition.* *Any continued oliguria or anuria should be reported to the physician to allow for modification of the treatment plan.*

THERAPEUTIC INTERVENTIONS	RATIONALE

Independent Actions
Implement measures to prevent urinary retention:
• Instruct client to urinate when the urge is first felt.
 	
• Perform actions to promote relaxation during voiding attempts:
  • Provide privacy, hold a warm blanket against abdomen, encourage client to read. **D ●**
• Perform actions that may help to trigger the micturition reflex and promote a sense of relaxation during voiding attempts:
  • Run water, place client's hands in warm water, pour warm water over perineum. **D ✦**
• Allow client to assume a normal position for voiding unless contraindicated. **D ●**
• Instruct client to lean upper body forward and/or gently press downward on lower abdomen during voiding attempts unless contraindicated.
	If the client feels the urge to urinate but suppresses it by contracting the external urinary sphincter, the urge will subside and not recur until the bladder fills more.
	If the client is relaxed when trying to urinate, he/she is better able to relax the pelvic floor muscles and external urinary sphincter, allowing voiding to occur.
	
	A sitting or standing position, if possible, uses gravity to facilitate bladder emptying.
	Proper positioning is necessary to put pressure on the bladder pressure helps create a sensation of bladder fullness, which stimulates the micturition reflex

THERAPEUTIC INTERVENTIONS	RATIONALE

Dependent/Collaborative Actions

Implement measures to prevent urinary retention:
- Perform actions to reduce postoperative pain.
- Encourage use of nonnarcotic rather than opioid analgesics once period of severe pain has subsided. **D** ✦

Narcotic analgesics may decrease the perception of a full bladder and promote urinary retention. The use of nonnarcotic analgesics may reduce this effect.

Consult physician regarding intermittent catheterization or insertion of an indwelling catheter if aforementioned actions fail to alleviate urinary retention.

If urinary catheter is present, **D** ✦
- Keep tubing free of kinks, and irrigate as ordered.

Prevents urinary retention by maintaining patency of the catheter.

Consult physician if there is no urine output within 6–8 hrs after surgery or if output continues to be less than intake 48 hrs after surgery.

For the first 48 hrs postoperatively, urine output is expected to be less than intake because of factors such as blood loss and increased secretion of ADH. Consulting the appropriate health care provider allows for modification of treatment plan.

- Administer cholinergic (parasympathomimetic) drugs to stimulate bladder contraction. **D** ✦

Cholinergic (parasympathomimetic) drugs promote urination by stimulating contraction of the bladder detrusor muscle.

Collaborative Diagnosis   # RISK FOR PARALYTIC ILEUS

Definition: Paralysis of the peristaltic activity resulting in blockage of the intestines.

CLINICAL MANIFESTATIONS

Subjective	Objective
Verbal self-report of persistent abdominal pain and cramping	Firm, distended abdomen; absent bowel sounds; failure to pass flatus; abdominal x-ray showing distended bowel

RISK FACTORS
- Manipulation of intestines during abdominal surgery, depressant effect of anesthesia and some medications (e.g., opioid analgesics, some antiemetics) on bowel motility, hypokalemia, and hypovolemia (can cause decreased blood supply to the intestine)

DESIRED OUTCOMES

The client will not develop a paralytic ileus, as evidenced by:
- a. Absence or resolution of abdominal pain and cramping
- b. Soft, nondistended abdomen
- c. Gradual return of bowel sounds
- d. Passage of flatus

NURSING ASSESSMENT	RATIONALE

Assess for and report signs and symptoms of paralytic ileus:
- Development of or persistent abdominal pain and cramping
- Firm, distended abdomen
- Absent bowel sounds
- Failure to pass flatus

Early recognition of signs and symptoms of a paralytic ileus allows for prompt intervention.

Monitor results of abdominal x-ray.

An abdominal x-ray that demonstrates distended bowel may be indicative of a paralytic ileus.

THERAPEUTIC INTERVENTIONS	RATIONALE

Independent Actions

Implement measures to prevent paralytic ileus:
- Increase activity as soon as allowed and tolerated. **D** ● ✦

Early ambulation in a postoperative client promotes the return of peristalsis.

NDx = NANDA Diagnosis   **D** = Delegatable Action   ● = UAP   ✦ = LVN/LPN   ⊖▶ = Go to ⊖volve for animation

Continued...

THERAPEUTIC INTERVENTIONS	RATIONALE

Dependent/Collaborative Actions

Implement measures to prevent paralytic ileus:

- Perform actions to maintain adequate tissue perfusion:
  - Administer gastrointestinal stimulants (e.g., metoclopramide) if ordered. **D** ✦

    Gastrointestinal stimulants help to maintain adequate blood supply to the bowel.

- Perform actions to prevent hypokalemia.
- Administer potassium supplements.

    Hypokalemia promotes atony of the intestinal wall, which results in a decrease in peristalsis.

If signs and symptoms of paralytic ileus occur: **D** ✦

- Withhold all oral intake.
- Insert nasogastric tube and maintain suction as ordered.

    Paralytic ileus results in cessation of normal peristalsis. The client should have nothing by mouth (NPO) with a nasogastric tube in place to facilitate gastric decompression until the ileus is resolved.

DISCHARGE TEACHING/CONTINUED CARE

Nursing Diagnosis **DEFICIENT KNOWLEDGE** NDx

Definition: Absence of cognitive information related to specific topic, or its acquisition.

CLINICAL MANIFESTATIONS

Subjective	Objective
Verbal self-report of not understanding postoperative instructions	Alteration in cognitive function; alteration in memory; inaccurate follow-through of instructions; inappropriate behaviors

RISK FACTORS

- Cognitive deficiency
- Misinterpretation of information
- Lack of interest in learning
- Language/cultural barriers

DESIRED OUTCOMES

The client will demonstrate an understanding of postoperative instructions as evidenced by:
a. Confirmation of understanding of postoperative instructions provided during the teach-back method of patient education

NOC OUTCOMES

Knowledge: treatment regimen

NIC INTERVENTIONS

Teaching: individual; teaching: prescribed exercise; teaching: prescribed medication; health system guidance

NURSING ASSESSMENT	RATIONALE
Assess client's ability and readiness to learn. Assess the client's understanding of teaching.	*Learning is more effective when the client is motivated and understands the importance of what is to be learned. Readiness to learn changes based on situations and physical and emotional challenges.*

THERAPEUTIC INTERVENTIONS	RATIONALE

Desired Outcomes: The client will identify ways to prevent postoperative infection.

Independent Actions

- Instruct client in ways to prevent postoperative respiratory infection:
  - Continue with coughing (unless contraindicated) and deep breathing every 2 hrs while awake.
  - Continue to use IS if activity is limited.

    Coughing and deep breathing exercises, as well as incentive spirometry, help to reduce atelectasis, reexpand alveoli, and decrease the risk of a postoperative pulmonary infection. Deep breathing helps to clear airways by loosening secretions and promoting a more effective cough.

THERAPEUTIC INTERVENTIONS	RATIONALE
• Increase activity as ordered.	*Activity helps to mobilize secretions and promotes deeper breathing.*
• Avoid contact with persons who have infections. • Avoid crowds during flu and cold seasons.	*During the healing process, while an individual's resistance to infection may be lowered, the client should avoid situations that increase the risk for infection. Protecting the client from others with infections reduces the risk of exposure to pathogens.*
• Decrease or stop smoking.	*Irritants in smoke increase mucus production and impair ciliary function, which can increase the risk for postoperative pulmonary infection.*
• Drink at least 10 glasses of liquid per day unless contraindicated.	*Proper hydration helps to thin pulmonary secretions, which facilitates mobilization and expectoration, reducing the risk of pulmonary infection. Proper hydration also helps maintain adequate blood flow and nutrient supply to healing tissues.*
• Maintain a balanced nutritional intake.	*Adequate nutrition is necessary for proper wound healing and maintenance of normal immune system function.*
• Maintain a proper balance of rest and activity.	*Rest helps the body to better use nutrients and oxygen for healing. Activity helps to reduce the risk of complications of prolonged immobility.*
• Maintain good personal hygiene, especially with oral care, hand washing, and perineal care.	*Good personal hygiene helps to maintain the integrity of protective mucosal linings (oral), reduce the amount of harmful organisms (perineal, oral, hand), and reduce the risk of colonization of organisms and subsequent infection.*
• Avoid touching any wound unless it is completely healed.	*Touching the wound may increase the transmission of pathogens, increasing the risk for infection.*
• Maintain sterile or clean technique as ordered during wound care.	*The use of sterile technique reduces the risk of introduction of pathogens into the body.*

THERAPEUTIC INTERVENTIONS	RATIONALE

Desired Outcomes: The client will demonstrate the ability to perform wound care.

Independent Actions

Discuss the rationale for, frequency of, and equipment necessary for the prescribed wound care.

Provide client with the necessary supplies (e.g., dressings, irrigating solution, tape) for wound care and with names and addresses of places where additional supplies can be obtained.

Assures client has what is needed at discharge.

Demonstrate wound care and proper cleansing of any reusable equipment. Allow time for questions, clarification, and return demonstration.

Return demonstration allows for the nurse to determine the client's comprehension of the task. Any deficiencies in performance can be addressed with further instruction.

THERAPEUTIC INTERVENTIONS	RATIONALE

Desired Outcomes: The client will state signs and symptoms to report to the health care provider.

Independent Actions

Instruct the client to report the following signs and symptoms:
• Persistent low-grade or significantly elevated (38.3°C [101°F]) temperature
• Difficulty breathing
• Chest pain
• Cough productive of purulent, green, or rust-colored sputum
• Increasing weakness or inability to tolerate prescribed activity level
• Increasing discomfort or discomfort not controlled by prescribed medications and treatments
• Continued nausea or vomiting

Signs and symptoms are indicative of potential infection and should be reported to the appropriate health care provider in a timely manner to avoid complications.

Recognition of signs and symptoms of infection allows for prompt intervention.

Continued...

THERAPEUTIC INTERVENTIONS	RATIONALE
• Increasing abdominal distention and/or discomfort • Separation of wound edges • Increasing redness, warmth, pain, or swelling around wound • Unusual or excessive drainage from any wound site • Pain or swelling in calf of one or both legs • Urine retention • Frequency, urgency, or burning on urination • Cloudy or foul-smelling urine	*Possible paralytic ileus, bowel obstruction, or constipation.* *Poor tissue healing.* *Possible thrombus development.* *Possible urinary tract infection.*

THERAPEUTIC INTERVENTIONS	RATIONALE
Desired Outcomes: The client will develop a plan for adhering to recommended follow-up care including future appointments with health care provider, dietary modifications, activity level, treatments, and medications prescribed.	*A written plan assures that client has considered all aspects of follow-up care and what support may be required to adhere to therapeutic regimen.*

Independent Actions

Reinforce importance of keeping scheduled follow-up appointments with the health care provider.

A follow-up appointment with the health care provider is important to monitor continued recovery.

Reinforce physician's instructions about dietary modifications. Obtain a dietary consult for client if needed.

A proper diet helps to enhance proper wound healing. Reinforcing instructions helps the nurse to both assess the client's level of understanding and determine the need for further instruction.

Reinforce physician's instructions on suggested activity level and treatment plan.

Activity levels must be maintained to ensure the proper balance between rest that aids in healing and activity that prevents complications.

Explain the rationale for, side effects of, and importance of taking medications prescribed. Inform client of pertinent food and drug interactions.

The client should be educated on how to take medications that are prescribed to be used as needed. It should be emphasized that the client should not increase the frequency or dosage of these medications without permission from the health care provider.

Implement measures to improve client compliance:
• Include significant others in teaching sessions if possible.

Involvement of significant others in patient teaching improves adherence to discharge instructions.

• Encourage questions and allow time for reinforcement and clarification of information provided.

Information is presented with time for questions to allow for clarification of information.

• Provide written instructions on scheduled appointments with health care provider, dietary modifications, activity level, treatment plan, medications prescribed, and signs and symptoms to report.

Written instructions allow the client to refer to instructions as needed.

ADDITIONAL CARE PLANS

RISK FOR CONSTIPATION NDx
Related to decreased gastrointestinal motility associated with manipulation of bowel during abdominal surgery, depressant effect of anesthesia and opioid analgesics, and decreased activity

DISTURBED SLEEP PATTERN NDx
Related to fear, anxiety, discomfort, inability to assume usual sleeping position, and frequent assessments and treatments

RISK FOR INFECTION NDx
Pneumonia related to stasis of pulmonary secretions and aspiration, if it occurs.
 Wound infection related to contamination associated with introduction of pathogens during or after surgery; decreased resistance to infection associated with factors such as diminished tissue perfusion of wound area and inadequate nutritional status
 Urinary tract infection related to increased growth and colonization of microorganisms associated with urinary stasis; introduction of pathogens associated with an indwelling catheter if present

RISK FOR FALLS NDx
Related to weakness and fatigue; dizziness or syncope associated with postural hypotension resulting from peripheral pooling of blood and blood loss during surgery; central nervous system depressant effect of some medications opioid analgesics, some antiemetics; presence of tubing or equipment

IMPAIRED PHYSICAL MOBILITY NDx
Related to weakness and fatigue associated with inadequate nutritional status, disturbed sleep pattern, pain, nausea, activity restrictions imposed by treatment plan

ACTIVITY INTOLERANCE NDx
Related to bed rest, immobility, and generalized weakness

RISK FOR ASPIRATION NDx
Related to decreased level of consciousness and absent or diminished gag reflex associated with depressant effect of anesthesia and narcotic (opioid) analgesics; supine positioning; increased risk for gastroesophageal reflux associated with increased gastric pressure resulting from decreased gastrointestinal motility

FEAR NDx/ANXIETY NDx
Related to unfamiliar environment; pain; lack of understanding of surgical procedure performed; diagnosis and postoperative treatment plan; possible change to body image and roles; and financial concerns

5

The Client With Alterations in Respiratory Function

ASTHMA

Asthma is a chronic disorder characterized by intermittent and reversible obstruction of the airways. This airflow obstruction is caused by bronchial hyperresponsiveness and inflammation of the airway mucous membranes. Allergens enter the airway and initiate the inflammatory cascade. Mast cells found in the basement membranes of the bronchial walls degranulate and release inflammation response mediators, which cause increased capillary permeability and vasodilation, and recruitment of eosinophils, lymphocytes, and neutrophils. The response leads to the production of thick, tenacious mucus that blocks the airways. Combined with the bronchial hyperresponsiveness and capillary vasodilation and permeability, intake of air significantly decreases, and air is trapped in the lungs below the obstruction. Chronic inflammation leads to remodeling of the bronchial walls. The bronchial walls show hypertrophy, and mucus-producing cells undergo hyperplasia.

There are two types of asthma: allergic (caused by exposure to an allergen) and nonallergic (caused by stress, exercise, illnesses, or exposure to extreme weather). Asthma attacks are variable and unpredictable, range from mild to severe, and differ from client to client. Clinical manifestations of an asthma attack include dyspnea, wheezing, chest tightness, tachycardia, sweating, cough, tightening of neck muscles, and the use of accessory muscles to breathe. The client may also have an audible wheezing or whistling on exhalation. Indications that asthma is becoming worse include an increase in the frequency and severity of asthma attacks and an increased need to use bronchodilators.

There is no clear indication why some people get asthma and others, exposed to the same conditions, do not. It is possibly due to a combination of environmental and genetic factors. Triggers for an asthma attack also vary from client to client and may include airborne allergens and air pollutants, viral respiratory infections, cold air, stress, medications (i.e., nonsteroidal anti-inflammatory drugs [NSAIDs]), exercise, gastroesophageal reflex disease, smoke, and occupational factors.

Treatment of asthma is focused on prevention of symptoms. Treatment consists of two types of medications: quick-relief or rescue medications (beta$_2$-agonists, anticholinergics) and long-term control medications (inhaled corticosteroids, immunomodulators, antileukotrienes, long-acting inhaled beta$_2$-agonists). Immunotherapy (allergy shots) may also be beneficial.

This care plan focuses on care of the adult client with asthma who is hospitalized during an exacerbation of the illness. Much of the information is applicable to clients receiving follow-up care in an extended care facility or home setting.

OUTCOME/DISCHARGE CRITERIA

The client will:
1. Have improved respiratory function
2. Have vital signs within client's normal range
3. Tolerate expected level of activity
4. Develop an education plan for ordered medications including rationale, food and drug interactions, side effects, methods of administering, and importance of taking as prescribed
5. Demonstrate appropriate use of inhalers

Nursing Diagnosis **IMPAIRED RESPIRATORY FUNCTION***

Definition: **Ineffective Breathing Pattern NDx:** Inspiration and/or expiration that does not provide adequate ventilation; **Ineffective Airway Clearance NDx:** Inability to clear secretions or obstructions from the respiratory tract to maintain a clear airway; **Impaired Gas Exchange NDx:** Excess or deficit in oxygenation and/or carbon dioxide elimination at the alveolar–capillary membrane.

---

*This diagnostic label contains the following nursing diagnoses: Inneffective breathing pattern; ineffective airway clearance; and impaired gas exchange.

Ineffective breathing pattern NDx

Related to:

* Increased rate of respirations associated with fear and anxiety, and feeling of "air hunger"
* Decreased depth of respirations associated with weakness, fatigue, fear, and anxiety

Ineffective airway clearance NDx

Related to:

* Narrowing of the airways associated with:
  * Excessive mucus production, inflammation, and bronchospasm
  * Bronchial wall remodeling with bronchial hypertrophy and hyperplasia of mucus-secreting cells
* Stasis of secretions associated with:
  * Difficulty in coughing up secretions resulting from fatigue, weakness, and presence of tenacious secretions if fluid intake is inadequate
  * Impaired ciliary function resulting from loss of ciliated epithelium (occurs with inflammation, destruction, and fibrosis of bronchial walls)

Impaired gas exchange NDx

Related to:

* Narrowing or obstruction of the small airways

CLINICAL MANIFESTATIONS

Subjective	Objective
Verbal self-report of restlessness; irritability; somnolence; chronic cough; chest tightness	Rapid, shallow respirations; abnormal breath sounds—wheezing; cough; use of accessory muscles when breathing; significant decrease in oximetry results; abnormal arterial blood gas values; reduced activity tolerance; tachycardia

RISK FACTORS

* Genetics
* Smoking
* Allergies
* Environmental factors

DESIRED OUTCOMES

The client will maintain adequate respiratory function as evidenced by:

a. Usual rate and depth of respiration
b. Usual or improved breath sounds
c. Usual mental status
d. Oximetry results within normal range for client
e. Arterial blood gas values within normal range for client

NURSING OUTCOME CLASSIFICATIONS (NOC)

Respiratory status; airway patency; respiratory status: ventilation; respiratory status: gas exchange

NURSING INTERVENTIONS CLASSIFICATIONS (NIC)

Respiratory monitoring; airway management; chest physiotherapy; cough enhancement; oxygen therapy; medication administration; ventilation assistance; fear and anxiety reduction

NURSING ASSESSMENT	RATIONALE
Assess for signs and symptoms of impaired respiratory function: <ul><li>Rapid, shallow respirations</li><li>Dyspnea, orthopnea</li><li>Use of accessory muscles when breathing</li><li>Abnormal breath sounds (e.g., wheezes, crackles)</li><li>Cough effectiveness</li><li>Restlessness, irritability</li><li>Confusion, somnolence</li><li>Central cyanosis (a late sign)</li></ul>	*Early recognition of signs and symptoms of ineffective breathing patterns allows for prompt intervention.*
Assess arterial blood gas and pulse oximetry values and report abnormal findings.	*Oximetry is a noninvasive method of measuring arterial oxygen saturation. Allows for evaluation of client's current oxygenation status, so that appropriate supplemental oxygen therapy can be implemented.*

NDx = NANDA Diagnosis   **D** = Delegatable Action   ● = UAP   ✦ = LVN/LPN   ⊖▶ = Go to ⊖volve for animation

THERAPEUTIC INTERVENTIONS	RATIONALE

Independent Actions

Implement measures to improve respiratory status.

Place client in a semi-Fowler's position. **D** ● ✦

Positioning in semi-Fowler's position promotes optimal gas exchange by enabling chest expansion and diaphragm excursion.

Instruct client in breathing exercises focusing on hypoventilation, breath holding after exhalation, and breathing through the nose.

These techniques help clients decrease the need for beta$_2$-agonists and inhaled corticosteroids.

Instruct client in exercises involving shoulder rotations and arm lifts performed in sync with breathing.

This technique helps expand the lungs.

Discourage smoking.

The irritants in smoke increase mucus production, impair ciliary function, and can cause inflammation and damage to the bronchial and alveolar walls; the carbon monoxide decreases oxygen availability.

Maintain activity restrictions and increase activity as allowed and tolerated.

Conservation of energy through activity restrictions allows energy to be focused on breathing. Increasing activity as tolerated helps to mobilize secretions and promotes deeper breathing.

Perform actions to reduce fear and anxiety (e.g., assure client that staff members are nearby; respond to call signal as soon as possible; provide calm, restful environment; instruct in relaxation techniques). **D** ● ✦

The experience of anxiety during an asthma attack can exacerbate the attack.

Maintain client fluid intake of at least 2500 mL/day unless contraindicated. **D** ✦

Maintaining adequate hydration decreases the viscosity of secretions and improves ciliary action in removing secretions.

Dependent/Collaborative Actions

Implement measures to improve respiratory status.

Administer beta$_2$-adrenergic agonists inhaled during an acute attack and oral for ongoing therapy. **D** ✦

Beta$_2$-agonists are the treatment of choice for an asthma attack because they relax airway smooth muscles and decrease bronchoconstriction.

Administer and monitor oxygen as ordered.

Provides support for the respiratory system until it is able to function appropriately.

Administer Heliox (a helium/oxygen mixture).

The combination of helium and oxygen is lighter than air and easier to breathe when gas flow is compromised by bronchospasms.

Administer corticosteroids both inhaled and oral.

Corticosteroids decrease airway inflammation and thereby improve bronchial airflow.

Consult appropriate health care providers (respiratory therapist and physician) if signs and symptoms of impaired respiratory function persist or worsen.

Notifying the appropriate health care professionals allows for a multifaceted approach to treatment.

Nursing Diagnosis ## ACTIVITY INTOLERANCE NDx

Definition: Insufficient physiological or psychological energy to endure or complete required or desired daily activities.

Related to:

- Tissue hypoxia associated with impaired gas exchange
- Inadequate nutrition status
- Difficulty resting and sleeping associated with dyspnea, excessive coughing, fear, anxiety, frequent assessment and treatments, and side effects of medication therapy (e.g., some bronchodilators, corticosteroids)
- Increased energy expenditure associated with strenuous breathing efforts and persistent coughing

CLINICAL MANIFESTATIONS

Subjective	Objective
Verbal self-report of fatigue or weakness	Abnormal heart rate or blood pressure (B/P) response to activity; exertional discomfort or dyspnea; electrocardiographic changes reflecting dysrhythmias or ischemia; unable to speak with physical activity

RISK FACTORS
- Smoking
- Malnutrition
- Allergens
- Insomnia

DESIRED OUTCOMES

The client will demonstrate an increased tolerance for activity as evidenced by:
a. Verbalization of feeling less fatigued and weak
b. Ability to perform ADL without exertional dyspnea, chest pain, diaphoresis, dizziness, and significant changes in vital signs

NOC OUTCOMES

Activity tolerance; endurance, fatigue level; vital signs

NIC INTERVENTIONS

Activity therapy; energy management; oxygen therapy; nutrition management; sleep enhancement; teaching: prescribed medication; teaching: prescribed treatment

NURSING ASSESSMENT	RATIONALE
Assess for signs and symptoms of activity intolerance: • Statements of fatigue or weakness • Exertional dyspnea, chest pain, diaphoresis, or dizziness • Abnormal heart rate response to activity (e.g., increase in rate of 20 beats/min above resting rate, rate not returning to preactivity level within 3 minutes after stopping activity, change from regular to irregular rate) • Significant change of 15 to 20 mm Hg in B/P with activity.	*Early recognition of signs and symptoms of activity intolerance allows for prompt intervention.*

THERAPEUTIC INTERVENTIONS	RATIONALE
Independent Actions Implement measures to promote rest and/or conserve energy (e.g., maintain prescribed activity restrictions, minimize environmental activity and noise, provide uninterrupted rest periods, assist with care, keep supplies and personal articles within easy reach, keep daily log of periods of high and low energy; limit the number of visitors, use shower chair when showering, sit to brush teeth or comb hair). **D** ● ✦	*Cells use oxygen and fat, protein, and carbohydrates to produce the energy needed for all body activities. Rest and activities that conserve energy result in a lower metabolic rate, which preserves nutrients and oxygen for necessary activities. Performing daily tasks during high energy periods allows for effectiveness and productivity while allowing for periods of needed rest.*
Implement measures to promote sleep (e.g., elevate head of bed and support arms on pillows to facilitate breathing, maintain oxygen therapy during sleep, discourage intake of fluids high in caffeine in the evening, reduce environmental stimuli). **D** ✦	*Sleep replenishes a client's energy and feelings of well-being.*
Implement measures to decrease excessive coughing and frequency of asthma attacks (e.g., protect client from exposure to irritants such as smoke, flowers, and powder; avoid extremely hot or cold foods/fluids). **D** ● ✦	*Altered respiratory function such as excessive coughing can lead to inadequate tissue oxygenation, which results in less efficient energy production and a reduced ability to tolerate activity. Improving respiratory status increases the amount of oxygen available for energy production.*
Discourage smoking and excessive intake of beverages high in caffeine such as coffee, tea, and colas.	*Excessive intake of nicotine and caffeine can increase cardiac workload and myocardial oxygen utilization, thereby decreasing oxygen availability.*
Perform actions to improve respiratory status (e.g., place client in semi- to high-Fowler's position; instruct client to deep breathe or use incentive spirometry every 1 to 2 hrs; maintain bedrest as ordered; and use oxygen as needed). **D** ✦	*Improvement of respiratory status is done to relieve dyspnea, decrease frequency of asthma attacks, and improve tissue oxygenation.*
Perform actions to maintain adequate nutritional status (e.g., increase activity as tolerated potentially improving appetite; encourage a rest period before meals to reduce fatigue; assist with oral hygiene before meals; maintain a clean environment and a relaxed, pleasant atmosphere). **D** ● ✦	*Adequate nutritional status is important in order to maintain ADL.*

Continued...

THERAPEUTIC INTERVENTIONS	RATIONALE
Instruct a client to: • Report a change in the frequency and consistency of asthma attacks. • Report a decreased tolerance for activity. • Stop any activity that causes increased chest pain, increased shortness of breath, dizziness, or extreme fatigue or weakness.	*Changes in a client's activity tolerance should be reported immediately. Assessment of the change will allow for timely diagnosis of the cause and subsequent treatment.*
Dependent/Collaborative Actions Consult appropriate health care providers (e.g., respiratory therapist, physician, dietitian) if signs and symptoms of activity intolerance persist or worsen.	*Notifying the appropriate health care provider allows for modification of the treatment plan.*

DISCHARGE TEACHING/CONTINUED CARE

Nursing Diagnosis **DEFICIENT KNOWLEDGE NDx; INEFFECTIVE HEALTH MAINTENANCE NDx; OR INEFFECTIVE HEALTH MANAGEMENT* NDx**

Definition: **Deficient Knowledge NDx**: Absence of cognitive information related to a specific topic, or its acquisition; **Ineffective Health Maintenance NDx**: Inability to identify, manage, and/or seek out help to maintain well-being; **Ineffective Health Management NDx**: Pattern of regulating and integrating into daily living a therapeutic regimen for the treatment of illness and its sequelae that is unsatisfactory for meeting specific health goals.

CLINICAL MANIFESTATIONS

Subjective	Objective
Verbal self-report of inability to manage illness; verbalizes inability to follow prescribed regimen	Increased frequency and intensity of asthma attacks

RISK FACTORS

- Cognitive deficit
- Financial concerns
- Smoking
- Inability to care for oneself
- Difficulty in modifying personal habits and integrating treatments into lifestyle

DESIRED OUTCOMES

The client will demonstrate an appropriate level of knowledge to maintain well-being as evidenced by:
a. Correctly stating the signs and symptoms to report to the health care provider
b. Ability to perform activities of daily living (ADL) without exertional dyspnea, chest pain, diaphoresis, dizziness, and significant changes in vital signs

NURSING ASSESSMENT	RATIONALE
Assess client readiness and ability to learn Assess meaning of illness to client	*Early recognition of client's readiness to learn and meaning of their illness allows for implementation of the appropriate teaching interventions.*

NOC OUTCOMES	NIC INTERVENTIONS
Knowledge: treatment regimen; energy conservation; treatment procedure(s); health resources; adherence behavior; health beliefs	Health system guidance; teaching: individual; teaching: disease process; teaching: prescribed activity/exercise; teaching: prescribed medication; self-modification assistance; values clarification; medication management; smoking cessation assistance

THERAPEUTIC INTERVENTIONS	RATIONALE

Independent Actions

Instruct client in ways to maintain respiratory health:

- Maintain overall general good health (e.g., reduce stress, eat a well-balanced diet, obtain adequate rest).
- Stop smoking.
- Avoid exposure to respiratory irritants such as smoke, dust, aerosol sprays, paint fumes, and solvents; wear a mask or scarf over nose and mouth if exposure to high levels of these irritants is unavoidable.
- Remain indoors as much as possible when air pollution levels are high.
- Avoid extremes in hot and cold weather.

- Avoid prolonged close contact with persons who have respiratory infection.
- Receive immunizations against influenza and pneumococcal pneumonia.

Have client keep a log/diary of the frequency, duration, and intensity of asthma attacks, and morning peak flow rates.

Include significant others in explanations and teaching sessions and encourage their support.

Good general health supports the individual's ability to fight off infection.

The irritants in smoke and respiratory irritants increase mucus production, impair ciliary function, and can cause inflammation and damage to the bronchial and alveolar walls.

Air pollution in high levels is harmful to persons with existing lung disease.

Exposure to extreme hot and cold air may cause bronchoconstriction, allowing less air into and out of the lungs.

Increases a client's potential for a respiratory infection

Immunizations help prevent further respiratory disease.

Changes in the incidence of asthma attacks should be reported to the client's health care provider because they may indicate a change in the disease process, effectiveness of medications, and/or a concurrent illness.

Involvement of the client's significant others contributes to adherence to the treatment regimen.

THERAPEUTIC INTERVENTIONS	RATIONALE

Independent Actions

Educate the patient about the disease process and treatment of asthma:

- Explain asthma in terms the client can understand; stress that adherence to the treatment plan is necessary in order to prevent complications and reactivation of the disease.
- Explain that asthma can be treated, but only if the client adheres to the prescribed medication regimen.
- Provide written instructions about and encourage client to participate in the treatment plan.
- Provide client with written instructions about disease process, signs and symptoms to report, medication therapy, and follow-up appointments.

Explain the rationale for side effects of drugs, food and drug interactions, the importance of taking medications as prescribed, and drugs to manage side effects.

Examples of asthma medications:
- Corticosteroids
- Mast cell stabilizers
- Anticholinergics
- IgE antagonists
- Leukotriene modifiers
- Beta₂-Adrenergic agonists
- Methylxanthines

Assist client to develop a method to promote adherence to the medication schedule.
- Assist client to identify ways the medication regimen can be incorporated into the client's lifestyle.

Understanding of the disease and its treatment plan provides patients with a sense of control, and they will be more likely to comply with the treatment regimen.

Written instructions allow the client to refer to them as needed. The instructions should include all information needed to understand disease processes and treatment.

Knowledge of medications and how they impact the system improves client adherence and helps enhance the client's understanding of the importance of adhering to the prescribed medication regimen. The client must be able to recognize alterations in functioning related to medication administration.

Corticosteroids suppress inflammation and the normal immune process. Mast cell stabilizers decrease the frequency and intensity of allergic reactions. Anticholinergics provide adjunctive management of bronchospasms caused by asthma. IgE antagonists prevent the release of mediators of the allergic response. Leukotriene modifiers decrease the inflammatory process.

Beta blockers can promote bronchodilation and reduce airway inflammation that improves asthma control and improve symptoms.

Methylxanthines promote bronchodilation through relaxing the airways.

Knowledge of the medication regimen and the impact of these medications on the body, as well as how the medication regimen can be incorporated into the client's lifestyle, allows the client some mechanism of control of his/her disease and the ability to have an active part in treatment and care.

Continued...

THERAPEUTIC INTERVENTIONS	RATIONALE
Instruct client to take all medications as often as prescribed and avoid skipping doses or altering the prescribed dose; if a dose is missed, instruct client to take it as soon as remembered unless it is almost time for the next dose of the same medication.	*Consistent use of medication(s) is important in preventing asthma attacks.*
Teach the client how to use the different types of inhalers.	*Medication is not delivered to the lungs and remains in the oral pharynx when inhalers are used incorrectly, leading to infections in the oral pharynx.*
Reinforce the need to consult physician before discontinuing any medication or taking additional prescription and nonprescription medications.	*This is important to prevent exacerbations in asthma attacks.*
Provide information about and encourage utilization of community resources and social services that can assist client to comply with the medication regimen or to provide financial support if needed (e.g., local Department of Health and Human Services, local chapter of the American Lung Association, support groups).	*Provides for continuum of care and can help improve client adherence with the medication regimen and possibly financial assistance for medications.*

THERAPEUTIC INTERVENTIONS	RATIONALE

Independent Actions

THERAPEUTIC INTERVENTIONS	RATIONALE
Instruct client to report the following to the health care provider: • Persistent or recurrent loss of appetite, nausea, weakness, fatigue, or weight loss • Fever, chills, continued or increased night sweats • Difficulty in breathing, continued or increased cough, or chest pain • Unusual color, amount, and odor of vaginal secretions; white patches or ulcerated areas in mouth; stiff neck and headache; hoarseness; persistent sore throat; bone pain; swollen, red, painful joints; swollen lymph nodes • Signs and symptoms of adverse effects of medications	*These clinical manifestations indicate an infection or super infection and should be reported to the health care provider.*

THERAPEUTIC INTERVENTIONS	RATIONALE
The client in collaboration with the nurse will develop a plan for adhering to recommended follow-up care, including future appointments with health care providers and graded exercise programs.	

Independent Actions

Reinforce the importance of keeping appointments for follow-up tests (e.g., blood work, chest radiographs) and physical examinations to determine effectiveness of the medication regimen and assess for side effects.	*Regular health care appointments are important to determine effectiveness of the medication regimen and assess for side effects.*

ADDITIONAL NURSING DIAGNOSES

DISTURBED SLEEP PATTERN NDx
Related to fear, anxiety, unfamiliar environment, excessive coughing, frequent assessments and treatments, side effects of medications (e.g., some bronchodilators, corticosteroids), and inability to assume usual sleep position associated with orthopnea

RISK FOR POWERLESSNESS NDx
Related to physical limitations; disease progression despite efforts to comply with treatment plan; dependence on others to meet self-care needs; and alterations in roles, lifestyle, and future plans

FEAR NDx AND ANXIETY NDx
Related to fear associated with difficulty breathing, fear of death during an asthma attack, potential changes in lifestyle

CHRONIC OBSTRUCTIVE PULMONARY DISEASE

Chronic obstructive pulmonary disease (COPD) is an inflammatory lung disease characterized by the presence of airflow obstruction in the lungs. The airflow obstruction is chronic, usually progressive, and may be accompanied by airway hyperactivity. Other terms sometimes used to describe this condition are chronic obstructive lung disease (COLD) and chronic airflow limitation (CAL). Signs and symptoms usually include dyspnea, cough, and sputum production that worsen over time and during periodic exacerbations.

The two most common conditions that contribute to COPD are chronic bronchitis and emphysema. Chronic bronchitis is characterized by a cough that persists at least 3 months of the year for 2 consecutive years and an excessive production of mucus in the bronchi due to inflammation of the bronchioles and hypertrophy and hyperplasia of the mucous glands. In contrast, emphysema is characterized by dyspnea and a mild cough. The impaired airflow that occurs with emphysema is related to loss of lung elasticity, narrowing of the terminal non-respiratory bronchioles, and destructive changes in the walls of the alveolar and/or respiratory bronchioles. Both chronic bronchitis and emphysema are usually present in the person with COPD, although one of the two usually predominates.

Causative factors of COPD include chronic irritation of the lungs by cigarette smoke, exposure to air pollution and chemical irritants, and recurrent respiratory tract infections. In a small percentage of cases of emphysema, the destruction of lung tissue by proteolytic enzymes is a result of a genetic deficiency of alpha1-antitrypsin.

This care plan focuses on care of the adult client with COPD who is hospitalized during an acute exacerbation. Much of the information is applicable to clients receiving follow-up care in an extended care facility or home setting.

OUTCOME/DISCHARGE CRITERIA

The client will:
1. Have improved respiratory function
2. Tolerate expected level of activity
3. Have no signs and symptoms of complications
4. Identify ways to prevent or minimize further respiratory problems
5. Verbalize ways to maintain an optimal nutritional status
6. Identify ways to conserve energy and/or reduce dyspnea and fatigue
7. Demonstrate proper chest physiotherapy and use of respiratory equipment
8. Verbalize an understanding of medications ordered, including rationale, food and drug interactions, side effects, methods of administering, and importance of taking as prescribed
9. Identify precautions that should be adhered to when using oxygen
10. State signs and symptoms to report to the health care provider
11. Share feelings and thoughts about the effects of COPD on lifestyle and roles
12. Identify resources that can assist with financial needs, home management, and adjustment to changes resulting from COPD
13. Develop a plan for adhering to recommended follow-up care, including future appointments with health care provider and graded exercise program.

Nursing Diagnosis **IMPAIRED RESPIRATORY FUNCTION***

Definition: **Ineffective Breathing Pattern NDx**: Inspiration and/or expiration that does not provide adequate ventilation; **Ineffective Airway Clearance NDx**: Inability to clear secretions or obstructions from the respiratory tract to maintain a clear airway; **Impaired Gas Exchange NDx**: Excess or deficit in oxygenation and/or carbon dioxide elimination at the alveolar-capillary membrane.

Related to:

Ineffective breathing pattern NDx
Related to:
- Increased rate of respirations associated with fear and anxiety
- Decreased depth of respirations associated with weakness, fatigue, fear, anxiety, and presence of a flattened diaphragm (a result of prolonged hyperinflation of the lungs)

Ineffective airway clearance NDx
Related to:
- Narrowing of the airways associated with:
  - Excessive mucus production and inflammation and hyperplasia of the bronchial walls (especially with chronic bronchitis)
  - Destruction of the elastic fibers in the walls of the small airways (with emphysema)
- Stasis of secretions associated with:
  - Difficulty coughing up secretions resulting from fatigue, weakness, and presence of tenacious secretions if fluid intake is inadequate
  - Impaired ciliary function resulting from loss of ciliated epithelium (occurs with inflammation, destruction, and fibrosis of bronchial walls)
  - Decreased mobility

NDx = NANDA Diagnosis   **D** = Delegatable Action   ● = UAP   ✦ = LVN/LPN   ⊖▶ = Go to ⊖volve for animation

Impaired gas exchange NDx
Related to:
- Narrowing or obstruction of the small airways
- A decrease in effective lung surface (occurs as a result of collapse or destruction of alveolar walls)

CLINICAL MANIFESTATIONS

Subjective	Objective
Verbal self-report of confusion; disorientation; restlessness; irritability; somnolence; chest tightness	Rapid, shallow respirations; abnormal breath sounds; chronic cough; use of accessory muscles when breathing; increased anterior-posterior diameter; dyspnea; nasal flaring; central cyanosis (late sign); decreased expiratory and inspiratory pressure; decreased minute ventilation and vital capacity; significant decrease in oximetry results; abnormal arterial blood gas values; reduced activity tolerance

RISK FACTORS
- Smoking
- Obstruction of airways
- Excessive mucous production
- Impaired ciliary function
- Occupational dust and chemicals
- Alpha$_1$-Antitrypsin deficiency

DESIRED OUTCOMES

The client will maintain adequate respiratory function as evidenced by:
a. Usual rate and depth of respiration
b. Decreased dyspnea
c. Usual or improved breath sounds
d. Usual mental status
e. Oximetry results within normal range for client
f. Arterial blood gas values within the normal range for client

NOC OUTCOMES

Respiratory status: airway patency; ventilation; gas exchange

NIC INTERVENTIONS

Respiratory monitoring; airway management; chest physiotherapy; cough enhancement; oxygen therapy; medication administration; ventilation assistance; fear and anxiety reduction

NURSING ASSESSMENT	RATIONALE
Assess for signs and symptoms of impaired respiratory function:	*Early recognition of signs and symptoms of ineffective breathing patterns allows for prompt intervention.*
• Rapid, shallow respirations • Dyspnea, orthopnea • Use of accessory muscles when breathing	*Rapid, shallow respirations do not provide adequate ventilatory support. Difficulty with breathing and the need to sit up to breathe, as well as use of accessory muscles, lead to client fatigue and further decline in respiratory status.*
• Abnormal breath sounds (e.g., diminished or absent, rhonchi, wheezes)	*Changes in the characteristics of breath sounds may be due to airway obstruction, mucus plugs, or retained secretions in larger airways.*
• Cough effectiveness	*Muscle fatigue/weakness may impair effective clearance of secretions.*
• Restlessness, irritability • Confusion, somnolence	*Restlessness, irritability, and change in mental status of level of consciousness indicate an oxygen deficiency and require immediate treatment.*
• Central cyanosis (a late sign)	*The bluish discoloration of the skin and mucous membranes occurs in the presence deoxygenated hemoglobin (Hgb). This occurs when arterial oxygen saturation falls below 85% to 90%.*
Assess arterial blood gas and pulse oximetry values and report abnormal findings.	*Oximetry is a noninvasive method of measuring arterial oxygen saturation. The results assist in evaluating respiratory status. Decreasing PaO$_2$ and increasing CO$_2$ are indicators of respiratory problems.*

THERAPEUTIC INTERVENTIONS	**RATIONALE**

Independent Actions

Implement measures to improve respiratory status:

- Reduce fear and anxiety.

  Fear and anxiety can lead to shallow, rapid breathing.
- Maintain supportive environment.

  The client's anxiety may increase if left alone during periods of respiratory distress.
- Don't leave client during periods of acute respiratory distress.

  Decreases client's feelings of being in an enclosed area, which can increase anxiety.
- Open curtains and doors.

Place client in a semi-Fowler's position, and position overbed table so client can lean on it if desired. **D** ● ✦

Positioning in semi-Fowler's position promotes optimal gas exchange by enabling chest expansion. Leaning on the overbed table decreases dyspnea through pressure on the gastric contents and diaphragmatic contraction.

- Instruct client in and assist with diaphragmatic and pursed-lip breathing techniques.

  These techniques help clients slow their pace of breathing, which makes each breath more effective.
- Instruct client to deep breathe or use incentive spirometer every 1 to 2 hrs. **D** ✦

  Forced deep breathing and use of incentive spirometry will increase expansion of the lungs and improve the client's ability to clear mucus from the lungs. The technique may also improve the amount of oxygen that is able to penetrate deep into the lungs.

- Maintain client's fluid intake of at least 2500 mL/day unless contraindicated. **D** ✦

  Increased fluid intake promotes thinning of secretions and reduces dryness of the respiratory mucous membranes.
- Perform suctioning if needed. **D** ✦

  Suctioning removes secretions from the large airways. It also stimulates coughing, which helps clear airways of mucus and foreign matter.

- Instruct client to avoid intake of large meals, gas-forming foods (i.e., cauliflower, beans, cabbage, onions, etc.), and carbonated beverages.

  Gas-forming foods and carbonated beverages can cause abdominal bloating, which places pressure on the diaphragm and reduces lung expansion.
- Discourage smoking.

  The irritants in smoke increase mucus production, impair ciliary function, and can cause inflammation and damage to the bronchial and alveolar walls; carbon monoxide decreases oxygen availability.

Maintain activity restrictions and increase activity as allowed and tolerated. **D** ● ✦

Conservation of energy through activity restrictions allows energy to be focused on breathing. Increasing activity as tolerated helps to mobilize secretions and promotes deeper breathing.

Dependent/Collaborative Actions

Implement measures to improve respiratory status:

⊖▶ • Assist with administration of mucolytics and diluent or hydrating agents via nebulizer if ordered. **D** ✦

- • *Mucolytics and diluent or hydrating agents help liquefy secretions for more effective removal.*
- Avoid use of central nervous system (CNS) depressants. **D** ✦

  • *CNS depressants further depress respiratory status, exacerbating the client's condition.*
- Administer and monitor oxygen as ordered. **D** ✦

  • *Oxygen should be administered at low doses. Question orders for high concentration, since many persons with COPD are depending on hypoxemia as a stimulus to breathe.*

- Administer the following medications if ordered:
  - Bronchodilators
  - Corticosteroids
  - Antimicrobials
  - *Alpha₁*-Proteinase inhibitor

  Bronchodilators relax smooth muscles of the airway, thus improving air exchange in the lungs. Corticosteroids decrease airway inflammation and thereby improve bronchial airflow. Antimicrobials may be given to prevent or treat pneumonia. Administration of alpha₁-proteinase inhibitor may be required if the cause of emphysema is a genetic deficiency of alpha₁-antitrypsin.

Consult appropriate health care providers (respiratory therapist and physician) if signs and symptoms of impaired respiratory function persist or worsen.

Notifying the appropriate health care professionals allows for a multidisciplinary approach to treatment.

NDx = NANDA Diagnosis   **D** = Delegatable Action   ● = UAP   ✦ = LVN/LPN   ⊖▶ = Go to ⊖volve for animation

Nursing Diagnosis	**IMBALANCED NUTRITION: LESS THAN BODY REQUIREMENTS** NDx

Definition: Intake of nutrients insufficient to meet metabolic needs.

Related to:
- Decreased oral intake associated with:
  - Dyspnea, weakness, and fatigue
  - Nausea (can occur in response to noxious stimuli such as the sight of expectorated sputum and as a side effect of some medications)
  - Early satiety resulting from compression of the stomach by flattened diaphragm
- Increased metabolic needs associated with increased energy expenditure resulting from strenuous breathing efforts and persistent coughing

CLINICAL MANIFESTATIONS

Subjective	Objective
Verbal self-report of aversion to food; alteration in taste sensation	Weight loss; weight less than normal for client's age, height, and body frame; abnormal blood urea nitrogen (BUN) and low serum prealbumin levels; inflamed mucous membranes; pale conjunctiva; excessive hair loss; poor muscle tone

RISK FACTORS
- Lack of appetite
- Shortness of breath causing difficulty with eating
- Poor diet
- Lack of resources

DESIRED OUTCOMES

The client will maintain adequate nutrition status as evidenced by:
a. Weight within normal range for client
b. Normal BUN and serum prealbumin and albumin levels
c. Usual strength and activity tolerance
d. Healthy oral mucous membrane

NOC OUTCOMES

Nutritional status

NIC INTERVENTIONS

Nutritional monitoring; nutrition management; nutrition therapy

NURSING ASSESSMENT	RATIONALE
Assess for and report signs and symptoms of malnutrition: • Weight significantly below a client's usual weight or less than normal for client's age, height, and body frame • Abnormal BUN and low serum prealbumin and albumin levels • Increased weakness and fatigue • Sore, inflamed oral mucous membranes • Pale conjunctiva	*Early recognition of signs and symptoms of malnutrition allows for prompt intervention.* *Inadequate nutritional intake may be exhibited by significant weight loss or a weight that is less than normal for a client's age, height, and body frame. If a significant amount of weight loss occurs in a short period of time, this may be an indication of another disease process occurring.*

THERAPEUTIC INTERVENTIONS	RATIONALE

Independent Actions
Monitor percentage of meals and snacks client consumes. Report a pattern of inadequate intake. **D** ✦
Implement measures to maintain an adequate nutritional status:
• Perform actions to improve oral intake.
  • Implement measures to improve respiratory status.
 	
  • Schedule treatments that assist in mobilizing mucus (e.g., aerosol treatments, postural drainage therapy) at least 1 hr before or after meals.
	Monitoring a client's intake helps to identify when a patient is at risk for inadequate nutrition.
	
	Interventions that relieve dyspnea allow the patient to eat a meal without interruption or need to rest.
	Appropriate scheduling of treatments assists in decreasing nausea.

THERAPEUTIC INTERVENTIONS	RATIONALE
• Increase activity as allowed and tolerated. **D** ✦	*Activity usually promotes a sense of well-being and can help improve an individual's appetite.*
• Encourage a rest period before meals. **D** ● ✦	*Rest before a meal helps to minimize fatigue during a meal.*
• Eliminate noxious sights and odors from the environment; provide client with an opaque, covered container for expectorated sputum. **D** ● ✦	*Noxious sites and odors can inhibit the feeding center in the hypothalamus. By eliminating them, the client's intake may improve.*
• Maintain a clean environment and a relaxed, pleasant atmosphere. **D** ● ✦	*An aesthetic pleasing and relaxed environment may help improve clients' intake.*
• Provide oral hygiene before meals. **D** ● ✦	*Oral hygiene moistens the mouth, which makes it easier to chew and swallow; it also removes unpleasant tastes, which often improves the taste of foods and fluids.*
• Assist the client who is dyspneic in selecting foods that require little or no chewing.	*Because a person cannot swallow and breathe at the same time, relief of dyspnea increases the likelihood of maintaining a good oral intake. Foods that require little or no chewing are easier to eat and help maintain a client's nutritional status.*
• Serve frequent, small meals rather than large ones if client is weak, fatigues easily, or has a poor appetite. **D** ✦	*Providing small rather than large meals can enable a client who is weak or fatigues easily to finish a meal. Also, a client who has a poor appetite is often more willing to attempt to eat smaller meals because they seem less overwhelming than larger ones. If smaller meals are served, the number of meals per day should be increased to help ensure adequate nutrition.*
• Place client in a high-Fowler's position for meals. **D** ● ✦	*Because a person cannot swallow and breathe at the same time, relief of dyspnea increases the likelihood of maintaining a good oral intake.*
• Allow adequate time for meals; reheat foods/fluids if necessary. **D** ● ✦	*Clients who feel rushed during meals tend to become anxious, lose their appetite, and stop eating. Appetite is also suppressed if foods/fluids normally served hot or warm become cold and do not appeal to the client.*
• Limit fluid intake with meals (unless the fluid has high nutritional value). **D** ✦	*When the stomach becomes distended, its volume receptors stimulate the satiety center in the hypothalamus and clients reduce their oral intake. Drinking liquids with meals distends the stomach and may cause satiety before an adequate amount of food is consumed.*
• Ensure that meals are well balanced and high in essential nutrients; offer dietary supplements if indicated.	*Clients must consume a diet that is well balanced and high in essential nutrients in order to meet their nutritional needs. Dietary supplements are often needed to help accomplish this.*

Dependent/Collaborative Actions
Implement measures to maintain an adequate nutritional status:
- Perform actions to improve oral intake:

• Provide supplemental oxygen during meals. **D** ✦	*Supplemental oxygen therapy relieves dyspnea and the client's anxiety about and preoccupation with breathing efforts and increases the ability to focus on eating and drinking.*
• Obtain a dietary consult to assist the client in selecting foods/fluids that meet nutritional needs, are appealing, and adhere to personal and cultural preferences.	*Notifying the appropriate health care professionals allows for a multidisciplinary approach to treatment.*
• Administer vitamins and minerals if ordered. **D** ✦	*Administration of vitamins and minerals helps maintain nutritional status.*
Perform a calorie count if ordered. Report information to dietitian and physician.	*A calorie count provides information about the caloric and nutritional value of the foods/fluids the client consumes. The information obtained helps the dietitian and physician determine whether an alternative method of nutritional support is needed.*
Consult physician about an alternative method of providing nutrition (e.g., parenteral nutrition, tube feedings) if client does not consume enough food or fluids to meet nutritional needs.	*If the client's oral intake is inadequate, an alternative method of providing nutrients needs to be implemented.*

NDx = NANDA Diagnosis   **D** = Delegatable Action   ● = UAP   ✦ = LVN/LPN   ⊜▶ = Go to ⊜volve for animation

Nursing Diagnosis **ACTIVITY INTOLERANCE** NDx

Definition: Insufficient physiological or psychological energy to endure or complete required or desired daily activities.

Related to:
- Tissue hypoxia associated with impaired gas exchange
- Inadequate nutrition status
- Difficulty resting and sleeping associated with dyspnea, excessive coughing, fear, anxiety, frequent assessment and treatments, and side effects of medication therapy (e.g., some bronchodilators, corticosteroids)
- Increased energy expenditure associated with strenuous breathing efforts and persistent coughing

CLINICAL MANIFESTATIONS

Subjective	Objective
Verbal self-report of fatigue or weakness	Abnormal heart rate or B/P response to activity; exertional discomfort or dyspnea; electrocardiographic changes reflecting dysrhythmias or ischemia; unable to speak with physical activity

RISK FACTORS
- Exertional dyspnea
- Dyspnea during rest and sleep
- Anxiety and fear
- Increased energy expenditure—coughing and breathing efforts

DESIRED OUTCOMES

The client will demonstrate an increased tolerance for activity as evidenced by:
a. Verbalization of feeling less fatigued and weak
b. Ability to perform activities of daily living without exertional dyspnea, chest pain, diaphoresis, dizziness, and significant changes in vital signs

NOC OUTCOMES

Activity tolerance; endurance; fatigue level; vital signs; self-care: activities of daily living; energy conservation

NIC INTERVENTIONS

Activity therapy; energy management; oxygen therapy; nutrition management; sleep enhancement; cardiac care; cardiac rehabilitation; teaching prescribed exercise

NURSING ASSESSMENT

Assess for signs and symptoms of activity intolerance:
- Statements of fatigue or weakness
- Exertional dyspnea, chest pain, diaphoresis, or dizziness
- Abnormal heart rate response to activity (e.g., increase in rate of 20 beats/min above resting rate, rate not returning to preactivity level within 3 minutes after stopping activity, change from regular to irregular rate)
- Significant change of 15 to 20 mm Hg in B/P with activity.

RATIONALE

Early recognition of signs and symptoms of activity intolerance allows for prompt intervention and treatment.

THERAPEUTIC INTERVENTIONS

Independent Actions
Implement measures to promote rest and/or conserve energy (e.g., maintain prescribed activity restrictions, minimize environmental activity and noise, provide uninterrupted rest periods, assist with care, keep supplies and personal articles within easy reach, limit the number of visitors, use shower chair when showering, sit to brush teeth or comb hair). **D** ● ✦

Implement measures to promote sleep (e.g., elevated head of bed and support arms on pillows to facilitate breathing, discourage intake of fluids high in caffeine in the evening, and reduce environmental stimuli). **D** ✦

RATIONALE

Cells use oxygen and fat, protein, and carbohydrates to produce the energy needed for all body activities. Rest and activities that conserve energy result in a lower metabolic rate, which preserves nutrients and oxygen for necessary activities.

Sleep replenishes a client's energy and feeling of well-being.

THERAPEUTIC INTERVENTIONS	**RATIONALE**
Implement measures to decrease excessive coughing (e.g., protect client from exposure to irritants such as smoke, flowers, and powder; avoid extremely hot or cold foods/fluids). **D** ● ✦	*Altered respiratory function such as excessive coughing can lead to inadequate tissue oxygenation, which results in less efficient energy production and a reduced ability to tolerate activity. Improving respiratory status increases the amount of oxygen available for energy production.*
Discourage smoking and excessive intake of beverages high in caffeine such as coffee, tea, and colas.	*Excessive intake of nicotine and caffeine can increase cardiac workload and myocardial oxygen utilization, thereby decreasing oxygen availability.*
Perform actions to improve respiratory status (e.g., place client in semi- to high-Fowler's position; assist client to deep breathe or use incentive spirometry every 1 to 2 hrs; maintain bedrest as ordered; and use oxygen as needed). **D** ● ✦	*Improvement of respiratory status through increased lung expansion.*
Perform actions to maintain adequate nutritional status (e.g., increase activity as tolerated, potentially improving appetite; encourage a rest period before meals to reduce fatigue; assist with oral hygiene before meals; maintain a clean environment and a relaxed pleasant atmosphere). **D** ✦	*Adequate nutritional status is important in order to maintain ADL.*
Increase client's activity gradually as allowed and tolerated. **D** ✦	*Gradual increase will slowly improve strength and ability in performance of activities.*
Instruct a client to: • Report a decreased tolerance for activity. • Stop any activity that causes increased chest pain, increased shortness of breath, dizziness, or extreme fatigue or weakness.	*Changes in a client's activity tolerance should be reported immediately. Assessment of the change will allow for timely diagnosis of the cause and subsequent treatment.*
Dependent/Collaborative Actions	
Consult appropriate health care providers (e.g., respiratory therapist, physician, dietitian) if signs and symptoms of activity intolerance persist or worsen.	*Notifying the appropriate health care provider allows for modification of the treatment plan.*

Nursing Diagnosis **RISK FOR INFECTION** NDx **(PNEUMONIA)**

Definition: Susceptible to invasion and multiplication of pathogenic organisms, which may compromise health.

Related to:
- Stasis of secretions in the lungs (secretions provide a good medium for bacterial growth)
- Inhalation of pathogens (especially if client is using respiratory equipment or medication delivery devices that are not being cleaned adequately or routinely)

CLINICAL MANIFESTATIONS

Subjective	**Objective**
Verbal self-report of pleuritic pain	Increased respiratory rate; dyspnea; abnormal breath sounds (crackles, rales); productive cough with purulent green or rust-colored sputum; chills and diaphoresis; fever; elevated white blood cell (WBC) count; significant decrease in pulse oximetry values; worsening arterial blood gas values

RISK FACTORS

- Stasis of secretions
- Inhalation of pathogens
- Debilitated state
- Smoking

DESIRED OUTCOMES

The client will not develop pneumonia as evidenced by:
a. Usual breath sounds and percussion note over lungs
b. Absence of tachypnea
c. Cough productive of clear mucus only
d. Afebrile status
e. WBC count within normal range
f. Arterial blood gas values within normal range for client
g. Negative sputum culture
h. Ability to perform ADL without increased dyspnea, chest pain, diaphoresis, dizziness, and a significant change in vital signs

NOC OUTCOMES

Infection severity; immune status

NIC INTERVENTIONS

Infection protection; infection control; cough enhancement; airway management

NURSING ASSESSMENT

Assess for and report signs and symptoms of pneumonia:
- Abnormal breath sounds (e.g., crackles [rales], pleural friction rub, bronchial breath sounds, diminished or absent breath sounds)
- Dull percussion note over the affected lung area
- Increase in respiratory rate
- Cough productive of purulent, green, or rust-colored sputum
- Chills and fever
- Pleuritic pain
- Elevated WBC count
- Significant decrease in oximetry results
- Worsening of arterial blood gas values
- Positive sputum culture results
- Chest radiograph results indicative of pneumonia

RATIONALE

Early recognition of signs and symptoms of pneumonia allows for prompt intervention.

THERAPEUTIC INTERVENTIONS

Independent Actions

Implement measures to prevent pneumonia:
- Perform actions to improve respiratory status (e.g., place client in semi- to high-Fowler's position; assist client to deep breathe or use incentive spirometer every 1 to 2 hrs; improve activity tolerance; maintain fluid intake of at least 2500 mL/day unless contraindicated). **D** ✦
- Protect client from persons with respiratory tract infections. **D** ✦
- Encourage and assist client to perform frequent oral hygiene. **D** ● ✦
- Replace or cleanse equipment used for respiratory care as often as needed.
- Instruct and assist client to rinse and clean medication delivery devices (e.g., dry powder inhaler, metered-dose inhaler, spacer) according to manufacturer's instructions.

Dependent/Collaborative Actions

If signs and symptoms of pneumonia occur, administer antimicrobials as ordered. **D** ✦

Consult other health care providers at the first signs and symptoms of an infection.

RATIONALE

Positioning the client in semi- to high-Fowler's position promotes optimal gas exchange by enabling chest expansion. Forced deep breathing and use of incentive spirometry will increase expansion of the lungs and improve the client's ability to clear mucus from the lungs. Maintaining fluid intake will help liquefy secretions for expectoration.

The potential for illness is decreased through avoidance of persons with respiratory infections and crowds during the cold and flu season.

Frequent oral hygiene helps to decrease the rate of infection through removal of pathogens and secretions that could be aspirated.

Equipment that is inadequately or incompletely cleaned after use harbors bacteria may lead to a respiratory infection.

Inhaled medication devices only deliver a certain percentage of the medication to the lungs. The rest of the medication is deposited in the oropharynx, which with some medications, increases the risk for infection, dysphonia, and/or candidiasis.

Early administration of antibiotics at the first sign of infection can decrease the impact and duration of the infection.

Notifying the appropriate health care provider allows for modification of the treatment plan.

Collaborative Diagnosis RISK FOR RIGHT-SIDED HEART FAILURE

Definition: A condition where the right side of the heart is unable to pump blood efficiently to meet the body's requirements.

Related to:
- Increased cardiac workload associated with:
  - Pulmonary hypertension (can result from pulmonary vasoconstriction that occurs in response to hypoxia and the release of vasoactive substances)
  - Compensatory response to decreased pulmonary blood flow that results from compression of the pulmonary capillaries by hyperinflated alveoli (with emphysema) and loss of large portions of the pulmonary vascular bed (occurs in emphysema as a result of destruction of the alveolar walls)

CLINICAL MANIFESTATIONS

Subjective	Objective
Reports of weakness and fatigue	Tachypnea; tachycardia; dyspnea; restlessness; confusion; irritability; peripheral edema; decreased urine output; distended neck veins

RISK FACTORS
- Hypertension
- Chronic respiratory disease
- Smoking
- Obesity

DESIRED OUTCOMES

The client will not develop right-sided heart failure as evidenced by:
a. Pulse rate of 60 to 100 beats/min
b. Usual mental status
c. Usual strength and activity tolerance
d. Adequate urine output
e. Stable weight
f. Absence of edema and distended neck veins

NURSING ASSESSMENT	RATIONALE
Assess for and report signs and symptoms of right-sided heart failure: • Further increase in pulse rate • Restlessness, confusion • Weakness and fatigue • Decreased urine output • Weight gain • Dependent peripheral edema • Distended neck veins • Chest radiograph results showing cardiomegaly	*Early recognition of signs and symptoms of right-sided heart failure allows for prompt intervention.*

THERAPEUTIC INTERVENTIONS	RATIONALE
Dependent/Collaborative Actions Implement measures to improve respiratory status (e.g., cough and deep breathe every 2–3 hrs, ambulate as tolerated, maintain fluid restriction).	*These interventions will reduce cardiac workload and the subsequent risk of right-sided heart failure by decreasing the pressure against which the heart must pump.*
If signs and symptoms of right-sided heart failure occur • Maintain oxygen therapy as ordered.	*Supplemental O_2 helps relieve dyspnea and improves gas exchange.*
Maintain client on strict bedrest in a semi-Fowler's to high-Fowler's position.	*Placing the client on strict bedrest will help conserve energy during periods of acute respiratory distress. Positioning the client in a semi- to high-Fowler's position promotes optimal gas exchange by enabling chest expansion.*
• Maintain fluid and sodium restrictions if ordered	*Restricting a client's sodium and fluid intake will help reduce fluid volume overload.*

Continued...

THERAPEUTIC INTERVENTIONS	RATIONALE
• Administer medications that may reduce vascular congestion and/or cardiac workload (e.g., diuretics, cardiotonics, vasodilators).	*Diuretics decrease fluid volume through inhibiting reabsorption of water, which decreases fluid volume.* *Cardiotonics increase the contractile force of the heart, which increases cardiac output.* *Vasodilators dilate the arterioles, which decreases B/P and decreases the work of the heart.*

Nursing Diagnosis **FEAR** NDx/**ANXIETY** NDx

Definition: Fear NDx: Response to perceived threat that is consciously recognized as a danger.

Anxiety NDx: Vague, uneasy feeling of discomfort or dread accompanied by an autonomic response (the source is often nonspecific or unknown to the individual); a feeling of apprehension caused by anticipation of danger. It is an alerting sign that warns of impending danger and enables the individual to take measures to deal with that threat.

Related to:
- Exacerbation of symptoms (e.g., increased dyspnea, feeling of suffocation), need for hospitalization, and concern about prognosis
- Lack of understanding of the diagnosis, diagnostic tests, treatments, and prognosis
- Financial concerns about hospitalization and lifelong treatment
- Feeling of lack of control over the progression of COPD and its effects on lifestyle and roles

CLINICAL MANIFESTATIONS

Subjective	Objective
Verbal self-report of anxiety and fear	Unusual sleep patterns; relaxed facial expressions and body movements; stable vital signs; restlessness; shakiness; diaphoresis; self-focused behavior

RISK FACTORS
- Shortness of breath
- Feelings of suffocation
- Fear of dying

DESIRED OUTCOMES

The client will experience a reduction in fear and anxiety as evidenced by:
a. Verbalization of feeling less anxious
b. Usual sleep pattern
c. Relaxed facial expression and body movements
d. Stable vital signs
e. Usual perceptual ability and interactions with others

NOC OUTCOMES

Anxiety level; fear level; anxiety self-control; fear self-control

NIC INTERVENTIONS

Anxiety reduction; calming technique; emotional support; presence; pain management

NURSING ASSESSMENT	RATIONALE
Assess client for signs and symptoms of fear and anxiety (e.g., verbalization of feeling anxious, insomnia, tenseness, shakiness, restlessness, diaphoresis, elevated B/P, tachycardia, self-focused behaviors). Validate perceptions carefully, remembering that some behavior may result from hypoxia and/or hypercapnia.	*Moderate anxiety enhances the client's ability to solve problems. With severe anxiety or panic, the client is not able to follow directions and may become hyperactive and extremely agitated.* *Assessment of the client's fear helps determine whether the coping mechanisms are effective and which need to be strengthened.*

THERAPEUTIC INTERVENTIONS	**RATIONALE**

Independent Actions

Implement measures to reduce fear and anxiety:

- Orient client to hospital environment, equipment, and routines. **D** ● ✦

Familiarity with the environment and usual routines reduces the client's anxiety about the unknown, provides a sense of security, and increases the client's sense of control, all of which help decrease anxiety.

- Introduce staff who will be participating in client's care. If possible, maintain consistency in staff assigned to client's care.

Introduction to staff familiarizes clients with those individuals who will be working with them, which provides clients with a feeling of stability, which reduces the anxiety that typically occurs with change.

- Assure client that staff members are nearby; respond to call signal as soon as possible. **D** ● ✦

Close contact and a prompt response to requests provide a sense of security and facilitate the development of trust, thus reducing the client's anxiety.

- Maintain a calm, supportive, confident manner when interacting with client; encourage verbalization of fear and anxiety.

A sense of calmness and confidence conveys to the client that someone is in control of the situation, which helps reduce anxiety.

- Reinforce physician's explanations and clarify misconceptions the client has about the disease process, treatment plan, and possible recurrence; encourage questions.

Factual information and an awareness of what to expect help decrease the anxiety that arises from uncertainty.

Implement measures to reduce respiratory distress if present:

- Elevate the head of the bed.
- Encourage the client to breathe deeply and more slowly. **D** ● ✦

Improvement of respiratory status helps relieve anxiety associated with the feeling of not being able to breathe.

- Implement measures to reduce pain:
  - Instruct client in relaxation techniques and encourage participation in diversional activities once the period of acute pain and respiratory distress has subsided.

Pain can create or increase anxiety because it is often perceived as a threat to well-being.

Pain also causes sympathetic nervous system stimulation with subsequent feelings of tenseness and increased anxiety.

- When appropriate, assist the client to meet spiritual needs (e.g., arrange for a visit from the clergy).

Spiritual support is a source of comfort and security for many people and can help reduce the client's fear and anxiety.

- Provide information based on current needs of client at a level that can be understood.
  - Encourage the client to ask questions and to seek clarification of information provided.

Providing information that the client is not ready to process or cannot understand tends to increase anxiety.

Making the client feel comfortable enough to ask questions or clarify information helps reduce anxiety.

- Provide a calm, restful environment. **D** ● ✦

A calm, restful environment facilitates relaxation and promotes a sense of security, which reduces fear and anxiety.

- Encourage significant others to project a caring, concerned attitude without obvious fear and anxiousness.

Anxiety is easily transferable from one person to another. If significant others convey empathy, provide reassurance, and do not appear anxious, they can help reduce the client's fear and anxiety.

Dependent/Collaborative Actions

Implement measures to reduce fear and anxiety:

- Administer oxygen via nasal cannula rather than mask if possible. **D** ✦

The use of a mask for some clients seems restrictive and suffocating. The use of a nasal cannula is more comfortable and less constraining. Improvement of respiratory status helps relieve anxiety associated with the feeling of not being able to breathe.

- Administer prescribed antianxiety agents if indicated. **D** ✦

Decreases anxiety.

Consult appropriate health care provider (e.g., psychiatric nurse clinician, physician) if the previously listed actions fail to control fear and anxiety.

Notifying the appropriate health care provider allows for modification of the treatment plan.

NDx = NANDA Diagnosis   **D** = Delegatable Action   ● = UAP   ✦ = LVN/LPN   ⊝▶ = Go to ⊝volve for animation

---

| Nursing Diagnosis | **INEFFECTIVE HEALTH MANAGEMENT** NDx |

Definition: Pattern of regulating and integrating into daily living a therapeutic regimen for the treatment of illness and its sequelae of illness that is unsatisfactory for meeting specific health goals.

CLINICAL MANIFESTATIONS

Subjective	Objective
Verbal self-report of inability to manage illness and/or follow prescribed regimen	Inaccurate follow-through with instructions; inappropriate behaviors; experience of preventable complications of COPD; frequent exacerbation of illness

RISK FACTORS
- Cognitive impairment
- Insufficient resources
- Feeling of lack of control over disease progression
- Difficulty modifying personal habits (e.g., smoking) and integrating necessary treatments into lifestyle

DESIRED OUTCOMES

The client will demonstrate the probability of effective self-health management as evidenced by:
a. Willingness to learn about and participate in treatments and care
b. Statements reflecting ways to modify personal habits and integrate treatments into lifestyle
c. Statements reflecting an understanding of the implications of not following the prescribed treatment plan

NOC OUTCOMES

Adherence behavior; health beliefs; knowledge: treatment regimen

NIC INTERVENTIONS

Self-modification assistance; values clarification; teaching: disease process; health system guidance; financial resource assistance; medication management; smoking cessation assistance

NURSING ASSESSMENT	RATIONALE

Assess client's knowledge base related to the disease process.

Assess for indications that the client may be unable to effectively manage the therapeutic regimen:
- Statements reflecting inability to manage care at home
- Failure to adhere to treatment plan (e.g., refusing to use proper breathing techniques, refusing medications)
- Statements reflecting a lack of understanding of factors that may cause further progression of COPD
- Statements reflecting an unwillingness or inability to modify personal habits and integrate necessary treatments into lifestyle
- Statements reflecting view that the COPD is incurable or that the situation is hopeless, and efforts to comply with the treatment plan are useless

The client's knowledge base provides the basis for education.

Early recognition of inability to understand disease process or self-care allows for change in teaching modality.

THERAPEUTIC INTERVENTIONS	RATIONALE

Independent Actions
Implement measures to promote effective therapeutic regimen management:
- Explain COPD in terms the client can understand; stress that COPD is a chronic condition, and adherence to the treatment program is necessary.
- Encourage questions and clarify misconceptions client has about COPD and its effects.

The client should understand that COPD is a chronic illness, and adherence to the treatment program is necessary in order to delay and/or prevent complications; however, caution client that some complications may occur despite strict adherence to treatment plan.

Everyone does not understand the information as presented. Questioning allows for clarification and for clients to put the information within a context they understand.

THERAPEUTIC INTERVENTIONS	RATIONALE
• Encourage client to participate in treatment plan (e.g., postural drainage therapy, breathing exercises).	*Client involvement in care helps reinforce the individual's understanding of lifestyle changes necessary to maintain health status.*
• Consult occupational and/or physical therapist if indicated about a home evaluation to identify assistive devices and necessary environmental modifications.	*Involvement of a variety of individuals on the health care team allows for a multifaceted plan of care and discharge planning that assists clients to be more independent in their living situation.*
• Assist client to develop a system for recording frequency of use of medications and respiratory treatments in order to avoid omission of those that should be used routinely and to avoid excessive use of those that should be used on an "as needed" basis (in times of respiratory distress, the client may tend to overuse medications because of fear, anxiety, and impaired cognition).	*Adherence to the medication regimen is required to improve and/or maintain the client's health status. Working with the client to develop a system for monitoring the medication regimen improves the potential for adherence.*
• Provide client with written instructions about chest physiotherapy, ways to prevent further respiratory problems, prescribed medications, signs and symptoms to report, where to obtain needed equipment and supplies, and future appointments with health care provider.	*Written instructions provide the client with information as a reference to use as needed.*
• Assist client to identify ways treatments can be incorporated into lifestyle; focus on modifications of lifestyle rather than complete change (e.g., statements reflecting plans for integrating treatments into lifestyle, active participation in treatment plan, changes in personal habits).	*To improve the potential for adherence to the treatment/medication regimen, the client must be actively involved in how/when and what lifestyle modifications are implemented. An individual's chance of success is decreased if one has to make a total lifestyle change.*
• Encourage client to discuss concerns regarding cost of hospitalization, medications, oxygen equipment, and follow-up care; obtain a social service consult to assist with financial planning and to obtain financial aid if indicated.	*Financial concerns play a large part in an individual's ability to adhere to a treatment regimen. Involvement of social services may be required to obtain financial assistance needed by the patient.*
• Provide information about and encourage utilization of community resources that can assist the client to make necessary lifestyle changes (e.g., American Lung Association; pulmonary rehabilitation groups; counseling, vocational, and social services; smoking cessation programs).	*Knowledge of community resources provides ongoing support and access to resources outside the acute care facility.*
• Include significant others in explanations and teaching sessions, and encourage their support; reinforce the need for the client to assume responsibility for managing as much of care as possible.	*Involvement of significant others in client teaching improves adherence to discharge instructions and lifestyle changes.*

Dependent/Collaborative Actions

Consult appropriate health care provider about referrals to community health agencies if continued instruction, support, or supervision is needed.	*Consult health care providers in the community for a continuum of care postdischarge.*

DISCHARGE TEACHING/CONTINUED CARE

Nursing Diagnosis **DEFICIENT KNOWLEDGE** NDx **OR INEFFECTIVE HEALTH MAINTENANCE*** NDx

Definition: **Deficient Knowledge NDx**: Absence of cognitive information related to a specific topic, or its acquisition.
Ineffective Health Maintenance NDx: Inability to identify, manage, and/or seek help to maintain well-being.

CLINICAL MANIFESTATIONS

Subjective	Objective
Verbal self-report of the problem	Inaccurate follow-through of instructions; inappropriate behaviors

*The nurse should set the diagnostic label that is most appropriate for the client's discharge teaching needs.

NDx = NANDA Diagnosis   **D** = Delegatable Action   ● = UAP   ✦ = LVN/LPN   ⊜▶ = Go to ⊖volve for animation

RISK FACTORS
- **Denial** of disease process
- **Cognitive** deficiency
- **Failure** to take action to reduce risk factors

NOC OUTCOMES	NIC INTERVENTIONS
Knowledge: treatment regimen; energy conservation; **treatment** procedure(s); health resources	Health system guidance; teaching: individual; teaching: disease process; teaching: prescribed activity/exercise; teaching: prescribed medication

NURSING ASSESSMENT	RATIONALE
Assess client understanding of illness and treatment plan. Assess client's ability and readiness to learn. Assess client's understanding of teaching.	*Learning is more effective when client is motivated and understands the importance of what is to be learned.* *Readiness to learn changes based on situations and physical and emotional challenges.*

THERAPEUTIC INTERVENTIONS	RATIONALE

Desired Outcome: The client will identify ways to prevent or minimize further respiratory problems.

Independent Actions

• Instruct client in ways to prevent or minimize further respiratory problems. • Maintain overall general good health (e.g., reduce stress, eat a well-balanced diet, obtain adequate rest, adhere to prescribed graded exercise program). • Stop smoking.	*There are a variety of ways a client can maintain general good health and support interventions focusing on the respiratory system.* *The irritants in smoke increase mucus production, impair ciliary function, and can cause inflammation and damage to the bronchial and alveolar walls; the carbon monoxide decreases oxygen availability.*
• Avoid exposure to respiratory irritants such as smoke, dust, some perfumes, aerosol sprays, paint fumes, and solvents; wear a mask or scarf over nose and mouth if exposure to high levels of irritants, such as smoke, fumes, and dust, is unavoidable.	*Exposure to respiratory irritants increases the risk of infection and impacts ciliary function.*
• Remain indoors when air pollution levels and/or pollen counts are high and/or outdoor temperatures are extremely hot or cold. • Exposure to extreme hot and cold air may cause broncho-constriction, allowing less air into and out of the lungs. • Avoid high altitudes; if air travel is required, consult physician about the need for supplemental oxygen.	*Air pollution in high levels is harmful to persons with existing lung disease.* *The oxygen content at high altitudes is decreased, which may cause significant dyspnea if supplemental oxygen is not available.*
• Adhere to chest physiotherapy (e.g., breathing exercises, postural drainage therapy) as ordered. • Take medications such as bronchodilators and mucolytics as prescribed. • Avoid contact with persons who have respiratory tract infections; avoid crowds and poorly ventilated areas; receive immunizations against influenza and pneumococcal pneumonia. • Drink at least 10 glasses of liquid per day unless contra-indicated. • Take antimicrobials as prescribed (some physicians instruct clients to begin antimicrobial therapy if sputum color becomes yellow or green).	*Chest physiotherapy is important to handle secretions and maintain positive respiratory status.* *Adherence to medication regimen is important to maintain and improve respiratory status.* *These actions decrease the client's risk of infection.* *Adequate fluid intake is necessary to liquefy secretions.* *Early treatment of infections may decrease the severity of the impact on the client with COPD.*

THERAPEUTIC INTERVENTIONS	RATIONALE
• Clean medication administration devices (e.g., metered-dose inhaler, dry powder inhaler, spacer, table-top nebulizer), oxygen delivery devices (e.g., mask, nasal cannula), humidifier, and air filters as instructed by health care provider and manufacturer.	*Equipment that is inadequately cleaned after use harbors bacteria, which may lead to an infection. Inhaled medication devices only deliver a certain percentage of the medication to the lungs. The rest of the medication is deposited in the oropharynx, which with some medications, increases the risk for infection, dysphonia, and/or candidiasis.*

THERAPEUTIC INTERVENTIONS	RATIONALE

Desired Outcome: The client will verbalize ways to maintain an optimal nutritional status.

Independent Actions
Provide instructions regarding ways to maintain an optimal nutritional status:

• Rest before meals; do the majority of food preparation in advance rather than just before eating.	*Preparing food in advance of eating and adequate rest before meals decrease fatigue that may occur when eating.*
• Perform good oral hygiene before meals.	*Good oral hygiene reduces unpleasant tastes in the mouth and moistens the mouth, making it easier to chew and swallow.*
• Eat sitting down in a pleasant environment.	*Eating in a pleasant environment helps increase a client's appetite.*
• Eat foods that require little or no chewing when energy is low and/or dyspnea is increased.	*Because a person cannot swallow and breathe at the same time, relief of dyspnea increases the likelihood of maintaining a good oral intake. Foods that require little or no chewing will be easier to eat and help maintain a client's nutritional status.*
• Eat meals that are well balanced; drink nutritional supplements if needed to maintain an adequate caloric intake.	*Clients must consume a diet that is well balanced and high in essential nutrients in order to meet their nutritional needs. Dietary supplements are often needed to help accomplish this.*

Dependent/Collaborative Actions
Provide instructions regarding ways to maintain an optimal nutritional status:

• Use supplemental oxygen via nasal cannula during meals if needed.	*Relief of dyspnea through the use of oxygen therapy decreases the client's anxiety about and preoccupation with breathing efforts and increases the ability to focus on eating and drinking.*
• Take vitamins and minerals as prescribed.	*Administration of vitamins and minerals helps maintain nutritional status.*
• Consult a dietician.	*To develop a nutritional plan that meets client's caloric needs.*

THERAPEUTIC INTERVENTIONS	RATIONALE

Desired Outcome: The client will identify ways to conserve energy and/or reduce dyspnea and fatigue.

Independent Actions
Instruct client in ways to conserve energy and/or reduce dyspnea and fatigue:

• Sit rather than stand during activities such as preparing food, rinsing dishes, ironing, showering, shaving, and talking on the phone.	*Each of these actions is a method of conserving energy during a variety of activities.*
• Have most frequently used food items, dishes, cleaning supplies, and clothing at waist level whenever possible rather than on high or low shelves.	
• Pace yourself during any activity; stop, relax your muscles, and take a few deep breaths as often as needed.	
• Simplify your life whenever possible; spread large projects over several days or weeks.	
• Allow others to assist you with or actually do strenuous or lengthy tasks.	

Continued...

THERAPEUTIC INTERVENTIONS	RATIONALE

- Modify activities to avoid bending, reaching, and raising arms whenever possible (e.g., use long-handled assistive devices, simplify hair style so that it does not need to be blow-dried or curled, sit with elbows resting on table while shaving).
- Do not try to carry on a conversation during activities that also require energy (e.g., walking, eating, cleaning, gardening).
- Use bronchodilators before activity as needed and prescribed.
- Use oxygen during activity as needed and prescribed; have portable oxygen system readily available.
- Use positions that minimize energy expenditure during sexual activity (e.g., side-lying).

THERAPEUTIC INTERVENTIONS	RATIONALE

Desired Outcome: The client will demonstrate proper chest physiotherapy and use of respiratory equipment.

Independent Actions

Reinforce instructions about proper breathing techniques (e.g., pursed-lip breathing, diaphragmatic breathing), postural drainage therapy (may be indicated if large amounts of mucus continue to be produced), and use of respiratory equipment (e.g., oxygen, incentive spirometer).

A variety of techniques and therapy are required for clients with COPD to maintain their health status.

Allow time for questions, clarification, and return demonstration.

Making the client feel comfortable enough to ask questions or clarify information and to provide a return demonstration will help improve adherence to treatment regimens.

THERAPEUTIC INTERVENTIONS	RATIONALE

Desired Outcome: The client will verbalize an understanding of medications ordered including rationale, food and drug interactions, side effects, methods of administration, and importance of taking as prescribed.

Independent Actions

Explain the rationale for, side effects of, and importance of taking medications prescribed.

A client's understanding of why medications are required, their side effects, and the importance of taking them as prescribed will promote adherence.

Inform client of pertinent food and drug interactions.

Clients need to understand what type of foods and other medications may impact their respiratory medications.

Have blood levels evaluated periodically, if indicated.

There are many medications where a blood level is required. The client needs to be aware of the importance of having these levels monitored to ensure appropriate dosing and to prevent toxic levels.

If client is discharged on medications via inhalation:

- Provide information about the proper use, cleaning, and replacement of the medication delivery devices (e.g., nebulizer, dry powder inhaler, metered-dose inhaler, spacer).

Equipment that is inadequately cleaned after use harbors bacteria, which may lead to an infection.

- Instruct to rinse mouth with water after using inhalers (removing remaining drug particles from the mouth helps reduce unpleasant tastes, dryness or irritation of the oral mucosa, and systemic absorption of the drug).

Inhaled medication devices only deliver a certain percentage of the medication to the lungs. The rest of the medication is deposited in the oropharynx. Rinsing the mouth after medication administration will remove remaining particles from the mouth.

- Instruct to observe for and report side effects such as persistent sore throat, increased cough, hoarseness, and/or white patches in mouth (could indicate candidiasis that can occur with corticosteroid use).

Some inhaled medications increase the risk for infection, dysphonia, and/or candidiasis.

THERAPEUTIC INTERVENTIONS	RATIONALE
• Instruct to use the prescribed bronchodilator before inhaling the corticosteroid and to wait 5 minutes between these two medications. (This maximizes the effectiveness of the corticosteroid.)	*Separation of inhaled medications by 5 minutes is important in maximizing the effectiveness of the medications, particularly corticosteroids.*
If client is discharged on a corticosteroid, instruct to:	
• Take oral preparations with food to reduce gastric irritation.	
• Expect that certain effects such as facial rounding, slight weight gain and swelling, increased appetite, and slight mood changes may occur.	*The client should be taught the correct method of administration to decrease the incidence of side effects and adverse reactions.*
• Report undesirable effects such as marked swelling in extremities, significant weight gain, extreme emotional and behavioral changes, extreme weakness, tarry stools, bloody or coffee-ground vomitus, frequent or persistent headaches, insomnia, lack of menses, and persistent gastric irritation.	*Clients should be educated about the physical changes that can occur while taking corticosteroids, and the importance of notifying their health care professional for treatment and potential readjustment of medication dosage.*
• Avoid contact with persons who have an infection.	*Corticosteroids reduce the ability of the body to fight off infection; therefore, it is important for the client to avoid contact with persons who have an infection*
• Follow recommendations about ways to reduce the risk for developing osteoporosis if long-term corticosteroid use is expected (e.g., take calcium and vitamin D supplements, stop smoking, do 30–60 minutes of weight-bearing exercise each day if able).	*Long-term use of corticosteroids increases the client's risk of developing osteoporosis. It is important to provide the client with methods of decreasing this risk.*
If client is discharged on a beta-adrenergic agonist (e.g., albuterol, metaproterenol, terbutaline, salmeterol), instruct to:	
• Take oral preparations with meals to reduce gastric irritation.	
• Expect that certain effects such as nervousness, restlessness, and slight tremor can occur.	*Clients need to be educated on the form of administration, side effects, and adverse reactions. Clients must also be informed that if undesirable effects occur, they should notify their health care provider.*
• Report undesirable effects such as persistent or excessive nervousness, restlessness, tremors, headache, and gastric irritation; chest pain; vomiting; irregular heart beat; and wheezing.	
Instruct client to take regularly scheduled medications as often as prescribed and to avoid skipping doses, altering the prescribed dose, making up for missed doses, and discontinuing medication without permission of the health care provider.	*Many medications require a blood level to be obtained in order for an appropriate client response. The client must be made aware of what to do when doses are missed, generic medications are used if they were not used initially when the medication was prescribed, and the importance of not discontinuing the medication without the permission of the health care provider.*
Reinforce instructions about the frequency and dosage of medications prescribed on an "as needed" basis.	*The client should be educated on how to take medications that are prescribed to be used as needed. It should be emphasized that the client should not increase the frequency or dosage of these medications without permission from the health care provider.*
Instruct client to inform all health care providers of medications and herbal supplements being taken.	*Many clients have more than one physician and should be educated to inform all health care providers of all medications and herbal supplements being taken. This is important so that the health care provider is aware of all medications and herbal supplements taken by the client so if new medications are ordered, the health care provider can determine the impact of drug-to-drug interactions.*
Reinforce the need to consult physician before taking nonprescription medications.	*Many over-the-counter (OTC) medications can cause significant drug-to-drug interactions.*

THERAPEUTIC INTERVENTIONS	RATIONALE

Desired Outcome: The client will identify precautions that should be adhered to when using oxygen.

Independent Actions

Instruct client about precautions that should be adhered to when using oxygen:

- Do not smoke.
- Do not set oxygen flow rate at a level higher than prescribed by physician.
- Do not allow the oxygen system to be within 10 feet of an open flame (e.g., gas stove, kerosene heater or lamp, fireplace, candle) or a source of sparks (e.g., electric razor, portable radio, wool blanket, hair dryer).
- Post "No Smoking" signs in and around areas of oxygen use.
- Ensure that all electrical equipment in the area of the oxygen source is grounded.
- Always have a battery-operated oxygen delivery system readily available.
- Demonstrate to the client how to recognize when the oxygen supply is low, and how to get the oxygen source refilled or replaced.
- Instruct client to have the oxygen delivery system checked regularly by the supplier.
- Always wear a medical alert identification bracelet or tag.

A client using oxygen outside the health care facility should be educated on its use and safety issues. Oxygen is not a combustible gas by itself, but when exposed to an open flame or a spark, it can exacerbate a fire.

Oxygen is highly flammable and should be placed at a safe distance from anything with an open flame. In the event of fire, the oxygen system should be shut off and removed from the area.

Prevents accidental smoking around oxygen

Decreases risk of oxygen-related fire

A backup battery-operated system is necessary for power failures and when away from a hardwired power source.

The client needs to be aware of how to assess the level of oxygen on hand and at what level to have it replenished to ensure it is available when it is required.

This check helps ensure it is working properly.

Wearing a medical alert identification bracelet provides information important to ensure that the appropriate oxygen flow rate for diagnosis is administered in emergency situations and to the client's history of COPD.

Instruct client on ways to prevent skin and mucous membrane irritation and breakdown resulting from the use of oxygen and/or oxygen delivery devices:

- Assess areas of skin and mucous membranes that are in contact with the oxygen mask or nasal cannula (e.g., nares, bridge of nose, tops of ears) a few times each day for redness and irritation.
- Pad areas of pressure and ensure that straps are not too tight.
- Keep skin areas under straps and mask clean and dry.
- Refill oxygen humidification reservoir as needed, perform frequent oral hygiene, and apply water-based gel to nares and lips to reduce dryness of the mucous membranes.

A client who continuously uses oxygen should be taught methods to prevent skin and mucous membrane irritation. Oxygen is a dry gas and can cause dryness of the skin and mucous membranes that may lead to skin breakdown.

Pressure areas not padded and/or straps that are too tight may lead to skin breakdown.

Helps reduce dryness and cracking of the mucous membranes.

THERAPEUTIC INTERVENTIONS	RATIONALE

Desired Outcome: The client will state signs and symptoms to report to the health care provider.

Independent Actions

Instruct the client to report:

- Changes in sputum characteristics (e.g., increase in volume or consistency, yellow or green color)
- Sputum that does not return to usual color after 3 days of antimicrobial therapy
- Cough that becomes worse
- Increased fatigue, weakness, and shortness of breath
- Increased need for medications and/or oxygen therapy
- Elevated temperature
- Drowsiness, confusion, new or increased irritability
- Chest pain
- Persistent weight loss or sudden weight gain
- Swelling in ankles and/or feet

A respiratory infection increases dyspnea and may precipitate respiratory failure.

Instruct the client on signs and symptoms of an infection. When these appear, the client is to contact the health care provider immediately. Prompt treatment may prevent the infection from becoming severe and precipitating respiratory infection.

May indicate cardiac complications of COPD and require medical treatment.

THERAPEUTIC INTERVENTIONS	**RATIONALE**

Desired Outcome: The client will identify resources that can assist with financial needs, home management, and adjustment to changes resulting from COPD.

Independent Actions

Provide information regarding resources that can assist client and significant others with financial needs, home management, and adjustment to changes resulting from COPD (e.g., American Lung Association; respiratory equipment suppliers; pulmonary rehabilitation programs; counseling, vocational, and social services; Meals on Wheels; transportation services; home health agencies).

Initiate a referral to community and home health agencies if indicated.

COPD is a chronic illness and can significantly impact an individual's and family's financial status. Providing information specific to community resources is important to provide a continuum of care and may impact the client's health status.

Provides for continuum of care postdischarge.

THERAPEUTIC INTERVENTIONS	**RATIONALE**

Desired Outcome: The client, in collaboration with the nurse, will develop a plan for adhering to recommended follow-up care including future appointments with health care provider and graded exercise program.

Independent Actions

Implement measures to promote effective therapeutic regimen management (adhere to an appropriate diet and an exercise plan; stop smoking and maintain medication regimen).

Reinforce importance of lifelong follow-up care.

Reinforce physician's instructions about a graded exercise program (e.g., walking for 20 minutes 3 times a week, stationary bicycling).

A chronic illness requires lifestyle changes. Client involvement in a comprehensive program of lifestyle changes (i.e., diet, exercise, stop smoking, etc.) has been shown to provide improved health status and slows the progression of the disease.

ADDITIONAL NURSING DIAGNOSES

SELF-CARE DEFICIT (BATHING, DRESSING, FEEDING, TOILETING) NDx
Related to weakness, fatigue, and dyspnea

DISTURBED SLEEP PATTERN NDx
Related to fear, anxiety, unfamiliar environment, excessive coughing, frequent assessments and treatments, side effects of medications (e.g., some bronchodilators, corticosteroids), and inability to assume usual sleep position associated with orthopnea

DISTURBED BODY IMAGE NDx
Related to:
- Change in appearance (e.g., "barrel" chest, clubbing of fingers, retraction of tissues around the neck and shoulders)

- Dependence on others to meet self-care needs
- Possible alteration in sexual functioning (may result from dyspnea, weakness, fatigue, and persistent cough)
- Stigma associated with chronic illness
- Possible changes in lifestyle and roles

RISK FOR POWERLESSNESS NDx
Related to physical limitations; disease progression despite efforts to comply with treatment plan; dependence on others to meet self-care needs; and alterations in roles, lifestyle, and future plans.

MECHANICAL VENTILATION

Mechanical ventilation, in an intervention intended for use as a temporary, life-saving therapy, is indicated for clients with acute respiratory failure who are unable to maintain normal gas exchange. Implemented using a variety of modes and techniques, methods of mechanical ventilation used in acute and long-term care settings are influenced by the type of underlying disease process and the need for an artificial airway.

Acute respiratory failure can be a result of either the failure to oxygenate, the failure to ventilate, or a combination of both. Two categories of respiratory failure influence the method of mechanical ventilation selected for ventilatory support. Type I, or hypoxemic respiratory failure, is defined as the inability to maintain a PaO_2 greater than 60 mm Hg with the client at rest and breathing room air. A variety of disease processes interfere with the normal exchange of oxygen and carbon dioxide across the alveolar membrane, leading to disturbances in diffusion. These processes include pulmonary fibrosis, pulmonary edema, acute respiratory distress syndrome (ARDS), and loss of functional lung tissue (pneumonectomy). Effective gas exchange is influenced by even distribution of gas (ventilation) and blood (perfusion) in all portions of the lung. Disturbances in the relationship between ventilation and perfusion also contribute to type I or hypoxemic respiratory failure and include pulmonary emboli, atelectasis, pneumonia, emphysema, and bronchitis, as well as ARDS. Type II failure, or the failure to ventilate, results from disease processes that interfere with a client's ability to effectively ventilate the waste products of respiration (CO_2). Characterized by a $PaCO_2$ greater than 50 mm Hg or a pH less than 7.35, type II respiratory failure, or hypercarbic respiratory failure, can occur as a result of disease processes that impair normal alveolar minute ventilation. These disease processes include COPD, restrictive pulmonary diseases (obesity, pneumothorax, diaphragmatic paralysis), neuromuscular defects (Guillain-Barré syndrome, myasthenia gravis, multiple sclerosis, muscular dystrophy, spinal cord injury), and chest trauma.

Invasive positive pressure ventilation is the most common method of mechanical ventilation used in the acute care setting. Invasive ventilation techniques require the use of an artificial airway (tracheostomy, endotracheal tube [ETT]). With this method of ventilation, the client's respiratory function is supported as positive pressure delivers the appropriate volume of air and concentration using the appropriate ventilator settings. The degree of mechanical support and the duration of therapy are determined by the client's underlying disease process and current state of health. As duration of mechanical support increases, the client is at increased risk for the development of complications associated with mechanical ventilation: tracheal damage, acid-base imbalances, aspiration pneumonia, nutritional imbalances, deep vein thrombosis (DVT), stress ulcers, immobility, and ventilator dependence.

To ensure the safe and effective care of a client requiring mechanical ventilation, a multidisciplinary approach is required. Collaboration among the physician provider, respiratory therapist, dietician, physical therapist, and nurse is essential in order to resolve the underlying disease process, prevent complications, and return the client to baseline pulmonary function. In addition, as with any artificial lifesaving or life-extending therapy, client and family choice must be respected if end-of-life issues arise.

This care plan focuses on the adult client hospitalized in an acute care setting with acute respiratory failure requiring support with mechanical ventilation.

OUTCOME/DISCHARGE CRITERIA

The client will:
1. Return to independent respiratory function
2. Tolerate an expected level of activity
3. Maintain a balanced nutritional state
4. Have no signs or symptoms of infection
5. Identify ways to maintain respiratory health
6. State signs and symptoms to report to health care provider
7. Develop a plan for adherence to the treatment regimen including prescribed medications, diet, and follow-up care

---

Nursing Diagnosis   **IMPAIRED RESPIRATORY FUNCTION***

Definition: **Impaired Spontaneous Ventilation NDx:** Inability to initiate and/or maintain independent breathing that is adequate to support life; **Ineffective Breathing Pattern NDx:** Inspiration and/or expiration that does not provide adequate ventilation; **Ineffective Airway Clearance NDx:** Inability to clear secretions or obstructions from the respiratory tract to maintain a clear airway; **Impaired Gas Exchange NDx:** Excess or deficit in oxygenation and/or carbon dioxide elimination at the alveolar-capillary membrane.

Impaired spontaneous ventilation NDx
Related to:
• Metabolic factors, respiratory muscle fatigue

Ineffective breathing pattern NDx
Related to:
• Cognitive impairment, neuromuscular dysfunction, respiratory muscle fatigue, spinal cord injury, obesity, hyperventilation/hypoventilation

Ineffective airway clearance NDx
Related to:
• Presence of an artificial airway, retained secretions, secretions in the bronchi, excessive mucus, infection

Impaired gas exchange NDx
Related to:
• Alveolar-capillary membrane changes, ventilation-perfusion imbalance

---

*This diagnostic label includes the following nursing diagnoses: impaired spontaneous ventilation, ineffective breathing pattern, ineffective airway clearance, and impaired gas exchange.

CLINICAL MANIFESTATIONS

Subjective	**Objective**
Verbal self-report of fatigue; confusion; restlessness; somnolence; shortness of breath	Dyspnea; orthopnea; use of accessory muscles; abnormal breath sounds; limited chest excursion; abnormal skin color; diaphoresis; decreased pulse oximetry values; abnormal arterial blood gas values

RISK FACTORS

- Apnea, or impending inability to breathe
- Acute respiratory failure
- Severe hypoxia
- Respiratory muscle fatigue

DESIRED OUTCOMES

The client will experience adequate respiratory function as evidenced by:
a. Normal rate and depth of breathing
b. Decrease or absence of dyspnea
c. Normal breath sounds
d. Usual mental status
e. Oximetry results within baseline range
f. Arterial blood gas values within baseline range

NOC OUTCOMES

Respiratory status: airway patency; gas exchange; ventilation; mechanical ventilation response: adult; vital signs

NIC INTERVENTIONS

Respiratory monitoring; ventilation assistance; artificial airway management; mechanical ventilation management: invasive; mechanical ventilatory weaning; acid-base management

NURSING ASSESSMENT	**RATIONALE**
Assess for and report signs and symptoms of impaired respiratory function: • Rapid, shallow, respirations • Dyspnea, orthopnea • Use of accessory muscles • Abnormal breath sounds • Limited chest excursion • Restlessness, irritability • Confusion • Somnolence	*Early recognition of signs and symptoms of impaired respiratory function allows for prompt intervention.*
Monitor arterial blood gas values/oximetry values.	*Allows for evaluation of therapy effectiveness.*
Monitor vital signs.	*Allows for assessment of client tolerance to ventilator settings. Changes in vital signs can indicate a decline in respiratory function.*
Assess proper functioning of equipment: • Ventilator connections • Artificial airway (presence of cuff leak)	*Any equipment malfunction can compromise safe and effective mechanical ventilation.*
Monitor chest radiograph results.	*Chest radiograph confirms proper position of ETT. Potential complications such as pneumothorax, right mainstem intubation, and infection can be assessed by assessing chest radiograph results.*

THERAPEUTIC INTERVENTIONS	**RATIONALE**

Independent Actions
Implement measures to ensure airway patency:
• Maintain position and patency of ETT or tracheostomy.
  • ETT-Provide oral airway or bite block to prevent biting on the ETT tube as appropriate.
  • Document centimeter reference marking for ETT tube to monitor for potential displacement.
  • Provide trach care every 4 to 8 hrs; cleaning the inner cannula while maintaining sterile technique.
	Actions that ensure airway patency contribute to adequate oxygenation and acid-base balance. An artificial airway must be maintained in proper position to ensure ventilation of both lung fields.

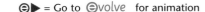

NDx = NANDA Diagnosis   **D** = Delegatable Action   ● = UAP   ✦ = LVN/LPN   ⊖▶ = Go to ⊖volve for animation

Continued...

THERAPEUTIC INTERVENTIONS	RATIONALE

⊖▶ • Perform endotracheal suctioning as appropriate.

  • Perform hand hygiene.
  • Use universal precautions.
  • Use personal protective equipment (e.g. gloves, goggles, mask) as appropriate.
  • Suction oropharynx before deflating cuff.

Reposition client every 1 to 2 hrs. **D** ●
Position client in a semi- to high-Fowler's position. **D** ●

Implement measures to reduce the risk for impaired skin integrity/pressure injuries around mouth (ETT), neck (trach), and oral mucosa.

  • Change endotracheal tapes/ties every 24 hrs, inspecting the skin and oral mucosa.
  • Reposition the ETT tube to other side of mouth.
  • Loosen commercial ETT holders at least once per day and provide skin care.
  • Inspect skin around tracheal stoma for drainage, redness/ irritation.
    • Clean and dry area around stoma.

Maintain appropriate emergency equipment at bedside— Ambu bag.

Suctioning should occur as needed to clear the large airways of accumulated secretions observing appropriate hand hygiene precautions and sterile suctioning technique helps reduce the risk for ventilator-acquired pneumonia.

Helps prevent aspiration/ventilator-acquired pneumonia.
Frequent repositioning helps loosen and mobilize secretions.
A semi- to high-Fowler's position allows for maximal diaphragmatic excursion and lung expansion.
The presence of an artificial airway increases the risk for development of pressure injuries/impaired skin integrity to the mouth, neck, and oral mucosa. Assessment of the skin around the affected areas along with routine skin care is necessary to prevent the development of a pressure-related injury.

An appropriate bag-valve device (Ambu) must be at the bedside of a client receiving mechanical ventilation in the event of equipment failure.

Dependent/Collaborative Actions

Maintain appropriate ventilator settings:
Oxygen concentration (fraction of inspired oxygen [FiO_2])
Tidal volume (Vt)
Ventilator rate (f)
Positive end-expiratory pressure (PEEP)

Adjustment of ventilator settings is accomplished collaboratively between the physician provider and the respiratory therapist.
Settings are adjusted to reduce the work of breathing and facilitate adequate ventilation and oxygenation. The nurse should always reassess the client's physiological response to ventilator changes through physical assessment and examination of arterial blood gas values.

Implement measures to ensure airway patency:
  • Monitor cuff pressure of ETT/tracheostomy tube.
    • Maintain cuff pressure at 15 to 25 mm Hg.

Inflating the cuff with the minimal amount of air needed to prevent leakage of air around the cuff ensures delivery of adequate Vt and prevents aspiration of oral secretions.

Implement measures to thin secretions and maintain adequate moisture of the respiratory mucous membranes:
  • Humidify inspired air.
  • Regulate fluid intake to optimize fluid balance.

Maintain integrity of ventilator circuit:
  • Keep ventilator circuit free of excess moisture.
  • Respond to ventilator alarms.
  • Monitor ventilator connections.

Adequate hydration and humidified inspired air help thin secretions, which facilitates the mobilization and expectoration of secretions. These actions also reduce dryness of the respiratory mucous membrane, which helps enhance mucociliary clearance.
These actions help maximize the effectiveness of mechanical ventilation, ensure a patent airway, and promote patient safety.

Assist with the administration of mucolytics as ordered:
  • Acetylcysteine
  • Water, saline

Mucolytics and diluent or hydrating agents are mucokinetic substances that reduce the viscosity of mucus, thus making it easier for the client to mobilize and clear secretions from the respiratory tract.

Administer the following medications if ordered:
  • Bronchodilators
  • Corticosteroids
  • Leukotriene modifiers

These medications increase the patency of the airways and enhance bronchial airflow. Bronchodilators produce bronchodilation by relaxing the bronchial smooth muscle. Corticosteroids and leukotriene modifiers reduce inflammation in the airways, which results in decreased bronchial hyperactivity and constriction, and decreased mucus production.

Collaborate with physician to develop a sedation plan:
  • Administer sedatives as ordered* (e.g., propofol [Diprivan]).
    • Administer neuromuscular blocking agents as ordered:
  • Cisatracurium besylate (Nimbex)

These strategies will help facilitate optimum ventilation and gas exchange, reducing ventilator asynchrony.

THERAPEUTIC INTERVENTIONS	RATIONALE
Implement measures to prevent spontaneous decannulation (e.g., secure airway with tapes/ties, administer sedatives, consider use of restraints).	
Consult appropriate health care provider if signs and symptoms of impaired respiratory function persist or worsen.	*Notifying the appropriate health care provider allows for modification of the treatment plan.*

Nursing Diagnosis IMBALANCED NUTRITION: LESS THAN BODY REQUIREMENTS NDx

Definition: Intake of nutrients insufficient to meet metabolic needs.

Related to: Inability to absorb nutrients and ingest food

CLINICAL MANIFESTATIONS

Subjective	Objective
Not evident in an intubated client	Evidence of lack of food; poor muscle tone; hyperactive bowel sounds; decreased subcutaneous fat; weight loss; sore, inflamed buccal cavity; low serum albumin and total protein levels, iron deficiency; electrolyte imbalances

RISK FACTORS

- Inadequate nutritional therapy
- Increased caloric requirements
- Altered gastrointestinal motility

DESIRED OUTCOMES

The client will maintain adequate nutrition status as evidenced by:
a. Consume adequate nourishment
b. Be free of signs of malnutrition
c. Weigh within normal range for height and age

NOC OUTCOMES

Nutritional status

NIC INTERVENTIONS

Nutritional monitoring; nutritional management; nutritional therapy

NURSING ASSESSMENT	RATIONALE
Assess for and report signs and symptoms of malnutrition: • Weight significantly below client's usual weight or below normal for client's age, height, and body frame • Weakness and fatigue • Sore, inflamed oral mucous membrane • Pale conjunctiva	*Early recognition of signs and symptoms of malnutrition allows for prompt intervention.*
Assess for return of bowel function every 2 to 4 hrs.	*Without bowel sounds, support for nutritional status must be accomplished with parenteral nutrition. When BS are re-established, recommend changing to tube feedings to support bowel health.*
Monitor serum albumin, prealbumin, total protein, ferritin, transferrin, Hgb, hematocrit (Hct), and serum electrolyte levels as indicated.	*Serum albumin levels less than 3.5 g/100 dL are considered a risk for poor nutritional status. Early recognition of abnormal lab values reflective of the client's overall nutritional state allows for prompt intervention.*

THERAPEUTIC INTERVENTIONS	RATIONALE
Dependent/Collaborative Actions Consult physician about an alternative method of providing nutrition: • Enteral nutrition • Parenteral nutrition	*Enteral feeding is the preferred method to meet the hypermetabolic nutritional needs of the ventilated client. If the client is unable to be fed enterally, nutritional support in the form of parenteral nutrition must be provided.*

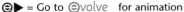

Nursing Diagnosis	**RISK FOR INFECTION NDx (VENTILATOR-ACQUIRED PNEUMONIA [VAP])**

Definition: Susceptible to invasion and multiplication of pathogenic organisms, which may compromise health.

Related to:
- Inadequate primary defenses
- Decrease in mucociliary action
- Stasis of pulmonary secretions
- Malnutrition
- Presence of invasive artificial airway
- Increased environmental exposure to pathogens

CLINICAL MANIFESTATIONS

Subjective	Objective
Not applicable	Increased temperature, tachypnea; increased or purulent secretions/hemoptysis, rhonchi, crackles, decreased breath sounds, bronchospasm; leukocytosis

RISK FACTORS
- Pooling of oropharyngeal secretions
- Immobility
- Malnutrition

DESIRED OUTCOMES

The client will remain free of infection as evidenced by:
a. No increase in temperature
b. Absence of purulent sputum
c. Normal breath sounds
d. Normal chest radiograph findings
e. WBC and differential counts returning to normal or within normal limits

NOC OUTCOMES

Immune status; infection severity

NIC INTERVENTIONS

Infection protection; infection control

NURSING ASSESSMENT	RATIONALE
Assess for signs and symptoms of ventilator-acquired pneumonia (VAP): • Elevated temperature • Purulent sputum • Odorous sputum • Abnormal breath sounds (crackles, rhonchi)	*Early recognition of signs and symptoms of VAP allows for prompt intervention.*
Assess WBC and differential cell counts for abnormalities.	*An increase in the WBC count above previous levels and/or a significant change in the differential may indicate the presence of an infection. Monitoring results allows for modification of treatment plan.*
Monitor chest radiograph results.	*The presence of pulmonary infiltrates on chest radiograph indicates the presence of pneumonia.*
Monitor results of sputum cultures.	*Monitoring results allows for modification of treatment plan.*

THERAPEUTIC INTERVENTIONS	RATIONALE
Independent Actions Implement measures to reduce the risk for VAP: • Elevate head of the bed a minimum of 30 to 45 degrees.	*Head of the bed elevation reduces the risk of aspiration of gastric secretions.*
• Perform hand hygiene: • Frequent hand washing before and after suctioning • Wear gloves when in contact with the patient and change gloves between activities.	*Prevents the transmission of bacteria to the patient*

THERAPEUTIC INTERVENTIONS	RATIONALE

• Drain excess condensation in ventilator circuit.
• Perform oral care every 2 to 4 hrs and prn.
  ○ Suction oropharyngeal secretions.
  ○ Brush teeth and surface of the tongue using suction toothbrush and small amounts of water and/or chlorhexidine solution.
  ○ Apply mouth moisturizer/lip balm if needed.
• Maintain integrity of ETT/tracheostomy cuff.
	Removes bacteria from the oropharynx, protects integrity of oral mucosal membranes, and prevents aspiration of bacteria-laden secretions.
	
	Prevents silent aspiration of oral/gastric secretions.

Dependent/Collaborative Actions

Monitor cuff pressures every 4 to 8 hrs using manometer. • Inflate cuff using minimal occlusive volume (MOV) technique. ○ Maintain cuff pressure at 15 to 25 mm Hg. Notify the appropriate health care provider if signs and symptoms of VAP develop. Obtain cultures as ordered.	*Adequate cuff pressure is necessary to prevent silent aspiration of oropharyngeal secretions, which may increase the risk of ventilator-acquired pneumonia.* *Notifying the appropriate health care provider allows for modification of the treatment plan.*

Nursing Diagnosis DYSFUNCTIONAL VENTILATORY WEANING RESPONSE NDx

Definition: Inability to adjust to lowered levels of mechanical ventilator support that interrupts and prolongs the weaning process.

Related to:
- **Physiological factors:** ineffective airway clearance; sleep disturbance; inadequate nutrition; uncontrolled pain or discomfort
- **Psychological factors:** knowledge deficient of the weaning process; moderate amount of anxiety or fear; hopelessness; powerlessness; insufficient trust in health care team
- **Situational factors:** uncontrolled energy demands; inappropriate pacing of diminished ventilator support; inadequate social support; adverse environment; low nurse-to-client ratio; history of ventilator dependence greater than 4; history of multiple unsuccessful weaning attempts

CLINICAL MANIFESTATIONS

Subjective	Objective
Not evident in an intubated client	Apprehension; agitation; baseline increase in respiratory rate (<5 breaths/min); diaphoresis; adventitious breath sounds; asynchronized breathing with the ventilator; cyanosis; decreased level of consciousness; use of respiratory accessory muscles; gasping breaths; increase from baseline blood pressure; inability to cooperate; inability to respond to coaching

RISK FACTORS
- Prolonged mechanical ventilation
- Muscle weakness
- Activity intolerance
- Debilitated state

DESIRED OUTCOMES

The client will wean from mechanical ventilation as evidenced by:
a. Arterial blood gas values within client's normal baseline
b. Absence of dyspnea
c. Absence of restlessness
d. Ability to effectively clear secretions
e. Tolerating and maintaining airway after extubation
f. Vital signs within normal limits

NOC OUTCOMES

Anxiety self-control; mechanical ventilation weaning response; adult; respiratory status: gas exchange; ventilation; vital signs

NIC INTERVENTIONS

Mechanical ventilatory weaning; mechanical ventilation management: invasive

NURSING ASSESSMENT

RATIONALE

Assess client's readiness for weaning:
- Resolution of underlying disease process
- Hemodynamic stability
- Absence of fever
- Normal state of consciousness
- Metabolic fluid balance
- Adequate nutritional status
- Adequate sleep

Assess client's psychological readiness to wean.

Assess client's tolerance of weaning process:
- Work of breathing
- Vital signs
- Pulse oximetry values
- Arterial blood gas values

Monitor Hgb/Hct; serum electrolyte levels; serum albumin/ prealbumin levels; chest radiograph for improvements.

Early recognition of readiness to wean allows for prompt intervention.

THERAPEUTIC INTERVENTIONS

RATIONALE

Independent Actions

Implement measures to facilitate the weaning process:
- **Provide a safe, comfortable environment.**
- Coordinate pain and sedation medications to minimize sedative effects.
- Schedule weaning periods for the time of the day when the client is **most rested.**
- Promote a normal sleep-wake cycle.
- Limit visitors to supportive persons.
- Coach client through periods of anxiety.
- Cluster care activities to promote successful weaning.
- Educate patient and family about the weaning process.

Evaluate patient tolerance of the weaning process.

Comfort will facilitate the weaning process.
Fatigued respiratory muscles require 12 to 24 hrs to recover.

Educating the client and family allows for the appropriate level of psychological support.
Allows for modification of the weaning plan.

Dependent/Collaborative Actions

Assist respiratory therapist in assessing readiness to wean by assessing:
- Minute ventilation
- Negative inspiratory force
- Vital capacity

Use evidence-based protocols for weaning.

Recommend a spontaneous breathing trial:
- 30 to 120 minutes with PEEP/continuous positive airway pressure (CPAP) or t-piece

Notify appropriate health care provider of signs and symptoms of dysfunctional weaning:
- Respiration rate less than 8 or greater than 30 breaths/min
- B/P changes greater than 20% of baseline
- Heart rate changes greater than 20% of baseline
- Pulse oximetry less than 90%
- Decrease in spontaneous tidal volume

Assessment of the mechanics of weaning allows for determination of the client's ability to support normal ventilation.

Protocol-driven weaning provides a standardized approach to the weaning process.
Tolerance of a weaning trial helps demonstrate readiness for extubation.

Notifying the appropriate health care provider allows for modification of the treatment plan.

THERAPEUTIC INTERVENTIONS	RATIONALE

- Labored respirations
- Diaphoresis
- Restlessness
- Anxiety

Collaborative/Nursing Diagnosis **RISK FOR DECREASED CARDIAC OUTPUT** NDx

Definition: Susceptible to inadequate blood pumped by the heart to meet metabolic demands of the body, which may compromise health.

Related to:
Altered hemodynamics related to increased intrathoracic pressure associated with positive pressure mechanical ventilation

CLINICAL MANIFESTATIONS

Subjective	Objective
Not evident in an intubated client	Hypotension; tachycardia; decreased level of consciousness

RISK FACTORS

- Large tidal volumes
- PEEP

DESIRED OUTCOMES

The client will maintain normal cardiac output as evidenced by:
a. B/P within baseline range
b. Heart rate within baseline range
c. Measured cardiac output/index within client's normal range

NURSING ASSESSMENT	RATIONALE
Assess for and report signs and symptoms of decreased cardiac output. Monitor vital signs frequently. Measure cardiac output/index if ordered.	*Early recognition of signs and symptoms of decreased cardiac output allows for prompt intervention.*

THERAPEUTIC INTERVENTIONS	RATIONALE
Independent Actions Monitor client's response to ventilator changes: • Adding of PEEP	*PEEP increases intrathoracic pressure, which may further decrease venous return, compromising cardiac output.*
Dependent/Collaborative Actions Administer intravenous fluids as ordered.	*Helps restore circulating volume, which helps minimize cardiovascular effects.*
Administer vasoactive infusions to restore normal cardiac output: • Inotropes • Vasopressors	*Helps maintain normal cardiac output.* *Inotropes increase the force of cardiac contractions, which increases cardiac output.* *Vasopressors should only be used if circulating volume has been restored.*
Notify physician provider if signs and symptoms of decreased cardiac output persist or worsen.	*Notifying the appropriate health care provider allows for modification of the treatment plan.*

NDx = NANDA Diagnosis   **D** = Delegatable Action   ● = UAP   ✦ = LVN/LPN   ⊖▶ = Go to ⊖volve for animation

Collaborative Diagnosis **RISK FOR GASTROINTESTINAL BLEEDING**

Definition: Bleeding within the gastrointestinal tract

Related to:
- Positive pressure ventilation
- Stress of critical illness/stress ulcers
- Atrophy of mucosal lining of stomach due to lack of enteral feeding

CLINICAL MANIFESTATIONS

Subjective	Objective
Not evident in an intubated client	Bleeding in stools; hematemesis

RISK FACTORS
- Stress of acute illness

DESIRED OUTCOMES

The client will not experience gastrointestinal bleeding.

NURSING ASSESSMENT	RATIONALE
Assess for and report signs and symptoms.	*Early recognition of signs and symptoms of gastrointestinal bleeding allows for prompt intervention.*

THERAPEUTIC INTERVENTIONS	RATIONALE
Dependent/Collaborative Actions	
Administer histamine (H_2) receptor blockers; proton pump inhibitors.	*Medications act to decrease gastric acidity and diminish the risk of stress ulcers.*
Administer enteral feedings as ordered.	*Stimulates the intestinal mucosa, preventing atrophy and disruption*
Notify physician provider if signs and symptoms persist or worsen.	*Notifying the appropriate health care provider allows for modification of the treatment plan.*

Collaborative Diagnosis **RISK FOR BAROTRAUMA**

Related to:
- Increased lung inflation pressures
- Noncompliant lungs

ADDITIONAL NURSING DIAGNOSES

FEAR NDx /ANXIETY NDx
Related to the perceived need for mechanical ventilation; inability to communicate effectively; psychological ventilator dependence

RISK FOR ASPIRATION NDx
Related to presence of an artificial airway that bypasses normal upper airway defenses

IMPAIRED PHYSICAL MOBILITY NDx
Related to mechanical ventilation

IMPAIRED VERBAL COMMUNICATION NDx
Related to artificial airway and mechanical ventilation

IMPAIRED ORAL MUCOUS MEMBRANE NDx
Related to the presence of an artificial airway; bypass of normal physiological humidification process

POWERLESSNESS NDx
Related to illness-related regimen; lifestyle of helplessness

RISK FOR INJURY NDx
Related to:

External factors: Use of restraints during mechanical ventilation; presence of artificial airway; malfunction of equipment. Internal factors: Agitation/confusion

RISK FOR IMBALANCED FLUID VOLUME NDx
Related to:

- Ventilator humidification
- Stimulation of the renin-angiotensin-aldosterone mechanism leading to retention of sodium and water

PNEUMONIA

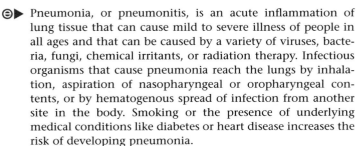 Pneumonia, or pneumonitis, is an acute inflammation of lung tissue that can cause mild to severe illness of people in all ages and that can be caused by a variety of viruses, bacteria, fungi, chemical irritants, or radiation therapy. Infectious organisms that cause pneumonia reach the lungs by inhalation, aspiration of nasopharyngeal or oropharyngeal contents, or by hematogenous spread of infection from another site in the body. Smoking or the presence of underlying medical conditions like diabetes or heart disease increases the risk of developing pneumonia.

Pneumonia may be classified according to the causative organism (e.g., pneumococcal pneumonia, staphylococcal pneumonia, viral pneumonia), the area of involvement (e.g., lobar pneumonia), or the etiological factor (e.g., aspiration pneumonia, radiation pneumonitis). Pneumonia may also be classified as community-acquired pneumonia (CAP) or hospital-acquired pneumonia (HAP), the latter often referred to as *nosocomial*.

Most persons hospitalized with pneumonia have bacterial pneumonia. The onset of bacterial pneumonia is often abrupt and manifested by chills, fever, a cough productive of purulent or blood-tinged sputum, and pleuritic chest pain (in some cases). Elderly persons, who often have impaired immune mechanisms, may present with a change in mental status and a recent history of weakness, fatigue, and a decline in appetite rather than the symptoms of typical pneumonia.

This care plan focuses on the adult client hospitalized with bacterial pneumonia. Much of the information is applicable to clients receiving follow-up care in an extended care facility or home setting.

OUTCOME/DISCHARGE CRITERIA

The client will:
1. Have improved respiratory function
2. Tolerate expected level of activity
3. Have no signs and symptoms of complications
4. State signs and symptoms to report to the health care provider
5. Develop a plan for adhering to recommended follow-up care, including future appointments with health care provider, medications prescribed, and activity limitations

---

Nursing Diagnosis ## IMPAIRED RESPIRATORY FUNCTION*

Definition: **Ineffective Breathing Pattern NDx**: Inspiration and/or expiration that does not provide adequate ventilation; **Ineffective Airway Clearance NDx**: Inability to clear secretions or obstructions from the respiratory tract to maintain a clear airway; **Impaired Gas Exchange NDx**: Excess or deficit in oxygenation and/or carbon dioxide elimination at the alveolar-capillary membrane.

Ineffective breathing pattern NDx
Related to:

- Decreased depth of respirations associated with:
  - Weakness, fatigue, and reluctance to breathe deeply because of chest pain
  - Decreased lung compliance (distensibility) if pleural effusion is present
- Increased rate of respirations associated with:
  - Compensation for hypoxia that results from impaired gas exchange
  - The increase in metabolic rate that occurs with an infectious process

Ineffective airway clearance NDx
Related to:

- Tracheobronchial inflammation and increased production of mucus associated with the infectious process
- Stasis of secretions associated with decreased activity, poor cough effort resulting from fatigue and chest pain, impaired ciliary function (results from increased viscosity and volume of mucus that occurs with the infectious process)

Impaired gas exchange NDx
Related to:

A decrease in effective lung surface associated with the accumulation of mucus and consolidation of lung tissue

---

NDx = NANDA Diagnosis   **D** = Delegatable Action   ● = UAP   ✦ = LVN/LPN   ◉▶ = Go to ⓔvolve for animation

CLINICAL MANIFESTATIONS

Subjective	Objective
Verbal self-report of shortness of breath and chest tightness	Tachypnea; pharyngitis; dullness on percussion over consolidated areas; abnormal breath sounds; productive cough; fever; irritability; confusion; disorientation; restlessness; somnolence; use of accessory muscles when breathing; pink, rusty, purulent, green, yellow, or white sputum; significant decrease in oximetry results; abnormal arterial blood gas values; abnormal chest radiograph results; declining results in pulmonary function tests; reduced activity tolerance; asymmetrical chest excursion

RISK FACTORS

- Smoking
- Outdoor/indoor pollutants
- Exposure to second-hand cigarette smoke
- Allergies
- Low birth weight
- Periodontal disease
- Individuals older than 60 years
- White male

DESIRED OUTCOMES

The client will maintain adequate respiratory function as evidenced by:
a. Normal rate and depth of respirations
b. Decreased dyspnea
c. Usual or improved breath sounds
d. Symmetrical chest excursion
e. Usual mental status
f. Oximetry results within normal range for client
g. Arterial blood gas values within normal range for client

NOC OUTCOMES

Respiratory status: airway patency; ventilation; gas exchange

NIC INTERVENTIONS

Respiratory monitoring; airway management; tube care: chest; cough enhancement; oxygen therapy; ventilation assistance; anxiety reduction

NURSING ASSESSMENT

Assess for signs and symptoms of impaired respiratory function:
- Dyspnea, orthopnea
- Use of accessory muscles when breathing
- Abnormal breath sounds (e.g., diminished, bronchial, crackles, wheezes)
- Asymmetrical or limited chest excursion
- Cough (usually a productive cough of rust-colored, purulent, or blood-tinged sputum)
- Restlessness, irritability
- Confusion, somnolence
- Central cyanosis (a late sign)
- Significant decrease in oximetry results

- Abnormal arterial blood gas values

- Changes in vital signs

Assess arterial blood gas values, oximetry values, and chest radiograph results. Report abnormal findings.

RATIONALE

Early recognition of signs and symptoms of ineffective breathing patterns allows for prompt intervention.

Changes in the characteristics of breath sounds may be due to airway obstruction, mucous plugs, or retained secretions in larger airways.

Restlessness, irritability, and changes in mental status or level of consciousness indicate an oxygen deficiency and require immediate treatment.

Oximetry is a noninvasive method of measuring arterial oxygen saturation. The results assist in evaluating respiratory status.

Decreasing PaO_2 and increasing $PaCO_2$ are indicators of respiratory problems.

Increased work of breathing or hypoxia may cause tachycardia and/or hypertension.

Changes in infiltrates noted in the lungs require prompt treatment.

THERAPEUTIC INTERVENTIONS

Independent Actions
Implement measures to improve respiratory status:
Place client in a semi-Fowler's position and position overbed table so client can lean on it if desired. **D** ● ✦

RATIONALE

Positioning in semi-Fowler's position promotes optimal gas exchange by enabling chest expansion. Leaning on the overbed table decreases dyspnea through pressure on the gastric contents and diaphragmatic contraction.

THERAPEUTIC INTERVENTIONS	RATIONALE
• Instruct client to breathe slowly if hyperventilating.	*Slowing the pace of breathing makes each breath more effective.*
• If client must remain flat in bed, assist with position change at least every 2 hrs. **D** ✦ ●	*Prevents consolidation of secretions.*
• Assist client to deep breathe or use incentive spirometer every 1 to 2 hrs. **D** ✦	*Forced deep breathing and use of incentive spirometry will increase expansion of the lungs and improve the client's ability to clear mucus from the lungs. The technique may also improve the amount of oxygen that is able to penetrate deep into the lungs.*
• Maintain client fluid intake of at least 2500 mL/day unless contraindicated. **D** ✦	*Increased fluid intake promotes thinning of secretions and reduces dryness of the respiratory mucous membranes.*
• Instruct client to avoid intake of large meals, gas-forming foods (i.e., cauliflower, beans, cabbage, onions, etc.), and carbonated beverages.	*Gas-forming foods and carbonated beverages can cause abdominal bloating, which places pressure on the diaphragm and reduces lung expansion.*
• Discourage smoking.	*The irritants in smoke increase mucus production, impair ciliary function, and can cause inflammation and damage to the bronchial and alveolar walls; the carbon monoxide decreases oxygen availability.*
• Maintain activity restrictions and increase activity as allowed and tolerated. **D** ● ✦	*Conservation of energy through activity restrictions allows energy to be focused on breathing. Increasing activity as tolerated helps mobilize secretions and promotes deeper breathing.*

Dependent/Collaborative Actions
Implement measures to improve respiratory status:

• Assist with or perform postural drainage therapy if ordered.	*Prevents consolidation of secretions.*
• Perform suctioning if ordered. **D** ✦	*Removes secretions from the large airways. It also stimulates coughing, which helps clear airways of mucus and foreign matter.*
• Humidify inspired air as ordered. **D** ✦	*Liquefies secretions, improving client's ability to eliminate them through expectoration*
• Assist with administration of mucolytics and diluent or hydrating agents via nebulizer if ordered. **D** ✦	*Mucolytics and diluent or hydrating agents help liquefy secretions for more effective removal.*
• Avoid use of CNS depressants.	*CNS depressants further depress respiratory status, exacerbating the client's condition.*
• Administer and monitor oxygen as ordered. **D** ✦	*Provides supplemental oxygen if required by client.*
• Administer bronchodilators, antimicrobials, expectorants. **D** ✦	*Bronchodilators relax smooth muscles of the airway, thus improving air exchange in the lungs. Antimicrobials may be given to prevent or treat pneumonia. Expectorants help the client remove secretions from the lungs.*
Consult appropriate health care providers—(respiratory therapist and physician) if signs and symptoms of impaired respiratory function persist or worsen.	*Notifying the appropriate health care professionals allows for a multidisciplinary approach to treatment.*

Nursing Diagnosis RISK FOR DEFICIENT FLUID VOLUME NDx

Definition: Susceptible to experiencing decreased intravascular, interstitial, and/or intracellular fluid volumes, which may compromise health.

Related to: Decreased oral intake and excessive fluid loss (occurs with profuse diaphoresis and hyperventilation if present)

CLINICAL MANIFESTATIONS

Subjective	Objective
Verbal self-report of thirst	Decreased B/P; decreased pulse pressure; decreased pulse volume; decreased skin turgor; decreased urine output; dry skin; elevated Hct; increased temperature; increased pulse rate; weakness

RISK FACTORS

- Active fluid volume loss
- Failure of regulatory mechanisms
- Decreased fluid volume intake
- Increased insensible loss of fluid

DESIRED OUTCOMES

The client will not experience a deficient fluid volume as evidenced by:
a. Normal skin turgor
b. Moist mucous membrane
c. Stable weight
d. B/P and pulse rate within normal range for client and stable with position change
e. Capillary refill time less than 2 to 3 seconds
f. Usual mental status
g. BUN and Hct within normal range
h. Balanced intake and output
i. Urine specific gravity within normal range

NOC OUTCOMES

Fluid balance; hydration; kidney function; vital signs

NIC INTERVENTIONS

Fluid management; fluid monitoring; fluid resuscitation; hypovolemia management; intravenous therapy

NURSING ASSESSMENT

Assess for signs and symptoms of deficient fluid volume:
- Decreased skin turgor
- Dry mucous membranes, thirst
- Weight loss of 2% or greater over a short period
- Postural hypotension and/or low B/P
- Weak, rapid pulse
- Capillary refill time greater than 2 to 3 seconds
- Neck veins flat when client is supine
- Change in mental status
- Elevated BUN and Hct
- Decreased urine output with increased specific gravity (reflects an actual rather than potential fluid volume deficit)

RATIONALE

Early recognition of signs and symptoms of deficient fluid volume allows for prompt intervention.

THERAPEUTIC INTERVENTIONS

Independent Actions
Implement measures to reduce nausea and vomiting if present:
- Instruct client to ingest food/fluid slowly.
- Eliminate noxious sights and odors. **D** ● ✦

Implement measures to control diarrhea if present:
- Discourage intake of spicy foods and foods high in fiber or lactose.

Implement measures to reduce fever if present:
- Sponge bath client with tepid water. **D** ● ✦
- Remove excessive clothing or bedcovers. **D** ● ✦

Carefully measure drainage:
- Nasogastric **D** ✦
- Wound **D** ✦
- Urine **D** ✦

Dependent/Collaborative Actions
Maintain a fluid intake of at least 2500 mL/day unless contraindicated. **D** ✦

Implement measures to reduce nausea and vomiting if present:
- Administer antiemetics as ordered. **D** ✦

Implement measures to control diarrhea if present:
- Administer antidiarrheal agents as ordered. **D** ✦

Implement measures to reduce fever if present:
- Administer antipyretics as ordered. **D** ✦

RATIONALE

Nausea often causes the client to have decreased fluid volume intake. Persistent vomiting results in excessive loss of fluid.

Persistent or severe diarrhea results in excessive loss of gastrointestinal fluid.

Fever may be accompanied by diaphoresis, which can result in excessive loss of fluid.

Accurate intake/output records must be maintained to ensure fluid loss is replaced appropriately.

Adequate fluid intake needs to be provided in order to ensure adequate hydration.

Nausea often causes the client to have decreased fluid volume intake. Persistent vomiting results in excessive loss of fluid.

Persistent or severe diarrhea results in excessive loss of gastrointestinal fluid.

Fever may be accompanied by diaphoresis, which can result in excessive loss of fluid.

THERAPEUTIC INTERVENTIONS	RATIONALE
Administer and maintain intravenous replacement fluids as ordered.	*Replacing fluid volume that is lost helps prevent/treat deficient fluid volume.*
Consult physician if signs and symptoms of deficient fluid volume persist or worsen.	*Notifying the physician allows for modification of the treatment plan.*

Nursing Diagnosis ## IMBALANCED NUTRITION: LESS THAN BODY REQUIREMENTS NDx

Definition: Intake of nutrients insufficient to meet metabolic needs.

Related to: Increased expenditure of energy to support the work of breathing

CLINICAL MANIFESTATIONS

Subjective	**Objective**
Verbal self-report of sore oral mucous membrane; altered taste sensations	Weight loss; weight less than normal for client's age, height, and body frame; abnormal BUN and low serum prealbumin and albumin levels; inflamed mucous membranes; pale conjunctiva; dyspnea on exertion

RISK FACTORS

- Smoking
- Aerosol treatments
- Productive cough
- Dyspnea
- Excessive coughing

DESIRED OUTCOMES

The client will maintain adequate nutrition status as evidenced by:
a. Weight within normal range for client
b. Normal BUN and serum prealbumin and albumin levels
c. Usual strength and activity tolerance
d. Healthy oral mucous membrane

NOC OUTCOMES

Nutritional status

NIC INTERVENTIONS

Nutritional monitoring; nutrition management; nutrition therapy

NURSING ASSESSMENT	RATIONALE
Assess for and report signs and symptoms of malnutrition: • Weight significantly below client's usual weight or less than normal for client's age, height, and body frame • Abnormal BUN and low serum prealbumin and albumin levels • Increased weakness and fatigue • Sore, inflamed oral mucous membrane • Pale conjunctiva	*Early recognition of signs and symptoms of malnutrition allows for prompt intervention.*

THERAPEUTIC INTERVENTIONS	RATIONALE
Independent Actions Monitor percentage of meals and snacks client consumes. Report inadequate intake. **D** ● ✦ Implement measures to maintain an adequate nutritional status: • Schedule treatments that assist in mobilizing mucus (e.g., aerosol treatments, postural drainage therapy) at least 1 hr before or after meals. **D** ✦	*Monitoring a client's intake helps identify when a patient is at risk for inadequate nutrition and allows for prompt intervention.* *The foul odor and taste of sputum and some aerosols are likely to decrease appetite. Appropriate scheduling of treatments also assists in decreasing nausea.*

Continued...

THERAPEUTIC INTERVENTIONS	RATIONALE
• Increase activity as tolerated. **D** ● ✦	Activity usually promotes a sense of well-being and can help improve an individual's appetite.
• Encourage a rest period before meals.	Rest before a meal helps minimize the fatigue that may occur when eating.
• Eliminate noxious sights and odors from the environment; provide client with an opaque, covered container for expectorated sputum. **D** ● ✦	Noxious sights and odors can decrease one's appetite. By eliminating them, the patient's intake may improve.
• Maintain a clean environment and a relaxed, pleasant atmosphere. **D** ● ✦	A clean environment and a relaxed atmosphere may increase intake.
• Provide oral hygiene before meals. **D** ● ✦	Oral hygiene moistens the mouth, which makes it easier to chew and swallow. It also removes unpleasant tastes, which often improves the taste of foods/fluids.
• Assist the client who is quite dyspneic in selecting foods that require little or no chewing.	Dyspnea decreases the ability of an individual to eat complete meals.
• Serve frequent, small meals rather than large ones if the client is weak, fatigues easily, or has a poor appetite. **D** ● ✦	Small, frequent meals decrease fatigue and help maintain an individual's nutritional status.
• Limit fluid intake with meals unless the fluid has high nutritional value. **D** ✦	Decreasing fluid intake during meals helps reduce early satiety and subsequent decreased food intake.
• Allow for adequate time for meals. **D** ● ✦	Clients who feel rushed during meals tend to become anxious, lose their appetite, and stop eating.
• Ensure that meals are well balanced and high in essential nutrients.	A diet that is well balanced and high in essential nutrients meets the client's nutritional needs.

Dependent/Collaborative Actions

Implement measures to maintain an adequate nutritional status:

• Place client in a high-Fowler's position for meals and provide supplemental oxygen therapy during meals if indicated. **D** ✦	Supplemental oxygen helps relieve dyspnea.
• Obtain a dietary consult to assist client in selecting foods/fluids that meet nutritional needs, are appealing, and adhere to personal and cultural preferences.	Notifying the appropriate health care professionals allows for a multifaceted approach to treatment.
• Perform a calorie count if ordered and report information to dietitian and physician.	A calorie count provides information about the caloric and nutritional value of the foods/fluids consumed. The information helps the dietitian and physician determine whether an alternative method of nutritional support is needed.
• Administer vitamins and minerals if ordered. **D** ✦	Administration of vitamins and minerals helps partially maintain nutritional status if dietary intake is not adequate.
Consult a physician about an alternative method of providing nutrition (e.g., parenteral nutrition, tube feedings) if client does not consume enough food or fluids to meet nutritional needs.	If a client is unable to eat, collaboration with the physician is required to determine alternative methods of maintaining nutritional status.

Nursing Diagnosis ACUTE PAIN NDx (CHEST)

Definition: Unpleasant sensory and emotional experience associated with actual or potential tissue damage, or described in terms of such damage (International Association for the Study of Pain); sudden or slow onset of any intensity from mild to severe with an anticipated or predictable end, and with a duration of less than 3 months.

Related to:

- Extension of the inflammatory/infection process to the pleura
- Muscle strain associated with excessive coughing

CLINICAL MANIFESTATIONS

Subjective	**Objective**
Verbal self-report of pain in chest with breathing and coughing	Increased blood pressure; increased heart rate; changes in respiratory rate; diaphoresis

RISK FACTORS

- Excessive coughing
- Increased sputum production
- Smoking and exposure to second-hand smoke

DESIRED OUTCOMES

The client will experience diminished chest pain as evidenced by:
a. Verbalization of a decrease in or absence of pain
b. Relaxed facial expression and body positioning
c. increased participation in activities

NOC OUTCOMES

Comfort level; pain control

NIC INTERVENTIONS

Pain management; environmental management; analgesic administration

NURSING ASSESSMENT	**RATIONALE**
Assess for signs and symptoms of pain (e.g., verbalization of pain, grimacing, reluctance to move, guarding of affected side of chest).	*Early recognition of signs and symptoms of pain allows for prompt intervention and improved pain control.*
Assess client's perception of the severity of pain using a pain intensity rating scale.	*An awareness of the severity of pain being experienced helps determine the most appropriate interventions for pain management. Use of a pain intensity scale gives the nurse a clearer understanding of the pain being experienced and promotes consistency when communicating with others about the client's pain experience.*
Assess the client's pain pattern (e.g., location, quality, onset, duration, precipitating factors, aggravating factors, alleviating factors).	*Knowledge of the client's pain pattern assists in the identification of effective pain management interventions.*
Ask the client to describe previous pain experiences and methods used to manage pain effectively.	*Many variables affect a client's response to pain (e.g., age, sex, coping style, previous experience with pain, culture, cause of pain). Knowledge of the client's usual response to pain and methods previously used to manage pain effectively enables the nurse to evaluate the client's pain more accurately and facilitates the identification of effective strategies for pain management.*

THERAPEUTIC INTERVENTIONS	**RATIONALE**
Independent Actions	
Implement measures to reduce fear and anxiety (e.g., assure client that chest pain is common with pneumonia and should subside with treatment of the pneumonia; assure the client that the need for pain relief is understood). **D** ✦	*Fear and anxiety can decrease the client's threshold and tolerance for pain and thereby heighten the perception of pain. In addition, pain management methods are not as effective if the client is tense and unable to relax.*
Implement measures to promote rest (e.g., minimize environmental activity and noise). **D** ● ✦	*Fatigue can decrease the client's threshold and tolerance for pain and thereby heighten the perception of pain. A client who is well rested often experiences decreased pain and increased effectiveness of pain management measures.*
Instruct and assist the client to splint the chest with hands or pillows when deep breathing, coughing, or changing position. **D** ✦	*Splinting the chest with deep breathing, coughing, or changing position reduces pain and promotes a more effective cough.*
Dependent/Collaborative Actions	
Administer analgesics before activities and procedures that can cause pain and before pain becomes severe. **D** ✦	*The administration of analgesics before a pain-producing event helps minimize the pain that may be experienced during a procedure.*

NDx = NANDA Diagnosis   **D** = Delegatable Action   ● = UAP   ✦ = LVN/LPN   ⓔ▶ = Go to ⓔvolve for animation

Continued...

THERAPEUTIC INTERVENTIONS	RATIONALE
Consult appropriate health care provider (e.g., physician, pharmacist, pain management specialist) if the provided measures fail to provide adequate pain relief.	*Notifying the appropriate health care provider allows for modification of the treatment plan.*

Nursing Diagnosis   HYPERTHERMIA NDx

Definition: Core body temperature above the normal diurnal range due to failure of thermoregulation.

Related to: Stimulation of the thermoregulatory center in the hypothalamus by endogenous pyrogens that are related to an infectious process

CLINICAL MANIFESTATIONS

Subjective	Objective
Verbal self-report of chills	Increased temperature; elevated heart rate; diaphoresis; elevated respiratory rate; flushed skin; skin warm to touch

RISK FACTORS

- Infection
- Smoking
- Smog
- Inadequate primary defenses
- Dehydration

DESIRED OUTCOMES

The client will experience resolution of hyperthermia as evidenced by:
a. Skin usual temperature and color
b. Pulse rate between 60 and 100 beats/min
c. Respiratory rate 12 to 20 breaths/min
d. Normal body temperature

NOC OUTCOMES

Thermoregulation

NIC INTERVENTIONS

Fever treatment

NURSING ASSESSMENT	RATIONALE
Assess for signs and symptoms of hyperthermia (e.g., warm, flushed skin; tachycardia; tachypnea; elevated temperature; chills; and excessive diaphoresis).	*Early recognition of signs and symptoms of a fever allows for prompt intervention.*

THERAPEUTIC INTERVENTIONS	RATIONALE

Independent Actions
Perform actions to resolve the infectious process:
- Assist client to cough and deep breathe frequently. **D** ● ✦
- Minimize environmental noise and activity. **D** ● ✦
- Organize nursing care to allow for periods of uninterrupted rest. **D** ● ✦
- Provide adequate caloric and protein intake.

Implement measures to reduce elevated temperature.
Administer tepid sponge bath and/or apply cold cloths to groin and axillae. **D** ● ✦
Use a room fan to provide cool circulating air. **D** ● ✦

Deep breathing and coughing will help remove secretions.
These actions promote rest and help conserve energy.

Adequate nutrition is needed to support functioning of the immune system.
These interventions will work to decrease the client's temperature.

Maintains air circulation and may decrease environmental temperature.

Dependent/Collaborative Actions
Implement measure to reduce elevated temperature.
Apply a cooling blanket if ordered. **D** ● ✦
Administer antipyretics and antimicrobials if ordered. **D** ✦

Consult physician if temperature remains elevated.

Helps decrease elevated temperature.

Antipyretics will help reduce elevated temperature. Appropriately prescribed anti-infectives can effectively treat the client's infection.
Notify the physician if a client's temperature does not respond to treatment.

Nursing Diagnosis **ACTIVITY INTOLERANCE** NDx

Definition: Insufficient physiological or psychological energy to endure or complete required or desired daily activities.

Related to:
- Tissue hypoxia associated with impaired gas exchange
- Difficulty resting and sleeping associated with excessive coughing, dyspnea, discomfort, unfamiliar environment, anxiety, and frequent assessments and treatments
- Inadequate nutritional status
- Increased energy expenditure associated with persistent coughing and the increased metabolic rate that is present in an infectious process

CLINICAL MANIFESTATIONS

Subjective	Objective
Verbal self-report of fatigue or weakness	Abnormal heart rate or B/P response to activity; exertional discomfort or dyspnea; electrocardiographic changes reflecting dysrhythmias or ischemia; unable to speak with physical activity

RISK FACTORS
- Bedrest or immobility
- Generalized weakness
- Sedentary lifestyle
- Imbalance between oxygen supply and demand

DESIRED OUTCOMES

The client will demonstrate an increased tolerance for activity as evidenced by:
a. Verbalization of feeling less fatigued and weak
b. Ability to perform ADL without dizziness, increased dyspnea, chest pain, diaphoresis, and a significant change in vital signs

NOC OUTCOMES

Energy conservation; rest; activity tolerance

NIC INTERVENTIONS

Energy management; oxygen therapy; sleep enhancement; nutrition management; infection control

NURSING ASSESSMENT

Assess for signs and symptoms of activity intolerance:
- Statements of fatigue or weakness
- Exertional dyspnea, chest pain, diaphoresis, or dizziness
- Abnormal heart rate response to activity (e.g., increase in rate of 20 beats/min above resting rate, rate not returning to preactivity level within 3 minutes after stopping activity, change from regular to irregular rate)
- Significant change of 15 to 20 mm Hg in B/P with activity.

RATIONALE

Early recognition of signs and symptoms of activity intolerance allows for prompt intervention.

THERAPEUTIC INTERVENTIONS

Independent Actions
Implement measures to promote rest and/or conserve energy (e.g., maintain prescribed activity restrictions, minimize environmental activity and noise, provide uninterrupted rest periods, assist with care, keep supplies and personal articles within easy reach, limit the number of visitors, use shower chair when showering, sit to brush teeth or comb hair). **D** ● ✦

Implement measures to promote sleep (e.g., elevated head of bed and support arms on pillows to facilitate breathing, maintain oxygen therapy during sleep, discourage intake of fluids high in caffeine in the evening, reduce environmental stimuli). **D** ✦

RATIONALE

Rest and activities that conserve energy result in a lower metabolic rate, which preserves nutrients and oxygen for necessary activities.

Sleep replenishes a client's energy and feeling of well-being.

NDx = NANDA Diagnosis   **D** = Delegatable Action   ● = UAP   ✦ = LVN/LPN   ⊝▶ = Go to ⊝volve for animation

Continued...

THERAPEUTIC INTERVENTIONS	RATIONALE
Implement measures to decrease excessive coughing (e.g., protect client from exposure to irritants such as smoke, flowers, and powder; avoid extremely hot or cold foods/fluids). **D** ● ✦	Excessive coughing can lead to inadequate tissue oxygenation, which results in less efficient energy production and a reduced ability to tolerate activity. Improving respiratory status increases the amount of oxygen available for energy production.
Discourage smoking and excessive intake of beverages high in caffeine such as coffee, tea, and colas. **D** ✦	Excessive intake of nicotine and caffeine can increase cardiac workload and myocardial oxygen utilization, thereby decreasing oxygen availability.
Perform actions to improve respiratory status (e.g., place client in semi- to high-Fowler's position; assist client to deep breathe or use incentive spirometry every 1 to 2 hrs; maintain bedrest as ordered; and use oxygen as needed). **D** ✦	Improvement of respiratory status is done to relieve dyspnea and improve tissue oxygenation.
Perform actions to maintain adequate nutritional status (e.g., increase activity as tolerated potentially improving appetite; encourage a rest period before meals to reduce fatigue; assist with oral hygiene before meals; maintain a clean environment and a relaxed, pleasant atmosphere). **D** ● ✦	Adequate nutritional status is important in order to maintain ADL.
Increase client's activity gradually as allowed and tolerated. **D** ● ✦	A gradual increase in activity will slowly improve strength and ability in performance of activities.
Instruct a client to:	Changes in a client's activity tolerance should be reported immediately.
• Report a decreased tolerance for activity.	Assessment of the change will allow for timely diagnosis of the cause and subsequent treatment.
• Stop any activity that causes increased chest pain, increased shortness of breath, dizziness, or extreme fatigue or weakness.	
Dependent/Collaborative Actions	
Consult appropriate health care providers (e.g., respiratory therapist, physician, dietitian) if signs and symptoms of activity intolerance persist or worsen.	Notifying the appropriate health care provider allows for modification of the treatment plan.

Nursing Diagnosis ## RISK FOR INFECTION NDx: (EXTRAPULMONARY (E.G., BACTEREMIA, PERICARDITIS, ENDOCARDITIS, MENINGITIS, SEPTIC ARTHRITIS) AND/OR SUPERINFECTION (E.G., CANDIDIASIS)

Definition: Susceptible to invasion and multiplication of pathogenic organisms, which may compromise health.

Related to:

- Spread of infecting organisms into the blood and to other sites associated with inadequate host defenses and resistance to antimicrobial agents
- Interruption in the balance of usual endogenous microbial flora associated with the administration of antimicrobial agents

CLINICAL MANIFESTATIONS

Subjective	Objective
Verbal self-report of chest pain, joint pain, fatigue, stiff neck, headache	Abnormal vital signs; unusual drainage from a body cavity; abnormal WBC and differential counts; white patches and/or ulcerations in the mouth; yeast infections

RISK FACTORS

- Smoking
- Hospitalization
- Exposure to infectious agents
- Overuse of antimicrobial agents

DESIRED OUTCOMES

The client will not develop an extrapulmonary infection or a superinfection as evidenced by:

a. Gradual return of vital signs to the client's normal range
b. Usual mental status
c. Absence of a pericardial friction rub, precordial pain, and a pathological murmur
d. Absence of joint pain and swelling
e. Absence of unusual drainage from any body cavity
f. Absence of white patches and ulcerations in the mouth
g. Absence of stiff neck and headache
h. WBC and differential counts returning toward normal range for the client

NOC OUTCOMES

Immune status; infection severity

NIC INTERVENTIONS

Infection protection; infection control

NURSING ASSESSMENT

Assess for and report signs and symptoms of an extrapulmonary infection or a superinfection:

- Increase in temperature and pulse rate above previous levels
- Change in mental status
- Pericardial friction rub, precordial pain, or development of a pathological murmur
- Swollen, red, painful joints
- Unusual color, amount, and odor of vaginal drainage (fungal infections are common superinfections with antimicrobial therapy); perineal itching; white patches or ulcerated areas in the mouth
- Stiff neck, headache, increase in WBC count above previous levels and/or significant change in differential

RATIONALE

Early recognition of signs and symptoms of an extrapulmonary or superinfection allows for prompt intervention.

THERAPEUTIC INTERVENTIONS

Independent Actions
Implement measures to prevent an extrapulmonary infection and/or a superinfection:

- Use good hand hygiene and encourage client to do the same. **D** ● ✦

- Maintain sterile technique during all invasive procedures (e.g., urinary catheterizations, venous and arterial punctures, injections). **D** ✦
- Change peripheral intravenous line sites according to hospital policy.

- Protect client from others with infection. **D** ● ✦

- Anchor catheters/tubings (e.g., urinary, intravenous) securely. **D** ✦
- Change equipment, tubings, and solutions used for treatments such as intravenous infusions and respiratory care according to hospital policy.

RATIONALE

Good hand hygiene removes transient flora, which reduces the risk of transmission of pathogens. Use of products such as an antibacterial soap, a chlorhexidine solution, or an alcohol-based hand rub agent can actually inhibit the growth of or kill microorganisms, which further reduces infection risks.

Use of sterile technique reduces the possibility of introducing pathogens into the body.

Peripheral intravenous line sites are changed routinely to reduce persistent irritation of one area of a vein wall and the resultant colonization of microorganisms at that site.

Protecting the client from others with infections reduces the client's risk of exposure to pathogens.

Trauma to the tissues and the risk for introduction of pathogens associated with in-and-out movement of the tubing are reduced.

The longer equipment, tubings, and solutions are in use, the greater the chance of colonization of microorganisms, which can then be introduced into the body.

Continued...

THERAPEUTIC INTERVENTIONS	RATIONALE
• Maintain a closed system for drains (e.g., urinary catheter) and intravenous infusions whenever possible. **D** ✦	*Each time a drainage or infusion system is opened, pathogens from the environment have an opportunity to enter the body. Maintaining a closed system decreases this risk, which reduces the possibility of infection.*
• Instruct and assist client to perform good perineal care routinely and after each bowel movement. **D** ✦	*Routine cleansing of the perineal area reduces the risk of colonization of organisms and subsequent perineal, urinary tract, and/or vaginal infection.*
• Reinforce importance of frequent oral hygiene. **D** ✦	*Frequent oral hygiene helps prevent infection by removing most of the food, debris, and many of the microorganisms that are present in the mouth. It also helps maintain the integrity of the oral mucous membranes, which provides a physical and chemical barrier to pathogens.*

Dependent/Collaborative Actions

If signs and symptoms of an extrapulmonary infection or a superinfection occur:	*An extrapulmonary and/or a superinfection should be addressed immediately. Preparation of the client for procedures that may be involved in the diagnostic process is important to alleviate associated fears and anxiety.*
• Prepare client for and/or assist with diagnostic tests (e.g., lumbar puncture, cultures, joint aspiration) if planned.	
• Administer antimicrobials as ordered.	*Antimicrobials should be administered as soon as a culture and sensitivity has been obtained.*

Collaborative Diagnosis ## RISK FOR PLEURAL EFFUSION

Definition: An abnormal accumulation of fluid in the pleural cavity that may compromise lung expansion.

Related to: Pulmonary infection; increased permeability of capillary beds

CLINICAL MANIFESTATIONS

Subjective	Objective
Verbal self-report of chest pain (pleural); dyspnea	Dull percussion note and diminished or absent breath sounds; chest radiograph showing pleural effusion; respiratory rate greater than 20 breaths/min; fever; night sweats; cough; weight loss

RISK FACTORS
- Pulmonary infection
- Increased permeability of capillary beds

DESIRED OUTCOMES

The client will not develop pleural effusion as evidenced by:
a. No increase in dyspnea
b. Symmetrical chest excursion
c. Improved breath sounds and percussion note throughout lung fields

NURSING ASSESSMENT	RATIONALE
Assess for and report signs and symptoms of pleural effusion (e.g., dyspnea, chest pain, decreased chest excursion on affected side, dull percussion note, decreased or absent breath sounds over the affected area, chest radiograph showing pleural effusion).	*Early recognition of signs and symptoms of pleural effusion allows for prompt intervention.*

THERAPEUTIC INTERVENTIONS	**RATIONALE**

Dependent/Collaborative Actions

Implement measures to resolve the infectious process:

Resolution of an infectious process reduces the risk for development of pleural effusion and/or atelectasis.

- Encourage coughing and deep breathing.

Helps expand lungs and mobilize secretions.

- Administer antimicrobials as ordered.

Treats infection.

If signs and symptoms of pleural effusion occur:

Continue with actions to improve respiratory status (e.g., increase activity tolerance; instruct client in and assist with diaphragmatic and pursed-lip breathing techniques; instruct client to deep breathe or use incentive spirometer every 1 to 2 hrs; encourage coughing and deep breathing; place client in high semi-Fowler's position).

Maintenance/improvement of the client's respiratory status and removal of secretions decrease the potential of infection or the occurrence of a pleural effusion.

- Prepare client for a thoracentesis if planned.

Removal of fluid from the lungs will help improve the client's ability to maintain adequate gas exchange.

Collaborative Diagnosis — RISK FOR ATELECTASIS

Definition: Collapse of lung tissue caused by hypoventilated alveoli.

Related to: Shallow respirations; stasis of secretion

CLINICAL MANIFESTATIONS

Subjective	**Objective**
Verbal self-report of dyspnea	Decreased breath sounds and/or crackles; cough; sputum production; low-grade fever; heart rate greater than 60 to 100 beats/min; increased respiratory rate above 20 breaths/min/effort Chest radiograph, ultrasound, or computed tomography results showing patchy infiltrates

RISK FACTORS

- Ineffective cough effort
- Immobility
- Smoking

DESIRED OUTCOMES

The client will not develop atelectasis as evidenced by:
a. Clear, audible breath sounds
b. Resonant percussion note over lungs
c. Unlabored respirations at 12 to 20 breaths/min
d. Pulse rate within normal range for client
e. Afebrile status

NURSING ASSESSMENT	**RATIONALE**

Assess for and report signs and symptoms of atelectasis:
- Diminished or absent breath sounds
- Dull percussion note over affected area
- Increased respiratory rate
- Dyspnea
- Tachycardia
- Elevated temperature

Early recognition of signs and symptoms of atelectasis allows for implementation of the appropriate interventions.

Monitor pulse oximetry results as indicated.

Pulse oximetry is an indirect measure of arterial oxygen saturation. Monitoring pulse oximetry (SaO_2) allows for early detection of hypoxia and implementation of the appropriate interventions.

Monitor chest radiograph results.

Chest radiograph provides radiographic confirmation of atelectasis.

THERAPEUTIC INTERVENTIONS	RATIONALE

Dependent/Collaborative Actions

Implement measures to prevent atelectasis:

* Perform actions to improve breathing pattern:
  * Encourage client to deep breathe.
  * Incentive spirometry
* Perform actions to promote effective airway clearance.
  * Turn, cough, and breathe deeply.

Administer antibiotics as ordered.

If signs and symptoms of atelectasis occur:

* Increase frequency of position change, coughing or "huffing," deep breathing, and use of incentive spirometer.

Consult physician if signs and symptoms of atelectasis persist or worsen.

Lack of movement places a client at risk for atelectasis. Changing positions frequently, coughing, and deep breathing help expand the lungs, enhancing alveolar expansion.
Helps mobilize secretions.

Treats infection.

Improves lung expansion and mobilization of secretions.

Allows for prompt alterations in interventions.

DISCHARGE TEACHING: CONTINUED CARE

Nursing Diagnosis **DEFICIENT KNOWLEDGE NDx, INEFFECTIVE HEALTH MAINTENANCE NDx, OR INEFFECTIVE HEALTH MANAGEMENT* NDx**

Definition: **Deficient Knowledge NDx**: Absence of cognitive information related to a specific topic, or its acquisition; **Ineffective Health Maintenance NDx**: Inability to identify, manage, and/or seek out help to maintain well-being; *Ineffective Health Management* **NDx**: Pattern of regulating and integrating into daily living a therapeutic regimen for the treatment of illness and its sequelae that is unsatisfactory for meeting specific health goals.

CLINICAL MANIFESTATIONS

Subjective	**Objective**
Verbal self-report of the problem	Inaccurate follow-through of instructions; inappropriate behaviors

RISK FACTORS

* Denial of disease process
* Cognitive deficiency
* Failure to take action to reduce risk factors

NOC OUTCOMES	NIC INTERVENTIONS
Knowledge: disease process; treatment regimen; infection control	Health system guidance; teaching: individual; teaching: disease process; teaching: prescribed medications

NURSING ASSESSMENT	RATIONALE
Assess client's ability and readiness to learn. Assess the client's understanding of teaching.	*Learning is more effective when the client is motivated and understands the importance of what is to be learned. Readiness to learn changes based on situations and physical and emotional challenges.*

THERAPEUTIC INTERVENTIONS	RATIONALE

Desired Outcome: The client will identify ways to maintain respiratory health.

THERAPEUTIC INTERVENTIONS	**RATIONALE**

Independent Actions

Instruct client in ways to maintain respiratory health:

- Consume a well-balanced diet.

- Drink at least 10 glasses of liquid per day unless contra-indicated.
- Maintain a balanced program of rest and exercise.

- Avoid crowds during flu and cold season.
- Avoid contact with persons who have respiratory infections.

- Consult physician about vaccinations available if at high risk for recurrent pneumonia.
- Continue coughing and deep breathing exercises for at least a few weeks after discharge and during any period of decreased physical activity or respiratory infection.
- Maintain good oral hygiene.

- Avoid excessive alcohol intake and stop smoking to prevent depression of pulmonary antimicrobial defenses.
- Avoid exposure to respiratory irritants (e.g., smoke and other environmental pollutants).

A well-balanced diet is important for the proper functioning of the immune system.

Adequate fluid intake is necessary to liquefy secretions.

Rest and exercise are important to maintain psychological and physical well-being.

The potential for illness is decreased through avoidance of persons with respiratory infections and of crowds during the cold and flu season.

Immunizations augment the client's immune system in fighting off infection.

Deep breathing and coughing will help remove secretions.

Good oral hygiene reduces the number of organisms in the oropharynx.

Avoidance of alcohol and smoking prevents depression of the pulmonary antimicrobial defenses.

Respiratory irritation caused by smoke and other environmental pollutants can cause changes in respiratory status in susceptible persons.

THERAPEUTIC INTERVENTIONS	**RATIONALE**

Desired Outcome: The client will state signs and symptoms to report to the health care provider.

Independent Actions

Instruct client to report the following signs and symptoms:

- Persistent or recurrent temperature elevation
- Chills
- Difficulty breathing
- Restlessness, irritability, drowsiness, or confusion
- Persistent or increased chest pain
- Persistent weight loss
- Persistent fatigue
- Persistent cough
- Unusual color, amount, and odor of vaginal secretions; white patches or ulcerated areas in the mouth; stiff neck and headache; or swollen, red, painful joints.

Reinforce the importance of keeping follow-up appointments with health care provider.

The patient's understanding of the signs and symptoms associated with infection, superinfection, extension of infection to another site, pleural effusion, and atelectasis is important for prompt identification, reporting, and treatment.

A follow-up appointment with the health care provider is important to monitor continued recovery.

THERAPEUTIC INTERVENTIONS	**RATIONALE**

Desired Outcome: The client in collaboration with the nurse, will develop a plan for adhering to recommended follow-up care including future appointment with health care provider, medications prescribed, and activity limitations.

Independent Actions

Explain the rationale for, side effects of, and importance of taking medications prescribed (e.g., antimicrobials). Inform client of pertinent food and drug interactions.

An informed client is more likely to adhere to medication regimens.

Continued...

THERAPEUTIC INTERVENTIONS	RATIONALE
Implement measures to improve client compliance: • Include significant others in all discharge teaching sessions if possible. • Encourage questions and allow time for reinforcement and clarification of information provided. Provide written instructions regarding scheduled appointments with health care provider, medications prescribed, fluid requirements, respiratory care, and signs and symptoms to report.	*Involvement of significant others in patient teaching improves adherence to discharge instructions.* *Everyone does not understand information as presented, so set aside time for questions to allow for clarification of information.* *Written instructions allow the client to refer to instructions as needed.*

ADDITIONAL NURSING DIAGNOSES

NAUSEA NDx
Related to stimulation of the vomiting center associated with noxious stimuli (e.g., foul taste of sputum and some aerosol treatments, sight of sputum)

DISTURBED SLEEP PATTERN NDx
Related to unfamiliar environment, discomfort, excessive coughing, anxiety, inability to assume usual sleep position because of dyspnea, and frequent assessments and treatments

FEAR NDx/ANXIETY NDx
Related to severity of symptoms (e.g., cough, chest pain, shortness of breath) and need for hospitalization, unfamiliar environment, and separation from significant others

PNEUMOTHORAX

Pneumothorax occurs when air accumulates in the pleural space and causes complete or partial collapse of a lung. Clinical manifestations vary with the degree of lung collapse but usually include sudden onset of unilateral sharp chest pain, tachypnea, dyspnea, anxiety, agitation, absent or diminished breath sounds, and tachycardia. When the pneumothorax is symptomatic and involves greater than 15% of the lung tissue, it is usually treated with placement of a chest tube into the intrapleural space. The tube is then connected to suction through a closed water-seal drainage system or, less frequently, to a flutter (Heimlich) valve to evacuate the intrapleural air, reestablish negative intrapleural pressure, and reexpand the lung. After lung reexpansion, obliteration of the pleural space may be necessary in some situations to minimize the risk of a recurrent pneumothorax. Methods for accomplishing this include chemical or mechanical pleurodesis, partial pleurectomy, or pleural stapling.

A pneumothorax can be classified in a variety of ways (e.g., open, closed, iatrogenic, spontaneous [primary, secondary], traumatic [penetrating, blunt]). An open pneumothorax occurs when air enters the pleural space through an opening in the chest wall. This opening can result from a penetrating injury (e.g., gunshot wound, stab wound), surgery involving the chest or diaphragm, or a complication of a diagnostic or therapeutic procedure (e.g., thoracentesis, lung biopsy, insertion of a pacemaker, subclavian venipuncture).

A closed pneumothorax occurs when air enters the pleural space without evidence of an external wound. The most common type of closed pneumothorax occurs in the absence of obvious respiratory disease and is often referred to as a primary spontaneous pneumothorax. Persons at greatest risk for this are men who are tall, 20 to 40 years of age, smokers, and have a family history of spontaneous pneumothorax. Other causes of a closed pneumothorax include damage to lung tissue as a result of a complication of pulmonary disease (e.g., COPD, cystic fibrosis, lung cancer, tuberculosis), mechanical ventilation, a fractured rib, and migration of a subclavian catheter or pacemaker lead.

This care plan focuses on the adult client hospitalized for diagnosis and treatment of a pneumothorax.

OUTCOME/DISCHARGE CRITERIA

The client will:
1. Experience reexpansion of affected lung
2. Have adequate respiratory function
3. Identify safety measures related to care of chest tube insertion site and flutter valve (if present)
4. Identify ways to reduce the risk of another pneumothorax
5. State signs and symptoms to report to the health care provider
6. Develop a plan for adhering to recommended follow-up care, including future appointments with a health care provider and activity restrictions

Nursing Diagnosis **INEFFECTIVE BREATHING PATTERN** NDx

Definition: Inspiration and/or expiration that does not provide adequate ventilation.

Related to:
- Increased rate of respirations associated with fear and anxiety
- Decreased rate of respirations associated with the depressant effect of some medications (e.g., narcotic [opioid] analgesics)
- Decreased depth of respirations associated with:
  - Reluctance to breathe deeply resulting from chest pain and fear of dislodging chest tube or experiencing another pneumothorax
  - Complete or partial collapse of the lung
  - Anxiety and the depressant effect of some medications (e.g., opioid analgesics)

CLINICAL MANIFESTATIONS

Subjective	Objective
Verbal self-report of pain, anxiety, fear/agitation, shortness of breath	Tachypnea; dyspnea; hypotension; impaired chest wall expansion; cough and/or hemoptysis; diaphoresis; diminished breath sounds; tachycardia; use of accessory muscles when breathing; significant decrease in oximetry results; abnormal arterial blood gas values; chest radiograph—collapsed lung

RISK FACTORS
- Fear
- Anxiety
- Pain

DESIRED OUTCOMES

The client will experience an effective breathing pattern as evidenced by:
a. Normal rate and depth of respirations
b. Decreased dyspnea
c. Symmetrical chest excursion

NOC OUTCOMES

Respiratory status: ventilation

NIC INTERVENTIONS

Respiratory monitoring; ventilation assistance; anxiety management; pain management

NURSING ASSESSMENT	RATIONALE
Assess for signs and symptoms of an ineffective breathing pattern (e.g., shallow respirations, tachypnea, dyspnea, asymmetrical chest excursion, use of accessory muscles when breathing).	*Early recognition of signs and symptoms of infective breathing patterns allows for prompt intervention.*

THERAPEUTIC INTERVENTIONS	RATIONALE

Independent Actions
Implement measures to improve breathing pattern:
- Perform actions to reduce chest pain (e.g., orient client to the hospital environment, equipment; maintain a calm, supportive, environment; instruct and assist client to splint chest when coughing or deep breathing). **D** ● ✦

  Reduction of chest pain increases the client's willingness to move and breathe more deeply.

- Perform actions to reduce fear and anxiety (e.g., assure client that staff members are nearby; respond to call signal as soon as possible; provide calm, restful environment; instruct in relaxation techniques; encourage family to project a supportive attitude without obvious anxiousness). **D** ✦

  Reduction of fear and anxiety assists in preventing the shallow and/or rapid breathing associated with these emotions.

Place the client in semi- to high-Fowler's position unless contraindicated; position with pillows to prevent slumping. **D** ● ✦

  Positioning the client in semi- to high-Fowler's position promotes optimal gas exchange by enabling chest expansion.
  Positioning with pillows prevents slumping.

NDx = NANDA Diagnosis   **D** = Delegatable Action   ● = UAP   ✦ = LVN/LPN   ⊜▶ = Go to ⊜volve for animation

Continued...

THERAPEUTIC INTERVENTIONS	RATIONALE
• Instruct client to breathe deeply or use incentive spirometer every 1 to 2 hrs. **D** ✦	*Forced deep breathing and use of incentive spirometry will increase expansion of the lungs and improve the client's ability to clear mucus from the lungs. The technique may also increase the amount of oxygen that is able to penetrate deep into the lungs.*
• Assure the client that deep breathing and turning should not dislodge the chest tube or increase the risk of another pneumothorax.	*This assurance will decrease the client's anxiety and fear associated with the chest tube and the original pneumothorax.*
• Instruct the client to breathe slowly, if hyperventilating.	*Hyperventilation is an ineffective breathing pattern that can eventually lead to respiratory alkalosis. Clients can often slow their breathing rate if they concentrate on doing so.*
• Increase activity as allowed and tolerated. **D** ● ✦	*During activity, especially ambulation, the client usually takes deeper breaths, thus increasing lung expansion.*

Dependent/Collaborative Actions

Implement measures to improve breathing pattern:

• Medicate with analgesics as needed. **D** ✦	*Pain relief increases client's willingness to take deep breaths and improve lung expansion.*
• Administer CNS depressants judiciously; hold medications and consult physician if respiratory rate is less than 12 breaths/min. **D** ✦	*CNS depressants cause depression of the respiratory center in the brainstem, which can result in a decreased rate and depth of respiration.*
Consult appropriate health care provider (e.g., respiratory therapist, physician) if ineffective breathing pattern continues.	*Notifying the appropriate health care provider allows for modifications of treatment.*

Nursing Diagnosis **IMPAIRED GAS EXCHANGE** NDx

Definition: Excess or deficit in oxygenation and/or carbon dioxide elimination at the alveolar-capillary membrane.

Related to: Loss of effective lung surface, associated with partial or complete lung collapse

CLINICAL MANIFESTATIONS

Subjective	Objective
Verbal self-report of restlessness, irritability, confusion, and somnolence	Tachypnea; dyspnea; significant decrease in oximetry results; decreased PaO_2 and/or increased $PaCO_2$; chest radiograph—presence of air or blood in the pleural space on the affected side and any mediastinal shift; abnormal arterial blood gases-oxygen saturation less than 90%; hypoxemia; hypercarbia; decreased Hgb and Hct associated with blood loss in a hemothorax; hypoxemia; hypocarbia; nasal flaring; tachycardia

RISK FACTORS

- Decreased lung expansion
- Pain
- Muscle fatigue
- Obesity

DESIRED OUTCOMES

The client will experience adequate O_2/CO_2 exchange as evidenced by:
a. Usual mental status
b. Unlabored respirations of 12 to 20 breaths/min
c. Oximetry results within normal range
d. Arterial blood gas values within normal range

NOC OUTCOMES

Respiratory status: gas exchange

NIC INTERVENTIONS

Respiratory monitoring; oxygen therapy; chest tube care; acid-base management

NURSING ASSESSMENT	**RATIONALE**
Assess for and report signs and symptoms of impaired gas exchange:	*Early recognition of signs and symptoms of ineffective gas exchange allows for prompt intervention.*
• Restlessness, irritability	
• Confusion, somnolence	
• Tachypnea, dyspnea	
• Significant decrease in oximetry results	
• Decreased PaO_2 and/or increased $PaCO_2$	

THERAPEUTIC INTERVENTIONS	**RATIONALE**

Independent Actions

Implement measures to improve gas exchange:

- Perform actions to promote lung reexpansion:
  - Prepare client for and assist with insertion of chest tube (the tube is then connected to a drainage system [with or without suction] or, less commonly, to a flutter valve).

    Provide client with information related to the procedure to decrease the experience of fear and anxiety.

  - After chest tube insertion, implement measures to maintain patency and integrity of chest drainage system:

    These actions help ensure maintenance of the chest tube drainage system and facilitate drainage.

  - Maintain fluid level in water seal and suction chambers as ordered.

    Fluid level determines the level of suction in a closed drainage system.

  - Maintain occlusive dressing over chest tube insertion site.

    Maintains a seal around the chest tube insertion site, preventing air leaks and loss of negative pressure

  - Tape all connections securely.

    Supports maintenance of a closed system and reduces the risk of air leaks

  - Tape the tubing to the chest wall close to insertion site.

    Taping the tubing to the chest wall close to the insertion site reduces the risk of inadvertent removal of the tube.

  - Position tubing to avoid kinks; coil excess tubing on the bed rather than allowing it to hang down below the collection device. **D** ✦

    Excess tubing hanging over the bed in a dependent loop allows drainage to collect in the loop and could occlude the drainage system. Kinked tubing blocks drainage and may promote fluid or blood accumulation in the pleural cavity.

  - Keep drainage collection device below level of client's chest at all times.

    The system must be lower than the level of the client's chest to promote chest tube drainage.

- Maintain suction as ordered; ensure that the air vent is open on the drainage collection device if the system is to water seal only; if a flutter valve is present, ensure that there is no fluid in the valve and that the distal end is open.

  These actions facilitate the escape of air from the pleural space.

- Avoid stripping or clamping a chest tube.

  Stripping a chest tube may cause high negative pressure in the pleural space and can potentially damage the lung tissue. Clamping a chest tube can block air from escaping the pleural space, which may lead to a tension pneumothorax.

  - Keep a petrolatum gauze dressing at the bedside.

    This dressing is applied to the insertion site if the chest tube becomes dislodged. This will maintain an airtight seal, preventing a recurrence of a pneumothorax.

  - Keep a bottle of sterile water at the bedside.

    If the chest tube becomes disconnected, submerging it in a bottle of sterile water will provide a temporary closed drainage system.

Perform actions to improve breathing patterns (e.g., place client in semi- to high-Fowler's position to improve air exchange; instruct client to breathe deeply or use incentive spirometer every 1 to 2 hrs).

Positioning the client in semi- to high-Fowler's position promotes optimal gas exchange by enabling chest expansion.

Forced deep breathing and use of incentive spirometry will increase expansion of the lungs and improve the client's ability to clear mucus from the lungs. The technique may also increase the amount of oxygen that is able to penetrate deep into the lungs.

- Discourage smoking.

  Smoking impairs gas exchange because it (1) reduces effective airway clearance by increasing mucus production and impairing ciliary function; (2) decreases oxygen availability (Hgb binds with the carbon monoxide in smoke rather than with oxygen); (3) causes damage to the bronchial and alveolar walls; and (4) causes vasoconstriction and subsequently reduces pulmonary blood flow.

NDx = NANDA Diagnosis   **D** = Delegatable Action   ● = UAP   ✦ = LVN/LPN   ⊜▶ = Go to ⊜volve for animation

Continued...

THERAPEUTIC INTERVENTIONS	RATIONALE
Dependent/Collaborative Actions Implement measures to improve gas exchange:	
• Maintain activity restrictions as ordered; increase activity gradually as allowed and tolerated. **D** ● ✦	*Conservation of energy through activity restrictions allows energy to be focused on breathing. Increasing activity as tolerated helps mobilize excretions and promotes deeper breathing and lung expansion.*
• Maintain oxygen therapy as ordered. **D** ✦	*Supplemental oxygen helps relieve dyspnea.*
Consult appropriate health care provider (e.g., respiratory therapist, physician) if signs and symptoms of impaired gas exchange persist or worsen.	*Notifying the appropriate health care professionals allows for a prompt and multifaceted approach to treatment.*

Nursing Diagnosis   ACUTE PAIN NDx (CHEST)

Definition: Unpleasant sensory and emotional experience associated with actual or potential tissue damage, or described in terms of such damage (International Association for the Study of Pain); sudden or slow onset of any intensity from mild to severe with an anticipated or predictable end, and a duration of less than 3 months.

Related to: Irritation of the parietal pleura and associated with:
• Stretching of the pleura resulting from air in the pleural space
• Tissue irritation associated with insertion and presence of a chest tube

CLINICAL MANIFESTATIONS

Subjective	Objective
Verbal self-report of chest pain with breathing and coughing	Grimacing; rubbing chest; reluctance to move; shallow respirations; restlessness; increased B/P; tachycardia

RISK FACTORS
• Excessive coughing
• Increased sputum production
• Chest tubes

DESIRED OUTCOMES

The client will experience diminished chest pain as evidenced by:
a. Verbalization of a decrease in or absence of pain
b. Relaxed facial expression and body positioning
c. Improve breathing pattern
d. Increased participation in activities
e. Stable vital signs

NOC OUTCOMES	NIC INTERVENTIONS
Pain control; comfort level	Pain management; environmental management; analgesic administration

NURSING ASSESSMENT	RATIONALE
Assess for signs and symptoms of chest pain (e.g., verbalization of pain, grimacing, rubbing chest, guarding of affected side of chest, reluctance to move, shallow respirations, restlessness, increased B/P, tachycardia).	*Early recognition of signs and symptoms of pain allows for prompt intervention and improved pain control.*
Assess client's perception of the severity of pain using a pain intensity rating scale.	*An awareness of the severity of pain being experienced helps determine the most appropriate interventions for pain management. Use of a pain intensity rating scale gives the nurse a clearer understanding of the pain being experienced and promotes consistency when communicating with others about the client's pain experience.*
Assess the client's pain pattern (e.g., location, quality, onset, duration, precipitating factors, aggravating factors, alleviating factors).	*Knowledge of the client's pain pattern assists in the identification of effective pain management interventions.*

NURSING ASSESSMENT	RATIONALE
Ask the client to describe previous pain experiences and methods used to manage pain effectively.	*Many variables affect a client's response to pain (e.g., age, sex, coping style, previous experience with pain, culture, cause of pain). Knowledge of the client's usual response to pain and methods previously used to manage pain effectively enables the nurse to evaluate the client's pain more accurately and facilitates the identification of effective strategies for pain management.*

THERAPEUTIC INTERVENTIONS	RATIONALE
Independent Actions	
Implement measures to reduce fear and anxiety (e.g., assure client that chest pain is common with pneumothorax and should subside with treatment; assure client that the need for pain relief is understood).	*Fear and anxiety can decrease the client's threshold and tolerance for pain and thereby heighten the perception of pain. In addition, pain management methods are not as effective if the client is tense and unable to relax.*
Implement measures to promote rest (e.g., minimize environmental activity and noise). **D** ● ✦	*Fatigue can decrease the client's threshold and tolerance for pain and thereby heighten the perception of pain. A client who is well rested often experiences decreased pain and increased effectiveness of pain management measures.*
Perform actions to facilitate the escape of air from the pleural space (e.g., maintain suction as ordered; ensure the air vent is open on the drainage collective device if system is to water seal only; if flutter valve is present, ensure that there is not fluid in the valve and that the distal end is open).	*These actions promote the removal of air from the pleural space and work to expand lung tissue.*
Instruct and assist the client to splint the chest with hands or pillows when deep breathing, coughing, or changing position.	*Splinting the chest with deep breathing, coughing, or changing position reduces pain and promotes a more effective cough.*
Provide or assist with nonpharmacological methods for pain relief (e.g., position change; progressive relaxation exercises; restful environment; diversional activities such as watching television, reading, or conversing).	*Nonpharmacological pain management includes a variety of interventions. It is believed that most of these are effective because they stimulate closure of the gating mechanism in the spinal cord and subsequently block the transmission of pain impulses. In addition, some interventions are thought to stimulate the release of endogenous analgesics (e.g., endorphins) that inhibit the transmission of pain impulses and/or alter the client's perception of pain. Many of the nonpharmacological interventions also help decrease pain by promoting relaxation.*
Securely anchor the chest tube.	*Limiting movement of the chest tube prevents resulting tissue irritation from the chest tube.*
Collaborative/Dependent Interventions	
Administer analgesics before activities and procedures that can cause pain and before pain becomes severe; and as ordered. **D** ✦	*The administration of analgesics before a pain-producing event helps minimize the pain that will be experienced. When given prior to a procedure, analgesics improve the client's ability to tolerate activities.*
Consult appropriate health care provider (e.g., pharmacist, pain management specialist, physician) if the provided measures fail to provide adequate pain relief.	*Notifying the appropriate health care professionals allows for a prompt and multifaceted approach to treatment.*

Collaborative Diagnosis · RISK FOR TENSION PNEUMOTHORAX WITH MEDIASTINAL SHIFT

Definition: Rapid accumulation of air in the pleural space causing severely high intrapleural pressures with resultant increased tension on the heart and great vessels; related to a significant increase in intrapleural pressure associated with inability of air to leave pleural space during expiration (can occur as a result of chest tube or flutter valve malfunction).

Related to: High intrapleural pressures, chest tube malfunction

NDx = NANDA Diagnosis   **D** = Delegatable Action   ● = UAP   ✦ = LVN/LPN   ⊝▶ = Go to ⊝volve for animation

CLINICAL MANIFESTATIONS

Subjective	Objective
Verbal self-report of pain; fear; anxiety	Lack of fluctuations in water seal chamber; dyspnea; subcutaneous emphysema; expanding area of absent breath sounds with hyperresonant percussion note; heart rate irregular and greater than 100 beats/min; low B/P; neck vein distention; hypoxemia ($PaO_2 < 80$ mm Hg); hypercarbia ($PaCO_2 > 45$ mm Hg); respiratory acidosis (pH < 7.35); chest radiograph—expanding size of the pneumothorax and mediastinal shift

RISK FACTORS

- Ineffective lung expansion
- Immobility
- Stasis of secretions

DESIRED OUTCOMES

The client will not develop tension pneumothorax with mediastinal shift as evidenced by:
a. No sudden increase in dyspnea
b. Vital signs within normal range for client
c. Usual mental status
d. Absence of neck vein distention
e. Trachea in midline position
f. Usual skin color
g. Arterial blood gas values returning toward normal

NURSING ASSESSMENT

Assess for and immediately report signs and symptoms of:
- Malfunction of chest drainage system (e.g., respiratory distress, lack of fluctuation in the water seal chamber without evidence of lung reexpansion, excessive bubbling in water seal chamber, significant increase in subcutaneous emphysema)
- Malfunction of the flutter valve if present (e.g., respiratory distress, abrupt cessation of air flow from the distal end of the valve during exhalation)
- Extended pneumothorax (e.g., extended area of absent breath sounds with hyperresonant percussion note, increased dyspnea, chest radiograph showing an increase in size of pneumothorax)
- Tension pneumothorax (e.g., severe dyspnea, rapid and/or irregular heart rate, hypotension, restlessness, agitation, confusion, neck vein distention, shift in trachea from midline, arterial blood gas values that have worsened, chest radiograph showing a mediastinal shift).

RATIONALE

Early recognition of signs and symptoms of a malfunction in the chest tube drainage system allows for prompt intervention and decreases the potential prevention of an extension of the pneumothorax.

THERAPEUTIC INTERVENTIONS

Dependent/Collaborative Actions

Implement measures to promote lung reexpansion (e.g., maintain proper functioning of the closed chest drainage system).

If signs and symptoms of tension pneumothorax with mediastinal shift occur:

Maintain client on bedrest in a semi- to high-Fowler's position.
- Maintain oxygen therapy as ordered.
- Assist with clearing existing chest tube or flutter valve, insertion of new tube, and/or needle aspiration of air from the pleural space.

RATIONALE

Proper functioning of a closed chest drainage system reduces the risk of tension pneumothorax with mediastinal shift.

Positioning the client in semi- to high-Fowler's position promotes optimal gas exchange by enabling chest expansion.
Supplemental oxygen helps relieve dyspnea and improves gas exchange.
By clearing existing chest tube/flutter valve, inserting a new tube, and/or performing needle aspiration, intrapleural pressure is reduced and lung expansion is promoted.

Nursing Diagnosis FEAR NDx/ANXIETY NDx

Definition: **Fear NDx:** Response to perceived threat that is consciously recognized as a danger.
Anxiety NDx: Vague, uneasy feeling of discomfort or dread accompanied by an autonomic response (the source is often nonspecific or unknown to the individual); a feeling of apprehension caused by anticipation of danger. It is an alerting signal that warns of impending danger and enables the individual to take measures to deal with the threat.

Related to:
- Exacerbation of symptoms (e.g., increased dyspnea, feeling of suffocation), need for hospitalization, and concern about prognosis
- Lack of understanding of the diagnosis, diagnostic tests, treatments, and prognosis
- Financial concerns about hospitalization

CLINICAL MANIFESTATIONS

Subjective	Objective
Verbal self-report of anxiety; usual perceptual ability and interactions with others	Unusual sleep patterns; unstable vital signs; restlessness; shakiness; diaphoresis; self-focused behavior

RISK FACTORS
- Pain
- Fear of unknown
- Fear of environment

DESIRED OUTCOMES

The client will experience a reduction in fear and anxiety as evidenced by:
a. Verbalization of feeling less anxious
b. Usual sleep pattern
c. Relaxed facial expression and body movements
d. Stable vital signs
e. Usual perceptual ability and interactions with others

NOC OUTCOMES

Anxiety level; fear level; anxiety self-control; fear self-control

NIC INTERVENTIONS

Anxiety reduction; calming technique; emotional support; presence; pain management

NURSING ASSESSMENT	RATIONALE
Assess client for signs and symptoms of fear and anxiety (e.g., verbalization of feeling anxious, insomnia, tenseness, shakiness, restlessness, diaphoresis, elevated B/P, tachycardia, self-focused behaviors).	*Moderate anxiety enhances the client's ability to solve problems. With severe anxiety or panic, the client is not able to follow directions and may become hyperactive and extremely agitated.*
Validate perceptions carefully, remembering that some behavior may result from hypoxia and/or hypercapnia.	*Assessment of the client's fear helps determine whether the coping mechanisms are effective and which need to be strengthened.*

THERAPEUTIC INTERVENTIONS	RATIONALE

Independent Actions
Implement measures to reduce fear and anxiety:

• Orient client to hospital environment, equipment, and routines. **D** ● ✦	*Familiarity with the environment and usual routines reduces the client's anxiety about the unknown, provides a sense of security, and increases the client's sense of control, all of which help decrease anxiety.*
• Introduce staff who will be participating in the client's care. If possible, maintain consistency in staff assigned to client's care.	*Introduction to staff familiarizes clients with those individuals who will be working with them, which provides clients with a feeling of stability, which reduces the anxiety that typically occurs with change.*
• Assure client that staff members are nearby; respond to call signal as soon as possible. **D** ● ✦	*Close contact and a prompt response to requests provide a sense of security and facilitate the development of trust, thus reducing the client's anxiety.*

Continued...

THERAPEUTIC INTERVENTIONS	RATIONALE
• Maintain a calm, supportive, confident manner when interacting with client; encourage verbalization of fear and anxiety. **D** ● ✦	A sense of calmness and confidence conveys to the client that someone is in control of the situation, which helps reduce anxiety.
• Reinforce physician's explanations and clarify misconceptions the client has about the pneumothorax, treatment plan, and possible recurrence; encourage questions.	Factual information and an awareness of what to expect help decrease the anxiety that arises from uncertainty.
• Implement measures to reduce respiratory distress if present:	Improvement of respiratory status helps relieve the anxiety associated with the feeling of not being able to breathe.
• Elevate the head of the bed.	
• Encourage the client to breathe deeply and more slowly. **D** ● ✦	
• Implement measures to reduce pain:	Pain can create or increase anxiety because it is often perceived as a threat to well-being.
• Instruct client in relaxation techniques and encourage participation in diversional activities once the period of acute pain and respiratory distress has subsided.	Pain also causes sympathetic nervous system stimulation with subsequent feelings of tenseness and increased anxiety.
• When appropriate, assist the client to meet spiritual needs (e.g., arrange for a visit from the clergy).	Spiritual support is a source of comfort and security for many people and can help reduce the client's fear and anxiety.
• Provide information based on current needs of client at a level that can be understood.	Providing information that the client is not ready to process or cannot understand tends to increase anxiety.
• Encourage the client to ask questions and to seek clarification of information provided.	Making the client feel comfortable enough to ask questions or clarify information helps reduce anxiety.
• Provide a calm, restful environment. **D** ● ✦	A calm, restful environment facilitates relaxation and promotes a sense of security, which reduces fear and anxiety.
• Encourage significant others to project a caring, concerned attitude without obvious fear and anxiousness. **D** ✦	Anxiety is easily transferable from one person to another. If significant others convey empathy, provide reassurance, and do not appear anxious, they can help reduce the client's fear and anxiety.
Dependent/Collaborative Actions	
• Implement measures to reduce fear and anxiety:	
• Administer oxygen via nasal cannula rather than mask if possible. **D** ✦	The use of a mask for some clients seems restrictive and suffocating. The use of a nasal cannula is more comfortable and less constraining. Improvement of respiratory status helps relieve anxiety associated with the feeling of not being able to breathe.
• Administer prescribed antianxiety agents if indicated. **D** ✦	Reduces client's fear and anxiety.
Consult appropriate health care provider (e.g., psychiatric nurse clinician, physician) if the provided actions fail to control fear and anxiety.	Notifying the appropriate health care provider allows for modification of the treatment plan.

DISCHARGE TEACHING/CONTINUED CARE

Nursing Diagnosis   ## DEFICIENT KNOWLEDGE NDx, INEFFECTIVE HEALTH MAINTENANCE NDx, OR INEFFECTIVE HEALTH MANAGEMENT* NDx

Definition: **Deficient Knowledge NDx:** Absence of cognitive information related to a specific topic, or its acquisition; **Ineffective Health Maintenance NDx:** Inability to identify, manage, and/or seek out help to maintain well-being; **Ineffective Health Management NDx:** Pattern of regulating and integrating into daily living a therapeutic regimen for the treatment of illness and its sequelae that is unsatisfactory for meeting specific health goals.

CLINICAL MANIFESTATIONS

Subjective	**Objective**
Verbal self-report of the problem	Inaccurate follow-through of instructions; inappropriate behaviors

RISK FACTORS

- Denial of disease process
- Fear and anxiety that blocks ability to understand

NOC OUTCOMES	**NIC INTERVENTIONS**
Knowledge: treatment regimen; health promotion	Health system guidance; teaching: individual; teaching: procedure/treatment

NURSING ASSESSMENT	**RATIONALE**
Assess client's readiness and ability to learn.	*Early recognition of readiness to learn and meaning of illness to client allows for implementation of the appropriate teaching interventions.*

THERAPEUTIC INTERVENTIONS	**RATIONALE**

Desired Outcome: The client will identify safety measures related to care of chest tube insertion site and flutter valve (if present).

Independent Actions

If the chest tube is removed before discharge, explain the importance of keeping a dressing over the insertion site until instructed by physician to remove it.	*The occlusive dressing over the insertion site maintains a seal to the area where the chest tube was removed, preventing potential air leaks and loss of negative pressure during healing. Removal of this by someone other than a physician may cause a recurrence of the pneumothorax.*
If client is discharged with a flutter valve in place, reinforce the following safety measures:	
• Maintain an occlusive dressing around the insertion site.	*The occlusive dressing around the insertion site prevents potential air leaks and loss of negative pressure.*
• Ensure that the connection between the chest tube and flutter valve is taped securely and anchored to the chest wall using tape.	*Supports maintenance of a closed system and reduces the risk of air leaks. Anchoring tubing to the chest wall close to the insertion site reduces the risk of inadvertent removal of the tube.*
• Maintain patency of the flutter valve (e.g., avoid occluding the distal end of the flutter valve, contact physician if fluid collects in the valve, avoid activities such as swimming and bathing [the valve should not be submerged in water]).	*A decrease in patency of the flutter valve causes a loss of negative pressure and may cause a recurrence of the pneumothorax.*
Allow time for questions and clarification of information provided.	*Everyone does not understand information as presented, so set aside time for questions to allow for clarification of information.*

THERAPEUTIC INTERVENTIONS	**RATIONALE**

Desired Outcome: The client will identify ways to reduce the risk of another pneumothorax.

Independent Actions

Caution client to avoid activities that involve experiencing marked changes in atmospheric pressure (e.g., scuba diving, flying in an unpressurized aircraft, mountain climbing).	*Changes in atmospheric pressure may cause a recurrence in an individual recovering from a pneumothorax.*

Continued...

THERAPEUTIC INTERVENTIONS	RATIONALE
Encourage client to stop smoking.	*Smoking impairs gas exchange because it (1) reduces effective airway clearance by increasing mucus production and impairing ciliary function; (2) decreases oxygen availability (Hgb binds with the carbon monoxide in smoke rather than with oxygen); (3) causes damage to the bronchial and alveolar walls; and (4) causes vasoconstriction and subsequently reduces pulmonary blood flow.*
Instruct client to continue treatment of any underlying lung disease (e.g., COPD, tuberculosis)	*Treatment of underlying lung disease helps prevent recurrence of a pneumothorax.*

THERAPEUTIC INTERVENTIONS	RATIONALE

Desired Outcome: The client will state signs and symptoms to report to the health care provider.

Independent Actions

Instruct client to report the following signs and symptoms: • Difficulty breathing • Chest pain • Elevated temperature • Chills • Increased redness and warmth at chest tube insertion site • Purulent drainage from chest tube insertion site or flutter valve	*Recognition of signs and symptoms of infection leads to early treatment of respiratory infections.*

THERAPEUTIC INTERVENTIONS	RATIONALE

Desired Outcome: The client, in collaboration with the nurse, will develop a plan for adhering to recommended follow-up care, including future appointments with the health care provider and activity restrictions.

Independent Actions

Reinforce importance of keeping follow-up appointments with health care provider.	*A follow-up appointment with the health care provider is important to monitor continued recovery.*
Instruct client to avoid excessive physical exertion and lifting objects over 10 lb until permitted by physician.	*Lifting an object over 10 lb and physical exertion may place the client at risk for recurrence of a pneumothorax.*
Reinforce physician's explanation about the possibility of another pneumothorax.	*Clients need to be aware that they are at risk for a recurrence of a pneumothorax.*
Assist client to develop a plan for obtaining emergency assistance if pneumothorax recurs.	*An informed client is more likely to adhere to medication regimens.*
Encourage client to continue with deep breathing exercises and use of incentive spirometer for the length of time recommended by physician.	*Forced deep breathing and use of incentive spirometry will increase expansion of the lungs and improve the client's ability to clear mucus from the lungs. The technique may also improve the amount of oxygen that is able to penetrate deep into the lungs.*
Implement measures to improve client compliance: • Include significant others in teaching sessions if possible.	*Involvement of significant others in patient teaching improves adherence to discharge instructions.*
• Encourage questions and allow time for reinforcement and clarification of information provided.	*Information is presented with time for questions to allow for clarification of information.*
• Provide written instructions about precautions related to chest tube insertion site and flutter valve (if present), signs and symptoms to report, future appointments with health care provider, and activity restrictions.	*Written instructions allow the client to refer to instructions as needed.*

ADDITIONAL NURSING DIAGNOSES

NAUSEA NDx

Related to stimulation of the vomiting center associated with noxious stimuli (e.g., foul taste of sputum and some aerosol treatments, sight of sputum)

DISTURBED SLEEP PATTERN NDx

Related to unfamiliar environment, discomfort, excessive coughing, anxiety, inability to assume usual sleep position because of dyspnea, and frequent assessments and treatments.

PULMONARY EMBOLISM

Pulmonary embolism is the partial or complete obstruction of one of the pulmonary arterial vessels by an embolus. The most common source of the embolus is a thrombus that originates in a deep vein of the lower extremities. The embolus can also originate in the right side of the heart, the upper extremities, and vessels that have sustained endothelial injury caused by factors such as trauma, surgery, or the presence of an indwelling central venous catheter. Non-thrombotic sources of pulmonary embolism include air, fat, amniotic fluid, tumor cells, and foreign material (e.g., broken intravenous catheter, talc [often used to "cut" drugs injected by intravenous drug abusers]).

The clinical manifestations of pulmonary embolism are varied and nonspecific. The extensiveness of the signs and symptoms depends on the size and number of emboli, size of the vessel that is occluded, extent of vessel occlusion, and presence of preexisting cardiac or pulmonary disease. The classic signs and symptoms of a moderate-size pulmonary embolism are sudden onset of dyspnea, tachypnea, tachycardia, hypoxia, and a feeling of apprehension or impending doom. The person may also experience pleuritic chest pain, cough, and low-grade fever.

Medical treatment varies depending on the source of the embolus and its effect on cardiopulmonary function. When the source is a thrombus, treatment usually consists of bedrest and immediate initiation of intravenous anticoagulant therapy. A thrombolytic agent might be administered if the thromboembolus is occluding a large vessel, cardiopulmonary status is severely compromised, or both. Anticoagulant therapy (subcutaneous and/or oral) often continues for 3 to 6 months after discharge. If thrombolytic agents and anticoagulant therapy are contraindicated or unsuccessful, or the source of the embolus is nonthrombotic, surgical removal of the embolus may be indicated.

This care plan focuses on the adult client hospitalized for treatment of a pulmonary embolism resulting from a deep vein thrombus. Much of the information is also applicable to clients receiving follow-up care at home.

OUTCOME/DISCHARGE CRITERIA

The client will:
1. Have adequate respiratory function
2. Have no signs and symptoms of complications
3. Identify ways to reduce the risk of recurrent thrombus formation and pulmonary embolism
4. Verbalize an understanding of medications ordered including rationale, food and drug interactions, side effects, schedule for taking, and importance of taking as prescribed
5. Demonstrate the ability to correctly draw up and administer anticoagulant medication subcutaneously if prescribed
6. Identify ways to prevent bleeding associated with anticoagulant therapy
7. State signs and symptoms to report to the health care provider
8. Develop a plan for adhering to recommended follow-up care, including future appointments with health care provider and activity level

---

Nursing Diagnosis **INEFFECTIVE BREATHING PATTERN** NDx

Definition: Inspiration and/or expiration that does not provide adequate ventilation.

Related to:
- Increased rate of respirations associated with fear, anxiety, and stimulant effects of hypoxia
- Decreased rate of respirations associated with the depressant effect of some medications (e.g., narcotic [opioid] analgesics)
- Decreased depth of respirations associated with:
  - Fear, anxiety, and reluctance to breathe deeply because of chest pain, if present
  - Depressant effect of some medications (e.g., narcotic [opioid] analgesics)
  - Decreased mobility

CLINICAL MANIFESTATIONS

Subjective	Objective
Verbal self-report of restlessness, anxiety, nausea, chest pain, shortness of breath	Dyspnea; tachypnea; tachycardia; hypotension; impaired chest wall expansion; cough and/or hemoptysis; transient pleural rub; jugular vein distention; diaphoresis; cyanosis; abnormal breath sounds—crackles; S1 and S4 gallop rhythms; transient pleural friction rub; fever; use of accessory muscles when breathing; significant decrease in oximetry results; abnormal arterial blood gas values; chest radiograph—normal or elevated hemidiaphragm; after 24 hrs—small infiltrates

RISK FACTORS

- DVT
- Pain
- Muscle fatigue
- Obesity
- Immobility

DESIRED OUTCOMES

The client will experience an effective breathing pattern as evidenced by:
a. Normal rate and depth of respirations
b. Absence of dyspnea

NOC OUTCOMES

Respiratory status; ventilation

NIC INTERVENTIONS

Respiratory monitoring; ventilation assistance; anxiety management; pain management

NURSING ASSESSMENT	RATIONALE
Assess for signs and symptoms of an ineffective breathing pattern: • Rapid, shallow respirations • Restlessness • Significant decrease in oximetry results • Abnormal arterial blood gas values • Assess for significant abnormalities in chest radiograph reports.	*Early recognition of signs and symptoms of ineffective breathing patterns allows for prompt intervention.*

THERAPEUTIC INTERVENTIONS	RATIONALE

Independent Actions

Implement measures to improve breathing pattern:
- Perform actions to reduce chest pain:
  - Splint chest with pillow or hands when deep breathing, coughing, and changing position. **D** ● ✦

  Splinting the chest with deep breathing, coughing, or changing position reduces pain and promotes a more effective respiratory effort.
  - Provide or assist with nonpharmacological methods for pain relief (e.g., relaxation techniques, restful environment, diversional activities).

  Relaxation and diversional activities help alleviate pain, fear, and anxiety. Pain causes sympathetic nervous system stimulation with subsequent feelings of tenseness and increased anxiety, and can increase respiratory distress.

- Perform actions to reduce fear and anxiety:
  - Remain with client during periods of respiratory distress.

  Reduction in fear and anxiety prevents the shallow and/or rapid breathing that can occur with fear and anxiety.
  - Provide a calm, restful environment. **D** ● ✦

  A calm, restful environment facilitates relaxation and promotes a sense of security, and reduces the rapid breathing associated with fear and anxiety.

- Elevate the head of the bed.

  Provides for improved expansion of the lungs.
- Encourage the client to breathe deeply and more slowly. **D** ● ✦

  Helps calm the client while improving ventilation.
- Perform actions to improve gas exchange:
  Place client in a semi- to high-Fowler's position unless contraindicated. **D** ● ✦

  Placing the client in a semi- to high-Fowler's position promotes optimal gas exchange by enabling chest expansion.
  - Position with pillows. **D** ● ✦

  Positioning with pillows helps prevent slumping.

THERAPEUTIC INTERVENTIONS	RATIONALE
• Instruct client to breathe slowly; if hyperventilating, instruct client to breathe deeply or use incentive spirometer every 1 to 2 hrs.	*Deep breathing and use of incentive spirometry help reduce dyspnea and improve tissue oxygenation.*
• Increase activity when allowed. **D** ● ✦	*Conservation of energy through activity restrictions allows energy to be focused on breathing. Increasing activity as tolerated helps mobilize excretions and promotes deeper breathing and lung expansion.*

Dependent/Collaborative Actions

Implement measures to improve breathing pattern:

• Perform actions to reduce chest pain: • Administer analgesics as needed.	*Pain relief increases client's willingness to take deep breaths and improves lung expansion.*
• Administer CNS depressants judiciously; hold medication and consult physician if respiratory rate is less than 12 breaths/min.	*CNS depressants cause depression of the respiratory center in the brainstem, which can result in a decreased rate and depth of respiration.*
Consult appropriate health care provider (e.g., respiratory therapist, physician) if ineffective breathing pattern persists or worsens.	*Notifying the appropriate health care professionals allows for a prompt and multidisciplinary approach to treatment.*

Nursing Diagnosis   **IMPAIRED GAS EXCHANGE** NDx

Definition: Deficit in oxygenation and/or carbon dioxide elimination at the alveolar-capillary membrane.

Related to:
- Decreased pulmonary perfusion associated with obstruction of pulmonary arterial blood flow by the embolus and vasoconstriction resulting from the release of vasoactive substances (e.g., serotonin, endothelin, some prostaglandins)
- Decreased bronchial airflow associated with bronchoconstriction resulting from:
  - The release of substances such as serotonin and some prostaglandins
  - A compensatory response to an increase in the amount of dead space in the underperfused lung area (the compensatory bronchoconstriction also affects airways in perfused lung areas)
  - Loss of effective lung surface associated with atelectasis if it occurs

CLINICAL MANIFESTATIONS

Subjective	Objective
Verbal self-report of restlessness; confusion; irritability; somnolence; shortness of breath	Tachypnea; dyspnea; diaphoresis; hypotension; decreased chest wall expansion; use of accessory muscles when breathing; significant decrease in oximetry results; abnormal arterial blood gas values; hypoxemia; hypocarbia; nasal flaring; tachycardia

RISK FACTORS

- DVT
- Pain
- Muscle fatigue
- Obesity
- Decreased lung expansion

DESIRED OUTCOMES

The client will experience adequate O_2/CO_2 exchange as evidenced by:

a. Usual mental status
b. Unlabored respirations at 12 to 20 breaths/min
c. Oximetry results within normal range
d. Arterial blood gas values within normal range

NOC OUTCOMES

Respiratory status: gas exchange

NIC INTERVENTIONS

Respiratory monitoring; oxygen therapy; airway management; ventilation assistance; acid-base management

---

NDx = NANDA Diagnosis   **D** = Delegatable Action   ● = UAP   ✦ = LVN/LPN   ⊖▶ = Go to ⊖volve for animation

NURSING ASSESSMENT	RATIONALE
Assess for and report signs and symptoms of impaired gas exchange: • Restlessness, irritability • Confusion, somnolence • Tachypnea, dyspnea • Abnormal arterial blood gas values • Significant decrease in oximetry results • Decreased PaO_2 and/or increased $PaCO_2$	Early recognition of signs and symptoms of impaired gas exchange allows for prompt intervention.

THERAPEUTIC INTERVENTIONS	RATIONALE

Independent Actions
Implement measures to improve gas exchange:

• Maintain client on bedrest; increase activity gradually as allowed and tolerated. **D** ● ✦	Placing the client on strict bedrest will help conserve energy during periods of acute respiratory distress. Increasing activity gradually will improve strength and ability to perform activities.
• Discourage smoking.	The carbon monoxide in smoke decreases oxygen availability, and the nicotine can cause vasoconstriction and further reduce pulmonary blood flow.

Dependent/Collaborative Actions
Implement measures to improve gas exchange:

• Maintain oxygen therapy as ordered. **D** ✦	Supplemental oxygen helps relieve dyspnea and improves gas exchange.
• Administer anticoagulants (e.g., continuous intravenous heparin, low-molecular-weight heparin, warfarin) as ordered.	Anticoagulants will prevent blood clotting, which will help improve pulmonary blood flow.
• Prepare client for the following if planned: • Injection of a thrombolytic agent (e.g., streptokinase, urokinase, alteplase)	Thrombolytics convert plasminogen to plasmin, which then degrades the fibrin in clots. The loss of the fibrin results in the lysis of a clot.
• Embolectomy	An embolectomy is the surgical removal of a blood clot. The patient should be educated about the procedure and postoperative care.
Consult appropriate health care provider (e.g., respiratory therapist, physician) if signs and symptoms of impaired gas exchange persist or worsen.	Notifying the appropriate health care provider allows for a multifaceted treatment plan.

Nursing Diagnosis **ACUTE PAIN** NDx **(CHEST)**

Definition: Unpleasant sensory and emotional experience associated with actual or potential tissue damage, or described in terms of such damage (International Association for the Study of Pain); sudden or slow onset of any intensity from mild to severe with an anticipated or predictable end, and a duration of less than 3 months.

Related to:
• Decreased pulmonary tissue perfusion associated with obstructed pulmonary blood flow
• Inflammation of the parietal pleura associated with tissue damage if infarction occurs

CLINICAL MANIFESTATIONS

Subjective	Objective
Verbal self-report of chest pain with breathing and coughing	Grimacing; rubbing chest; reluctance to move; shallow respiration; tachycardia; increased B/P

RISK FACTORS
- DVT
- Excessive coughing
- Increased sputum production

DESIRED OUTCOMES

The client will experience diminished chest pain as evidenced by:
a. Verbalization of a decrease in or absence of pain
b. Relaxed facial expression and body positioning
c. Increased participation in activities when allowed
d. Pulse and B/P within normal range for client

NOC OUTCOMES

Pain control; pain level

NIC INTERVENTIONS

Analgesic administration; pain management; environmental management: comfort; analgesic administration

NURSING ASSESSMENT	RATIONALE
Assess for signs and symptoms of pain (e.g., verbalization of pain, grimacing, reluctance to move, rubbing chest, guarding of affected side of chest, shallow respirations, increased B/P, tachycardia).	*Early recognition of signs and symptoms of pain allows for prompt intervention and improved pain control.*
Assess client's perception of the severity of pain using a pain intensity rating scale.	*An awareness of the severity of pain being experienced helps determine the most appropriate interventions for pain management. Use of a pain intensity scale gives the nurse a clearer understanding of the pain being experienced and promotes consistency when communicating with others about the client's pain experience.*
Assess the client's pain pattern (e.g., location, quality, onset, duration, precipitating factors, aggravating factors, alleviating factors).	*Knowledge of the client's pain pattern assists in the identification of effective pain management interventions.*
Ask the client to describe previous pain experiences and methods used to manage pain effectively.	*Many variables affect a client's response to pain (e.g., age, sex, coping style, previous experience with pain, culture, cause of pain). Knowledge of the client's usual response to pain and methods previously used to manage pain effectively enables the nurse to evaluate the client's pain more accurately and facilitates the identification of effective strategies for pain management.*

THERAPEUTIC INTERVENTIONS	RATIONALE

Independent Actions

Implement measures to reduce fear and anxiety (e.g., assure client that chest pain is common with embolism and should subside with treatment; assure the client that the need for pain relief is understood).	*Fear and anxiety can decrease the client's threshold and tolerance for pain and thereby heighten the perception of pain. In addition, pain management methods are not as effective if the client is tense and unable to relax.*
Implement measures to improve gas exchange:	
• Maintain client on bedrest and increase activity gradually as allowed and tolerated. **D** ● ✦	*Placing the client on strict bedrest will help conserve energy during periods of acute respiratory distress. Increasing activity gradually will improve strength and ability to perform activities.*
Place client in a semi- to high-Fowler's position unless contraindicated. **D** ● ✦	*Positioning the client in semi- to high-Fowler's position promotes optimal gas exchange by enabling chest expansion.*
• Position with pillows. **D** ● ✦	*Positioning with pillows helps prevent slumping.*
• Instruct and assist the client to splint the chest with hands or pillows when deep breathing, coughing, or changing position. **D** ● ✦	*Splinting the chest with deep breathing, coughing, or changing position reduces pain and promotes a more effective cough.*
• Instruct client to breathe slowly if hyperventilating.	
• Instruct client to breathe deeply or use incentive spirometer every 1 to 2 hrs. **D** ✦	*Deep breathing and use of incentive spirometry help expand the lungs and improve oxygenation.*
• Provide or assist with nonpharmacological methods for pain relief (e.g., relaxation techniques, restful environment, diversional activities).	*Relaxation and diversional activities help alleviate pain, fear, and anxiety, which in turn will decrease dyspnea.*

Continued...

THERAPEUTIC INTERVENTIONS	RATIONALE
• Implement measures to promote rest (e.g., minimize environmental activity and noise). **D** ● ✦	*A calm, restful environment facilitates relaxation and promotes a sense of security, and reduces rapid breathing associated with fear and anxiety.*

Dependent/Collaborative Actions
Implement measures to improve gas exchange:

• Maintain oxygen therapy as ordered. **D** ✦	*Supplemental oxygen helps relieve dyspnea and improves gas exchange.*
Administer analgesics before activities and procedures that can cause pain and before pain becomes severe. **D** ✦	*The administration of analgesics before a pain-producing event helps minimize the pain that will be experienced. Analgesics are also more effective if given before a procedure and will improve the client's ability to tolerate the procedure.*
Consult appropriate health care provider (e.g., physician, pharmacist, pain management specialist) if the provided measures fail to provide adequate pain relief.	*Notifying the appropriate health care provider allows for a multifaceted treatment plan.*

Nursing Diagnosis: **RISK FOR BLEEDING** NDx

Definition: Susceptible to a decrease in blood volume, which may compromise health.

Related to: Excessive use of thrombolytics and anticoagulants

CLINICAL MANIFESTATIONS

Subjective	**Objective**
Verbal self-report of excessive or unusual bruising	Petechiae; bruises easily; prolonged bleeding from puncture sites; unusual joint pain; hypotension; tachycardia; decreases in Hgb and Hct

RISK FACTORS

• Treatment regimen

DESIRED OUTCOMES

The client will not experience unusual bleeding as evidenced by:
a. Skin and mucous membranes free of petechiae, purpura, ecchymoses, and active bleeding
b. Absence of unusual joint pain
c. No increase in abdominal girth
d. Absence of frank and occult blood in stool, urine, and vomitus
e. Usual menstrual flow
f. Vital signs within normal range for client
g. Stable Hct and Hgb

NOC OUTCOMES

Blood coagulation; blood loss severity

NIC INTERVENTIONS

Bleeding precautions; bleeding reduction; blood product administration

NURSING ASSESSMENT	RATIONALE
Assess client for and report signs and symptoms of unusual bleeding: • Petechiae, purpura, ecchymoses • Gingival bleeding • Prolonged bleeding from puncture sites • Epistaxis, hemoptysis • Unusual joint pain • Increase in abdominal girth	*Early recognition of signs and symptoms of unusual bleeding, which may occur as part of the infarction process and from medications (i.e., thrombolytics and anticoagulants) during treatment of a thrombus or pulmonary embolism, allows for implementation of the appropriate interventions.*

NURSING ASSESSMENT	RATIONALE

- Frank or occult blood in stool, urine, or vomitus
- Menorrhagia
- Restlessness, confusion
- Decreasing B/P and increased pulse rate
- Decrease in Hct and Hgb levels

THERAPEUTIC INTERVENTIONS	RATIONALE

Dependent/Collaborative Actions

Monitor platelet count and coagulation test results (e.g., prothrombin time or international normalized ratio [INR], activated partial thromboplastin time). Report a low platelet count and coagulation test results that exceed the therapeutic range.

Monitoring effectiveness and dosage requirements of heparin and warfarin is done via prothrombin time/INR/activated partial thromboplastin time. Platelet counts should be monitored every 2 to 3 days because these medications may cause mild thrombocytopenia.

If platelet count is low, coagulation test results are abnormal, or Hct and Hgb levels decrease, test all stools, urine, and vomitus for occult blood. Report positive results.

Increased bleeding may occur when a patient is receiving anticoagulant therapy. Reporting any signs of bleeding, including a positive result for occult blood, allows for timely treatment and changes in medication dosage as needed.

Implement measures to prevent bleeding:

- Avoid giving injections whenever possible; consult a physician about prescribing an alternative route for medications ordered to be given intramuscularly or subcutaneously.

It is important to prevent bleeding while the patient is receiving anticoagulants. Injections may cause increased bleeding and oozing from the injection sites.

  - When giving injections or performing venous or arterial punctures, use the smallest gauge needle possible and apply gentle, prolonged pressure to the site after the needle is removed. **D** ✦

Use of the smallest needle possible and application of gentle, prolonged pressure at the puncture site will help prevent excessive bleeding.

- Caution client to avoid activities that increase the risk for trauma (e.g., shaving with a straight-edge razor, using stiff bristle toothbrush or dental floss).

These activities increase the risk of trauma and associated bleeding.

- Whenever possible, avoid intubations (e.g., nasogastric) and procedures that can cause injury to the rectal mucosa (e.g., taking temperature rectally, inserting a rectal suppository, administering an enema).

Procedures that may cause injury to the mucous membranes may cause excessive bleeding. If the client must undergo one of these procedures, the nurse must monitor the client closely for bleeding.

- Perform actions to reduce the risk for falls (e.g., keep bed in low position with side rails up when client is in bed, avoid unnecessary clutter in room, instruct client to wear slippers/shoes with nonslip soles when ambulating). **D** ● ✦
- Pad side rails if client is confused or restless.

Falls are another way that a client who is receiving anticoagulants may experience increased bleeding. Mechanisms should be put in place to decrease the risk of falls.

- Instruct client to avoid blowing nose forcefully or straining to have a bowel movement; consult physician about an order for a decongestant and/or laxative if indicated.

Forcefully blowing one's nose or straining with a bowel movement should be avoided during anticoagulant therapy because these actions may increase bleeding.

If bleeding occurs and does not subside spontaneously:

- Apply firm, prolonged pressure to bleeding areas if possible.

Pressure at the site helps promote clotting.

If epistaxis occurs, place client in a high-Fowler's position and apply pressure and ice pack to nasal area.

Placing the client in high-Fowler's and applying pressure and ice to the nasal area helps promote clotting.

- Maintain oxygen therapy as ordered. **D** ✦

Oxygen therapy will assist in maintaining oxygen saturation if bleeding occurs.

- Administer protamine sulfate (antidote for heparin), vitamin K (e.g., phytonadione), and/or whole blood or blood products (e.g., fresh frozen plasma, platelets) as ordered.

Administration of the antidotes for heparin and warfarin will reverse the effects of these medications and decrease bleeding.

Collaborative Diagnoses **RISK FOR RIGHT-SIDED HEART FAILURE**

Definition: A condition where the right side of the heart is unable to pump blood efficiently.

Related to:
Increased cardiac workload associated with:
- Pulmonary hypertension (can result from pulmonary vasoconstriction that occurs in response to hypoxia and the release of vasoactive substances)
- Compensatory response to decreased pulmonary blood flow that results from obstruction of multiple and/or large pulmonary vessels

CLINICAL MANIFESTATIONS

Subjective	Objective
Verbal self-report of weakness and fatigue	Tachypnea; tachycardia; dyspnea; restlessness; confusion; irritability; peripheral edema; decreased urine output; distended neck veins

RISK FACTORS
- Smoking
- Chronic respiratory disease
- Obesity
- Hypertension

DESIRED OUTCOMES

The client will not develop right-sided heart failure as evidenced by:
a. Pulse rate of 60 to 100 beats/min
b. Usual mental status
c. Usual strength and activity tolerance
d. Adequate urine output
e. Stable weight
f. Absence of edema and distended neck veins

NURSING ASSESSMENT	RATIONALE
Assess for and report signs and symptoms of right-sided heart failure: • Further increase in pulse rate • Restlessness, confusion • Weakness and fatigue • Decreased urine output • Weight gain • Dependent peripheral edema • Distended neck veins • Chest radiograph results showing cardiomegaly	*Early recognition of signs and symptoms of right-sided heart failure allows for prompt intervention.*

THERAPEUTIC INTERVENTIONS	RATIONALE

Dependent/Collaborative Actions
Implement measures to improve pulmonary blood flow:
 	
• Administer anticoagulants (e.g., continuous intravenous heparin, low-molecular-weight heparin, warfarin [as ordered]).
 	
• Prepare client for the following if planned:
  • Injection of a thrombolytic agent (e.g., streptokinase, urokinase, alteplase)
  • Embolectomy
 	
If signs and symptoms of right-sided heart failure occur:
• Maintain oxygen therapy as ordered.
Maintain client on strict bedrest in a semi- to high-Fowler's position
	These interventions will reduce cardiac workload and the subsequent risk of right-sided heart failure by decreasing the pressure against which the heart must pump.
	Anticoagulants will prevent blood clotting, which will help improve pulmonary blood flow and decrease the potential of an extension or recurrence of a pulmonary embolism.
	
	Thrombolytics convert plasminogen to plasmin, which then degrades the fibrin in clots. The loss of the fibrin results in the lysis of a clot.
	An embolectomy is the surgical removal of a blood clot. The patient should be educated about the procedure and postoperative care.
	
	Supplemental oxygen helps relieve dyspnea and improves gas exchange.
	Placing the client on strict bedrest will help conserve energy during periods of acute respiratory distress. Positioning the client in a semi- to high-Fowler's position promotes optimal gas exchange by enabling chest expansion.

THERAPEUTIC INTERVENTIONS	RATIONALE
• Maintain fluid and sodium restrictions if ordered.	*Restricting a client's sodium and fluid will help reduce fluid volume overload.*
• Administer medications that may reduce vascular congestion and/or cardiac workload (e.g., diuretics, cardiotonics, vasodilators)	*Diuretics decrease fluid volume through inhibiting reabsorption of water, which decreases fluid volume.*
	Cardiotonics increase the contractile force of the heart, which increases cardiac output.
	Vasodilators dilate the arterioles, which decreases B/P and decreases the work of the heart.

Collaborative Diagnosis ## RISK FOR ATELECTASIS

Definition: Collapse of lung tissue caused by hypoventilated alveoli.

Related to:
• Shallow respirations
• Stasis of secretions in alveoli and bronchioles
• Decreased surfactant production (results from inadequate deep breathing and changes in regional blood flow in the lungs)

CLINICAL MANIFESTATIONS

Subjective	Objective
Verbal self-report of difficulty breathing	Diminished or absent breath sounds; dull percussion over affected area; increased respiratory rate; dyspnea; tachycardia; elevated temperature

RISK FACTORS
• Immobility
• Ineffective airway clearance
• Smoking
• Obesity

DESIRED OUTCOMES
The client will not develop atelectasis as evidenced by:
a. Clear, audible breath sounds
b. Resonant percussion note over lungs
c. Unlabored respirations at 12 to 20 breaths/min
d. Pulse rate within normal range for client
e. Afebrile status

NURSING ASSESSMENT	RATIONALE
Assess for and report signs and symptoms of atelectasis: • Diminished or absent breath sounds • Dull percussion noted over affected area • Increased respiratory rate • Dyspnea • Tachycardia • Elevated temperature	*Early recognition of signs and symptoms of atelectasis allows for implementation of the appropriate interventions.*
Monitor pulse oximetry results as indicated.	*Pulse oximetry is an indirect measure of arterial oxygen saturation. Monitoring pulse oximetry (SaO_2) allows for early detection of hypoxia and implementation of the appropriate interventions.*
Monitor chest radiograph results.	*Chest radiograph provides radiographic confirmation of atelectasis.*

THERAPEUTIC INTERVENTIONS	RATIONALE

Independent Actions
 Implement measures to prevent atelectasis: **D** ✦
 • Perform actions to improve breathing pattern:
   • Encourage client to breathe deeply.
   • Incentive spirometry
 • Perform actions to promote effective airway clearance.
   • Turn, cough, and breathe deeply.
	Improves client ability to expand lung tissue and improve oxygenation and clearance of mucous

Continued...

THERAPEUTIC INTERVENTIONS	RATIONALE
If signs and symptoms of atelectasis occur: • Increase frequency of position change, coughing or "huffing," deep breathing, and use of incentive spirometer. Consult physician if signs and symptoms of atelectasis persist or worsen.	*Lack of movement places a client at risk for atelectasis. Changing positions frequently, coughing, and deep breathing help expand the lungs, enhancing alveolar expansion.* *Notifying the appropriate health care provider will allow for modification of the treatment plan.*

Nursing Diagnosis   **FEAR** NDx/**ANXIETY** NDx

Definition: Fear NDx: Response to perceived threat that is consciously recognized as a danger.

Anxiety NDx: Vague, uneasy feeling of discomfort or dread accompanied by an autonomic response (the source often nonspecific or unknown to the individual); a feeling of apprehension caused by anticipation of danger. It is an alerting signal that warns of impending danger and enables the individual to take measures to deal with a threat.

Related to:
• Exacerbation of symptoms (e.g., increased dyspnea, feeling of suffocation)
• Lack of understanding of the diagnosis, diagnostic tests, treatments, and prognosis
• Unfamiliar environment
• Possibility of recurrent embolism; threat of death

CLINICAL MANIFESTATIONS

Subjective Verbal self-report of fear and/or anxiety	**Objective** Unusual sleep patterns; unstable vital signs; restlessness; shakiness; diaphoresis; self-focused behavior

RISK FACTORS	**DESIRED OUTCOMES**
• Fear of the unknown • Fear of death • Pain • Unknown environment • Fear of recurrence of embolism	The client will experience a reduction in fear and anxiety as evidenced by: a. Verbalization of feeling less anxious b. Usual sleep pattern c. Relaxed facial expression and body movements d. Stable vital signs e. Usual perceptual ability and interactions with others

NOC OUTCOMES	**NIC INTERVENTIONS**
Anxiety level; fear level; anxiety self-control; fear self-control	Anxiety reduction; calming technique; emotional support; presence; pain management

NURSING ASSESSMENT	RATIONALE
Assess client for signs and symptoms of fear and anxiety (e.g., verbalization of feeling anxious, insomnia, tenseness, shakiness, restlessness, diaphoresis, elevated B/P, tachycardia, self-focused behaviors). Validate perceptions carefully, remembering that some behavior may result from hypoxia and/or hypercapnia.	*Moderate anxiety enhances the client's ability to solve problems. With severe anxiety or panic, the client is not able to follow directions and may become hyperactive and extremely agitated.* *Assessment of the client's fear helps determine whether the coping mechanisms are effective and which need to be strengthened.*

THERAPEUTIC INTERVENTIONS	RATIONALE
Independent Actions Implement measures to reduce fear and anxiety: • Orient client to hospital environment, equipment, and routines. **D** ● ✦	*Familiarity with the environment and usual routines reduces the client's anxiety about the unknown, provides a sense of security, and increases the client's sense of control, all of which help decrease anxiety.*

THERAPEUTIC INTERVENTIONS	RATIONALE
• Introduce staff who will be participating in the client's care. If possible, maintain consistency in staff assigned to client's care.	*Introduction to staff familiarizes clients with those individuals who will be working with them, which provides clients with a feeling of stability, which reduces the anxiety that typically occurs with change.*
• Assure client that staff members are nearby; respond to call signal as soon as possible. **D** ● ✦	*Close contact and a prompt response to requests provide a sense of security and facilitate the development of trust, thus reducing the client's anxiety.*
• Maintain a calm, supportive, confident manner when interacting with client; encourage verbalization of fear and anxiety. **D** ● ✦	*A sense of calmness and confidence conveys to the client that someone is in control of the situation, which helps reduce anxiety.*
• Reinforce physician's explanations and clarify misconceptions the client has about the pulmonary embolus, treatment plan, and possible recurrence; encourage questions.	*Factual information and an awareness of what to expect help decrease the anxiety that arises from uncertainty.*

• Implement measures to reduce respiratory distress if present:
  • Elevate the head of the bed.
  • Encourage the client to breathe deeply and more slowly. **D** ● ✦
	Improvement of respiratory status helps relieve anxiety associated with the feeling of not being able to breathe.

• Implement measures to reduce pain: • Instruct the client in relaxation techniques and encourage participation in diversional activities once the period of acute pain and respiratory distress has subsided.	*Pain can create or increase anxiety because it is often perceived as a threat to well-being.* *Pain also causes sympathetic nervous system stimulation with subsequent feelings of tenseness and increased anxiety.*
• When appropriate, assist the client to meet spiritual needs (e.g., arrange for a visit from the clergy).	*Spiritual support is a source of comfort and security for many people and can help reduce the client's fear and anxiety.*
• Provide information based on current needs of the client at a level that can be understood. • Encourage the client to ask questions and to seek clarification of information provided.	*Providing information that the client is not ready to process or cannot understand tends to increase anxiety.* *Making the client feel comfortable enough to ask questions or clarify information helps reduce anxiety.*
• Provide a calm, restful environment. **D** ● ✦	*A calm, restful environment facilitates relaxation and promotes a sense of security, which reduces fear and anxiety.*
• Encourage significant others to project a caring, concerned attitude without obvious fear and anxiousness.	*Anxiety is easily transferable from one person to another. If significant others convey empathy, provide reassurance, and do not appear anxious, they can help reduce the client's fear and anxiety.*

Dependent/Collaborative Actions

Implement measures to reduce fear and anxiety:

• Administer oxygen via nasal cannula rather than mask if possible. **D** ✦	*The use of a mask for some clients seems restrictive and suffocating. The use of a nasal cannula is more comfortable and less constraining. Improvement of respiratory status helps relieve anxiety associated with the feeling of not being able to breathe.*
• Administer prescribed antianxiety agents if indicated. **D** ✦	*Decreasing anxiety may improve respiratory status.*
Consult appropriate health care provider (e.g., psychiatric nurse clinician, physician) if the provided actions fail to control fear and anxiety.	*Notifying the appropriate health care provider allows for modification of the treatment plan.*

DISCHARGE TEACHING/CONTINUED CARE

Nursing Diagnosis **DEFICIENT KNOWLEDGE NDx, INEFFECTIVE HEALTH MAINTENANCE NDx, OR INEFFECTIVE HEALTH MANAGEMENT* NDx**

Definition: **Deficient Knowledge NDx**: Absence of cognitive information related to a specific topic, or its acquisition; **Ineffective Health Maintenance NDx**: Inability to identify, manage, and/or seek out help to maintain well-being; **Ineffective Health Management NDx**: Pattern of regulating and integrating into daily living a therapeutic regimen for the treatment of illness and its sequelae that is unsatisfactory for meeting specific health goals.

NDx = NANDA Diagnosis   **D** = Delegatable Action   ● = UAP   ✦ = LVN/LPN   ⊜▶ = Go to ⊜volve for animation

CLINICAL MANIFESTATIONS

Subjective	**Objective**
Verbal self-report of the problem	Inaccurate follow-through of instructions; inappropriate behaviors

RISK FACTORS
* Denial of disease process
* Fear and anxiety that blocks ability to understand

NOC OUTCOMES	NIC INTERVENTIONS
Knowledge: disease process; treatment regimen	Health system guidance; teaching: individual; teaching: prescribed medication; teaching: prescribed activity/exercise; teaching: psychomotor skill

NURSING ASSESSMENT	RATIONALE
Assess client readiness to learn Assess meaning of illness to client	*Early recognition of readiness to learn and meaning of illness to client allows for appropriate teaching interventions.*

THERAPEUTIC INTERVENTIONS	RATIONALE

Desired Outcome: The client will identify ways to reduce the risk of recurrent thrombus formation and pulmonary embolism.

Independent Actions
Provide the following instructions on ways to promote venous blood flow and reduce the risk of thrombus recurrence:

* Avoid wearing constrictive clothing (e.g., garters, girdles, narrow-banded knee-high hose).

  Wearing constrictive clothing decreases blood flow from the lower extremities, increasing the risk of a thrombus.

* Avoid sitting and standing in one position for long periods.

  Decreases the ability of veins to prevent stasis of blood.

* Avoid crossing legs and lying or sitting with pillows under knees.

  Decreases blood flow and increases the risk of developing a thrombus.

* Wear graduated compression stockings or support hose during the day.

  Compression stockings and support hose prevent venous dilation and increase blood flow to the heart.

* Engage in regular aerobic exercise (e.g., swimming, walking, cycling)

  Each of these activities stimulates venous blood return to the heart, decreasing the incidence of a thrombus.

* Elevate legs periodically, especially when sitting.
* Dorsiflex feet regularly.
* Maintain recommended weight for age, height, and body frame.

  Overweight individuals are at a higher risk for development of a thrombus because of increased endothelial fibrinolytic dysfunction and an increased risk for atherothrombotic events.

* Inform client that smoking and the use of estrogen or oral contraceptives can increase the risk for recurrent thrombus formation.

  Smoking and the use of estrogens or oral contraceptives have been associated with thrombus formation and pulmonary embolism.

* Instruct client to avoid trauma to or massage of any area of suspected thrombus formation in order to decrease the risk of pulmonary embolism.

  Trauma or massage to an area of suspected thrombus may dislodge the thrombus into the vascular system and place the patient at risk for a pulmonary embolism.

* Provide information regarding exercise programs and support groups that can assist the client to stop smoking and/or lose weight.

  Providing information on community resources provides a continuum of care.

THERAPEUTIC INTERVENTIONS	RATIONALE

Desired Outcome: The client will verbalize an understanding of medications ordered, including rationale, food and drug interactions, side effects, schedule for taking, and importance of taking as prescribed.

Independent Actions

Explain the rationale for, side effects of, and importance of taking medications prescribed.

Understanding of the impact of medications improves adherence.

If client is discharged on warfarin (e.g., Coumadin), instruct to:

• Keep scheduled appointments for periodic blood studies to monitor coagulation time.

Appropriate dosing of warfarin is based on monitoring of lab values (INR) and bleeding time. If these values are not monitored, the client's dosage may become too high, increasing the risk of bleeding, or too low, increasing the risk of thrombus.

• Take medication at the same time each day, do not stop taking medication abruptly, and do not attempt to make up for missed doses.

Appropriate medication administration is important to obtain the most beneficial effects.

• Avoid regular and/or excessive intake of alcohol (may alter responsiveness to warfarin).

Alcohol intake beyond 1 to 2 drinks per day decreases the effects of warfarin; in clients with liver disease, alcohol will increase the effects of warfarin.

• Avoid significantly increasing or decreasing consumption of foods high in vitamin K (e.g., green leafy vegetables).

Increasing the amount of foods high in vitamin K will antagonize warfarin's anticoagulant effects.

• Report prolonged or excessive bleeding from skin, nose, or mouth; red, rust-colored, or smoky urine; bloody or tarry stools; blood in vomitus or sputum; prolonged or excessive menses; excessive bruising; severe or persistent headache; or sudden abdominal or back pain.

Increased incidence of bleeding must be reported to the client's health care provider for appropriate intervention.

• Inform physician immediately if pregnancy is suspected or if breastfeeding (warfarin crosses the placental barrier and enters the breast milk).

Warfarin is contraindicated in pregnancy because it crosses the placenta and is found in breast milk.

• Wear a medical alert identification bracelet or tag identifying self as being on anticoagulant therapy.

This allows health care providers to be aware of health conditions and prescribed medications if the client is unable to provide this information.

• Inform physician of any other medications being taken because there are some that affect the anticoagulant activity of warfarin (e.g., NSAIDs, various antimicrobials, phenytoin).

There are some medications that affect the anticoagulant activity of warfarin (e.g., NSAIDs, various antimicrobials, phenytoin).

• Notify health care provider immediately of any sudden changes in the skin, such as bruised, darkened, or painful areas.

Warfarin can cause necrosis of the skin.

• Instruct client to inform all health care providers of medications and herbal supplements being taken.

Health care providers must be aware of all medications and herbal supplements taken because they can interact with prescribed medications.

THERAPEUTIC INTERVENTIONS	RATIONALE

Desired Outcome: The client will demonstrate the ability to correctly draw up and administer heparin subcutaneously if prescribed.

Independent Actions

If client is to be discharged on subcutaneous heparin, provide instructions about subcutaneous injection technique.

The client should be instructed on the proper method of medication administration.

Allow time for questions, practice, and return demonstration.

Allowing for questioning, practice, and return demonstration of proper medication administration helps clients feel confident that they can perform this once they are at home.

THERAPEUTIC INTERVENTIONS	**RATIONALE**

Desired Outcome: The client will identify ways to prevent bleeding associated with anticoagulant therapy.

Independent Actions

Instruct client about ways to minimize the risk of bleeding while receiving anticoagulant therapy:

- Use an electric rather than a straight-edge razor.
- Floss and brush teeth; use waxed floss and a soft bristle toothbrush.
- Avoid putting sharp objects (e.g., toothpicks) in mouth.
- Do not walk barefoot.
- Cut nails carefully.
- Avoid situations that could result in injury (e.g., contact sports).
- Do not blow nose forcefully.
- Avoid straining to have a bowel movement.

Instruct client to control any bleeding by applying firm, prolonged pressure to the area if possible.

All of these mechanisms will help minimize the risk of bleeding.

Application of firm, prolonged pressure will promote clotting.

THERAPEUTIC INTERVENTIONS	**RATIONALE**

Desired Outcome: The client will state signs and symptoms to report to the health care provider.

Independent Actions

Stress the importance of reporting the following:

- Tenderness, swelling, or pain in extremity
- Sudden chest pain
- New or increased shortness of breath
- Extreme anxiousness or restlessness
- Cough productive of blood-tinged sputum
- Unusual bleeding
- Fever

These symptoms are indicative of an embolism or increased bleeding from the use of anticoagulants. Immediate reporting allows for prompt treatment.

THERAPEUTIC INTERVENTIONS	**RATIONALE**

Desired Outcome: The client will, in collaboration with the nurse, develop a plan for adhering to recommended follow-up care, including future appointments with the health care provider and activity level.

Independent Actions

Reinforce the importance of keeping follow-up appointments with the health care provider.

Reinforce the physician's instructions regarding activity limitations.

Implement measures to improve client compliance:

- Include significant others in teaching sessions if possible.

- Encourage questions and allow time for reinforcement and clarification of information provided.

- Provide written instructions regarding future appointments with health care provider, medications prescribed, activity restrictions, signs and symptoms to report, and future laboratory studies.

Follow-up appointments are important to monitor the client's recovery and medication regimen.

Clients may not fully understand the instructions regarding activity limitations, as they are feeling better and may increase activities prematurely.

Involvement of significant others in patient teaching improves adherence to discharge instructions.

Everyone does not understand information as presented, so set aside time for questions to allow for clarification of information.

Written instructions allow the client to refer to instructions as needed.

THORACIC SURGERY

Thoracic surgery is a term used to refer to surgical procedures that involve entry into the thoracic cavity to gain access to the lungs, heart, aorta, or esophagus. Types of thoracic surgery performed to treat pulmonary disorders include pneumonectomy, lobectomy, segmental resection, and wedge resection. The surgery may be performed to repair lung damage resulting from trauma and to remove benign or malignant tumors; areas of bronchiectasis, fungal infection, or tuberculosis; abscesses; blebs; and bullae. Although some thoracic surgery can be accomplished using an intercostally inserted endoscope, an open thoracic approach is needed to treat conditions requiring surgery deep in the lung, extensive removal of lung tissue, or both.

This care plan focuses on the adult client hospitalized for thoracic surgery to remove a portion or all of a lung. Much of the information is applicable to clients receiving follow-up care in an extended care facility or home setting.

OUTCOME/DISCHARGE CRITERIA

The client will:
1. Have optimal respiratory function
2. Have evidence of normal healing of surgical wound
3. Have surgical pain controlled
4. Have no signs and symptoms of postoperative complications
5. Identify ways to promote optimal respiratory health
6. Demonstrate the ability to perform prescribed arm and shoulder exercises
7. State signs and symptoms to report to the health care provider
8. Identify community resources that can assist with home management and adjustment to the diagnosis, effects of surgery, and subsequent treatment if planned
9. Develop a plan for adhering to recommended follow-up care, including future appointments with health care providers, medications prescribed, activity level, pain management, wound care, and subsequent treatment of the underlying disorder

POSTOPERATIVE CARE PLAN TO USE IN CONJUNCTION WITH THE PREOPERATIVE CARE PLAN

Nursing Diagnosis **IMPAIRED RESPIRATORY FUNCTION***

Definition: **Ineffective Breathing Pattern NDx**: Inspiration and/or expiration that does not provide adequate ventilation; **Ineffective Airway Clearance NDx**: Inability to clear secretions or obstructions from the respiratory tract to maintain a clear airway; **Impaired Gas Exchange NDx**: Excess or deficit in oxygenation and/or carbon dioxide elimination at the alveolar-capillary membrane.

Ineffective breathing pattern NDx
Related to:
- Increased rate of respirations associated with fear and anxiety
- Decreased rate of respirations associated with the depressant effect of anesthesia and some medications (e.g., narcotic [opioid] analgesics, some antiemetics)
- Decreased depth of respirations associated with:
- Reluctance to breathe deeply resulting from incisional pain and fear of dislodging chest tube(s) if in place
- Weakness, fatigue, fear, and anxiety
- Depressant effect of anesthesia and some medications (e.g., narcotic [opioid] analgesics, some antiemetics)
- Limited chest expansion resulting from positioning and elevation of the diaphragm (can occur if abdominal distention is present or if the phrenic nerve was injured during surgery)

Ineffective airway clearance NDx
Related to:
- Occlusion of the pharynx in the immediate postoperative period associated with relaxation of the tongue resulting from the effect of anesthesia and some medications (e.g., narcotic [opioid] analgesics)
- Stasis of secretions associated with:
- Decreased activity
- Depressed ciliary function resulting from effects of anesthesia
- Difficulty coughing up secretions resulting from the depressant effect of anesthesia and some medications (e.g., narcotic [opioid] analgesics, some antiemetics), pain, weakness, fatigue, and presence of tenacious secretions (can occur as a result of deficient fluid volume)
- Increased secretions associated with irritation of the respiratory tract (can result from inhalation anesthetics, endotracheal intubation, and surgically induced lung tissue injury and inflammation)

*This diagnostic label includes the following nursing diagnoses: ineffective breathing pattern, ineffective airway clearance, and impaired gas exchange.

NDx = NANDA Diagnosis   **D** = Delegatable Action   ● = UAP   ✦ = LVN/LPN   ⊖▶ = Go to ⊖volve for animation

Impaired gas exchange NDx
Related to:
A decrease in alveolar surface area and pulmonary vasculature associated with the extensive removal of lung tissues

CLINICAL MANIFESTATIONS

Subjective	Objective
Verbal self-report of pain; anxiety; fear/agitation; restlessness; irritability; confusion	Tachypnea; orthopnea; dyspnea; diminished breath sounds; tachycardia; productive cough; significant decrease in oximetry values; abnormal arterial blood gas values; chest radiograph changes

RISK FACTORS

- Increased secretions
- Postoperative incision pain
- Anxiety
- Analgesics
- Potential immobility
- Anesthesia

DESIRED OUTCOMES

The client will experience adequate respiratory function as evidenced by:
a. Normal rate and depth of respirations
b. Absence of dyspnea
c. Normal breath sounds over remaining lung tissue
d. Usual mental status
e. Usual skin color
f. Oximetry results within normal range
g. Arterial blood gas values within normal range

NOC OUTCOMES

Respiratory status: gas exchange; ventilation; airway patency

NIC INTERVENTIONS

Respiratory monitoring; airway management; chest physiotherapy; cough enhancement; oxygen therapy; medication administration; ventilation assistance; fear and anxiety reduction

NURSING ASSESSMENT	RATIONALE
Assess for signs and symptoms of impaired respiratory function:	*Early recognition of signs and symptoms of infective breathing patterns allows for prompt intervention.*
• Rapid, shallow respirations • Dyspnea, orthopnea • Use of accessory muscles when breathing • Abnormal breath sounds (e.g., diminished or absent over remaining lung tissue)	*Changes in the characteristics of breath sounds may be due to airway obstruction, mucous plugs, or retained secretions in larger airways.*
• Development of or increase in cough	*Muscle fatigue/weakness may impair effective clearance of secretions.*
• Restlessness, irritability • Confusion, somnolence	*Restlessness, irritability, and changes in mental status or level of consciousness indicate an oxygen deficiency and require immediate treatment.*
• Significant decrease in oximetry results	*Oximetry is a noninvasive method of measuring arterial oxygen saturation. The results assist in evaluating respiratory status.*
• Abnormal arterial blood gas values	*Decreasing PaO_2 and increasing $PaCO_2$ are indicators of respiratory problems.*
• Changes in vital signs	*Increased work of breathing or hypoxia may cause tachycardia and/or hypertension.*
• Significant abnormalities in chest radiograph reports	*Changes in infiltrates noted in the lungs require prompt treatment.*

THERAPEUTIC INTERVENTIONS	RATIONALE
Independent Actions Implement measures to maintain adequate respiratory function: • Perform actions to reduce chest pain (e.g., orient client to the hospital environment, equipment; maintain a calm, supportive environment; instruct and assist client to splint chest when coughing or deep breathing). **D** ✦	*Reduction of chest pain increases the client's willingness to move and breathe more deeply.*

THERAPEUTIC INTERVENTIONS	RATIONALE
• Perform actions to reduce fear and anxiety (e.g., assure client that staff members are nearby; respond to call signal as soon as possible; provide calm, restful environment; instruct in relaxation techniques; encourage family to project a supportive attitude without obvious anxiousness). **D** ✦	*Reduction of fear and anxiety assists in preventing the shallow and/or rapid breathing associated with these emotions.*
• Perform actions to reduce the accumulation of gas and fluid in the gastrointestinal tract (e.g., ambulate as early as possible, progress to solid foods slowly).	*This helps decrease the pressure on the diaphragm, allowing the individual to have greater lung expansion.*
• Position client as ordered (e.g., usually on back or operative side after pneumonectomy, on back or either side after removal of a portion of the lung).	*Proper positioning after surgery allows for full expansion of the remaining lung tissue.*
• When positioning clients on their side, use a 30 to 45 degrees "tip" position (rather than complete lateral positioning).	*This position helps minimize lateral compression of lung tissue.*
• Instruct client to breathe deeply or use incentive spirometer every 1 to 2 hrs. **D** ● ✦	*Forced deep breathing and use of incentive spirometry will increase expansion of the lungs and improve the client's ability to clear mucus from the remaining lung tissue. The technique may also improve the amount of oxygen that is able to penetrate deep into the lungs.*
• Assure the client that deep breathing and turning should not dislodge the chest tube.	*This assurance will decrease the client's anxiety and fear associated with the chest tube.*
• Maintain activity restrictions as ordered; increase activity gradually as allowed and tolerated. **D** ● ✦	*During activity, especially ambulation, the client usually takes deeper breaths, thus increasing expansion of remaining lung tissue.*

Dependent/Collaborative Actions

Implement measures to maintain adequate respiratory function:

• Administer bronchodilators (e.g., methylxanthines, sympathomimetics) if ordered.	*These medications will dilate the bronchioles, improve the volume of air reaching the lungs, and improve arterial blood gas values.*
• Administer pain medications as ordered.	*Reduction of chest pain increases the client's willingness to move and breathe more deeply.*
• Maintain oxygen therapy as ordered. **D** ✦	*Improves oxygenation of body tissues.*
Consult appropriate health care provider (e.g., respiratory therapist, physician) if signs and symptoms of impaired respiratory function persist or worsen.	*Notifying the appropriate health care provider allows for modifications of treatment.*

Nursing Diagnosis ## ACUTE PAIN NDx (CHEST)

Definition: Unpleasant sensory and emotional experience associated with actual potential tissue damage, or described in terms of such damage (International Association for the Study of Pain); sudden or slow onset of any intensity from mild to severe with an anticipated or predictable end, and a duration of less than 3 months.

Related to:

- Tissue trauma, reflex muscle spasm, and disruption of intercostal nerves associated with the surgery
- Irritation of the parietal pleura associated with surgical trauma and stretching of the pleura (occurs if there is an accumulation of blood or air in the pleural space)
- Tissue irritation associated with the presence of chest tubes
- Stress on surgical area associated with deep breathing

CLINICAL MANIFESTATIONS

Subjective	Objective
Verbal self-report of pain in chest with breathing and coughing and pain around the chest tube insertion site	Increased B/P; tachycardia; shallow respirations; grimacing with movement

RISK FACTORS
- Frequent coughing
- Suture line pain
- Chest tubes
- Anxiety

DESIRED OUTCOMES

The client will experience diminished chest pain as evidenced by:
a. Verbalization of a decrease in or absence of pain
b. Relaxed facial expression and body positioning
c. Increased participation in activities
d. Stable vital signs

NOC OUTCOMES

Pain control; comfort level

NIC INTERVENTIONS

Pain management; analgesic administration; environmental management: comfort

NURSING ASSESSMENT	RATIONALE
Assess for signs and symptoms of pain (e.g., verbalization of pain, grimacing, reluctance to move, guarding of affected side of chest, shallow respirations, increased B/P, tachycardia).	*Early recognition of signs and symptoms of pain allows for prompt intervention and improved pain control.*
Assess client's perception of the severity of pain using a pain intensity rating scale.	*An awareness of the severity of pain being experienced helps determine the most appropriate interventions for pain management. Use of a pain intensity scale gives the nurse a clearer understanding of the pain being experienced and promotes consistency when communicating with others about the client's pain experience.*
Assess the client's pain pattern (e.g., location, quality, onset, duration, precipitating factors, aggravating factors, alleviating factors).	*Knowledge of the client's pain pattern assists in the identification of effective pain management interventions.*
Ask the client to describe previous pain experiences and methods used to manage pain effectively.	*Many variables affect a client's response to pain (e.g., age, sex, coping style, previous experience with pain, culture, cause of pain). Knowledge of the client's usual response to pain and methods previously used to manage pain effectively enables the nurse to evaluate the client's pain more accurately and facilitates the identification of effective strategies for pain management.*

THERAPEUTIC INTERVENTIONS	RATIONALE
Independent Actions	
Implement measures to reduce fear and anxiety (e.g., assure client that chest pain is expected postoperatively, and assure the client that the need for pain relief is understood).	*Fear and anxiety can decrease the client's threshold and tolerance for pain and thereby heighten the perception of pain. In addition, pain management methods are not as effective if the client is tense and unable to relax.*
Perform actions to promote rest (e.g., minimize environmental activity and noise). **D** ● ✦	*A restful environment reduces fatigue and subsequently increases the client's threshold and tolerance for pain.*
Provide or assist with nonpharmacologic methods for pain relief (e.g., relaxation techniques, restful environment, watching television, reading).	*Relaxation and diversional activities help alleviate pain, fear, and anxiety, which may increase tolerance for pain.*
Instruct and assist client to support chest incision with a pillow or hands when turning, coughing, and deep breathing. **D** ● ✦	*Supporting the chest incision with a pillow or hands when turning, coughing, and deep breathing supports the incision and makes the activity less painful.*
Securely anchor chest tubes.	*Anchoring of chest tubes decreases irritation from the movement of the tubes.*
Dependent/Collaborative Actions	
Administer analgesics before activities and procedures that can cause pain and before pain becomes severe. **D** ✦	*The administration of analgesics before a pain-producing event helps minimize the pain that will be experienced. Analgesics given before procedures will improve the client's ability to tolerate the procedures before the pain becomes severe.*

THERAPEUTIC INTERVENTIONS	RATIONALE
Encourage client to use the patient-controlled analgesia device as instructed.	*Patient-controlled analgesia allows the client to control pain medication administration. Clients using patient-controlled analgesia have been shown to use less medication and ambulate more quickly after surgery than patients receiving nurse-controlled analgesia.*
Maintain integrity of analgesia delivery system (epidural, intravenous, subcutaneous, transdermal).	
Consult appropriate health care provider (e.g., physician, pharmacist, pain management specialist) if the provided measures fail to provide adequate pain relief.	*Notifying the appropriate health care provider allows for a multifaceted treatment plan.*

Collaborative Diagnosis ## RISK FOR INEFFECTIVE LUNG EXPANSION

Definition: Inability to expand the lung to provide adequate oxygenation to the body.

Extended pneumothorax
Related to:
An increase in intrapleural pressure associated with accumulation of air in pleural space (can occur if the chest drainage system malfunctions and/or air leaks into the pleural space through the incision)

Hemothorax
Related to:
Intraoperative or postoperative bleeding and/or malfunction of the chest drainage system

Mediastinal shift
Related to:
- A significant increase in intrapleural pressure on the operative side after a lobectomy associated with an accumulation of fluid and air in the pleural space
- Excessive negative pressure on the operative side after pneumonectomy associated with inadequate serous fluid accumulation in the empty thoracic space (the position of the mediastinum is maintained by accumulation of serous fluid in the empty thoracic space)

CLINICAL MANIFESTATIONS

Subjective	Objective
Verbal self-report of shortness of breath	Absent breath sounds; hyperresonant percussion with pneumothorax; dull percussion with hemothorax; rapid, shallow, and/or labored respirations; restlessness; agitation; confusion; arterial blood gas values that have worsened; chest radiograph results showing a lung collapse; further decrease in Hct and Hgb

RISK FACTORS
- Surgery
- Smoking
- Pain
- Anesthetics

DESIRED OUTCOMES

The client will experience normal lung reexpansion as evidence by:
a. Audible breath sounds and resonant percussion note over remaining lung tissue by third or fourth postoperative day
b. Unlabored respirations at 12 to 20 breaths/min
c. Arterial blood gas values within normal range
d. Absence of or no sudden increase in dyspnea
e. Vital signs within normal limits
f. Usual mental status
g. Trachea in midline position
h. Absence of neck vein distention
i. Chest radiograph showing lung reexpansion

NDx = NANDA Diagnosis   **D** = Delegatable Action   ● = UAP   ✦ = LVN/LPN   ⊙▶ = Go to ⊖volve for animation

NURSING ASSESSMENT	RATIONALE
Assess for and immediately report signs and symptoms of: • Malfunction of chest drainage system (e.g., respiratory distress, lack of fluctuation in water seal chamber without evidence of lung reexpansion, excessive bubbling in water seal chamber, significant increase in subcutaneous emphysema) • Extended pneumothorax (e.g., extended area of absent breath sounds with hyperresonant percussion note; rapid, shallow, and/or labored respirations; restlessness; agitation; confusion; arterial blood gas values that have worsened; chest radiograph results showing delayed lung reexpansion or further lung collapse). • Mediastinal shift (e.g., severe dyspnea, rapid and/or irregular pulse rate, hypotension, restlessness, agitation, confusion, shift in trachea from midline, neck vein distention, arterial blood gas values that have worsened, chest radiograph results showing a deviation of trachea from midline)	*Early recognition of signs and symptoms of respiratory problems after thoracic surgery allows for prompt intervention.*

THERAPEUTIC INTERVENTIONS	RATIONALE
Independent Actions Implement measures to promote lung reexpansion and prevent further lung collapse: • Perform actions to maintain patency and integrity of chest drainage system:	
• Maintain fluid levels in the water seal and suction chambers as ordered.	*Maintains negative pressure within the lungs*
• Maintain occlusive dressing over chest tube insertion site.	*Maintains negative pressure seal*
• Tape all connections securely.	*Prevents tubing from being disconnected and maintains a closed drainage system*
• Tape the tubing to the chest wall close to insertion site.	*Reduces the risk of inadvertent removal of the chest tube*
• Position tubing to promote optimum drainage (e.g., coil excess tubing on bed rather than allowing it to hang down below the collection device, keep tubing free of kinks). **D** ✦	*Promotes drainage*
• Drain fluid that accumulates in tubing into the collection chamber.	*Maintains patency of the drainage system*
• Avoid stripping of chest tubes. If ordered, milk tubing using a hand over hand method while moving along the drainage tube.	*Chest tube stripping increases high negative pressures in the pleural space and may damage lung tissues.*
• Keep drainage collection device below level of client's chest at all times. **D** ✦	*Prevents backflow of drainage into the lungs*
• Perform actions to facilitate the escape of air from the pleural space (e.g., maintain suction as ordered, ensure that the air vent is open on the drainage collection device if system is to water seal only).	*Improves lung expansion and removal of secretions*
• Perform actions to improve breathing pattern and facilitate airway clearance (e.g., encourage client to cough and breathe deeply every 1 to 2 hrs; use incentive spirometry every 2 hrs; ambulate as ordered and as tolerated). **D** ✦	
Dependent/Collaborative Actions If signs and symptoms of further lung collapse or a hemothorax or mediastinal shift occur:	
• Maintain client on bedrest in a semi- to high-Fowler's position.	*Improves client's ability to expand the lungs*
• Maintain oxygen therapy as ordered. **D** ✦	*Helps maintain tissue oxygenation*
• Assess for and immediately report signs and symptoms of tension pneumothorax (e.g., severe dyspnea, increased restlessness and agitation, rapid and/or irregular pulse rate, hypotension, neck vein distention, shift in trachea from midline).	*Emergency treatment is required to prevent further respiratory difficulty.*

THERAPEUTIC INTERVENTIONS	RATIONALE
• Assist with clearing of existing chest tube and/or insertion of a new tube.	*Reestablishes a closed drainage system*
• Assist with autotransfusion of blood from chest tube and/or administer blood products and/or volume expanders if ordered.	*Addresses decreased Hct and Hgb*
• Assist with clearing of existing chest tubes, thoracentesis, or insertion of chest tube if not already present.	*Prevents drainage from accumulating in the lungs*
• Prepare client for surgical intervention to ligate bleeding vessels if indicated.	*Decreases anxiety*

Collaborative Diagnosis RISK FOR CARDIAC DYSRHYTHMIAS

Definition: A disturbance of the heart's normal rhythm. Dysrhythmias can range from missed or rapid beats to serious disturbances that impair the pumping ability of the heart.

Related to: Altered nodal function and myocardial conductivity associated primarily with myocardial hypoxia (may result from impaired gas exchange and diminished myocardial blood flow that can occur with hypovolemia and sympathetic nervous system–medicated vasoconstriction in the immediate postoperative period)

CLINICAL MANIFESTATIONS

Subjective	Objective
Verbal self-report of palpitations or "skipped beats"	Irregular apical pulse; heart rate less than 60 or greater than 100 beats/min; apical-radial pulse deficit; syncope; palpitations; abnormal rate, rhythm, or configuration on electrocardiogram (ECG)

RISK FACTORS
- Electrolyte imbalance
- Activity intolerance
- Myocardial hypoxia
- Hypovolemia

DESIRED OUTCOMES

The client will maintain normal sinus rhythm as evidenced by:
a. Regular apical pulse rate at 50 to 100 beats/min
b. Equal apical and radial pulse rates
c. Absence of syncope and palpitations
d. ECG showing normal sinus rhythm

NURSING ASSESSMENT	RATIONALE
Assess for and report signs and symptoms of cardiac dysrhythmias (e.g., irregular apical pulse; pulse rate less than 60 and greater than 100 beats/min; apical-radial pulse deficit; syncope; palpitations; abnormal rate, rhythm, or configurations on ECG).	*Early recognition of signs and symptoms of cardiac dysrhythmias after thoracic surgery allows for prompt intervention.*

THERAPEUTIC INTERVENTIONS	RATIONALE
Independent Actions Implement measures to prevent cardiac dysrhythmias: • Reduce pain, fear, and anxiety (e.g., assure client need for pain relief is understood, and plan methods for achieving pain control with client; orient client to environment, equipment, and routines; maintain a calm, supportive environment; encourage/instruct client in use of relaxation techniques; allow client to discuss anxiety and fears). **D** ✦	*Pain, anxiety, and fear cause stimulation of the sympathetic nervous system, which increases the heart rate and causes vasoconstriction, both of which increase cardiac workload and decrease oxygen availability to the myocardium.*

Continued...

THERAPEUTIC INTERVENTIONS	RATIONALE

Dependent/Collaborative Actions

If cardiac dysrhythmias occur:

- Administer antidysrhythmics (e.g., digoxin) as ordered.
- Restrict client's activity based on client's tolerance and severity of the dysrhythmia.
- Maintain oxygen therapy as ordered.
- Assess cardiovascular status frequently and report signs and symptoms of inadequate tissue perfusion (e.g., decrease in B/P, cool skin, cyanosis, diminished peripheral pulses, urine output less than 30 mL/h, restlessness and agitation, increased shortness of breath).

Prevention of dysrhythmias
Reduces client's potential for injury

Provides supplemental oxygenation, which may decrease dysrhythmias
Provides for prompt treatment of dysrhythmias
Indications of decreased cardiac output

Collaborative Diagnosis   **RISK FOR ACUTE PULMONARY EDEMA**

Definition: Accumulation of fluid in the lungs that leads to impaired O_2/CO_2 exchange.

Related to:
- Increased pulmonary capillary permeability associated with hypoxia
- Increased hydrostatic pressure in the remaining pulmonary vessels associated with reduced size of the pulmonary vascular bed and decreased effectiveness of lymphatic drainage resulting from extensive removal of pulmonary tissue (especially if pneumonectomy was performed).

CLINICAL MANIFESTATIONS

Subjective	Objective
Verbal self-report of shortness of breath and difficulty breathing	Adventitious breath sounds (e.g., rales), productive cough (e.g. blood tinged, frothy sputum; increased work of breathing, increased respiratory rate; decreased oxygen saturation; diaphoresis; dyspnea; tachypnea; auscultated; wheezes; decreasing pulse oximetry; abnormal arterial blood gases

RISK FACTORS

- Increased pulmonary hydrostatic pressure
- Decreased effectiveness of the lymph drainage
- Smoking

DESIRED OUTCOMES

The client will not develop pulmonary edema as evidenced by:
a. Unlabored respirations at 12 to 20 breaths/min
b. Clear breath sounds and resonant percussion note over nonoperated lung tissue
c. Absence of productive, persistent cough
d. Usual skin color
e. Oximetry results within normal range
f. Arterial blood gas values within normal range

NURSING ASSESSMENT	RATIONALE

Pulmonary edema (e.g., severe dyspnea, tachycardia, development of or increase in crackles [rales] or wheezes, dull percussion note over remaining lung tissue, persistent cough productive of frothy and/or blood-tinged sputum, cyanosis, significant decrease in oximetry results, decrease in PaO_2 and/or increase in $PaCO_2$, chest radiograph results showing pulmonary edema)

Early recognition of signs and symptoms of pulmonary edema allows for prompt intervention.

THERAPEUTIC INTERVENTIONS	RATIONALE

Independent Actions

Implement measures to maintain adequate respiratory function (e.g., encourage use of incentive spirometry every 2 to 3 hrs; ambulate as tolerated; provide supplemental oxygen as needed; maintain patency of chest tube).

Improves lung expansion and mobilization of secretions

Dependent/Collaborative Actions

If signs and symptoms of pulmonary edema occur, administer bronchodilators and agents to reduce pulmonary vascular congestion (e.g., diuretics and morphine sulfate).

Improves bronchial airflow and decreases pulmonary congestion

---

Collaborative Diagnosis RISK FOR BRONCHOPLEURAL FISTULA

Definition: A fistula between the lungs and the pleural space.

Related to: Inadequate bronchial closure and healing after a partial or complete resection of the lungs (most often associated with preoperative radiation to the lungs and/or residual cancer of the bronchial stump).

CLINICAL MANIFESTATIONS

Subjective	**Objective**
Verbal self-report of pain; shortness of breath, difficulty breathing	Hyperthermia; cough with purulent sputum; continuous bubbling of chest drainage system; increasing subcutaneous emphysema around neck and incision; elevated WBC count; chest radiograph with presence of bronchopleural fistula

RISK FACTORS

- Surgery
- Radiation

DESIRED OUTCOMES

The client will experience resolution of a bronchopleural fistula if it occurs as evidenced by:
a. Afebrile status
b. Absence of cough
c. Absence of continuous bubbling in water seal chamber of chest drainage system
d. Unlabored respirations at 12 to 20 breaths/min
e. WBC and differential counts returning toward normal

NURSING ASSESSMENT	RATIONALE

Assess for and report signs and symptoms of bronchopleural fistula (e.g., fever, cough, purulent sputum, continuous bubbling in water seal chamber of chest drainage system, increasing subcutaneous emphysema around incision and neck, respiratory distress, persistent elevation of WBC count and significant change in differential, chest radiograph results showing presence of bronchopleural fistula).

Early recognition of the signs and symptoms of bronchopleural fistula allows for prompt intervention.

THERAPEUTIC INTERVENTIONS	RATIONALE

Independent Actions

If signs and symptoms of a bronchial fistula occur:
- Turn client to operative side unless contraindicated.
- Have tracheostomy tray readily available.

- Prepare client for chest tube insertion, thoracentesis, and surgical repair of bronchial stump if planned.

Reduces risk for aspiration of pleural fluid
Severe subcutaneous emphysema in the neck can compress trachea and obstruct the airway.
Decreases client anxiety

NDx = NANDA Diagnosis   **D** = Delegatable Action   ● = UAP   ✦ = LVN/LPN   ⊖▶ = Go to ⊖volve for animation

Collaborative Diagnosis RESTRICTED ARM AND SHOULDER MOVEMENT

Definition: Decreased movement of the upper limbs.

Related to: Decreased activity of the arm and shoulder on the operative side associated with weakness, fatigue, pain, and adhesion formation between incised muscles

CLINICAL MANIFESTATIONS

Subjective	Objective
Verbal self-report of difficulty/inability in moving arm and shoulder, pain with movement	Limited range of motion of arm and shoulder

RISK FACTORS

- Limited movement
- Fatigue
- Pain
- Weakness

DESIRED OUTCOMES

The client will maintain normal arm and shoulder function as evidenced by the ability to move the arm and shoulder on the operative side through the usual range of motion.

NURSING ASSESSMENT	RATIONALE
Assess for and report signs and symptoms of restricted arm and shoulder movement on operative side (e.g., inability to move arm and shoulder through usual range of motion, inability to use arm in ADL).	*Early recognition of signs and symptoms of reduced arm and shoulder movement allows for prompt intervention.*

THERAPEUTIC INTERVENTIONS	RATIONALE
Dependent/Collaborative Actions Implement measures to prevent restriction of arm and shoulder movement on operative side:	
• Instruct client in and assist with arm and shoulder exercises ordered (usually passive range of motion is started the evening of surgery, and active range of motion exercises are started by the second postoperative day).	*Early intervention and movement of the arms and shoulders are important in preventing restricted movement.*
• Perform actions to reduce pain (e.g., administer analgesics). **D ✦**	*Reduction of pain will increase client's ability and willingness to move arm and shoulder.*
• Encourage client to use arm on operative side to perform self-care activities. **D ● ✦**	*Use of the arm on the operative side by the client helps maintain movement.*
• Place frequently used articles and bed stand on operative side. **D ● ✦**	*Place articles on the operative side of the bed so that client will be more likely to use that arm.*
• Anchor pull rope at foot of bed. **D ● ✦**	

DISCHARGE TEACHING/CONTINUED CARE

Nursing Diagnosis DEFICIENT KNOWLEDGE, NDx INEFFECTIVE HEALTH MAINTENANCE NDx, OR INEFFECTIVE HEALTH MANAGEMENT* NDx

Definition: Deficient Knowledge NDx: Absence of cognitive information related to a specific topic, or its acquisition; **Ineffective Health Maintenance NDx:** Inability to identify, manage, and/or seek out help to maintain well-being; **Ineffective Health Management NDx:** Pattern of regulating and integrating into daily living a therapeutic regimen for the treatment of illness and its sequelae that is unsatisfactory for meeting specific health goals.

CLINICAL MANIFESTATIONS

Subjective	Objective
Verbal self-report of the problem	Inaccurate follow-through of instructions; inappropriate behaviors

RISK FACTORS
- Denial of disease process
- Cognitive deficiency
- Failure to take action to reduce risk factors

NOC OUTCOMES

Knowledge: health promotion; health resources; treatment regimen

NIC INTERVENTIONS

Health system guidance; teaching: individual; teaching: prescribed activity/exercise; teaching: disease process

NURSING ASSESSMENT	RATIONALE
Assess client readiness to learn. Assess meaning of illness to client.	*Early recognition of readiness to learn and meaning of illness to client allows for appropriate teaching interventions.*

THERAPEUTIC INTERVENTIONS	RATIONALE

Desired Outcome: The client will identify ways to promote optimal respiratory health.

Independent Actions
Instruct client in ways to promote optimal respiratory health:

- Maintain overall general good health (e.g., reduce stress, eat a well-balanced diet, obtain adequate rest, obtain adequate exercise).

Maintenance of good general health helps fight off respiratory infections and maintain adequate respiratory status.

- Stop smoking.
- Avoid exposure to respiratory irritants such as smoke, dust, aerosol sprays, paint fumes, and solvents.

The irritants in smoke and other respiratory irritants increase mucus production, impair ciliary function, and can cause inflammation and damage to the bronchial and alveolar walls; the carbon monoxide decreases oxygen availability.

- Remain indoors as much as possible when air pollution levels are high.

High levels of air pollution are lung irritants and impair ciliary function.

- Wear a mask or scarf over nose and mouth if exposure to high levels of irritants such as smoke, fumes, and dust is unavoidable.

Wearing a mask or scarf decreases the level of exposure to irritants in the air.

- Take medications as prescribed to treat any underlying respiratory disease such as COPD, cancer of the lung, or tuberculosis.

Helps maintain adequate lung functioning and oxygenation of body tissues.

- Decrease the risk of respiratory tract infections:
  - Avoid contact with persons who have respiratory tract infections.
  - Avoid crowds and poorly ventilated areas.

Each of these actions helps decrease the incidence of infections and maintain good lung health.

- Drink at least 10 glasses of liquid/day unless contraindicated.

Maintains adequate circulatory volume.

- Receive immunizations against influenza and pneumococcal pneumonia.

Improves client's resistance to influenza and pneumococcal pneumonia.

THERAPEUTIC INTERVENTIONS	RATIONALE

Desired Outcome: The client will demonstrate the ability to perform prescribed arm and shoulder exercises.

Instruct client regarding the importance of exercising the arm and shoulder on the operative side. Emphasize that the exercises should be performed at least 5 times per day for several weeks.

Exercise of the arm and shoulder on the operative side prevents restriction of arm and shoulder movement.

Demonstrate appropriate arm and shoulder exercises (e.g., shoulder shrugs, arm circles).

The client's ability to perform the exercises should be evaluated before leaving the health care facility.

NDx = NANDA Diagnosis   **D** = Delegatable Action   ● = UAP   ✦ = LVN/LPN   ⊖▶ = Go to ⊖volve for animation

Continued...

THERAPEUTIC INTERVENTIONS	RATIONALE
Allow time for questions, clarification, and return demonstration.	*Everyone does not understand information as presented; allowing time for questioning helps clients assimilate the information in terms they can understand. Return demonstration allows the nurse to verify client's ability to perform exercises.*

THERAPEUTIC INTERVENTIONS	RATIONALE
Desired Outcome: The client will state signs and symptoms to report to the health care provider. Instruct the client to report these signs and symptoms: • Increased discomfort in or decreased ability to move arm and shoulder on operative side • Increased shortness of breath • Persistent cough • Persistent low-grade fever • Difficulty breathing • Chest pain • Increasing weakness or inability to tolerate prescribed activity level • Separation of wound edges • Increased redness, warmth, pain, or swelling around the wound • Unusual or excessive drainage from any wound site	*Clients need to be aware of the signs and symptoms that should be reported to their health care provider to allow for prompt treatment of complications.*

THERAPEUTIC INTERVENTIONS	RATIONALE
Desired Outcome: The client will identify community resources that can assist with home management and adjustment to the diagnosis, effects of surgery, and subsequent treatment if planned. Provide information about community resources that can assist the client and significant others with home management and adjustment to the diagnosis, effects of surgery, and subsequent treatment if planned (e.g., American Lung Association, American Cancer Society, smoking cessation program, Meals on Wheels, counselors, support groups, home health agencies).	*Information on how to access community resources and information related to home management is important to maintain client's recovery.*

THERAPEUTIC INTERVENTIONS	RATIONALE
Desired Outcome: The client, in collaboration with the nurse, will develop a plan for adhering to recommended follow-up care, including future appointments with health care provider, medications prescribed, activity level, pain management, wound care, and subsequent treatment of the underlying disorder. Reinforce physician's instructions about activity level: • Gauge activity according to tolerance and ensure adequate rest periods. • Stop any activity that causes excessive fatigue, dyspnea, or chest pain. • Avoid lifting heavy objects and doing strenuous upper body exercises until complete healing of chest muscles has occurred (usually 3–6 months). Inform client that numbness and discomfort in the operative area can persist for several weeks but are usually temporary. Clarify plans for subsequent treatment of underlying disorder (e.g., chemotherapy, radiation therapy) if appropriate.	*Reinforcement of instructions and providing written instructions for the client provide a reference for questions once the client is home.* *The client should be aware of when numbness and discomfort in the operative area will resolve, so they won't become anxious if pain and numbness persist.* *Client should be aware that the surgery may not completely remove the necessity of treatment of the underlying condition.*

TUBERCULOSIS

Tuberculosis (TB) is an infectious disease caused by *Mycobacterium tuberculosis,* a gram-positive, acid-fast bacillus. It is spread by airborne droplets released when a person with active TB disease coughs, sneezes, or speaks. These droplets can cause infection in others if contact with the infected person is close and repeated or prolonged. The inhaled tubercle bacilli implant themselves in the lung, multiply, and can spread to other areas of the body through the lymphatic channels (lymphatic dissemination) and blood (hematogenous dissemination).

Most people who are infected with tubercle bacilli do not develop an active form of TB. Those who do are usually part of high-risk populations that include persons who are immunosuppressed, persons in continued close contact with people with active untreated TB, and those who have been exposed to virulent strains of multidrug-resistant tuberculosis (MDR-TB). In addition, TB that has previously been inactive (latent, dormant) in a person with an effective immune system can become active if that person experiences situations that suppress the immune response (e.g., chemotherapy treatment, long-term corticosteroid use, malnutrition, human immunodeficiency virus [HIV] infection, advanced age).

Signs and symptoms of active TB can include fatigue, anorexia, weight loss, night sweats, fever (usually low grade), cough (usually progresses from a dry cough to one that is productive of mucopurulent or blood-tinged sputum), dyspnea, and/or pleuritic pain (in some cases).

A person with suspected active TB is placed on precautions to prevent airborne transmission of the tubercle bacilli and started on a regimen of multiple antitubercular/antimicrobial medications while awaiting results of sputum cultures. If the diagnosis is confirmed, a major health care focus becomes one of promoting compliance with the lengthy (usually 6–18 months), multiple-drug treatment regimen.

This care plan focuses on the adult client hospitalized with signs and symptoms of active pulmonary tuberculosis. Much of the information presented here is applicable to clients receiving follow-up care in an extended care facility or home setting.

OUTCOME/DISCHARGE CRITERIA

The client will:
1. Have an adequate respiratory status
2. Tolerate expected level of activity
3. Have no signs and symptoms of complications
4. Identify ways to maintain respiratory health
5. Identify ways to prevent the spread of TB to others
6. Verbalize an understanding of medications ordered including rationale, food and drug interactions, side effects, and importance of taking as prescribed
7. State signs and symptoms to report to the health care provider
8. Develop a plan for adhering to recommended follow-up care, including future appointments with health care providers.

Nursing Diagnosis ## IMPAIRED RESPIRATORY FUNCTION*

Definition: **Ineffective Breathing Pattern NDx** : Inspiration and/or expiration that does not provide adequate ventilation; **Ineffective Airway Clearance NDx**: Inability to clear secretions or obstructions from the respiratory tract to maintain a clear airway; **Impaired Gas Exchange NDx**: Excess or deficit in oxygenation and/or carbon dioxide elimination at the alveolar-capillary membrane.

Ineffective breathing pattern NDx
Related to:
- Decreased depth of respirations associated with weakness, fatigue, and reluctance to breathe deeply if chest pain is present
- Increased rate of respirations associated with the increase in metabolic rate that occurs with an infectious process

Ineffective airway clearance NDx
Related to:
- Tracheobronchial inflammation
- Increase in secretions associated with the infectious process and the necrosis and subsequent liquefaction of tubercle nodules (the nodules, or caseations, are lesions that consist of tubercle bacilli surrounded by a fibrous capsule)
- Stasis of secretions associated with decreased activity; poor cough effort resulting from weakness, fatigue, and chest pain (if present); and impaired ciliary function (results from the increased viscosity and volume of mucus that occurs with the infectious process)

Impaired gas exchange NDx
Related to:
- A decrease in effective lung surface associated with the accumulation of secretions
- Destruction of normal lung tissue that occurs with the presence of the tubercle nodules

---

*This diagnostic label includes the following nursing diagnoses: ineffective breathing pattern, ineffective airway clearance, and impaired gas exchange.

CLINICAL MANIFESTATIONS

Subjective	Objective
Verbal self-report of fatigue, pleuritic pain, confusion, restlessness, and somnolence	Dyspnea; orthopnea; use of accessory muscles; fever (usually low grade); cough—progressive from a dry cough to one that is productive of mucopurulent or blood-tinged sputum; decreased expiratory and inspiratory pressures; abnormal breath sounds; limited chest excursion; significantly decreased oximetry results; abnormal arterial blood gas values; sputum positive for acid-fast stain; chest radiograph—nodular calcification, enlargement of hilar lymph nodes, parenchymal infiltrate, pleural effusion, and cavitation

RISK FACTORS

- Exposure to someone who has TB
- Increased secretions
- Smoking and exposure to second-hand smoke
- Ineffective medication regimen

DESIRED OUTCOMES

The client will experience adequate respiratory function as evidenced by:
a. Normal rate and depth of respirations
b. Absence of dyspnea
c. Normal breath sounds over remaining lung tissue
d. Usual mental status
e. Usual skin color
f. Oximetry results within normal range
g. Arterial blood gas values within normal range

NOC OUTCOMES

Respiratory status: gas exchange; ventilation; airway patency

NIC INTERVENTIONS

Respiratory monitoring; airway management; chest physiotherapy; cough enhancement; oxygen therapy; medication administration; ventilation assistance

NURSING ASSESSMENT	RATIONALE
Assess for and report signs and symptoms of impaired respiratory function: • Rapid, shallow respirations • Dyspnea, orthopnea • Use of accessory muscles when breathing • Abnormal breath sounds (e.g., diminished, crackles [rales], rhonchi) • Cough (usually a productive cough of mucopurulent or blood-tinged sputum) • Limited chest excursion • Restlessness, irritability • Confusion, somnolence Assess arterial blood gas values, oximetry values, and chest radiograph results. Report abnormal findings.	*Early recognition of signs and symptoms of impaired respiratory function allows for prompt intervention.*

THERAPEUTIC INTERVENTIONS	RATIONALE
Independent Actions Implement measures to improve respiratory status: • Perform actions to reduce chest pain if present (e.g., splint chest with pillow when coughing and deep breathing). **D** ✦ Place client in a semi- to high-Fowler's position unless contraindicated; position with pillows. **D** ● ✦	*These actions increase the client's willingness to move, cough, and breathe deeply.* *Positioning in semi- to high-Fowler's position promotes optimal gas exchange by enabling chest expansion. Positioning with pillows prevents slumping.*

THERAPEUTIC INTERVENTIONS	**RATIONALE**
• If client must remain flat in bed, assist with position change at least every 2 hrs. **D ● ✦**	*Changing positions every 2 hrs helps mobilize secretions for expectoration.*
• Instruct client to breathe deeply or use inspiratory exercises every 1 to 2 hrs. **D ● ✦**	*Forced deep breathing and use of incentive spirometry will increase expansion of the lungs and improve the client's ability to clear mucus from the lungs. The technique may also improve the amount of oxygen that is able to penetrate deep into the lungs.*
• Perform actions to promote removal of pulmonary secretions: • Assist client to cough or "huff" every 1 to 2 hrs. **D ● ✦**	*Coughing or "huffing" every 1 to 2 hrs will help remove secretions.*
• Implement measures to thin tenacious secretions and reduce dryness of the respiratory mucous membrane: • Maintain a fluid intake of at least 2500 mL/day unless contraindicated. **D ● ✦**	*Increasing fluid intake will help liquefy secretions.*
• Increase activity as allowed and tolerated. **D ● ✦**	*Conservation of energy through activity restrictions allows energy to be focused on breathing. Increasing activity as tolerated helps mobilize secretions and promotes deeper breathing.*
• Discourage smoking.	*Irritants in smoke increase mucus production, impair ciliary function, and can cause inflammation and damage to the bronchial and alveolar walls; the carbon monoxide decreases oxygen availability.*

Dependent/Collaborative Actions

Implement measures to improve respiratory status:

• Assist with positive airway pressure techniques (e.g., CPAP, bilevel positive airway pressure [BiPAP], flutter/positive expiratory pressure [PEP] device) if ordered.	*Improves volume of air that is breathed into the lungs.*
• Maintain oxygen as ordered. **D ✦**	*Supplemental oxygen helps relieve dyspne.*
• Humidify air as ordered. **D ✦**	*Humidity will help liquefy secretions.*
• Administer CNS depressants judiciously; hold medication and consult physician if respiratory rate is less than 12 breaths/min. **D ✦**	*CNS depressants may significantly decrease respiratory rate, leading to respiratory acidosis and hypoxemia.*
• Administer the following medications as ordered: • Bronchodilators (e.g., methylxanthines, sympathomimetic [adrenergic] agents).	*Bronchodilators open bronchioles and allow for improved ventilation of the lungs.*
• Antitubercular/antimicrobial agents	*Antitubercular agents impact the active infection.*
Consult appropriate health care provider (e.g., respiratory therapist, physician) if signs and symptoms of impaired respiratory function persist or worsen.	*Notifying the appropriate health care professionals allows for a prompt and multifaceted approach to treatment.*

Nursing Diagnosis **IMBALANCED NUTRITION: LESS THAN BODY REQUIREMENTS NDx**

Definition: Intake of nutrients insufficient to meet metabolic needs.

Related to:
• Decreased oral intake associated with dyspnea, weakness, fatigue, excessive coughing, and the foul order and taste of sputum and some aerosol treatments
• Nausea (can occur in response to noxious stimuli such as the sight of expectorated sputum and as a side effect of some medications)
• Increased nutritional needs associated with the increase in metabolic rate that occurs with an infectious process

---

CLINICAL MANIFESTATIONS

Subjective	Objective
Verbal self-report of sore buccal membranes; report of altered taste sensation	Weight loss; weight less than normal for client's age, height, and body frame; abnormal BUN and low serum prealbumin and albumin levels; inflamed mucous membranes; pale conjunctiva; poor muscle tone; excessive hair loss

RISK FACTORS

- Shortness of breath
- Lack of appetite
- Inappropriate diet
- Nausea
- Respiratory treatments
- Productive cough

DESIRED OUTCOMES

The client will maintain adequate nutrition status as evidenced by:
a. Weight within normal range for clients
b. Normal BUN and serum prealbumin and albumin levels
c. Usual strength and activity tolerance
d. Healthy oral mucous membrane

NOC OUTCOMES

Nutritional status

NIC INTERVENTIONS

Nutritional monitoring; nutrition management; nutrition therapy

NURSING ASSESSMENT

Assess for and report signs and symptoms of malnutrition:
- Weight significantly below client's usual weight or less than normal for client's age, height, and body frame
- Abnormal BUN and low serum prealbumin and albumin levels
- Increased weakness and fatigue
- Sore, inflamed oral mucous membrane
- Pale conjunctiva
- Sore buccal membranes
- Excessive hair loss
- Poor muscle tone

RATIONALE

Early recognition of signs and symptoms of malnutrition allows for prompt intervention.

THERAPEUTIC INTERVENTIONS

Independent Actions

Monitor percentage of meals and snacks client consumes. Report inadequate intake. **D** ✦

Implement measures to maintain an adequate nutritional status:
- Schedule treatments that assist in mobilizing mucus (e.g. aerosol treatments, postural drainage therapy) at least 1 hr before or after meals.
- Increase activity as tolerated. **D** ● ✦

- Encourage a rest period before meals. **D** ● ✦

- Eliminate noxious sights and odors from the environment; provide client with an opaque, covered container for expectorated sputum. **D** ● ✦
- Maintain a clean environment and a relaxed, pleasant atmosphere. **D** ● ✦
- Provide oral hygiene before meals. **D** ● ✦

RATIONALE

Monitoring a client's intake helps identify when a patient is at risk for inadequate nutrition and allows for prompt intervention.

The foul odor and taste of sputum and some aerosols are likely to decrease appetite. Appropriate scheduling of treatments also assists in decreasing nausea.

Activity usually promotes a sense of well-being and can help improve an individual's appetite.

Rest before a meal helps minimize fatigue that may occur when eating.

Noxious sights and odors can decrease one's appetite. By eliminating them, the patient's intake may improve.

A clean environment and a relaxed atmosphere may increase intake.

Oral hygiene moistens the mouth, which makes it easier to chew and swallow. It also removes unpleasant tastes, which often improves the taste of foods/fluids.

THERAPEUTIC INTERVENTIONS	RATIONALE
• Assist the client who is quite dyspneic in selecting foods that require little or no chewing.	*Dyspnea decreases the ability of an individual to eat complete meals.*
• Serve frequent, small meals rather than large ones if the client is weak, fatigues easily, or has a poor appetite. **D ● ✦**	*Small, frequent meals decrease fatigue and help maintain an individual's nutritional status.*
Place client in a high-Fowler's position for meals. **D ✦**	*The high-Fowler's position improves lung expansion and helps relieve dyspnea.*
• Limit fluid intake with meals unless the fluid has high nutritional value. **D ● ✦**	*Decreasing fluid intake during meals helps reduce early satiety and subsequent decreased food intake.*
• Allow for adequate time for meals. **D ● ✦**	*Clients who feel rushed during meals tend to become anxious, lose their appetite, and stop eating.*
• Ensure that meals are well balanced and high in essential nutrients.	*A diet that is well balanced and high in essential nutrients meets the client's nutritional needs.*

Dependent/Collaborative Actions
Implement measures to maintain an adequate nutritional status:

• Administer dietary supplements as needed. **D ✦**	*If dietary intake does not provide the recommended daily allowances of vitamins and minerals, supplements may be necessary. Dietary supplements are often needed to accomplish appropriate nutritional status.*
• Administer supplemental oxygen while eating. **D ✦**	*Maintains appropriate oxygenation while client is eating, which may improve intake*
• Obtain a dietary consult to assist client in selecting foods/fluids that meet nutritional needs, are appealing, and adhere to personal and cultural preferences.	*Provides client an additional resource in determining which preferred fluids and foods that are best for meeting the client's nutritional needs.*
• Perform a calorie count if ordered and report information to dietitian and physician.	*A calorie count provides information about the caloric and nutritional value of the foods/fluids consumed. The information helps the dietitian and physician determine whether an alternative method of nutritional support is needed.*
Consult a physician about an alternative method of providing nutrition (e.g., parenteral nutrition, tube feedings) if client does not consume enough food or fluids to meet nutritional needs.	*If a client is unable to eat, collaboration with the physician is required to determine alternative methods of maintaining nutritional status.*

Nursing Diagnosis   ## ACTIVITY INTOLERANCE NDx

Definition: Insufficient physiological or psychological energy to endure or complete required or desired daily activities.

Related to:
• Tissue hypoxia associated with impaired gas exchange
• Difficulty resting and sleeping associated with frequent coughing, dyspnea, and frequent assessments and treatment
• Inadequate nutritional status
• Increased energy expenditure associated with persistent coughing and the increased metabolic rate that is present in an infectious process

CLINICAL MANIFESTATIONS

Subjective	Objective
Verbal self-report of fatigue, weakness, and/or dizziness	Abnormal heart rate or B/P response to activity; exertional discomfort or dyspnea; electrocardiographic changes reflecting dysrhythmias or ischemia; unable to speak during physical activity

---

NDx = NANDA Diagnosis   **D** = Delegatable Action   ● = UAP   ✦ = LVN/LPN   ⊖▶ = Go to ⊖volve for animation

RISK FACTORS

- Generalized weakness
- Imbalance between oxygen supply/demand
- Debilitated condition
- Immobility
- Sedentary lifestyle

DESIRED OUTCOMES

The client will demonstrate an increased tolerance for activity as evidenced by:
a. Verbalization of feeling less fatigued and weak
b. Ability to perform ADL without exertional dyspnea, chest pain, diaphoresis, dizziness, and significant changes in vital signs

NOC OUTCOMES

Activity tolerance, endurance: fatigue level; vital signs; energy conservation; symptom severity

NIC INTERVENTIONS

Activity therapy; energy management; oxygen therapy; nutrition management; sleep enhancement; cardiac care; cardiac rehabilitation; teaching regarding prescribed activity

NURSING ASSESSMENT

Assess for signs and symptoms of activity intolerance:
- Statements of fatigue or weakness
- Exertional dyspnea, chest pain, diaphoresis, or dizziness
- Abnormal heart rate response to activity (e.g., increase in rate of 20 beats/min above resting rate, rate not returning to preactivity level within 3 minutes after stopping activity, change from regular to irregular rate)
- Significant change of 15 to 20 mm Hg in B/P with activity.

RATIONALE

Early recognition of signs and symptoms of activity intolerance allows for prompt intervention.

THERAPEUTIC INTERVENTIONS

Independent Actions
Implement measures to improve activity tolerance:
- Conserve energy.
- Maintain prescribed activity restrictions.
- Minimize environmental activity and noise.
- Provide uninterrupted rest periods.
- Assist with care.
- Keep supplies and personal articles within easy reach.
- Limit the number of visitors.
- Assist client in energy-saving techniques (e.g., using a shower chair when showering, sitting to brush teeth or comb hair).
- Implement measures to promote sleep (e.g., maintain a quiet, restful environment; discourage client from napping during the day, participating in group care activities to allow for periods of rest).
- Increase client's activity gradually as allowed and tolerated. **D** ● ✦
- Discourage smoking and excessive intake of beverages high in caffeine such as coffee, tea, and colas.

- Implement measures to improve respiratory status (e.g., encourage use of incentive spirometer; elevate head of bed; assist with turning, coughing, and deep breathing) if ineffective breathing pattern, ineffective airway clearance, or impaired gas exchange is contributing to client's activity intolerance. **D** ✦
Instruct client to report a decreased tolerance for activity and to stop any activity that causes chest pain, shortness of breath, dizziness, or extreme fatigue or weakness.

RATIONALE

Cells use oxygen and fat, protein, and carbohydrates to produce the energy needed for all body activities. Rest and activities that conserve energy result in a lower metabolic rate, which preserves nutrients and oxygen for necessary activities.

Progressive increase in activity helps strengthen the myocardium, which enhances cardiac output and improves activity tolerance.
Both nicotine and excessive caffeine intake can increase cardiac workload and myocardial oxygen utilization, thereby decreasing the amount of oxygen necessary for energy production.
Improving respiratory status increases the amount of oxygen available for energy production. It also eases the work of breathing, which reduces energy expenditure.

These symptoms indicate that insufficient oxygen is reaching the tissues and that activity has been increased beyond a therapeutic level.

THERAPEUTIC INTERVENTIONS	RATIONALE

Dependent/Collaborative Actions
Implement measures to improve activity tolerance:

- Implement measures to increase cardiac output (e.g., administer positive inotropic agents, vasodilators, or anti-dysrhythmics as ordered; elevate the head of the bed) if decreased cardiac output is contributing to the client's activity intolerance.

  Sufficient cardiac output is necessary to maintain an adequate blood flow and oxygen supply to the tissues. Adequate tissue oxygenation promotes more efficient energy production, which subsequently improves client's activity tolerance.

- Implement measures to reduce fever if present (e.g., administer tepid sponge bath, administer antipyretics as ordered). **D** ✦

  An elevated temperature increases the metabolic rate with subsequent depletion of available energy and a decrease in the ability to tolerate activity.

- Maintain oxygen therapy as ordered. **D** ✦

  Supplemental oxygen helps alleviate hypoxia and restore the more efficient aerobic metabolism, thereby improving energy levels and activity tolerance.

- Implement measures to maintain an adequate nutritional status (e.g., provide a diet high in essential nutrients, provide dietary supplements as indicated, administer vitamins and minerals as ordered).

  Metabolism is the process by which nutrients are transformed into energy. If nutrition is inadequate, energy production is decreased, which subsequently reduces one's ability to tolerate activity.

- Implement measures to treat anemia if present (e.g., administer prescribed iron, folic acid, and/or vitamin B12; administer packed red blood cells as ordered).

  Anemia reduces the blood's oxygen-carrying capacity. Resolution of anemia increases oxygen availability to the cells, which increases the efficiency of energy production and subsequently improves activity tolerance.

Consult physician if signs and symptoms of activity intolerance persist.

Notifying the physician allows for modification of the treatment plan.

Nursing Diagnosis

RISK FOR INFECTION NDx (EXTRAPULMONARY (E.G., PERICARDIAL, LARYNGEAL, SKELETAL, JOINT, RENAL, BRAIN, ADRENAL, LYMPHATIC) AND/OR SUPERINFECTION (E.G., CANDIDIASIS)

Definition: Susceptible to invasion and multiplication of pathogenic organisms, which may compromise health.

Related to:
- Spread of the tubercle bacilli into the lymph nodes (lymphatic dissemination) and blood (hematogenous dissemination)
- Decreased resistance to infection associated with inadequate nutritional status and/or presence of other disease (e.g., HIV infection, COPD) and side effects of the treatment of those diseases
- Interruption in the balance of usual endogenous microbial flora associated with the administration of antitubercular/antimicrobial agents

CLINICAL MANIFESTATIONS

Subjective	Objective
Verbal self-report of precordial pain; bone pain; painful joints; headache	Increase in temperature; increased pulse rate; pericardial friction rub and/or precordial pain; swollen lymph nodes; swollen, reddened joints; unusual color, amount, and odor of vaginal drainage; perineal itching; white patches or ulcerated areas in the mouth; increased weakness or fatigue; hoarseness, sore throat; increase in WBC count above previous levels and/or significant change in differential

---

RISK FACTORS

- Inadequate primary defenses
- Inadequate secondary defenses (decreased Hgb level, leukopenia, suppressed inflammatory response)
- Inadequate acquired immunity
- Malnutrition
- Ineffective pharmaceutical agents
- Insufficient knowledge to avoid exposure to pathogens

DESIRED OUTCOMES

The client will not develop extrapulmonary infection or superinfection as evidenced by:
a. No increase in temperature
b. Pulse rate within client's normal range
c. Absence of a pericardial friction rub and precordial pain
d. Absence of heat, pain, redness, swelling, and unusual drainage in any area
e. Absence of white patches and ulcerations in mouth
f. No reports of increased weakness and fatigue
g. Normal voice quality
h. Absence of headache
i. WBC and differential counts returning toward normal

NOC OUTCOMES

Immune status; infection severity

NIC INTERVENTIONS

Infection protection; infection control

NURSING ASSESSMENT

Assess for and report signs and symptoms of extrapulmonary infection or superinfection:
- Further increase in temperature
- Increased pulse rate
- Pericardial friction rub and/or precordial pain
- Bone pain
- Swollen, red, painful joints
- Swollen lymph nodes
- Unusual color, amount, and odor of vaginal drainage; perineal itching
- White patches or ulcerated areas in the mouth
- Increased weakness or fatigue
- Hoarseness, sore throat
- Headache
- Increase in WBC count above previous levels and/or significant change in differential

RATIONALE

Early recognition of signs and symptoms of infection allows for prompt treatment.
Fungal infections are common superinfections with antimicrobial therapy.

THERAPEUTIC INTERVENTIONS

Independent Actions
Implement measures to reduce the risk for extrapulmonary infection and/or superinfection:
- Use good hand hygiene and encourage client to do the same. **D** ● ✦
- Perform actions to maintain an adequate nutritional status (provide frequent meals, provide oral hygiene before meals, decrease fluid intake with meals).
- Maintain sterile technique during all invasive procedures (e.g., venous and arterial punctures, injections, urinary catheterization).
- Change peripheral intravenous line sites, and change equipment, tubing, and solutions used for treatments such as intravenous infusions and respiratory care according to hospital policy.

Protect client from others with an infection. **D** ● ✦
- Anchor catheters/tubings (e.g., urinary, intravenous) securely.

- Maintain a closed system for drains (e.g., urinary catheter) and intravenous infusions whenever possible.

RATIONALE

Good hand washing prevents the spread of infection.

Adequate nutritional status is important to prevent infections.

Sterile technique during invasive procedures is important to prevent exposure to infectious agents.

Changing intravenous line sites, equipment, tubings, etc. helps prevent infection.

Exposure to others with infection increases the client's risk.
Securing catheters/tubing reduces trauma to the tissues and the risk for introduction of pathogens associated with the in-and-out movement of the tubing.
Closed drainage systems prevent the introduction of infectious agents into the system.

THERAPEUTIC INTERVENTIONS	RATIONALE
• Assist client to perform good perineal care routinely and after each bowel movement. **D** ● ✦	*Good perineal care and hygiene prevent skin breakdown and exposure to potential infectious agents.*
• Reinforce importance of frequent oral hygiene. **D** ✦	*Good oral hygiene prevents accumulation of infectious agents.*

Dependent/Collaborative Actions

If signs and symptoms of an extrapulmonary infection or superinfection occur:

• Prepare client for and/or assist with diagnostic tests (e.g., blood, vaginal, pleural fluid, and urine cultures; lumbar puncture; aspiration of joint fluid; bone marrow aspiration).	*If an infection occurs, a culture and sensitivity of the infected area allow for prescription of appropriate antibiotics.*
• Administer additional or alternative antitubercular/ antimicrobial medications as ordered.	*Antitubercular and antimicrobial agents help resolve the infectious process.*

Collaborative Diagnosis **RISK FOR PLEURAL EFFUSION**

Definition: An abnormal accumulation of fluid in the pleural cavity.

Related to: An increase in capillary permeability of the pulmonary and pleural vessels associated with the inflammatory response to the presence of tubercle bacilli in the lung and pleural space

CLINICAL MANIFESTATIONS

Subjective	Objective
Verbal self-report of dyspnea; chest pain (pleural)	Dull percussion note and diminished or absent breath sounds; chest radiograph showing pleural effusion; respiratory rate greater than 20 breaths/min; fever; night sweats; cough; weight loss

RISK FACTORS
- Pulmonary infection
- Increased permeability of capillary beds

DESIRED OUTCOMES

The client will not develop pleural effusion as evidenced by:
a. No increase in dyspnea
b. Symmetrical chest excursion
c. Improved breath sounds and percussion note throughout lung fields

NURSING ASSESSMENT	RATIONALE
Assess for and report signs and symptoms of pleural effusion (e.g., dyspnea, chest pain, decreased chest excursion on affected side, dull percussion note, decreased or absent breath sounds over the affected area, chest radiograph showing pleural effusion)	*Early recognition of signs and symptoms of pleural effusion allows for prompt intervention.*

THERAPEUTIC INTERVENTIONS	RATIONALE
Dependent/Collaborative Actions	
Implement measures to resolve the infectious process:	*Resolution of an infectious process reduces the risk for development of pleural effusion and/or atelectasis.*
• Encourage coughing and deep breathing.	
• Administer antimicrobials as ordered.	*Treats infection*

NDx = NANDA Diagnosis   **D** = Delegatable Action   ● = UAP   ✦ = LVN/LPN   ⊖▶ = Go to ⊖volve for animation

Continued...

THERAPEUTIC INTERVENTIONS	RATIONALE
If signs and symptoms of pleural effusion occur: Continue with actions to improve respiratory status (e.g., increase activity tolerance; instruct client in and assist with diaphragmatic and pursed-lip breathing techniques; instruct client to breathe deeply or use incentive spirometer every 1–2 hrs; encourage coughing and deep breathing; place client in semi- to high-Fowler's position).	*Maintenance/improvement of the client's respiratory status and removal of secretions decrease the potential of infection or the occurrence of a pleural effusion.*
• Prepare client for a thoracentesis if planned.	*Removal of fluid from the lungs will help improve the client's ability to maintain adequate gas exchange.*

Collaborative Diagnosis   # RISK FOR ATELECTASIS

Definition: Collapse of lung tissue caused by hypoventilated alveoli.

Related to:
- Consolidation of lung tissue
- Proliferation of the infection
- Stasis of secretions

CLINICAL MANIFESTATIONS

Subjective	Objective
Verbal self-report of dyspnea	Decreased breath sounds and/or crackles; cough; sputum production; low-grade fever; heart rate greater than 60 to 100 beats/min; increased respiratory rate >20 breaths/min; increased work of breathing; chest radiograph, ultrasound, or computed tomography results showing patchy infiltrates

RISK FACTORS
- Ineffective treatment regimen
- Smoking
- Immobility

DESIRED OUTCOMES

The client will not develop atelectasis as evidenced by:
a. Clear, audible breath sounds
b. Resonant percussion note over lungs
c. Unlabored respirations at 12 to 20 breaths/min
d. Pulse rate within normal range for client
e. Afebrile status

NURSING ASSESSMENT	RATIONALE
Assess for and report signs and symptoms of atelectasis: • Diminished or absent breath sounds • Dull percussion note over affected area • Increased respiratory rate • Dyspnea • Tachycardia • Elevated temperature	*Early recognition of signs and symptoms of atelectasis allows for implementation of the appropriate interventions.*
Monitor pulse oximetry results as indicated.	*Pulse oximetry is an indirect measure of oxygen saturation. Monitoring pulse oximetry (SaO_2) allows for early detection of hypoxia and implementation of the appropriate interventions.*
Monitor chest radiograph results.	*Chest radiograph provides radiographic confirmation of atelectasis.*

THERAPEUTIC INTERVENTIONS	RATIONALE

Dependent/Collaborative Actions

Implement measures to prevent atelectasis:

- Perform actions to improve breathing pattern:
  - Encourage client to breathe deeply.
  - Use of incentive spirometry.
  - Perform actions to promote effective airway clearance:
  - Turn, cough, and breathe deeply.

Administer antibiotics as ordered.

If signs and symptoms of atelectasis occur:

- Increase frequency of position change, coughing or "huffing," deep breathing, and use of incentive spirometer.

Consult physician if signs and symptoms of atelectasis persist or worsen.

Lack of movement places a client at risk for atelectasis. Changing positions frequently, coughing, and deep breathing help expand the lungs, enhancing alveolar expansion.

Treats infection
Improves lung expansion and mobilization of secretions

Allows for prompt alterations in interventions

PATIENT AND DISCHARGE TEACHING/CONTINUED CARE

Nursing Diagnosis # DEFICIENT KNOWLEDGE, NDx INEFFECTIVE HEALTH MAINTENANCE NDx, OR INEFFECTIVE HEALTH MANAGEMENT* NDx

Definition: Deficient Knowledge NDx: Absence of cognitive information related to a specific topic, or its acquisition; **Ineffective Health Maintenance NDx:** Inability to identify, manage, and/or seek out help to maintain well-being; **Ineffective Health Management NDx:** Pattern of regulating and integrating into daily living a therapeutic regimen for the treatment of illness and its sequelae that is unsatisfactory for meeting specific health goals.

CLINICAL MANIFESTATIONS

Subjective	**Objective**
Verbal self-report of the problem	Inaccurate follow-through of instructions; inappropriate behaviors

RISK FACTORS

- Denial of disease process
- Cognitive deficiency
- Failure to take action to reduce risk factors

NOC OUTCOMES	NIC INTERVENTIONS
Knowledge: medication; health promotion; disease process; infection control; treatment behavior: illness or injury; compliance behavior; health beliefs: perceived resources; health beliefs: perceived ability to perform; health beliefs: perceived control	

NURSING ASSESSMENT	RATIONALE
Assess client readiness and ability to learn. Assess meaning of illness to client.	*Early recognition of readiness to learn and meaning of illness to client allows for implementation of the appropriate teaching interventions.*

THERAPEUTIC INTERVENTIONS	RATIONALE

Desired Outcome: The client will identify ways to maintain respiratory health and ways to prevent the spread of TB to others.

Dependent/Collaborative Actions
Instruct client in ways to maintain respiratory health:

- Maintain overall general good health (e.g., reduce stress, eat a well-balanced diet, obtain adequate rest).
- Stop smoking.
- Avoid exposure to respiratory irritants such as smoke, dust, aerosol sprays, paint fumes, and solvents; wear a mask or scarf over nose and mouth if exposure to high levels of these irritants is unavoidable.
- Remain indoors as much as possible when air pollution levels are high.

Good general health supports the individual's ability to fight off infection.
The irritants in smoke and respiratory irritants increase mucus production, impair ciliary function, and can cause inflammation and damage to the bronchial and alveolar walls; the carbon monoxide decreases oxygen availability

Air pollution in high levels is harmful to persons with existing lung disease.
Exposure to extreme hot and cold air may cause bronchoconstriction, allowing less air into and out of the lungs and decreasing oxygen/CO_2 exchange.

- Avoid prolonged close contact with persons who have active TB or any other respiratory infection.
- Avoid crowds and poorly ventilated areas.
- Drink at least 10 glasses of liquid per day unless contraindicated.

Leads to increased potential for an infection and the spread of TB

Increased fluid intake is necessary with many of the medications used in the treatment of TB to maintain adequate hydration. Increased fluid intake is important to thin or liquefy secretions making them easier to expectorate.

- Receive immunizations against influenza and pneumococcal pneumonia.

Immunizations help prevent further respiratory disease.

Educate the patient on the disease process and treatment of TB:

- Explain TB in terms the client can understand; stress that TB is an infectious disease and that adherence to the treatment plan is necessary in order to prevent transmission to others, complications, and reactivation of the disease.
- Explain that active TB can be treated successfully but only if the client adheres to the prescribed multiple drug therapy.
- Provide written instructions about and encourage the client to participate in the treatment plan (e.g., protecting others from the infection, adhering to medication regimen, participating in respiratory care treatments).
- Provide client with written instructions about disease transmission, signs and symptoms to report, medication therapy, and follow-up appointments.

Understanding of the disease and its treatment plan provides the patient with a sense of control and makes it more likely that the patient will be adherent to the treatment regimen.

The client must understand that TB can be successfully treated only with a multiple drug regimen.
Written instructions allow the client to refer to them as needed. The instructions should include all information needed to understand disease processes and treatment.

Educate the patient on ways to prevent the spread of TB to others:

- Cover nose and mouth with a tissue when coughing, sneezing, and laughing.
- Refrain from spitting or do so into a tissue.
- Practice good hand hygiene (e.g., wash hands using an antimicrobial soap, use an alcohol-base hand rub), especially after placing hands over mouth or nose and handling soiled tissues.
- Dispose of soiled tissues properly (e.g., place in paper or plastic bag, flush down toilet).
- Avoid close contact with people who are at high risk for infection (e.g., those who are very young or elderly, those with HIV infection); wear a mask if close contact is unavoidable.
- Adhere strictly to the prescribed medication regimen for the treatment of TB.

These actions are important to prevent the spread of TB. TB is an airborne bacteria and is spread through close contact with someone who is infected.

Appropriate hand washing and care of soiled tissues helps prevent spread of infection.
Individuals who are at high risk for infection are at high risk for contracting TB.
Medications require an adequate blood level to be effective

THERAPEUTIC INTERVENTIONS	RATIONALE
• Inform clients that they will continue to be infectious until three consecutive sputum cultures show absence of the tubercle bacilli (this usually occurs after a couple of weeks of taking the antitubercular/antimicrobial agents) and that in order to not become infectious again, they must continue with the medication regimen for the prescribed length of time (usually 6–18 months).	*Clients need to know that they will be infectious for an extended period even though they continue taking medications. The longer the medication regimen, the greater the incidence of nonadherence.*

THERAPEUTIC INTERVENTIONS	RATIONALE

Desired Outcome: The client will verbalize an understanding of medications ordered including rationale, food and drug interactions, side effects, and importance of taking as prescribed.

Dependent/Collaborative Actions	
Explain the rationale for, side effects of, and importance of taking medications prescribed, as well as food and drug interactions, and drugs to manage side effects.	*Knowledge of the medication regimen and the impact of these medications on the body, as well as how the medication regimen can be incorporated into the client's lifestyle, allows the client some mechanism of control of his/her disease and the ability to have an active part in treatment and care.*
Examples of TB drugs: isoniazid, rifampin, ethambutol, pyrazinamide, and streptomycin	*Treatment failures often result from clients not taking their medications correctly or prematurely stopping their medications. Clients must understand that they increase their chance of developing a "drug-resistant" strain of TB if the medications are not taken as prescribed.*
Assist client to identify ways the medication regimen can be incorporated into the client's lifestyle.	
Assist client to develop a method to promote adherence to the medication schedule (e.g., filling a pill box or empty egg carton with the medications that need to be taken that day/week, setting a timer or alarm as a reminder of when to take medications, using a checklist to document when each medication is due and taken).	
Remind client of the consequences of not adhering to the multiple drug regimen.	*Nonadherence to the multiple drug regimen may cause spread of TB from lungs to other parts of the body, development of a strain of TB that will be very difficult to treat, and transmission of TB to others.*
Reinforce the need to consult a physician before discontinuing any medication or taking additional prescription and nonprescription medications.	*There may be drug-drug interactions that occur when taking TB prescriptions. A physician should approve of any medications taken to alleviate potential negative effects.*
Instruct client to take all medications as often as prescribed and avoid skipping doses or altering the prescribed dose; if a dose is missed, instruct client to take it as soon as remembered unless it is almost time for the next dose of the same medication.	*Proper treatment occurs when medications are taken as prescribed. If the clients are unable to take medications as prescribed, it may prolong treatment time and lead to exacerbation of the disease.*
Instruct client to consult health care provider if considering becoming pregnant, if pregnancy occurs, and if breastfeeding.	*Some of the medications used to treat TB are contraindicated in pregnancy and if breastfeeding.*

THERAPEUTIC INTERVENTIONS	RATIONALE

Desired Outcome: The client will state signs and symptoms to report to the health care provider.

Continued...

THERAPEUTIC INTERVENTIONS	RATIONALE

Dependent/Collaborative Actions

Instruct client to report the following:

- Persistent or recurrent loss of appetite, nausea, weakness, fatigue, or weight loss
- Fever, chills, continued or increased night sweats
- Difficulty breathing, continued or increased cough, or chest pain
- Unusual color, amount, and odor of vaginal secretions; white patches or ulcerated areas in mouth
- Stiff neck and headache
- Hoarseness; persistent sore throat
- Bone pain; swollen, red, painful joints
- Swollen lymph nodes

These signs and symptoms may indicate a superinfection or spread of infection to another site, ineffectiveness of medications, inadequate nutrition, and/or adverse effects of medication regimen.

THERAPEUTIC INTERVENTIONS	RATIONALE

Desired Outcome: The client, in collaboration with the nurse, will develop a plan for adhering to recommended follow-up care, including future appointments with health care providers.

Dependent/Collaborative Actions

Reinforce the importance of keeping appointments for follow-up tests (e.g., blood work, hearing tests, sputum cultures, chest radiographs) and physical examinations to determine the effectiveness of the medication regimen and assess for side effects such as liver and kidney damage.

Monitoring of TB is critical in maintaining client's health and the effectiveness of the medication regimen.

Provide information about and encourage utilization of community resources and social services that can assist the client to comply with the medication regimen or to provide financial support if needed (e.g., home health agencies, local Department of Health and Human Services, directly observed therapy [DOT] programs, local chapter of the American Lung Association, support groups).

Provide for continuum of care and can help client's adherence with the medication regimen and possibly financial assistance for medications

Include significant others in explanations and teaching sessions and encourage their support.

Involvement of the client's significant others contributes to treatment regimen adherence and may help with medication administration, if needed.

ADDITIONAL NURSING DIAGNOSES

FEAR NDx/ANXIETY NDx

Related to unfamiliar environment, separation from significant others, financial concerns, and fear of transmitting disease to others

RISK FOR DEFICIENT FLUID VOLUME NDx

Related to decreased oral fluid intake and excessive fluid loss (can occur with night sweats and profuse diaphoresis)

ACUTE PAIN: CHEST NDx

Related to extension of the inflammatory/infectious process to the pleura and muscle strain (can result from excessive coughing)

DISTURBED SLEEP PATTERN NDx

Related to an unfamiliar environment, night sweats, persistent coughing, anxiety, and frequent assessments and treatments

The Client With Alterations in Cardiovascular Function

ABDOMINAL AORTIC ANEURYSM

An abdominal aortic aneurysm (AAA) is an abnormal dilation of the wall of the abdominal aorta. The aneurysm usually develops in the segment of the vessel that is between the renal arteries and the iliac branches of the aorta. The most common cause of an AAA is atherosclerosis. The plaque that forms on the wall of the artery causes degenerative changes in the medial layer of the vessel. These changes lead to loss of elasticity, weakening, and eventual dilation of the affected segment. Additional factors that may play a role in the development of an AAA include inflammation (arteritis), trauma, infection, congenital abnormalities of the vessel, connective tissue disorders that cause vessel wall weakness, tobacco use, and high blood pressure. AAAs also may be hereditary with the likelihood of developing a AAA 12 times greater in individuals with a first-degree relative with the condition.

Most AAAs are asymptomatic and are discovered during a routine physical examination (signs include palpation of a pulsatile mass in the abdomen and/or auscultation of a bruit over the abdominal aorta) or during a review of x-ray results of the abdomen or lower spine. The presence of symptoms such as mild to severe abdominal, lumbar, or flank pain and/or lower extremity arterial insufficiency is usually indicative of a large aneurysm that is exerting pressure on surrounding tissues or an aneurysm that is leaking.

Surgical repair of an aneurysm is usually performed if the aneurysm is growing rapidly and/or reaches a size of 5 to 6 cm or larger, or if the client experiences symptoms. Repair of an AAA can be accomplished in one of two ways: open repair through a large incision in the abdomen followed by insertion of a synthetic graft to replace or support the weakened vessel, or by endovascular repair, a minimally invasive option through a small incision in the groin threading a stent and graft up to the aneurysm for support.

This care plan focuses on the adult client hospitalized for open surgical repair of an AAA. Much of the postoperative information is applicable to clients receiving follow-up care in an extended care facility or home setting.

OUTCOME DISCHARGE CRITERIA

The client will:
1. Tolerate prescribed diet
2. Tolerate expected level of activity
3. Have surgical pain controlled
4. Have clear, audible breath sounds throughout lungs
5. Have evidence of normal healing of surgical wounds
6. Have no signs and symptoms of postoperative complications
7. Identify ways to prevent or slow the progression of atherosclerosis
8. State signs and symptoms to report to the health care provider
9. Develop a plan for adhering to recommended follow-up care including future appointments with health care provider, medications prescribed, activity level, and wound care

PREOPERATIVE: USE IN CONJUNCTION WITH THE STANDARDIZED PREOPERATIVE CARE PLAN

Related Preoperative Nursing/Collaborative Diagnoses **ANXIETY** NDx **/FEAR** NDx

Definition: **Anxiety NDx:** Vague, uneasy feeling of discomfort or dread accompanied by an autonomic response (the source is often nonspecific or unknown to the individual); a feeling of apprehension caused by anticipation of danger. It is an alerting sign that warns of impending danger and enables the individual to take measures to deal with that threat. **Fear NDx:** Response to perceived threat that is consciously recognized as a danger.

Related to:
- Unfamiliar environment and separation from significant others
- Lack of understanding of diagnostic tests, surgical procedure, and postoperative care
- Anticipated loss of control associated with effects of anesthesia risk of disease if blood transfusions are necessary
- Anticipated postoperative discomfort and potential change in sexual functioning
- Possibility of death

NDx = NANDA Diagnosis   **D** = Delegatable Action   ● = UAP   ✦ = LVN/LPN   ⊝▶ = Go to ⊝volve for animation

POSTOPERATIVE NURSING/COLLABORATIVE DIAGNOSIS*

| Nursing/Collaborative Diagnosis | **RISK FOR IMBALANCED FLUID VOLUME** NDx **AND RISK FOR ELECTROLYTE IMBALANCE** NDx |

Definition: Risk for Imbalanced Fluid Volume NDx: Susceptible to a decrease, increase, or rapid shift from one to the other of intravascular, interstitial and/or intracellular fluid, which may compromise health. This refers to body fluid loss, gain, or both; **Risk for Electrolyte Imbalance NDx:** Susceptible to changes in serum electrolyte levels, which may compromise health.

Related to:
- **Third-spacing of fluid** related to:
  - Increased capillary permeability in surgical area associated with the inflammation that occurs after extensive dissection of tissue during major abdominal surgery
  - Increased vascular hydrostatic pressure associated with excess fluid volume if present
  - Hypoalbuminemia associated with the escape of proteins from the vascular space into the peritoneum (a result of increased capillary permeability in the surgical area)
- **Excess fluid volume NDx** related to:
  - Vigorous fluid replacement
  - Fluid retention associated with increased secretion of antidiuretic hormone (ADH; output of ADH is stimulated by trauma, pain, and anesthetic agents) and/or renal insufficiency (can occur if there is inadequate blood flow to the kidneys during or after surgery)
  - Reabsorption of third-space fluid (occurs about the third postoperative day)
- **Deficient fluid volume NDx** related to restricted oral fluid intake before, during, and after surgery; blood loss; and loss of fluid associated with nasogastric tube drainage
- **Hypokalemia, hypochloremia, and metabolic alkalosis** related to loss of electrolytes and hydrochloric acid associated with nasogastric tube drainage

CLINICAL MANIFESTATIONS

Subjective	Objective
Excessive fluid volume: Not applicable	**Excessive fluid volume:** Weight gain of 2% or greater in a short period; elevated B/P (B/P may not be elevated if cardiac output is poor or fluid has shifted out of the vascular space); presence of an S_3 heart sound; intake greater than output; change in mental status; crackles (rales); dyspnea, orthopnea; edema, distended neck veins; elevated central venous pressure (CVP) (use internal jugular vein pulsation method to estimate CVP if monitoring device is not present)
Deficient fluid volume: Verbal self-report of thirst	**Deficient fluid volume:** Hypotension; tachycardia; decreased urine output; tenting skin turgor; dry mucous membranes; thick, tenacious pulmonary secretions
Hypokalemia: Verbal self-report of muscular weakness, leg cramps; paresthesia; palpitations	**Hypokalemia:** Decreased or absent deep tendon reflexes; anorexia; nausea; vomiting; rhabdomyolysis; orthostatic hypotension; ventricular arrhythmias; cardiac arrest
Hypochloremia: Verbal self-report of muscle cramps, weakness, and/or twitching; irritability	**Hypochloremia:** Tetany; hyperactive deep tendon reflexes; arrhythmias; seizures, coma
Metabolic alkalosis: Verbal self-report of muscle cramps, weakness, and/or twitching; irritability; complaints of numbness and tingling of fingers, nose, and/or mouth	**Metabolic alkalosis:** Apathy; confusion; slow, shallow respirations; hyperactive reflexes; seizures; stupor; anorexia; nausea; vomiting

*Use in conjunction with the Standardized Postoperative Care Plan.

RISK FACTORS

* Aneurysm rupture resulting in hypovolemic shock
* Excessive volume replacement during resuscitation
* Excessive electrolyte loss through nasogastric drainage

DESIRED OUTCOMES

The client will experience resolution of third-spacing as evidenced by:
a. Absence of ascites
b. B/P and pulse rate within normal range for client and stable with position changes

The client will not experience excess fluid volume as evidenced by:
a. Stable B/P
b. Absence of an S_3 heart sound
c. Balanced intake and output
d. Normal breath sounds

The client will experience fluid and electrolyte balance as evidenced by:
a. B/P and pulse rate within normal range for client and stable with position change
b. Balanced intake and output within 48 hrs after surgery
c. Absence of cardiac dysrhythmias, muscle weakness, paresthesias, twitching, spasms, and dizziness
d. Blood urea nitrogen (BUN), serum electrolytes, and arterial blood gas values within normal range

NURSING OUTCOMES INTERVENTIONS (NOC)

Fluid balance; fluid overload severity; electrolyte and acid-base balance

NURSING INTERVENTIONS CLASSIFICATIONS (NIC)

Fluid monitoring; fluid/electrolyte management; electrolyte monitoring; acid-base management

NURSING ASSESSMENT	RATIONALE
Assess for and report signs and symptoms of third-spacing: • Ascites (e.g., increase in abdominal girth, dull percussion note over abdomen with finding of shifting dullness) • Evidence of vascular depletion (e.g., postural hypotension; weak, rapid pulse).	*Early recognition of signs and symptoms of third-spacing allows for prompt intervention.*
Monitor serum albumin levels. Report below-normal levels.	*Low serum albumin levels result in fluid shifting out of vascular space because albumin normally maintains plasma colloid osmotic pressure.*
Monitor serum electrolyte values. Report abnormal values.	*Early recognition of signs of electrolyte imbalances allows for prompt intervention.*
Assess quantity of nasogastric tube drainage.	*Excessive nasogastric tube drainage can lead to hypokalemia, hypochloremia, and metabolic alkalosis.*

THERAPEUTIC INTERVENTIONS	RATIONALE
Dependent/Collaborative Actions Implement measures to prevent further third-spacing of fluid/fluid volume overload: • Administer fluid replacement judiciously. • Maintain fluid restrictions as ordered.	*Actions help to reduce the risk of fluid volume overload.*
• If client is receiving intravenous fluids that contain sizeable amounts of sodium (e.g., 0.9% sodium chloride [NaCl] or lactated Ringer's), consult the physician about a change in solution or a decrease in the rate of infusion.	*Actions help to reduce the risk of third-spacing and electrolyte imbalances.*
• Administer albumin infusions if ordered.	*Administration of albumin helps to increase colloid osmotic pressure, promoting mobilization of fluid back into the vascular space.*
• Administer diuretics if ordered. **D** ✦	*Diuretics help to increase excretion of water.* *Diuretics should only be administered if signs and symptoms of fluid volume overload are evident.*

NDx = NANDA Diagnosis   **D** = Delegatable Action   ● = UAP   ✦ = LVN/LPN   ⊜▶ = Go to ⊜volve for animation

Continued...

THERAPEUTIC INTERVENTIONS	RATIONALE
Implement measures to prevent or treat deficient fluid volume, hypokalemia, hypochloremia, and metabolic alkalosis: • Administer fluid and electrolytes as ordered. • Carefully measure all drainage (e.g., wound, nasogastric) and administer fluid replacement as ordered. **D** ✦	
Consult physician if signs and symptoms of third-spacing, fluid volume deficit, fluid volume overload, or electrolyte imbalances persist or worsen.	*Consulting the appropriate health care provider allows for modification of the treatment plan.*

Nursing Diagnosis **RISK FOR SHOCK** NDx

Definition: Susceptible to an inadequate blood flow to the body's tissues that may lead to life-threatening cellular dysfunction, which may compromise health.

Related to:
• Hypovolemia associated with blood loss during surgery
• Third-space fluid shift
• Hemorrhage (can occur as a result of inadequate wound closure and/or stress on and subsequent leakage or rupture of anastomotic sites)

CLINICAL MANIFESTATIONS

Subjective	Objective
Verbal self-report of anxiety; confusion; agitation	Tachypnea; hypotension; tachycardia; decreased urine output; pallor; cool, clammy skin, observable bleeding

RISK FACTOR	DESIRED OUTCOMES
• Aneurysm rupture • Coagulopathy • Inadequate volume replacement during surgical procedure	The client will not develop hypovolemic shock as evidenced by: a. Usual mental status b. Stable vital signs c. Skin warm and usual color d. Palpable peripheral pulses e. Urine output at least 30 mL/h f. Absence of bleeding

NOC OUTCOMES	NIC INTERVENTIONS
Shock severity: hypovolemic; fluid balance; fluid overload severity; electrolyte and acid-base balance; vital signs	Shock prevention; shock management: volume; electrolyte management; fluid/electrolyte management; fluid monitoring; acid-base management; vital sign monitoring

NURSING ASSESSMENT	RATIONALE
Assess for and report signs and symptoms of leakage at anastomotic sites: • New or expanding hematoma at incision site and/or ecchymosis of flank or perineal area • Increased abdominal girth (can also occur with third-spacing) • New or increased reports of lumbar, flank, abdominal, pelvic, or groin pain • Increasing feeling of abdominal and/or gastric fullness unrelated to oral intake • Diminishing or absent peripheral pulses • Decreased motor or sensory function in lower extremities • Decreasing B/P, increasing pulse rate.	*Early recognition of signs and symptoms of hypovolemic shock allows for prompt intervention.*

NURSING ASSESSMENT	**RATIONALE**

Assess for and report signs and symptoms of hypovolemic shock:
- Restlessness, agitation, changes in mental status
- Significant decrease in B/P
- Postural hypotension
- Rapid, weak pulse
- Rapid respirations
- Cool skin
- Pallor, cyanosis
- Diminished or absent peripheral pulses
- Urine output less than 30 mL/h

Monitor red blood cell (RBC) count, hematocrit (Hct), and hemoglobin (Hgb) values for abnormal trends.

While decreasing values may be indicative of hemorrhage, lab value trends should be evaluated in light of overall fluid status because fluid volume overload may dilute actual Hgb values.

Monitor serum electrolyte values for abnormal trends.

Decreased perfusion that occurs with shock can contribute to abnormal serum electrolyte values which may further compromise the health status of the client.

THERAPEUTIC INTERVENTIONS	**RATIONALE**

Independent Actions
- Maintain accurate intake and output (I/O) record:
  - Oral intake
  - Enteral intake
  - IV intake (e.g., fluids/antibiotics)
  - Urine output
  - Drain output (e.g., NG tube)
- Maintain large bore IV access—consider more than one site as available.
- Perform actions to reduce stress on and separation of anastomotic sites: **D** ✦
  - Instruct client to avoid positions that compromise peripheral blood flow (use of knee gatch, crossing legs).
  - Instruct client to avoid activities that create a Valsalva response (e.g., straining to have a bowel movement, holding breath while moving up in bed).
  - Instruct client to avoid vigorous coughing.

Accurate I/O records are necessary to direct appropriate fluid management.

Appropriate IV access is necessary in clients at risk for shock in the event that rapid fluid resuscitation becomes necessary.

Stress on anastomotic sites increases the risk for disruption of suture lines, which may lead to hemorrhage and/or hypovolemic shock due to blood loss.

THERAPEUTIC INTERVENTIONS	**RATIONALE**

Dependent/Collaborative Actions
Implement measures to prevent hypovolemic shock:
- Perform actions to prevent or treat hypovolemia:
  - If bleeding occurs, apply firm pressure to area if possible.
  - Administer blood and/or volume expanders (colloids/crystalloids) as ordered.
  - Provide maximum fluid intake allowed.
  - Implement measures to reduce the accumulation of gas and fluid in the gastrointestinal tract (e.g., insert nasogastric tube).

  - Administer fluid replacement therapy judiciously.
  - Maintain fluid restrictions if ordered.
  - Administer antihypertensives if ordered. **D** ✦

Blood replaces loss of cells, volume expanders maintain vascular fluid volume.

Interstitial fluid accumulation in the gastrointestinal tract along with excessive gas accumulation can result in excessive stress on anastomotic sites, increasing the risk of disruption of suture lines and subsequent hemorrhage.

Interstitial fluid accumulation in the gastrointestinal tract can lead to excessive stress on anastomotic sites, increasing the risk of disruption of suture lines and subsequent hemorrhage.

Elevated B/P must be reduced to a level that does not stress vascular anastomotic sites. Medications must be administered to keep a client's B/P within an acceptable range, especially within the immediate postoperative period.

NDx = NANDA Diagnosis **D** = Delegatable Action ● = UAP ✦ = LVN/LPN ⊜▶ = Go to ℯvolve for animation

Continued...

THERAPEUTIC INTERVENTIONS	RATIONALE
If signs and symptoms of hypovolemic shock occur: • Place client flat in bed unless contraindicated. • Monitor vital signs frequently. • Administer oxygen as ordered. Prepare client for surgery if signs and symptoms of hypovolemic shock occur, persist, or worsen.	*Surgical exploration will aid in identifying and controlling suspected sources of hemorrhage.*

Nursing Diagnosis   RISK FOR VENOUS THROMBOEMBOLIZATION NDx

Definition: Susceptible to the development of a blood clot in a deep vein, commonly in the thigh, calf, or upper extremity, which can break off and lodge in another vessel, which may compromise health.

Related to: Dislodgment of necrotic debris or clot from surgical site

CLINICAL MANIFESTATIONS

Subjective	Objective
Verbal self-report of sudden, severe pain in affected limb; numbness in affected limb	Diminished or absent pulses in affected limb; pale, cool, mottled extremity Six P's of acute arterial ischemia: pain, pallor, pulselessness, paresthesia, paralysis, poikilothermia

RISK FACTORS

- Virchow's triad: venous stasis, hypercoagulability of blood, endothelial damage at surgical site
- History of previous thromboembolism
- Surgery and total anesthesia time > 90 minutes

DESIRED OUTCOMES

The client will not experience venous thromboembolism as evidenced by:
a. No reports of pain or diminished sensation in lower extremities
b. Palpable peripheral pulses
c. Usual temperature and color of extremities

NURSING ASSESSMENT	RATIONALE
Assess for and report signs and symptoms of lower extremity arterial embolization: • Sudden, severe onset of pain in extremity • Diminishing or absent peripheral pulses (pulses may be absent for a few hours after surgery as a result of vasospasm) • Cool, pale, or mottled extremities.	*Early recognition of signs and symptoms of arterial embolization allows for prompt intervention.*

NOC OUTCOMES

Tissue perfusion: peripheral

NIC INTERVENTIONS

Embolus precautions; embolus care: peripheral

THERAPEUTIC INTERVENTIONS	RATIONALE
Independent Actions • Implement measures to prevent venous thromboembolism. • Assist patient with passive or active range of motion as appropriate. • Encourage flexion and extension of feet and legs at least 10 times per hour. • Change client position every 2 hrs.	*Range of motion exercises, including flexion and extension of the feet and legs, promote reduced venous stasis by promoting venous return to the heart.*

THERAPEUTIC INTERVENTIONS	RATIONALE
• Instruct patient on strategies to prevent venous thrombo-embolism:	
• Refrain from crossing legs and to avoid sitting for long periods with legs dependent.	*Crossing legs and sitting for long periods of time increases venous stasis/pooling of blood in the extremities.*
• Avoid activities that result in the Valsalva maneuver (e.g., straining during bowel movement).	*Valsalva maneuver will change pressures in the body and affect venous blood flow in the system.*

THERAPEUTIC INTERVENTIONS	RATIONALE

Dependent/Collaborative Actions

Implement measures to prevent venous thromboembolism:

- Apply intermittent pneumatic compression device stockings/graduated elastic compression stockings per organizational policy and protocol.
  - Remove stockings for 15 to 20 minutes every 8 hrs or per organizational policy and protocol.

Application of intermittent pneumatic compression stockings and/or graduated elastic stockings promotes the return of blood to the heart and prevents the pooling of blood in the legs which increases the risk of clot formation.

Encourage early mobilization or ambulate as tolerated as ordered by physician.

Early mobilization improves venous return from the lower extremities, reducing the risk of thromboembolism.

If signs and symptoms of lower extremity arterial embolization occur:

- Maintain client on bed rest. **D** ✦
- Prepare client for the following if planned:
  - Diagnostic studies (e.g., Doppler ultrasound, arteriography)
  - Embolectomy

In order to prevent dislodgment of existing thrombi.
To restore blood flow, an embolus should be removed as soon as possible after identification/location of the obstruction.

Nursing Diagnosis # RISK FOR DECREASED CARDIAC OUTPUT NDx

Definition: Susceptible to inadequate blood pumped by the heart to meet metabolic demands of the body, which may compromise health.

Related to: Altered nodal function and myocardial conductivity associated with:
- Alteration in heart rate
- Alteration in heart rhythm

Alteration in myocardial contractility due to diminished myocardial blood flow/damage

CLINICAL MANIFESTATIONS

Subjective	Objective
Verbal self-report of chest pain and/or shortness of breath; verbalization of syncope, dizziness, palpitations; and/or abdominal pain	Irregular apical pulse; pulse rate less than 60 or greater than 100 beats/min; electrocardiogram (ECG) tracing abnormalities; ischemic changes on ECG tracing (e.g., dysrhythmias, elevated or depressed T-wave); hypotension/hypertension; decreased or absent urine output; diminished peripheral pulses, cool clammy skin; auscultated rales/crackles in lung fields; decreased oxygen saturation; distended neck veins

RISK FACTORS

- Stress associated with general anesthesia
- Preexisting cardiovascular disease
- Electrolyte imbalances

DESIRED OUTCOMES

The client will maintain normal cardiac output as evidenced by:
a. Regular apical pulse at 60 to 100 beats/min
b. Normal sinus rhythm or return to client's baseline rhythm
c. Blood pressure within client's normal range
d. Normal respiratory rate/clear breath sounds
e. Oxygen saturation within client's baseline
f. Balanced fluid intake/output
g. Presence of bowel sounds/bowel movements

NDx = NANDA Diagnosis **D** = Delegatable Action ● = UAP ✦ = LVN/LPN ⊝▶ = Go to ⊝volve for animation

NURSING ASSESSMENT	RATIONALE
Assess for and report signs and symptoms of decreased cardiac perfusion: • Alterations in heart rate/rhythm • Irregular apical pulse • Pulse rate less than 60 or greater than 100 beats/min • Abnormal rhythms, or configurations on ECG • Verbalization of chest pain Assess for signs and symptoms of decreased cardiac output • Decreased blood pressure below client's baseline • Verbalization of shortness of breath • Auscultation of crackles in lungs • Decreased oxygen saturation • Decreased urine output • Abdominal pain/absence of bowel sounds • Decreased strength and quality of peripheral pulses • Cool, clammy skin Assess baseline vital signs for symptoms of decreased cardiac output: • Increased or decreased heart rate • Decreased blood pressure • Decreased oxygen saturation Assess baseline serum electrolytes, BUN, creatinine, brain natriuretic peptide (BNP), cardiac enzymes for abnormalities that may contribute to alterations in normal cardiac rhythm and cardiac output. Assess baseline radiographic studies (e.g., CXR) for abnormalities indicating alterations in normal cardiac output.	*Early recognition of signs and symptoms of decreased cardiac output allows for prompt intervention.*

NOC OUTCOMES	NIC INTERVENTIONS
Cardiac pump effectiveness; cardiopulmonary status; gastrointestinal function; tissue perfusion abdominal organs; tissue perfusion cardiac; tissue perfusion cellular	Cardiac care acute; dysrhythmia management; fluid/electrolyte management; hypotension management; hypovolemia management

THERAPEUTIC INTERVENTIONS	RATIONALE
Independent Actions • Perform actions to maintain an adequate respiratory status. • Assist client in performing incentive spirometry Q2h. • Assist client in turning, coughing, and deep breathing Q2h until ambulating.	*Actions help to maintain adequate myocardial tissue oxygenation.*

• Perform actions to decrease stimulation of the sympathetic nervous system:
  • Implement measures to reduce pain and anxiety.
  • Perform relaxation therapy if appropriate (e.g., music therapy, meditation).
  • Implement measures to keep client from getting cold.
	Sympathetic stimulation increases the heart rate and causes vasoconstriction, both of which increase cardiac workload and decrease oxygen availability to the myocardium.

• Ensure activity level does not compromise cardiac output or provoke cardiac events. • Provide frequent rest periods/avoid fatigue.	*Ensures myocardial oxygen demand does not exceed supply.*

THERAPEUTIC INTERVENTIONS	RATIONALE

Dependent/Collaborative Actions
• Perform actions to prevent or treat hypokalemia:
  • Prevent nausea and vomiting.
  • Administer fluid and electrolyte replacements as ordered.
	Electrolyte imbalances, particularly hypokalemia and hypocalcemia, can contribute to cardiac dysrhythmias.

THERAPEUTIC INTERVENTIONS	RATIONALE

• Perform actions to prevent or treat hypotension:
  • Consult physician before giving negative inotropic agents, diuretics, and vasodilating agents if systolic B/P is below 90 to 100 mm Hg.
  • Administer opioid analgesics judiciously, being alert to the synergistic effect of the narcotic ordered and the anesthetic that was used during surgery.
  • Gradually bring client's body temperature to normal if hypothermic.
  • Administer sympathomimetics (e.g., dopamine) if ordered.
	Actions help to ensure adequate vascular volume, tissue perfusion, and delivery of oxygen to the myocardial tissue.
	
	Rapid warming results in vasodilation, which may reduce B/P and tissue perfusion.
	Sympathomimetics mimic the action of the sympathetic nervous system, causing vasoconstriction, which elevates B/P.

If cardiac dysrhythmias occur: • Administer antidysrhythmics as ordered. • Restrict client's activity based on his/her tolerance and severity of the dysrhythmia. • Maintain oxygen therapy as ordered. • Assess cardiovascular status frequently and report signs and symptoms of inadequate tissue perfusion (e.g., decrease in B/P, cool skin, cyanosis, diminished peripheral pulses, urine output less than 30 mL/h, restlessness and agitation, shortness of breath). • Have emergency cart readily available for cardioversion, defibrillation, or cardiopulmonary resuscitation (CPR). • Consult physician if signs and symptoms of decreased cardiac output persist.	*Cardiac dysrhythmias may deteriorate and become life-threatening. Life-threatening dysrhythmias or those that render the client unstable are treated with electrical therapy.* *Allows for modification of the treatment plan.*

DISCHARGE TEACHING/CONTINUED CARE

Nursing Diagnosis **DEFICIENT KNOWLEDGE NDx; INEFFECTIVE HEALTH MAINTENANCE NDx; OR INEFFECTIVE HEALTH MANAGEMENT* NDx**

Definition: **Deficient Knowledge NDx:** Absence of cognitive information related to a specific topic, or its acquisition; **Ineffective Health Maintenance NDx:** Inability to identify, manage, and/or seek out help to maintain well-being; **Ineffective Health Management NDx:** Pattern of regulating and integrating into daily living a therapeutic regimen for the treatment of illness and its sequelae that is unsatisfactory for meeting specific health goals.

CLINICAL MANIFESTATIONS

Subjective	Objective
Verbal self-report of the problem	Inaccurate follow-through of instructions; inappropriate behaviors

RISK FACTORS
• Denial of disease process
• Cognitive deficiency
• Failure to take action to reduce risk factors

NOC OUTCOMES	NIC INTERVENTIONS
Knowledge: treatment regimen; cardiac disease management	Health system guidance; teaching: individual; teaching: disease process; teaching: prescribed diet

*The nurse should select the diagnosis that is most appropriate for the client's discharge teaching needs.

NURSING ASSESSMENT	RATIONALE
Assess client's readiness and ability to learn. Assess meaning of illness to client.	*Early recognition of readiness to learn and meaning of illness to client allows for implementation of the appropriate teaching interventions.*

THERAPEUTIC INTERVENTIONS	RATIONALE

Desired Outcome: The client will identify ways to prevent or slow the progression of atherosclerosis.

Independent Actions

Inform the client that certain modifiable factors such as elevated serum lipid levels, a sedentary lifestyle, smoking, and hypertension have been shown to increase the risk of atherosclerosis.	*After vascular surgery, clients should be educated as to health promotion activities that slow the progression of atherosclerosis. Clients should be encouraged to control B/P, increase physical activity, stop smoking, and maintain normal body weight and serum lipid levels.*
Assist client to identify changes in lifestyle that could reduce the risk for atherosclerosis: • Dietary modifications • Smoking cessation • Physical exercise on a regular basis	*Appropriate modifications of diet, exercise, and smoking cessation can modify the progression of coronary artery disease (CAD).*
Provide instructions on ways the client can reduce intake of saturated fat and cholesterol: • Reduce intake of meat fat (e.g., trim visible fat off meat; replace fatty meats such as fatty cuts of steak, hamburger, and processed meats with leaner products). • Reduce intake of milk fat (e.g., avoid dairy products containing more than 1% fat). • Reduce intake of *trans* fats (e.g., avoid stick margarine and shortening and foods such as commercial baked goods that are prepared with these products). • Use vegetable oil rather than coconut or palm oil in cooking and food preparation. • Use cooking methods such as steaming, baking, broiling, poaching, microwaving, and grilling rather than frying. • Restrict intake of eggs (recommendations about the number of whole eggs allowed per week vary depending on the client's lipid levels).	*Decreasing intake of saturated fat and cholesterol and increasing complex carbohydrates can reduce the risk of CAD by lowering low-density lipoprotein (LDL) cholesterol.*
Instruct client to take lipid-lowering agents (e.g., HMG-CoA [3-hydroxy-3-methylglutaryl-coenzyme A] reductase inhibitors ["statins"], ezetimibe, gemfibrozil, niacin) as prescribed.	*Lipid-lowering agents inhibit the synthesis of cholesterol in the liver. The result of this inhibition is an increase in hepatic LDL receptors. This results in the liver being able to remove more LDLs from the blood.*

THERAPEUTIC INTERVENTIONS	RATIONALE

Desired Outcome: The client will state signs and symptoms to report to the health care provider.

Independent Actions

Instruct client to report these additional signs and symptoms: • Sudden or gradual increase in lower back, flank, groin, or abdominal pain • Chest pain • Coolness, pallor, or blueness of lower extremities • Increased weakness and fatigue • Decreased urine output • Bloody or persistent diarrhea • Increased bruising of incision site, flank area, or perineum • Impotence	*Additional signs and symptoms indicate internal bleeding. Prompt treatment for the client exhibiting signs and symptoms of internal bleeding from graft site reduces the risk of life-threatening complications.*

THERAPEUTIC INTERVENTIONS	**RATIONALE**

Desired Outcome: The client, in collaboration with the nurse, will develop a plan for adhering to recommended follow-up care including future appointments with health care provider, medications prescribed, activity level, and wound care.

Independent Actions
Reinforce the physician's instructions regarding:
- Importance of scheduling adequate rest periods
- Ways to prevent constipation and subsequent straining to have a bowel movement (e.g., drink at least 10 glasses of liquid per day unless contraindicated, increase intake of foods high in fiber, take stool softeners if necessary)
- The need to avoid sexual intercourse, isometric exercise/activity (e.g., lifting objects over 10 lb, pushing heavy objects), and strenuous exercise for specified length of time (usually 4–12 weeks depending on the activity)
- The need to take prophylactic antimicrobials before any dental work or invasive procedure
- Collaborate with the client to develop a plan for success following discharge from the acute care facility.

The nurse should reinforce the need to follow up with the physician/surgeon provider as instructed to ensure adherence to all aspects of the treatment plan.

Some physicians recommend this for the first 6–12 months after surgical placement of a synthetic graft.

ADDITIONAL NURSING DIAGNOSIS

SEXUAL DYSFUNCTION

Related to:
- Decreased libido associated with operative site discomfort and fear of surgical site bleeding
- Impotence associated with prolonged reduction in blood flow in the mesenteric or internal iliac arteries (can occur

as a result of prolonged aortic clamp time during surgery, persistent hypovolemia, embolization, or graft occlusion) and/or nerve damage (can occur during surgery)

RELATED CARE PLANS

Standardized Preoperative Care Plan
Standardized Postoperative Care Plan

ANGINA PECTORIS

Angina pectoris is transient chest pain or discomfort that is caused by an imbalance between myocardial oxygen supply and demand. The discomfort typically occurs in the retrosternal area; may or may not radiate; and is described as a tight, heavy, squeezing, burning, or choking sensation. The most common cause of angina pectoris is decreased coronary blood supply due to atherosclerosis of a major coronary artery. The atherosclerosis causes narrowing of the vessel lumen and an inability of the vessel to dilate and supply sufficient blood to the myocardium at times when myocardial oxygen needs are increased. Other conditions that can compromise coronary blood flow (e.g., spasm and/or thrombosis of a coronary artery, hypovolemia) and conditions that reduce oxygen availability and/or increase myocardial workload and oxygen demands (e.g., anemia, smoking, exercise, heavy meals, increased altitude, exposure to cold, stress) may precipitate or increase the frequency of angina attacks by widening the gap between oxygen needs and availability.

The two major types of angina are stable angina (angina pectoris) and unstable angina (acute coronary syndrome). Stable angina, the most common type, is usually precipitated by physical exertion or emotional stress, but can be triggered by exposure to very hot or very cold temperatures, heavy meals, or smoking. Stable angina typically lasts a short time (5 minutes or less), may feel like gas or indigestion, may spread to arms, back or other areas, and is relieved by rest and nitroglycerin. Unstable angina is characterized by an increasing frequency and/or severity of attacks that occur with less provocation or at rest. It is considered to be an acute coronary syndrome, which is associated with thrombus formation in a coronary artery. Persons with unstable angina are usually hospitalized and treated with heparin and antiplatelet agents while decisions regarding medical versus surgical treatment are made. A third type of angina is Prinzmetal variant angina. It is less common than stable or unstable angina, almost always occurs at rest usually between midnight and early morning, and is due to severe focal spasm of a coronary artery.

Angina symptoms can differ by gender. Angina symptoms in men are often to due blockages in the coronary arteries referred to as CAD. In women, symptoms are more frequently associated with disease within the very small arteries that branch out from the coronary arteries referred to as microvascular disease (MVD). While angina is most often associated with a heart attack, women are warned that they may experience symptoms not related to angina at all and include unusual fatigue, sweating, and/or shortness of breath, and neck, jaw, or back pain

This care plan focuses on the adult client hospitalized during an episode of chest pain/discomfort suspected to be unstable angina.

OUTCOME/DISCHARGE CRITERIA

The client will:
1. Perform activities of daily living and ambulate without angina
2. Have angina controlled by oral medication
3. Have no signs and symptoms of complications
4. Verbalize a basic understanding of angina pectoris
5. Identify factors that may precipitate angina attacks and ways to control these factors

6. Identify modifiable cardiovascular risk factors and ways to alter these factors
7. Verbalize an understanding of the rationale for and components of a diet designed to lower serum cholesterol and triglyceride levels
8. Demonstrate accuracy in counting pulse
9. Verbalize an understanding of medications ordered including rationale, food and drug interactions, side effects, schedule for taking, and importance of taking as prescribed
10. State signs and symptoms to report to the health care provider
11. Identify community resources that can assist in making necessary lifestyle changes and adjusting to the effects of angina pectoris
12. Develop a plan for adhering to recommended follow-up care including future appointments with health care provider.

Nursing Diagnosis RISK FOR DECREASED CARDIAC OUTPUT NDx

Definition: Susceptible to inadequate blood pumped by the heart to meet metabolic demands of the body, which may compromise health.

Related to: Mechanical and/or electrical dysfunction of the heart associated with severe or prolonged myocardial ischemia

CLINICAL MANIFESTATIONS

Subjective	Objective
Verbal self-report of palpitations; fatigue; shortness of breath/dyspnea; orthopnea; anxiety	Dysrhythmias; ECG changes; altered preload (jugular venous distention [JVD], edema, weight gain, increased CVP, murmurs); altered afterload (cold, clammy skin; cyanosis; prolonged capillary refill time; decreased peripheral pulses); altered contractility (crackles, cough, decreased cardiac output); restlessness

RISK FACTORS
- Altered heart rate
- Altered heart rhythm
- Altered stroke volume

DESIRED OUTCOMES

The client will maintain adequate cardiac output as evidenced by:
a. B/P within client's normal range
b. Apical pulse regular and between 60 and 100 beats/min
c. Absence of S_3, S_4 heart sounds (gallop)
d. Absence of fatigue and weakness
e. Unlabored respirations at 12 to 20 breaths/min
f. Clear, audible breath sounds
g. Usual mental status
h. Absence of dizziness and syncope
i. Palpable peripheral pulses
j. Capillary refill time less than 2 to 3 seconds
k. Urine output of at least 30 mL/h
l. Absence of edema and JVD

NOC OUTCOMES

Circulation status; cardiac pump effectiveness; tissue perfusion: cardiac; peripheral

NIC INTERVENTIONS

Cardiac care: acute; hemodynamic regulation; cardiac risk management; cardiac care: rehabilitative

NURSING ASSESSMENT	RATIONALE
Assess for and report signs and symptoms of decreased cardiac output: • Variations in B/P • Tachycardia • Presence of extra heart sounds (gallop) • Fatigue and weakness • Dyspnea, tachypnea • Crackles (rales) • Restlessness, change in mental status • Dizziness, syncope • Diminished or absent peripheral pulses • Cool extremities • Capillary refill time greater than 2 to 3 seconds • Oliguria • Edema • JVD	*Early recognition of signs and symptoms of decreased cardiac output allows for prompt intervention.*
Monitor and report abnormal chest radiograph, arterial blood gas, or pulse oximetry values.	*Diagnostic tests may demonstrate vascular congestion (pulmonary edema) indicative of decreased cardiac output. Arterial blood gas/pulse oximetry values may indicate hypoxia as cardiac output decreases and pulmonary congestion worsens.*
Monitor and report abnormal ECG readings.	*May demonstrate findings associated with ischemia such as dysrhythmias, ST-segment depression/elevation, or inverted T waves.*
Monitor and report elevated cardiac enzymes (i.e., creatine kinase–MB [CK-MB]; troponin).	*Elevated values may indicate myocardial ischemia/damage. Extensive damage may further decrease cardiac output.*

THERAPEUTIC INTERVENTIONS	RATIONALE

Independent Actions

Implement measures to improve cardiac output: • Maintain a calm, quiet environment, limit the number of visitors, and maintain activity restrictions. **D** ✦	*Actions promote emotional and physical rest and help to reduce cardiac workload.*
Instruct client to avoid activities that create a Valsalva response: • Straining to have a bowel movement • Holding breath while moving up in bed	*Excessive straining can increase cardiac workload.*
Discourage excessive intake of beverages high in caffeine such as coffee, tea, and colas.	*Caffeine is a myocardial stimulant and can increase myocardial oxygen consumption.*
Discourage smoking.	*Nicotine has a cardiostimulatory effect and causes vasoconstriction; the carbon monoxide in smoke reduces oxygen availability.*

Dependent/Collaborative Actions

Maintain oxygen therapy as ordered. **D** ✦	*Oxygen helps to improve oxygenation and reduce damage to the myocardium.*
Administer the following medications if ordered:	*Medications act to improve blood flow to the coronary arteries helping to maintain adequate cardiac output.*
• Nitrates	*Nitrates dilate the coronary and peripheral (primarily venous) blood vessels, thereby improving myocardial blood flow and reducing cardiac workload and myocardial oxygen consumption.*
• Beta-adrenergic blockers	*Beta blockers reduce myocardial oxygen requirements by decreasing the heart rate and force of myocardial contractility.*
• Calcium channel blockers (CCBs)	*CCBs dilate the coronary arteries and also reduce cardiac workload by dilating peripheral vessels.*
• Anticoagulants	*Anticoagulants prevent obstruction of the coronary arteries by thrombosis.*

Continued...

THERAPEUTIC INTERVENTIONS	RATIONALE
Prepare client for percutaneous coronary intervention if planned: • Balloon angioplasty • Atherectomy • Intracoronary stenting • Coronary artery bypass grafting (CABG) Increase activity as allowed and tolerated. **D** ✦	*Providing information to a client about what will occur during a procedure may increase client's participation in the procedure and decrease anxiety.*

Nursing Diagnosis ACUTE PAIN NDx (RADIATING OR NONRADIATING CHEST PAIN/DISCOMFORT)

Definition: Unpleasant sensory and emotional experience associated with actual or potential tissue damage, or described in terms of such damage (International Association for the Study of Pain); sudden or slow onset of any intensity from mild to severe with an anticipated or predictable end, and with a duration of less than 3 months.

Related to: Decreased myocardial oxygenation (an insufficient oxygen supply forces the myocardium to convert to anaerobic metabolism; the end products of anaerobic metabolism act as irritants to myocardial neural receptors)

CLINICAL MANIFESTATIONS

Subjective	Objective
Verbal self-report of chest discomfort or pain over the sternal border, radiating to the neck, jaw, left arm; indigestion	ECG changes (ST-segment depression/elevation); dysrhythmias

RISK FACTORS
• Arteriosclerosis
• Increased oxygen demand
• Decreased oxygen supply
• Hypertension

DESIRED OUTCOMES

The client will experience relief of chest pain/discomfort as evidenced by:
a. Verbalization of the same
b. Relaxed facial expression and body positioning
c. Increased participation in activities
d. Stable vital signs

NOC OUTCOMES

Comfort status; pain control

NIC INTERVENTIONS

Pain management acute; medication administration; analgesic administration

NURSING ASSESSMENT	RATIONALE
Assess for signs and symptoms of pain/discomfort: • Verbalization of pain • Grimacing • Rubbing neck, jaw, or arm • Reluctance to move • Clutching chest • Restlessness • Diaphoresis • Increased B/P • Tachycardia Assess client's perception of the severity of the pain/discomfort using an intensity rating scale. Assess the client's pattern of pain/discomfort (location, quality, onset, duration, precipitating factors, aggravating factors, alleviating factors).	*Early recognition and reporting of signs and symptoms of ischemic chest pain allow for prompt intervention.*

NURSING ASSESSMENT	RATIONALE
Monitor and report abnormal ECG readings.	*May demonstrate findings associated with ischemia such as dysrhythmias, ST-segment depression/elevation, or inverted T waves.*
Monitor and report elevated cardiac enzymes (CK-MB; troponin).	*Elevated values may indicate myocardial ischemia.*

THERAPEUTIC INTERVENTIONS	RATIONALE

Independent Actions

| Provide or assist with nonpharmacological measures for relief of discomfort: **D** ✦ <ul><li>Position change</li><li>Relaxation techniques</li><li>Restful environment</li></ul> | *Activities that promote rest help to reduce myocardial oxygen consumption.* |

Dependent/Collaborative Actions

Administer nitroglycerin as ordered. Maintain oxygen therapy as ordered. **D** ✦	*Nitrates dilate the coronary and peripheral (primarily venous) blood vessels, thereby improving myocardial blood flow and reducing cardiac workload and myocardial oxygen consumption.*
Administer a opioid analgesic (e.g., morphine sulfate) as ordered if pain/discomfort is unrelieved by rest and nitroglycerin within 15 to 20 minutes (narcotic analgesics are usually administered intravenously).	*Narcotic analgesics help to alleviate pain and anxiety, lower B/P, and decrease myocardial oxygen consumption.*
Consult physician if pain/discomfort persists or worsens. Prepare client for percutaneous coronary intervention if planned: <ul><li>Balloon angioplasty</li><li>Atherectomy</li><li>Intracoronary stenting</li><li>CABG</li></ul>	*Consulting the appropriate health care provider allows for modification of the treatment plan.*

Collaborative Diagnosis **RISK FOR CARDIAC DYSRHYTHMIAS**

Definition: A disturbance of the heart's normal rhythm. Dysrhythmias can range in severity from missed or rapid beats to serious disturbances that impair the pumping ability of the heart.

Related to: Myocardial irritability associated with myocardial hypoxia

CLINICAL MANIFESTATIONS

Subjective	Objective
Verbal self-report of palpitations or skipped beats; syncope	ECG rate or rhythm abnormalities

RISK FACTORS
- Myocardial ischemia
- Electrolyte disturbances
- Coronary artery disease

DESIRED OUTCOMES

The client will maintain normal sinus rhythm as evidenced by:
a. Regular apical pulse at 60 to 100 beats/min
b. Equal apical and radial pulse rates
c. Absence of syncope and palpitations
d. ECG showing normal sinus rhythm

NURSING ASSESSMENT	RATIONALE
Assess for and report signs and symptoms of cardiac dysrhythmias: • Irregular apical pulse • Pulse rate less than 60 or greater than 100 beats/min • Apical-radial pulse deficit • Syncope • Palpitations • Abnormal rate, rhythm, or configurations on ECG Assess cardiovascular status frequently and report signs and symptoms of inadequate cardiac output. Assess ECG tracing.	*Early recognition of signs and symptoms of dysrhythmias allows for prompt intervention.*

THERAPEUTIC INTERVENTIONS	RATIONALE
Independent Actions Restrict client's activity based on his/her tolerance and severity of the dysrhythmia. **D** ✦	*Decreases myocardial workload thus improving cardiac oxygenation.*
Have emergency cart readily available for cardioversion, defibrillation, or CPR.	*Many dysrhythmias can be lethal and may only respond to electrical therapy.*
Dependent/Collaborative Actions Maintain oxygen therapy as ordered. **D** ✦	*Oxygen helps to improve oxygenation and reduce myocardial ischemia.*
Implement measures to help maintain an adequate cardiac output: • Antidysrhythmics • Add the following categories of medications: nitrates, beta-adrenergic blocking agents; CCBs, anticoagulants	*Classes of medications are administered in order to improve myocardial blood flow and oxygenation, reducing the risk for dysrhythmias. Antidysrhythmics help to reduce myocardial irritability.*

Collaborative Diagnosis   RISK FOR MYOCARDIAL INFARCTION

Definition: Irreversible myocardial damage.

Related to: Persistent ischemia or complete occlusion of a coronary artery

CLINICAL MANIFESTATIONS

Subjective	Objective
Verbal self-report of sudden, severe chest pain; nausea	Q-wave tracing on ECG; diaphoresis; variations in B/P; increased heart rate; abnormal or extra heart sounds; pericardial friction rub; increased CK-MB level; elevated tropin level

RISK FACTORS

• Coronary artery disease
• Hypertension
• Hyperlipidemia
• Smoking
• Diabetes

DESIRED OUTCOMES

The client will not experience a myocardial infarction (MI) as evidenced by:
a. Resolution of chest pain within 15 to 20 minutes
b. Stable vital signs
c. Cardiac enzyme levels within normal range
d. Absence of ST-segment depression or elevation, T-wave inversion, and abnormal Q waves on ECG

NURSING ASSESSMENT	RATIONALE
Assess for and report signs and symptoms of an MI: • Chest pain that lasts longer than 20 minutes • Increase in pulse rate • Significant change in B/P • Labored respirations Assess for elevation of cardiac enzymes: • CK-MB • Troponin Assess ECG tracing for abnormalities: • ST-segment depression or elevation • T-wave inversion • Abnormal Q waves on ECG	*Early recognition of signs and symptoms of an MI allows for prompt intervention.*

THERAPEUTIC INTERVENTIONS	RATIONALE
Independent Actions Maintain client on strict bed rest in a semi- to high-Fowler's position. **D** ✦	*Reduces myocardial oxygen consumption.*
Dependent/Collaborative Actions Maintain oxygen therapy as ordered. **D** ✦ Administer the following medications if ordered: • Morphine sulfate • Nitrates Beta-adrenergic blockers Prepare client for the following procedures that may be performed: • Injection of a thrombolytic agent (e.g., streptokinase, alteplase [tissue-type plasminogen activator; tPA], anistreplase [APSAC, Eminase], reteplase, tenecteplase [TNK-tPA]) • Percutaneous coronary intervention • Insertion of an intra-aortic balloon pump (IABP)	*Oxygen helps to improve oxygenation and reduce myocardial ischemia.* *Reduces pain and anxiety and decreases cardiac workload.* *Improve myocardial blood flow and reduce myocardial oxygen requirements.* *Reduce myocardial oxygen requirements by decreasing heart rate and force of myocardial contraction.* *Procedures may be performed to improve myocardial blood flow.*

DISCHARGE TEACHING/CONTINUED CARE

Nursing Diagnosis **DEFICIENT KNOWLEDGE** NDx; **INEFFECTIVE FAMILY HEALTH MANAGEMENT** NDx; **OR INEFFECTIVE HEALTH MAINTENANCE** NDx*

Definition: **Deficient Knowledge NDx**: Absence of cognitive information related to specific topic, or its acquisition; **Ineffective Family Health Management NDx**: A pattern of regulating and integrating into family processes a program for the treatment of illness and its sequelae that is unsatisfactory for meeting specific health goals of the family unit; **Ineffective Health Maintenance NDx**: Inability to identify, manage, and/or seek out help to maintain well-being.

CLINICAL MANIFESTATIONS

Subjective	Objective
Verbal self-report of unfamiliarity with information resources; collateral report of exaggerated behaviors	Inaccurate follow-through of instructions; inaccurate performance of a test; lack of recall

*The nurse should select the diagnostic label that is most appropriate for the client's discharge teaching needs.

NDx = NANDA Diagnosis **D** = Delegatable Action ● = UAP ✦ = LVN/LPN ⊜▶ = Go to ⊜volve for animation

RISK FACTORS

- Denial of disease process
- Cognitive deficiency
- Failure to take action to reduce risk factors

NOC OUTCOMES	NIC INTERVENTIONS
Knowledge: treatment regimen; cardiac disease management	Teaching: individual; teaching: disease process; teaching: prescribed activity/exercise; teaching: prescribed medication; health system guidance

NURSING ASSESSMENT	RATIONALE
Assess client's readiness and ability to learn. Assess meaning of illness to client.	*Early recognition of readiness to learn and meaning of illness to client allows for implementation of the appropriate teaching interventions.*

THERAPEUTIC INTERVENTIONS	RATIONALE

Desired Outcome: The client will verbalize a basic understanding of angina pectoris.

Independent Actions

Explain angina pectoris in terms that client can understand:
- Use teaching aids (e.g., pamphlets, diagrams) whenever possible.

Clients vary in physical and cognitive ability to learn. When educating clients, nurses need to determine their ability to read and understand written materials. If literacy barriers are present, alternative educational materials should be provided.

THERAPEUTIC INTERVENTIONS	RATIONALE

Desired Outcome: The client will identify factors that may precipitate an angina attack and ways to control these factors.

Independent Actions

Provide the following instructions regarding ways to reduce risk of precipitating an angina attack:
- Take nitroglycerin before strenuous activity or sexual intercourse and during times of high emotional stress.
- Gradually increase activity by engaging in a regular aerobic exercise program (e.g., walking, biking, swimming).
- Avoid strenuous exercise and activities that involve pushing or lifting heavy objects (e.g., weightlifting).
- Avoid exercising for at least an hour after eating, and exercise with caution at higher altitude and when the environmental temperature is extremely hot or cold.
- Avoid tobacco use before exercise.
- Rest between activities.
- Stop any activity that causes shortness of breath, palpitations, dizziness, or extreme fatigue or weakness.
- Begin a cardiovascular fitness program if recommended by physician.
- Adhere to the following precautions regarding sexual activity:
  - Avoid intercourse for at least 1 to 2 hrs after a heavy meal or alcohol consumption and when fatigued or stressed.
  - Engage in sexual activity in a familiar environment and in a position that minimizes exertion (e.g., side-lying, partner on top).
  - Recognize that a new sexual relationship can be started but may result in greater energy expenditure initially.
  - Avoid hot or cold showers just before and after intercourse.

Clients with diagnosed cardiovascular disease should be educated to learn what may precipitate angina and ways to decrease the risk for angina. In addition, clients should be taught to recognize that changes in their individual pattern of angina may indicate advancing disease, and if changes occur, prompt treatment should occur.

Activities eliciting these responses may lead to angina and should be discontinued.

Physical activity, if recommended, should be regular, rhythmic, and repetitive.

Resumption of sexual activity should be based on the physiological status of the patient.

THERAPEUTIC INTERVENTIONS	RATIONALE

Desired Outcome: The client will identify modifiable cardiovascular risk factors and ways to alter these factors.

Independent Actions

Inform client that certain modifiable factors such as elevated serum lipid levels, a sedentary lifestyle, hypertension, and smoking have been shown to increase the risk for CAD.

A person with modifiable risk factors should be encouraged to make lifestyle changes to reduce the risk for CAD. For the motivated client, knowing how to reduce the risk may be all the information that is needed.

Assist client to identify changes in lifestyle that can help to eliminate or reduce the above risk factors and help to manage angina:
- Dietary modification
- Physical exercise on a regular basis
- Moderation of alcohol intake
- Smoking cessation

Encourage client to limit daily alcohol consumption. Current recommendations:
- No more than two drinks per day for men
- No more than one drink per day for women and lighter-weight persons.

Daily alcohol intake exceeding 1 oz of ethanol may contribute to the development of hypertension and some forms of heart disease.
A "drink" is considered to be ½ oz of ethanol [e.g., 1½ oz of 80-proof whiskey, 12 oz of beer, 5 oz of wine].

THERAPEUTIC INTERVENTIONS	RATIONALE

Desired Outcome: The client will verbalize an understanding of the rationale for and components of a diet designed to lower serum cholesterol and triglyceride levels.

Independent Actions

Explain the rationale for a diet low in saturated fat and cholesterol.

Fat intake should be approximately 30% of calories with most coming from monosaturated fats found in nuts and oils such as olive oil or canola oil.
Dietary modifications that reduce LDLs help reduce the risk of CAD.

Provide instructions on ways the client can reduce intake of saturated fat and cholesterol:
- Reduce intake of meat fat (e.g., trim visible fat off meat; replace fatty meats such as fatty cuts of steak, hamburger, and processed meats with leaner products).
- Reduce intake of milk fat (e.g., avoid dairy products containing more than 1% fat).
- Reduce intake of *trans* fats (e.g., avoid stick margarine and shortening and foods such as commercial baked goods that are prepared with these products).
- Use vegetable oil rather than coconut or palm oil in cooking and food preparation.
- Use cooking methods such as steaming, baking, broiling, poaching, microwaving, and grilling rather than frying.
- Restrict intake of eggs

Recommendations about the number of whole eggs allowed per week vary depending on the client's lipid levels.
Omega-3 fatty acids have been shown to reduce the risk for CAD if consumed regularly.

Encourage client to increase intake of omega-3 fatty acids (e.g., flaxseed, cold water ocean fish such as salmon and halibut) to help lower triglyceride levels and increase high-density lipoprotein (HDL) levels.

THERAPEUTIC INTERVENTIONS	RATIONALE

Desired Outcome: The client will demonstrate accuracy in counting pulse.

Independent Actions

Teach clients how to count their pulse, being alert to the regularity of the rhythm.

Allow time for return demonstration and accuracy check.

Educating clients to their baseline rhythm allows for early detection of irregularities warranting immediate attention from a health care provider. Early detection may reduce the incidence of sudden death.

THERAPEUTIC INTERVENTIONS	RATIONALE

Desired Outcome: The client will verbalize an understanding of medications ordered including rationale, food and drug interactions, side effects, schedule for taking, and importance of taking as prescribed.

Independent Actions

Explain the rationale for, side effects of, and importance of taking the medications prescribed. Inform client of pertinent food and drug interactions.

- Nitrates
- Nitroglycerin skin patches
- Beta-adrenergic blockers
- CCBs
- Lipid-lowering agents

Instruct client to consult physician before taking other prescription and nonprescription medications.

Instruct client to inform all health care providers of medications being taken.

Taking medications as prescribed ensures that therapeutic drug levels will be maintained.

Clients should be instructed not to discontinue taking medications if they feel better. Clients without financial resources should be assisted in accessing appropriate resources to obtain needed medications (e.g., pharmacy assistance programs).

Drug-drug interactions may render medications inactive or result in life-threatening side effects.

Continuity of health care information is critical to reduce the incidence of prescribing medications with potential adverse drug-drug interactions.

THERAPEUTIC INTERVENTIONS	RATIONALE

Desired Outcome: The client will state signs and symptoms to report to the health care provider.

Independent Actions

Stress the importance of reporting the following signs and symptoms:

- Chest, arm, neck, or jaw discomfort unrelieved by rest and/or nitroglycerin taken every 5 minutes for 15 minutes
- Shortness of breath
- Irregular pulse or a resting pulse less than 56 or greater than 100 beats/min (the rate the client should report may vary depending on the medications prescribed, the client's baseline pulse rate, and physician's preference)
- Fainting spells
- Diminished activity tolerance
- Swelling of feet or ankles
- Increase in severity or frequency of angina attacks

Early identification of signs and symptoms of advancing coronary disease allows for prompt intervention by the appropriate health care provider.

THERAPEUTIC INTERVENTIONS	RATIONALE

Desired Outcome: The client will identify community resources that can assist in making necessary lifestyle changes and adjusting to the effects of angina pectoris.

Independent Actions

Provide information about community resources that can assist client in making lifestyle changes and adjusting to effects of angina pectoris (e.g., weight loss, smoking cessation, and stress management programs; American Heart Association; counseling services).

Cardiac disease can significantly impact an individual's and family's socioeconomic status. Providing information specific to community resources is important to provide a necessary continuum of care and may impact the client's health status preventing future hospitalizations.

THERAPEUTIC INTERVENTIONS	RATIONALE

Desired Outcome: The client, in collaboration with the nurse, will develop a plan for adhering to recommended follow-up care including future appointments with health care provider.

Independent Actions

Collaborate with the client to develop a plan specific to treatment regimen.

Reinforce the importance of keeping follow-up appointments with health care provider.

Implement measures to improve client compliance:
- Include significant others in teaching sessions if possible.
- Encourage questions and allow time for reinforcement and clarification of information provided.

- Provide written instructions regarding future appointments with health care provider, dietary modifications, activity level, medications prescribed, and signs and symptoms to report.

Regular health care appointments are important to determine the effectiveness of the prescribed treatment plan.

Involvement of significant others in patient teaching improves adherence to discharge instructions.

Everyone does not understand information as presented, so set aside time for questions to allow for clarification of information.

Written instructions allow the client to refer to instructions as needed.

ADDITIONAL NURSING DIAGNOSES

FEAR/ANXIETY NDx
Related to:
- Discomfort during angina attack and threat of recurrent attacks

- Lack of understanding of diagnostic tests, diagnosis, and treatment plan
- Unfamiliar environment
- Effect of angina pectoris on future lifestyle and roles

NDx = NANDA Diagnosis   **D** = Delegatable Action   ● = UAP   ✦ = LVN/LPN   ⊖▶ = Go to ⊖volve for animation

CAROTID ENDARTERECTOMY

Carotid endarterectomy is the surgical removal of atherosclerotic plaque from the intima of the carotid artery. The most common site of plaque formation in the carotid artery is the bifurcation. Access to this extracranial area is gained through an incision along the anterior sternocleidomastoid muscle. Surgery is performed to improve carotid artery blood flow and to reduce the risk of cerebral embolization and stroke.

This care plan focuses on the adult client hospitalized for a carotid endarterectomy. Much of the postoperative information is applicable to clients receiving follow-up care in an extended care facility or home setting.

OUTCOME/DISCHARGE CRITERIA

The client will:
1. Have adequate cerebral blood flow
2. Have surgical pain controlled
3. Have evidence of normal wound healing
4. Identify ways to prevent or slow the progression of atherosclerosis
5. Identify ways to manage signs and symptoms resulting from cranial nerve damage if it has occurred
6. State signs and symptoms to report to the health care provider
7. Develop a plan for adhering to recommended follow-up care including future appointments with health care provider, medications prescribed, activity level, and wound care

---

Nursing/Collaborative Diagnosis ## PREOPERATIVE

Use in conjunction with the Standardized Preoperative Care Plan.

Nursing Diagnosis ## RISK FOR INEFFECTIVE CEREBRAL TISSUE PERFUSION NDx

Definition: Susceptible to a decrease in cerebral tissue circulation, which may compromise health.

Related to:
- Partial or complete occlusion of the carotid artery by atherosclerotic plaque and/or a thrombus
- A cerebral embolus associated with dislodgment of atherosclerotic plaque or a thrombus from the carotid artery

CLINICAL MANIFESTATIONS

Subjective	Objective
Verbal self-report of behavioral changes; changes in motor response	Altered mental status; changes in pupillary reactions; difficulty swallowing; extremity weakness; paralysis; speech abnormalities

RISK FACTORS
- Arterial fibrillation
- Carotid stenosis
- Hypertension
- Hypercholesterolemia
- Embolism

DESIRED OUTCOMES

The client will maintain adequate cerebral tissue perfusion as evidenced by:
a. Mentally alert and oriented
b. Absence of dizziness, visual disturbances, and speech impairments
c. Normal motor and sensory function

NOC OUTCOMES

Tissue perfusion: cerebral; neurological status; cognition

NIC INTERVENTIONS

Cerebral perfusion promotion; neurological monitoring

NURSING ASSESSMENT	RATIONALE
Assess for and report signs and symptoms of carotid artery occlusion and/or cerebral embolization: • Agitation • Lethargy • Confusion • Dizziness • Diplopia • Ipsilateral blindness • Homonymous hemianopsia • Slurred speech	*Early recognition and reporting of signs and symptoms of ineffective cerebral tissue perfusion allow for prompt intervention.*

NURSING ASSESSMENT	RATIONALE

- Expressive aphasia
- Paresthesias
- Hemiparesis
- Hemiplegia

THERAPEUTIC INTERVENTIONS	RATIONALE

Independent Actions

Implement measures to maintain adequate cerebral tissue perfusion:
- Caution client to avoid activities that create a Valsalva response.
  - Straining to have a bowel movement
  - Holding breath while moving up in bed

Perform actions to prevent hypertension in order to reduce the risk of cerebral embolism:
- Implement measures to reduce stress (e.g., explain procedures, maintain calm environment).

If signs and symptoms of decreased cerebral tissue perfusion persist or worsen:
- Provide emotional support to client and significant others; be aware that the development of signs and symptoms usually necessitates postponement or cancellation of planned surgery.

Actions help to prevent dislodgment of existing thrombi.

Dependent/Collaborative Actions

Implement measures to maintain adequate cerebral tissue perfusion:
- Administer anticoagulants if ordered:
  - Heparin
  - Warfarin
  - Antiplatelet agents

Perform actions to prevent hypertension in order to reduce the risk of cerebral embolism:
- Administer antihypertensives as ordered.

If signs and symptoms of decreased cerebral tissue perfusion persist or worsen:
- Administer anticoagulants if ordered.
- Maintain client on bed rest with head of bed flat unless contraindicated.
- Notify the appropriate health care provider.

Anticoagulants act to prevent new or extended thrombus formation and further occlusion of the carotid artery. NOTE: These medications might be discontinued before surgery to reduce the risk of intraoperative and postoperative hemorrhage.

These medications are sometimes discontinued before surgery to reduce the risk of a critical drop in B/P during and immediately after surgery.

Notification of the appropriate health care provider allows for modification of the treatment plan.

POSTOPERATIVE

Use in conjunction with the Standardized Postoperative Care Plan.

Nursing Diagnosis RISK FOR INNEFFECTIVE CEREBRAL TISSUE PERFUSION

Definition: Susceptible to a decrease in cerebral tissue circulation, which may compromise health.

Related to:
- Prolonged carotid artery clamp time during surgery and/or vasospasm associated with clamping and manipulation of cerebral vessels
- Compression of carotid vessels associated with inflammation, edema, and/or development of a hematoma in the operative area
- Hypotension associated with:
  - Hypovolemia resulting from intraoperative and/or postoperative blood loss

NDx = NANDA Diagnosis   **D** = Delegatable Action   ● = UAP   ✦ = LVN/LPN   ⊝▶ = Go to ⊝volve for animation

- Stimulation of the carotid sinus baroreceptors resulting from surgical manipulation and/or improved blood flow in the carotid artery after surgery
- Increased cerebral vascular dilation and pressure associated with inability of the autoregulatory system to adjust to increased blood flow in cerebral vessels distal to the surgical site (this hyperperfusion syndrome can occur in the initial postoperative period in clients who have had a high-grade, long-term carotid artery blockage that has resulted in chronic cerebral vessel dilation)
- Embolization during or after surgery and/or formation of a thrombus at surgical site

CLINICAL MANIFESTATIONS

Subjective	Objective
Verbal self-report of dizziness	Agitation; lethargy; confusion; visual disturbances (e.g., blurred or dimmed vision, diplopia, ipsilateral blindness, homonymous hemianopsia); speech impairments (e.g., slurred speech, expressive aphasia); paresthesias, paresis, paralysis

RISK FACTORS

- Arteriosclerosis
- Hypertension

DESIRED OUTCOMES

The client will maintain adequate cerebral blood flow as evidenced by:
a. Mentally alert and oriented
b. Absence of dizziness, visual disturbances, and speech impairments
c. Normal sensory and motor function

NOC OUTCOMES

Tissue perfusion: cerebral; neurological status; cognition

NIC INTERVENTIONS

Cerebral perfusion promotion; neurological monitoring

NURSING ASSESSMENT

Assess for and report signs and symptoms of:
- Cerebral ischemia
- Excessive operative site bleeding
- New or expanding hematoma
- Continued bright red bleeding from incision or wound drain
- Hypovolemic shock

Assess RBC count, Hct and Hgb levels for abnormalities.

RATIONALE

Early recognition and reporting of signs and symptoms of cerebral ischemia allow for prompt intervention.

THERAPEUTIC INTERVENTIONS

Independent Actions

Implement measures to prevent cerebral ischemia:
- Perform actions to reduce pressure on carotid vessels:
  - Implement measures to reduce operative site inflammation and/or edema:
  - Keep head of bed elevated 30 degrees unless contraindicated.
  - Maintain patency of wound drain (e.g., keep tubing free of kinks, empty collection device as often as necessary) if present.
  - Instruct client to support head and neck with hands during position changes and to avoid turning head abruptly or hyperextending neck.
- Caution client to avoid activities that create a Valsalva response (e.g., straining to have a bowel movement, holding breath while moving up in bed)

RATIONALE

Interventions that focus on maintaining adequate cerebral blood flow and vessel patency help to prevent cerebral ischemia.
Corticosteroids help reduce operative site inflammation and/or edema reducing pressure on carotid vessels.

Action helps to reduce stress on the suture line and prevent subsequent bleeding and hematoma formation.

Action helps to prevent dislodgment of existing thrombi and reduce stress on and subsequent bleeding from the suture line.

THERAPEUTIC INTERVENTIONS

Dependent/Collaborative Actions
Implement measures to prevent cerebral ischemia:
- **Perform actions to prevent** or treat hypovolemic shock.
- Apply cooling pad or ice pack to incisional area as ordered.
- Administer corticosteroids if ordered.
- Administer the following medications if ordered:
  - Antihypertensives
  - Sympathomimetics

RATIONALE

Interventions that focus on maintaining adequate cerebral blood flow and vessel patency help to prevent cerebral ischemia.

Corticosteroids help reduce operative site inflammation and/or edema reducing pressure on carotid vessels.

Medications help to maintain B/P within a safe range, preventing either hypotension, which can reduce cerebral blood flow, or hypertension, which can stress and disrupt the operative vessel leading to hemorrhage.

Collaborative Diagnosis RISK FOR RESPIRATORY DISTRESS

Definition: Inability of a client to get enough oxygen to support respiration; can result from upper airway obstruction or lung disease.

Related to: Airway obstruction associated with tracheal compression (can occur as a result of inflammation, edema, and/or hematoma formation in the surgical area)

CLINICAL MANIFESTATIONS

Subjective	Objective
Verbal self-report of difficulty getting "air" or breathing	Agitation; restlessness; rapid/labored respirations; stridor; sternocleidomastoid muscle retraction

RISK FACTOR
- Surgical manipulation in close proximity to airway

DESIRED OUTCOMES
The client will not experience respiratory distress as evidenced by:
a. Usual mental status
b. Unlabored respirations at 12 to 20 breaths/min
c. Absence of stridor and sternocleidomastoid muscle retraction
d. Oximetry results within normal range
e. Arterial blood gas values within normal range

NURSING ASSESSMENT

Assess for and report:
- Increased edema or expanding hematoma in surgical area
- Deviation of trachea from midline
- New or increased difficulty swallowing
- Signs and symptoms of respiratory distress:
  - Restlessness
  - Agitation
  - Rapid and/or labored respirations
  - Stridor
  - Sternocleidomastoid muscle retraction
Monitor arterial blood gas values and pulse oximetry values for abnormalities.

RATIONALE

Early recognition of signs and symptoms of respiratory distress allows for prompt intervention.

THERAPEUTIC INTERVENTIONS	RATIONALE

Dependent/Collaborative Actions

Have tracheostomy and suction equipment readily available.

Implement measures to prevent compression of the trachea:
- Perform actions to prevent inflammation, edema, and hematoma formation in the operative area (e.g., maintain head and neck in alignment, place client in semi- to high-Fowler's, apply ice to operative area as ordered).
- Perform actions to prevent excessive pressure:
  - Caution client to avoid activities that create a Valsalva response (e.g., straining to have a bowel movement, holding breath while moving up in bed)
  - Administer antihypertensives if ordered.

If signs and symptoms of respiratory distress occur:
- Place client in a high-Fowler's position unless contraindicated.
- Loosen neck dressing if it appears tight.
- Administer oxygen as ordered.
- Assist with intubation or tracheostomy if performed.
- Prepare client for evacuation of hematoma or surgical repair of the bleeding vessel if planned.

An emergency tracheostomy may be necessary if a client's airway becomes compromised.

Compression of the trachea can result in respiratory distress. During the postoperative period, frequent assessment of the position of the trachea (midline, shifted to the left or right) is critical.

Interventions and medications help to prevent excessive pressure in the operative vessel and subsequent bleeding and hematoma formation.

Identification of signs and symptoms of respiratory distress allows for modification of the treatment plan and initiation of emergency measures if indicated.

Collaborative Diagnosis | # RISK FOR CRANIAL NERVE DAMAGE (FACIAL, HYPOGLOSSAL, GLOSSOPHARYNGEAL, VAGUS, AND/OR ACCESSORY NERVES)

Definition: Damage to cranial nerve(s).

Related to: Surgical trauma and/or compression of the nerves (can occur as a result of inflammation, edema, and/or hematoma formation)

CLINICAL MANIFESTATIONS

Subjective	Objective
Facial: Verbal self-report of altered taste sensations	**Facial:** Difficulty raising eyebrows, closing eyes tightly, pursing lips, and/or smiling.
Hypoglossal: Not applicable	**Hypoglossal:** Inability to protrude tongue or move tongue side to side
Glossopharyngeal/vagus: Not applicable	**Glossopharyngeal/vagus:** Absence of gag reflex; difficulty in swallowing
Accessory nerves: Not applicable	**Accessory nerves:** Inability to shrug shoulders against resistance.

RISK FACTOR
- Surgical retraction

DESIRED OUTCOMES

The client will experience beginning resolution of cranial nerve damage if it occurs as evidenced by:
a. Gradual return of facial symmetry and usual taste sensation
b. Increased ability to chew and swallow
c. Improved speech
d. Return of usual shoulder movements

NURSING ASSESSMENT	**RATIONALE**
Assess for and report signs and symptoms of the following: • Facial nerve damage (e.g., facial ptosis on affected side, impaired sense of taste) • Vagus and glossopharyngeal nerve damage (e.g., loss of gag reflex, difficulty swallowing, hoarseness, inability to speak clearly) • Hypoglossal nerve damage (e.g., tongue biting when chewing, tongue deviation toward affected side, difficulty swallowing and speaking). • Accessory nerve damage (e.g., unilateral shoulder sag, difficulty raising shoulder against resistance)	*Early recognition and reporting of signs and symptoms of nerve damage allow for prompt intervention.*

THERAPEUTIC INTERVENTIONS	**RATIONALE**
Dependent/Collaborative Actions Implement measures to prevent compression of the cranial nerves at the operative site: • Keep head of bed elevated 30 degrees unless contraindicated. • Apply ice pack to incisional area. • Maintain patency of wound drain. • Avoid Valsalva maneuvers. **D** ✦	*These actions decrease edema at the surgical site.*

If signs and symptoms of cranial nerve damage occur:
  • If the facial, hypoglossal, vagus, and/or glossopharyngeal nerves are affected:
  • Withhold oral foods/fluids until gag reflex returns and client is better able to chew and swallow; provide parenteral nutrition or tube feeding if indicated.
• When oral intake is allowed and tolerated:
  • Implement measures to improve client's ability to chew and/or swallow:
    • Place client in high-Fowler's position for meals and snacks.
    • Assist client to select foods that require little or no chewing and are easily swallowed (e.g., custard, eggs, canned fruits, mashed potatoes).
    • Avoid serving foods that are sticky (e.g., peanut butter, soft bread, honey).
    • Serve thick rather than thin fluids or add a thickening agent (e.g., "Thick-It," gelatin, baby cereal) to thin fluids.
	Actions help to reduce the risk of aspiration.

• Instruct client to add extra sweeteners or seasonings to foods/fluids if desired.	*Action helps to compensate for impaired sense of taste.*
• Implement measures to facilitate communication (e.g., maintain quiet environment; provide pad and pencil, Magic Slate, or word cards; listen carefully when client speaks). • Consult speech pathologist about additional ways to facilitate swallowing and communication.	
• If the accessory nerve is affected, instruct client in and assist with exercises (e.g., range of motion of affected shoulder, wall climbing with fingers, shoulder shrugs). • Provide emotional support to client and significant others; assure them that the nerve damage is usually not permanent, but caution them that the symptoms may take months to resolve.	*Exercises help to prevent atrophy of trapezius and sternocleidomastoid muscles.*

DISCHARGE TEACHING/CONTINUED CARE

Nursing Diagnosis **DEFICIENT KNOWLEDGE NDx; INEFFECTIVE HEALTH MAINTENANCE NDx; OR INEFFECTIVE HEALTH MANAGEMENT NDx***

Definition: **Deficient Knowledge NDx:** Absence of cognitive information related to a specific topic, its acquisition;
Ineffective Health Maintenance NDx: Inability to identify, manage, and/or seek out help to maintain well-being;
Ineffective Health Management NDx: Pattern of regulating and integrating into daily living a therapeutic regimen for the treatment of illness and its sequelae that is unsatisfactory for meeting specific health goals.

CLINICAL MANIFESTATIONS

Subjective	Objective
Verbal self-report of unfamiliarity with information resources	Inaccurate follow-through of instructions

RISK FACTORS
- Denial of disease process
- Cognitive deficiency
- Failure to take action to reduce risk factors

NOC OUTCOMES	NIC INTERVENTIONS
Knowledge: treatment regimen; cardiac disease management	*Health system guidance; teaching: disease process; teaching: individual; teaching: prescribed diet*

NURSING ASSESSMENT	RATIONALE
Assess client's readiness and ability to learn. Assess meaning of illness to client.	*Early recognition of readiness to learn and meaning of illness to client allows for implementation of the appropriate teaching interventions.*

THERAPEUTIC INTERVENTIONS	RATIONALE

Desired Outcome: The client will identify ways to prevent or slow the progression of atherosclerosis.

Independent Actions
Inform the client that certain modifiable factors such as elevated serum lipid levels, a sedentary lifestyle, cigarette smoking, and hypertension have been shown to increase the risk of atherosclerosis.

Assist client to identify changes in lifestyle that could reduce the risk for atherosclerosis (e.g., smoking cessation, dietary modifications, physical exercise on a regular basis).

Provide instructions on ways the client can reduce intake of saturated fat and cholesterol:
- Reduce intake of meat fat (e.g., trim visible fat off meat; replace fatty meats such as fatty cuts of steak, hamburger, and processed meats with leaner products).
- Reduce intake of milk fat (e.g., avoid dairy products containing more than 1% fat).
- Reduce intake of *trans* fats (e.g., avoid stick margarine and shortening and foods such as commercial baked goods that are prepared with these products).

A person with modifiable risk factors should be encouraged to make lifestyle changes to reduce the risk for atherosclerosis in order to prevent progression of the disease.

*The nurse should select the diagnostic label that is most appropriate for the client's discharge teaching needs.

THERAPEUTIC INTERVENTIONS	**RATIONALE**

- Use vegetable oil rather than coconut or palm oil in cooking and food preparation.
- Use cooking methods such as steaming, baking, broiling, poaching, microwaving, and grilling rather than frying.
- Restrict intake of eggs.

Instruct client to take lipid-lowering agents (e.g., HMG-CoA reductase inhibitors ["statins"], ezetimibe, gemfibrozil, niacin) and antiplatelet agents (e.g., low-dose aspirin) as prescribed.

Recommendations about the number of whole eggs allowed per week vary depending on the client's lipid levels

THERAPEUTIC INTERVENTIONS	**RATIONALE**

Desired Outcome: The client will identify ways to manage signs and symptoms resulting from cranial nerve damage if it has occurred.

Independent Actions

If signs and symptoms of hypoglossal, facial, vagus, and/or glossopharyngeal nerve damage are present:
- Reinforce techniques to improve swallowing and speaking.
- Assist client in identifying foods that are nutritious and easy to chew and swallow; obtain a dietary consult if needed.
- Instruct client to increase the amount of sweeteners and seasonings usually used and/or to try different seasonings in foods and beverages if sense of taste is altered.

If signs and symptoms of accessory nerve damage are present, reinforce exercises that should be performed to maintain shoulder muscle tone and prevent contractures.

Educating the client as to normal nerve function allows for early detection of irregularities warranting immediate attention from a health care provider. Early detection may reduce the incidence of permanent nerve damage.

THERAPEUTIC INTERVENTIONS	**RATIONALE**

Desired Outcome: The client will state signs and symptoms to report to the health care provider.

Independent Actions

Instruct client to also report any of the following signs and symptoms to the health care provider:
- Increased swelling or purple discoloration at wound site
- New or increased difficulty chewing, swallowing, or speaking
- Any loss of or change in vision
- Dizziness
- Numbness, tingling, or weakness of arms or legs
- Increasing irritability
- Lethargy, confusion
- Failure of signs and symptoms of cranial nerve damage to resolve as expected; remind client that it can take months for reversible signs and symptoms to resolve.

Early identification of signs and symptoms of complications associated with surgery allows for prompt intervention.

THERAPEUTIC INTERVENTIONS	**RATIONALE**

Desired Outcome: The client, in collaboration with the nurse, will develop a plan for adhering to recommended follow-up care including future appointments with health care provider, medications prescribed, activity level, and wound care.

Continued...

THERAPEUTIC INTERVENTIONS	RATIONALE

Independent Actions

Collaborate with the client to develop a plan to adhere to the treatment regimen including:

Reinforce the physician's instructions regarding:

- Ways to prevent constipation and subsequent straining to have a bowel movement (e.g., drink at least 10 glasses of liquid per day unless contraindicated, increase intake of foods high in fiber, take stool softeners if necessary)
- The need to avoid isometric exercise/activity (e.g., lifting objects over 10 lb, pushing heavy objects) and strenuous exercise for specified length of time (usually 4–12 weeks depending on the activity)

Actions help to prevent increased straining, which may lead to wound or vascular graft dehiscence.

RELATED CARE PLANS

Standardized Preoperative Care Plan
Standardized Postoperative Care Plan

DEEP VEIN THROMBOSIS

Venous thrombosis occurs when a thrombus forms in a superficial or deep vein. This condition is often called thrombophlebitis because of the associated inflammation in the involved vessel wall. The predisposing factors for venous thrombus formation are venous stasis, damage to the endothelium of the vein wall, and/or hypercoagulability. Conditions/factors associated with a high risk for venous thrombosis include surgery (especially orthopedic and abdominal surgery), immobility, advanced age, heart failure, certain malignancies, fractures or other injuries of the pelvis or lower extremities, varicose veins, pregnancy, obesity, estrogen and oral contraceptive use, sepsis, venous cannulation, administration of vessel irritants (e.g., hypertonic solutions, chemotherapeutic agents, high-dose antibiotics), history of deep vein thrombosis (DVT), and inherited coagulation abnormalities.

DVT usually develops in a lower extremity; however, the incidence of subclavian venous thrombosis is rising because of the increased use of central venous catheters. Clinical manifestations of DVT are often not distinctive and, in many cases, the client is asymptomatic. Signs and symptoms that may be present include pain, tenderness, swelling, unusual warmth, and/or increase in calf circumference comparison (with unaffected extremity). The greatest danger associated with DVT is that the clot, or parts of it, will detach and cause embolic occlusion of a pulmonary vessel.

Diagnosis of a DVT is accomplished through physical exam, including symptom and medical history. A D-dimer blood test along with an ultrasound may be performed. Persons with DVT are usually treated medically rather than surgically unless there is massive occlusion of a vessel and anticoagulation and thrombolytic therapy are contraindicated. With the increasing use of thrombolytic therapy, thrombectomies and embolectomies are rarely performed. Medical treatment varies depending on the location of the thrombus, the person's risk for bleeding and history of previous thrombus, and whether a coagulation abnormality exists. Anticoagulant therapy is not universally used to treat calf vein thrombosis because the incidence of

pulmonary embolism is low if there is no proximal vein involvement. However, there is a risk of extension of calf vein thrombi into a proximal venous segment if untreated, and because of this risk, many persons with calf vein thrombosis are treated with anticoagulants. There is also some variation in the anticoagulant regimen in relation to the time that oral anticoagulants are initiated and the route and type of heparin ordered (e.g., continuous intravenous heparin, intermittent intravenous heparin, adjusted-dose subcutaneous heparin, low-molecular-weight heparin [LMWH]).

This care plan focuses on the adult client hospitalized for treatment of DVT in a lower extremity. The information is also applicable to clients receiving follow-up care at home.

OUTCOME DISCHARGE CRITERIA

The client will:

1. Have adequate tissue perfusion in affected extremity
2. Have no evidence of tissue irritation or breakdown
3. Have no signs and symptoms of complications
4. Identify ways to promote venous blood flow and reduce the risk of chronic venous insufficiency and recurrent thrombus formation
5. Verbalize an understanding of medications ordered including rationale, food and drug interactions, side effects, schedule for taking, and importance of taking as prescribed
6. Demonstrate the ability to correctly draw up and administer heparin subcutaneously if prescribed
7. Identify precautions necessary to prevent bleeding associated with anticoagulant therapy
8. State signs and symptoms to report to the health care provider
9. Develop a plan for adhering to recommended follow-up care including future appointments with health care provider and activity level

Nursing Diagnosis INEFFECTIVE PERIPHERAL TISSUE PERFUSION NDx

Definition: Decrease in blood circulation to the periphery, which may compromise health.

Related to:
- Obstructed venous blood flow in affected extremity associated with the presence of a thrombus and inflammation of the vessel
- Venous stasis associated with decreased mobility

CLINICAL MANIFESTATIONS

Subjective	Objective
Verbal self-report of tenderness/pressure over involved vein; extremity pain	Edema; brawny hemosideric skin discoloration; dependent blue or purple skin color; positive Homans' sign; slow healing of lesions; skin temperature changes; altered sensations; weak or absent pulses

RISK FACTORS
- Virchow's triad: venous stasis, endothelial damage due to trauma or inflammation, blood hypercoagulability

DESIRED OUTCOME

The client will have improved venous blood flow in the affected extremity as evidenced by diminished pain, tenderness, swelling, and distention of superficial blood vessels in extremity.

NOC OUTCOMES

Tissue perfusion: peripheral

NIC INTERVENTIONS

Embolus care: peripheral; circulatory care: venous insufficiency; lower extremity monitoring

NURSING ASSESSMENT

Assess for signs and symptoms of impaired venous blood flow in the affected extremity:
- Pain or tenderness in extremity
- Increase in circumference of extremity
- Distention of superficial blood vessels in extremity

Assess activated clotting time (ACT), activated partial thromboplastin time (aPTT), bleeding time, Hgb level, Hct, international normalized ratio (INR), platelet count, and D-dimer for abnormalities.

RATIONALE

Early recognition of signs and symptoms of altered peripheral tissue perfusion allows for prompt intervention.

Alterations in lab values may indicate risk factors for the formation of DVT. D-dimer elevation is suggestive of DVT.

THERAPEUTIC INTERVENTIONS

Independent Actions

Elevate affected extremity 10 to 20 degrees above the level of the heart. **D** ✦

Maintain the client on bed rest.

Discourage positions that compromise blood flow (e.g., pillows under knees, crossing legs, sitting or standing for long periods). **D** ✦

Dependent/Collaborative Actions

Perform actions to treat the thrombosis:
- Administer medications as ordered.
  - Indirect thrombin inhibitors
  - Direct thrombin inhibitors
  - Factor Xa inhibitors
  - Anticoagulants
  - Vitamin K antagonists

RATIONALE

Actions help to reduce venous stasis.

Bed rest until the thrombus is considered stable helps to reduce the risk of dislodgment.

Administration of identified medications helps to improve venous blood flow.
Indirect thrombin inhibitors are divided into two classes: unfractionated heparin, which acts upon both intrinsic and extrinsic pathways, and LMWH, which acts as an antithrombin.
Direct thrombin inhibitors bind with thrombin, inhibiting its function.
Factor Xa inhibitors inhibit factor Xa directly or indirectly.

Continued...

THERAPEUTIC INTERVENTIONS	RATIONALE
• Prepare client for intravenous injection of a thrombolytic agent or catheter-directed fibrinolysis.	*Anticoagulants act by inhibiting clotting factors.* *Vitamin K antagonists inhibit vitamin K-dependent clotting factors II, VII, IX, and X.*
Maintain a minimum fluid intake of 2500 mL (unless contra-indicated). **D** ✦	*Ensuring adequate fluid intake helps to prevent increased blood viscosity.*
Apply antiembolism stockings or intermittent compression devices if ordered. **D** ● ✦	*Actions help to reduce venous stasis.*
Consult physician if signs and symptoms of impaired venous blood flow in affected extremity persist or worsen.	*Notification of the appropriate health care provider allows for modification of the treatment plan. Clients may require surgical intervention to remove an embolus (embolectomy) or prevent a pulmonary embolus (vena caval interruption device—Greenfield filter).*

Nursing Diagnosis ACUTE PAIN NDx (AFFECTED EXTREMITY)

Definition: Unpleasant sensory and emotional experience associated with actual or potential tissue damage, or described in terms of such damage (International Association for the Study of Pain); sudden or slow onset of any intensity from mild to severe with an anticipated or predictable end, and with a duration of less than 3 months.

Related to:
• Decreased tissue perfusion and swelling associated with obstructed venous blood flow
• Inflammation of vein

CLINICAL MANIFESTATIONS

Subjective	Objective
Verbal self-report of pain in the affected extremity	Diaphoresis, B/P and heart rate changes; increased respiratory rate

RISK FACTORS
• Arteriosclerosis
• Venous stasis
• Immobility

DESIRED OUTCOMES

The client will experience diminished pain in the affected extremity as evidenced by:
a. Verbalization of a decrease in pain
b. Relaxed facial expression and body positioning
c. Increased participation in activities when allowed

NOC OUTCOMES

Comfort level; pain control

NIC INTERVENTIONS

Pain management; analgesic administration; heat/cold application

NURSING ASSESSMENT	RATIONALE
Assess for signs and symptoms of pain (e.g., verbalization of pain, grimacing, rubbing affected area, restlessness, reluctance to move).	*Early recognition of signs and symptoms of pain allows for prompt intervention.*
Assess client's perception of the severity of pain using a pain intensity rating scale.	
Assess client's pain pattern (e.g., location, quality, onset, duration, precipitating factors, aggravating factors, alleviating factors).	

THERAPEUTIC INTERVENTIONS	RATIONALE
Dependent/Collaborative Actions	
Implement measures to reduce pain:	
• Perform actions to protect the affected extremity from trauma, pressure, or excessive movement: **D ✦**	*Bed cradles help to relieve pressure from bed linens.*
• Avoid jarring the bed.	
• Use a bed cradle or footboard.	
• Support extremity during position changes.	
• Maintain activity restrictions as ordered.	
• Instruct client to move affected extremity slowly and cautiously.	
• Provide or assist with nonpharmacological methods for pain relief: **D ● ✦**	
• Position change	
• Relaxation techniques	
• Restful environment	
• Diversional activities	
• Instruct client and significant others that the painful extremity should not be rubbed to relieve pain.	*Rubbing the affected extremity could dislodge the thrombus, resulting in a thromboembolism.*
Independent Actions	
Implement measures to reduce pain:	
• Administer analgesics and anti-inflammatory agents if ordered. **D ✦**	
Consult physician if above measures fail to provide adequate pain relief.	*Notification of the appropriate health care provider allows for modification of the treatment plan.*

Nursing Diagnosis RISK FOR IMPAIRED TISSUE INTEGRITY NDx

Definition: Susceptible to damage to the mucous membrane, cornea, integumentary system, muscular fascia, muscle, tendon, bone, cartilage, joint capsule, and/or ligament, which may compromise health.

Related to:
• Accumulation of waste products and decreased oxygen and nutrient supply to the skin and subcutaneous tissue associated with prolonged pressure on tissues as a result of decreased mobility
• Damage to the skin and/or subcutaneous tissue associated with friction or shearing that can occur with movement while on bed rest
• Increased skin fragility in affected extremity associated with insufficient blood flow and edema

CLINICAL MANIFESTATIONS

Subjective	Objective
Verbal self-report of pain or altered sensation at site of tissue impairment	Color changes; redness; swelling; warmth of skin areas demonstrating impairment

RISK FACTORS
• Altered circulation
• Impaired mobility
• Mechanical factors: shear

DESIRED OUTCOMES
The client will maintain tissue integrity as evidenced by:
a. Absence of redness and irritation
b. No skin breakdown

NOC OUTCOMES
Tissue integrity: skin and mucous membranes

NIC INTERVENTIONS
Skin surveillance; pressure management; pressure ulcer prevention

---

NDx = NANDA Diagnosis   **D** = Delegatable Action   ● = UAP   ✦ = LVN/LPN   ⊖▶ = Go to ⊖volve for animation

NURSING ASSESSMENT	RATIONALE
Inspect the skin (especially bony prominences, dependent areas, and affected extremity) for pallor, redness, and breakdown.	*Early recognition of impaired skin integrity allows for prompt intervention.*

THERAPEUTIC INTERVENTIONS	RATIONALE

Dependent/Collaborative Actions

Implement measures to prevent tissue breakdown: **D** ●

- Assist client with turning every 2 hrs.
- Use pressure-relieving devices to position client properly:
  - Pillows, gel or foam cushions
- Keep client's skin dry.
- Keep bed linens dry and wrinkle free.

Implement measures to prevent tissue breakdown in involved extremity:

- Perform actions to protect affected extremity from trauma and/or excessive pressure: **D** ✦
  - Use a bed cradle or footboard to relieve pressure from bed linens.
  - Keep heel off bed by elevating extremity on foam block or pillows or using heel protector.
  - Instruct and assist client to move affected extremity cautiously.
  - Remove antiembolism stockings for 30 to 60 minutes at least twice daily.
  - Use caution when applying heat to extremity.

Prolonged pressure on the skin obstructs capillary blood flow.

Excessive moisture on the skin softens epidermal cells and makes them less resistant to damage.

Dependent/Collaborative Actions

If tissue breakdown occurs:

- Notify appropriate health care provider (e.g., wound care specialist, physician).
- Perform care of involved areas as ordered or per standard hospital procedure.

Notification of the appropriate health care provider allows for modification of the treatment plan.

Collaborative Diagnosis RISK FOR PULMONARY EMBOLISM

Definition: Occlusion of a portion of the pulmonary vascular bed by an embolus, which can be a thrombus (blood clot).

Related to: Dislodgment of thrombus

CLINICAL MANIFESTATIONS

Subjective	Objective
Verbal self-report of chest or pleural pain	Pleural friction rub; pleural effusion; tachycardia; tachypnea; dyspnea; unexplained anxiety

RISK FACTORS

- Virchow's triad: venous stasis, endothelial trauma or inflammation, blood hypercoagulability

DESIRED OUTCOMES

The client will not experience a pulmonary embolism as evidenced by:
a. Absence of sudden chest pain
b. Unlabored respirations at 12 to 20 breaths/min
c. Pulse rate 60 to 100 beats/min
d. Arterial blood gas values within normal range

NURSING ASSESSMENT	RATIONALE
Assess for and report signs and symptoms of a pulmonary embolism: • Sudden chest pain • Dyspnea • Tachypnea • Tachycardia • Apprehension Assess pulse oximetry and arterial blood gas values for abnormalities.	*Early recognition of signs and symptoms of a pulmonary embolism allows for prompt intervention.*
Assess vital signs for signs of shock associated with massive pulmonary embolism.	*Clinical stability of the client is dependent upon the degree of obstruction associated with the embolism (e.g., massive occlusion, embolus with infarction, embolus without infarction, or chronic/recurrent pulmonary embolism).*

THERAPEUTIC INTERVENTIONS	RATIONALE
Dependent/Collaborative Actions	
Implement measures to prevent a pulmonary embolism: **D** ✦ • Maintain client on bed rest as ordered. • Do not exercise or check for Homans' sign in affected extremity during acute phase of DVT. • Never massage affected extremity, and caution client not to allow significant others to massage extremity. • Caution client to avoid activities that create a Valsalva response (e.g., straining to have a bowel movement, blowing nose forcefully, holding breath while moving up in bed).	*Actions help to prevent dislodgment of thrombus.*
• Administer anticoagulants as ordered. **D** ✦	*While anticoagulants will not dissolve clots, they will prevent development of new thrombi.*
• Prepare client for a vena caval interruption (e.g., insertion of an intracaval filtering device) if planned.	*These devices allow for filtration of clots without interruption of blood flow, reducing the risk of an embolus.*
If signs and symptoms of a pulmonary embolism occur: • Maintain client on bed rest in a semi- to high-Fowler's position.	*Semi- to high-Fowler's position facilitates adequate lung expansion.*
• Maintain oxygen therapy as ordered. • Prepare client for diagnostic tests (e.g., arterial blood gases, D-dimer level, ventilation-perfusion lung scan, pulmonary angiography). • Administer anticoagulants as ordered. • Prepare client for the following if planned:	
• Injection of a thrombolytic agent (e.g., streptokinase, urokinase, tissue plasminogen activator [tPA])	*Anticoagulants (e.g., heparin) prevent the formation of new clots, while thrombolytic agents dissolve pulmonary embolism.*
• Vena caval interruption (e.g., insertion of an intracaval filtering device)	*Vena caval interruption techniques assist in preventing further pulmonary embolization.*
• Embolectomy	*Primary indication for surgery is to prevent the recurrence of a pulmonary embolism.*

Nursing Diagnosis · RISK FOR BLEEDING NDx

Definition: Susceptible to a decrease in blood volume, which may compromise health.

Related to: Prolonged coagulation time associated with anticoagulant therapy and possible heparin-induced thrombocytopenia

NOC OUTCOMES	NIC INTENTIONS
Bleeding status	Bleeding precautions

CLINICAL MANIFESTATIONS

Subjective	Objective
Verbal self-report of bleeding	Petechiae, purpura, ecchymoses; gingival bleeding; prolonged bleeding from puncture sites; epistaxis, hemoptysis; unusual joint pain; increase in abdominal girth; frank or occult blood in stool, urine, or vomitus; menorrhagia; restlessness, confusion; decreasing B/P and increased pulse rate; decrease in Hct and Hgb levels

RISK FACTORS

- Anticoagulant therapy
- Prolonged clotting times
- Heparin-induced thrombocytopenia

DESIRED OUTCOMES

The client will not experience unusual bleeding as evidenced by:
a. Skin and mucous membranes free of petechiae, purpura, ecchymoses, and active bleeding
b. Absence of unusual joint pain
c. No increase in abdominal girth
d. Absence of frank and occult blood in stool, urine, and vomitus
e. Usual menstrual flow
f. Vital signs within normal range for client
g. Stable Hct and Hgb

NURSING ASSESSMENT

Assess client for and report signs and symptoms of unusual bleeding:
- Petechiae, purpura, ecchymoses
- Gingival bleeding
- Prolonged bleeding from puncture sites
- Epistaxis, hemoptysis
- Unusual joint pain
- Increase in abdominal girth
- Frank or occult blood in stool, urine, or vomitus
- Menorrhagia
- Restlessness, confusion
- Decreasing B/P and increased pulse rate
- Decrease in Hct and Hgb levels
Monitor Hct, platelet count, and coagulation test results (e.g., prothrombin time [PT], INR, aPTT, partial thromboplastin time [PTT]), and report abnormal values.
Assess stool, urine, and vomitus for blood.
Monitor and assess vital signs.

RATIONALE

Early recognition of signs and symptoms of bleeding allows for prompt intervention.

THERAPEUTIC INTERVENTIONS

Dependent/Collaborative Actions

Implement measures to prevent bleeding:
- Avoid giving injections whenever possible; consult physician for alternative routes.
- When giving injections or performing venous or arterial punctures, use the smallest gauge needle possible and apply gentle, prolonged pressure to the site after the needle is removed. **D** ✦
- Caution client to avoid activities that increase the risk for trauma (e.g., shaving with a straight-edge razor, using a stiff bristle toothbrush or dental floss).
- Pad side rails if client is confused or restless.

RATIONALE

Nursing activities should be adjusted to reduce the risk of bleeding while a client is undergoing anticoagulation therapy.

THERAPEUTIC INTERVENTIONS	RATIONALE
• Whenever possible, avoid intubations (e.g., nasogastric) and procedures that can cause injury to rectal mucosa (e.g., inserting a rectal suppository or tube, administering an enema).	
• Perform actions to reduce the risk for falls (e.g., keep bed in low position with side rails up when client is in bed, avoid unnecessary clutter in room, instruct client to wear shoes with nonslip soles when ambulating). **D** ✦	
• Instruct client to avoid blowing nose forcefully or straining to have a bowel movement; consult physician about an order for a decongestant and/or laxative if indicated.	
If bleeding occurs and does not subside spontaneously:	*If bleeding occurs, efforts must be directed at controlling active bleeding, replacing blood products as needed, and reversing anticoagulant therapy effects.*
• Apply firm, prolonged pressure to bleeding areas if possible.	
• If epistaxis occurs, place client in a high-Fowler's position and apply pressure and ice pack to nasal area.	
• Maintain oxygen therapy as ordered.	
• Administer protamine sulfate (antidote for heparin), vitamin K (e.g., phytonadione), and/or whole blood or blood products (e.g., fresh frozen plasma, platelets) as ordered.	

DISCHARGE TEACHING/CONTINUED CARE

Nursing Diagnosis | ## DEFICIENT KNOWLEDGE NDx; INEFFECTIVE HEALTH MAINTENANCE NDx; OR INEFFECTIVE HEALTH MANAGEMENT NDx*

Definition: Deficient Knowledge NDx: Absence of cognitive information related to a specific topic, or its acquisition;
Ineffective Health Maintenance NDx: Inability to identify, manage, and/or seek out help to maintain well-being;
Ineffective Health Management NDx: Pattern of regulating and integrating into daily living a therapeutic regimen for the treatment of illness and its sequelae that is unsatisfactory for meeting specific health goals.

NOC OUTCOMES	NIC INTERVENTIONS
Knowledge: disease process; treatment regimen	Health system guidance; teaching: individual; teaching: prescribed medication; teaching: prescribed activity/exercise

CLINICAL MANIFESTATIONS

Subjective	**Objective**
Verbal self-report of unfamiliarity with information	Demonstrated lack of understanding of disease process and/or the collaborative plan of care; inaccurate follow-through of instructions

RISK FACTORS
• Denial of disease process
• Cognitive deficiency
• Failure to take action to reduce risk factors

NURSING ASSESSMENT	RATIONALE
Assess client's readiness and ability to learn. Assess meaning of illness to client.	*Early recognition of readiness to learn and meaning of illness to client allows for implementation of the appropriate teaching interventions.*

*The nurse should select the diagnostic label that is most appropriate for the client's discharge teaching needs.

NDx = NANDA Diagnosis **D** = Delegatable Action ● = UAP ✦ = LVN/LPN ⊖▶ = Go to ⊖volve for animation

THERAPEUTIC INTERVENTIONS	RATIONALE

Desired Outcome: The client will identify ways to promote venous blood flow and reduce the risk of chronic venous insufficiency and recurrent thrombus formation.

Independent Actions
Educate the client regarding interventions to reduce the risk of DVT:
- Avoid wearing constrictive clothing (e.g., garters, girdles, narrow-banded knee-high hose).
- Avoid sitting and standing in one position for long periods.
- Wear graduated compression stockings or support hose during the day.
- Avoid crossing legs and lying or sitting with pillows under knees.
- Engage in regular aerobic exercise (e.g., swimming, walking, bicycling).
- Elevate legs periodically, especially when sitting.
- Dorsiflex feet regularly.
- Maintain an ideal body weight for age, height, and body frame.

Inform client that smoking and the use of estrogen or oral contraceptives can increase the risk for recurrent thrombus formation.

Clients identified as at risk for the development of DVT should be educated as to what may precipitate embolic events. In addition, clients should be taught to recognize that vascular changes may indicate serious problems that require prompt treatment.

THERAPEUTIC INTERVENTIONS	RATIONALE

Desired Outcome: The client will verbalize an understanding of medications ordered including rationale, food and drug interactions, side effects, schedule for taking, and importance of taking as prescribed.

Independent Actions
Educate the client regarding prescribed medications including rationale, food and drug interactions, side effects, dosing schedule, and importance of taking medications as prescribed.
- Coumadin
- Heparin

Taking medications as prescribed ensures that therapeutic drug levels will be maintained and adverse reactions avoided.
Clients should be instructed not to discontinue taking medications if they feel better. Clients without financial resources should be assisted in accessing appropriate resources to obtain needed medications (e.g., pharmacy assistance programs).

THERAPEUTIC INTERVENTIONS	RATIONALE

Desired Outcome: The client will demonstrate the ability to correctly draw up and administer heparin subcutaneously if prescribed.

Independent Actions
Provide instructions on subcutaneous injection techniques as needed.
Assess understanding through return demonstration.

Return demonstration of skill allows the nurse to evaluate client's understanding and implement additional education if necessary.

THERAPEUTIC INTERVENTIONS	RATIONALE

Desired Outcome: The client will identify precautions necessary to prevent bleeding associated with anticoagulant therapy.

THERAPEUTIC INTERVENTIONS	**RATIONALE**

Independent Actions

Instruct client about ways to minimize risk of bleeding:

- Use an electric rather than straight-edge razor.
- Floss and brush teeth gently; use waxed floss and a soft bristle toothbrush.
- Avoid putting sharp objects (e.g., toothpicks) in mouth.
- Do not walk barefoot.
- Cut nails carefully.
- Avoid situations that could result in injury (e.g., contact sports).
- Avoid blowing nose forcefully.
- Avoid straining to have a bowel movement.

Instruct client to control any bleeding by applying firm, prolonged pressure to the area if possible.

Actions that reduce the risk of bleeding prevent the development of complications.

THERAPEUTIC INTERVENTIONS	**RATIONALE**

Desired Outcome: The client will state signs and symptoms to report to the health care provider.

Independent Actions

Instruct the client to report the following signs and symptoms to the appropriate health care provider:

- Recurrent tenderness, pain, distention of superficial veins, or swelling in extremity
- Sudden chest pain accompanied by shortness of breath
- Unusual bleeding
- Discoloration or itching of affected extremity (indicative of stasis dermatitis associated with chronic venous insufficiency)
- Skin breakdown on affected extremity

Reinforce importance of keeping follow-up appointments with health care provider.

Reinforce physician's instructions regarding activity limitations.

Implement measures to improve client compliance:

- Include significant others in teaching sessions if possible.
- Encourage questions and allow time for reinforcement and clarification of information provided.
- Provide written instructions regarding future appointments with health care provider, medications prescribed, activity restrictions, signs and symptoms to report, and future laboratory studies.

Early identification of signs and symptoms of bleeding associated with drug therapy or the development of DVT allows for prompt intervention by the appropriate health care provider.

Regular health care appointments are important to determine effectiveness of the prescribed treatment plan.

Involvement of significant others in patient teaching improves adherence to discharge instructions.

Everyone does not understand information as presented, so set aside time for questions to allow for clarification of information.

Written instructions allow the client to refer to instructions as needed.

FEMOROPOPLITEAL BYPASS

Lower extremity arterial bypass is performed to treat peripheral artery insufficiency that has not responded well to conservative management. The impaired blood flow can occur as a result of acute conditions (e.g., trauma, embolization), but most often is caused by atherosclerotic changes in the vessels. The femoropopliteal arterial segment is the most common site of occlusion in persons with lower extremity arterial disease. Surgical intervention is usually indicated when the client experiences signs and symptoms of severe occlusion (e.g., intermittent claudication that has become disabling, foot pain that is present at rest, presence of lower extremity ischemic ulcers) and/or when more conservative invasive treatment measures such as balloon angioplasty, laser angioplasty, stent placement, or percutaneous atherectomy have been unsuccessful.

Surgical treatment of the diseased femoropopliteal arterial segment can be accomplished by endarterectomy or removal of the segment and replacement with a synthetic graft, but the most commonly performed procedure is to bypass the segment using a synthetic or an autogenous vein graft. The saphenous vein is the preferred autogenous graft for femoropopliteal bypass because it is thick walled and has an adequate lumen diameter. Before grafting the saphenous vein proximal and distal to the occluded arterial segment, reversal of the vein or division of its valve cusps is done to allow unimpeded arterial blood flow.

NDx = NANDA Diagnosis   **D** = Delegatable Action   ● = UAP   ✦ = LVN/LPN   ⊖▶ = Go to ⊖*volve* for animation

This care plan focuses on the adult client with atherosclerotic occlusion of the femoropopliteal arterial segment who is hospitalized for a femoropopliteal bypass. Much of the postoperative information is applicable to clients receiving follow-up care in an extended care facility or home setting.

OUTCOME/DISCHARGE CRITERIA

The client will:
1. Have adequate circulation in the operative extremity
2. Have surgical pain controlled
3. Tolerate expected level of activity
4. Have evidence of normal wound healing
5. Have no signs and symptoms of postoperative complications
6. Identify ways to prevent or slow the progression of atherosclerosis
7. Identify ways to promote blood flow in the operative extremity
8. State signs and symptoms to report to the health care provider
9. Develop a plan for adhering to recommended follow-up care including future appointments with health care provider, medications prescribed, activity level, and wound care

PREOPERATIVE: USE IN CONJUNCTION WITH THE STANDARDIZED PREOPERATIVE CARE PLAN

Nursing Diagnosis **INEFFECTIVE PERIPHERAL TISSUE PERFUSION** NDx

Definition: Decrease in blood circulation to the periphery, which may compromise health.

Related to: Diminished blood flow in the affected lower extremity associated with:
- Atherosclerotic changes in the femoral and popliteal arteries
- Thrombus formation in the affected vessel

CLINICAL MANIFESTATIONS

Subjective	Objective
Verbal self-report of altered sensation to the affected extremity; intermittent claudication; slow healing of lesions	Altered skin characteristics (hair, moisture) or nails; cold extremities; diminished arterial pulses; pale skin upon leg elevation; pallor; shiny, waxy skin; weak or absent pulses

RISK FACTORS
- Virchow's triad: venous stasis, endothelial trauma (surgery), blood hypercoagulability

DESIRED OUTCOMES

The client will not experience further reduction in arterial blood flow in the affected lower extremity as evidenced by:
a. No increase in lower extremity pain
b. No further decrease in peripheral pulses
c. No increase in capillary refill time
d. Usual temperature and color of extremity

NOC OUTCOMES

Tissue perfusion: peripheral

NIC INTERVENTIONS

Circulatory care: arterial insufficiency; circulatory care: venous insufficiency; lower extremity monitoring

NURSING ASSESSMENT	RATIONALE
Assess for and report signs and symptoms of a further reduction in arterial blood flow in the affected lower extremity: - Intermittent claudication occurring with increased intensity and/or with less activity than previously	*Early recognition of signs and symptoms of altered peripheral tissue perfusion allows for prompt intervention.*

NURSING ASSESSMENT	RATIONALE
• Development of or increase in intensity of rest pain (the foot and toe pain that occurs when the client is in a horizontal position results from decreased blood flow to the skin and subcutaneous tissue; because it occurs in the absence of lower extremity muscle activity, it reflects a severe reduction in the femoropopliteal arterial blood flow)	
• Diminishing peripheral pulses	
• Increase in usual capillary refill time	
• Increased coolness and numbness of foot and lower leg	
• Increased pallor or blanching of foot and lower leg when extremity is elevated	
• More rapid appearance of rubor or cyanosis in foot and lower leg when extremity is in a dependent position	

THERAPEUTIC INTERVENTIONS	RATIONALE
Independent Actions	
Implement measures to prevent further reduction in and/or improve blood flow in the affected lower extremity: **D** ✦	
• Discourage positions that compromise blood flow in lower extremities (e.g., crossing legs, pillows under knees, use of knee gatch, elevating legs when in bed, sitting for long periods).	*Prevents pooling of blood in the extremities.*
• Perform actions to prevent vasoconstriction:	*Reduces vascular response to the neuroendocrine stimulation.*
• Implement measures to reduce stress (e.g., maintain a calm environment, control pain, explain preoperative and postoperative care).	
• Discourage smoking.	*Stimulates release of norepinephrine.*
• Implement measures to keep client from getting cold (e.g., maintain a comfortable room temperature; provide adequate clothing, warm socks, and blankets).	
• Encourage short walks unless contraindicated.	*Promotes venous return.*
Dependent/Collaborative Actions	
Administer the following medications if ordered:	*Hemorrheologic agents help to improve the flow of blood to the ischemic area. Anticoagulants help to prevent or treat thrombi.*
• A hemorrheologic agent	
• Anticoagulants	
Consult physician if signs and symptoms of further reduction in lower extremity tissue perfusion occur.	*Notification of the appropriate health care provider allows for modification of the treatment plan.*

Nursing Diagnosis | ACUTE/CHRONIC PAIN NDx (INTERMITTENT CLAUDICATION AND REST PAIN)

Definitions: **Acute Pain NDx:** Unpleasant sensory and emotional experience associated with actual or potential tissue damage, or described in terms of such damage (International Association for the Study of Pain); sudden or slow onset of any intensity from mild to severe with an anticipated or predictable end, and with a duration of less than 3 months
Chronic Pain NDx: Unpleasant sensory and emotional experience associated with actual or potential tissue damage, or described in terms of such damage (International Association for the Study of Pain); sudden or slow onset of any intensity from mild to severe without an anticipated or predicable end and a duration of greater than 3 months.

Related to: Diminished arterial blood flow in the affected lower extremity (ischemia results in the release of anaerobic metabolites that irritate the nerve endings of the affected lower extremity)

CLINICAL MANIFESTATIONS

Subjective	**Objective**
Verbal-self report of pain; helplessness; anxiety	Expressions of pain are variable; diaphoresis, B/P and pulse changes

NDx = NANDA Diagnosis   **D** = Delegatable Action   ● = UAP   ✦ = LVN/LPN   ⊖▶ = Go to ⊖volve for animation

RISK FACTORS
- Immobility
- Blood hypercoagulability
- Peripheral vascular disease

DESIRED OUTCOMES

The client will experience diminished lower extremity pain as evidenced by:
a. Verbalization of same
b. Relaxed facial expression and body positioning

NOC OUTCOMES

Comfort level; pain control

NIC INTERVENTIONS

Pain management

NURSING ASSESSMENT

Assess for and report signs and symptoms of pain in the affected lower extremity:
- Intermittent claudication (e.g., verbalization of pain, aching, and/or cramping [usually in the calf muscle] during ambulation)
- Rest pain (e.g., awakening at night with reports of severe burning or aching in foot or toes)
- Grimacing, restlessness, reluctance to move, and/or rubbing leg or foot

Assess client's perception of the severity of pain using a pain intensity rating scale.

Assess the client's pain pattern (e.g., location, quality, onset, duration, precipitating factors, aggravating factors, alleviating factors).

RATIONALE

Early recognition of signs and symptoms of acute/chronic pain allows for prompt intervention.

THERAPEUTIC INTERVENTIONS

Independent Actions
Implement measures to reduce pain in the affected extremity: **D** ✦
- Perform actions to prevent further reduction in and/or improve blood flow in the affected lower extremity:
  - Discourage positions that compromise blood flow in lower extremities (e.g., crossing legs, pillows under knees, use of knee gatch, elevating legs when in bed, sitting for long periods).
- Perform actions to reduce fear and anxiety about the pain experience (e.g., assure client that the need for pain relief is understood, plan methods for achieving pain control with client).
- Perform actions to reduce the number of episodes of intermittent claudication:
  - Encourage client to stop activity minutes before symptoms are usually experienced (intermittent claudication is predictable, and clients are often aware of how far or how long they can ambulate before the discomfort begins or intensifies).
  - Maintain client on bed rest if experiencing severe intermittent claudication.
- If client is experiencing rest pain in the affected extremity, perform actions to facilitate gravity flow of arterial blood to the ischemic area: **D** ✦
  - Allow client to sleep in a recliner with legs in a dependent position or, if in bed, to hang affected lower leg over the side of bed.
  - Instruct client to avoid horizontal positioning and elevation of affected extremity for prolonged periods.

RATIONALE

Improves blood flow from the lower extremities.

Fear and anxiety can decrease the client's threshold and tolerance for pain and thereby heighten the perception of pain.

Limiting activity decreases muscle contractions in and subsequent ischemia of the affected lower extremity.

THERAPEUTIC INTERVENTIONS	RATIONALE
• Provide lightweight blankets or a foot cradle if external pressure aggravates lower extremity pain. • Provide or assist with nonpharmacological measures for relief of pain (e.g., relaxation techniques; position change; diversional activities such as conversing, watching television, or reading). **D** ✦	

Dependent/Collaborative Actions

Implement measures to reduce pain in the affected extremity:
• Administer analgesics (if ordered). **D** ✦
Consult physician if above measures fail to provide adequate pain relief.

Notification of the appropriate health care provider allows for modification of the treatment plan.

POSTOPERATIVE: USE IN CONJUNCTION WITH THE STANDARDIZED POSTOPERATIVE CARE PLAN

Nursing Diagnosis **RISK FOR INEFFECTIVE PERIPHERAL TISSUE PERFUSION** NDx

Definition: Susceptible to a decrease in blood circulation to the periphery, which may compromise health.

Related to: Diminished blood flow in the operative extremity associated with:
• Inflammation of the femoral and popliteal arteries at the sites of graft anastomoses
• Pressure on vessels in the operative extremity resulting from edema that can occur as a result of decreased venous return and dissection of tissue around perivascular lymphatics
• Venous stasis resulting from decreased mobility and decreased venous return if the saphenous vein was used for the bypass graft (can result in impaired venous return until collateral venous circulation improves)
• Graft occlusion
• Hypovolemia resulting from blood loss during surgery and decreased fluid intake

CLINICAL MANIFESTATIONS

Subjective Verbal self-report of pain unrelieved by analgesics; numbness	**Objective** Diminished or absent pulses; diminished or absent Doppler flow; coolness/cyanosis of foot; increased edema in operative extremity; capillary refill time greater than 2 to 3 seconds

RISK FACTORS	**DESIRED OUTCOMES**
• Virchow's triad: venous stasis, endothelial trauma (surgery), blood hypercoagulability	The client will maintain adequate tissue perfusion in the operative extremity as evidenced by: a. Resolution of leg and foot pain b. Palpable peripheral pulses c. Adequate Doppler flow readings in operative extremity d. Absence of coolness, numbness, and cyanosis in foot and lower leg e. Resolution of edema in operative extremity f. Capillary refill time less than 2 to 3 seconds

NOC OUTCOMES	**NIC INTERVENTIONS**
Tissue perfusion: peripheral	Circulatory care: arterial insufficiency; circulatory care: venous insufficiency; lower extremity monitoring

NDx = NANDA Diagnosis   **D** = Delegatable Action   ● = UAP   ✦ = LVN/LPN   ⊝▶ = Go to ⊝volve for animation

NURSING ASSESSMENT	RATIONALE
Assess for and report signs and symptoms of ineffective tissue perfusion in operative extremity: • Pain unrelieved by prescribed analgesics • Diminished or absent pulses (the pulses may be difficult to palpate for 4–12 hrs after surgery because of vasospasm that can occur in the operative extremity) • Diminished or absent Doppler flow readings over operative extremity • Coolness, numbness, or cyanosis of foot and lower leg • Increase in edema in the operative extremity • Capillary refill time greater than 2 to 3 seconds	*Early recognition and reporting of signs and symptoms of ineffective peripheral tissue perfusion allow for prompt intervention.*

THERAPEUTIC INTERVENTIONS	RATIONALE

Independent Actions

Implement measures to promote adequate tissue perfusion in operative extremity: **D** ✦	
• Avoid 90-degree flexion of the hip as much as possible (e.g., place client in high-Fowler's position for meals only, limit length of time that client is in straight-back chair, provide recliner for client's use when sitting up).	*Extensive flexing of the hip can reduce perfusion to the operative limb.*
• Limit length of time that operative leg is in dependent position (e.g., allow client to sit up for meals only; encourage short, frequent walks rather than long walks).	*Sitting for an extended period with legs in a dependent position may increase peripheral edema, stressing suture line.*
• Instruct client to keep knee in a neutral or slightly flexed position.	
• Perform actions to prevent graft occlusion.	
• If lower extremity edema is present, elevate foot of bed 15 degrees as ordered.	*Elevation of the edematous operative extremity helps to promote venous return without compromising arterial flow.*
• Place a bed cradle over lower extremities.	*Bed cradles help to minimize pressure from bed linens.*
• Instruct client to perform active foot and leg exercises every 1 to 2 hrs while awake.	
• Perform actions to prevent vasoconstriction:	*Vasoconstriction narrows vessel lumens, which results in diminished blood flow through affected vessels.*
• Implement measures to reduce stress (e.g., control pain, maintain a calm environment, explain postoperative care).	*Stress stimulates the sympathetic nervous system, which results in vasoconstriction.*
• Discourage smoking.	*Nicotine increases catecholamine output, which subsequently causes vasoconstriction.*
• Implement measures to keep client from getting cold (e.g., maintain a comfortable room temperature; provide adequate clothing, warm socks, and blankets).	*When the body is cold, peripheral vasoconstriction occurs in an attempt to conserve heat.*

Dependent/Collaborative Actions

Implement measures to promote adequate tissue perfusion in operative extremity:	
• Maintain a minimum fluid intake of 2500 mL/day unless contraindicated; if oral intake is inadequate or contraindicated, maintain intravenous fluid therapy as ordered.	*Intravenous fluids and/or blood help maintain vascular volume, which is essential for adequate tissue perfusion.*
• Administer blood and blood products as ordered.	
Consult physician if signs and symptoms of diminished tissue perfusion in the operative extremity persist or worsen.	*Notification of the appropriate health care provider allows for modification of the treatment plan.*

Collaborative Diagnosis | **RISK FOR COMPARTMENT SYNDROME**

Definition: Elevated intracompartmental pressure within a confined myofascial compartment compromises the neurovascular function of tissues within that space

Related to: Severe edema of the operative extremity (an infrequent but serious complication that can occur as a result of surgical site inflammation, reperfusion of the ischemic muscles, or dissection of tissue around the perivascular lymphatics)

CLINICAL MANIFESTATIONS

Subjective	Objective
Verbal self-report of increasing leg pain; new onset or increasing numbness of affected extremity; difficulty moving foot	Diminished or absent peripheral pulses; cyanotic, cool leg

RISK FACTORS

- Acute arterial occlusion
- Prolonged ischemia to tissues

DESIRED OUTCOMES

The client will not experience compartment syndrome in the operative extremity as evidenced by:
a. No complaints of increasing leg pain
b. No statements of new or increasing numbness and tingling in foot or leg, or tightness and tenseness of thigh or calf muscle
c. Ability to move leg and foot
d. No decrease in or absence of peripheral pulses
e. Absence of cyanosis and coldness of leg and foot

NURSING ASSESSMENT	RATIONALE
Assess for and report signs and symptoms of compartment syndrome in the operative extremity: • Sudden, severe pain in toes or foot • Diminishing or absent peripheral pulses • Capillary refill time greater than 2 to 3 seconds • Cyanosis, coolness, or diminished sensation in the foot	*Early recognition of signs and symptoms of compartment syndrome allows for prompt intervention.*
Assess for and report reddish-brown discoloration of urine.	*Assessment finding of reddish-brown urine discoloration could indicate myoglobinuria resulting from the release of myoglobin from the damaged muscle cells. If an excessive amount of myoglobin is released, it can get trapped in the renal tubules and cause renal failure.*

THERAPEUTIC INTERVENTIONS	RATIONALE
Dependent/Collaborative Actions Limit length of time that operative leg is in a dependent position (e.g., limit sitting and walking as ordered). Elevate operative extremity 15 degrees if ordered. Administer osmotic diuretics if ordered.	*Measures help to prevent an increase in edema in operative leg in order to reduce the risk of development of compartment syndrome.*
If signs and symptoms of compartment syndrome occur: • Maintain client on bed rest. • Prepare client for a fasciotomy if planned.	*Surgical decompression (fasciotomy) may be necessary to decompress soft tissue and improve circulation.*

Collaborative Diagnosis | **RISK FOR SAPHENOUS NERVE DAMAGE**

Definition: Damage to the saphenous nerve

Related to:
- Inadvertent or unavoidable dissection of the nerve during surgery
- Trauma to the nerve during surgery

NDx = NANDA Diagnosis **D** = Delegatable Action ● = UAP ✦ = LVN/LPN ⊖▶ = Go to ⊖*volve* for animation

CLINICAL MANIFESTATIONS

Subjective	Objective
Verbal self-report of numbness and tingling in affected extremity; heightened sensitivity to affected extremity	Not applicable

RISK FACTOR	DESIRED OUTCOME
• Vascular surgery	The client will have resolution of or adapt to operative extremity saphenous nerve damage if it has occurred.

NURSING ASSESSMENT	RATIONALE
Assess for and report signs and symptoms of saphenous nerve damage: • Numbness, tingling • Hypersensitivity of the operative extremity	*Early recognition of signs and symptoms of saphenous nerve damage allows for prompt intervention.*

THERAPEUTIC INTERVENTIONS	RATIONALE

Dependent/Collaborative Actions
If signs and symptoms of saphenous nerve damage are present:
• Adhere to and instruct client in the following safety precautions:
  • Wear shoes or slippers whenever out of bed.
  • Do not apply heat or cold to the affected extremity.
  • Test temperature of bath water before use.
  • Protect operative extremity from trauma.
• Reinforce information from physician regarding permanence of numbness, tingling, or hypersensitivity.
 	
• Consult physician if signs and symptoms increase in severity.
	
	Nerve damage eliminates ability to sense temperature changes which can lead to tissue damage.
	These symptoms are permanent if the nerve was severed during surgery; if the nerve was just traumatized, the symptoms are temporary and expected to resolve within 1 year.
	Notification of the appropriate health care provider allows for modification of the treatment plan.

DISCHARGE TEACHING/CONTINUED CARE

Nursing Diagnosis   **DEFICIENT KNOWLEDGE** NDx; **INEFFECTIVE FAMILY HEALTH MANAGEMENT** NDx; **OR INEFFECTIVE HEALTH MANAGEMENT** NDx*

Definition: **Deficient Knowledge NDx:** Absence of cognitive information related to a specific topic, or its acquisition; **Ineffective Family Health Management NDx:** A pattern of regulating and integrating into family processes a program for the treatment of illness and its sequelae that is unsatisfactory for meeting specific health goals of the family unit; **Ineffective Health Management NDx:** Inability to identify, manage, and/or seek out help to maintain well-being.

CLINICAL MANIFESTATIONS

Subjective	Objective
Verbal self-report of unfamiliarity with information	Inaccurate follow-through of instructions

*The nurse should select the diagnostic label that is most appropriate for the client's discharge teaching needs.

NOC OUTCOMES

Knowledge: treatment regimen; cardiac disease management

NIC INTERVENTIONS

Health system guidance; teaching: individual; teaching: disease process; teaching: prescribed diet; teaching: prescribed activity/exercise

RISK FACTORS

- Denial of disease process
- Cognitive deficiency
- Failure to take action to reduce risk factors

NURSING ASSESSMENT

Assess client's readiness and ability to learn.
Assess meaning of illness to client.

RATIONALE

Early recognition of readiness to learn and meaning of illness to client allows for implementation of the appropriate teaching interventions.

THERAPEUTIC INTERVENTIONS

RATIONALE

Desired Outcome: The client will identify ways to prevent or slow the progression of atherosclerosis.

Independent Actions

Inform the client that certain modifiable factors such as elevated serum lipid levels, a sedentary lifestyle, smoking, and hypertension have been shown to increase the risk of atherosclerosis.

Assist client to identify changes in lifestyle that could reduce the risk for atherosclerosis (e.g., smoking cessation, dietary modifications, physical exercise on a regular basis).

Provide instructions on ways the client can reduce intake of saturated fat and cholesterol:
- Reduce intake of meat fat (e.g., trim visible fat off meat; replace fatty meats such as fatty cuts of steak, hamburger, and processed meats with leaner products).
- Reduce intake of milk fat (e.g., avoid dairy products containing more than 1% fat).
- Reduce intake of *trans* fats (e.g., avoid stick margarine and shortening and foods such as commercial baked goods that are prepared with these products).
- Use vegetable oil rather than coconut or palm oil in cooking and food preparation.
- Use cooking methods such as steaming, baking, broiling, poaching, microwaving, and grilling rather than frying.
- Restrict intake of eggs.

Instruct client to take lipid-lowering agents as prescribed.

After vascular surgery, clients should be educated as to health promotion activities that slow the progression of atherosclerosis.

Making these changes will decrease the incidence of hypertension and improve circulatory status to the lower extremities.

Dietary modifications that reduce saturated fat and cholesterol intake may slow the progression of arteriosclerosis.

Recommendations about the number of whole eggs allowed per week vary depending on the client's lipid levels
Lipid-lowering agents help to keep cholesterol within normal limits, reducing the risk of atherosclerosis.

THERAPEUTIC INTERVENTIONS

RATIONALE

Desired Outcome: The client will identify ways to promote blood flow in the operative extremity.

Continued...

THERAPEUTIC INTERVENTIONS	RATIONALE

Independent Actions

Provide the following instructions about ways to promote blood flow in the operative extremity:

- Avoid wearing constrictive clothing (e.g., garters, girdles, narrow-banded knee-high stockings).
- Avoid positions that compromise blood flow (e.g., pillows under knees, crossing legs, sitting or standing for prolonged periods).
- Do active foot and leg exercises for 5 minutes every hour while awake.
- Maintain a regular exercise program (walking and swimming are recommended).
- Stop smoking.
- Drink at least 10 glasses of liquid per day unless contraindicated.

Actions reduce the risk of compression of vessels, which may compromise blood flow.

Dorsiflexion/plantar extension exercises help to stimulate blood flow to the extremities.

Proper hydration thins circulating blood volume, allowing for optimum flow-through vessels.

THERAPEUTIC INTERVENTIONS	RATIONALE

Desired Outcome: The client will state signs and symptoms to report to the health care provider.

Independent Actions

Instruct client to report these additional signs and symptoms:

- Sudden or gradual increase in operative leg or foot pain
- Increased swelling or purple discoloration at incision sites
- Pallor, coldness, or bluish color of the operative extremity
- Diminishing or sudden absence of peripheral pulses (client may be instructed to monitor his/her peripheral pulses)
- Significant increase in swelling of operative extremity (edema is expected to resolve gradually within the first 2–8 weeks after surgery)
- Difficulty moving foot on operative side
- Increasing numbness and/or tingling sensation of operative lower leg or foot
- Any area of persistent skin irritation or breakdown of foot on operative side

Early identification of signs and symptoms of bleeding associated with drug therapy or the development of arterial or venous thrombosis allows for prompt intervention by the appropriate health care provider.

THERAPEUTIC INTERVENTIONS	RATIONALE

Desired Outcome: The client, in collaboration with the nurse, will develop a plan for adhering to recommended follow-up care including future appointments with health care provider, medications prescribed, activity level, and wound care.

Independent Actions

Collaborate with the client to develop a plan for adherence to the treatment regimen including:

Reinforce the physician's instructions regarding:

- Importance of scheduling adequate rest periods
- Need to avoid sitting or standing for long periods
- Need to take prophylactic antimicrobials before any dental work or invasive procedure.

Promotes healing.
Decreases pooling of blood in the lower extremities.
Prevents infection.
Some physicians recommend this for the first 6–12 months after surgical placement of a synthetic graft.

RELATED CARE PLANS

Standardized Preoperative Care Plan
Standardized Postoperative Care Plan

HEART FAILURE

Heart failure is a syndrome in which the heart is unable to pump an adequate supply of blood to meet the body's metabolic needs. To compensate for decreased cardiac output, there is an increase in sympathetic nervous system activity and stimulation of renin-angiotensin-aldosterone output and ADH release. These neurohormonal compensatory mechanisms temporarily aid in maintaining an adequate cardiac output but are thought to contribute to cardiac remodeling (changes in the structure of the ventricle [e.g., dilation, hypertrophy]). The increase in fluid volume that results from increased aldosterone and ADH causes elevated pressure in the cardiac chambers, which stimulates the release of natriuretic peptides (atrial natriuretic factor [ANF] and BNP). These hormones counteract the effects of the increased levels of norepinephrine, renin, angiotensin II, and aldosterone and promote sodium and water excretion and vasodilation. Chronic distention of the heart chambers eventually exhausts stores of these natriuretic hormones and the effects of norepinephrine, renin, aldosterone, and ADH prevail, leading to heart failure.

Numerous conditions can lead to heart failure including CAD, MI, cardiomyopathy, cardiac valve malfunction, hypertension, congenital heart defects, and systemic conditions that increase the metabolic rate (e.g., thyrotoxicosis, infection) or cause prolonged or severe hypoxia. Heart failure can be classified in a number of ways. It is often classified as left-sided or right-sided, backward or forward, and/or systolic or diastolic failure. A functional classification system based on the relationship between symptoms and the amount of activity needed to provoke the symptoms was developed by the New York Heart Association and is commonly used by many practitioners. In this system, which has four levels or classes, a person is said to have class I (mild) heart failure if no symptoms are experienced with ordinary physical activity and class IV (severe) failure when symptoms occur with any physical activity and possibly at rest. The American Heart Association and American College of Cardiology classify heart failure by stages from stage A (at risk but without structural heart disease or symptoms) to stage D or refractory heart failure requiring advanced care measures (e.g., heart transplant). Current algorithms combine both classification systems when recommending treatment by classification/stage.

Signs and symptoms of heart failure are dependent on which side of the heart is failing as well as whether there is forward or backward failure. Symptoms of forward failure are caused by low cardiac output. Symptoms of backward failure are associated with the ventricle failing to empty completely, which results in blood flow backup. In left-sided failure, there is reduced emptying of the left ventricle, which results in decreased systemic tissue perfusion as well as blood flow

backup in the left atrium and pulmonary vasculature. Pulmonary vascular congestion leads to pulmonary edema with symptoms such as tachypnea, dyspnea, cough, and abnormal breath sounds. In right-sided failure, the effect of reduced function and emptying of the right ventricle is decreased pulmonary blood flow and backup of blood in the right atrium. This results in systemic venous congestion, which is manifested by peripheral edema and signs of major organ enlargement and dysfunction. Initially only one side of the heart may fail (more commonly the left side), but as failure progresses, both sides are usually affected.

Biomarkers used in initial and serial evaluation of the presence and severity of heart failure include B-type natriuretic peptide (BNP) and N-terminal pro-B-type natriuretic peptide (NT-proBNP). BNP is a hormone produced in the heart while NT-proBNP is a non-active prohormone released from the same molecule as BNP. Both biomarkers are released in response to changes in pressure inside the heart that occur in the presence of heart failure and are elevated in patients with heart failure.

The treatment of heart failure is dependent upon the classification of heart failure with the overall goal to improve performance of the failing heart. Pharmacological treatment consists of renin-angiotensin system inhibition with angiotensin converting enzyme inhibitors (ACE-I) or angiotensin receptor blockers (ARNI). A positive inotropic agent (e.g., digitalis) may be used in selected patients to ameliorate symptoms. Additional medications that may be used in symptomatic patients include beta blockers (e.g., carvedilol) and aldosterone inhibitors (e.g., spironolactone). Recent studies have shown that the addition of a beta-adrenergic blocking agent and spironolactone also improve the clinical status of many persons with chronic heart failure. It is thought that ACE inhibitors, beta blockers, and spironolactone interfere with the compensatory neurohormonal activity that occurs with heart failure and alter the course of cardiac remodeling, subsequently slowing disease progression. The pharmacological treatment of heart failure varies somewhat depending on whether the client has systolic failure (an impaired inotropic state characterized by inadequate ventricular emptying) or diastolic failure (impaired filling of the ventricle). Positive inotropic agents are contraindicated for treatment of diastolic failure.

As long as the body's compensatory mechanisms and/or treatment measures are able to maintain cardiac output that is sufficient to prevent or relieve symptoms, a state of compensated heart failure exists. If the myocardium is severely damaged and intrinsic compensatory mechanisms and treatment measures fail to maintain adequate cardiac output and tissue perfusion, a state of decompensated heart failure exists. When this state persists and is no longer responsive to medical treatment, it is termed intractable or refractory heart failure.

This care plan focuses on the adult client hospitalized for management of heart failure. Much of the information is applicable to clients receiving follow-up care in an extended care facility or home setting.

OUTCOME/DISCHARGE CRITERIA

The client will:
1. Have vital signs within a safe range and evidence of adequate peripheral circulation
2. Tolerate expected level of activity without undue fatigue or dyspnea
3. Have achieved dry weight and have minimal or no edema
4. Have clear, audible breath sounds throughout lungs
5. Have oxygen saturation within normal limits for client's age
6. Identify modifiable cardiovascular risk factors and ways to alter these factors
7. Verbalize an understanding of the rationale for and components of a diet low in sodium
8. Demonstrate accuracy in counting pulse
9. Verbalize an understanding of medications ordered including rationale, food and drug interactions, side effects, schedule for taking, and importance of taking as prescribed
10. State signs and symptoms to report to the health care provider
11. Identify community resources that can assist with home management and adjustment to changes resulting from heart failure
12. Share feelings and concerns about changes in body functioning and usual roles and lifestyle
13. Develop a plan for adhering to recommended follow-up care including future appointments with health care provider and activity limitations.

USE IN CONJUNCTION WITH THE CARE PLAN ON IMMOBILITY

Nursing Diagnosis **DECREASED CARDIAC OUTPUT** NDx

Definition: Inadequate blood pumped by the heart to the meet metabolic demands of the body.

Related to:
- Alterations in preload, afterload, and myocardial contractility associated with the cardiac condition causing the heart failure (e.g., ischemia of the myocardium, valve malfunction, cardiomyopathy)
- The effects of sympathetic nervous system and renin-angiotensin-aldosterone stimulation that occur in response to decreased cardiac output
- Structural changes in the heart (e.g., dilation, hypertrophy) that occur with prolonged activation of neurohormonal adaptive responses

CLINICAL MANIFESTATIONS

Subjective	Objective
Verbal self-report of fatigue; weakness; dyspnea; orthopnea; dizziness	Variations in B/P; tachycardia; pulsus alternans; S_3 heart sounds; tachypnea; dry, hacking cough; productive cough with pink, frothy sputum; abnormal breath sounds (e.g., crackles/rales, wheezes); syncope; diminished or absent pulses; cool extremities; capillary refill time greater than 3 seconds; decreased urine output; nocturia; edema; JVD; elevated serum levels of BNP and ANF; increased (CVP; chest radiograph evidence of pulmonary vascular congestion or pulmonary edema

DESIRED OUTCOMES

The client will have improved cardiac output as evidenced by:
a. B/P within normal range for client
b. Apical pulse between 60 and 100 beats/min and regular
c. Resolution of gallop rhythm
d. Verbalization of feeling less fatigued and weak
e. Unlabored respirations at 12 to 20 breaths/min
f. Improved breath sounds
g. Usual mental status
h. Absence of dizziness and syncope
i. Palpable peripheral pulses
j. Skin warm and usual color
k. Capillary refill time less than 2 to 3 seconds
l. Urine output at least 30 mL/h
m. Decrease in edema and jugular vein distention
n. CVP within normal range

NOC OUTCOMES

Cardiac pump effectiveness; circulation status; tissue perfusion: peripheral

NIC INTERVENTIONS

Cardiac care: acute; invasive hemodynamic monitoring; hemodynamic regulation; cardiac risk management; dysrhythmia management; hypervolemia management; cardiac care: rehabilitative

NURSING ASSESSMENT

Assess for signs and symptoms of heart failure and decreased cardiac output:
- Dyspnea, orthopnea
- Variations in B/P
- Tachycardia
- Pulsus alternans
- S_3 heart sounds
- Tachypnea
- Dry, hacking cough
- Productive cough with pink, frothy sputum
- Abnormal breath sounds (e.g., crackles/rales, wheezes)
- Syncope
- Diminished or absent pulses
- Cool extremities
- Capillary refill time greater than 3 seconds
- Decreased urine output
- Nocturia
- Edema
- JVD

Assess chest radiograph results for abnormalities (e.g., pulmonary vascular congestion or pulmonary edema).

Assess serum levels of BNP and NT-proBNP for abnormalities.

RATIONALE

Early recognition of signs and symptoms of heart failure and decreased cardiac output allows for prompt intervention.

THERAPEUTIC INTERVENTIONS

Independent Actions

Implement measures to improve cardiac output:
- Perform actions to reduce cardiac workload:
  - Place client in a semi- to high-Fowler's position. **D** ● ✦
  - Instruct client to avoid activities that create a Valsalva response (e.g., straining to have a bowel movement, holding breath while moving up in bed).
  - Implement measures to promote emotional and physical rest:
    - Maintain a calm, quiet environment.
    - Limit the number of visitors.
    - Maintain activity restrictions. **D** ● ✦
- Implement measures to improve respiratory status:
  - Position in semi- to high-Fowler's position
  - Administer supplemental oxygen
- Discourage smoking. **D** ✦

- Provide small meals rather than large ones. **D** ✦

- Discourage excessive intake of beverages high in caffeine such as coffee, tea, and colas. **D** ✦
- Increase activity gradually as allowed and tolerated. **D** ● ✦

RATIONALE

Measures that impact preload, afterload, and contractility help to improve cardiac performance, resulting in increased cardiac output.

Actions help improve alveolar gas exchange and promote adequate tissue oxygenation to the heart, improving performance.

Nicotine has a cardiostimulatory effect and causes vasoconstriction; the carbon monoxide in smoke reduces oxygen availability.

Large meals can increase cardiac workload because they require a greater increase in blood supply to gastrointestinal tract for digestion.

Caffeine is a myocardial stimulant and can increase myocardial oxygen consumption.

THERAPEUTIC INTERVENTIONS	RATIONALE

Dependent/Collaborative Actions
Implement measures to improve cardiac output:

• Perform actions to reduce cardiac workload: • Implement measures to reduce excess fluid volume.	*Decreasing circulating fluid volume reduces preload, thus reducing the workload of the heart.*
• Administer diuretics (e.g., Lasix)	*In addition, reducing excess fluid volume helps to decrease pulmonary vascular congestion.*
• Administer the following medications if ordered: • Diuretics	*Reduce sodium and water retention and subsequently reduce cardiac workload.*
• ACE inhibitors—angiotensin-converting enzyme inhibitors	*Reduce vascular resistance and subsequently decrease cardiac workload; they also alter the course of cardiac remodeling and slow disease progression.*
• ARBs—angiotensin blockers	*Block the action of angiotensin II by preventing it from binding to angiotensin II receptors on the blood vessels. Associated with a much lower incidence of cough and angioedema than ACE inhibitors.*
• Positive inotropic agents	*To improve myocardial contractility.*
• Beta-adrenergic blocking agents	*To blunt the effects of sympathetic nervous system stimulation on the heart and kidney.*
• B-type natriuretic peptide (nesiritide)	*To promote diuresis and vasodilation.*
• Vasodilators	*To reduce cardiac workload.*
Consult physician if signs and symptoms of decreased cardiac output persist or worsen.	*Consulting the appropriate health care provider allows for modification of the treatment plan.*

Nursing Diagnosis   IMPAIRED RESPIRATORY FUNCTION*

Definition: **Ineffective Breathing Pattern NDx:** Inspiration and/or expiration that does not provide adequate ventilation; **Ineffective Airway Clearance NDx:** Inability to clear secretions or obstructions from the respiratory tract to maintain a clear airway; **Impaired Gas Exchange NDx:** Excess or deficient in oxygenation and/or carbon dioxide elimination at the alveolar–capillary membrane.

Ineffective breathing pattern NDx related to:
• Increased rate of respirations associated with fear and anxiety
• Decreased depth of respirations associated with:
   • Weakness, fatigue, and decreased mobility
   • Decreased lung compliance (distensibility) as a result of pleural effusion or accumulation of fluid in the pulmonary interstitium
   • Pressure on the diaphragm if ascites is present

Ineffective airway clearance NDx related to:
• Increased airway resistance associated with edema of the bronchial mucosa and pressure on the airways resulting from engorgement of the pulmonary vessels
• Stasis of secretions associated with decreased mobility and poor cough effort

Impaired gas exchange NDx related to:
• Impaired diffusion of gases associated with accumulation of fluid in the pulmonary interstitium and alveoli
• Decreased pulmonary tissue perfusion associated with decreased cardiac output

CLINICAL MANIFESTATIONS

Subjective	Objective
Verbal self-reports of dyspnea; orthopnea; restlessness; irritability	Rapid, shallow, slow, or irregular respirations; use of accessory muscles when breathing; adventitious breath sounds (e.g., crackles [rales], wheezes); diminished or absent breath sounds; dry, hacking cough or cough productive of frothy or blood-tinged sputum; limited chest excursion; confusion, somnolence; central cyanosis (a late sign); significant decrease in oximetry results; abnormal arterial blood gas values; abnormal chest radiograph results

*This diagnostic label includes the following nursing diagnoses: ineffective breathing pattern, ineffective airway clearance, and impaired gas exchange.

RISK FACTORS

- Fluid volume overload
- Structural valve defects
- MI

DESIRED OUTCOMES

The client will experience adequate respiratory function as evidenced by:
a. Normal rate, rhythm, and depth of respirations
b. Decreased dyspnea
c. Usual or improved breath sounds
d. Symmetrical chest excursion
e. Usual mental status
f. Oximetry results within normal range
g. Arterial blood gas values within normal range

NOC OUTCOMES

Respiratory status: ventilation; airway patency; gas exchange

NIC INTERVENTIONS

Respiratory monitoring; airway management; chest physiotherapy; cough enhancement; ventilation assistance; oxygen therapy; anxiety reduction

NURSING ASSESSMENT

Assess for signs and symptoms of impaired respiratory function:
- Dyspnea, orthopnea
- Restlessness, irritability
- Rapid, shallow, slow, or irregular respirations
- Use of accessory muscles when breathing
- Adventitious breath sounds (e.g., crackles [rales], wheezes)
- Diminished or absent breath sounds
- Dry, hacking cough or cough productive of frothy or blood-tinged sputum
- Limited chest excursion
- Confusion, somnolence
- Central cyanosis (a late sign)

Assess results of chest radiograph, pulse oximetry, and arterial blood gases for abnormalities.

RATIONALE

Early recognition of signs and symptoms of impaired respiratory dysfunction allows for prompt intervention.

THERAPEUTIC INTERVENTIONS

Independent Actions

Implement measures to improve respiratory status:

- Perform actions to reduce fear and anxiety:
  - Maintain a calm, supportive, confident manner when interacting with the client.
- Instruct client to breathe slowly if hyperventilating.
- Place client in a semi- to high-Fowler's position unless contraindicated; position overbed table so client can lean forward on it if desired. **D** ● ✦
- Instruct client to change position and deep breathe or use incentive spirometer every 1 to 2 hrs.
- Perform actions to increase strength and activity tolerance.

- Perform actions to promote removal of pulmonary secretions:
  - Instruct and assist client to cough or "huff" every 1 to 2 hrs.
  - Humidify inspired air as ordered. **D** ✦
- Instruct client to avoid intake of gas-forming foods (e.g., beans, cauliflower, cabbage, onions), carbonated beverages, and large meals.

RATIONALE

To improve pulmonary tissue perfusion and reduce fluid accumulation in the lungs.
Decreases respiratory rate and anxiety.

Improves lung expansion and decreases stasis of secretions.

Increasing strength and activity help with mobilization and removal of secretions.

To keep secretions thin.
In order to prevent gastric distention and an increase in pressure on the diaphragm.

NDx = NANDA Diagnosis   **D** = Delegatable Action   ● = UAP   ✦ = LVN/LPN   ⊜▶ = Go to ⊜volve for animation

THERAPEUTIC INTERVENTIONS	RATIONALE
• Discourage smoking.	*The irritants in smoke increase mucus production, impair ciliary function, and can cause damage to the bronchial and alveolar walls; the carbon monoxide in smoke decreases oxygen availability.*
• Maintain activity restrictions; increase activity gradually as allowed and tolerated. **D** ● ✦	*Improves strength.*

Dependent/Collaborative Actions
Implement measures to improve respiratory status:
• Perform actions to improve cardiac output:

• Administer positive inotropic agents.	*Positive inotropic agents increase cardiac output by improving myocardial contractility.*

• Maintain oxygen therapy as ordered.   *Improves tissue oxygenation.*
• Assist with positive airway pressure techniques (e.g., continuous positive airway pressure [CPAP], bilevel positive airway pressure [BiPAP], flutter/positive expiratory pressure [PEP] device) if ordered.

    Positive airway pressure techniques help to improve oxygenation by keeping terminal airways and alveoli open. The more alveoli that remain open, the better the gas exchange.

• Administer central nervous system depressants judiciously; hold medication and consult physician if respiratory rate is less than 12 breaths/min.
• Administer the following medications if ordered:

• Diuretics **D** ✦	*Diuretics help to decrease pulmonary vascular congestion.*
• Theophylline **D** ✦	*Theophylline helps to dilate the bronchioles.*
• Morphine sulfate	*Morphine has a vasodilatory action that helps to reduce myocardial workload; morphine also reduces apprehension associated with dyspnea.*

• Assist with thoracentesis/paracentesis if performed.	*Removes excess fluid to allow increased lung expansion.*
Consult appropriate health care provider (e.g., physician, respiratory therapist) if signs and symptoms of impaired respiratory function persist or worsen.	*Allows for multidisciplinary client care.*

Collaborative Diagnosis   # RISK FOR IMBALANCED FLUID NDx AND RISK FOR ELECTROLYTE IMBALANCE NDx

Definition: Risk for Imbalanced Fluid NDx: Susceptible to a decrease, increase, or rapid shift from one to the other of intravascular, interstitial, and/or intracellular fluid which may compromise health. This refers to body fluid loss, gain, or both; **Risk for Electrolyte Imbalance NDx:** Susceptible to changes in serum electrolyte levels, which may compromise health.

Related to:
• **Excess fluid volume NDx** related to:
  • Retention of sodium and water associated with a decreased glomerular filtration rate (GFR) and activation of the renin-angiotensin-aldosterone mechanism (both are a result of the reduced renal blood flow that occurs with decreased cardiac output)
  • Decreased excretion of water associated with increased ADH output (a compensatory response to decreased cardiac output)
• **Third-spacing of fluid** related to:
  • Increased intravascular pressure associated with excess fluid volume
  • Low plasma colloid osmotic pressure if serum albumin is decreased as a result of malnutrition or impaired liver function (occurs with hepatic venous congestion)
• **Hyponatremia** related to:
  • Hemodilution associated with excess fluid volume
  • Sodium loss associated with diuretic therapy and increased release of natriuretic peptide hormones

CLINICAL MANIFESTATIONS

Subjective	Objective
Fluid overload: Verbal self-report of dyspnea; orthopnea	**Fluid overload**: Weight gain of 2% or greater in a short period; elevated B/P (B/P may not be elevated if cardiac output is poor or fluid has shifted out of the vascular space); presence of an S_3 heart sound; intake greater than output; change in mental status; crackles (rales); low Hct (may be normal or even increased if fluid has shifted out of the vascular space); edema; distended neck veins; elevated CVP (use internal jugular vein pulsation method to estimate CVP if monitoring device not present)
Third-spacing: Verbal self-reports of increased dyspnea	**Third-spacing**: Ascites; diminished or absent breath sounds; evidence of vascular depletion (e.g., postural hypotension; weak, rapid pulse; decreased urine output)
Hyponatremia: Verbal self-reports of nausea; weakness	**Hyponatremia**: Vomiting; abdominal cramps; confusion; seizures; low serum sodium level

DESIRED OUTCOMES

The client will experience resolution of fluid imbalance as evidenced by:
a. Decline in weight toward client's normal
b. B/P and pulse within normal range for client and stable with position change
c. Resolution of S_3 heart sound
d. Balanced intake and output
e. Usual mental status
f. Improved breath sounds
g. Hct returning toward normal range
h. Decreased dyspnea and orthopnea
i. Decrease in edema and ascites
j. Resolution of neck vein distention
k. CVP within normal range

The client will maintain a safe serum sodium level as evidenced by:
a. Usual mental status
b. Usual muscle strength
c. Absence of seizure activity
d. Serum sodium level within normal range

NOC OUTCOMES

Fluid balance; fluid overload severity; electrolyte and acid-base balance

NIC INTERVENTIONS

Fluid monitoring; fluid/electrolyte management; electrolyte management: hyponatremia; hypervolemia management

NURSING ASSESSMENT	RATIONALE

Assess for signs and symptoms of fluid and electrolyte imbalance:
 • Fluid overload
   • Dyspnea, orthopnea
   • Weight gain of 2% or greater in a short period
   • Elevated B/P (B/P may not be elevated if cardiac output is poor or fluid has shifted out of the vascular space)
   • Presence of an S_3 heart sound
   • Intake greater than output
   • Change in mental status
   • Crackles (rales)
   • Low Hct (may be normal or even increased if fluid has shifted out of the vascular space)
   • Edema
   • Distended neck veins
   • Elevated CVP (use internal jugular vein pulsation method to estimate CVP if monitoring device not present)
	Early recognition of signs and symptoms of fluid and electrolyte imbalance allows for prompt intervention.

Continued...

NURSING ASSESSMENT	RATIONALE

- Third-spacing
  - Increased dyspnea
  - Ascites
  - Diminished or absent breath sounds
  - Evidence of vascular depletion (e.g., postural hypotension; weak, rapid pulse; decreased urine output)
- Hyponatremia
  - Nausea, weakness
  - Vomiting
  - Abdominal cramps
  - Confusion
  - Seizures
  - Low serum sodium level

Monitor chest x-ray results for indications of pulmonary vascular congestion, pleural effusion, or pulmonary edema.

Monitor serum albumin levels for abnormalities.

Low serum albumin levels result in fluid shifting out of the vascular space because albumin normally maintains plasma colloid osmotic pressure.

THERAPEUTIC INTERVENTIONS	RATIONALE

Dependent/Collaborative Actions

Implement measures to restore fluid balance:
- Perform actions to reduce excess fluid volume:
  - Restrict sodium intake as ordered.
  - Maintain fluid restrictions if ordered.
  - Implement measures to improve cardiac output.
  - If client is receiving numerous and/or large-volume intravenous medications, consult pharmacist about ways to prevent excessive fluid administration (e.g., stop primary infusion during administration of intravenous medications, dilute medications in the minimum amount of solution).
  - Administer diuretics as ordered.
- Perform actions to prevent further third-spacing and promote mobilization of fluid back into the vascular space:
  - Administer albumin infusions if ordered.

  - Assist with thoracentesis or paracentesis if performed.

Implement measures to treat hyponatremia:
- Maintain fluid restrictions if ordered.
- Administer intravenous saline solution if ordered (if client's hyponatremia is thought to be due to "salt wasting," treatment includes administration of saline and discontinuation of diuretics).
- Consult physician about a decrease in or discontinuation of diuretics and temporary discontinuation of dietary sodium restriction if sodium level is significantly reduced.

Consult physician if signs and symptoms of imbalanced fluid and/or hyponatremia persist or worsen.

All actions help to reduce circulating fluid volume, helping to decrease preload and reduce the workload of the heart. Decreasing circulating fluid volume and implementing measures to optimize cardiac output help to restore circulation and improve oxygenation and tissue perfusion to the vital organs.

Diuretics help increase excretion of water.

Increasing colloid osmotic pressure with the infusion of protein-based fluids pulls accumulated third-spaced fluid back into the vascular space, reducing edema.

Remove excess fluid from the pleural space or peritoneal cavity.

For hyponatremia induced by water excess, fluid restrictions are implemented to treat the problem.

If hyponatremia is severe and associated with neurological symptoms, 3% saline may be administered to restore sodium levels while the body is returning to a normal fluid balance.

Diuretic therapy causes loss of sodium.

Consulting the appropriate health care provider allows for modification of the treatment plan.

Collaborative Diagnosis | RISK FOR RENAL INSUFFICIENCY

Definition: A deficiency in the kidney's ability to clear waste products; a sign of inadequate glomerular filtration.

Related to: A prolonged or severe decrease in renal blood flow associated with low cardiac output, volume depletion (may result from third-spacing, increased output of natriuretic hormones, and/or excessive diuretic use), and vasodilator-induced hypotension

CLINICAL MANIFESTATIONS

Subjective	**Objective**
Not applicable	Urine output less than 30 mL/h; urine specific gravity fixed at or less than 1.010; elevated BUN and serum creatinine levels; decreased creatinine clearance

RISK FACTORS
- Decreased cardiac output
- Volume depletion

DESIRED OUTCOMES

The client will maintain adequate renal function as evidenced by:
a. Urine output at least 30 mL/h
b. BUN, serum creatinine, and creatinine clearance values within normal range

NURSING ASSESSMENT	**RATIONALE**
Assess for and report signs and symptoms of impaired renal function: • Urine output < 30 mL/h • Urine specific gravity ≤ 1.010 • Elevated BUN/serum creatinine • Decreased creatinine clearance Monitor serum electrolyte, BUN/creatinine results for abnormalities.	*Early recognition and reporting of signs and symptoms of renal insufficiency allow for prompt intervention.*

THERAPEUTIC INTERVENTIONS	**RATIONALE**
Dependent/Collaborative Actions Implement measures to maintain adequate renal blood flow: • Perform actions to improve cardiac output. • Perform actions to reduce third-spacing. • Ensure a minimum fluid intake of 1000 mL/day unless ordered otherwise. • Consult physician before giving vasodilators and diuretics if client is hypotensive. If signs and symptoms of impaired renal function occur: • Consult physician about possible need to reduce the digitalis dosage. • Consult physician about lowering the dose of or discontinuing angiotensin-converting enzyme (ACE) inhibitors and diuretics if BUN and serum creatinine levels continue to rise significantly. • Assess for and report signs of acute renal failure (e.g., oliguria or anuria; further weight gain; increasing edema; increased B/P; lethargy and confusion; increasing BUN and serum creatinine, phosphorus, and potassium levels). • Prepare client for dialysis if indicated.	*Prerenal causes of renal insufficiency/renal failure include factors such as decreased cardiac output and hypovolemia, which can reduce blood flow to the kidneys, decreasing the glomerular perfusion and filtration.* *Digitalis is excreted by the kidney and will quickly reach toxic levels when renal function is impaired.* *ACE inhibitors and many diuretics should be used cautiously in persons with impaired renal function because they can have an adverse effect on renal function.*

NDx = NANDA Diagnosis   **D** = Delegatable Action   ● = UAP   ✦ = LVN/LPN   ⊖▶ = Go to ⊖volve for animation

⊖▶ Collaborative Diagnosis   # RISK FOR CARDIAC DYSRHYTHMIAS

Definition: Irregularities of the heart rate or rhythm.

Related to:
- Impaired nodal function and/or altered myocardial conductivity associated with:
  - Hypoxia
  - Sympathetic nervous system stimulation (a compensatory response to low cardiac output)
  - Structural changes in the myocardium (e.g., dilation, hypertrophy)
  - Imbalanced electrolytes (particularly the magnesium and potassium depletion that can result from diuretic therapy)

CLINICAL MANIFESTATIONS

Subjective	Objective
Verbal self-report of lightheadedness/dizziness	Irregular apical pulse; pulse rate below 60 or above 100 beats/min; apical-radial pulse deficit; syncope; palpitations; abnormal rate, rhythm, or configurations on ECG

RISK FACTORS
- Diuretic administration
- MI

DESIRED OUTCOMES

The client will maintain normal sinus rhythm as evidenced by:
a. Regular apical pulse at 60 to 100 beats/min
b. Equal apical and radial pulse rates
c. Absence of syncope and palpitations
d. ECG reading showing normal sinus rhythm

NURSING ASSESSMENT	RATIONALE
Assess for and report signs and symptoms of cardiac dysrhythmias: • Subjective • Objective Monitor ECG for abnormalities. Monitor serum electrolyte levels for abnormalities.	*Early recognition of signs and symptoms of cardiac dysrhythmias allows for prompt intervention.*

THERAPEUTIC INTERVENTIONS	RATIONALE
Dependent/Collaborative Actions Implement measures to prevent cardiac dysrhythmias: • Perform actions to improve cardiac output.	*Adequate cardiac output helps to promote adequate myocardial tissue perfusion and oxygenation. Myocardial ischemia can lead to dysrhythmias.*
• Perform actions to improve respiratory status.	*Optimum respiratory function helps to improve tissue oxygenation, reducing the potential for myocardial ischemia.*
• Consult physician regarding an order for a potassium (K⁺) or magnesium (Mg⁺) replacement if serum levels of either are below normal.	K^+ and Mg^+ *abnormalities can cause cardiac dysrhythmias.*
If cardiac dysrhythmias occur: • Initiate cardiac monitoring if not already being done. • Administer antidysrhythmics if ordered. • Restrict client's activity based on client's tolerance and severity of the dysrhythmia.	*Decreases stress on the heart.*
• Maintain oxygen therapy as ordered.	*Increases tissue oxygenation.*
• Assess cardiovascular status frequently and report signs and symptoms of a further decline in cardiac output and tissue perfusion.	
• Prepare client for catheter ablation or insertion of a pacemaker or ICD if planned.	*Decreases fear and anxiety.*

THERAPEUTIC INTERVENTIONS	RATIONALE
• Have emergency cart readily available for cardioversion, defibrillation, or CPR.	

Collaborative Diagnosis **RISK FOR ACUTE PULMONARY EDEMA**

Definition: Excess water in the lungs, usually a result of heart failure.

Related to: Accumulation of fluid in the lungs associated with increased hydrostatic pressure in the pulmonary vessels as a result of blood flow backup in the left ventricle

CLINICAL MANIFESTATIONS

Subjective	Objective
Verbal self-report of shortness of breath	Increased crackles (rales) or wheezes; disorientation; increased restlessness and anxiousness; cough productive of frothy or blood-tinged sputum; significant decrease in oximetry results; worsening arterial blood gas results; chest radiograph showing pulmonary edema

RISK FACTORS	DESIRED OUTCOMES
• Acute MI • Decreased cardiac output • High afterload	The client will not develop acute pulmonary edema as evidenced by: a. Decreased dyspnea b. Usual or improved breath sounds c. Usual mental status d. Arterial blood gas values within normal range

NURSING ASSESSMENT	RATIONALE
Assess for and report signs and symptoms of acute pulmonary edema: • Subjective • Objective Monitor pulse oximetry and arterial blood gas values and chest radiograph results for abnormalities.	*Early recognition of signs and symptoms of acute pulmonary edema allows for prompt intervention.*

THERAPEUTIC INTERVENTIONS	RATIONALE

Dependent/Collaborative Actions
Implement measures to improve cardiac output.
 	
If signs and symptoms of pulmonary edema occur:
• Place client in a high-Fowler's position unless contraindicated.
• Maintain oxygen therapy as ordered.
• Administer the following medications if ordered:
  • Diuretics
  • Theophylline
  • Morphine sulfate
 	
• Vasodilators
	Improving cardiac output results in a decrease in pulmonary vascular congestion as the left side of the heart improves performance.
	Interventions for acute pulmonary edema focus on the immediate improvement of oxygenation and relief of pulmonary vascular congestion by improving cardiac output and diuresis to reduce fluid accumulation in the lungs.
	
	Morphine sulfate is very beneficial in acute pulmonary edema because it helps to reduce anxiety and decrease pulmonary vascular congestion (increases venous capacitance, which lowers venous return to the heart).
	Vasodilators help to reduce afterload and improve left ventricular emptying, which reduces pulmonary blood flow backup.

Collaborative Diagnosis   **RISK FOR THROMBOEMBOLISM**

Definition: A clot attached to a vessel wall that detaches and circulates within the blood.

Related to:
- Venous stasis in the periphery associated with decreased cardiac output and decreased mobility
- Stasis of blood in the heart associated with decreased ventricular emptying (risk increases if dysrhythmias are present)

CLINICAL MANIFESTATIONS

Subjective	Objective
Verbal self-reports of deep vein thrombus: Pain, tenderness	**Deep vein thrombus:** Swelling, unusual warmth, and/or positive Homans' sign in extremity
Verbal self-reports of arterial thrombus: Numbness and/or pain in extremity	**Arterial thrombus:** Diminished or absent peripheral pulses; pallor, coolness
Cerebral ischemia: Not applicable	**Cerebral ischemia:** Decreased level of consciousness; alteration in usual sensory and motor function
Verbal self-reports of pulmonary embolism: Sudden onset of chest pain; increased dyspnea	**Pulmonary embolism:** Increased restlessness and apprehension; significant decrease in arterial oxygen saturation (SaO_2)

RISK FACTORS
- Venous stasis
- Atrial fibrillation
- Mural thrombus

DESIRED OUTCOMES

The client will not develop a thromboembolism as evidenced by:
a. Absence of pain, tenderness, swelling, and numbness in extremities
b. Usual temperature and color of extremities
c. Palpable and equal peripheral pulses
d. Usual mental status
e. Usual sensory and motor function
f. Absence of sudden chest pain and increased dyspnea

NURSING ASSESSMENT

Assess for and report signs and symptoms of deep vein thrombus, arterial embolus in an extremity, cerebral ischemia, or pulmonary embolism:
- Pain/tenderness in extremity
- Chest pain
- Shortness of breath
- Altered mental status
- Diminished/absent pulses

RATIONALE

Early recognition of signs and symptoms of thromboembolism allows for prompt intervention.

THERAPEUTIC INTERVENTIONS

Dependent/Collaborative Actions

Implement additional measures to prevent the development of thromboemboli:
- Perform actions to improve cardiac output.
- Perform actions to treat cardiac dysrhythmias if present.
- Administer anticoagulants or antiplatelet agents if ordered.

If signs and symptoms of an arterial embolus in an extremity occur:
- Maintain client on bed rest with affected extremity in a level or slightly dependent position.

RATIONALE

Adequate cardiac output ensures that blood flow continues to the extremities without pooling. Dysrhythmias, especially atrial fibrillation, allow blood to pool in the atria, leading to clot formation. Anticoagulant therapy is used to prevent clot formation.

Improves arterial blood flow.

THERAPEUTIC INTERVENTIONS	RATIONALE
• Prepare client for the following if planned: • Diagnostic studies (e.g., Doppler or duplex ultrasound, arteriography)	*Decreases fear and anxiety.*
• Injection of a thrombolytic agent • Embolectomy	*Anticoagulants work to prevent a thrombus from increasing in size.*
• Administer anticoagulants as ordered.	
If signs and symptoms of cerebral ischemia occur: • Maintain client on bed rest; keep head and neck in neutral, midline position.	*Actions help to reduce intracranial pressure (ICP) that accompanies cerebral ischemia.*
• Administer anticoagulants as ordered.	

Collaborative Diagnosis # RISK FOR CARDIOGENIC SHOCK

Definition: Decreased cardiac output and evidence of tissue hypoxia in the presence of adequate intravascular volume.

Related to: Inability of heart, intrinsic compensatory mechanisms, and treatments to maintain adequate tissue perfusion to vital organs

CLINICAL MANIFESTATIONS

Subjective	Objective
Verbal self-report of increased restlessness, lethargy, or confusion	Systolic B/P below 80 mm Hg; rapid, weak pulse; diminished or absent peripheral pulses; increased coolness and duskiness or cyanosis of skin; urine output less than 30 mL/h

RISK FACTORS
- Acute MI
- Cardiomyopathy

DESIRED OUTCOMES

The client will not develop cardiogenic shock as evidenced by:
a. Stable or improved mental status
b. Systolic B/P greater than 80 mm Hg
c. Palpable peripheral pulses
d. Stable or improved skin temperature and color
e. Urine output at least 30 mL/h

NURSING ASSESSMENT	RATIONALE
Assess for and immediately report signs and symptoms of cardiogenic shock: • Confusion • Hypertension • Rapid, weak pulse • Diminished/absent pulse • Urine output < 30 mL/h	*Early recognition of signs and symptoms of cardiogenic shock allows for prompt intervention.*

THERAPEUTIC INTERVENTIONS	RATIONALE
Dependent/Collaborative Actions Implement measures to prevent cardiogenic shock: • Perform actions to improve cardiac output. • Perform actions to treat cardiac dysrhythmias if present.	*Treating dysrhythmias and restoring a stable cardiac rhythm improves filling time of the ventricles, enhancing cardiac output.*
If signs and symptoms of cardiogenic shock occur: • Maintain oxygen therapy as ordered.	*Increases tissue oxygenation.*
• Administer the following medications if ordered: • Sympathomimetics	*Sympathomimetics increase cardiac output and maintain arterial pressure.*

NDx = NANDA Diagnosis   **D** = Delegatable Action   ● = UAP   ✦ = LVN/LPN   ⊖▶ = Go to ⊖volve for animation

Continued...

THERAPEUTIC INTERVENTIONS	RATIONALE
• Vasodilators	*If the client's B/P is not too low, vasodilators can be used to decrease afterload, reducing cardiac workload.*
• Assist with intubation and insertion of hemodynamic monitoring device (e.g., Swan-Ganz catheter) and IABP if indicated.	*Cardiogenic shock unresponsive to drug therapy requires more invasive intervention to obtain numeric values that guide treatment or to assist the heart if function continues to deteriorate.*

DISCHARGE TEACHING/CONTINUED CARE

Nursing Diagnosis | ## DEFICIENT KNOWLEDGE NDx; INEFFECTIVE FAMILY HEALTH MANAGEMENT NDx; OR INEFFECTIVE HEALTH MANAGEMENT NDx*

Definition: **Deficient Knowledge NDx:** Absence of cognitive information related to a specific topic, or its acquisition; **Ineffective Family Health Management NDx:** A pattern of regulating and integrating into family processes a program for the treatment of illness and its sequelae that is unsatisfactory for meeting specific health goals of the family unit; **Ineffective Health Management NDx:** Pattern of regulating and integrating into daily living a therapeutic regimen for the treatment of illness and its sequelae that is unsatisfactory for meeting specific health goals.

CLINICAL MANIFESTATIONS

Subjective	Objective
Verbal self-report of unfamiliarity with information	Inability to follow-through with instructions

RISK FACTORS
• Denial of disease process
• Cognitive deficiency
• Failure to take action to reduce risk factors

NOC OUTCOMES	NIC INTERVENTIONS
Knowledge: treatment regimen; cardiac disease management; disease process; medication	Health system guidance; teaching: individual; teaching: disease process; teaching: prescribed diet; teaching: prescribed medication; teaching: prescribed activity/exercise

NURSING ASSESSMENT	RATIONALE
Assess client's readiness and ability to learn. Assess meaning of illness to client.	*Early recognition of readiness to learn and meaning of illness to client allows for implementation of the appropriate teaching interventions.*

THERAPEUTIC INTERVENTIONS	RATIONALE

Desired Outcome: The client will identify modifiable cardiovascular risk factors and ways to alter these factors.

Independent Actions
Inform client that certain modifiable factors such as elevated serum lipid levels, excessive alcohol intake, a sedentary lifestyle, hypertension, and smoking have been shown to increase the risk for CAD and certain forms of heart disease. | *Thorough education is a critical component of the care of a client with heart failure. The client must have a thorough understanding of the importance of adhering to diet, medication, activity/exercise, and nutritional recommendations to prevent an exacerbation and control the disease.*

Assist client to identify changes in lifestyle that can help the client manage the above risk factors (e.g., dietary modification, physical exercise on a regular basis, moderation of alcohol intake, smoking cessation). | *Improves client's ability to maintain or improve state of health.*

---

*The nurse should select the diagnostic label that is most appropriate for the client's discharge teaching needs.

THERAPEUTIC INTERVENTIONS	RATIONALE
Encourage client to limit daily alcohol consumption. Current recommendations are no more than two drinks per day for men and no more than one drink per day for women and lighter-weight persons. A "drink" is considered to be ½ oz of ethanol (e.g., 1½ oz of 80-proof whiskey, 12 oz of beer, 5 oz of wine).	*Daily alcohol intake exceeding 1 oz of ethanol may contribute to the development of hypertension and some forms of heart disease.*

THERAPEUTIC INTERVENTIONS	RATIONALE

Desired Outcome: The client will verbalize an understanding of the rationale for and components of a diet low in sodium.

Independent Actions

Explain the rationale for a diet low in sodium.

Provide the following information about decreasing sodium intake:

- Read labels on foods/fluids and calculate sodium content of items; avoid those products that tend to have a high sodium content (e.g., canned soups and vegetables, tomato juice, commercial baked goods, commercially prepared frozen or canned entrees and sauces).
- Do not add salt when cooking foods or to prepared foods; use low-sodium herbs and spices if desired.
- Avoid cured and smoked foods.
- Avoid salty snack foods (e.g., crackers, nuts, pretzels, potato chips).
- Avoid commercially prepared fast foods.
- Avoid routine use of over-the-counter medications with a high sodium content (e.g., Alka-Seltzer, some antacids).

Obtain a dietary consult to assist client in planning meals that will meet prescribed dietary modifications.

The edema associated with chronic heart failure is often treated with a reduction in dietary sodium. The degree of sodium restriction depends on the severity of heart failure and the effectiveness of diuretic therapy.

THERAPEUTIC INTERVENTIONS	RATIONALE

Desired Outcome: The client will demonstrate accuracy in counting pulse.

Independent Actions

Teach clients how to count their pulse, being alert to the regularity of the rhythm.

Allow time for return demonstration and accuracy check.

Educating clients to their baseline heart rate allows for early detection of irregularities that warrant immediate attention from a health care provider. Early detection may reduce the incidence of exacerbation of heart failure.

THERAPEUTIC INTERVENTIONS	RATIONALE

Desired Outcome: The client will verbalize an understanding of medications ordered including rationale, food and drug interactions, side effects, schedule for taking, and importance of taking as prescribed.

Independent Actions

Explain the rationale for, side effects of, and importance of taking the medications prescribed. Inform client of pertinent food and drug interactions.

- Digitalis preparations

Digitalis is a positive inotrope that improves cardiac contractility, increasing cardiac output.

Continued...

THERAPEUTIC INTERVENTIONS	RATIONALE
• Diuretics	*Diuretics help to mobilize edematous fluid, reducing pulmonary venous pressure and preload.*
• ACE inhibitors	*ACE inhibitors block the effects of ACE, which facilitates the conversion of angiotensin I to angiotensin II, a potent vasoconstrictor.*
• Beta-adrenergic blockers	*Beta-blockers reduce the effects of the sympathetic nervous system on the failing heart by slowing the heart rate.*
• ARBs—angiotensin blockers	*Block the action of angiotensin II by preventing it from binding to angiotensin II receptors on the blood vessels. Associated with a much lower incidence of cough and angioedema than ACE inhibitors.*
Instruct client to take medications on a regular basis and avoid skipping doses, altering prescribed dose, making up for missed doses, and discontinuing medication without permission of health care provider.	*Taking medications as prescribed ensures that therapeutic drug levels will be maintained.*
Instruct client to consult physician before taking other prescription and nonprescription medications. Instruct client to inform all health care providers of medications being taken.	*Clients should be instructed not to discontinue taking medications if they feel better. Clients without financial resources should be assisted in accessing appropriate resources to obtain needed medications (e.g., pharmacy assistance programs).*

THERAPEUTIC INTERVENTIONS	RATIONALE

Desired Outcome: The client will state signs and symptoms to report to the health care provider.

Independent Actions

Instruct client to report: • Weight gain of more than 2 lb in a day or 4 lb in a week • Increased swelling of ankles, feet, or abdomen • Persistent cough • Increasing shortness of breath • Chest discomfort/pain • Increased weakness and fatigue • Frequent nighttime urination • Signs and symptoms of digitalis toxicity • Side effects of diuretic therapy	*Reporting signs and symptoms of heart failure to the appropriate provider allows for modification of the treatment plan and possibly can prevent a client's readmission to the hospital.*

THERAPEUTIC INTERVENTIONS	RATIONALE

Desired Outcome: The client will identify community resources that can assist with home management and adjustment to changes resulting from heart failure.

Independent Actions

Provide information regarding community resources that can assist with home management and adjustment to changes resulting from heart failure (e.g., Meals on Wheels, home health agencies, transportation services, American Heart Association, counseling services).	*Heart failure can significantly impact an individual's and family's socioeconomic status. Providing information specific to community resources is important to provide a necessary continuum of care and may impact the client's health status, preventing future hospitalizations.*

THERAPEUTIC INTERVENTIONS	RATIONALE

Desired Outcome: The client, in collaboration with the nurse, will develop a plan for adhering to recommended follow-up care including future appointments with health care provider and activity limitations.

THERAPEUTIC INTERVENTIONS	RATIONALE

Independent Actions

Collaborate with the client to develop a plan to adhere to the treatment regimen that includes:

Reinforce the importance of keeping follow-up appointments with health care provider.

Provide the following instructions regarding activity:

- Increase activity gradually and only as tolerated.
- Stop any activity that causes chest pain, dizziness, or a significant increase in shortness of breath or fatigue.
- Plan and adhere to rest periods during the day.
- Adhere to physician's recommendations about activities that should be avoided.
- Notify physician if activity tolerance declines.
- Reduce dyspnea and fatigue during sexual activity by:
  - Avoiding sexual activity when unusually fatigued
  - Waiting 1 to 2 hrs after a heavy meal or alcohol intake before engaging in sexual activity
  - Identifying and using positions that minimize energy expenditure
  - Using portable oxygen during sexual activities

Implement measures to improve client adherence:

- Include significant others in teaching sessions if possible.

- Encourage questions and allow time for reinforcement and clarification of information provided.
- Provide written instructions regarding scheduled appointments with health care provider, medications prescribed, dietary sodium restrictions, and signs and symptoms to report.
- Ensure client has the necessary financial or social support resources to meet the conditions of the treatment plan.

Regular health care appointments are important to determine effectiveness of the prescribed treatment plan.

Involvement of significant others in patient teaching improves adherence to discharge instructions.

Everyone does not understand information as presented, so set aside time for questions to allow for clarification of information.

Written instructions allow the client to refer to instructions as needed.

ADDITIONAL NURSING DIAGNOSES

RISK FOR FALLS NDx

Related to:

- Weakness
- Dizziness and syncope associated with inadequate cerebral blood flow resulting from decreased cardiac output and the hypotensive effect of some medications (e.g., ACE inhibitors, diuretics)
- Getting up without assistance as a result of restlessness, agitation, forgetfulness, and confusion (can result from cerebral hypoxia and imbalanced fluid and electrolytes)

DISTURBED SLEEP PATTERN NDx

Related to: Unfamiliar environment, frequent assessments and treatments, decreased physical activity, fear, anxiety, and inability to assume usual sleep position associated with orthopnea

ACTIVITY INTOLERANCE NDx

Related to:

- Tissue hypoxia associated with impaired alveolar gas exchange and decreased cardiac output
- Inadequate nutritional status

- Difficulty resting and sleeping associated with dyspnea, frequent assessments and treatments, fear, and anxiety

RISK FOR IMPAIRED TISSUE INTEGRITY NDx

Related to:

- Damage to the skin and/or subcutaneous tissue associated with prolonged pressure on the tissues, friction, and/or shearing if mobility is decreased
- Increased fragility of the skin associated with edema, poor tissue perfusion, and inadequate nutritional status

IMBALANCED NUTRITION: LESS THAN BODY REQUIREMENTS NDx

Related to:

- Decreased oral intake associated with:
  - Anorexia and nausea (result from venous congestion in the gastrointestinal tract and can occur if digitalis levels exceed a therapeutic level)
  - Weakness, fatigue, dyspnea, and dislike of prescribed diet
- Elevated metabolic rate associated with the increased oxygen needs of the heart and the increased work of breathing
- Impaired absorption of nutrients associated with poor tissue perfusion

FEAR/ANXIETY NDx
Related to:
- Exacerbation of symptoms and need for hospitalization
- Lack of understanding of diagnostic tests, the diagnosis, and treatments
- Cost of hospitalization and lifelong treatment
- Possibility of early disability and death

NAUSEA NDx
Related to: Stimulation of the vomiting center associated with:
- Stimulation of the visceral afferent pathways resulting from vascular congestion in the heart and gastrointestinal tract
- Stimulation of the cerebral cortex resulting from stress
- Stimulation of the chemoreceptor trigger zone by certain medications (e.g., digitalis preparations)

DISTURBED THOUGHT PROCESSES NDx
Related to:
- Cerebral hypoxia associated with impaired alveolar gas exchange and inadequate cerebral tissue perfusion (a result of decreased cardiac output)
- Imbalanced fluid and electrolytes

INEFFECTIVE COPING NDx
Related to: Fear, anxiety, possible need to alter lifestyle, and knowledge that condition is chronic and will require life-long medical supervision and medication therapy

HEART SURGERY: CORONARY ARTERY BYPASS GRAFTING OR VALVE REPLACEMENT

Heart surgery is performed for a variety of reasons including myocardial revascularization, valve repair or replacement, repair of congenital or acquired structural abnormalities, placement of a mechanical assist device, and heart transplantation. Two common heart surgeries are CABG, which is done to treat severe CAD, and heart valve replacement. CABG involves removing a segment of a vein from a leg (e.g., saphenous, cephalic) or an artery from the chest (e.g., internal mammary, radial, gastroepiploic) to create an anastomosis between the aorta or other major artery and a point on the coronary artery distal to the obstruction. Heart valve replacement involves replacing the stenotic or regurgitant valve with a mechanical prosthesis or a biological (tissue) valve (porcine or bovine valve, human valve).

Heart surgery is usually performed through a median sternotomy. Cardiopulmonary bypass (CPB; extracorporeal circulation) is maintained during surgery by a machine that diverts the blood from the heart and lungs, oxygenates the blood and removes carbon dioxide, maintains the desired body temperature, filters the blood, and then recirculates the blood into the arterial system. Systemic hypothermia (provided by the CPB machine) can reduce tissue oxygen requirements to 50% of normal, which affords the major organs additional protection from ischemic injury. Cold cardioplegia (infusion of a cold alkaline solution containing potassium into the coronary circulation) is used to precipitate cardiac arrest and provide additional protection to the myocardium during surgery. An isotonic crystalloid solution is used to prime the bypass machine. This dilutes the client's blood, which improves blood flow and reduces the risk of microemboli formation. Before closing the chest, pacing electrodes are usually placed on the epicardial surface of the heart and brought out through the chest wall to be used for temporary pacing if needed. A chest tube is placed in the mediastinum to drain blood, and if needed, one is also placed in the pleural space to promote lung reexpansion.

In addition to the traditional sternotomy approach performed on CPB, heart surgery may be performed "off pump" (referred to as off pump coronary bypass [OPCAB]) or using a minimally invasive approach (e.g., small incision in left sternal border, a series of holes or "ports" using video-assisted equipment). Minimally invasive procedures such as a MIDCAB (minimally invasive direct coronary artery bypass) can be performed without CPB or with a less invasive, catheter-based system of CPB. Several techniques are used to stabilize the operative area during a beating heart procedure (stabilizer device to "still" certain areas of the heart while the rest keeps beating, drugs that decrease the heart rate or cause transient asystole). Because "off pump" and minimally invasive approaches reduce the risk for some of the major complications (e.g., mediastinitis, emboli associated with cross-clamping the aorta) and shorten hospitalization and rehabilitation time, they promise to become more common.

This care plan focuses on the adult client hospitalized for either CABG or valve replacement surgery. Much of the postoperative information is applicable to clients receiving follow-up care in an extended care facility or home setting.

OUTCOME/DISCHARGE CRITERIA

The client will:
1. Have adequate cardiac output and tissue perfusion
2. Have clear, audible breath sounds throughout lungs
3. Have evidence of normal healing of surgical wound(s)
4. Have oxygen saturation within normal limits for client's age
5. Tolerate expected level of activity
6. Have surgical pain controlled
7. Have no signs and symptoms of complications
8. Identify modifiable cardiovascular risk factors and ways to alter these factors
9. Verbalize an understanding of the rationale for and components of a diet restricted in sodium, saturated fat, and cholesterol
10. Verbalize an understanding of activity restrictions and the rate of activity progression
11. Verbalize an understanding of medications ordered including rationale, food and drug interactions, side effects, schedule for taking, and importance of taking as prescribed
12. State signs and symptoms to report to the health care provider
13. Identify community resources that can assist with cardiac rehabilitation and adjustment to having had heart surgery
14. Develop a plan for adhering to recommended follow-up care including future appointments with health care provider, wound care, and pain management

PREOPERATIVE: USE IN CONJUNCTION WITH THE STANDARDIZED PREOPERATIVE CARE PLAN

Related Preoperative Nursing/Collaborative Diagnoses   **FEAR** NDx**/ANXIETY** NDx

Definition: **Fear NDx:** Response to perceived threat that is recognized as danger; **Anxiety NDx:** Vague, uneasy feeling of discomfort or dread accompanied by an autonomic response (the source is often nonspecific or unknown to the individual); a feeling of apprehension caused by anticipation of danger. It is an alerting sign that warns of impending danger and enables the individual to take measures to deal with that threat.

Related to:
- Unfamiliar environment and separation from significant others
- Lack of understanding of diagnostic tests, preoperative procedures/preparation, planned surgery, and postoperative course
- Anticipated loss of control associated with effects of anesthesia
- Financial concerns associated with surgery and hospitalization
- Anticipated postoperative discomfort and alterations in lifestyle and roles
- Risk of disease if blood transfusions are necessary
- Potential embarrassment or loss of dignity associated with body exposure
- Possibility of death

POSTOPERATIVE: USE IN CONJUNCTION WITH THE STANDARDIZED POSTOPERATIVE CARE PLAN

Nursing Diagnosis   **DECREASED CARDIAC OUTPUT** NDx

Definition: Inadequate blood pumped by the heart to meet the metabolic demands of the body.

Related to:
- Preexisting compromise in cardiac function
- Trauma to the heart during surgery
- Increased afterload associated with:
  - Vasoconstriction resulting from hypothermia and an increase in catecholamine output and plasma renin levels (these increases occur with CPB and the effect of stressors [e.g., pain, anxiety])
  - Fluid overload
- Decreased preload associated with:
  - Hypovolemia (can result from blood loss, fluid shifting from the intravascular to interstitial space, loss of fluid from nasogastric tube, fluid intake, and excessive diuresis)
- Hypotension (can occur if body is warmed rapidly after surgery and as a result of the effect of anesthesia and certain medications [e.g., narcotic analgesics, beta-adrenergic blockers, vasodilators])
- Effects of anesthesia, hypothermia, hypoxemia, and acid-base and/or electrolyte imbalances on contractility and conductivity of the heart

CLINICAL MANIFESTATIONS

Subjective	Objective
Verbal self-reports of fatigue and weakness	Low B/P; resting pulse rate greater than 100 beats/min; postural hypotension; cool, pale, or cyanotic skin; capillary refill time greater than 2 to 3 seconds; diminished or absent peripheral pulses; urine output less than 30 mL/h; low CVP; crackles (rales); presence of gallop rhythm; dyspnea, tachypnea; restlessness, change in mental status; edema; JVD; chest radiograph results showing pulmonary vascular congestion, pulmonary edema, or pleural effusion; abnormal arterial blood gas values; significant decrease in oximetry results; dysrhythmias

DESIRED OUTCOMES

The client will maintain adequate cardiac output as evidenced by:
a. B/P within range of 100/60 to 130/80 mm Hg
b. Apical pulse regular and between 60 and 100 beats/min
c. Absence of or no increase in intensity of gallop rhythm
d. Increased strength and activity tolerance
e. Unlabored respirations at 12 to 20 breaths/min
f. Absence of adventitious breath sounds

g. Usual mental status
h. Absence of dizziness and syncope
i. Palpable peripheral pulses
j. Skin warm and usual color
k. Capillary refill time less than 2 to 3 seconds
l. Urine output at least 30 mL/h
m. Absence of edema and JVD

NOC OUTCOMES

Cardiac pump effectiveness; circulation status; tissue perfusion: peripheral; cardiac

NIC INTERVENTIONS

Cardiac care: acute; invasive hemodynamic monitoring; hemodynamic regulation; cardiac risk management; dysrhythmia management; cardiac care: rehabilitative

NURSING ASSESSMENT

Assess for and report signs and symptoms of decreased cardiac output:
• Hypotension
• Cool, pale, cyanotic skin
• Diminished/absent pulses
• Urine output < 30 mL/h
• Jugulovenous distention
• Tachypnea
• Dyspnea
Monitor ECG for dysrhythmias.

Monitor chest radiograph, pulse oximetry, and arterial blood gas values for abnormalities.

RATIONALE

Early recognition of signs and symptoms of decreased cardiac output allows for prompt intervention.

THERAPEUTIC INTERVENTIONS

Independent Actions
Implement measures to maintain an adequate cardiac output:
• Perform actions to prevent or treat hypotension:
  • Avoid rapid rewarming; gradually bring client's body temperature to normal if client is hypothermic.
• Perform actions to reduce cardiac workload:
  • Place client in a semi- to high-Fowler's position. **D** ● ✦
  • Instruct client to avoid activities that create a Valsalva response (e.g., straining to have a bowel movement, holding breath while moving up in bed).
  • Implement measures to promote rest (e.g., maintain activity restrictions, limit the number of visitors, reduce anxiety).
• Discourage smoking.

• Discourage excessive intake of beverages high in caffeine such as coffee, tea, and colas.

Dependent/Collaborative Actions
Administer prescribed pain medications.
Implement measures to maintain an adequate cardiac output:
• Perform actions to prevent or treat hypovolemia:
  • Administer blood and/or colloid or crystalloid solutions as ordered.
  • Maintain a minimum fluid intake of 1000 mL/day unless ordered otherwise.
  • Implement measures to prevent and control bleeding.

RATIONALE

Vasodilation occurs with warming. Warming measures should be gradual to prevent hypotension.

Decreasing cardiac workload will help to improve or maintain cardiac output.

Nicotine has a cardiostimulatory effect and causes vasoconstriction; the carbon monoxide in smoke reduces oxygen availability.
Caffeine is a myocardial stimulant and can increase myocardial oxygen consumption.

Actions help to maintain or restore circulating blood volume. An adequate circulating blood volume is necessary to achieve the optimum preload necessary for effective cardiac output.

THERAPEUTIC INTERVENTIONS	RATIONALE
• Perform actions to prevent or treat hypotension: • Consult physician before giving negative inotropic agents, diuretics, and vasodilating agents if client is hypotensive. • Administer narcotic (opioid) analgesics judiciously; in the immediate postoperative period, be alert to the synergistic effect of the narcotic ordered and the anesthetic that was used during surgery. • Administer sympathomimetics if ordered.	*Opioids promote vasodilation.* *Sympathomimetics may be administered as a temporary measure to improve B/P if adequate circulating fluid volume has been restored.*

• Administer positive inotropic agents (e.g., dopamine, dobutamine, digitalis preparations) if ordered.
• Perform actions to prevent or treat cardiac dysrhythmias.
• Administer antidysrhythmic medications.
• Replace K$^+$, Mg$^+$ electrolytes.
• Perform actions to reduce cardiac workload:
  • Perform actions to prevent or treat hypertension:
    • Implement measures to gradually rewarm client (e.g., increased room temperature, radiant heat lamp, warm blankets) if client is hypothermic.
    • Implement measures to reduce stress (e.g., initiate pain relief measures, reduce fear and anxiety).
    • Administer vasodilators if ordered.
  • Implement measures to maintain adequate respiratory function.
  • Implement measures to prevent or treat excess fluid volume:
    • Administer diuretics.
    • Limit excess fluid intake.
  • Increase activity gradually as allowed and tolerated.
Consult physician if signs and symptoms of decreased cardiac output persist or worsen.
	Positive inotropic agents increase myocardial contractility, improving cardiac output.
	Cardiac dysrhythmias can alter ventricular filling time and significantly reduce cardiac output.
	
	Actions help to prevent vasoconstriction associated with hypothermia and also prevent shivering, which elevates the metabolic rate and increases cardiac workload.
	
	Reduces vasoconstriction.
	
	Promotes adequate tissue oxygenation.
	
	Use of diuretics and limiting fluid intake will help to maintain appropriate vascular volume.
	
	Consulting the appropriate health care provider allows for modification of the treatment plan.

Nursing Diagnosis RISK FOR IMPAIRED RESPIRATORY FUNCTION*

Definition: **Ineffective Breathing Pattern NDx**: Inspiration and/or expiration that does not provide adequate ventilation; **Ineffective Airway Clearance NDx**: Inability to clear secretions or obstructions from the respiratory tract to maintain a clear airway; **Impaired Gas Exchange NDx**: Excess or deficient in oxygenation and/or carbon dioxide elimination at the alveolar-capillary membrane.

Related to:

Ineffective breathing pattern NDx related to:
• Increased rate of respirations associated with fear and anxiety
• Decreased rate of respirations associated with the depressant effect of anesthesia and some medications (e.g., opioid analgesics)
• Decreased depth of respirations associated with:
  • Weakness, fatigue, and decreased mobility
  • Depressant effect of anesthesia and some medications (e.g., opioid analgesics)
  • Reluctance to breathe deeply because of chest incision and fear of dislodging chest tube
  • Hemiparesis of the diaphragm if the phrenic nerve was injured
  • Decreased lung compliance (distensibility) if pleural effusion is present

Ineffective airway clearance NDx related to:
• Stasis of secretions associated with decreased activity, depressed ciliary function resulting from the effect of anesthesia, and a weak cough effort
• Increased secretions associated with irritation of the respiratory tract (can result from inhalation anesthetics and endotracheal intubation)

---

*This diagnostic label includes the following nursing diagnoses: ineffective breathing pattern, ineffective airway clearance, and impaired gas exchange.

NDx = NANDA Diagnosis   **D** = Delegatable Action   ● = UAP   ✦ = LVN/LPN   ⊙▶ = Go to ⊖volve for animation

Impaired gas exchange NDx related to ventilation/perfusion imbalances associated with:
- Atelectasis resulting from:
  - Deflation of the alveoli while on the CPB machine
  - Decreased surfactant production/function (occurs because of lack of alveolar expansion and decreased pulmonary blood flow during CPB and as a result of a systemic inflammatory response to the bypass machine)
  - Postoperative hypoventilation or ineffective clearance of secretions
  - Accumulation of fluid in the pulmonary interstitium and alveoli (can occur as a result of excess fluid volume)
  - Decreased pulmonary blood flow resulting from decreased cardiac output

CLINICAL MANIFESTATIONS

Subjective	Objective
Verbal self-report of restlessness; irritability	Rapid, shallow, or slow respirations; dyspnea, orthopnea; use of accessory muscles when breathing; adventitious breath sounds (e.g., crackles [rales], rhonchi); diminished or absent breath sounds; asymmetrical chest excursion; cough; confusion, somnolence; abnormal arterial blood gas values; significant decrease in oximetry results; abnormal chest radiograph results

RISK FACTORS
- Immobility
- Atelectasis
- Ineffective clearance of secretions

DESIRED OUTCOMES

The client will experience adequate respiratory function as evidenced by:
a. Normal rate and depth of respirations
b. Absence of dyspnea
c. Normal breath sounds by third to fourth postoperative day
d. Symmetrical chest excursion
e. Usual mental status
f. Oximetry results within normal range
g. Arterial blood gas values within normal range

NOC OUTCOMES

Respiratory status: ventilation; airway patency; gas exchange

NIC INTERVENTIONS

Respiratory monitoring; airway management; chest physiotherapy; cough enhancement; ventilation assistance; oxygen therapy; anxiety reduction

NURSING ASSESSMENT

Assess for and report signs and symptoms of impaired respiratory function:
- Rapid, shallow, or slow respirations
- Dyspnea, orthopnea
- Use of accessory muscles when breathing
- Adventitious breath sounds (e.g., crackles [rales], rhonchi)
- Diminished or absent breath sounds
- Asymmetrical chest excursion
- Cough
- Confusion, somnolence

Monitor pulse oximetry and arterial blood gas values, and chest radiograph results for abnormalities.

RATIONALE

Early recognition of signs and symptoms of impaired respiratory function allows for prompt intervention.

THERAPEUTIC INTERVENTIONS	**RATIONALE**

Independent Actions

Implement measures to maintain adequate respiratory function:

- Perform actions to decrease fear and anxiety (e.g., explain procedures, interact with client in a confident manner, initiate pain relief measures).

  Actions that decrease fear and anxiety help to prevent the shallow and/or rapid breathing that can occur with fear and anxiety.

- Place client in a semi- to high-Fowler's position unless contraindicated.

  Improves lung expansion.

- If client must remain flat in bed, assist with position change at least every 2 hrs.

  Actions help to mobilize secretions and prevent alveolar collapse associated with immobility.

- Instruct and assist client to cough and deep breathe or use incentive spirometer every 1 to 2 hrs; assure client that chest tube is sutured in place and that these activities should not dislodge the tube.

  Improves lung expansion and prevents stasis of secretions.

- Instruct client to avoid intake of gas-forming foods (e.g., beans, cauliflower, cabbage, onions), carbonated beverages, and large meals.

  Helps to prevent gastric distention and subsequent pressure on the diaphragm.

- Discourage smoking.

  The irritants in smoke increase mucus production, impair ciliary function, and can cause damage to the bronchial and alveolar walls; the carbon monoxide in smoke decreases oxygen availability.

Dependent/Collaborative Actions

Implement measures to maintain adequate respiratory function:

- Monitor mechanical ventilation carefully to ensure that ventilatory rate and pressures are correct.

  The nurse collaborates with the respiratory therapist to ensure that mechanical ventilation is delivered therapeutically without adverse outcomes.

- Perform actions to decrease pain and increase strength and activity (e.g., administer analgesics before activities that can cause pain).

  Providing adequate pain relief helps to increase client's willingness and ability to move, cough, deep breathe, and use incentive spirometer.

- Perform actions to maintain an adequate cardiac output.

  Adequate cardiac output ensures pulmonary blood flow, facilitating gas exchange.

- Administer blood and blood products as ordered.
- Perform actions to prevent or treat excess fluid volume and third-spacing (e.g., administer diuretics as ordered).

  Actions help to reduce the risk for pleural effusion and pulmonary edema.

- Maintain an adequate fluid intake and humidify inspired air if ordered.

  Actions help to thin tenacious secretions and reduce dryness of the respiratory mucous membrane.

- Maintain oxygen therapy as ordered.

  Maintains tissue oxygenation.

- Maintain activity restrictions as ordered; increase activity gradually as allowed and tolerated.
- Administer central nervous system depressants judiciously; hold medication and consult physician if respiratory rate is less than 12 breaths/min.

  Prevents decreased tissue oxygenation.

Consult appropriate health care provider (e.g., respiratory therapist, physician) if signs and symptoms of impaired respiratory function persist or worsen.

Consulting the appropriate health care provider allows for modification of the treatment plan.

Nursing/Collaborative Diagnosis | ## RISK FOR IMBALANCED FLUID VOLUME NDx AND RISK FOR ELECTROLYTE IMBALANCE NDx

Definition: Risk for Imbalanced Fluid Volume NDx: Susceptible to a decrease, increase, or rapid shift from one to the other of intravascular, interstitial, and/or intracellular fluid, which may compromise health. This refers to body fluid loss, gain, or both; **Risk for Electrolyte Imbalance NDx:** Susceptible to changes in serum electrolyte levels, which may compromise health.

Related to:

Excess fluid volume NDx related to:
- Vigorous fluid therapy during and immediately after surgery (the CPB machine is primed with a large amount of crystalloid solution to decrease blood viscosity and the risk for embolic complications, decrease hemolysis of cells, and help maintain adequate circulation throughout the body)
- Increased production of ADH (output of ADH is stimulated by trauma, pain, and anesthetic agents)
- Reshifting of fluid from the interstitial space back into the intravascular space approximately 3 days after surgery
- Decreased GFR and activation of the renin-angiotensin-aldosterone mechanism (a result of nonpulsatile renal perfusion while on the bypass machine and the decreased renal blood flow that can occur with decreased cardiac output)
- Presence of preexisting heart failure

Third-spacing of fluid related to:
- Increased capillary permeability (a result of the systemic inflammatory response that occurs with CPB) and the subsequent low plasma colloid osmotic pressure associated with decreased plasma proteins

Deficient fluid volume NDx related to:
- Restricted oral intake before, during, and after surgery
- Blood loss during surgery and via chest tube after surgery
- Loss of fluid associated with nasogastric tube drainage and excessive diuresis
- Third-spacing of intravascular fluid

Hypokalemia, hypochloremia, and/or metabolic alkalosis related to:
- Loss of electrolytes and hydrochloric acid associated with nasogastric tube drainage (diuretic therapy and the hemodilution created by priming the bypass machine with large amounts of fluid also contribute to the imbalanced electrolytes)

CLINICAL MANIFESTATIONS

Subjective	Objective
Excess fluid volume: Not applicable	**Excess fluid volume:** Weight gain of 2% or greater in a short period; elevated B/P (B/P may not be elevated if cardiac output is poor or fluid has shifted out of the vascular space); presence of an S_3 heart sound; intake greater than output; change in mental status; crackles (rales); dyspnea, orthopnea; edema, distended neck veins; elevated CVP (use internal jugular vein pulsation method to estimate CVP if monitoring device is not present)
Third-spacing: Not applicable	**Third-spacing:** Ascites; increased dyspnea and diminished or absent breath sounds; evidence of vascular depletion (e.g., postural hypotension; weak, rapid pulse; decreased urine output)
Deficient fluid volume: Verbal self-report of thirst	**Deficient fluid volume:** Hypotension; tachycardia; decreased urine output; tenting skin turgor; dry mucous membranes; thick, tenacious pulmonary secretions

DESIRED OUTCOMES

The client will experience resolution of excess fluid volume and third-spacing as evidenced by:
a. Decline in weight toward client's normal
b. B/P and pulse within normal range for client and stable with position change
c. Resolution of S_3 heart sound
d. Balanced intake and output
e. Usual mental status
f. Improved breath sounds
g. Decreased dyspnea and orthopnea
h. Decrease in edema and ascites
i. Resolution of neck vein distention
j. CVP within normal range

The client will not experience deficient fluid volume, hypokalemia, hypochloremia, or metabolic alkalosis.

NOC OUTCOMES

Fluid balance; fluid overload severity; electrolyte and acid-base balance

NIC INTERVENTIONS

Fluid monitoring; electrolyte monitoring; acid-base monitoring; fluid/electrolyte management: hypokalemia; acid-base management: metabolic alkalosis

NURSING ASSESSMENT	RATIONALE
Assess for and report signs and symptoms of excess fluid volume and third-spacing.	Early recognition of signs and symptoms of excess fluid volume and third-spacing allows for prompt intervention.
Monitor chest radiograph for abnormal findings: • Pulmonary vascular congestion • Pleural effusion • Pulmonary edema	
Monitor serum albumin levels for abnormal values.	Low serum albumin levels result in fluid shifting out of the vascular space because albumin normally maintains plasma colloid osmotic pressure.
Monitor postoperative drains (mediastinal tubes/chest tubes) for amount and consistency of drainage.	Excessive postoperative drainage can lead to deficient circulating fluid volume.

THERAPEUTIC INTERVENTIONS	RATIONALE

Dependent/Collaborative Actions

Implement measures to restore fluid balance: • Perform actions to reduce excess fluid volume: • Perform actions to maintain adequate renal blood flow.	Adequate renal blood flow helps to maintain normal glomerular filtration with subsequent fluid removal.
• Maintain adequate blood pressure within client's baseline normal values.	
• Administer diuretics if ordered.	Decreases fluid volume excess.
• Maintain fluid and sodium restrictions as ordered (2500 mL fluid and 3–4 g sodium restrictions are common).	High sodium levels cause fluid retention.
• Perform actions to prevent further third-spacing and promote mobilization of fluid back into the vascular space: • Administer albumin infusions if ordered.	Albumin helps to increase colloid osmotic pressure, pulling fluid back into the vascular space and helping to reduce third-spacing.
• Administer the following if ordered to treat deficient fluid volume and hypokalemia: • Blood and/or colloid or crystalloid solutions	Colloid solutions may be used rather than crystalloid solutions because they help maintain colloid osmotic pressure and subsequently reduce shifting of fluid from the intravascular to the interstitial space.
• Potassium supplements	Keeping the serum potassium at 4.0 to 4.5 mEq/L reduces the risk for dysrhythmias.
Consult physician if signs and symptoms of excess fluid volume and third-spacing persist or worsen.	Allows for prompt alterations in interventions.

Nursing Diagnosis **RISK FOR INFECTION** NDx

Definition: Susceptible to invasion and multiplication of pathogenic organisms, which may compromise health.

Related to:

Pneumonia related to:

- Stasis of pulmonary secretions associated with decreased activity
- Depressed ciliary function resulting from the effect of anesthesia
- A poor cough effort resulting from weakness, surgical site pain, and fear of dislodging chest tube

Wound infection and mediastinitis related to:

- Wound contamination associated with introduction of pathogens during or after surgery
- Decreased resistance to infection associated with factors such as inadequate nutritional status and diminished tissue perfusion to wound area (an increased risk if client is elderly or has diabetes or if on CPB a prolonged time or cardiac output is low for a prolonged time)

CLINICAL MANIFESTATIONS

Subjective	Objective
Verbal self-report of increased pain at wound site	Increased temperature; redness; warmth, discharge in close proximity to wound; thick, malodorous pulmonary secretions

DESIRED OUTCOMES

The client will not develop pneumonia.
The client will remain free of wound infection and mediastinitis.

NOC OUTCOMES	NIC INTERVENTIONS
Immune status; infection severity; wound healing: primary intention	Infection protection; infection control; cough enhancement; airway management; incision site care

NURSING ASSESSMENT	RATIONALE
Assess for and report signs and symptoms of sternal wound infection and mediastinitis: • Fever persisting beyond the fourth postoperative day • Grating sound and/or movement of sternum when client moves or coughs Monitor chest radiograph results for abnormalities.	*Early recognition of signs and symptoms of pneumonia or sternal wound infection/mediastinitis allows for prompt intervention. Signs and symptoms of sternal infection and mediastinitis are often not manifested until the second week after surgery.*

THERAPEUTIC INTERVENTIONS	RATIONALE

Independent Actions
 Implement additional measures to reduce the risk for pneumonia:
 • Perform actions to maintain adequate respiratory function:
   • Encourage cough and deep breathing.
   • Increase activity as tolerated.
	Improves lung expansion and decreases stasis of secretions.

• Have client splint chest incision with a pillow when turning, coughing, and deep breathing.	*Splinting the incision helps increase client's willingness to move, cough, and deep breathe.*
Dependent/Collaborative Actions If signs and symptoms of a sternal wound infection and mediastinitis occur: • Administer antimicrobial agents as ordered.	*Treats infection.*
• Prepare client for surgical debridement, drainage, and antibiotic irrigation of wound if planned.	*Decreases fear and anxiety.*

Collaborative Diagnosis RISK FOR CARDIAC DYSRHYTHMIAS

Definition: Disturbance of the heart rhythm

Related to: Impaired nodal function and/or altered myocardial conductivity associated with trauma to the heart during surgery, hypothermia, hypoxia, sympathetic stimulation (can result from anxiety, volume depletion, and pain), or electrolyte and acid-base imbalances

CLINICAL MANIFESTATIONS

Subjective	Objective
Verbal self-report of palpitations; lightheadedness	Irregular apical pulse; pulse rate below 60 or above 100 beats/min; apical-radial pulse deficit; syncope; palpitations; abnormal rate, rhythm, or configurations on ECG

RISK FACTORS
- Electrolyte imbalances
- Myocardial ischemia

DESIRED OUTCOMES

The client will maintain normal sinus rhythm as evidenced by:
a. Regular apical pulse at 60 to 100 beats/min
b. Equal apical and radial pulse rates
c. Absence of syncope and palpitations
d. ECG showing normal sinus rhythm

NURSING ASSESSMENT	RATIONALE
Assess for and report signs and symptoms of cardiac dysrhythmias: • Irregular apical • Pulse rate < 60 or > 100 beats/min • Palpitations Monitor ECG, levels of serum cardiac enzymes/troponin for abnormalities.	*Early recognition of signs and symptoms of excess of cardiac dysrhythmias allows for prompt intervention.*

THERAPEUTIC INTERVENTIONS	RATIONALE
Dependent/Collaborative Actions Implement measures to prevent cardiac dysrhythmias: • Perform actions to maintain adequate cardiac output and myocardial blood flow. • Maintain oxygen therapy as ordered. • Monitor serum electrolyte levels; consult physician about administration of a potassium or magnesium supplement if serum levels of either are low. • Perform actions to maintain adequate respiratory function.	*Optimum respiratory function helps to improve tissue oxygenation and prevent respiratory acidosis or alkalosis (myocardial conductivity is altered by hypoxia and acid-base imbalance).*
• Administer prophylactic antidysrhythmic agents if ordered. If cardiac dysrhythmias occur: • Initiate cardiac monitoring if not still being done. • Administer antidysrhythmics if ordered. • Maintain temporary pacemaker function as ordered. • Restrict client's activity based on client's tolerance and severity of the dysrhythmia. • Maintain oxygen therapy as ordered. • Assess cardiovascular status frequently and report signs and symptoms of inadequate tissue perfusion (e.g., decrease in B/P, cool skin, cyanosis, diminished peripheral pulses, urine output less than 30 mL/h, restlessness and agitation, shortness of breath). • Have emergency cart readily available for cardioversion, defibrillation, or CPR.	*Administration of prophylactic antidysrhythmic agents decrease incidence of cardiac dysrhythmias and help to maintain adequate cardiac output.* *Allows for prompt changes in treatment regimen.*

Collaborative Diagnosis **RISK FOR CARDIAC TAMPONADE**

Definition: Pericardial effusion that creates sufficient pressure to cause cardiac compression.

Related to: Accumulation of fluid (usually blood) in the pericardial sac and/or mediastinum associated with excessive bleeding and/or obstructed drainage of the mediastinal tube

CLINICAL MANIFESTATIONS

Subjective	Objective
Not applicable	Sudden decrease in chest tube drainage; chest radiograph report of widening mediastinum; decreased B/P; narrowed pulse pressure; pulsus paradoxus; distant muffled heart sounds

RISK FACTORS

- Cardiac surgery
- Obstructed postsurgical draining

DESIRED OUTCOMES

The client will not experience cardiac tamponade as evidenced by:
a. Stable vital signs
b. Audible heart sounds
c. Absence of JVD
d. Absence of pulsus paradoxus
e. CVP within normal limits

NURSING ASSESSMENT	RATIONALE
Assess for and report signs and symptoms of cardiac tamponade: • Decreased blood pressure • Pulsus paradoxus • Muffled heart sounds	*Early recognition of signs and symptoms of cardiac tamponade allows for prompt intervention.*

THERAPEUTIC INTERVENTIONS	RATIONALE
Dependent/Collaborative Actions Implement measures to reduce the risk of cardiac tamponade: • Perform actions to maintain patency and integrity of chest drainage system.	*Prevents pressure buildup on the heart.*
• If chest tube becomes obstructed, assist with clearing of existing tube and/or insertion of a new tube.	*Maintains patency.*
• When removing the pacemaker catheter(s), do it carefully. If signs and symptoms of cardiac tamponade occur:	*Avoid trauma to the surrounding vessels and subsequent bleeding.*
• Prepare client for echocardiography.	*Decreases fear and anxiety.*
• Administer intravenous fluids and/or vasopressors if ordered.	*Maintains mean arterial pressure.*
• Prepare client for surgical drainage of pericardial fluid.	*Decreases fear and anxiety.*

Nursing Diagnosis **RISK FOR BLEEDING** NDx

Definition: Susceptible to a decrease in blood volume, which may compromise health.

Related to:

- Impaired platelet function associated with mechanical damage to the platelets by the bypass machine and possible heparin-induced thrombocytopenia
- Incomplete neutralization of the heparin used during surgery to prevent thrombus formation in the bypass machine
- Decreased release and function of clotting factors associated with systemic hypothermia during surgery
- Anticoagulant therapy (relevant primarily for clients who have had valve replacement and are taking warfarin)
- Inadequate surgical hemostasis or disruption of suture lines associated with hypertension if it occurs

CLINICAL MANIFESTATIONS

Subjective	Objective
Verbal self-report of unusual bruising or bleeding; dizziness	Excessive amount of bloody drainage from chest tube; continuous oozing of blood from incisions; prolonged bleeding from puncture sites; gingival bleeding; petechiae, purpura, ecchymoses; epistaxis, hemoptysis; increase in abdominal girth; frank or occult blood in stool, urine, or vomitus; menorrhagia; restlessness, confusion; significant drop in B/P accompanied by an increased pulse rate; decrease in Hct and Hgb levels

DESIRED OUTCOMES

The client will not experience unusual bleeding as evidenced by:
a. Gradual decrease in amount of bloody drainage from chest tube
b. Skin and mucous membranes free of active bleeding, petechiae, purpura, and ecchymoses
c. Absence of unusual joint pain
d. No increase in abdominal girth
e. Absence of frank and occult blood in stool, urine, and vomitus
f. Usual menstrual flow
g. Usual mental status
h. Vital signs within normal range for client
i. Stable or improved Hct and Hgb levels

NURSING ASSESSMENT	RATIONALE
Assess for and report signs and symptoms of unusual bleeding: • Excessive amounts of bleeding from chest tubes • Decreased B/P • Increased heart rate Monitor platelet count and coagulation tests for abnormal results or results that exceed the therapeutic range for clients receiving anticoagulant therapy.	*Early recognition of signs and symptoms of unusual bleeding allows for prompt intervention.*

NOC OUTCOMES	NIC INTERVENTIONS
Blood coagulation; blood loss severity	Bleeding reduction; bleeding precautions; bleeding reduction: wound

THERAPEUTIC INTERVENTIONS	RATIONALE

Independent Actions
Implement measures to prevent bleeding:
• When giving injections or performing venous and arterial punctures, use the smallest gauge needle possible and apply gentle, prolonged pressure to the site after the needle is removed.
• Educate client to avoid activities that increase the risk for trauma (e.g., shaving with a straight-edge razor, using stiff bristle toothbrush or dental floss).
• Pad side rails if client is confused or restless.
• Perform actions to reduce the risk for falls (e.g., keep bed in low position with side rails up when client is in bed, avoid unnecessary clutter in room, instruct client to wear shoes/slippers with nonslip soles when ambulating).
• Instruct client to avoid blowing nose forcefully or straining to have a bowel movement; consult physician regarding order for a decongestant and/or laxative if indicated.
 	
Dependent/Collaborative Actions
Test all stools, urine, and vomitus for occult blood if platelet count and coagulation tests are abnormal.
• If bleeding occurs and does not subside spontaneously:
  • Apply firm, prolonged pressure to bleeding area(s) if possible.
  • Maintain oxygen therapy as ordered.
  • Autotransfuse blood from the chest drainage device if ordered.
	In order to maintain systolic B/P at a level less than 140 mm Hg and subsequently decrease the risk for disruption of suture lines.
	
	Prevents injury and potential for increased bleeding.
	
	Early detection of abnormal bleeding and allows for prompt treatment regimen changes.

NDx = NANDA Diagnosis   **D** = Delegatable Action   ● = UAP   ✦ = LVN/LPN   ⓔ▶ = Go to ⓔvolve for animation

Continued...

THERAPEUTIC INTERVENTIONS	RATIONALE

• Administer the following if ordered:
  • Vitamin K or protamine sulfate
  • Whole blood or packed RBCs
  • Blood products
• Prepare client for return to surgery.
	Promotes blood clotting.
	Vitamin K counteracts the effect of warfarin therapy.
	Protamine sulfate further neutralizes the heparin used to prime the bypass machine.
	Decreases fear and anxiety.

Collaborative Diagnosis RISK FOR NEUROLOGICAL DYSFUNCTION

Definition: Decreased level of consciousness and client's normal cognitive, sensory, and motor function.

Related to:
- Inadequate cerebral blood flow associated with:
  - Decreased systemic arterial pressure while on CPB
  - An embolus (can result from dislodgment of atherosclerotic plaque during cross-clamping of the aorta and cannulation for bypass, dislodgment of debris from calcified valve, incomplete filtration of air by bypass machine, or cardiac thrombus formation on prosthetic valve or as a result of dysrhythmias)
  - Hypotension or low cardiac output postoperatively
- Cerebral edema initiated by a systemic inflammatory response to the CPB machine
- Possible poor cerebral protection during CPB from inadequate temperature regulation (hypothermia must be adequate to help protect the central nervous system)

CLINICAL MANIFESTATIONS

Subjective	Objective
Verbal self-report of visual disturbances; swallowing difficulties; paresthesias	Slurred speech, expressive or receptive aphasia; decreased level of consciousness, delirium, hallucinations, confusion; impaired memory, lack of ability to concentrate, difficulty problem-solving; weakness of extremity, facial droop, ptosis, paralysis Decline in client's normal sensory and motor function

RISK FACTORS
- Thromboembolism
- Altered cerebral perfusion during bypass

DESIRED OUTCOMES

The client will maintain usual neurological function as evidenced by:
a. Absence of visual disturbances, swallowing difficulties, and speech impairments
b. Mentally alert and oriented
c. Usual memory and problem-solving abilities
d. Normal sensory and motor function

NURSING ASSESSMENT	RATIONALE
Assess for and report signs and symptoms of neurological dysfunction: • Slurred speech • Expressive/receptor dysphagia • Decreased level of consciousness • Weakness of extremity • Facial droop • Ptosis • Swallowing difficulties	*Early recognition of signs and symptoms of neurological dysfunction allows prompt intervention.*

THERAPEUTIC INTERVENTIONS	RATIONALE

Dependent/Collaborative Actions

Implement measures to promote adequate cerebral blood flow and reduce the risk for neurological dysfunction:

- Keep head of bed flat until B/P is stabilized at a satisfactory level (at least 90 mm Hg systolic).
- Keep head and neck in neutral, midline position.
- Perform actions to maintain adequate cardiac output (e.g., administer positive inotropic medications as ordered).
- Perform actions to prevent thrombi and microemboli formation in the heart.
- Perform actions to reduce the risk for increased ICP:
  - Limit activities that can increase ICP (e.g., excessive suctioning, instruct client to avoid excessive coughing and straining to have a bowel movement).
  - Implement measures to maintain adequate respiratory function and gas exchange.

If signs and symptoms of neurological dysfunction occur:

- Maintain client on bed rest until physician evaluates symptoms.
- Maintain oxygen therapy as ordered.
- Administer anticoagulants if ordered.

Improves blood flow to the central nervous system.
To prevent dilation of the cerebral vessels associated with hypoxia and hypercapnia.

Maintains tissue oxygenation.
Decreases potential for thrombi.

Collaborative Diagnosis # RISK FOR IMPAIRED RENAL FUNCTION

Definition: Renal insufficiency refers to a decline in renal function to about 25% of normal.

Related to: Deposit of hemolyzed RBC products in renal tubules or inadequate renal blood flow associated with CPB, low cardiac output, hypotension, an embolus, or effect of vasopressor drugs (risk is increased if client is elderly or has preexisting renal disease)

CLINICAL MANIFESTATIONS

Subjective	Objective
Verbal self-report of confusion	Urine output less than 30 mL/h; urine specific gravity fixed at or less than 1.010; elevated BUN and serum creatinine levels; decreased creatinine clearance

RISK FACTORS

- Decreased cardiac output
- Thromboembolism

DESIRED OUTCOMES

The client will maintain adequate renal function as evidenced by:
a. Urine output at least 30 mL/h
b. BUN, serum creatinine, and creatinine clearance values within normal range

NURSING ASSESSMENT	RATIONALE

Assess for and report signs and symptoms of impaired renal function:
- Urine output > 30 mL/h
- Elevated BUN, creatinine values

Monitor serum creatinine levels for abnormalities.

Early recognition of signs and symptoms of impaired renal function allows prompt intervention.

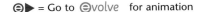

THERAPEUTIC INTERVENTIONS	RATIONALE

Dependent/Collaborative Actions

Implement measures to maintain adequate renal blood flow:

- Maintain a minimum fluid intake of 1000 mL/day unless ordered otherwise.

  Maintains adequate fluid volume.

- Perform actions to maintain adequate cardiac output.
- Perform actions to prevent thrombi and microemboli formation in the heart.

  To reduce the risk for occlusion of the renal artery by an embolus.

If signs and symptoms of impaired renal function occur:

- Administer diuretics.

  To increase urine output and subsequently reduce further accumulation of hemolyzed RBC products in the renal tubules.

- Consult physician about discontinuing any potentially nephrotoxic medications.

  Potentially improves renal functioning.

- Assess for and report signs of acute renal failure (e.g., oliguria or anuria; weight gain; edema; elevated B/P; lethargy and confusion; increasing BUN and serum creatinine, phosphorus, and potassium levels).

  Allows for prompt alteration in interventions.

- Prepare client for dialysis if indicated.

  Decreases fear and anxiety.

Collaborative Diagnosis   RISK FOR PNEUMOTHORAX

Definition: Presence of air or gas in the pleural space caused by rupture of the visceral pleural or the parietal pleura and chest wall.

Related to: The accumulation of air in the pleural space if the pleura was opened during surgery

CLINICAL MANIFESTATIONS

Subjective	Objective
Verbal self-report of sudden pleural pain; verbalization of shortness of breath	Tachypnea; dyspnea; absent or decreased breath sounds; hyperresonance to percussion on affected side; chest radiograph abnormalities; abnormal arterial blood gas values

RISK FACTORS

- Surgical procedures within the chest cavity
- Invasive line placement in great vessels (e.g., subclavian)

DESIRED OUTCOMES

The client will experience normal lung re-expansion as evidenced by:
  a. Audible breath sounds and a resonant percussion note over lungs by third to fourth postoperative day
  b. Unlabored respirations at 12 to 20 breaths/min
  c. Arterial blood gas values returning toward normal
  d. Chest radiograph showing lung reexpansion

NURSING ASSESSMENT	RATIONALE

Assess for and immediately report signs and symptoms of pneumothorax:

Early recognition of signs and symptoms of a pneumothorax allows prompt intervention.

- Subjective
- Objective

Assess for malfunction of chest drainage system:

- Respiratory distress
- Excessive bubbling in water seal chamber
- Significant increase in subcutaneous emphysema

Monitor chest radiograph results.

THERAPEUTIC INTERVENTIONS	RATIONALE

Dependent/Collaborative Actions

Perform actions to maintain patency and integrity of chest drainage system:

- Maintain fluid level in the water seal and suction chambers as ordered.
- Maintain occlusive dressing over chest tube insertion site.
- Tape all connections securely.
- Tape the tubing to the chest wall close to insertion site.
- Position tubing to promote optimum drainage (e.g., coil excess tubing on bed rather than allowing it to hang down below the collection device, keep tubing free of kinks).
- Drain any fluid that accumulates in tubing into the collection chamber and milk tube gently if indicated to dislodge clots.
- Keep drainage collection device below level of client's chest at all times.

Perform actions to facilitate the escape of air from the pleural space (e.g., maintain suction as ordered, ensure that the air vent is open on the drainage collection device if system is to water seal only).

Perform actions to maintain adequate respiratory function:

- Encourage use of incentive spirometer every 2 hrs.
- Increase activity as tolerated.

If signs and symptoms of further lung collapse occur:

- Maintain client on bed rest in a semi- to high-Fowler's position.
- Maintain oxygen therapy as ordered.
- Assess for and immediately report signs and symptoms of tension pneumothorax (e.g., severe dyspnea, increased restlessness and agitation, rapid and/or irregular pulse rate, hypotension, neck vein distention, shift in trachea from midline).
- Assist with clearing of existing chest tube and/or insertion of a new tube.

Measures help to promote lung reexpansion and prevent further lung collapse.
Maintains negative pressure.
To reduce the risk of inadvertent removal of the tube.

Dislodges clots.

Prevents backflow and stasis of drainage.

Promotes full lung expansion.

Promotes lung expansion and prevents stasis of secretions.

Improves ability for lung expansion.
Maintains tissue oxygenation.
Allows for prompt alterations in interventions.

DISCHARGE TEACHING/CONTINUED CARE

Nursing Diagnosis

DEFICIENT KNOWLEDGE NDx; INEFFECTIVE FAMILY HEALTH MANAGEMENT NDx; OR INEFFECTIVE HEALTH MANAGEMENT NDx*

Definition: Deficient Knowledge NDx: Absence of cognitive information related to specific topic, or its acquisition; **Ineffective Family Health Management NDx:** A pattern of regulating and integrating into family processes a program for the treatment of illness and its sequelae that is unsatisfactory for meeting specific health goals of the family unit; **Ineffective Health Management NDx:** Inability to identify, manage, and/or seek out help to maintain well-being.

CLINICAL MANIFESTATIONS

Subjective	Objective
Verbal self-report of unfamiliarity with information	Inability to follow instructions

RISK FACTORS

- Denial of disease process
- Cognitive deficiency
- Failure to take action to reduce risk factors

*The nurse should select the nursing diagnostic label that is most appropriate for the client's discharge teaching needs.

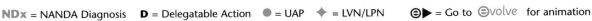

NDx = NANDA Diagnosis   **D** = Delegatable Action   ● = UAP   ✦ = LVN/LPN   ⊖▶ = Go to ⊖volve for animation

NOC OUTCOMES	NIC INTERVENTIONS
Knowledge: treatment regimen; cardiac disease management; disease process	Health system guidance; teaching: individual; teaching: disease process; teaching: prescribed diet; teaching: prescribed medication; teaching: prescribed activity/exercise

NURSING ASSESSMENT	RATIONALE
Assess client's readiness and ability to learn. Assess meaning of illness to client.	*Early recognition of readiness to learn and meaning of illness to client allows for implementation of the appropriate teaching interventions.*

THERAPEUTIC INTERVENTIONS	RATIONALE

Desired Outcome: In collaboration with the nurse, client will identify modifiable cardiovascular risk factors and ways to alter these factors.

Independent Actions

Inform client that certain modifiable factors such as elevated serum lipid levels, a sedentary lifestyle, hypertension, excessive alcohol intake, and smoking have been shown to increase the risk for CAD and certain forms of heart disease.	*Thorough education is a critical component of the care of a client after open heart surgery. Continued lifestyle modifications consistent with recommendations for clients with cardiovascular disease are necessary to maintain patency of vessel grafts. The client must have a thorough understanding of the importance of adhering to diet, medication, activity/exercise, and nutritional recommendations to prevent an exacerbation and control the disease.*
Assist clients to identify changes in lifestyle that can help them to eliminate or reduce the above risk factors (e.g., dietary modification, physical exercise on a regular basis, moderation of alcohol intake, smoking cessation).	
Encourage client to limit daily alcohol consumption. Current recommendations are no more than two drinks per day for men and no more than one drink per day for women and lighter-weight persons.	*Daily alcohol intake exceeding 1 oz of ethanol may contribute to the development of hypertension and some forms of heart disease.* *A "drink" is considered to be ½ oz of ethanol (e.g., 1½ oz of 80-proof whiskey, 12 oz of beer, 5 oz of wine).*

THERAPEUTIC INTERVENTIONS	RATIONALE

Desired Outcome: The client will verbalize an understanding of the rationale for and components of a diet restricted in sodium, saturated fat, and cholesterol.

Independent Actions

Explain the rationale for a diet restricting sodium, saturated fat, and cholesterol intake.	*Current daily dietary sodium intake is less than 2400 mg. Excessive sodium intake causes water to be retained, resulting in increased circulating fluid volume, increased cardiac workload, and hypertension.*
Provide the following information about decreasing sodium intake:	*Understanding of disease limitations improves client adherence to treatment regimen.*

- Read labels on foods/fluids and calculate sodium content of items; avoid those products that tend to have a high sodium content (e.g., canned soups and vegetables, tomato juice, commercial baked goods, commercially prepared frozen or canned entrees and sauces).
- Do not add salt when cooking foods or to prepared foods; use low-sodium herbs and spices if desired.
- Avoid cured and smoked foods.

THERAPEUTIC INTERVENTIONS	**RATIONALE**

- Avoid salty snack foods (e.g., crackers, nuts, pretzels, potato chips).
- Avoid commercially prepared fast foods.
- Avoid routine use of over-the-counter medications with a high sodium content (e.g., Alka-Seltzer, some antacids).

Provide instructions on ways the client can reduce intake of saturated fat and cholesterol:

- Reduce intake of meat fat (e.g., trim visible fat off meat; replace fatty meats such as fatty cuts of steak, hamburger, and processed meats with leaner products).
- Reduce intake of milk fat (e.g., avoid dairy products containing more than 1% fat).
- Reduce intake of *trans* fats (e.g., avoid stick margarine and shortening and foods such as commercial baked goods that are prepared with these products).
- Use vegetable oil rather than coconut or palm oil in cooking and food preparation.
- Use cooking methods such as steaming, baking, broiling, poaching, microwaving, and grilling rather than frying.
- Restrict intake of eggs.

Obtain a dietary consult to assist client in planning meals that will meet the prescribed restrictions of sodium, saturated fat, and cholesterol.

The risk of CAD is associated with a serum cholesterol level of more than 200 mg/dL or a fasting triglyceride level of more than 150 mg/dL. Elevated serum lipid levels are one of the most firmly established risk factors for CAD.

Recommendations about the number of whole eggs allowed per week vary depending on the client's lipid levels.

THERAPEUTIC INTERVENTIONS	**RATIONALE**

Desired Outcome: The client will verbalize an understanding of activity restrictions and the rate of activity progression.

Independent Actions

Reinforce physician's instructions regarding activity. Instruct client to:

- Gradually rebuild activity level by adhering to a planned exercise program (often begins with walking and light household activities).
- Take frequent rest periods for 4 to 6 weeks after surgery.
- Avoid lifting heavy objects in order to allow incision to heal and prevent a sudden increase in cardiac workload.
- Avoid driving a car and riding a bicycle, motorcycle, lawn mower, tractor, or a horse for 4 to 6 weeks; if minimally invasive surgery was performed, these activities will probably be allowed much sooner.
- Check with physician or cardiac rehabilitation therapist before resuming sexual activity (usually permitted 3–4 weeks after surgery once able to walk two blocks or climb two flights of stairs without shortness of breath).
- Stop any activity that causes chest pain, shortness of breath, palpitations, dizziness, or extreme fatigue or weakness.
- Participate in a cardiac rehabilitation program if recommended by physician.

While the benefits of physical activity are an integral part of cardiac rehabilitation, the level of activity should be increased gradually. Physical activity guidelines after acute coronary syndromes focus on frequency, intensity, type, and time of activity.

THERAPEUTIC INTERVENTIONS	**RATIONALE**

Desired Outcome: The client will verbalize an understanding of medications ordered including rationale, food and drug interactions, side effects, schedule for taking, and importance of taking as prescribed.

NDx = NANDA Diagnosis   **D** = Delegatable Action   ● = UAP   ✦ = LVN/LPN   ⊖▶ = Go to ⊖volve for animation

Continued...

THERAPEUTIC INTERVENTIONS	RATIONALE
Independent Actions Explain the rationale for, side effects of, and importance of taking medications prescribed. Inform client of pertinent food and drug interactions. • Warfarin (Coumadin) Instruct client to inform physician before taking other prescription and nonprescription medications. Instruct client to inform all health care providers of medications being taken.	*Taking medications as prescribed ensures that therapeutic drug levels will be maintained. Clients should be instructed not to discontinue taking medications if they feel better. Clients without financial resources should be assisted in accessing appropriate resources to obtain needed medications (e.g., pharmacy assistance programs).*

THERAPEUTIC INTERVENTIONS	RATIONALE
Desired Outcome: The client will state signs and symptoms to report to the health care provider.	
Independent Actions Instruct client to report these additional signs and symptoms: • Chest pain that seems unrelated to incisional discomfort • Development of or increased shortness of breath • Dizziness, fainting • Increased fatigue and weakness • Weight gain of more than 2 lb in a day or 4 lb in a week • Swelling of feet or ankles • Persistent cough, especially if productive of yellow, green, rust-colored, or frothy sputum • Significant change in pulse rate or rhythm (check with physician about client's need to monitor pulse at home) • Persistent low-grade fever or temperature above 101°F (38.3°C) for more than 1 day • Depression or problems with concentration or memory that last more than 6 weeks • A fever in combination with chest pain and malaise occurring 1 week to 1 month after surgery	*Reporting concerning signs and symptoms to the appropriate provider allows for modification of the treatment plan.* *May indicate a pulmonary embolism.* *May indicate decreased cardiac output.* *May indicate decreased renal function.* *May indicate infection or pulmonary embolism.* *May indicate decreased cardiac output.* *May indicate dehydration and/or infection.* *A common feature after bypass surgery, but it should be resolved by 6 weeks.* *May be indicative of postpericardiotomy syndrome and require treatment with anti-inflammatory agents.*

THERAPEUTIC INTERVENTIONS	RATIONALE
Desired Outcome: The client will identify community resources that can assist with cardiac rehabilitation and adjustment to having had heart surgery.	
Independent Actions Provide information about community resources that can assist client with cardiac rehabilitation and adjustment to having had heart surgery (e.g., American Heart Association, Mended Hearts Club, counseling services).	*Cardiac disease can significantly impact an individual's and family's socioeconomic status. Providing information specific to community resources is important to provide a necessary continuum of care and may impact the client's health status, preventing future hospitalizations.*

THERAPEUTIC INTERVENTIONS	RATIONALE
Desired Outcome: The client, in collaboration with the nurse, will develop a plan for adhering to recommended follow-up care including future appointments with health care provider, wound care, and pain management.	

THERAPEUTIC INTERVENTIONS	RATIONALE

Independent Actions

Collaborate with the client to develop a plan for adherence with the medial regimen that includes:

Provide the client with routine postoperative instructions and measures to improve adherence.

If valve replacement surgery was done, instruct the client to:
- Not have dental work for 6 months.
- Inform health care providers of valve surgery so prophylactic antimicrobials may be started before any dental work, invasive diagnostic procedures, or surgery.
- Perform good oral hygiene in order to reduce the risk for infective endocarditis.

Regular health care appointments are important to determine effectiveness of the prescribed treatment plan.

Actions are important to prevent the development of endocarditis.

ADDITIONAL NURSING DIAGNOSES

ACTIVITY INTOLERANCE NDx
Related to:
- Tissue hypoxia associated with decreased cardiac output, impaired alveolar gas exchange, and anemia (results from hemodilution, blood loss, and red cell hemolysis [red cells are traumatized by the CPB machine])
- Difficulty resting and sleeping associated with frequent assessments and treatments, discomfort, fear, and anxiety

RELATED CARE PLANS

Standardized Preoperative Care Plan
Standardized Postoperative Care Plan

HYPERTENSION

High blood pressure is categorized by the American College of Cardiology and the American Heart Association as normal, elevated, or stage 1 or stage 2 hypertension on the basis of average BP measured in a healthcare setting. In adults, normal blood pressure is classified as a systolic BP < 120 mm Hg and a diastolic BP < 80 mm Hg. Elevated blood pressure in adults is defined as a systolic BP between 120 and 129 mm Hg and a diastolic BP < 80 mm Hg. Hypertension is categorized into two stages with stage 1 hypertension defined as a systolic BP between 130 and 139 mm Hg or diastolic BP between 80 and 89 mm Hg. Stage 2 hypertension is defined as a systolic BP ≥ 140 mm Hg or a diastolic ≥ 90 mm Hg. Hypertensive crisis, defined as a systolic BP > 180 mm Hg and/or a diastolic BP > 120 mm Hg, is a medical emergency and requires immediate medical attention.

Based on current definitions, approximately 46% of the US general adult population (≥20 years of age) have stage 1 or stage 2 hypertension with the prevalence higher in males, higher in African Americans than in whites, Asians, and Hispanic Americans, and rising dramatically with increasing age. In the landmark Framingham Heart Study, approximately 90% of adults free of hypertension at age 55 or at age 65 developed hypertension during their lifetimes (prevalence based on earlier definitions of hypertension). Additional risk factors associated with the development of hypertension include family history, obesity, sedentary lifestyle, tobacco use, heavy use of alcohol, stress, and certain chronic conditions such as kidney disease, diabetes, and sleep apnea.

The two major types of hypertension are primary (essential) hypertension and secondary hypertension. Primary hypertension, which constitutes approximately 95% of the cases, has an unknown etiology. Secondary hypertension tends to appear suddenly and has identifiable causes, which include renal parenchymal or vascular disease, Cushing syndrome, certain neurological disorders, pheochromocytoma, primary aldosteronism, coarctation of the aorta, and use of certain drugs (e.g., adrenal steroids, oral contraceptives, nonsteroidal anti-inflammatories, cyclooxygenase-2 inhibitors, sympathomimetics such as decongestants and anorexiants, amphetamines, cocaine).

The pathological hallmark of hypertension is an increase in systemic vascular resistance. In order to sustain adequate tissue perfusion when vascular resistance is increased, the heart must pump harder. A prolonged increase in cardiac workload eventually leads to ventricular hypertrophy and heart failure. The prolonged increase in vascular pressure causes widespread pathological changes in the blood vessels. The end result of all the changes in the cardiovascular system is a decreased blood supply to the tissues, with target organ damage occurring most often in the eyes, kidneys, brain, and heart. This target organ damage is often what causes the initial symptoms in the person with hypertension.

Initial treatment of hypertension may be nonpharmacologic and consists of lifestyle modifications such as weight reduction, regular aerobic exercise, and moderation of dietary sodium and alcohol intake. If these measures do not achieve the desired control of blood pressure, pharmacological therapy is initiated. Primary pharmacological agents used to treat hypertension include thiazide diuretics, ACE inhibitors, angiotensin II receptor blockers (ARBs), and CCBs. If the person's blood pressure is inadequately controlled by the initial drug, a second drug from another class is added or another drug is substituted until the desired control of blood pressure is achieved with a minimum of side effects.

This care plan focuses on the adult client hospitalized with severe hypertension that is either newly diagnosed or uncontrolled.

OUTCOME/DISCHARGE CRITERIA

The client will:
1. Have B/P within a safe range
2. Have evidence of adequate tissue perfusion
3. Have no signs and symptoms of complications
4. Verbalize a basic understanding of hypertension and its effects on the body
5. Identify modifiable risk factors for hypertension and ways to alter these factors
6. Verbalize an understanding of medications ordered including rationale, food and drug interactions, side effects, schedule for taking, and importance of taking as prescribed
7. Verbalize an understanding of the rationale for and components of the recommended diet
8. State signs and symptoms to report to the health care provider
9. Identify community resources that can assist in making lifestyle changes necessary for effective control of hypertension
10. Develop a plan for adhering to recommended follow-up care including future appointments with health care provider

Nursing Diagnosis   INEFFECTIVE PERIPHERAL TISSUE PERFUSION NDx

Definition: Decrease in blood circulation to the periphery, which may compromise health.

Related to:
- Increased peripheral vascular resistance
- Atherogenic changes in the blood vessels associated with the effects of prolonged or excessive elevation of B/P
- Possible decrease in cardiac output associated with the increased cardiac workload and eventual myocardial hypertrophy that result from elevated B/P
- Excessive lowering of B/P by antihypertensive medications

CLINICAL MANIFESTATIONS

Subjective	Objective
Verbal self-report of pain, numbness, or tingling in the extremities at rest or while walking.	Altered mental status, restlessness, confusion, cold extremities, diminished pulses, pallor in extremities, absent bowel sounds, abdominal pain, anemia, elevated BUN

RISK FACTORS
- Peripheral vascular disease
- Atherosclerosis
- Decreased hemoglobin
- Interruption of blood flow

DESIRED OUTCOMES

The client will maintain adequate tissue perfusion as evidenced by:
a. B/P declining toward normal range for client
b. Usual mental status
c. Extremities warm with absence of pallor and cyanosis
d. Palpable peripheral pulses
e. Capillary refill time less than 2 to 3 seconds
f. Absence of exercise-induced pain
g. Urine output at least 30 mL/h

NOC OUTCOMES	NIC INTERVENTIONS
Circulation status; tissue perfusion	Vital signs monitoring; hypertension management

NURSING ASSESSMENT	RATIONALE

Assess for and report the following:
• Further increase in B/P, failure of B/P to decline in response to antihypertensive agents, or rapid or excessive decline in B/P.
• Signs and symptoms of diminished tissue perfusion:
  • Restlessness
  • Confusion
  • Cool extremities
  • Pallor or cyanosis of extremities
  • Diminished or absent peripheral pulses
  • Low capillary refill
  • Angina
  • Increasing BUN and serum creatinine levels
  • Oliguria
Assess and monitor B/P.
	Early recognition of signs and symptoms of ineffective tissue perfusion allows for prompt intervention.

THERAPEUTIC INTERVENTIONS	RATIONALE
Independent Actions Implement measures to reduce anxiety (e.g., provide a calm, restful environment). Implement measures to relieve headache (e.g., minimize environmental stimulation). Implement measures to promote rest: **D** ● ✦ • Maintain a calm environment. • Limit the number of visitors. • Maintain activity restrictions.	*Identified independent nursing actions help to reduce sympathetic nervous system stimulation, which could increase B/P and heart rate.*
Discourage excessive intake of beverages high in caffeine such as coffee, tea, and colas. **D** ✦	*Caffeine has a vasoconstrictive effect.* *Vasoconstriction reduces the size/diameter of arterial vessel walls, increasing systemic vascular resistance or afterload. As a result of an increase in afterload, B/P must be increased to maintain adequate tissue perfusion.*
Discourage smoking.	*Nicotine causes vasoconstriction, which elevates B/P by increasing afterload/systemic vascular resistance.*
Maintain dietary sodium restrictions as ordered. **D** ✦	*Restricting sodium intake helps to reduce fluid retention, which can increase preload and B/P.*
Dependent/Collaborative Actions Administer the following medications if ordered: **D** ✦ • Adrenergic inhibiting agents • Centrally acting adrenergic inhibitors • Alpha-adrenergic blockers • Peripheral adrenergic inhibitors • Beta-adrenergic blockers • Combined alpha-adrenergic and beta-adrenergic blockers • Vasodilators for immediate reduction in B/P • ACE inhibitors • Calcium-channel blocking agents • Angiotensin II receptor antagonists • Diuretics	*Medications are administered to reduce B/P in order to improve tissue perfusion.* *Persistent, untreated hypertension leads to myocardial hypertrophy and possibly heart failure.*
Consult physician: • Before administering antihypertensive medications if client has an excessive or rapid drop in B/P • If signs and symptoms of diminished tissue perfusion persist or worsen.	*A rapid drop in B/P of more than 20% to 25% in a person with severe hypertension can reduce perfusion to vital organs.* *Notification of the appropriate health care provider allows for modification of the treatment plan.*

NDx = NANDA Diagnosis   **D** = Delegatable Action   ● = UAP   ✦ = LVN/LPN   ⊝▶ = Go to ⊝volve for animation

Nursing Diagnosis **ACUTE PAIN NDx (HEADACHE)**

Definition: Unpleasant sensory and emotional experience associated with actual or potential tissue damage, or described in such terms of such damage (International Association for the Study of Pain); sudden or slow onset of any intensity from mild to severe with an anticipated or predictable end, and with a duration of less than 3 months.

Related to: Distention of the cerebral blood vessels associated with increased vascular pressure

CLINICAL MANIFESTATIONS

Subjective	Objective
Verbal self-report of pain such as "pressure," "squeezing tightness" in the skull, face, or both	Increased B/P; increased heart rate

RISK FACTORS

- Increased B/P
- Increased cerebral blood flow

DESIRED OUTCOMES

The client will obtain relief of headache as evidenced by:
a. Verbalization of same
b. Relaxed facial expression and body positioning
c. Increased participation in activities

NOC OUTCOMES

Comfort level; pain control

NIC INTERVENTIONS

Pain management; environmental management: comfort; analgesic administration

NURSING ASSESSMENT	**RATIONALE**
Assess for signs and symptoms of headache: • Statements of same • Restlessness • Irritability • Grimacing • Rubbing head • Avoidance of bright lights and noises • Reluctance to move Assess client's perception of the severity of the headache using a pain intensity rating scale. Assess the client's pain pattern (e.g., location, quality, onset, duration, precipitating factors, aggravating factors, alleviating factors).	*Early recognition of signs and symptoms of acute headache pain allows for prompt intervention.*

THERAPEUTIC INTERVENTIONS	**RATIONALE**
Independent Actions Perform actions to reduce fear and anxiety about the pain experience. Provide a quiet environment. **D ● ✦** Avoid jarring bed or startling client to minimize risk of sudden movements. **D ● ✦** Provide or assist with nonpharmacological measures for headache relief: **D ✦** • Cool cloth to forehead • Back and neck massage • Elevation of head • Relaxation exercises • Diversional activities	*Fear and anxiety can stimulate the sympathetic nervous system, causing an increase in B/P and heart rate.* *Decreasing fear and anxiety helps to promote relaxation and increase the client's threshold and tolerance for pain.* *Patients with migraine-type headaches can benefit from a dimly lit environment.*

THERAPEUTIC INTERVENTIONS	RATIONALE
Dependent/Collaborative Actions	
Perform actions to reduce B/P:	*Elevated B/P, if extreme, can cause headaches in some individuals.*
• Administer ordered antihypertensive medications. **D** ✦	
Administer analgesics as ordered and before headache becomes severe. **D** ✦	
Consult appropriate health care provider (e.g., pharmacist, physician) if above measures fail to relieve headache.	*Notification of the appropriate health care provider allows for modification of the treatment plan.*

Collaborative Diagnosis | RISK FOR CEREBROVASCULAR ACCIDENT/ HYPERTENSIVE ENCEPHALOPATHY

Definition: Death of brain cells due to ischemia (lack of blood flow) to a part of the brain, or hemorrhage into the brain.

Related to:

Cerebrovascular accident related to cerebral thrombosis, embolism, or hemorrhage associated with injury to the arterial walls resulting from atherosclerosis and/or a prolonged increase in pressure in the cerebral vessels

Hypertensive encephalopathy related to cerebral edema associated with hyperperfusion of the brain (excessive cerebral blood flow results from decompensation of the cerebral blood flow autoregulatory mechanism in response to markedly elevated B/P)

CLINICAL MANIFESTATIONS

Subjective	Objective
Verbal self-report of difficulty swallowing	Speech difficulty, impaired mobility, decreased level of consciousness, facial droop, ptosis

RISK FACTORS
- Hypertension
- Cerebrovascular disease
- Smoking
- Obesity
- Metabolic syndrome

DESIRED OUTCOMES

The client will not experience a cerebrovascular accident or hypertensive encephalopathy as evidenced by:
a. Absence of dizziness, syncope, visual disturbances, and speech impairments
b. Absence or resolution of headache
c. Absence of vomiting
d. Mentally alert and oriented
e. Pupils equal and normally reactive to light
f. Normal sensory and motor function

NURSING ASSESSMENT	RATIONALE
Assess for signs and symptoms of cerebrovascular accident/ hypertensive encephalopathy:	*Early recognition of signs and symptoms of cerebrovascular accident and/or hypertensive encephalopathy allows for prompt intervention.*
• Dizziness, syncope	
• Visual disturbances (e.g., diplopia, blurred vision, loss of vision)	
• Slurred speech, aphasia	
• Persistent or increasing headache	
• Vomiting	
• Decreased level of consciousness	
• Unequal pupils or a sluggish or absent pupillary reaction to light	
• Paresthesias, facial droop, ptosis, weakness of extremity, paralysis	
• Seizures	

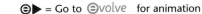

NDx = NANDA Diagnosis   **D** = Delegatable Action   ● = UAP   ✦ = LVN/LPN   ⊖▶ = Go to ⊖volve for animation

THERAPEUTIC INTERVENTIONS	RATIONALE

Dependent/Collaborative Actions

Perform actions to reduce B/P:
- Administer medications as ordered. **D** ✦

Instruct client to avoid activities that create a Valsalva response (e.g., straining to have a bowel movement, holding breath while moving up in bed).

Keep head of bed elevated at least 30 degrees and encourage client to keep head and neck in neutral, midline position. **D** ● ✦

If signs and symptoms of a cerebrovascular accident or hypertensive encephalopathy occur:
- Administer antihypertensive agents if ordered:
  - Vasodilators
- Maintain client on bed rest.
- Initiate appropriate safety measures (e.g., side rails up, seizure precautions).
- Administer osmotic diuretics and corticosteroids if ordered.

Collectively, all collaborative actions help to reduce the risk of a cerebrovascular accident and hypertensive encephalopathy.

Actions help to prevent a sudden increase in ICP and dislodgment of an existing thrombus.

Actions help to promote adequate venous return from the cerebral vessels.

Provides for rapid B/P reduction.
Medications help to reduce ICP.

Collaborative Diagnosis   # RISK FOR IMPAIRED RENAL FUNCTION

Definition: Renal insufficiency refers to a decline in renal function to about 25% of normal.

Related to: Vascular changes in the kidneys associated with effects of prolonged or severe hypertension

CLINICAL MANIFESTATIONS

Subjective	Objective
Verbal self-report of shortness of breath	Oliguria; fluid and electrolyte imbalances; weight gain; elevated B/P; crackles/rales

RISK FACTORS
- MI
- Hypertension
- Arteriosclerosis

DESIRED OUTCOMES

The client will maintain adequate renal function as evidenced by:
a. Urine output at least 30 mL/h
b. Absence of proteinuria
c. BUN, serum creatinine, and creatinine clearance values within normal range

NURSING ASSESSMENT	RATIONALE

Assess for signs and symptoms of impaired renal function:
- Nocturia
- Urine output less than 30 mL/h
- Urine specific gravity fixed at or less than 1.010
- Proteinuria

Assess BUN/serum creatinine levels for abnormalities.

Early recognition of signs and symptoms of impaired renal function allows for prompt intervention.

THERAPEUTIC INTERVENTIONS	RATIONALE

Dependent/Collaborative Actions

Perform actions to reduce B/P:
- Administer antihypertensive agents.
- Maintain an adequate fluid intake to reduce risk of dehydration.
  - Encourage oral fluid intake.
  - Administer intravenous fluids as ordered.

Collaborative actions help to improve renal blood flow.

THERAPEUTIC INTERVENTIONS	RATIONALE
If signs and symptoms of impaired renal function occur: • Consult physician about lowering the dose of or discontinuing ACE inhibitors if BUN and serum creatinine levels continue to rise significantly. • Prepare client for dialysis if indicated.	*ACE inhibitors should be used cautiously in persons with impaired renal function because they can have an adverse effect on renal function.* *Decreases fear and anxiety.*

Collaborative Diagnosis | RISK FOR AORTIC DISSECTION

Definition: A tear in the wall of the aorta that allows blood to flow between the layers of the wall of the aorta, forcing the layers apart.

Related to: Weakening and degeneration of the aortic media associated with a severe or prolonged increase in pressure in the aorta

CLINICAL MANIFESTATIONS

Subjective	Objective
Verbal self-report of tearing, stabbing, or shearing-type pain that is severe with sudden onset	Widening of the mediastinum; hemodynamic instability; lack of peripheral pulses

RISK FACTOR

• Hypertension

DESIRED OUTCOMES

The client will not experience dissection of the aorta as evidenced by:
a. Absence of sudden, severe chest pain
b. Palpable peripheral pulses with no change in pulse pattern
c. Usual sensory and motor function
d. Usual mental status
e. Stable vital signs
f. Skin warm and usual color

NURSING ASSESSMENT	RATIONALE
Assess for signs and symptoms of aortic dissection: • Sudden, severe chest pain that may radiate to back • Abnormal pulse pattern in extremities • Sudden lack of pulse in an extremity Assess for signs and symptoms of hypovolemic shock: • Restlessness • Agitation • Significant decrease in B/P • Rapid, weak pulse • Cool skin • Pallor • Diminished or absent pulses	*Early recognition of signs and symptoms of aortic dissection allows for prompt intervention.*

THERAPEUTIC INTERVENTIONS	RATIONALE
Dependent/Collaborative Actions Perform actions to reduce B/P: • Administer antihypertensives. • Alleviate pain. • Alleviate anxiety.	*Actions help to prevent aortic dissection.*

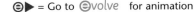

Continued...

THERAPEUTIC INTERVENTIONS	RATIONALE
Instruct client to avoid activities that create a Valsalva response (e.g., straining to have a bowel movement, holding breath while moving up in bed).	*Increases intrathoracic pressure.*
If signs and symptoms of aortic dissection occur:	
• Maintain client on strict bed rest.	*Helps to maintain B/P.*
• Monitor vital signs frequently.	
• Administer oxygen as ordered.	*Maintains tissue oxygenation.*
• Prepare client for diagnostic studies (e.g., transesophageal echocardiogram, computed tomography) if planned.	*Decreases fear and anxiety.*
• Administer antihypertensive agents.	*Decreases B/P.*
• Prepare client for surgery if planned.	*Decreases fear and anxiety.*

Nursing Diagnosis **INEFFECTIVE FAMILY HEALTH MANAGEMENT** NDx

Definition: A pattern of regulating and integrating into family processes a program for the treatment of illness and its sequelae that is unsatisfactory for meeting specific health goals of the family unit.

Related to:
- Lack of understanding of the implications of not following the prescribed treatment plan
- Difficulty modifying personal habits (e.g., alcohol intake, dietary preferences)
- Undesirable side effects of some antihypertensive agents
- Insufficient financial resources

CLINICAL MANIFESTATIONS

Subjective	Objective
Verbal self-report of difficulty with regulating one or more prescribed regimens for treatment and illness; not taking action to include treatment regimen in daily routines	Acceleration of illness symptoms; choice of daily living ineffective for meeting goals of a treatment program

RISK FACTORS
- Complex therapeutic regimen
- Excessive demands

DESIRED OUTCOMES

The client will demonstrate the probability of effective management of the therapeutic regimen as evidenced by:
a. Willingness to learn about and participate in treatments and care
b. Statements reflecting ways to modify personal habits
c. Statements reflecting an understanding of the implications of not following the prescribed treatment plan

NOC OUTCOMES

Compliance behavior; treatment behavior: illness or injury; knowledge: treatment regimen; health beliefs: perceived resources; knowledge: cardiac disease management; health beliefs: perceived ability to perform

NIC INTERVENTIONS

Self-modification assistance; medication management; values clarification; exercise promotion; smoking cessation assistance; teaching: prescribed diet; weight reduction assistance; financial resource assistance

NURSING ASSESSMENT	RATIONALE
Assess for indications that the client may be unable to effectively manage the therapeutic regimen:	*Identification of indications of the inability to effectively manage a therapeutic regimen allows for implementation of the appropriate support/interventions.*
• Statements reflecting inability to manage care at home	
• Failure to adhere to treatment plan (e.g., not adhering to dietary modifications, refusing medications)	
• Statements reflecting a lack of understanding of factors that may cause progression of hypertension	
• Statements reflecting an unwillingness or inability to modify personal habits	

NURSING ASSESSMENT	RATIONALE

- Statements reflecting view that hypertension will reverse itself or that the situation is hopeless and efforts to comply with the therapeutic regimen are useless
- Statements reflecting that the side effects of medications are too uncomfortable and that the client feels better when not taking medication
- Statements reflecting that medications are too expensive

THERAPEUTIC INTERVENTIONS	RATIONALE

Independent Actions

Implement measures to promote effective management of the therapeutic regimen:

- Explain hypertension in terms the client can understand; stress that hypertension is a chronic condition and that adherence to the treatment plan is necessary in order to delay and/or prevent complications.
- Encourage questions and clarify misconceptions client has about hypertension and its effects, and the side effects of medications.
- Provide instructions on and encourage client to participate in the treatment plan (e.g., calculating sodium intake, monitoring B/P); determine areas of misunderstanding and reinforce teaching as necessary.
- Provide client with written instructions about dietary modifications, signs and symptoms to report, medication therapy, B/P monitoring, and exercise regimen.
- Assist client to identify ways medication regimen, exercise, and dietary modifications can be incorporated into lifestyle; focus on modifications of lifestyle rather than complete change.
- Assist client to identify a reward system for self that will assist him/her to effect necessary change(s).
- Initiate and reinforce discharge teaching.
- Provide information about and encourage utilization of community resources that can assist client to make necessary lifestyle changes (e.g., cardiovascular fitness, weight loss, and smoking cessation programs; stress management classes).
- Encourage client to discuss concerns about the cost of medications and visits with health care provider; obtain a social service consult to assist with financial planning and to obtain financial aid if indicated.
- Encourage client to attend follow-up educational classes
- Reinforce behaviors suggesting future compliance with the therapeutic regimen (e.g., statements reflecting plan for adhering to treatment plan, statements reflecting an understanding of hypertension and its long-term effects).
- Include significant others in explanations and teaching sessions and encourage their support; reinforce the need for client to assume responsibility for managing as much of care as possible.

Dependent/Collaborative Actions

Consult appropriate health care provider (e.g., social worker, physician) regarding referrals to community health agencies if continued instruction or support is needed.

To promote effective management of a therapeutic regimen, the nurse must ensure that the client understands expectations. In addition, the nurse must ensure that the client has the appropriate resources to adhere to the treatment plan (e.g., financial, social support).

Consulting the appropriate health care provider allows for modification of discharge teaching/continued care.

DISCHARGE TEACHING/CONTINUED CARE

Nursing Diagnosis **DEFICIENT KNOWLEDGE NDx OR INEFFECTIVE HEALTH MAINTENANCE NDx***

Definition: Deficient Knowledge NDx: Absence of cognitive information related to a specific topic, or its acquisition; **Ineffective Health Maintenance NDx:** Inability to identify, manage, and/or seek out help to maintain well-being.

CLINICAL MANIFESTATIONS

Subjective	Objective
Verbal self-report of unfamiliarity with information	Inability to accurately follow instructions

NOC OUTCOMES

Knowledge: treatment regimen; cardiac disease management

NIC INTERVENTIONS

Health system guidance; teaching: individual; teaching: prescribed diet; teaching: prescribed medication

NURSING ASSESSMENT	RATIONALE
Assess client's readiness and ability to learn. Assess meaning of illness to client.	*Early recognition of readiness to learn and meaning of illness to client allows for implementation of the appropriate teaching interventions.*

THERAPEUTIC INTERVENTIONS	RATIONALE

Desired Outcome: The client will verbalize a basic understanding of hypertension and its effects on the body.

Independent Actions

Explain hypertension and its effects in terms client can understand. Use available teaching aids (e.g., pamphlets, videotapes).

Inform client that hypertension is often asymptomatic and that absence of symptoms is not a reliable indication that B/P is within a safe range.

Educating clients in terms they understand regarding their underlying disease process can facilitate understanding as to the importance of adhering to a treatment plan.

THERAPEUTIC INTERVENTIONS	RATIONALE

Desired Outcome: The client will identify modifiable risk factors for hypertension and ways to alter these factors.

Independent Actions

Inform client that certain modifiable factors such as elevated serum lipid levels, excessive alcohol intake, a sedentary lifestyle, smoking, and excess body weight have been shown to increase the risk for cardiovascular disease and hypertension.

Assist client to identify changes in lifestyle that can help the client to manage hypertension (e.g., dietary modification, physical exercise on a regular basis, smoking cessation, moderation of alcohol intake, weight loss if overweight).

Encourage client to limit daily alcohol consumption (daily alcohol intake exceeding 1 oz of ethanol may contribute to the development of hypertension).

Thorough education is a critical component of the care of a client with hypertension. The client must have a thorough understanding of the importance of adhering to diet, medication, activity/exercise, and nutritional recommendations to prevent an exacerbation and control the disease.

Current recommendations are no more than two drinks per day for men and no more than one drink per day for women and lighter-weight persons. A "drink" is considered to be ½ oz of ethanol (e.g., 1½ oz of 80-proof whiskey, 12 oz of beer, 5 oz of wine).

---

*The nurse should select the nursing diagnostic label that is most appropriate for the client's discharge teaching needs.

THERAPEUTIC INTERVENTIONS	RATIONALE
Instruct client to participate in a regular aerobic exercise program (e.g., walking, swimming) and avoid isometric exercise (e.g., weight training). Caution client to consult physician before beginning an exercise program.	*Decreases weight and improves cardiovascular stamina.*

THERAPEUTIC INTERVENTIONS	RATIONALE

Desired Outcome: The client will verbalize an understanding of medications ordered including rationale, food and drug interactions, side effects, schedule for taking, and importance of taking as prescribed.

Independent Actions

Explain the rationale for, side effects of, and importance of taking medications prescribed. Inform client of pertinent food and drug interactions. • Diuretics • Beta-adrenergic blockers • ACE inhibitors	*Taking medications as prescribed ensures that therapeutic drug levels will be maintained.* *Clients should be instructed not to discontinue taking medications if they feel better. Clients without financial resources should be assisted in accessing appropriate resources to obtain needed medications (e.g., pharmacy assistance programs).*

THERAPEUTIC INTERVENTIONS	RATIONALE

Desired Outcome: The client will verbalize an understanding of the rationale for and components of the recommended diet.

Independent Actions

Explain the rationale for the recommended dietary modifications: • Reduced sodium intake • Reduced intake of saturated fat and cholesterol • Include the recommended daily allowances of potassium, calcium, and magnesium in diet.	*Reducing sodium intake to a recommended 2.4 g/day can help control hypertension by reducing the fluid retention associated with increased intake.*

THERAPEUTIC INTERVENTIONS	RATIONALE

Desired Outcome: The client will state signs and symptoms to report to the health care provider.

Independent Actions

Instruct the client to report: • Persistent headache or headache present upon awakening • Sudden and continued increase in B/P (if B/P is monitored at home) • Chest pain • Shortness of breath • Significant weight gain or swelling of feet or ankles • Changes in vision • Frequent or uncontrollable nosebleeds • Persistent dizziness, lightheadedness, or fainting • Persistent side effects experienced from use of antihypertensive medications (e.g., impotence; dry mouth; depression; persistent dry cough; swelling of the tongue, face, or neck) • Side effects of diuretic therapy	*Reporting signs and symptoms indicative of hypertension to the appropriate provider allows for modification of the treatment plan and may prevent complications.*

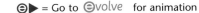

THERAPEUTIC INTERVENTIONS	RATIONALE

Desired Outcome: The client will identify community resources that can assist in making lifestyle changes necessary for effective control of hypertension.

Independent Actions

Provide information regarding community resources and support groups that can assist client in making lifestyle changes that are necessary for effective control of hypertension (e.g., cardiovascular fitness, weight loss, and smoking cessation programs; stress management classes).

Hypertension can significantly impact an individual's and family's socioeconomic status. Providing information specific to community resources is important to provide a necessary continuum of care and may impact the client's health status, preventing future hospitalizations.

THERAPEUTIC INTERVENTIONS	RATIONALE

Desired Outcome: The client, in collaboration with the nurse, will develop a plan for adhering to recommended follow-up care including future appointments with health care provider.

Independent Actions

Reinforce the importance of keeping follow-up appointments with health care provider and continuing lifelong medical supervision.

Regular health care appointments are important to determine effectiveness of the prescribed treatment plan.

RELATED NURSING DIAGNOSES

FEAR/ANXIETY NDX

Related to:
- Necessity for urgent treatment
- Possibility of severe disability or sudden death
- Unfamiliar environment
- Persistent or severe headache
- Lack of understanding of diagnostic tests, diagnosis, and treatment plan

IMPLANTABLE CARDIAC DEVICES

Implantable cardiac devices are surgically implanted for use in rhythm control. Pacemakers and ICDs are small battery-powered devices that monitor the heart rate and deliver electrical impulses to the heart to help correct dysrhythmias. Both pacemakers and ICDs consist of a pulse generator (contains the battery and electronic circuitry) and electrode catheters (leads). Both devices can be implanted during a minor surgical procedure under local anesthesia. The leads are inserted into the heart transvenously via the subclavian, jugular, or cephalic vein. The leads are then tunneled under the skin and attached to the pulse generator that is implanted in a subcutaneous pocket created in the subclavicular area or, less commonly, in the abdomen. A combined pacemaker and cardioverter-defibrillator is also available.

A pacemaker is used to stimulate the heart electrically when the heart fails to initiate or conduct intrinsic electrical impulses at a rate that is sufficient to maintain adequate perfusion. Pacemaker insertion is indicated for treatment of symptomatic bradydysrhythmias (e.g., sinus bradycardia, second- and third-degree heart block, sick sinus syndrome)

and on some occasions, for treatment of tachydysrhythmias that have been unresponsive to other forms of therapy.

Pacemakers are either temporary or permanent. Temporary pacemakers are used to regulate the heart rate in emergency or short-term situations. In most instances, temporary pacing is done using external transcutaneous pacing electrodes or using temporary pacemaker electrodes that have been placed on the epicardium during thoracic surgery (e.g., heart surgery). Temporary pacemakers are attached to and regulated by an external power source. Permanent pacemakers are used for long-term management of certain dysrhythmias. There are a number of permanent pacemakers available. Their functional capabilities are described by a three- or five-letter code that specifies the chamber being paced, the chamber being sensed, mode of response, programmability/rate responsiveness, and antitachycardia functions.

Most pacemakers used now are dual-chambered pacemakers with leads in both the atrium and ventricle. Dual-chamber pacing allows for the physiological timing between atrial systole and ventricular systole to be maintained, which improves cardiac output. Present-day pacemakers can also be programmed externally, and most operate in a synchronous mode (a chamber of the heart is triggered to fire or is inhibited by the intrinsic activity of the heart) or a rate-responsive mode. The most frequently used rate-responsive systems have an activity sensor in the pulse generator that detects movement and then appropriately increases or decreases the pacing rate.

ICDs are used to treat life-threatening dysrhythmias. They are indicated for persons who have survived one or more incidents of sudden cardiac death, persons with recurrent ventricular tachycardia or ventricular fibrillation, and for persons with demonstrated risk factors for sudden cardiac death. The sensing lead of an ICD monitors the heart's electrical activity and if the heart rate exceeds the generator's programmed rate, the generator delivers a burst of antitachycardia pacing (ATP) to override the heart's pacemaker. If after a programmed number of ATP therapies the rate continues to exceed the desired rate, the ICD device then delivers low-energy and high-energy cardioversion shocks. If ventricular fibrillation is present, defibrillation shocks are delivered.

This care plan focuses on the adult client with a symptomatic dysrhythmia hospitalized for implantation of either a cardioverter-defibrillator or permanent pacemaker.

OUTCOME/DISCHARGE CRITERIA

The client will:
1. Have adequate cardiac output
2. Have no signs and symptoms of postoperative complications
3. Verbalize a basic understanding of the rationale for and function of an ICD/pacemaker
4. Demonstrate knowledge of how to monitor ICD function
5. Verbalize an understanding of appropriate actions to take if the ICD delivers a shock
6. Verbalize an understanding of recommended activity restrictions
7. Identify appropriate safety precautions associated with having an ICD/pacemaker
8. State signs and symptoms to report to the health care provider
9. Develop a plan for adhering to recommended follow-up care including future appointments with health care provider, medications prescribed, and wound care

---

Nursing/Collaborative Diagnosis | # PREOPERATIVE USE IN CONJUNCTION WITH THE STANDARDIZED PREOPERATIVE CARE PLAN

Nursing Diagnosis | ## RISK FOR DECREASED CARDIAC OUTPUT NDx

Definition: Susceptible to inadequate blood pumped by the heart to meet metabolic demands of the body, which may compromise health.

Related to:
- A slow heart rate (if client has a bradydysrhythmia)
- Decreased diastolic filling time associated with a rapid and/or irregular heart rate (if client has a tachydysrhythmia)
- Decreased diastolic filling time and ineffective ventricular contractions if client has sustained ventricular tachycardia or ventricular fibrillation
- Related factors will depend upon the type of device implanted and underlying dysrhythmias

CLINICAL MANIFESTATIONS

Subjective	Objective
Verbal self-report of anxiety; fatigue; weakness; dizziness; syncope; exertional dyspnea	Change in mental status; B/P less than 90 mm Hg systolic or below normal for patient; irregular or absent pulses; diminished peripheral pulses; tachypnea; cool, pale skin; cool extremities; increased capillary refill time

RISK FACTOR

- Cardiac dysrhythmias

DESIRED OUTCOMES

The client will maintain an adequate cardiac output as evidenced by:
a. Systolic B/P of at least 90 mm Hg
b. Palpable peripheral pulses
c. No increase in number or duration of dizziness or syncopal episodes
d. Baseline mental status
e. Absence of cyanosis
f. Urine output at least 30 mL/h

NOC OUTCOMES

Circulation status; cardiac pump effectiveness

NIC INTERVENTIONS

Cardiac care; cardiac risk management; dysrhythmia management; tissue perfusion: cardiac

NURSING ASSESSMENT

Assess client upon admission for baseline data regarding status of cardiac output.
Assess for and report signs and symptoms of decreased cardiac output:
- Change in mental status
- B/P less than 90 mm Hg systolic or below normal for patient
- Irregular or absent pulses
- Diminished peripheral pulses
- Tachypnea
- Cool, pale skin
- Cool extremities
- Increased capillary refill time
- Verbal reports of anxiety, fatigue, weakness, dizziness, syncope, exertional dyspnea
Assess for and report ECG rhythm abnormalities that may alter cardiac output:
- Bradydysrhythmias
- Tachydysrhythmias
- Ventricular tachycardia/fibrillation

RATIONALE

Early recognition and reporting of signs and symptoms of decreased cardiac output allow for prompt intervention.

THERAPEUTIC INTERVENTIONS

Independent Actions

Implement measures to maintain an adequate cardiac output before surgery:
- Perform actions to reduce cardiac workload:
  - Place client in a semi- to high-Fowler's position unless systolic B/P is less than 90 mm Hg (then head of bed should be flat).
  - Implement measures to promote rest (e.g., reduce fear and anxiety, maintain activity restrictions, limit the number of visitors).
  - Discourage smoking.

- Instruct client to avoid activities that create a Valsalva response (e.g., straining to have a bowel movement, holding breath while moving up in bed).
- Notify physician if serum potassium level is abnormal.

RATIONALE

Nicotine has a cardiostimulatory effect and causes vasoconstriction; the carbon monoxide in smoke reduces oxygen availability.
Valsalva maneuvers can increase vagal stimulation, resulting in slowing of the heart rate. In addition, Valsalva maneuvers can also lead to a sudden increase in cardiac workload.
Abnormal potassium levels affect myocardial conductivity.

THERAPEUTIC INTERVENTIONS	RATIONALE
Dependent/Collaborative Actions Implement measures to maintain an adequate cardiac output before surgery: • Perform actions to reduce cardiac workload: • Maintain oxygen therapy as ordered. • Administer the following medications if ordered: • Antidysrhythmics • Anticholinergics • Consult physician before giving prescribed digitalis preparations if client has heart block or ventricular dysrhythmias. • Prepare for and assist with cardioversion or defibrillation if performed. • Maintain temporary pacing if ordered.	 *Anticholinergic drugs increase the heart rate by blocking the action of the vagal nerve in patients with symptomatic bradycardia.* *Digitalis preparations can increase ventricular irritability.* *Prevents further compromise of cardiac output by decreasing heart rate.* *Decreases fear and anxiety.* *Maintains cardiac output.*

NURSING/COLLABORATIVE DIAGNOSIS: POSTOPERATIVE

USE IN CONJUNCTION WITH THE STANDARDIZED POSTOPERATIVE CARE PLAN

Collaborative Diagnoses **RISK FOR PACEMAKER/IMPLANTABLE CARDIOVERTER-DEFIBRILLATOR MALFUNCTION**

Definition: Failure of the implanted device to maintain cardiac output.

Related to: Improper placement or dislodgment of the leads, break in or faulty attachment of the leads, or pulse generator malfunction

CLINICAL MANIFESTATIONS

Subjective	Objective
Verbal self-report of receiving multiple shocks without ECG evidence of tachydysrhythmia; dizziness; lightheadedness	ECG showing rapid and/or irregular rate without accompanying ATP; presence of sustained ventricular tachycardia or fibrillation on ECG; absence of pacer spikes when heart rate falls below the programmed pacing rate; pacer spikes present with normal P waves and QRS complexes; absence of P wave or QRS complex after a pacer spike; presence of ectopic beats; apical pulse less than programmed pacing rate; significant decrease in B/P; syncope; dyspnea

DESIRED OUTCOMES

The client will experience normal cardioverter-defibrillator function as evidenced by:
a. Absence of sustained ventricular dysrhythmias on ECG
b. Client reports of receiving internal shocks when ventricular tachycardia or fibrillation is evident on the ECG
The client will experience normal pacemaker function as evidenced by:
a. Regular pulse at a rate equal to or greater than the programmed pacing rate

b. Stable B/P
c. Absence of dizziness, syncope, and dyspnea
d. ECG showing pacer spikes before the P wave and/or QRS complex when the pulse rate falls below the programmed pacing rate

NURSING ASSESSMENT	RATIONALE
Assess for and report signs and symptoms of cardioverter-defibrillator/pacemaker malfunction: • Multiple shocks without ECG evidence of tachydysrhythmia; dizziness; lightheadedness; significant decrease in BP; syncope; dyspnea • ECG with regular/irregular pulse rate without pacing spikes • Symptoms will depend upon type of implantable device. Ascertain the type of ICD/pacemaker the client has and how it is programmed (including the rate at which pacing should occur if a combination pacemaker cardioverter-defibrillator was implanted). Have information available about problem-solving techniques and activation and deactivation of the specific device.	*Early recognition and reporting of signs and symptoms of device malfunction allow for prompt intervention.*

THERAPEUTIC INTERVENTIONS	RATIONALE
Independent Actions Implement measures to reduce the risk for breakage and dislodgment of the ICD leads in order to prevent ICD malfunction: • Maintain activity restrictions as ordered. • Instruct client to limit movement of the arm and shoulder on the side that the ICD was inserted for the first 48 hrs after surgery. If signs and symptoms of pacemaker malfunction occur: • Turn the client to either side.	*Limiting movements during the first 48 hrs after surgery allows for leads to embed in the myocardium.* *In the event of a pacemaker malfunction, such as failure to capture, turning the client to the left side may help facilitate placement of the lead(s) against the myocardium.*

Dependent/Collaborative Actions
If signs and symptoms of ICD malfunction occur:
• If the device is activated and ventricular fibrillation or pulseless ventricular tachycardia occurs:
  • Notify the physician.
  • Proceed with external defibrillation (the defibrillation paddles should be positioned at least 3–4 inches away from the pulse generator).
  • Administer antidysrhythmics.
• If the device is activated and delivering inappropriate shocks:
  • Notify the physician.
If signs and symptoms of pacemaker malfunction occur:
• Follow manufacturer's suggestions for problem solving:
  • Have a pacemaker magnet available.
  • If client has a temporary pacemaker, adjust sensitivity and/or output (milliamperes [mA]) within prescribed limits until capture occurs.
• Prepare client for chest radiograph to check placement of leads.
• Prepare client for surgical repair or replacement of pulse generator if indicated.
	Allows for prompt intervention and prevention of a deleterious outcome.
	
	The physician or other trained personnel may need to deactivate the device.
	
	Increasing the sensitivity or output (mA) may help improve pacer capture of the myocardial wall, producing ventricular or atrial contraction.
	Decreases fear and anxiety.

Collaborative Diagnoses | # RISK FOR CARDIAC TAMPONADE

Definition: Rapid collection of blood in the pericardial sac that compresses the myocardium, preventing the heart from pumping effectively.

Related to: Perforation of the atria or ventricle by the pacemaker leads

CLINICAL MANIFESTATIONS

Subjective	Objective
Verbal self-report of pericardial pain; sense of fullness in chest	Pericardial friction rub; significant decrease in B/P; narrowed pulse pressure; pulsus paradoxus; distant or muffled heart sounds; JVD

RISK FACTOR

- Lead malposition

DESIRED OUTCOMES

The client will not experience cardiac tamponade as evidenced by:
a. Stable vital signs
b. Audible heart sounds
c. Absence of JVD

NURSING ASSESSMENT	**RATIONALE**
Assess for and report signs and symptoms of cardiac perforation/cardiac tamponade: • Decrease in B/P • Pulsus paradoxus • Narrow pulse pressure • Muffled heart sounds Assess chest radiograph results/echocardiogram results for abnormalities.	*Early recognition and reporting of signs and symptoms of cardiac tamponade allow for prompt intervention.*

THERAPEUTIC INTERVENTIONS	**RATIONALE**
Independent Actions Implement measures to prevent dislodgment of the pacemaker/ICD leads: • Maintain activity restrictions as ordered. • Instruct client to limit movement of the arm and shoulder on the side that the ICD was inserted for the first 48 hrs after surgery. **Dependent/Collaborative Actions** If signs and symptoms of cardiac perforation or tamponade occur: • Prepare client for chest radiograph and echocardiogram. • Prepare client for repositioning or replacement of the lead(s), repair of perforation, and/or pericardiocentesis if planned.	*Actions reduce the risk for perforation of the heart wall.*

Collaborative Diagnoses **RISK FOR PNEUMOTHORAX**

Definition: Air in the pleural space with resulting collapse of the lung.

Related to: Accumulation of air in the pleural space associated with accidental puncture of the pleura during subclavian insertion of the cardioverter-defibrillator leads

CLINICAL MANIFESTATIONS

Subjective	Objective
Verbal self-report of sudden onset of chest pain	Absent breath sounds with hyperresonant percussion note over involved area; rapid, shallow, and/or labored respirations; tachycardia; restlessness; confusion; significant decrease in oximetry results; abnormal arterial blood gas values; chest radiograph results showing lung collapse

RISK FACTOR

- Surgical implantation in close proximity to lung

DESIRED OUTCOMES

The client will have resolution of pneumothorax if it occurs as evidenced by:
a. Audible breath sounds and a resonant percussion note over lungs
b. Normal respiratory rate and pattern
c. Usual mental status
d. Arterial blood gas values returning to normal range

NURSING ASSESSMENT	RATIONALE
Assess for and immediately report signs and symptoms of pneumothorax: • Absent breath sounds • Dyspnea • Tachycardia • Restlessness • Confusion	*Early recognition and reporting of signs and symptoms of a pneumothorax allow for prompt intervention.*
Assess for and immediately report signs and symptoms of tension pneumothorax with mediastinal shift: • Severe dyspnea • Increased restlessness and agitation • Rapid and/or irregular heart rate • Hypotension • Neck vein distention • Shift in trachea from midline	*A tension pneumothorax is a rapid accumulation of air in the pleural space that can result from a pneumothorax.* *Compression of the great vessels can result in altered cardiac output. This complication is a medical emergency.*

THERAPEUTIC INTERVENTIONS	RATIONALE
Independent Actions If signs and symptoms of pneumothorax occur: • Maintain client on bed rest in a semi- to high-Fowler's position	*Promotes lung expansion.*
Dependent/Collaborative Actions If signs and symptoms of pneumothorax occur: • Maintain oxygen therapy as ordered. • Prepare client for insertion of chest tube if indicated.	*Maintains tissue oxygenation.* *A chest tube will evacuate accumulated air from the pleural space and reexpand the lung.*

Collaborative Diagnoses **RISK FOR UNDESIRED STIMULATION OF THE HEART AND/OR CERTAIN NERVES AND MUSCLES**

Definition: Adverse stimulation of the heart and nerves which may cause dysrhythmias, pain, or breathing problems.

Related to: The presence of a foreign body in the heart and the emission of electrical impulses from the pacemaker lead(s) to nearby muscles and nerves such as the diaphragm, intercostal muscles, and phrenic nerve

CLINICAL MANIFESTATIONS

Subjective	Objective
Verbal self-report of abdominal or chest wall twitching	Ventricular ectopic beats on ECG; hiccups

RISK FACTOR

- Malposition of leads

DESIRED OUTCOMES

The client will have resolution of ventricular irritability and undesired nerve and muscle stimulation as evidenced by:
a. Absence of ventricular ectopic beats
b. Absence of hiccups
c. Absence of abdominal and intercostal muscle twitching

NURSING ASSESSMENT	**RATIONALE**
Assess for and report signs and symptoms of ventricular irritability and undesired nerve or muscle stimulation.	*Early recognition and reporting of signs and symptoms of ventricular irritability and undesired nerve or muscle stimulation allow for prompt intervention.*

THERAPEUTIC INTERVENTIONS	**RATIONALE**

Dependent/Collaborative Actions
If signs and symptoms persist:
- Consult physician.
- Turn client to left side.
- Prepare client for the following procedures if planned:
  - Chest x-ray to determine placement of lead(s)
  - Repositioning of the lead(s)
	Turning the client to the left side may help facilitate placement of the lead(s) against the myocardium.

DISCHARGE TEACHING/CONTINUED CARE

Nursing Diagnosis **DEFICIENT KNOWLEDGE NDx; INEFFECTIVE FAMILY HEALTH MANAGEMENT NDx; OR INEFFECTIVE HEALTH MANAGEMENT NDx***

Definition: **Deficient Knowledge NDx:** Absence of cognitive information related to a specific topic, or its acquisition; **Ineffective Family Health Management NDx:** Pattern of regulating and integrating into family processes a therapeutic regimen for the treatment of illness and its sequelae that is unsatisfactory for meeting specific health goals of the family unit; **Ineffective Health Management NDx:** Inability to identify, manage, and/or seek out help to maintain well-being.

---

*The nurse should select the diagnosis that is most appropriate for the client's discharge teaching needs.

NDx = NANDA Diagnosis   **D** = Delegatable Action   ● = UAP   ✦ = LVN/LPN   ⊝▶ = Go to ⊝volve for animation

CLINICAL MANIFESTATIONS

Subjective	Objective
Verbal self-report of unfamiliarity with information	Inability to accurately follow instructions

RISK FACTORS

- Denial of disease process
- Cognitive deficiency
- Failure to take action to reduce risk factors

NOC OUTCOMES	NIC INTERVENTIONS
Knowledge: treatment regimen	Teaching: individual; teaching: prescribed activity/exercise

NURSING ASSESSMENT	RATIONALE
Assess client's readiness and ability to learn.	*Early recognition of readiness to learn and meaning of illness to client allows for implementation of the appropriate teaching interventions.*
Assess meaning of treatment plan with client.	

THERAPEUTIC INTERVENTIONS	RATIONALE

Desired Outcome: The client will verbalize a basic understanding of the rationale for and function of an ICD/pacemaker.

Independent Actions

Reinforce preoperative teaching regarding the rationale for and basic function of an ICD/pacemaker.	*Ensuring client's understanding preoperatively helps to reinforce necessity of the treatment plan and allows for additional client concerns to be addressed.*

THERAPEUTIC INTERVENTIONS	RATIONALE

Desired Outcome: The client will demonstrate knowledge of how to monitor ICD/pacemaker function.

Independent Actions

Inform the client with a combined pacemaker/cardioverter-defibrillator device of the pacemaker's programmed pacing rate and, if appropriate, provide instructions about how to take pulse and monitor both the rate and regularity. (Many physicians prefer that their clients not monitor their own pulse because of the confusion between paced beats and spontaneous beats.)	*Proper education enables the client to monitor for possible device malfunction and seek out the appropriate health care provider if concerning signs and symptoms develop.*
Instruct client with an ICD to monitor for and report the following:	
• Signs of a heart rhythm disturbance such as dizziness, fainting, shortness of breath, unexplained fatigue, or feeling that heart is fluttering.	*May indicate malfunction of the ICD.*

THERAPEUTIC INTERVENTIONS	**RATIONALE**

Instruct the client with a pacemaker to have pulse generator function checked regularly per physician's instructions or if experiencing symptoms such as dizziness, fainting, unexplained fatigue, or shortness of breath. Inform the client that monitoring may be done at the physician's office or by telephone monitoring device.

Decreases potential for malfunction and allows for alterations in settings as indicated.

THERAPEUTIC INTERVENTIONS	**RATIONALE**

Desired Outcome: The client will identify appropriate safety precautions associated with having an ICD/pacemaker.

Independent Actions

Instruct client to adhere to the following safety precautions:

- Inform all health care providers about the device (certain medical equipment such as a magnetic resonance imaging [MRI] machine, radiation therapy machine, and electrocautery equipment may actually damage the pulse generator and/or interfere with normal function of these devices).
- Avoid close proximity with strong magnets (e.g., MRI machine, large industrial magnets), high-voltage electrical equipment (e.g., arc welder, running car engine), and large electromagnetic fields (e.g., radio and television transmitters).
- Move away from any electrical device if dizziness or light-headedness occurs.
- If planning to travel, obtain name of a physician and/or pacemaker/ICD clinic at point(s) of destination.
- Alert airport personnel to device (it may set off the security alarm).
- Always wear a medical alert bracelet or tag and carry an identification card that includes the name of the manufacturer, model number, mode of operation, and insertion date of the device.
- Clients with ICDs should adhere to restrictions on driving; typically, clients are not allowed to drive until they have had a 6-month discharge-free period (this is a law in some states for persons with ICDs).

Safety precautions are necessary to maintain proper functioning of device at all times.

THERAPEUTIC INTERVENTIONS	**RATIONALE**

Desired Outcome: The client will verbalize an understanding of appropriate actions to take if the ICD delivers a shock.

Independent Actions

- Instruct client to call an ambulance or emergency rescue service and then to lie down if the ICD delivers a shock.
- Instruct family members to call the client's physician and the ambulance or emergency rescue service if the client's ICD delivers a shock while they are present. Instruct them to get CPR training and to initiate CPR if the client is having symptoms such as an irregular and rapid pulse along with dizziness, shortness of breath, chest pain, sweatiness, or loss of consciousness and the device fails to fire after 30 seconds or if the device fires unsuccessfully 4 to 7 times.

Delivery of a shock indicates a potentially life-threatening dysrhythmia has occurred. The appropriate health care provider should be notified for possible alteration of the treatment plan or hospitalization for further evaluation and stabilization of client's condition.

THERAPEUTIC INTERVENTIONS	RATIONALE

Desired Outcome: The client will verbalize an understanding of recommended activity restrictions.

Independent Actions

Provide the following instructions about activity restrictions after ICD/pacemaker insertion:
- Limit movement of the arm and shoulder on the operative side for the first 48 hrs after surgery.
- Limit activities that put undue stress on the incision site (e.g., using arms over head, bowling, racquetball, tennis, lifting over 25 lb) until cleared by physician (usual time is 1–2 months).
- Avoid letting anything rub on or hit the device.
- Do not rub or "play with" the device under the skin.
- Avoid immersing the device insertion site in water for at least 3 days after surgery.
- Avoid activities that can cause blunt trauma to the pulse generator (e.g., contact sports, firing a rifle with the butt end of the gun against affected shoulder).

Activity restrictions serve to ensure that the service wires embed in the appropriate position in the myocardium to achieve maximum device function. Additional restrictions serve to prevent the formation of a wound hematoma, wound infection, or device damage.

THERAPEUTIC INTERVENTIONS	RATIONALE

Desired Outcome: The client will state signs and symptoms to report to the health care provider.

Independent Actions

Instruct client to report these additional signs and symptoms to health care provider:
- Increased irregularity of pulse (if self-monitoring is being done) or episodes of feeling that heart is fluttering
- Unexplained fatigue
- Lightheadedness, dizziness, fainting
- Shortness of breath
- Redness, swelling, drainage, or increased soreness at implant site
- Unexplained fever
- Swelling of arm on the side of the device

Reporting signs and symptoms of device malfunction to the appropriate provider allows for modification of the treatment plan and may prevent life-threatening complications.

May indicate infection.

May indicate venous thrombosis associated with insertion/presence of leads in vein.

THERAPEUTIC INTERVENTIONS	RATIONALE

Desired Outcome: The client, in collaboration with the nurse, will develop a plan for adhering to recommended follow-up care including future appointments with health care provider, medications prescribed, and wound care.

Independent Actions

Collaborate with the client to develop a plan for adherence including:

The importance of keeping scheduled appointments with pacemaker/ICD clinic and for chest radiograph verification of lead placement.

Allow adequate time for questions and clarification of information provided.

Regular health care appointments are important to determine effectiveness of the prescribed treatment plan.

ADDITIONAL NURSING DIAGNOSES

FEAR NDx /ANXIETY NDx
Related to unfamiliar environment, lack of understanding of surgical procedure, anticipated postoperative discomfort, possibility of ICD/pacemaker malfunction, and possible changes in lifestyle as a result of having an ICD/pacemaker

RELATED CARE PLANS

Standardized Preoperative Care Plan
Standardized Postoperative Care Plan

MYOCARDIAL INFARCTION

An MI is an acute coronary syndrome resulting from prolonged ischemia of the heart muscle and occurs when blood flow to an area of the myocardium is insufficient to meet the myocardial oxygen requirements. Sustained ischemia causes tissue necrosis and irreversible cellular damage, which results in disturbances in mechanical, biochemical, and electrical function in the necrotic or infarcted area. The degree of altered function depends on the area of the heart involved and the size of the infarct.

MIs may be classified in a number of ways. A transmural MI is characterized by ischemic necrosis of the full thickness of the myocardium. A nontransmural MI is characterized by ischemic necrosis that is limited to the endocardium or to the endocardium and myocardium. A more common classification distinguished MI types based on electrocardiographic findings with one type marked by ST elevation (STEMI) and one that is not (NSTEMI). In addition to these classification systems, many practitioners also describe an MI by the area of the heart that has been damaged (e.g., anterior MI, lateral MI, inferior MI). Across MI types, the presence of Q waves or ST-segment elevation is associated with higher early mortality and morbidity.

Most MIs are caused by rupture of atherosclerotic plaque in a coronary artery, which leads to the release of substances that activate platelet aggregation and clotting factors and cause local vasoconstriction. Other less common causes include severe, persistent spasm of a coronary artery; severe or prolonged hypotension; a rapid ventricular rate; and cocaine use.

The classic symptom of an MI is intense retrosternal chest pain/discomfort. It is often described as a tight, heavy, squeezing, or crushing sensation or "heartburn," may radiate to the left arm, neck, jaw, or back; lasts longer than 20 minutes; and is unrelieved by nitroglycerin and rest. However, 15% to 25% of infarctions go unrecognized because clients have only mild or no chest discomfort or may be asymptomatic. Asymptomatic MIs are more likely to be experienced by diabetic patients. Other signs and symptoms may include shortness of breath, diaphoresis, dizziness, weakness, pallor, nausea, and vomiting. As with men, women most commonly experience some chest pain or discomfort, however, women are more likely than men to experience other common symptoms particularly shortness of breath, nausea/vomiting, and back or jaw pain.

The extent of myocardial damage can be limited by early (within 4–6 hrs of the onset of symptoms) restoration of coronary blood flow. This can be accomplished by injection of a thrombolytic agent to dissolve the clot obstructing the coronary artery or by a coronary angioplasty. In addition to early restoration of coronary blood flow, treatment with an antiplatelet agent, a beta blocker, an ACE inhibitor, and an HMG-CoA (3-hydroxy-3-methylglutaryl-coenzyme A) reductase inhibitor has been found to significantly reduce mortality after an MI. The prognosis for a client who has had an MI is largely influenced by size and location of the infarct, concurrent cardiovascular status, and promptness and effectiveness of treatment.

This care plan focuses on the adult client hospitalized during an episode of intense chest pain for definitive diagnosis and management of a MI.

OUTCOME/DISCHARGE CRITERIA

The client will:
1. Have adequate cardiac output and tissue perfusion
2. Tolerate prescribed activity without a significant change in vital signs, chest pain, dyspnea, dizziness, or extreme fatigue or weakness
3. Verbalize a basic understanding of an MI
4. Demonstrate accuracy in counting pulse
5. Identify modifiable cardiovascular risk factors and ways to alter these factors
6. Verbalize an understanding of the rationale for and components of a diet designed to lower serum cholesterol and triglyceride levels
7. Verbalize an understanding of medications ordered including rationale, food and drug interactions, side effects, schedule for taking, and importance of taking as prescribed
8. Verbalize an understanding of activity restrictions and the rate at which activity can be progressed
9. State signs and symptoms to report to the health care provider
10. Identify community resources that can assist with cardiac rehabilitation and adjustment to the effects of an MI
11. Share feelings and concerns about changes in body functioning and usual roles and lifestyle
12. Develop a plan for adhering to recommended follow-up care including future appointments with health care provider

---

Nursing Diagnosis **RISK FOR DECREASED CARDIAC OUTPUT** NDx

Definition: Susceptible to inadequate blood pumped by the heart to meet metabolic demands of the body, which may compromise health.

Related to: Possible decreased contractility and altered conductivity of the heart associated with the myocardial damage that has occurred with infarction

---

NDx = NANDA Diagnosis   **D** = Delegatable Action   ● = UAP   ✦ = LVN/LPN   ⊕▶ = Go to ⊜volve for animation

CLINICAL MANIFESTATIONS

Subjective	Objective
Verbal self-report of anxiety; fatigue; weakness; dizziness; syncope; exertional dyspnea	Change in mental status; B/P less than 90 mm Hg systolic or below normal for patient; irregular or absent pulses; diminished peripheral pulses; tachypnea; cool, pale skin; cool extremities; increased capillary refill time

DESIRED OUTCOMES

The client will have adequate cardiac output as evidenced by:
a. B/P within normal range for client
b. Apical pulse between 60 and 100 beats/min and regular
c. Resolution of gallop rhythm(s)
d. No reports of fatigue and weakness
e. Unlabored respirations at 12 to 20 breaths/min
f. Clear, audible breath sounds
g. Usual mental status
h. Absence of dizziness and syncope
i. Palpable peripheral pulses
j. Skin warm and usual color
k. Capillary refill time less than 2 to 3 seconds
l. Urine output at least 30 mL/h
m. Absence of edema and JVD

NOC OUTCOMES

Cardiac pump effectiveness; circulation status; tissue perfusion: peripheral; cardiac

NIC INTERVENTIONS

Cardiac care: acute; hemodynamic regulation; cardiac risk management; dysrhythmia management; cardiac care: rehabilitative

NURSING ASSESSMENT

Assess for signs and symptoms of decreased cardiac output:
- Variations in B/P (may be increased because of pain or compensatory vasoconstriction; may be decreased when compensatory mechanisms and pump fail)
- Tachycardia
- Presence of gallop rhythm(s)/S_4 heart sound
- Fatigue and weakness
- Dyspnea, orthopnea, tachypnea
- Crackles (rales)
- Restlessness, anxiousness, confusion, or other change in mental status
- Dizziness, syncope
- Diminished or absent peripheral pulses
- Cool extremities
- Pallor or cyanosis of skin
- Capillary refill time greater than 2 to 3 seconds
- Oliguria
- Edema
- JVD
- Chest radiograph results showing pulmonary vascular congestion, pulmonary edema, or pleural effusion
- Abnormal arterial blood gas values
- Significant decrease in oximetry results

Assess for diagnostic findings indicative of an MI:
- Elevated serum creatine kinase (CK)-MB level
- Elevated serum troponin level
- Elevated serum lactate dehydrogenase (LDH) level with an LDH_1 level that is higher than the LDH_2 (a reliable indicator of an acute MI)
- ECG showing ST-segment elevation or depression, inversion of T waves, and/or presence of abnormal Q waves (there may be no Q waves if client has had a subendocardial infarction)

RATIONALE

Early recognition and reporting of signs and symptoms of an MI allow for prompt intervention.

THERAPEUTIC INTERVENTIONS	RATIONALE

Independent Actions

Perform actions to reduce cardiac workload:

- Place client in a semi- to high-Fowler's position. **D** ✦

- Instruct client to avoid activities that create a Valsalva response (e.g., straining to have a bowel movement, holding breath while moving up in bed).

- Implement measures to promote rest and conserve energy. **D** ● ✦

- Discourage smoking.

- Provide small meals rather than large ones.

- Discourage excessive intake of beverages high in caffeine such as coffee, tea, and colas.

- Restrict sodium intake if ordered.

- Increase activity gradually as allowed and tolerated.

Elevation of client's upper body reduces cardiac workload by decreasing venous return from the periphery and subsequently reducing preload.

When a client exhales after the Valsalva maneuver, the intrathoracic pressure falls, causing a sudden increase in venous return and a subsequent increase in preload and cardiac workload.

Physical rest reduces cardiac workload by lowering the body's energy requirements and subsequent need for oxygen.

Nicotine has a cardiostimulatory effect and causes vasoconstriction; the carbon monoxide in smoke reduces oxygen availability.

Large meals require a greater increase in blood supply to the gastrointestinal tract for digestion.

Caffeine is a myocardial stimulant and can increase myocardial oxygen consumption.

Restricting sodium helps to prevent fluid retention.

A gradual increase in activity prevents a sudden increase in cardiac workload.

Dependent/Collaborative Actions

Implement measures to maintain an adequate cardiac output

- Prepare client for procedures that may be performed to improve coronary blood flow:
  - Injection of a thrombolytic agent
  - Percutaneous coronary intervention
  - Insertion of an IABP
- Maintain oxygen therapy as ordered. **D** ✦
- Administer the following medications if ordered:

  - Nitrates

  - Beta-adrenergic blocking agents

  - ACE inhibitors

  - Antidysrhythmics

  - Anticoagulants

Consult physician if signs and symptoms of decreased cardiac output persist or worsen.

Decreases fear and anxiety.

When tissue oxygenation is adequate, the heart does not need to work as hard to supply oxygen to the tissues; thus more oxygen is available for myocardial use.

Nitrates decrease cardiac workload and myocardial oxygen demands by relaxing peripheral veins and, to a lesser extent, arterioles.

Beta-adrenergic blockers reduce cardiac workload by blocking sympathetic nervous system stimulation of beta receptors in the heart.

ACE inhibitors/angiotensin II receptor antagonists block the vasoconstrictor effect of angiotensin II, which causes a decrease in aldosterone output.

Antidysrhythmics improve cardiac output by correcting automaticity and/or conduction abnormalities in the heart.

Anticoagulants help to restore/improve coronary blood flow.

Notifying the physician allows for modification of the treatment plan.

Nursing Diagnosis   **ACUTE PAIN NDx (CHEST PAIN/DISCOMFORT THAT MAY RADIATE TO ARM, NECK, JAW, OR BACK)**

Definition: Unpleasant sensory and emotional experience associated with actual on potential tissue damage, or described in terms of such damage (International Association for the Study of Pain); sudden or slow onset of any intensity from mild to severe with an anticipated or predictable end, and with a duration of less than 3 months.

Related to: Myocardial ischemia (a decreased oxygen supply forces the myocardium to convert to anaerobic metabolism; the end products of anaerobic metabolism act as irritants to myocardial neural receptors)

CLINICAL MANIFESTATIONS

Subjective	Objective
Verbal self-report of pain	Grimacing; rubbing neck, jaw, or arm; reluctance to move; clutching chest; restlessness; diaphoresis; increased B/P and/or tachycardia

RISK FACTORS

- Coronary artery disease
- Increase in oxygen demand

DESIRED OUTCOMES

The client will experience relief of chest pain/discomfort as evidenced by:
a. Verbalization of same
b. Relaxed facial expression and body positioning
c. Increased participation in activities
d. Stable vital signs

NOC OUTCOMES

Comfort level; pain control

NIC INTERVENTIONS

Pain management; analgesic administration; oxygen therapy

NURSING ASSESSMENT

Assess signs and symptoms of chest pain/discomfort:
- Verbalization of pain
- Grimacing
- Rubbing neck, jaw, or arm
- Reluctance to move
- Clutching chest
- Restlessness
- Diaphoresis
- Increased B/P
- Tachycardia

Assess client's perception of the severity of the pain/discomfort using an intensity rating scale.

Assess the client's pattern of pain/discomfort (e.g., location, quality, onset, duration, precipitating factors, aggravating factors, alleviating factors).

RATIONALE

Early recognition and reporting of signs and symptoms of chest pain allow for prompt intervention.

THERAPEUTIC INTERVENTIONS

Independent Actions
Implement measures to relieve pain/discomfort:
- Maintain client on bed rest in a semi- to high-Fowler's position. **D** ● ✦
- Provide or assist with nonpharmacological measures for pain relief (e.g., relaxation techniques, restful environment). **D** ✦

Dependent/Collaborative Actions
Implement measures to relieve pain/discomfort:
- Administer the following medications if ordered:
  - Intravenous narcotis opioid analgesics
  - Nitrates

- Maintain oxygen therapy as ordered. **D** ✦

RATIONALE

Bed rest helps to reduce myocardial oxygen demands by reducing cardiac workload.
Nonpharmacological interventions are effective because they stimulate closure of the gating mechanism in the spinal cord and subsequently block the transmission of pain impulses.

Intravenous rather than an intramuscular route should be used because intramuscular injections are poorly absorbed if tissue perfusion is decreased; intramuscular injections also elevate some serum enzyme levels, which may interfere with assessment of myocardial damage.
- *Oxygen therapy helps to increase the myocardial oxygen supply.*

THERAPEUTIC INTERVENTIONS	RATIONALE
Implement measures to maintain an adequate cardiac output: Prepare client for procedures that may be performed to improve coronary blood flow: • Injection of a thrombolytic agent • Percutaneous coronary intervention • Insertion of an IABP	*Decreases fear and anxiety.*
Consult physician if pain/discomfort persists or worsens.	*Notifying the physician allows for modification of the treatment plan.*

Nursing Diagnosis RISK FOR ACTIVITY INTOLERANCE NDx

Definition: Susceptible to experiencing insufficient physiological or psychological energy to endure or complete required or desired daily activities, which may compromise health.

Related to:
• Tissue hypoxia if cardiac output is decreased
• Difficulty resting and sleeping associated with discomfort, frequent assessments and treatments, fear, and anxiety

CLINICAL MANIFESTATIONS

Subjective	Objective
Verbal self-report of fatigue or weakness	Abnormal heart rate or B/P response to activity; exertional discomfort or dyspnea; ECG changes reflecting ischemia

RISK FACTORS	DESIRED OUTCOMES
• Increased oxygen demand • Immobility • Generalized weakness	The client will not experience activity intolerance as evidenced by: a. No reports of fatigue or weakness b. Ability to perform activities of daily living without exertional dyspnea, chest pain, diaphoresis, dizziness, and a significant change in vital signs

NOC OUTCOMES	NIC INTERVENTIONS
Activity tolerance; energy conservation; self-care: activities of daily living	Energy management; oxygen therapy; cardiac care: rehabilitative; sleep enhancement

NURSING ASSESSMENT	RATIONALE
Assess for signs and symptoms of activity intolerance: • Statements of fatigue or weakness • Exertional dyspnea, chest pain, diaphoresis, or dizziness • Abnormal heart rate response to activity (e.g., increase in rate of 20 beats/min above resting rate, rate not returning to preactivity level within 3 minutes after stopping activity, change from regular to irregular rate) • Significant change of 15–20 mm Hg in B/P with activity.	*Early recognition and reporting of signs and symptoms of activity intolerance allow for prompt intervention.*

THERAPEUTIC INTERVENTIONS	RATIONALE

Independent Actions

Implement measures to prevent activity intolerance:

- Perform actions to promote rest and/or conserve energy:
  - Maintain activity restrictions as ordered.
  - Minimize environmental activity and noise. **D** ✦
  - Organize nursing care to allow for periods of uninterrupted rest.
  - Limit the number of visitors and their length of stay.
  - Assist client with self-care activities as needed. **D** ✦
  - Keep supplies and personal articles within easy reach.
  - Instruct client in energy-saving techniques (e.g., using shower chair when showering, sitting to brush teeth or comb hair).
  - Implement measures to reduce fear and anxiety.
  - Implement measures to promote sleep:
  - Encourage relaxing diversional activities in the evening.
  - Allow client to continue usual sleep practices unless contraindicated.
  - Reduce environmental distractions.
  - Implement nonpharmacological measures to relieve pain/discomfort. **D** ✦

Instruct client to:

- Report a decreased tolerance for activity.
- Stop any activity that causes chest pain, shortness of breath, dizziness, or extreme fatigue or weakness.

Cells use oxygen and fat, protein, and carbohydrates to produce the energy needed for all body activities. Rest and activities that conserve energy result in a lower metabolic rate, which preserves nutrients and oxygen for necessary activities.

Dependent/Collaborative Actions

Implement measures to prevent activity intolerance:

- Perform actions to promote rest and/or conserve energy:
  - Implement measures to promote sleep:
  - Administer prescribed sedative-hypnotics.
  - Administer prescribed analgesics.
- Perform actions to maintain an adequate cardiac output if decreased cardiac output is contributing to client's activity intolerance.

- Maintain oxygen therapy as ordered.
- Increase client's activity gradually as allowed and tolerated.

Consult appropriate health care provider (e.g., cardiac rehabilitation therapist, physician) if signs and symptoms of activity intolerance persist or worsen.

Conservation of energy allows the patient to rest and improve ability to increase activity.

Sufficient cardiac output is necessary to maintain an adequate blood flow and oxygen supply to the tissues. Adequate tissue oxygenation promotes more efficient energy production, which subsequently improves the client's activity tolerance.

Maintains tissue oxygenation.

Improves cardiac stamina.

Notifying the physician allows for modification of the treatment plan.

Collaborative Diagnosis   # RISK FOR CARDIAC DYSRHYTHMIAS

Definition: Disturbance of heart rhythm.

CLINICAL MANIFESTATIONS

Subjective	Objective
Verbal self-report of palpitations; lightheadedness	Irregular apical pulse; pulse rate below 60 or above 100 beats/min; apical-radial pulse deficit; syncope; palpitations; abnormal rate, rhythm, or configurations on ECG

RISK FACTORS
- Electrolyte abnormalities
- Drug toxicities
- Myocardial ischemia

DESIRED OUTCOMES

The client will maintain normal sinus rhythm as evidenced by:
a. Regular apical pulse at 60 to 100 beats/min
b. Equal apical and radial pulse rates
c. Absence of syncope and palpitations
d. ECG showing normal sinus rhythm

NURSING ASSESSMENT

Assess frequently for and report signs and symptoms of cardiac dysrhythmias:
- Irregular apical pulse
- Syncope
- Palpitations

RATIONALE

Early recognition of dysrhythmias allows for prompt intervention.

THERAPEUTIC INTERVENTIONS

Independent Actions
If cardiac dysrhythmias occur:
- Initiate cardiac monitoring if not currently being done.
- Restrict client's activity based on client's tolerance and severity of the dysrhythmia.

Dependent/Collaborative Actions
Implement measures to maintain an adequate cardiac output.

If cardiac dysrhythmias occur:
- Administer antidysrhythmics if ordered.
- Maintain oxygen therapy as ordered.
- Prepare client for the following if planned:
  - Cardioversion
  - Insertion of a pacemaker or ICD
  - Catheter ablation of irritable site
- Have emergency cart readily available for defibrillation or CPR.

RATIONALE

Monitoring should be implemented in order to identify dysrhythmias that could cause further deterioration of the client's condition.
Rest reduces the workload of the injured heart.

Adequate cardiac output promotes adequate myocardial tissue perfusion and oxygenation and reduces the risk of cardiac dysrhythmias.
The most common complication after an MI is dysrhythmias due to the irritability of the heart muscle. Dysrhythmias are not usually treated unless they are life-threatening.

Collaborative Diagnosis **RISK FOR THROMBOEMBOLISM**

Definition: A clot attached to a vessel/cardiac chamber wall that becomes dislodged, circulating within the blood. After an acute MI, a thromboembolism may result from debris and clots that collect inside dilated aneurismal sacs in the ventricle or from infarcted endocardium.

Related to:
- Venous stasis in the periphery associated with decreased cardiac output and decreased mobility
- Stasis of blood in the heart associated with decreased ventricular emptying (risk increases if dysrhythmias are present)

CLINICAL MANIFESTATIONS*

Subjective	Objective
Verbal self-report of pain; apprehension; anxiety	**Deep vein:** Tenderness; swelling; positive Homans' sign; increased warmth **Arterial:** Diminished or absent peripheral pulses; pallor, coolness, numbness, and/or pain in extremity **Cerebral:** Decreased level of consciousness; alteration in usual sensory and motor function **Pulmonary:** Sudden onset of chest pain, dyspnea, increased restlessness, and significant decrease in arterial oxygen saturation (SaO_2)

*Clinical manifestations vary depending upon the location of the embolus and may occur in the veins and arteries located in the legs, brain, and pulmonary system.

NDx = NANDA Diagnosis   **D** = Delegatable Action   ● = UAP   ✦ = LVN/LPN   ⊝▶ = Go to ⊝volve for animation

RISK FACTORS

- Immobility
- Ventricular aneurysms
- MIs
- Hypercoagulability

DESIRED OUTCOMES

The client will not develop a thromboembolism as evidenced by:
a. Absence of pain, tenderness, swelling, and numbness in extremities
b. Usual temperature and color of extremities
c. Palpable and equal peripheral pulses
d. Usual mental status
e. Usual sensory and motor function
f. Absence of sudden chest pain and dyspnea

NURSING ASSESSMENT

Assess for and report signs and symptoms of deep vein, arterial, cerebral, or pulmonary thromboembolism:
Monitor results of echocardiogram and report findings of a cardiac thrombus.

RATIONALE

Early recognition of signs and symptoms of thromboembolism allows for prompt intervention.

THERAPEUTIC INTERVENTIONS

Independent Actions

If signs and symptoms of an arterial embolus in an extremity occur:
- Maintain client on bed rest with affected extremity in a level or slightly dependent position.

If signs and symptoms of cerebral ischemia occur:
- Maintain client on bed rest; keep head and neck in neutral, midline position.

Dependent/Collaborative Actions

Implement measures to prevent the development of thromboemboli:
- Perform actions to reduce the risk of thrombus formation in the heart:
  - Implement measures to maintain an adequate cardiac output.
  - Prepare client for procedures to improve coronary blood flow (e.g., PCTA, insertion of IABP—intraaortic balloon pump).
  - Implement measures to treat dysrhythmias if present.
  - Administer antiarrhythmic medications.
  - Administer anticoagulants and antiplatelet agents if ordered.

If signs and symptoms of an arterial embolus in an extremity occur:
- Prepare client for diagnostic studies.
  - Doppler or duplex ultrasound
  - Arteriography
- Prepare client for the following if planned:
  - Injection of a thrombolytic agent
  - Embolectomy
- Administer anticoagulants as ordered.

RATIONALE

Positioning helps to improve arterial blood flow.

Bed rest should be maintained until it is determined that clot is stable and solidified.
Positioning helps to facilitate venous drainage of the head, reducing the risk of increased ICP.

The goal of dependent nursing actions is to prevent the formation of a thrombus by maintaining adequate blood flow and preventing venous stasis, reducing hypercoagulability of the blood, and limiting damage to the vessel linings.
Procedures will help improve coronary blood flow and improve cardiac output.
Reduces the risk of dysrhythmias that allow pooling of blood in the heart (e.g., atrial fibrillation).

Procedures act to restore blood flow to affected vessel.

Collaborative Diagnosis | RISK FOR RUPTURE OF A PORTION OF THE HEART (E.G., VENTRICULAR FREE WALL, INTERVENTRICULAR SEPTUM, PAPILLARY MUSCLE)

Definition: Tearing of cardiac tissues within the heart.

Related to: Weakening of cardiac tissue from ischemia and/or necrosis

CLINICAL MANIFESTATIONS*

Subjective	Objective
Not applicable	**Papillary muscle rupture:** Holosystolic murmur; dyspnea; evidence of papillary muscle rupture on echocardiography or cardiac catheterization **Ventricular septal defect:** Holosystolic murmur; parasternal thrill; finding of septal defect on echocardiography or cardiac catheterization **Cardiac tamponade:** Significant decrease in B/P; narrowed pulse pressure; pulsus paradoxus; distant or muffled heart sounds; JVD; increased CVP

RISK FACTOR

- MI or damage

DESIRED OUTCOME

The client will not experience rupture of any portion of the heart as evidenced by absence of signs of acute heart failure and/or cardiogenic shock.

NURSING ASSESSMENT

Assess for and report signs and symptoms of papillary muscle rupture, ventricular septal defect, and cardiac tamponade:
- Holosystolic murmurs
- Dyspnea

Assess for and immediately report signs and symptoms of acute heart failure and/or cardiogenic shock:
- Increased restlessness/confusion
- Systolic B/P less than 80 mm Hg
- Rapid, weak pulse
- Diminished or absent pulses
- Increase coolness and duskiness of skin
- Urine output less than 30 mL/h

RATIONALE

Early recognition of signs and symptoms of rupture of heart structures allows for prompt intervention.

THERAPEUTIC INTERVENTIONS

Independent Actions

Implement measures to reduce cardiac workload and increase activity as allowed. Add the following actions:
- Place client in semi-Fowler's position.
- Instruct client to avoid activities that create a Valsalva response (e.g., straining).
- Discourage smoking.

If signs and symptoms of rupture of a portion of the heart occur:
- Maintain client on bed rest.

Dependent/Collaborative Actions

If signs and symptoms of rupture of a portion of the heart occur:
- Assist with pericardiocentesis if performed.
- Assist with measures to treat heart failure or cardiogenic shock.

RATIONALE

Reducing cardiac workload helps to reduce risk of rupture of the papillary muscle and ventricular free wall or septum.

Nicotine increases vasoconstriction and increases cardiac workload.
The client may become hemodynamically unstable and therefore should be maintained on bed rest.

Cardiac tamponade is treated with pericardiocentesis.

*Clinical manifestations will vary depending upon which structures are affected.

Continued...

THERAPEUTIC INTERVENTIONS	RATIONALE

• Prepare client for surgical intervention if planned:
  • Valve replacement
  • Repair of ventricular septal defect
	Decreases fear and anxiety.

Collaborative Diagnosis **RISK FOR PERICARDITIS**

Definition: Inflammation of the pericardium.

Related to:
• Exposure to pathogens
• Death of tissue

CLINICAL MANIFESTATIONS

Subjective	Objective
Verbal self-report of precordial pain that frequently radiates to shoulder, neck, back, and arm; is intensified during deep inspiration, movement, and coughing; and usually is relieved by sitting up and leaning forward	Pericardial friction rub; persistent temperature elevation; further increase in white blood cell (WBC) count and sedimentation rate

RISK FACTORS
• MI
• Myocardial necrosis
• Infection

DESIRED OUTCOMES

The client will experience resolution of pericarditis if it develops as evidenced by:
a. Fewer reports of pericardial pain
b. Absence of pericardial friction rub
c. Temperature declining toward normal
d. WBC count and sedimentation rate declining toward normal range

---

NURSING ASSESSMENT	RATIONALE
Assess for and report signs and symptoms of pericarditis: • Pericardial friction rub • Elevated temperature • Pericardial pain Monitor erythrocyte sedimentation rate, WBC and differential cell counts for abnormalities.	*Early recognition of signs and symptoms of pericarditis allows for prompt intervention.*

THERAPEUTIC INTERVENTIONS	RATIONALE
Independent Actions If signs and symptoms of pericarditis occur: • Allay client's anxiety. • Assist client to assume position of comfort.	 *The client may believe that symptoms indicate recurrent MI.* *Pericarditic pain is best relieved with the patient sitting or leaning forward.*
Dependent/Collaborative Actions If signs and symptoms of pericarditis occur: • Administer anti-inflammatory agents if ordered.	 *Pain and inflammation associated with pericarditis are usually treated with anti-inflammatory agents.*

Collaborative Diagnosis · **RISK FOR INFARCTION EXTENSION OR RECURRENCE**

Definition: Expansion of tissue death from the MI and/or secondary MI.

Related to: Inadequate treatment of original MI

CLINICAL MANIFESTATIONS

Subjective	Objective
Verbal self-report of chest pain	Changes in vital signs; increase in cardiac enzyme levels; increase in ECG abnormalities (ST-segment elevation/ Q waves)

RISK FACTOR

- Previous MI

DESIRED OUTCOMES

The client will not experience infarct extension or recurrence as evidenced by:
a. No further episodes of persistent chest pain
b. Stable vital signs
c. Cardiac enzyme levels declining toward normal range
d. Improved ECG readings

NURSING ASSESSMENT	RATIONALE
Assess for and report signs and symptoms of infarct extension or recurrence (e.g., changes in vital signs; increase in cardiac enzyme levels; ECG changes [ST-segment elevation/ Q waves]).	*Early recognition of signs and symptoms of reinfarction allows for prompt intervention.*

THERAPEUTIC INTERVENTIONS	RATIONALE
Dependent/Collaborative Actions If client experiences signs and symptoms of infarct extension or recurrence: - Administer medications ordered: - Medications such as nitrates, ACE inhibitors, beta-blocking agents, aspirin, and heparin. - Prepare the client for coronary angiogram, thrombolytic therapy, or revascularization procedure (e.g., percutaneous transluminal coronary angioplasty [PTCA], CABG) if planned.	*The goal of dependent nursing actions is to reduce the workload of the heart, optimize function, and improve perfusion to the myocardium.* *Act to optimize cardiac performance and reduce the risk of reinfarction* *These medications optimize cardiac performance, reduce blood clotting activity and reduce the risk for reinfarction.* *Decreases fear and anxiety.*

Collaborative Diagnosis · **RISK FOR CARDIOGENIC SHOCK**

Definition: Decreased cardiac output and evidence of tissue hypoxia in the presence of adequate intravascular volume.

Related to:
- Inability of the heart to effectively provide perfusion to the tissues
- Cardiac tissue ischemia and/or necrosis

CLINICAL MANIFESTATIONS

Subjective	Objective
Verbal self-report of lethargy; restlessness	Systolic B/P below 80 mm Hg; rapid, weak pulse; diminished or absent peripheral pulses; increased coolness and duskiness or cyanosis of skin; urine output less than 30 mL/h

RISK FACTORS

- Myocardial ischemia
- MI
- Heart failure
- Pericardial infections

DESIRED OUTCOMES

The client will not develop cardiogenic shock as evidenced by:
a. Stable or improved mental status
b. Systolic B/P greater than 80 mm Hg
c. Palpable peripheral pulses
d. Stable or improved skin temperature and color
e. Urine output at least 30 mL/h

NURSING ASSESSMENT

Assess for and report signs and symptoms of cardiogenic shock:
- Systolic B/P <80 mm Hg
- Weak pulse
- Diminished peripheral pulses
- Cyanosis of skin
- Urine output <30 mL/h

RATIONALE

Early recognition of signs and symptoms of cardiogenic shock allows for prompt intervention.

THERAPEUTIC INTERVENTIONS

Dependent/Collaborative Actions

Implement measures to prevent cardiogenic shock:
- Perform actions to maintain an adequate cardiac output (e.g., administer inotropic agents).
- Perform actions to treat cardiac dysrhythmics if present (e.g., administer antiarrhythmics).
- Perform actions to treat heart failure if it occurs.
- Perform actions to treat rupture of any portion of the heart if it occurs.

If signs and symptoms of cardiogenic shock occur:
- Maintain oxygen therapy as ordered.
- Administer medications:
  - Positive inotropic agents
- Administer the following if ordered:
  - Sympathomimetics
  - Vasodilators
  - Intravenous fluids
- Assist with intubation and insertion of hemodynamic monitoring devices and/or cardiac assist devices:
  - Swan Ganz
  - IABP

RATIONALE

Cardiogenic shock that is unresponsive to therapy has a high mortality rate.

Medications geared toward optimizing cardiac performance and improving cardiac output are necessary. Cardiac assist devices support the failing heart when medication therapy is ineffective.

Inotropic agents act to increase myocardial contractility and improve heart failure.

DISCHARGE TEACHING/CONTINUED CARE

Nursing Diagnosis ## DEFICIENT KNOWLEDGE NDx OR INEFFECTIVE S-HEALTH MANAGEMENT NDx*

Definition: Deficient Knowledge NDx: Absence of cognitive information related to a specific topic, or its acquisition; **Ineffective Health Management NDx:** Pattern of regulating and integrating into daily living a therapeutic regimen for the treatment of illness and its sequelae that is unsatisfactory for meeting specific health goals.

CLINICAL MANIFESTATIONS

Subjective	Objective
Verbal self-report of unfamiliarity with information	Inability to follow-through with instructions

*The nurse should select the nursing diagnostic label that is most appropriate for the client's discharge teaching needs.

RISK FACTORS
- Denial of disease process
- Cognitive deficiency
- Failure to take action to reduce risk factors

NOC OUTCOMES	NIC INTERVENTIONS
Knowledge: treatment regimen; disease process; cardiac disease management	Health system guidance; teaching: individual; teaching: disease process; teaching: prescribed activity/exercise; teaching: prescribed medication

NURSING ASSESSMENT	RATIONALE
Assess client's readiness and ability to learn. Assess meaning of illness to client.	*Early recognition of readiness to learn and meaning of illness to client allows for implementation of the appropriate teaching interventions.*

THERAPEUTIC INTERVENTIONS	RATIONALE

Desired Outcome: The client will verbalize a basic understanding of an MI.

Independent Actions

Explain an MI in terms the client can understand. Use appropriate teaching aids (e.g., pictures, videotapes, heart models). Inform client that it takes approximately 6 to 8 weeks for the heart to heal after an MI.	*Clients vary in physical and cognitive ability to learn. When educating clients, nurses need to determine a client's ability to read and understand written materials. If literacy barriers are present, alternative educational materials should be provided. Better understanding of the clinical problem may enhance adherence.*

THERAPEUTIC INTERVENTIONS	RATIONALE

Desired Outcome: The client will demonstrate accuracy in counting pulse.

Independent Actions

Teach client how to count his/her pulse, being alert to the regularity of the rhythm. Allow time for return demonstration and accuracy check.	*Educating clients to assess their baseline pulse allows for early detection of irregularities warranting immediate attention from a health care provider. Early detection may reduce the incidence of sudden death.*

THERAPEUTIC INTERVENTIONS	RATIONALE

Desired Outcome: The client will identify modifiable cardiovascular risk factors and ways to alter these factors.

Independent Actions

Inform client that certain modifiable factors such as elevated serum lipid levels, a sedentary lifestyle, hypertension, and smoking have been shown to increase the risk for CAD.	*Thorough education is a critical component of the care of a client after an MI. Continued lifestyle modifications consistent with recommendations for clients with cardiovascular disease are necessary to prevent coronary reocclusion. The client must have a thorough understanding of the importance of adhering to diet, medication, activity/exercise, and nutritional recommendations to prevent an exacerbation and control the disease.*

NDx = NANDA Diagnosis   **D** = Delegatable Action   ● = UAP   ✦ = LVN/LPN   ⊖▶ = Go to ⊖volve for animation

Continued...

THERAPEUTIC INTERVENTIONS	RATIONALE
Assist client to identify changes in lifestyle that can help the client to eliminate or reduce the above risk factors and to help prevent a recurrent MI (e.g., dietary modification, physical exercise on regular basis, moderation of alcohol intake, smoking cessation). Encourage client to limit daily alcohol consumption. Daily alcohol intake exceeding 1 oz of ethanol may contribute to the development of hypertension and some forms of heart disease.	*Current recommendations are no more than two drinks per day for men and no more than one drink per day for women and lighter-weight persons. A "drink" is considered to be ½ oz of ethanol (e.g., 1½ oz of 80-proof whiskey, 12 oz of beer, 5 oz of wine).*

THERAPEUTIC INTERVENTIONS	RATIONALE

Desired Outcome: The client will verbalize an understanding of the rationale for and components of a diet designed to lower serum cholesterol and triglyceride levels.

Independent Actions

Provide instructions on ways the client can reduce intake of saturated fat and cholesterol:

- Reduce intake of meat fat (e.g., trim visible fat off meat; replace fatty meats such as fatty cuts of steak, hamburger, and processed meats with leaner products).
- Reduce intake of milk fat (e.g., avoid dairy products containing more than 1% fat).
- Reduce intake of *trans* fats (e.g., avoid stick margarine and shortening and foods such as commercial baked goods that are prepared with these products).
- Use vegetable oil rather than coconut or palm oil in cooking and food preparation.
- Use cooking methods such as steaming, baking, broiling, poaching, microwaving, and grilling rather than frying.
- Restrict intake of eggs.
- Encourage client to increase intake of omega-3 fatty acids (e.g., flaxseed, cold water ocean fish such as salmon and halibut) to help lower triglyceride levels and increase HDL levels.

The risk of CAD is associated with a serum cholesterol level of more than 200 mg/dL or a fasting triglyceride level of more than 150 mg/dL. Elevated serum lipid levels are one of the most firmly established risk factors for CAD.

Recommendations about the number of whole eggs allowed per week vary depending on the client's lipid levels.

THERAPEUTIC INTERVENTIONS	RATIONALE

Desired Outcome: The client will verbalize an understanding of medications ordered including rationale, food and drug interactions, side effects, schedule for taking, and importance of taking as prescribed.

Independent Actions

Explain the rationale for, side effects of, and importance of taking the medications prescribed. Inform client of pertinent food and drug interactions.

Taking medications as prescribed ensures that therapeutic drug levels will be maintained. Clients should be instructed not to discontinue taking medications if they feel better. Clients without financial resources should be assisted in accessing appropriate resources to obtain needed medications (e.g., pharmacy assistance programs).

THERAPEUTIC INTERVENTIONS	RATIONALE

Educate the client on the proper administration, dosing regimen, side effects, precautions, and storage of the following medications if ordered:
- Nitrates/nitrate patches/nitrate paste
- Beta-adrenergic blockers
- ACE inhibitors
- Lipid-lowering agents

Instruct the client to notify physician provider before taking other prescription medications and to inform all health care providers of medications being taken.

THERAPEUTIC INTERVENTIONS	RATIONALE

Desired Outcome: The client will state signs and symptoms to report to the health care provider.

Independent Actions

Instruct the client to report:
- Chest, arm, neck, jaw, or back discomfort unrelieved by nitroglycerin
- Shortness of breath
- Significant weight gain or swelling of feet or ankles
- Irregular pulse or a significant unexpected change in the pulse rate
- Persistent impotence or decreased libido (can be a side effect of certain medications or result from anxiety, depression, or fatigue)
- Inability to tolerate prescribed activity
- Increase in severity or frequency of episodes of angina

Reporting concerning signs and symptoms to the appropriate provider allows for modification of the treatment plan.

THERAPEUTIC INTERVENTIONS	RATIONALE

Desired Outcome: The client will verbalize an understanding of activity restrictions and the rate at which activity can be progressed.

Independent Actions

Reinforce physician's instructions about activity. Instruct client to:
- Gradually increase activity by adhering to a regular aerobic exercise program (often begins with walking).
- Take frequent rest periods for about 4 to 8 weeks after discharge.
- Avoid physical conditioning programs such as jogging and aerobic dancing until advised by physician.
- Avoid strenuous exercise and activities that involve pushing or lifting heavy objects (e.g., weightlifting).
- Avoid exercising for at least an hour after eating and when the environmental temperature is extremely hot or cold.
- Avoid tobacco use before exercise.
- Stop any activity that causes chest pain, shortness of breath, palpitations, dizziness, or extreme fatigue or weakness.
- Begin a cardiovascular fitness program if recommended by physician.

While the benefits of physical activity are an integral part of cardiac rehabilitation, the level of activity should be increased gradually. Physical activity guidelines after acute coronary syndromes focus on frequency, intensity, type, and time of activity.

Continued...

THERAPEUTIC INTERVENTIONS	RATIONALE
Reinforce instructions regarding sexual activity: • Sexual activity with usual partner can be resumed after the prescribed length of time (many physicians consider a client ready to resume sexual activity when the client is able to climb two flights of stairs briskly without dyspnea or angina). • Assume a comfortable and unstrenuous position for intercourse (e.g., side-lying, partner on top). • A new sexual relationship can be started but may result in greater energy expenditure until it becomes a more familiar or usual experience. • Take nitroglycerin before sexual activity if angina occurs with sexual activity. • Avoid intercourse for at least 1 to 2 hrs after a heavy meal or alcohol consumption. • Avoid sexual activity when fatigued or stressed. • Avoid hot or cold showers just before and after intercourse.	

THERAPEUTIC INTERVENTIONS	RATIONALE
Desired Outcome: The client will identify community resources that can assist with cardiac rehabilitation and adjustment to the effects of an MI. **Independent Actions** Provide information on community resources and support groups that can assist client with cardiac rehabilitation and adjustment to the effects of an MI (e.g., American Heart Association, "coronary clubs," counseling services).	*Cardiac disease can significantly impact an individual's and family's socioeconomic status. Providing information specific to community resources is important to provide a necessary continuum of care and may impact the client's health status, preventing future hospitalizations.*

THERAPEUTIC INTERVENTIONS	RATIONALE
Desired Outcome: The client, in collaboration with the nurse, will develop a plan for adhering to recommended follow-up care including future appointments with health care provider. **Independent Actions** Collaborate with the client to develop a plan for adherence to treatment regimen that includes: The importance of keeping follow-up appointments with health care provider and for exercise stress testing and laboratory studies to monitor serum lipid levels. Implement measures to improve client adherence: • Include significant others in teaching sessions if possible. • Encourage questions and allow time for reinforcement and clarification of information provided. • Provide written instructions on future appointments with health care provider, dietary modifications, activity progression, medications prescribed, and signs and symptoms to report. • Obtain social service consult as needed to help client obtain financial assistance.	*Regular health care appointments are important to determine effectiveness of the prescribed treatment plan.* *Involvement of significant others in patient teaching improves adherence to discharge instructions.* *Everyone does not understand information as presented, so set aside time for questions to allow for clarification of information.* *Written instructions allow the client to refer to instructions as needed.*

ADDITIONAL NURSING DIAGNOSES

DISTURBED SLEEP PATTERN NDx
Related to:
- Symptoms being experienced with the MI (e.g., chest discomfort, shortness of breath)
- Frequent assessments and treatments
- Fear and anxiety

FEAR/ANXIETY NDx
Related to:
- Symptoms being experienced with the MI (e.g., chest discomfort, arm pain, and/or shortness of breath)
- Possible future disability, change in roles and lifestyle, and/or death associated with severe damage to the heart
- Unfamiliar environment and separation from significant others
- Lack of understanding of diagnostic tests, diagnosis, and treatment
- Financial concerns about the cost of hospitalization and future treatment

GRIEVING NDx
Related to:
- Loss of normal function of the heart
- Possible changes in lifestyle, occupation, and roles
- Uncertainty of prognosis

See Bibliography at the back of the book.

The Client With Alterations in Neurological Function

ALZHEIMER'S DISEASE/DEMENTIA

Alzheimer's disease is a slow, progressive, degenerative brain disease that is characterized by difficulty with memory, language, problem solving, and other cognitive skills that affect the ability to perform everyday activities. More than 5 million Americans are currently living with Alzheimer's disease, with a predicted increase to 16 million by 2050. It is the most common cause of dementia and affects more women than men (possibly because women live longer), and older African Americans and Hispanics are more likely than older whites to have Alzheimer's.

Although the cause of disease is unknown, multiple nonmodifiable and modifiable factors are associated with the development of the disease. The greatest risk factors for late-onset Alzheimer's are older age, family history, and carrying the APOE-e4 gene.

Age is one of the most important factors in the development of Alzheimer's disease with the vast majority of people with Alzheimer's being over the age of 65 years. Though not considered a normal part of aging, the percentage of Alzheimer's dramatically increases with age: 3% of people ages 65 to 74; 17% of people ages 75 to 84; and 32% of people 85 years of age or older.

The second greatest risk factor is family history. An individual who has a first-degree relative—a sister, brother, or parent—with Alzheimer's is at a greater risk for developing the disease. The risk increases even more if more than one family member has the illness.

The third greatest risk factor is carrying the apolipoprotein E-e4 gene (APOE-e4). This form of APOE gene is one of three in the body (e2, e3, or e4) and is responsible for the development of proteins in the blood that carry cholesterol. The presence of APOE-e4 increases the risk of developing the disease, including developing the disease at an earlier age; however, the presence of this gene does not mean development of the disease is certain. Individuals who inherit a copy of the APOE-e4 gene are simply at increased risk for developing Alzheimer's. If the individual inherits two copies of the gene (one from each parent), he or she has an even greater risk of developing the disease; however, again inheriting the APOE-e4 gene is not a guarantee that the individual will develop Alzheimer's disease.

Additional risk factors, modifiable in nature, have been identified as increasing the risk for the development of Alzheimer's disease. Modifiable risk factors include the presence of cardiovascular disease risk factors (e.g., smoking, obesity in midlife, and diabetes), traumatic brain injury (TBI), and chronic traumatic encephalopathy (CTE). Other modifiable risk factors known to decrease risk include more formal years of education, and remaining socially and cognitively engaged.

Alzheimer's disease affects the brain structures. Changes that occur in the brain are the development of neurofibrillary tangles, amyloid or neurotic plaques, and the loss of connection between neurons. The plaques develop initially in the areas of the brain responsible for memory and cognitive functioning. Over time, the plaques develop in the cerebral cortex in the areas that control language and reasoning.

Research suggests that the brain changes associated with Alzheimer's may begin 20 years or more before the first symptoms occur. Based on the patterns of symptom progression, several methods of staging have been developed to help families and health care professionals make better care decisions. The Global Deterioration Scale (GDS) outlines key symptoms in seven stages, ranging from unimpaired to very severe cognitive decline.

In the early stages of Alzheimer's disease (stages 1 to 4), the individual may appear healthy, but experiences forgetfulness, short-term memory loss, mild impairment in judgment, and becoming progressively moody and withdrawn with greater difficulty performing complex tasks such as managing finances or paying bills. Loss of initiative and interest, decreased ability to make judgment, and geographic disorientation are also experienced. These clinical manifestations develop over time; the initial memory deterioration is so subtle that it may not be noticed. The timeframe for the early stages is 2 to 4 years.

In the middle stages (5 to 6), the clinical manifestations of the disease become more pronounced with moderate to severe cognitive decline. The client may experience inability to recognize close family or friends, impairment of cognitive functions, disorientation to person, place, and time, agitation, confusion, possible paranoia hallucinations, and delusions. Affected individuals may wander away from their regular environment and become lost; they may experience mood swings and exhibit aggressive behaviors. The individual's lack of concern about personal hygiene and appearance also become more noticeable.

In the final late stage (stage 7), impairment is severe. Clients are unable to interact with or respond to their environment.

They become bedridden and are totally dependent upon others for activities of daily living. They are unable to carry on a conversation and have no recognition of self or others. This stage lasts until the individual dies. On average, people with Alzheimer's live 8 years after diagnosis but may survive anywhere from 3 to 20 years.

There is no cure for Alzheimer's disease. Treatment focuses on retaining memory, cognitive and physical functioning, and slowing the progression of the disease. Drug therapy consists of five medications that have been approved by the US Food and Drug Administration: donepezil (Aricept), rivastigmine (Exelon), galantamine (Razadyne), memantine (Namenda), and the combination memantine + donepezil (Namzaric). Three of the five available medications are cholinesterase inhibitors (donepezil, galantamine, rivastigmine) that prevent the breakdown of a chemical messenger in the brain important for learning and memory. Both galantamine (Razadyne) and rivastigmine (Exelon) are approved for the treatment of mild to moderate stages of Alzheimer's while donepezil (Aricept) is approved for use in the treatment of all stages. Memantine regulates the activity of a different chemical messenger also important for learning and memory and is approved for use in moderate to severe stages. The fifth medication, memantine + donepezil, approved for use in moderate to severe Alzheimer's combines a cholinesterase inhibitor with memantine. Other medications may be used in conjunction with these medications to control the symptoms of insomnia, agitation, depression, and anxiety.

This care plan focuses on the adult client with Alzheimer's disease who has been hospitalized. However, much of the information is also applicable to clients with dementia who are receiving follow-up care in an extended care facility or home setting.

OUTCOME/DISCHARGE CRITERIA

The client will:
1. Maintain cognitive functioning as long as possible
2. Have a decline in number of wandering incidents
3. Have minimal episodes of aggressive behavior
4. Avoid behaviors that may harm self or others
5. Participate in activities of daily living
6. Engage in appropriate social interaction with others
7. Engage in a regular exercise program

Nursing Diagnosis **CHRONIC CONFUSION** NDx

Definition: Irreversible, progressive, insidious, and long-term alteration of intellect, behavior, and personality, manifested by impairment in cognitive functions (memory, speech, language, decision making, and executive function), and dependency in execution of daily activities.

Related to: Degeneration of the CNS and cognitive functioning

CLINICAL MANIFESTATIONS

Subjective	Objective
N/A	Inaccurate interpretation of environment and time; short-term/long-term memory loss; alteration in behavior (e.g., lability, hostility, irritability, inappropriate affect); inability to make decisions or problem solve; changes in attention span; disorientation; inappropriate social behavior; progressive cognitive impairment

RISK FACTORS
- Physiologic changes from progression of Alzheimer's disease

DESIRED OUTCOMES
The client will:
a. Remain calm and display minimal aggressive behaviors
b. Have limited disorientation to person, place, and time

NOC OUTCOMES
Agitation level; cognition; cognitive orientation; distorted thought self-control; safe wandering; information processing

NIC INTERVENTIONS
Calming technique; memory training; reality orientation; environmental management; behavioral management

NURSING ASSESSMENT
Assess for episodes of disorientation to person, place, and time, episodes of inappropriate behavior, impaired decision-making ability, impaired memory and judgment, delusions, impaired attention span.

RATIONALE
Early recognition of signs and symptoms of confusion allows for prompt intervention.

THERAPEUTIC INTERVENTIONS	RATIONALE

Independent Actions

Implement measures to maintain client orientation to person, place, and time:

- Maintain a structured environment with routine activities, while continuing to monitor the client.
- Orient to person, place, and time frequently. **D** ● ✦
- When speaking to the client, use his/her name. **D** ● ✦

- Place familiar objects and personal belongings of the client in his/her room. **D** ●/✦
- When interacting with the client, maintain a calm demeanor, speak slowly, and maintain eye contact. **D** ● ✦
- Give client information and/or directions in a simple manner. Provide only one piece of information at a time.

- Refer to current events when interacting with the client. **D** ● ✦
- Allow client time to formulate responses to questions and during interactions. Allow for periods of silence by the client. **D** ● ✦

- Use attentive listening when interacting with the client even when what is being said is confusing or gibberish. **D** ● ✦
- Allow hoarding of objects as long as they will not be harmful to the client. **D** ● ✦
- Allow client to interact with other patients, while monitoring client for inappropriate behavior.
- Monitor for cyclic changes in cognition and behaviors (e.g., wandering, hoarding items, evening confusion, picking at clothing).
- Maintain client on an appropriate schedule for sleep and rest. Turn off lights when client is in bed. Use a nightlight if needed. **D** ● ✦

A predictable environment helps client maintain a sense of security.

Frequent orientation may help improve client's sense of orientation.
Use of the client's name during communication decreases potential for misunderstanding.
Having familiar objects in the client's room increases client's sense of security and comfort level in a strange environment.
These actions improve potential for client understanding and demonstrates respect.
Clients' ability to process information decreases as the disease progresses. They are unable to process more than one piece of information at a time.
Discussion of current events grounds client in the present and helps decrease disorientation, because client is not focusing on unreal events.
Allowing time for client responses demonstrates respect, encourages a response, and helps improve communication.
With progression of the disease, the client may have difficulty processing information and formulating an appropriate response.

Allowing client to horde objects provides a sense of security.

Allows the nurse to observe client's social interaction.

Cyclic changes in cognition indicate client may be experiencing "sundowner" syndrome.

Maintaining a schedule for the client decreases incidence of fatigue and promotes a sense of well-being.

Nursing Diagnosis   WANDERING   NDx

Definition: Meandering, aimless, or repetitive locomotion that exposes the individual to harm; frequently incongruent with boundaries, limits, or obstacles.

Related to:
- Alteration in cognitive function

CLINICAL MANIFESTATIONS

Subjective	Objective
Verbal self-report of "wanting to go home" and or threatening to leave	Appears frightened; weeping; pacing; searching behaviors; shadowing a caregiver's locomotion; long periods of locomotion without an apparent destination; impaired ability to locate landmarks in a familiar setting; hyperactivity; continuous movement from place to place

RISK FACTORS

- Alteration in sleep-wake cycle
- Overstimulating environment
- Desire to go home
- Separation from familiar environment

DESIRED OUTCOMES

The client will not experience wandering as evidenced by:
a. No reported occurrences of leaving institution/ residence unattended
b. No reported attempts to leave secure area

NOC OUTCOMES

Elopement occurrence; elopement propensity risk

NIC INTERVENTIONS

Elopement precautions; environmental management safety

NURSING ASSESSMENT	RATIONALE
Assess client's cognitive functioning (e.g., disorientation)	*Early recognition of signs and symptoms of altered cognitive function (e.g. confusion, identity confusion, impaired judgement, loss of short-term or long-term memory) allows for prompt intervention.*
Assess client's potential for elopement: • Verbal indicators • Loitering near exits • Wearing of multiple layers of clothing • Packing belongings • Homesickness	*Early recognition of elopement behaviors allows for prompt intervention.*

THERAPEUTIC INTERVENTIONS	RATIONALE

Independent Actions

Implement measures to decrease client anxiety. • Familiarize client with the environment. • Provide reassurance/comfort. • Encourage client to seek care providers for assistance when experiencing feelings that may lead to elopement (e.g., anxiety, anger, fear).	*Familiarizing client with the environment and related routines can reduce anxiety associated with risk for elopement.* *Discussing feelings the client may be experiencing may decrease anxiety/fear and reduce the risk of elopement.*
Implement measures to decrease the risk of elopement: • Limit client to a physically secure environment as needed. • Provide appropriate level of supervision to monitor client. Increasing supervision when client is outside the secure environment. • Provide adaptive devices (e.g., side rails, restraints) while maintaining the least restrictive environment as possible.	*Implementing measures to reduce risk for elopement may also prevent client injury/harm.* *Reduces the risk for elopement.* *Use of adaptive devices such as restraints help limit client's exposure to harmful situations. When using restraints, appropriate justification must be documented including efforts to use alternative measures (e.g., sitters) before the decision to implement restraints.*
• Provide adaptive devices that monitor client's remote location (e.g., electronic sensors that trigger alarms or locks).	
Record client physical descriptors: • Height/weight • Hair/eye/skin color	*Physical descriptors will be helpful to reference in the event of elopement.*
Engage the client in structured activities appropriate for setting (e.g., music therapy, reading, painting, drawing).	
Educate family/caregivers regarding risk factor for patient elopement and strategies to reduce risk for wandering in the home environment. • Identify times of day wandering most likely to occur. • Avoid busy places that may cause confusion. • Place locks out of the line of site. • Use motion detectors/devices that trigger when a door or window is opened. • Keep car keys out of sight.	*Client's with memory problems are at risk for wandering—even in the early stages of dementia.*
Assist family/caregivers in the development of a plan to be implemented in the event of elopement: • Keep emergency list of who to call for help. • Ask neighbors, friends, or family to call if they see client alone. • Keep a recent, close-up photo and updated medical information on hand. • Know the local neighborhood/areas where client may be easily lost. • Keep a list of the places the client may wander (e.g., past jobs, former homes, place of worship, restaurants). • Know client's dominant hand. • Provide client with ID jewelry. • If elopement occurs, search area for no more than 15 minutes before contacting 911.	*The stress experienced by family members/caregivers during a wandering episode is significant. Having a plan in place in advance will help focus recovery efforts potentially reducing the risk for injury/harm.*

NDx = NANDA Diagnosis   **D** = Delegatable Action   ● = UAP   ✦ = LVN/LPN   ⊖▶ = Go to ⊖volve for animation

| Nursing Diagnosis | **SELF-CARE DEFICIT: DRESSING, BATHING, FEEDING, AND TOILETING** NDx |

Definition: **Self-Care Deficit:** Dressing **NDx:** Inability to independently put on or remove clothing; **Self-Care Deficit: Bathing NDx:** Inability to independently complete cleansing activities; **Self-Care Deficit: Feeding NDx:** Inability to eat independently; **Self-Care Deficit: Toileting NDx:** Inability to independently perform tasks associated with bowel and bladder elimination.

Related to:
- Inability to make decisions
- Loss of cognitive understanding
- Altered thought processes
- Difficulty in processing information

CLINICAL MANIFESTATIONS

Subjective	Objective
Verbal self-report of problem	Inability to determine what to wear; inability to feed self; inability to run bath water or clean self after micturition or defecation

RISK FACTORS
- Neuromuscular impairment
- Altered cognitive functioning
- Impaired ability to perceive spatial relationships

DESIRED OUTCOMES

The client will be able to perform activities of daily living as evidenced by:
a. Ability to appropriately dress and groom self with no or minimal assistance
b. Ability to feed self with no or minimal assistance
c. Ability to care for personal hygiene with no or minimal assistance

NOC OUTCOMES

Self-care: activities of daily living; bathing, dressing, eating, hygiene, toileting

NIC INTERVENTIONS

Self-care assistance: bathing, dressing/grooming, feeding, toileting

NURSING ASSESSMENT	RATIONALE
Assess client's current self-care habits.	*Provides a baseline of client's ability and where interventions should be implemented.*
Assess client's cognitive and physical ability to perform self-care habits.	*When a client's cognitive abilities are impaired, the client is unable to determine self-care needs.*

THERAPEUTIC INTERVENTIONS	RATIONALE

Independent Actions
Implement measures to involve client in activities of daily living: **D** ● ✦

- Allow client time for dressing and bathing in a quiet environment.

Allowing a client time for ADLS in a quite environment decreases the client's stress and frustration.

- Follow a consistent routine for bathing, dressing, and grooming.

Routines may prevent confusion, require less decision-making, and may decrease client's frustration.

- Assist as needed in bathing and perineal care.

Appropriate bathing and perineal care helps prevent skin breakdown.

- Limit clothing choices by putting together complete outfits that are easy to put on and to take off.

Limiting choices decreases frustration if clothing is easy to put on and remove.

- Lay out or give client clothing in the order in which it will be put on. Start with the bottom half and then top half.

When helping a client dress, this establishes a routine and simplifies the dressing process.

THERAPEUTIC INTERVENTIONS	RATIONALE
• Encourage client independence when dressing; provide assistance as needed.	*Preserves client's independence as long as possible.*
• Assist client in selecting foods that will provide appropriate nutrients. Allow client to choose foods he/she likes.	*Client self-selection of food helps maintain client's nutritional status and decreases frustration if client receives foods he/she likes.*
• If assisting client, serve only two foods at a time.	*Keeping food selections to a minimum decreases frustration because client may not be able to decide which food to eat first.*
• Place food in a bowl rather than on a plate, or offer finger foods if client has impaired coordination.	*A bowl is easier for the client to eat from and helps maintain client's independence and decreases frustrations in trying to feed self.*

Nursing Diagnosis IMPAIRED HOME MAINTENANCE NDx

Definition: Inability to independently maintain a safe and growth-promoting immediate environment.

Related to:
• Alteration in cognitive functioning

CLINICAL MANIFESTATIONS

Subjective	Objective
Verbal self-report of difficulty in maintaining household; family member request for assistance in caring for the client in their home	Impaired ability to maintain home; unsanitary/unhygienic environment

RISK FACTORS
• Insufficient support systems
• Financial crisis
• Insufficient knowledge of neighborhood resources
• Insufficient knowledge of home maintenance

DESIRED OUTCOMES

The client will not experience impaired home maintenance as evidenced by:
a. Maintains a clean and safe home
b. Use of neighborhood resources
c. Engaged support systems (family/friends)

NOC OUTCOMES

Family functioning; safe home environment; social support

NIC INTERVENTIONS

Family involvement promotion; home maintenance assistance

NURSING ASSESSMENT	RATIONALE
Assess client's sensory, motor, and cognitive functioning. Assess client's ability to maintain a safe household (e.g., ability to lock doors at night, smell smoke, recognize safety hazards). Assess ability of family to support client in the home environment.	*Early recognition of signs and symptoms that client is not able to independently maintain his/her household without assistance allows for prompt intervention.*

THERAPEUTIC INTERVENTIONS	RATIONALE
Independent Actions Develop a plan for home maintenance with family and client:	
• Implement measures to maintain client safety in his/her home:	*This equipment provides security and may decrease wandering activities.*
◦ Encourage family to install smoke detectors, a security system, and easy-to-use door locks.	
◦ Encourage client to wear a medic alert bracelet.	*Helps client be quickly identified if client becomes lost.*
• Assist client and family to develop a sleep/rest schedule.	*Schedules help decrease client's fatigue, which may increase client's coping abilities.*

Continued...

THERAPEUTIC INTERVENTIONS	RATIONALE
• Encourage client and family members to identify safety concerns in the home (e.g., lots of throw rugs, poor lighting).	*These actions help protect the client from injury.*
• Install child safety devices to prevent client from wandering into areas where injury might occur (e.g., decks, swimming pools, stairs).	
• Assist family in identifying community support services (e.g., Meals on Wheels, adult day care, support groups, respite services).	*Community support assists caregivers in caring for the client and promotes client independence.*

Susceptibility to difficulty in fulfilling care responsibilities, expectations, and/or behaviors for family or significant others, which may compromise health.

ADDITIONAL NURSING DIAGNOSES

IMPAIRED SOCIAL INTERACTIONS NDx
Related to:
• Alterations in cognition
• Memory deficits
• Impaired judgment
• Inappropriate, hostile, and bizarre behaviors

RISK FOR INJURY NDx
Related to:
• Alteration in cognitive functioning
• Alteration in psychomotor functioning

GRIEVING NDx
Related to:
• Awareness of disease and disease progression

CEREBROVASCULAR ACCIDENT

A cerebrovascular accident (CVA, stroke, brain attack) is the result of an interruption in the blood flow in areas of the brain and is characterized by the sudden development of neurological deficits. These deficits range from mild symptoms such as tingling, weakness, and slight speech impairment to more severe symptoms such as hemiplegia, aphasia, dysphagia, loss of portions of the visual field, spatial-perceptual changes, altered cognitive function, and loss of consciousness. Clinical manifestations depend on factors such as the area(s) of the brain affected, the adequacy of collateral cerebral circulation, and the extensiveness of subsequent cerebral edema.

CVAs are classified according to etiology. The major classifications are ischemic and hemorrhagic. Ischemic CVAs are most frequently the result of a thrombosis (which is usually associated with atherosclerosis) or an embolus. Conditions most often associated with a hemorrhagic CVA are extreme hypertension, cerebral aneurysm, or arteriovenous malformation. Treatment after a CVA is determined by the etiology and the neurological deficits that are present. Transient ischemic attacks (TIAs), sometimes referred to as "mini strokes," differ from major types of cerebrovascular accidents in that blood flow to the brain is interrupted for a short time usually no more than 5 minutes. More than one-third of people that experience a TIA and do not get treatment experience a major

stroke within 1 year. As many as 10% to 15% of people will have a major stroke within 3 months of experiencing a TIA.

This care plan focuses on the adult client hospitalized with signs and symptoms of a CVA. Much of the information is also applicable to clients receiving follow-up care in an extended care or rehabilitation facility or home setting. This care plan focuses on the more common problems that occur as a result of a CVA. The reader should refer to neurological texts for additional information about specific speech, motor, and sensory deficits that can occur.

OUTCOME/DISCHARGE CRITERIA

The client will:
1. Have improved or stable neurological function
2. Have no signs or symptoms of complications
3. Identify ways to manage sensory and speech impairments and disturbed thought processes
4. Identify ways to improve ability to swallow
5. Identify ways to manage urinary incontinence
6. Demonstrate measures to facilitate the performance of activities of daily living and increase physical mobility

7. Communicate an awareness of signs and symptoms to report to the health care provider and share thoughts and feelings about the effects of the CVA on lifestyle, roles, and self-concept
8. Communicate knowledge of community resources that can assist with home management and adjustment to changes resulting from the CVA

9. Develop a plan for adhering to recommended follow-up care including regular laboratory studies, future appointments with health care providers, and medications prescribed.

Collaborative Diagnosis | # DECREASED INTRACRANIAL ADAPTIVE CAPACITY NDx

Definition: Compromise in intracranial fluid dynamic mechanisms that normally compensate for increases in intracranial volumes, resulting in repeated disproportionate increases in intracranial pressure (ICP) in response to a variety of noxious and non-noxious stimuli.

Related to: Changes in the CNS blood flow associated with thrombus, bleeding, alterations in blood pressure, and/or hypoxia

CLINICAL MANIFESTATIONS

Subjective	**Objective**
Verbal self-report of headache	Increases in ICP for greater than 5 minutes after stimuli; baseline ICP greater than 10 mm Hg; altered level of consciousness (early); changes in vital signs/cardiac rhythm (late), changes in papillary response, generalized weakness; Positive Babinski sign, seizures

RISK FACTORS

- Brain injury
- Decreased cerebral perfusion <50 to 60 mmHg
- Sustained increase in ICP of 10 to 15 mm Hg
- Systemic hypotension with intracranial hypertension

DESIRED OUTCOMES

The client will demonstrate improved neurological status as evidenced by:
a. Stable/normalized ICP
b. Absence of seizures

NOC OUTCOMES

Neurological status: autonomic; central motor control; consciousness

NIC INTERVENTIONS

ICP monitoring; cerebral perfusion promotion; cerebral edema management; tube care: ventriculostomy; seizure precautions

NURSING ASSESSMENT	**RATIONALE**
Assess client for signs and symptoms of increased intracranial pressure:	*As ICP increases, neurological assessment will change.*
	Most sensitive indicator of increased ICP is level of consciousness.
• Self-report of headache	
• Changes in level of consciousness	
• Changes in pupillary response	
• Positive Babinski	*Reveals upper motor neuron lesion indicating corticospinal tract injury.*
• Generalized weakness	
• Seizures	
• Assess vital signs for the presence of Cushing triad	
• Assess ICP and cerebral perfusion pressure (CPP)	*Irregular breathing, widening pulse pressure, and decreased heart rate (Cushing triad) are late signs of increased ICP.*
	Assessing for values indicating elevation of ICP and decreases in cerebral perfusion pressure allow for prompt intervention. Elevations of ICP can indicate deterioration in neurological status.

THERAPEUTIC INTERVENTIONS	RATIONALE
Independent Actions	
Implement measures to maintain or decrease increased intracranial pressure.	Elevations in $PaCO_2$ can lead to cerebral vasodilation, which further increases ICP.
• Maintain patent airway.	
• Maintain neutral neck position. Elevate head of bed no more than 30 degrees avoiding extreme hip flexion. **D** ✦	Neutral head position and head elevation both facilitate venous drainage of head and aid in lowering ICP.
• Do not group caregiving activities such as bathing, suctioning, and dressing changes. **D** ● ✦	Spacing activities minimizes sustained elevations in ICP.
• Institute seizure precautions:	Seizures are possible with elevated ICP, and client safety must be considered.
• Keep Ambu bag at bedside	
• Keep oral/nasopharyngeal airway at bedside	
• Keep side rails up	
Dependent/Collaborative Actions	
Administer medications such as osmotic diuretics, loop diuretics, and corticosteroids.	Medications act to reduce swelling of cerebral tissues or volume of cerebrospinal fluid (CSF), thereby decreasing ICP.
Administer anticonvulsants as ordered.	In the presence of increased ICP, anticonvulsants may be ordered to prevent seizures.
Drain CSF fluid via ventriculostomy as ordered.	Draining CSF fluid via ventriculostomy reduces the volume of CSF fluid in the head, lowering ICP. CSF fluid should be clear presence of blood or cloudy appearance can indicate further complications and/or the presence of infection.
• Monitor amount, rate, and characteristics of CSF drainage.	
Consult physician if signs and symptoms of increased intracranial pressure persist.	Notifying the physician allows for modification of the treatment plan

---

Nursing Diagnosis ## RISK FOR INEFFECTIVE CEREBRAL TISSUE PERFUSION NDx

Definition: Susceptible to a decrease in cerebral tissue circulation, which may compromise health.

Related to:
• Embolism
• Coagulopathy
• Cerebral aneurysm
• Carotid stenosis
• Hypertension

CLINICAL MANIFESTATIONS

Subjective	Objective
May not be able to self-report symptoms; verbal self-report of headache	Altered neurological status; altered level of consciousness; changes in motor response; behavioral changes; changes in pupillary reactions; difficulty swallowing

RISK FACTORS	DESIRED OUTCOMES
• Trauma	The client will improve cerebral tissue perfusion as evidenced by:
• Recent myocardial infarction	a. Improved or return to client's baseline neurological status
	b. Improved or return to client's baseline sensory and motor function

NOC OUTCOMES	NIC INTERVENTIONS
Neurological status: consciousness; cranial sensory/motor function; tissue perfusion: cerebral	Cerebral perfusion promotion; neurological monitoring; seizure precautions

NURSING ASSESSMENT	RATIONALE
Assess neurological status hourly (or more frequently as condition warrants) during acute phase (e.g., dizziness, visual disturbances, aphasia, irritability, restlessness, decreased level of consciousness, paresthesias, weakness, paralysis, seizure activity).	*Provides baseline assessment data and determines signs of decreased tissue perfusions. Changes may be reflective of increased intracranial pressure.*
Assess vital signs hourly or more frequently as indicated during the acute phase.	*Vitals signs must be maintained at a level that supports adequate oxygenation and perfusion of cerebral tissues.*
Assess baseline prothrombin time (PT) and partial thromboplastin time (PTT).	*Assessment of baseline values allows for modification of the treatment plan.*

THERAPEUTIC INTERVENTIONS	RATIONALE
Independent Actions	
Perform actions to promote increased cerebral tissue perfusion (e.g., encourage client to not cough, avoid neck flexion or extreme hip or knew flexion).	*Increased intracranial pressure reduces blood flow to the brain because of the closed nature of the skull. Coughing causes an increase in intracranial pressure while extreme neck flexion prevents venous drainage from the brain further risking increased intracranial pressure decreasing cerebral tissue perfusion.*
Ensure client positioning facilitates a patent airway and optimum gas exchange.	*Client positioning should ensure patent airway and effective gas exchange. Optimum elimination of carbon dioxide with effective ventilation/patent airway is necessary to prevent vasoconstriction, further reducing perfusion to the brain.*
Dependent/Collaborative Actions	
Implement measures to improve cerebral tissue perfusion:	
• Maintain blood pressure (B/P) within optimum range using antihypertensive, sympathomimetics, and/or fluid therapy (volume expansion).	*B/P must be maintained within optimum range to keep cerebral perfusion pressure at a level that promotes oxygenation of cerebral tissues. Exact values may vary.*
• Administer calcium channel blockers.	*Calcium channel blockers reduce cerebral vasospasm, which improves perfusion to the cerebral tissues.*
• Administer anticoagulant, antiplatelet and/or thrombolytic therapy.	*Anticoagulant, antiplatelet, and/or thrombolytic therapy reduces or prevents clot formation, which restores blood flow to the brain.*
• Consult with physician to determine optimal head of bed (placement).	*Elevation of the HOB improves venous drainage and reduces intracranial pressure. Type of injury and location in the brain determines optimum head elevation and should be determined by the physician.*

Nursing Diagnosis **RISK FOR ASPIRATION** NDx

Definition: Susceptible to entry of gastrointestinal secretions, oropharyngeal secretions, solids, or fluids to the tracheobronchial passages, which may compromise health.

Related to: Changes in neuromuscular functioning

CLINICAL MANIFESTATIONS

Subjective	Objective
N/A	Cough; tachypnea; dyspnea; tachycardia; dull percussion noted over affected lung area; presence of food in aspirate

RISK FACTORS
- Reduced level of consciousness
- Depressed cough and gag reflexes
- Impaired swallowing in an acute neurological insult

DESIRED OUTCOMES

The client will not aspirate secretions or foods/fluids as evidenced by:
a. Clear breath sounds
b. Resonant percussion over lungs
c. Absence of cough, tachypnea, and dyspnea

NOC OUTCOMES	NIC INTERVENTIONS
Respiratory status	Aspiration precautions; respiratory monitoring; swallowing therapy

NURSING ASSESSMENT	RATIONALE
Assess level of consciousness.	*Alterations in level of consciousness place a patient at risk for aspiration.*
Assess for the presence of a cough or gag reflex.	*Lack of protective reflexes places patient at risk for aspiration.*
Assess for the presence of nausea or vomiting.	*Increases the risk of aspiration of gastric contents in the setting of an acute neurological event.*
Assess respiratory system for signs and symptoms of aspiration of secretions or foods/fluids:	*Early recognition of objective assessment findings allows for prompt treatment and recognition.*
• Auscultate breath sounds for wheezes or crackles.	
Monitor chest radiograph results.	*Evidence of pulmonary infiltrates on chest radiograph results can indicate that aspiration has occurred.*

THERAPEUTIC INTERVENTIONS	RATIONALE

Independent Actions

Implement measures to reduce the risk for aspiration:

• Keep suction equipment readily available at bedside.	*Necessary to maintain patency of airway.*
• Place conscious, impaired patient in a side-lying position unless contraindicated. **D** ● ✦	*Oral secretions accumulate in the mouth, allowing for easier expectoration or removal by suctioning.*
• Position patient in high-Fowler's positions before initiating feeding. Maintain patient in an upright position 30 to 45 minutes after eating. **D** ● ✦	*This position uses gravity to facilitate movement of food/fluids through the pharynx into the esophagus.*
• Supervise administration of oral intake. **D** ✦	*Supervision allows for observation of potential swallowing difficulty and implementation of actions to improve swallowing.*
• Offer foods with a thicker consistency, which facilitates swallowing. **D** ✦	*Semisolid foods are more readily swallowed. Thin fluids are difficult for patients with dysphagia to manage.*
• Place foods/medications on unaffected side of the mouth. **D** ● ✦	*Chewing on the unaffected side of the mouth facilitates effective swallowing of food.*
• Encourage eat slowly and to client to thoroughly chew food. **D** ✦	*Taking adequate time to eat, thoroughly chewing food, makes food easier to swallow, and decreases incidence of aspiration.*
• Provide oral care after feedings.	*Good oral hygiene and inspection of the oral cavity after meals results in removal of any remaining food that could enter the pharynx and be aspirated into the lungs.*
• Inspect for "pocketing" of food. **D** ● ✦	

Dependent/Collaborative Actions

Administer prokinetic agents as ordered. **D** ✦	*Prokinetic agents enhance gastric motility.*
Consult appropriate health care provider for swallowing difficulties.	*Dysphagia assessment can establish techniques to prevent aspiration in patients with impaired swallowing.*

Nursing Diagnosis   **UNILATERAL NEGLECT** NDx

Definition: Impairment in sensory and motor response, mental representation, and spatial attention of the body, and the corresponding environment, characterized by inattention to one side and overattention to the opposite side. Left-side neglect is more severe and persistent than right-side neglect.

Related to: Ischemia primarily of the parietal lobe of the nondominant cerebral hemisphere

CLINICAL MANIFESTATIONS

Subjective	Objective
Verbal self-report of feeling as though one part of the body does not belong to own self	Inattention to stimuli applied to affected side; lack of awareness of affected side/inattention to safety; failure to use the affected side after being reminded to do so; failure to notice people approaching from the neglected side; marked deviation of the eyes to the non-neglected side to stimuli and activities on that side

RISK FACTORS

- Stroke
- Smoking
- Hypertension

DESIRED OUTCOMES

The client will experience a reduction in and/or demonstrate beginning adaptation to unilateral neglect as evidenced by:
a. Awareness of stimuli on affected side
b. Awareness of the affected side of the body

NOC OUTCOMES

Sensory function: proprioception; self-care activities of daily living; body positioning: self-initiated

NIC INTERVENTIONS

Unilateral neglect management; self-care assistance; self-care assistance: transfer

NURSING ASSESSMENT	RATIONALE
Assess baseline mental status including comprehension.	*Determines ability of client to understand information and follow instructions.*
Assess for presence of unilateral neglect:	*Determines extent of impairment and how the patient acknowledges senses on the affected side.*
• Client responses to sensory stimuli bilaterally (visual, tactile)	
• Distorted spatial-perceptual relationships	
• Denial of body parts (have client point to body parts)	*Determines the lack of recognition of body parts or distorted awareness of body parts; important to identify plan safe care of the patient.*

THERAPEUTIC INTERVENTIONS	RATIONALE

Independent Actions
If unilateral neglect is present:
- Ensure affected extremities are positioned properly at all times. **D** ● ✦ — *Protects extremities from development of contractures.*
- Protect affected extremities from pressure/injury/burns. **D** ● ✦ — *Lack of extremity recognition increases risk of injury.*

Provide active/passive range of motion. — *Range-of-motion activities promote circulation in affected extremities.*
- Touch and move affected extremities. **D** ● ✦

Encourage client to touch and use affected body part. — *Provision of sensory stimulation can help client experience normal movement patterns.*

- Approach patient from unaffected side during acute phase. **D** ● ✦ — *Diminishes fear and anxiety in a client with difficulty in interpreting the environment in its entirety.*

Provide mirror for client during self-care activities. **D** ● ✦ — *Use of a mirror helps improves recognition of affected side.*

Gradually focus client's attention to affected side as client demonstrates ability to compensate for neglect: — *Following the acute phase, to enhance recovery and improve awareness of the client's recovering side, begin activities to increase awareness of the neglected side.*
- Gradually move personal items to affected side. **D** ● ✦
- Stand on affected side when ambulating with client. **D** ● ✦
- Assist with activities of daily living from affected side including bathing and grooming. **D** ● ✦ — *Placing items on the affected side assists the client to recognize that the extremities are part of his/her body.*
- Assist patient to groom on affected side.
- Focus tactile and verbal stimulation on affected side. **D** ● ✦

Dependent/Collaborative Actions
Consult physical therapy/occupational therapy as appropriate. — *PT/OT can prescribe exercises that aid the client in client development of adaptive skills.*

Nursing Diagnosis   IMPAIRED VERBAL COMMUNICATION NDx

Definition: Decreased, delayed, or absent ability to receive, process, transmit, and/or use a system of symbols.

Related to: Damage to Broca motor (expressive) or Wernicke (receptive) speech centers in the brain

CLINICAL MANIFESTATIONS

Subjective	Objective
Verbal self-report of difficulty expressing self	Unable to speak dominant language; speaks or verbalizes with difficulty; cannot speak; slurring/stuttering; difficulty forming words and sentences; difficulty in comprehending statements

RISK FACTOR	DESIRED OUTCOME
• Central nervous system impairment	The client will communicate needs and desires effectively.

NOC OUTCOMES	NIC INTERVENTIONS
Communication: receptive; communication: expressive	Communication enhancement: speech deficit; active listening

NURSING ASSESSMENT	RATIONALE
Assess for motor speech impairment or difficulty forming words (expressive).	*Provides a baseline assessment of client's impairment.*
Assess for inability to understand words (receptive).	*Type of impairment will depend on area of the brain involved.*
Assess for total loss of ability to comprehend and speak (global aphasia).	

THERAPEUTIC INTERVENTIONS	RATIONALE

Independent Actions
Implement measures to facilitate communication:

- Approach communication with client as an adult. **D** ● ✦ — *Approaching the client in this manner prevents startling the client.*
- Ask questions that require short answers and allow time for the patient to respond. **D** ● ✦ — *The client will need more time to process information. Short, simple answers will reduce client's frustration, allowing for easier communication.*

- Face client when speaking, using short statements, speaking slowly, and presenting one thought at a time. **D** ● ✦ — *Facing the client when speaking enhances understanding and allows client to concentrate on one thing at a time.*
- Create a calm, quiet environment. **D** ● ✦ — *In a quiet environment, the client can concentrate on communication efforts, does not have to speak loudly, and is able to hear others more clearly.*
- Provide rest periods before speech therapy. — *Rest periods help conserve client's energy to maximize communication ability during therapy.*

- Provide assistive communication aids such as pad/pencil, computer, word cards, or picture boards. **D** ● ✦ — *Communication aids help facilitate communication.*
- Encourage family to communicate with patient. **D** ✦ — *Family involvement will reinforce consistency of communication measures.*

Dependent/Collaborative Actions
Consult speech pathologist. — *Multidisciplinary plan of care can be developed.*

Nursing Diagnosis   SELF-CARE DEFICIT NDx (BATHING, FEEDING, DRESSING, TOILETING)

Definition: **Self-Care Deficit: Bathing NDx:** Inability to independently complete cleansing activities; **Self-Care Deficit: Feeding NDx:** Inability to eat independently; **Self-Care Deficit: Dressing NDx:** Inability to independently put on or remove clothing; **Self-Care Deficit: Toileting NDx:** Inability to independently perform tasks associated with bowel and bladder elimination.

Related to:
- Impaired physical mobility
- Visual and spatial-perceptual impairments
- Apraxia
- Unilateral neglect
- Disturbed thought processes

CLINICAL MANIFESTATIONS

Subjective	Objective
Verbal self-report of inability to independently bath, feed, dress, or complete tasks associated with toileting.	Inability to prepare food, handle or use containers and/or utensils; inability to handle a glass or cup; inability to bathe or access the bathtub or shower; inability to dress self, use button closures; inability to get to the toilet or manipulate clothing; inability to provide appropriate personal hygiene

RISK FACTORS

- Weakness
- Loss of neuromuscular activity
- Bed rest

DESIRED OUTCOME

The client will perform self-care activities within cognitive and physical limitations.

NOC OUTCOMES

Self-care: activities of daily living

NIC INTERVENTIONS

Self-care assistance; self-care assistance: bathing, dressing/grooming, feeding, toileting; exercise therapy: ambulation, balance, joint mobility, muscle control

NURSING ASSESSMENT	RATIONALE
Assess the client's ability to perform activities of daily living: - Dressing - Toileting - Preparing food - Eating - Providing hair and/or nail care	*Identification of client's self-care deficits will guide the nurse in the development of the plan of care.*

THERAPEUTIC INTERVENTIONS	RATIONALE

Independent Interventions

Implement additional measures to facilitate client's ability to perform self-care activities:

- If apraxia is present, explain and demonstrate use of items such as toothbrush, comb, and washcloth as often as necessary.

  Demonstrating the skill while explaining it will help the client in relearning skills for activities of daily living.

- Encourage client to wear eyepatch or opaque lens if diplopia is present.

  Without an eyepatch, client will be unable to correctly focus on and/or have difficulty in using objects necessary for activities of daily living.

- Perform actions to enable client to feed self:
  - Place foods/fluids within client's visual field until client learns to effectively use scanning techniques. **D** ● ✦

    Food/fluids should be placed where client can easily see it.

  - Place only a few items on the tray at one time if spatial-perceptual deficits are present. **D** ● ✦

    When there are too many items on the tray, the client is unable to focus on a specific item.

  - Identify where items are placed on the plate and tray and open containers, cut meat, and butter bread as indicated. **D** ● ✦

    The client should know where each item is placed. Cutting food into small sizes helps prevent overfilling of the mouth, thus reducing the risk for choking.

- Perform actions to enable client to dress self:

  These actions help the client maintain a degree of independence.

  - Encourage use of assistive devices such as button hooks, long-handled shoehorns, and pull loops for pants.
  - Encourage client to select clothing that is easy to put on and remove (e.g., shirts with zippers or Velcro closures rather than buttons, loose-fitting clothing, pants with an elastic waistband or Velcro closures, shoes with Velcro fasteners or elastic laces).
  - If client has difficulty distinguishing right from left, mark outer aspect of shoes with tape.

NDx = NANDA Diagnosis   **D** = Delegatable Action   ● = UAP   ✦ = LVN/LPN   ⊖▶ = Go to ⊖*volve* for animation

Continued...

THERAPEUTIC INTERVENTIONS	RATIONALE
• Perform actions to increase mobility (e.g., turn every 2 hrs, perform active and passive range of motion, ambulate client as able). **D ● ✦**	*Increasing mobility and exercise further facilitates the client's ability to perform self-care activities.*
• Reinforce exercises and activities recommended by the occupational therapist to improve fine motor skills. Assist the client with activities he/she is unable to perform independently. **D ● ✦**	
Inform significant others of client's abilities to perform own care. Explain importance of encouraging and allowing client to maintain an optimal level of independence.	*Encouraging client's family to allow the client to care for his or her self helps the client maintain some degree of independence.*

Dependent/Collaborative Interventions

Implement additional measures to facilitate client's ability to perform self-care activities:	
• Consult with occupational therapist about assistive devices available (e.g., broad-handled utensils, rocker knife, non-slip tray mat, plate guard); reinforce use of these devices.	*Provides multidisciplinary approach to care.*

Nursing Diagnosis # ACUTE CONFUSION NDx ; CHRONIC CONFUSION NDx

Definition: Acute NDx: Reversable disturbances of consciousness, attention, cognition and perception that develop over a short period of time, and which last less than 3 months; **Chronic NDx:** Irreversible, progressive, insidious, and long-term alteration of intellect, behavioral and personality, manifested by impairment in cognitive functions (memory, speech, language, decision-making, and executive function), and dependency in execution of daily activities.

Related to: Cerebral vascular accident

CLINICAL MANIFESTATIONS

Subjective	Objective
N/A	Inaccurate interpretation of environment and time; memory loss; altered mood states (e.g., lability, hostility, irritability, inappropriate affect); inability to make decisions or problem solve; changes in attention span; disorientation; inappropriate social behavior

RISK FACTOR	DESIRED OUTCOMES
• Cerebral edema	The client will experience less confusion as evidence by: a. Improved attention span, memory, and problem-solving abilities b. Improved level of orientation c. Reduction in instances of inappropriate responses

NOC OUTCOMES	NIC INTERVENTIONS
Information processing; neurological status: consciousness; cognitive orientation; memory	Reality orientation; cognitive stimulation; presence; behavior management

NURSING ASSESSMENT	RATIONALE
Assess client for changes in level of confusion and orientation (e.g., shortened attention span, impaired memory, decreased ability to problem solve, confusion, inappropriate response, mood changes).	*Early recognition of signs and symptoms of confusion allows for prompt intervention.*
Ascertain from significant others client's usual level of cognitive and emotional functioning.	

THERAPEUTIC INTERVENTIONS	RATIONALE

Independent Actions

If client shows evidence of confusion and/or disorientation:

- Reorient to person, place, and time as necessary. **D** ● ✦

- Address client by name. **D** ● ✦
- Place familiar objects, clock, and calendar within client's view. **D** ● ✦
- Face client when conversing with client. **D** ● ✦
- Approach client in a slow, calm manner; allow adequate time for communication. **D** ● ✦
- Repeat instructions as necessary using clear, simple language and short sentences. **D** ● ✦
- Keep environmental stimuli to a minimum but avoid sensory deprivation. **D** ● ✦
- Maintain a consistent and fairly structured routine. **D** ● ✦

- Provide written or audio recorded information whenever possible for client to review as often as necessary.
- Have client perform only one activity at a time and allow adequate time for performance of activities. **D** ● ✦
- Encourage client to make lists of planned activities, questions, and concerns.
- Implement measures to stop emotional outbursts and inappropriate responses if they occur (e.g., provide distraction by clapping hands, handing client an object to look at or hold, or turning on the radio or television). **D** ✦
- Maintain realistic expectations of client's ability to learn, comprehend, and remember information provided.
- Encourage significant others to be supportive of client; instruct them in methods of dealing with client's disturbed thought processes.
- Discuss physiological basis for disturbed thought processes with client and significant others; inform them that cognitive and emotional functioning may improve gradually during the next 6 to 12 months.

These techniques help keep client oriented to environment, self, others, and current reality.
Helps client recognize self.
Having familiar things surrounding the client increases his/her comfort level.
These techniques will help decrease client's frustration when communicating with others.

Repetition of information helps client process information when thinking is impaired.
Overstimulation may cause the client to become anxious or aggressive.
Maintenance of a structured routine helps the client maintain orientation and sense of reality.
Written or audio recorded instructions provide a resource for the client concerning appropriate care.
Prevents client from being frustrated with many activities at one time.
Provides a mechanism for the client to organize thoughts.

These techniques help the client refocus and decreases inappropriate responses.

Don't ask clients to do things beyond their ability. Reinforce information as needed.
Significant others need to learn coping mechanisms and how to work with client.

Understanding what occurred helps the client and significant others work toward improving cognitive and emotional functioning.

Dependent/Collaborative Interventions

- Consult physician if disturbed thought processes worsen.

Notifying the physician allows for modification of the treatment plan.

DISCHARGE TEACHING/CONTINUED CARE

Nursing Diagnosis **DEFICIENT KNOWLEDGE** NDx; **INEFFECTIVE FAMILY HEALTH MANAGEMENT** NDx; **OR INEFFECTIVE HEALTH MAINTENANCE*** NDx

Definition: Deficient Knowledge NDx: Absence of cognitive information related to a specific topic, or its acquisition;
Ineffective Family Health Management NDx: A pattern of regulating and integrating into family processes a program for the treatment of illness and its sequelae that is unsatisfactory for meeting specific health goals of the family unit;
Ineffective Health Maintenance NDx: Inability to identify, manage, and/or seek out help to maintain well-being.

CLINICAL MANIFESTATIONS

Subjective	Objective
Verbal requests for information; client statements reflect misunderstanding	Inadequate follow-through of instruction; inappropriate or exaggerated behaviors

*The nurse should select the diagnostic label that is most appropriate for the client's discharge teaching.

NDx = NANDA Diagnosis   **D** = Delegatable Action   ● = UAP   ✦ = LVN/LPN   ⊖▶ = Go to ⊖volve for animation

RISK FACTOR
- Cognitive limitations or unfamiliarity of situation

NOC OUTCOMES	NIC INTERVENTIONS
Knowledge: disease process; treatment regimen; health resources	Teaching: individual; teaching: disease process; teaching: psychomotor skills; teaching: prescribed activity

NURSING ASSESSMENT	RATIONALE
Assess for stroke-related factors that may impede the learning process. Assess client/family understanding of disease process.	*Client may not be emotionally or physically able to learn.* *The nurse's understanding of the client's and significant other's knowledge-based aids in formulating an educational plan.*

THERAPEUTIC INTERVENTIONS	RATIONALE

Desired Outcome: The client will communicate an awareness of ways to decrease the risk of a recurrent CVA.

Independent Actions

Assist client in recognizing factors that contributed to the stroke (e.g., hypertension, elevated serum lipids, diabetes, atrial fibrillation, use of oral contraceptives). Identify appropriate actions that client can take to decrease risk of a recurrent CVA (e.g., take medications as prescribed, decrease stress, stop smoking, modify diet, adhere to medical treatment, plan to control hypertension and diabetes, use another form of birth control if taking oral contraceptives).	*Knowledge of disease process and how to decrease the impact of risk factors helps the client and family understand what lifestyle changes decrease the incidence of a recurrent CVA.*

THERAPEUTIC INTERVENTIONS	RATIONALE

Desired Outcome: The client will identify ways to manage sensory and speech impairments and disturbed thought processes.

Independent Actions

Instruct client regarding ways to adapt to visual impairments: • Use scanning techniques if visual field cut is present. • Arrange home setting so that when in favorite chair or bed, stimuli other than wall or furniture are within visual fields. • Wear eye patch or opaque lens if double vision persists. Reinforce use of established communication techniques and continuation with speech therapy if indicated. If client is experiencing spatial perceptual deficits and/or unilateral neglect, stress need for assistance with usual daily activities and strict adherence to safety measures. Reinforce methods of adapting to impaired memory and shortened attention span (e.g., make lists of planned activities, review taped or written instructions frequently).	*These interventions reduce the risk of injury from a visual deficit.* *Continued use of established communication techniques helps the client maintain current level of functioning.* *Decreases client frustration and risk for injury.* *This helps foster independence and decreases client's frustration with changes due to illness.*

THERAPEUTIC INTERVENTIONS	RATIONALE

Desired Outcome: The client will identify ways to improve ability to swallow.

Independent Actions

Reinforce instructions regarding appropriate swallowing techniques: • Sit upright for meals and snacks. • Tilt head and neck forward slightly when eating. • Place food on unaffected side of mouth.	*These techniques promote effective swallowing and reduce the risk of aspiration.*

THERAPEUTIC INTERVENTIONS	RATIONALE

- Do not put a lot of food in the mouth at one time.
- Thicken foods to promote ease of swallowing.

Reinforce food selection/preparation of foods and fluids (e.g., avoid sticky foods, use "Thick It," gelatin, or baby cereal to thicken liquids that are thin; moisten dry foods with gravy or sauces).

THERAPEUTIC INTERVENTIONS	RATIONALE

Desired Outcome: The client will identify ways to manage urinary incontinence.

Independent Actions

Reinforce instructions regarding client's bladder training program, stressing the importance of adhering to the program.

Continue implementation of the bladder training program reduces the risk of incontinence and allows client a sense of independence.

Demonstrate procedures that are included in client's bladder training program (e.g., intermittent catheterization, application of an external catheter).

Improves self-care abilities of the patient.

THERAPEUTIC INTERVENTIONS	RATIONALE

Desired Outcome: The client will demonstrate measures to facilitate the performance of activities of daily living and increase physical mobility.

Independent Actions

Instruct on measures to increase ability to perform activities of daily living:

Increases client muscle tone and ability to perform activities of daily living.

- Use of assistive devices and mobility aids
- Continue concentration on body positioning, balance, and movement
- Participation in an exercise program

THERAPEUTIC INTERVENTIONS	RATIONALE

Desired Outcome: The client will communicate an awareness of signs and symptoms to report to the health care provider.

Independent Actions

- Instruct client to report the development of or increase in these signs and symptoms:

  These clinical manifestations may indicate a subsequent stroke.

  - Weakness or loss of sensation in extremities
  - Visual disturbances such as tunnel vision, blurred vision, or transient blindness
  - Lethargy, irritability, or confusion
  - Difficulty chewing or swallowing
  - Difficulty speaking or understanding verbal and non-verbal communication
  - Difficulty maintaining balance
- Seizures

  Seizures can begin to occur months after the CVA as scar tissue forms in the ischemic area.

NDx = NANDA Diagnosis   **D** = Delegatable Action   ● = UAP   ✦ = LVN/LPN   ⊖▶ = Go to ⊖volve for animation

Continued...

THERAPEUTIC INTERVENTIONS	RATIONALE

Desired Outcome: The client will communicate knowledge of community resources that can assist with home management and adjustment to changes resulting from the CVA.

Independent Actions

Provide information about community resources that can assist client and significant others with home management and adjustment to impairments in motor and sensory function and disturbed thought processes resulting from the CVA (e.g., home health agencies, stroke support groups, Meals on Wheels, social and financial services, local chapter of the American Heart Association, local service groups that can help obtain assistive devices, individual and family counselors).

Most stroke clients and significant others have some degree of disability that requires additional support.

THERAPEUTIC INTERVENTIONS	RATIONALE

Desired Outcome: Develop, in collaboration with the nurse, a plan for adhering to recommended follow-up care including regular laboratory studies, future appointments with healthcare providers, and medications prescribed.

Independent Actions

Reinforce the importance of keeping follow-up appointments with health care provider and physical, occupational, and speech therapy.

Recovery from a stroke requires long-term activities to restore and improve health status.

Teach client the rationale for, side effects of, drug-to-drug interactions, food-drug interactions, and importance of taking prescribed medications (e.g., anticoagulants, platelet aggregation inhibitors, antihypertensives).

Client's and significant others' understanding of medication regimen helps improve regimen adherence and reduces the risk of a subsequent stroke.

ADDITIONAL NURSING DIAGNOSES

IMBALANCED NUTRITION: LESS THAN BODY REQUIREMENTS NDx
Related to:
- Decreased oral intake associated with difficulty chewing, swallowing, and feeding self

RISK FOR CONSTIPATION NDx
Related to:
- Decreased GI motility associated with decreased activity
- Decreased intake of fluids and foods high in fiber associated with difficulty chewing, swallowing, and feeding self
- Failure to respond to the urge to defecate associated with decreased level of consciousness or inability to recognize sensation of rectal fullness

SEXUAL DYSFUNCTION NDx
Related to:
- Alteration in usual sexual activities associated with impaired motor function
- Decreased libido and/or impotence associated with impaired motor and sensory function, fear of urinary incontinence, depression, disturbed self-concept, and fear of rejection by partner

FEAR/ANXIETY NDx
Related to:
- Impaired verbal communication and/or motor and sensory function unfamiliar environment
- Lack of understanding of diagnosis, diagnostic tests, and treatments
- Uncertain prognosis
- Disturbed thought processes
- Financial concerns
- Anticipated effect of the CVA on future lifestyle and roles

GRIEVING NDx
Related to changes in motor and sensory function and thought processes, and the effect of these changes on future lifestyle and roles

IMPAIRED SWALLOWING NDx
Related to weakness or paralysis of the swallowing muscles on the affected side and diminished or absent swallowing reflex

IMPAIRED PHYSICAL MOBILITY NDx
Related to:
- Activity limitations associated with decreased motor function and spatial-perceptual impairments
- Loss of muscle tone during period of flaccidity of affected extremities (flaccid paralysis is usually present during the first few days after a CVA)
- Hypertonia of affected extremities (as muscle tone returns after period of flaccidity, it often progresses to spasticity within about 6–8 weeks)
- Reluctance to move associated with fear of injuring self (occurs mainly with ischemia of the dominant hemisphere)
- Loss of muscle mass, tone, and strength associated with prolonged disuse

IMPAIRED URINARY ELIMINATION NDx
Related to:
- Increased reflex activity of the bladder and loss of voluntary control of urinary elimination associated with upper motor neuron involvement if it has occurred
- Decreased ability to control urination associated with decreased level of consciousness or inability to recognize sensation of bladder fullness
- Inability to get to bedside commode or bathroom in a timely manner associated with:
  - Delay in obtaining assistance resulting from inability to communicate the urge to urinate
  - Impaired physical mobility

DISTURBED BODY IMAGE NDx
Related to:
- Change in appearance (e.g., hemiplegia, facial droop, ptosis)
- Lifestyle and role changes associated with motor and spatial-perceptual impairments and disturbed thought processes
- Impaired verbal communication
- Loss of self-control (e.g., automatic speech, emotional lability, inappropriate behavior) or exaggerated emotional responses
- Urinary incontinence
- Dependence on others to meet basic needs

INEFFECTIVE COPING NDx
Related to:
- Fear
- Anxiety
- Depression
- Decreased ability to communicate verbally
- Changes in motor and sensory function, thought processes, and future lifestyle and roles
- Need for lengthy rehabilitation

INTERRUPTED FAMILY PROCESSES NDx
Related to:
- Change in family roles and structure associated with a family member's verbal, motor, and sensory impairments
- Disturbed thought processes
- Need for lengthy rehabilitation

TRAUMATIC BRAIN INJURY/CRANIOTOMY

Traumatic brain injury (TBI) is defined as an alteration in brain function, or other evidence of brain pathology caused by an external force. The leading causes of traumatic brain injury are falls, being struck by or against an object, motor vehicle or traffic accidents, and assault/self-harm events. Additional injuries that can result from traumatic brain injury include skull fracture, dural tear, cerebral contusion, concussion, and laceration, diffuse axonal injury (DAI), brainstem damage, and intracranial hemorrhage. Brain damage can occur during the initial injury and/or as a result of subsequent cerebral damage resulting from factors such as cerebral hematoma, infection, and edema; seizure activity; and/or obstruction of the flow of CSF.

There are several different systems used to classify traumatic brain injuries. The Mayo system classifies TBI into one of three categories: Definite Moderate–Severe TBI, Probable Mild TBI, and Possible TBI. To classify TBI, multiple indicators are evaluated including loss of consciousness, Glasgow Coma Scale score, length of posttraumatic amnesia (PTA), presence of abnormalities on neuroimaging, and the presence of skull

fractures. A classification of Definite Moderate–Severe TBI is made if one of the following were present: death due to this TBI, loss of consciousness of 30 minutes or more, PTA of 24 hrs or more, worst Glasgow Coma Scale score in the first 24 hrs of <13 as well as evidence of hematoma, contusion, penetrating TBI, hemorrhage, or brain stem injury on neuroimaging. Probable Mild TBI is made if one or more of the following were present: momentary loss of consciousness to 30 minutes with PTA not extending beyond 24 hrs. If neuroimaging identifies a depressed, basilar, or linear skull fracture, TBI is still classified as probable. Finally, TBI is classified as possible is made if one or more of the following were present: blurred vision, confusion, dizziness, focal neurological symptoms, headache, and/or nausea.

To repair additional injuries associated with TBI, surgery may be required via a craniotomy or surgical opening of the skull to gain access to the brain. Reasons for the surgery include removing a hematoma, bone fragments, or foreign object (e.g., bullet); controlling cerebrovascular bleeding associated with TBI. In addition, a craniotomy may be performed for conditions other than TBI including removing a tumor or abscess, repairing a vascular abnormality (e.g., aneurysm, arteriovenous malformation), and improving ventricular drainage.

Decompressive craniectomy (excision of a portion of the skull) may be performed for the purpose of relieving elevated intracranial pressure in an effort to improve outcomes in patients with TBI. The portion of the removed skull is replaced (using the preserved bone or a synthetic substance), sometime in the future after there are no longer concerns about increased ICP and/or cerebral infection.

After traumatic brain injury, a person may have a disturbance in consciousness ranging from a brief loss of consciousness to persistent coma. As the level of consciousness improves, clients often experience headache, dizziness, and alterations in thought processes. These signs and symptoms tend to subside gradually but can persist for weeks to years. Additional signs and symptoms after craniocerebral trauma vary depending on the area of the brain that has been affected. For example, tissue damage in the frontal lobe could result in loss of voluntary motor control, personality changes, and/or expressive aphasia; damage to the occipital lobe could cause visual disturbances; and damage to the temporal lobe could result in receptive aphasia and/or hearing impairment. Many of the disturbances noted above may also occur after a craniotomy.

This care plan focuses on the adult client hospitalized after craniocerebral trauma and/or surgery. It deals mainly with nursing and collaborative diagnoses appropriate for a client who has regained consciousness after sustaining a moderate injury or undergoing an uncomplicated craniotomy. Much of the information is also applicable to clients receiving follow-up care in an extended care or rehabilitation facility or home setting. Nursing care and discharge teaching need to be individualized according to the areas of the brain affected and the extensiveness of the tissue damage. Use in conjunction with Preoperative and Postoperative Care Plan if the patient underwent surgery. If the client has sustained more severe craniocerebral trauma, refer also to the Care Plan on Cerebrovascular Accident.

OUTCOME/DISCHARGE CRITERIA

The client will:
1. Have improved cerebral tissue perfusion
2. Have improved or stable neurological function
3. Have an adequate nutritional status
4. Have no signs or symptoms of complications
5. Identify ways to adapt to neurological deficits that may persist after craniocerebral trauma and/or surgery
6. Identify ways to reduce headache
7. State signs and symptoms to report to the health care provider
8. Share thoughts and feelings about residual neurological impairments
9. Identify community resources that can assist with home management and adjustment to changes resulting from craniocerebral trauma and/or craniotomy
10. Develop a plan of care for adhering adhering to recommended follow-up care including future appointments with health care provider and therapists and medications prescribed

---

Nursing Diagnosis **DECREASED INTRACRANIAL ADAPTIVE CAPACITY** NDx

Definition: Compromise in intracranial fluid dynamic mechanisms that normally compensate for increases in intracranial volumes, resulting in repeated disproportionate increases in intracranial pressure (ICP) in response to a variety of noxious and non-noxious stimuli.

Related to:
- Cerebral hemorrhage resulting from laceration of blood vessels at the time of injury or loss of integrity of the ligated vessels
- Compression of cerebral vessels resulting in hematoma formation, cerebral edema, or accumulation of blood in cerebral hemispheres
- Spasm of the cerebral vessels resulting from trauma to and/or stretching of the vessels during surgery
- Hypotension resulting from hypovolemia and peripheral pooling of blood

CLINICAL MANIFESTATIONS

Subjective	Objective
Verbal self-report of headache	Decreased level of consciousness; baseline ICP >10 mm Hg; repeated increases in ICP >10 mm Hg for 5 minutes following external stimuli; vomiting; confusion; agitation; inappropriate affect; lethargy; speech impairment; pupil changes and asymmetry; cerebral perfusion pressure <50 to 60 mm Hg

RISK FACTORS
* Traumatic brain injury
* Hypertension
* Smoking

DESIRED OUTCOME

The client will maintain adequate cerebral adaptation as evidenced by:
a. Absence or reduction of neurological deficits
b. Improved sensory and motor function
c. Improved mental status

NOC OUTCOMES

Neurological status; consciousness; cranial/sensory

NIC INTERVENTIONS

Cerebral edema management; neurological monitoring; ICP monitoring; seizure precautions;

NURSING ASSESSMENT	RATIONALE
Assess client for signs and symptoms of changes in cerebral perfusion:	*Early recognition of signs and symptoms of changes in cerebral perfusion allows for prompt intervention.*
Alterations in: • Level of consciousness • Orientation to person, place, and time • Pupil size and reaction to light • Motor function • Paresthesias • Decreased motor movement • Altered reflexes • Posturing	*Use a coma scale such as the Glasgow Coma Scale to assess eye opening, position and movement, pupil size and changes, and consciousness/mental status. Low scores in persons with severe head injury indicate impaired cerebral perfusion requiring prompt intervention.* *Abnormal movements, posturing, and abnormal flexion of extremities indicate diffuse cerebral damage.*
• Variability in B/P	*Changes in B/P impact cerebral perfusion pressure. Maintain systolic BP >100 mm Hg for clients 50 to 69 years of age or >110 for clients 15 to 49 years or over 70 years of age.*
• ICP	*Normal ICP ranges between 0 and 10 mm Hg. Treatment of ICP values >10 mm Hg are based upon individualized values (rather than generic values) that consider client characteristics, pathology, and a risk-benefit analysis of treating ICP.*
• Speech and thought processes • PaO$_2$ less than 70 mm Hg	*Impaired thought processes indicate damage to the cerebral cortex.* *Hypoxemia causes cerebrovascular dilation further increasing cerebral blood flow which may reduce cerebral perfusion.*

THERAPEUTIC INTERVENTIONS	RATIONALE
Independent Actions Implement measures to improve cerebral tissue perfusion: • Elevate head of bed 30 degrees unless contraindicated.	*Elevating head of bed 30 degrees decreases ICP while maintaining adequate cerebral pressure.*
• **Note:** If surgery was performed using the infratentorial approach, head of bed is usually kept flat postoperatively.	*Keeping the head of bed flat after surgery reduces the pressure on the brainstem.*
• Position client on side not operated on if bone flap and/or large mass was removed.	*This helps prevent an increase in ICP and venous congestion in the operative area.*
• Align head and neck in the midline position; avoid flexion, extension, and rotation of head and neck.	*Maintaining the head in midline position maximizes venous return.*
• Prevent hip flexion of 90 degrees or more.	*Hip flexion of 90 degrees or greater may maintain blood in the abdominal space, thus increasing abdominal and intrathoracic pressure, which reduces venous outflow from the head.*
Perform actions to prevent cerebral hypoxia and the subsequent vasodilation and cerebral edema: • Implement measures to maintain patent airway and suction if necessary.	*A patent airway is necessary for optimum ventilation necessary for both oxygen delivery and the prevention of hypoxia.*
Implement measures to decrease ICP: • Reorient to staff and environment. **D** ● ✦	*Relieves anxiety and helps maintain or lower ICP.*

Continued...

THERAPEUTIC INTERVENTIONS	RATIONALE
• Instruct client to avoid activities that result in isometric muscle contractions (e.g., pushing feet against footboard, tightly gripping side rails).	*Isometric exercises increase ICP.*

Dependent/Collaborative Actions

Implement measures to improve cerebral tissue perfusion:

• Administer osmotic and/or loop diuretics.	*Osmotic diuretics lower ICP by creating an osmotic force in the cerebral vasculature that draws edematous fluid out of the brain. Loop diuretics decrease body fluid volume, which helps decrease cerebral edema. Corticosteroids decrease inflammation.*
• Administer a laxative, antitussive, and/or antiemetic if ordered.	*Prevents straining, coughing, or vomiting that can increase the intrathoracic pressure, which subsequently impedes venous return from the brain.*
• Administer central nervous system depressants judiciously; hold medication and consult physician if respiratory rate is less than 12 breaths/min.	*Hypoxemia increases cerebral vasodilation causing increased ICP.*
• Administer calcium channel blockers if ordered.	*Reduces cerebral vasospasm (the calcium that is released by the injured neural cells can cause vasospasm).*
• Administer oxygen as ordered and before and after tracheal suctioning.	*Administration of oxygen decreases cerebral hypoxia. It is not routine to hyperventilate the client before suctioning; however, hyperventilation that maintains $PaCO_2$ between 30 and 35 mm Hg may be used to prevent cerebral hypoxia.*
• If the client is hypotensive, administer sympathomimetic agents and maintain intravenous fluid therapy.	*Sympathomimetics and IV fluid therapy help maintain adequate blood pressure, which is required to maintain cerebral perfusion. Improves cerebral blood flow.*

If signs and symptoms of increased ICP are present:

• Initiate seizure precautions.	*Protects client from injury.*

Prepare client for:

• Insertion of ICP monitoring device	*Provides direct measurement of ICP, which guides treatment plan.*
• Surgical intervention (i.e., ligation of bleeding vessels, repair of blocked shunt, removal of bone flap or hematoma)	*Decreases ICP and prevents further compromise of cerebral tissue.*

Nursing Diagnosis ACUTE PAIN NDx (HEADACHE)

Definition: Unpleasant sensory and emotional experience associated with actual or potential tissue damage, or described in terms of such damage (International Association for the Study of Pain); sudden or slow onset of any intensity from mild to severe with an anticipated or predictable end, and a duration of less than 3 months.

Related to:
• Trauma to the cerebral tissue associated with the surgical procedure
• Stretching or compression of cerebral vessels and tissue associated with increased ICP if it occurs
• Irritation of the meninges associated with bleeding from meningeal vessels into the CSF and/or inflammation of the meninges

CLINICAL MANIFESTATIONS

Subjective	Objective
Verbal self-report of pain.	Restlessness; irritability; grimacing; rubbing source of pain; avoidance of bright lights and noises; reluctance to move

RISK FACTORS
• Edema
• Positioning
• Hypertension
• Trauma

DESIRED OUTCOMES
The client will obtain relief from pain as evidenced by:
a. Verbalization of pain relief
b. Relaxed facial expression and body positioning

NOC OUTCOMES	NIC INTERVENTIONS
Comfort level; pain control	Pain management: acute; analgesic administration

NURSING ASSESSMENT	RATIONALE
Assess for signs and symptoms of pain: • Verbalization of pain • Restlessness • Irritability • Grimacing • Rubbing affected area • Avoidance of bright lights and noises • Reluctance to move	*Early recognition of signs and symptoms of a pain allows for prompt interventions.*
Assess client's perception of the severity of the pain using a pain intensity rating scale.	*An awareness of the severity of pain being experienced helps determine the most appropriate interventions for pain management. Use of a pain intensity rating scale gives the nurse a clearer understanding of the pain being experienced and promotes consistency when communicating with others about the client's pain experience.*
Assess the client's pain pattern (e.g., location, quality, onset, duration, precipitating factors, aggravating factors, alleviating factors).	*Knowledge of the client's pain pattern assists in the identification of effective pain management interventions.*

THERAPEUTIC INTERVENTIONS	RATIONALE
Independent Actions Implement measures to relieve pain • Perform actions to reduce fear and anxiety about the pain experience (e.g., assure client that the need for headache relief is understood, plan methods for relieving pain with client). Assure client that staff members are nearby; respond to call signal as soon as possible.	*Fear and anxiety decrease a client's threshold for pain.*
• Perform actions to minimize environmental stimuli (e.g., provide a quiet environment, limit number of visitors and their length of stay, dim lights).	*Decreased environmental stimuli promotes relaxation and subsequently increases the client's threshold and tolerance for pain.*
• Avoid jarring bed or startling client.	*Minimizes risk of sudden movements.*
• Provide or assist with nonpharmacologic measures for pain relief (e.g., cool cloth to forehead, progressive relaxation exercise, repositioning).	*Nonpharmacologic measures provide relief of pain without sedation.*
Dependent/Collaborative Actions Implement measures to relieve pain: • Administer analgesics before activities and procedures that can cause pain and before pain becomes severe.	*Analgesics prevent pain from becoming too severe, which may prevent client from participating in activities and procedures.*
• Administer nonnarcotic analgesics or codeine if ordered.	*Opioid narcotics are usually contraindicated because they have a greater depressant effect on the central nervous system.*
Consult appropriate health care provider (e.g., physician, pharmacist, pain management specialist) if above measures fail to provide adequate pain relief.	*Notifying the appropriate health care provider allows for modification of the treatment plan.*

Nursing Diagnosis   **RISK FOR ACUTE CONFUSION** NDx

Definition: Susceptible to reversible disturbances of consciousness, attention, cognition and perception that develop over a short period of time, which may compromise health.

Related to: Damage to cerebral tissue associated with cerebral edema

CLINICAL MANIFESTATIONS

Subjective	Subjective
N/A	Inaccurate interpretation of environment and time; memory loss; altered mood states (e.g., lability, hostility, irritability, inappropriate affect); inability to make decisions or problem solve; changes in attention span; disorientation; inappropriate social behavior

RISK FACTOR

- Trauma

DESIRED OUTCOMES

The client will experience less confusion as evidence by:
a. Improved attention span, memory, and problem-solving abilities
b. Improved level of orientation
c. Reduction in instances of inappropriate responses

NOC OUTCOMES

Information processing; neurological status cognitive ability; memory

NIC INTERVENTIONS

Reality orientation; cognitive stimulation; dementia management; presence; behavior management

NURSING ASSESSMENT	RATIONALE
Assess client for changes in level of confusion and orientation (e.g., shortened attention span, impaired memory, decreased ability to problem solve, confusion, inappropriate response. mood changes). Ascertain from significant others client's usual level of cognitive and emotional functioning.	*Early recognition of signs and symptoms of confusion allows for prompt intervention.*

THERAPEUTIC INTERVENTIONS	RATIONALE

Independent Actions

If client shows evidence of confusion and/or disorientation:

- Reorient to person, place, and time as necessary. **D** ● ✦
- Address client by name. **D** ● ✦
- Place familiar objects, clock, and calendar within client's view. **D** ● ✦
- Face client when conversing with client. **D** ● ✦
- Approach client in a slow, calm manner; allow adequate time for communication. **D** ● ✦
- Repeat instructions as necessary using clear, simple language and short sentences. **D** ● ✦
- Keep environmental stimuli to a minimum but avoid sensory deprivation. **D** ● ✦
- Maintain a consistent and fairly structured routine. **D** ● ✦

- Provide written or taped information whenever possible.

- Have client perform only one activity at a time and allow adequate time for performance of activities. **D** ● ✦
- Encourage client to make lists of planned activities, questions, and concerns.
- Implement measures to stop emotional outbursts and inappropriate responses if they occur (e.g., provide distraction by clapping hands, handing client an object to look at or hold, or turning on the radio or television). **D** ● ✦
- Maintain realistic expectations of client's ability to learn, comprehend, and remember information provided.

These techniques help keep client oriented to environment, self, others, and current reality.

Facing the client when speaking helps improve communication with the client and decreases the client's stress concerning communication.

Repeating information helps client process information when thinking is impaired.

Overstimulation may cause the client to become anxious or aggressive and can block communication.

A structured routine helps client maintain orientation to place and time, and provides a sense of reality.

Written or taped instructions allow client to review information as often as necessary.

Prevents client from being frustrated with having to perform many activities at one time

Making lists provides a mechanism with which the client can organize thoughts.

Distraction helps client refocus and decreases inappropriate responses.

Don't ask clients to do things beyond their ability.

THERAPEUTIC INTERVENTIONS	RATIONALE
• Encourage significant others to be supportive of client; instruct them in methods of dealing with client's disturbed thought processes.	*Significant others need to learn coping mechanisms and how to deal with psychological change.*
• Discuss physiological basis for disturbed thought processes with client and significant others; inform them that cognitive and emotional functioning may improve gradually during the next 6 to 12 months.	*Understanding what occurred helps the client and significant others work toward improving cognitive and emotional functioning.*

Dependent/Collaborative Actions

Consult physician if symptoms worsen.	*Notifying the physician allows for modification of the treatment plan.*

Collaborative Diagnosis RISK FOR MENINGITIS

Definition: Infection of the meninges.

Related to:
• Irritation of the meninges associated with trauma to the meningeal vessels or presence of blood in the CSF
• Introduction of pathogens into the meninges or CSF associated with a tear in the dura (more likely to occur with a compound fracture of the skull, a linear fracture of the frontal or temporal bone, and/or penetration of the skull by an object such as a bullet) and presence of an intracranial monitoring devices and/or external ventricular drain

CLINICAL MANIFESTATIONS

Subjective	Objective
Verbal self-report of persistent headache	Fever; chills; nuchal rigidity; photophobia; positive Kernig sign (inability to straighten knee when hip is flexed); positive Brudzinski sign (flexion of hip and knee in response to forward flexion of the neck); cloudy CSF; elevated CSF pressure; CSF analysis showing increased white blood cell (WBC) count and protein levels

RISK FACTOR	DESIRED OUTCOMES
• Exposure to pathogens as a result of trauma	The client will not develop meningitis as evidenced by: a. Absence of fever and chills b. Absence of nuchal rigidity and photophobia c. Negative Kernig and Brudzinski signs d. Normal CSF analysis

NURSING ASSESSMENT	RATIONALE
Assess for and report signs and symptoms of CSF leak:	*CSF leak indicates a tear in the dura and should be reported immediately.*
• Presence of glucose in clear drainage from nose, ear, or wound as shown by positive results on a glucose reagent strip	*This is one method of determining origin of the fluid draining from the nose.*
• Yellowish ring ("halo") around bloody serosanguineous drainage on dressing or pillowcase	*Yellowish ring indicates cerebrospinal fluid.*
• Constant swallowing	*May indicate increased post nasal drip which may be composed of CSF.*
Assess for and report signs and symptoms of meningitis:	*Early recognition of signs and symptoms of meningitis allows for prompt intervention.*
• Fever, chills	
• Increasing or persistent headache	
• Nuchal rigidity	
• Photophobia	
• Positive Kernig sign (inability to straighten knee when hip is flexed)	
• Positive Brudzinski sign (flexion of hip and knee in response to forward flexion of the neck)	
• The presence of cloudy CSF following a spinal tap or insertion of a drain.	

Continued...

NURSING ASSESSMENT	RATIONALE
• Elevated CSF pressure	*Pressure is often elevated with meningitis.*
• CSF analysis showing increased WBC count and protein levels	*Indicates possible infection of the CSF.*

THERAPEUTIC INTERVENTIONS	RATIONALE

Independent Actions

Implement measures to prevent meningitis:

These techniques and interventions prevent the introduction of bacteria into the brain tissue.

- Assist with thorough cleansing and debridement of head wound if indicated.
- Use sterile technique when changing dressings and working with ICP monitoring device and external ventricular drain.
- Instruct client to keep hands away from head wound, drainage tube(s), and dressing; apply wrist restraints or mittens if necessary.
- If a CSF leak is present:
  - Instruct client to avoid excessive movement and activity (bed rest is usually ordered). — *Prevention of excessive movement prevents further stress on the torn dura.*
  - Instruct client to avoid coughing, blowing nose, or straining to have a bowel movement). — *These activities raise ICP and can cause extension of the dural tear.*
  - If CSF is leaking from nose: — *Elevating the head of the bed facilitates venous drainage.*
    1. Position client with head of bed elevated at least 20 degrees unless contraindicated.
    2. If client needs to sneeze, instruct to do so with mouth open. — *Withholding a sneeze can force the bacteria backward through the torn dura and into the brain tissue.*
    3. Instruct client to avoid putting finger in nose. — *These actions potentially introduce bacteria into the brain tissue.*
    4. Do not perform nasal suctioning or insert a nasogastric tube.
    5. Do not attempt to clean nose unless ordered by physician.
  - If CSF is leaking from ear:
    1. Position client on side of CSF leakage unless contraindicated. — *This position allows the fluid to drain.*
    2. Instruct client to avoid putting finger in ear. — *These actions potentially introduce bacteria into the brain tissue.*
    3. Do not attempt to clean ear unless ordered by physician.
  - Do not pack dressing into area of CSF leakage (nose, ear, or wound). — *Packing the wound interferes with drainage of fluid.*
  - Place a sterile pad over area of CSF leakage to absorb drainage and change pad as soon as it becomes damp. — *This helps prevent bacteria from being introduced into the brain tissues.*

If signs and symptoms of meningitis occur:

- Initiate seizure precautions. — *Cerebral irritation can cause seizures. Seizure precautions help prevent client injury if a seizure does occur.*
- Provide a quiet environment with dim lighting. — *This reduces headaches and photophobia.*

Dependent/Collaborative Actions

Implement measures to prevent meningitis:

- Assist with thorough cleansing and debridement of head wound if indicated. — *It is important to remove dead tissue so the wound does not become infected.*
- If a CSF leak is present:
  - Consult physician regarding an order for an antitussive, decongestant, and laxative if indicated. — *These medications decrease potential coughing, blowing the nose, and straining, which can increase ICP.*
  - Prepare client for surgical repair of the torn dura if the leak does not heal spontaneously. — *Prevents introduction of pathogens into the CNS.*

If signs and symptoms of meningitis occur:

- Administer antimicrobials as ordered. — *Treats and/or prevents infection.*

Collaborative Diagnosis **RISK FOR SEIZURES**

Definition: Transient, uncontrolled electrical activity in the brain that may be exhibited in physical and/or psychological signs and symptoms.

Related to: Altered activity of the cerebral neurons associated with irritation of the brain tissue resulting from the injury, surgery, increased ICP, and/or meningitis

CLINICAL MANIFESTATIONS

Subjective	Objective
Verbal self-report of feelings of general discomfort and feeling "out of sorts" (i.e., malaise), headache, or sense of depression (prodromal)	Dependent upon the type of seizure: focal/motor; temporal lobe or psychomotor; grand mal Excessive muscle tone phase (tonic); alternating contraction/relaxation of muscles (clonic)

RISK FACTORS
- Edema
- Tissue irritation

DESIRED OUTCOME

The client will not experience seizure activity or injury if seizures occur.

NURSING ASSESSMENT	**RATIONALE**
Assess for and report signs and symptoms of seizure activity (e.g., twitching [usually of face or hands], clonic-tonic movements).	*Cerebral irritation places the patient at risk for seizure activity. Risks for seizures are greater with head injuries.*

THERAPEUTIC INTERVENTIONS	**RATIONALE**

Independent Actions
Implement measures to prevent seizures:
- Perform actions to prevent and treat increased ICP and meningitis (e.g., maintain fluid restrictions, elevated head of bed 30 degrees, keep head and neck in neutral position).

Increased ICP and meningitis are associated with seizures.

Initiate and maintain seizure precautions:
- Have oral airway and suction equipment readily available.
- Pad side rails with blankets or soft pads.
- Keep bed in low position with side rails up when client is in bed.

Placing the client on seizure precautions helps prevent injury if and when seizures occur.

If seizures do occur:
- Implement measures to decrease risk of injury:
  - Ease client to the floor if client is sitting in chair or ambulating at onset of seizure.
  - Remain with but do not restrain client during seizure activity.
  - Do not force any object between clenched teeth or try to pry mouth open.
  - Clear area of objects that may cause injury.
  - Place towel under client's head if client is on floor.
  - As seizure activity subsides, perform actions to maintain a client's airway (e.g., turn client on side, insert an oral airway, suction as needed).
- Observe for and report characteristics of seizures (e.g., progression, time elapsed).

These measures help protect the client from further injury.

Dependent/Collaborative Actions
Implement measures to prevent/treat seizures:
- If seizures are occurring, administer IV anticonvulsants (i.e., benzodiazepines or diazepam).
- To prevent reoccurrence of seizures:
- Administer antiepileptic medications (i.e., carbamazepine, phenytoin, valproic acid).

IV anticonvulsants decrease seizure activity.

Medication prescribed depends on the type of seizures experienced by the client.

NDx = NANDA Diagnosis   **D** = Delegatable Action   ● = UAP   ✦ = LVN/LPN   ⊖▶ = Go to ⊖volve for animation

RISK FOR DIABETES INSIPIDUS

Definition: A condition in which kidneys are unable to conserve water from impaired release of antidiuretic hormone (ADH).

Related to: Decreased production and/or impaired release of ADH associated with trauma to the hypothalamus and/or the posterior lobe of the pituitary gland (can occur as a result of trauma or postoperative edema or hematoma in that area)

CLINICAL MANIFESTATIONS

Subjective	Objective
Verbal self-report of extreme/continuous thirst and frequent urination	Polyuria; nocturia; polydipsia; low urine specific gravity; low urine osmolality; high serum plasma osmolality

RISK FACTORS

- Trauma
- Edema

DESIRED OUTCOMES

The client will not experience diabetes insipidus as evidenced by:
a. Absence of polyuria
b. Absence of intense thirst (polydipsia)

NURSING ASSESSMENT

Assess for and report signs and symptoms of diabetes insipidus:
- Polyuria (urine output can range from 4 to 10 L/day or more)
- Reports of intense thirst (if oral fluids are allowed and tolerated, the client's intake is often an amount that corresponds to the high volume of urine output)
- A decrease in urine specific gravity (often 1.005 or less)

Assess for and report signs and symptoms of water deficit:
- Decreased skin turgor
- Dry mucous membranes
- Weight loss of 2% or greater over a short period
- Postural hypotension and/or low B/P
- Weak, rapid pulse
- Elevated serum sodium level and osmolality

RATIONALE

Signs and symptoms of hypovolemia and decreased urine specific gravity indicate diabetes insipidus and require prompt treatment to prevent further impact on other systems in the body.

Early recognition of signs and symptoms of water deficit allows for prompt intervention.

THERAPEUTIC INTERVENTIONS

Dependent/Collaborative Actions
If signs and symptoms of diabetes insipidus occur:
- Maintain fluid intake equal to output.

- Administer an ADH replacement (e.g., vasopressin, desmopressin [DDAVP]) if ordered.

RATIONALE

Decreases edema of the hypothalamus, pituitary gland, and surrounding tissue and subsequently reduces the risk of the development of diabetes insipidus

Administration of vasopressin and desmopressin provides replacement for absent endogenous ADH.

RISK FOR SYNDROME OF INAPPROPRIATE ANTIDIURETIC HORMONE

Definition: A condition in which ADH is not released appropriately.

Related to:
- Increased production and/or release of ADH associated with altered function of the hypothalamus or the posterior lobe of the pituitary gland as a result of trauma and/or postoperative edema or hematoma in that area
- Stimulation of ADH output associated with pain, trauma, and/or stress

CLINICAL MANIFESTATIONS

Subjective	Objective
Verbal self-report of loss of appetite, headaches, nausea	Hyponatremia; hypoosmolarity; concentrated urine; anorexia; dyspnea on exertion; fatigue, vomiting; diarrhea; cramping; hostility, confusion; lethargy; muscle twitching, change in level of consciousness, and/or convulsions

RISK FACTORS

- Pain
- Trauma
- Stress

DESIRED OUTCOMES

The client will not develop SIADH as evidenced by:
a. Stable weight
b. Balanced intake and output
c. Stable or improved mental status
d. Stable or improved muscle strength
e. Absence of cellular edema, abdominal cramping, nausea, vomiting, and seizure activity
f. Urine and serum sodium and osmolality levels within normal limits

NURSING ASSESSMENT

Assess for and report signs and symptoms of SIADH:
- Weight gain of 2% or greater over a short period
- Intake greater than output
- Increased irritability or confusion
- Increasing muscle weakness
- Reports of persistent or increased headache
- Fingerprint edema over sternum (reflects cellular edema)
- Abdominal cramping, nausea, or vomiting
- Seizures
- Elevated urine sodium and osmolality levels
- Low serum sodium and osmolality levels

RATIONALE

Early recognition of the signs and symptoms of SIADH allows for prompt intervention.

THERAPEUTIC INTERVENTIONS

Independent Actions
Implement measures to reduce the risk for the development of SIADH:
- Perform actions to reduce pain.
- Perform actions to reduce fear and anxiety (e.g., assure client that staff members are nearby, respond to call signal as soon as possible).

Dependent/Collaborative Actions
Implement measures to reduce the risk for the development of SIADH:
- Administer osmotic diuretics (e.g., mannitol), loop diuretics (e.g., furosemide), and/or corticosteroids (e.g., dexamethasone) if ordered.

If signs and symptoms of SIADH occur:
- Maintain fluid restrictions if ordered (typically this is a restriction of free water).
- Encourage intake of foods/fluids high in sodium (e.g., tomato juice, cured meats, processed cheese, canned soups, ketchup, canned vegetables, dill pickles, bouillon) if oral intake is allowed and tolerated.

RATIONALE

Pain, fear, and anxiety increase the production of ADH.

Osmotic diuretics decrease cerebral edema, which may decrease pressure on the pituitary and hypothalamus, thus decreasing SIADH; loop diuretics decrease circulating fluid volume; corticosteroids decrease swelling reducing pressure on the hypothalamus, pituitary gland, and surrounding tissue.

Fluid restriction helps decrease vascular fluid volume.

A high sodium intake improves the sodium and vascular fluid (water) balance and increases fluid osmolality.

Continued...

THERAPEUTIC INTERVENTIONS	RATIONALE
● Initiate seizure precautions.	
● Administer the following if ordered:	
● Diuretics (usually furosemide)	*Loop diuretics promote water excretion and retention of sodium, thus improving the sodium/vascular fluid (water) balance.*
● Intravenous infusion of a hypertonic saline solution	*Improves vascular fluid (water)/sodium balance.*
● Demeclocycline	*Demeclocycline increases urine output, thus decreasing free water and improving sodium/vascular fluid (water) balance.*

Collaborative Diagnosis   RISK FOR GASTROINTESTINAL BLEEDING

Definition: Bleeding in the esophagus, stomach, or duodenum.

Related to:
● The development of an ulcer (often referred to as a stress-induced ulcer, stress-related mucosal damage, or Cushing ulcer) associated with:
● Gastric ischemia resulting from vasoconstriction (occurs with sympathetic nervous system stimulation that can result from cerebral injury)
● Hypersecretion of hydrochloric acid resulting from parasympathetic nervous system stimulation that can occur with cerebral injury and stress

CLINICAL MANIFESTATIONS

Subjective	Objective
Verbal self-report of abdominal pain and fullness	Bloody vomitus (bright red or coffee ground); black, tarry stools; frank bright red blood from the rectum; trace amounts of blood in gastric secretions

RISK FACTORS	DESIRED OUTCOMES
● Trauma	The client will not experience GI bleeding as evidenced by:
● Stress	a. No reports of epigastric discomfort and fullness
	b. Absence of frank and occult blood in stool and gastric contents
	c. B/P and pulse within normal range for client
	d. Red blood cell (RBC) count, hematocrit (Hct), and hemoglobin (Hgb) levels within normal range

NURSING ASSESSMENT	RATIONALE
Assess for and report signs and symptoms of GI bleeding (e.g., reports of epigastric discomfort or fullness; frank or occult blood in stool or gastric contents; decreased B/P; increased pulse; decreasing RBC count, Hct, and Hgb levels).	*Early recognition of signs and symptoms of GI bleeding allows for prompt intervention.*

THERAPEUTIC INTERVENTIONS	RATIONALE
Independent Actions Implement measures to prevent ulceration of the gastric and duodenal mucosa:	
● Perform actions to decrease fear and anxiety (e.g., assure client that staff members are nearby, respond to call signal as soon as possible).	*Fear and anxiety increase gastric acid production.*
● When oral intake is allowed:	
● Instruct client to avoid coffee; caffeine-containing tea and colas; spices such as black pepper, chili powder, and nutmeg.	*These foods/fluids stimulate hydrochloric acid secretion or directly irritate the gastric mucosa.*

THERAPEUTIC INTERVENTIONS	RATIONALE

Dependent/Collaborative Actions
Implement measures to prevent ulceration of the gastric and
   duodenal mucosa:

- When oral intake is allowed:
  - Administer ulcerogenic medications (e.g., corticosteroids, phenytoin) with meals or snacks.
  - Administer histamine₂-receptor antagonists (e.g., ranitidine, famotidine), proton-pump inhibitors (e.g., omeprazole, rabeprazole), antacids, and/or cytoprotective agents (e.g., sucralfate)if ordered. **D** ✦

Decreases gastric irritation, which can occur when taking certain medications on an empty stomach.

Histamine receptor antagonists and proton-pump inhibitors suppress secretion of gastric acid. Antacids neutralize stomach acid and cytoprotective agents create a protective barrier against stomach acid and pepsin.

If signs and symptoms of GI bleeding occur:
- Insert nasogastric tube and maintain suction as ordered. **D** ✦

Insertion of an HG tube and suction removes gastric acid and pressure on the gastric lining.

- Administer blood products and/or volume expanders if ordered.

Hypotension may occur. Administration of blood and/or volume expanders may be needed to maintain adequate blood pressure and tissue perfusion.

- Assist with measures to control bleeding (e.g., gastric lavage, endoscopic electrocoagulation) if planned.

These interventions decrease or stop GI bleeding.

DISCHARGE TEACHING/CONTINUED CARE

Nursing Diagnosis **DEFICIENT KNOWLEDGE** NDx**; INEFFECTIVE HEALTH MAINTENANCE** NDx**; OR INEFFECTIVE FAMILY HEALTH MANAGEMENT** NDx*****

Definition: **Deficient Knowledge NDx:** Absence of cognitive information related to a specific topic, or its acquisition;
   Ineffective Health Maintenance NDx: Inability to identify, manage, and/or seek out help maintain well-being;
   Ineffective Family Health Management NDx: A pattern of regulating and integrating into family processes a
   program for the treatment of illness and its sequelae that is unsatisfactory for meeting specific health goals of the
   family unit.

CLINICAL MANIFESTATIONS

Subjective	Objective
Verbal self-report of inability to manage illness; inability to follow prescribed regimen	Inaccurate follow-through with instructions; inappropriate behaviors; experience of preventable complications of spinal cord injury

RISK FACTORS

- Cognitive deficit
- Financial concerns
- Failure to take action to reduce risk factors

- Inability to care for oneself
- Difficulty in modifying personal habits and integrating treatments into lifestyle

NOC OUTCOMES

Knowledge: treatment regimen; health behavior; health
resources

NIC INTERVENTIONS

Health system guidance; teaching: individual; teaching: prescribed activity/exercise; teaching: prescribed medications

NURSING ASSESSMENT	RATIONALE
Assess client's willingness to learn and knowledge related to the disease process.	*The client's willingness to learn and knowledge base provides the basis for education.*
Assess for indications that the client may be unable to effectively manage the therapeutic regimen.	*Early recognition of inability to understand disease process or self-care allows for change in the teaching plan.*

*The nurse should select the diagnostic label that is most appropriate for the client's discharge teaching.

NDx = NANDA Diagnosis   **D** = Delegatable Action   ● = UAP   ✦ = LVN/LPN   ⊖▶ = Go to ⊖volve for animation

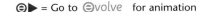

THERAPEUTIC INTERVENTIONS	**RATIONALE**

Desired Outcome: The client will identify ways to adapt to neurological deficits that may persist after craniocerebral trauma and/or surgery.

Independent Actions

Instruct client in ways to adapt to neurological deficits resulting from craniocerebral trauma:

- Wear an eye patch or opaque lens if double vision is a problem.
- Use scanning techniques if visual field cut is present.

- Use paper and pencil, Magic Slate, computer, pictures, and gestures to express self if verbal communication is impaired.
- Make lists, write or record messages and reminders, and refer to written instructions repeatedly if experiencing difficulty concentrating or remembering.
- Request assistance when problem solving and setting priorities, and seek validation of decisions if reasoning ability is impaired.
- Continue with techniques and exercises to improve swallowing if indicated.
- Prepare meals that are visually appealing to help stimulate appetite if senses of smell and/or taste are impaired.
- Use assistive devices (e.g., broad-handled eating utensils, plate guard) and mobility aids (e.g., wheelchair, cane, walker) if motor function is impaired.
- Plan daily activities to allow for adequate rest periods.

These techniques provide a mechanism that helps the client adapt to neurological changes while maintaining as much independence as possible.
Eye patch alleviates double vision.

Visual scanning techniques provide a more complete view of the environment for a client with a visual deficit.
These techniques help improve communication.

Helps maintain activities of daily living when client experiences difficulty in concentrating and remembering.

Client is able to validate decision making.

Improves swallowing ability and decreases risk of aspiration.

This helps maintain adequate nutritional status when sense of smell and/or taste are impaired.
Use of assistive devices helps client maintain as much independent functioning as possible.

Planning daily activities reduces irritability that often occurs after craniocerebral trauma and/or surgery.

THERAPEUTIC INTERVENTIONS	**RATIONALE**

Desired Outcome: The client will identify ways to protect the surgical site from injury (if required).

Independent Actions

Instruct the client in ways to protect the surgical site from injury:
- Wear a scarf, turban, hat, or cap until hair has grown back.
- Do not shampoo hair until the incision has healed (usually 7 to 10 days after surgery).
- When shampooing hair, avoid vigorous scrubbing; pat surgical site dry rather than rubbing.
- Avoid use of hair dryer on hot setting, curling iron, and hot curlers at or near surgical site until hair has grown back.
- Avoid scratching the surgical site; if it itches as the incision heals and the hair grows back, apply light pressure to the surgical site or distract self with activities like taking a walk or watching television.
- If the bone flap was not replaced, avoid bumping or putting excessive pressure on the surgical site (if the skull depression is large, client may need to wear a protective helmet as level of activity increases).

These techniques aid in the promotion of healing and decrease the potential of infection.
Prevents sunburn and irritation to the scalp.
Prevents fluid and soap from getting into the surgical area.

Vigorous scrubbing may irritate and scratch scalp.

Direct heat can burn the unprotected scalp.

Scratching the surgical site can increase risk of infection. Use of light surgical site pressure and distractions can help decrease urge to scratch the surgical site.

Prevents further client injury.

THERAPEUTIC INTERVENTIONS	RATIONALE

Desired Outcome: The client will identify ways to reduce headaches.

Independent Actions

Instruct client in ways to reduce headache, which may persist for months after injury/surgery:

- Dim environmental lighting if possible or wear sunglasses when light is bright.
- Reduce environmental noise whenever possible (e.g., lower volume on TV and radio).
- Avoid situations that increase stress.
- Advise client to take analgesics as prescribed.

These techniques decrease incidence of headaches and pain experienced.

THERAPEUTIC INTERVENTIONS	RATIONALE

Desired Outcome: The client will state signs and symptoms to report to the health care provider.

Independent Actions

- Instruct client to report the following signs and symptoms:
  - Increased drowsiness unrelated to a significant increase in activity or decrease in amount of sleep obtained
  - Increased irritability or restlessness
  - Changes in behavior, increased difficulty remembering or concentrating
  - New or increased weakness of extremities
  - Decreased sensation in extremities
  - Severe headache
  - Difficulty speaking or understanding what others are saying
  - Difficulty chewing or swallowing
  - Changes in vision (e.g., double vision, blurred vision, visual field cut)
  - Increased dizziness, difficulty maintaining balance
  - Seizures
  - Bloody, yellowish, or clear drainage from nose or ear
  - Stiff neck
  - Sudden weight gain or loss, excessive thirst, and/or unusual increase or decrease in amount of urination
  - Unexplained fever
  - Exaggerated startle response; angry outbursts; diminished interest or participation in significant activities; feeling of detachment from others; and recurrent, intrusive, disturbing images and thoughts of the event that resulted in the craniocerebral trauma/surgery

All of these signs may indicate increased ICP and should be reported to a health care provider immediately.

May indicate a leak of CSF.
May indicate an irritation of the meninges.
Indicative of SIADH or diabetes insipidus.

May indicate an infection.
These are signs and symptoms of posttraumatic stress disorder (PTSD) that may occur for weeks to months after involvement in a traumatic event.

THERAPEUTIC INTERVENTIONS	RATIONALE

Desired Outcome: The client will identify community resources that can assist with home management and adjustment to changes resulting from craniocerebral trauma or surgery.

Continued...

THERAPEUTIC INTERVENTIONS	RATIONALE

Independent Actions

Inform client and significant others of community resources that can assist with home management and adjustment to changes resulting from craniocerebral trauma (e.g., home health agencies, Meals on Wheels, social and financial services, brain injury support groups, local service groups that can help obtain assistive devices, individual and family counseling services).
Initiate a referral if indicated.

Provides for continuum of care postdischarge from the acute care facility.

THERAPEUTIC INTERVENTIONS	RATIONALE

Desired Outcome: In collaboration with the nurse, develop a plan for adhering to recommend follow-up care including future appointments with health care provider, therapists, and prescribed medication regimen.

Independent Actions

Reinforce the importance of keeping follow-up appointments with health care provider and physical, occupational, and speech therapists.

Teach client the rationale for, side effects of, schedule for taking, and importance of taking medications prescribed (e.g., anticonvulsants, analgesics, antimicrobials). Inform client of pertinent food and drug interactions.

Implement measures to improve client compliance:

- Include significant others in teaching sessions if possible.
- Encourage questions and allow time for reinforcement and clarification of information provided.
- Provide written instructions on scheduled appointments with health care provider and occupational, physical, and speech therapists; medications prescribed; and signs and symptoms to report.

Keeping follow-up appointments helps the client have continued progress in improving health status.

Knowledge of the medication regimen and the impact of these medications on the system, as well as how the medication regimen can be incorporated into the client's lifestyle, allows the client some mechanism of control of his/her disease and the ability to have an active part in treatment and care.

Significant others may be able to assist client as needed.
Helps significant others learn what ways they can assist the client.

An informed client and family are better able to adhere to a treatment regimen.

ADDITIONAL NURSING DIAGNOSES

RISK FOR INEFFECTIVE AIRWAY CLEARANCE
Related to:

- Alteration in consciousness
- Alteration in respiratory ineffective cough
- Excessive sputum
- Presence of an artificial airway

INEFFECTIVE THERMOREGULATION NDx
Related to direct trauma to the hypothalamus and/or pressure on the hypothalamus associated with hematoma formation or edema of the surrounding tissue

IMPAIRED PHYSICAL MOBILITY NDx
Related to:

- Motor and spatial-perceptual impairments if present
- Activity restrictions imposed by the treatment plan
- Reluctance to move because of headache

BATHING SELF-CARE DEFICIT; DRESSING SELF-CARE DEFICIT; TOILETING SELF-CARE DEFICIT NDx
Related to:

- Impaired physical mobility
- Disturbed thought processes
- Visual impairments if present

FEAR/ANXIETY* NDx
Related to:

- Impaired motor and/or sensory function
- Disturbed thought processes
- Uncertainty as to permanence of neurological deficits
- Unfamiliar environment
- Lack of understanding of diagnostic tests, diagnosis, and treatments

RISK FOR POST-TRAUMA SYNDROME NDx
Related to having experienced a situation that resulted in physical injury and involved intense feelings of fear and helplessness

RISK FOR INJURY NDx: (FALLS, BURNS, AND LACERATIONS)
Related to:

- Dizziness
- Motor, visual, and/or spatial-perceptual impairments if present
- Quick, impulsive behavior (can occur with injury involving the nondominant cerebral hemisphere)
- Ataxia (can occur with cerebellar injury)

*The nurse should select the diagnostic label that is most appropriate based on the client's clinical manifestations.

DISTURBED BODY IMAGE NDx
Related to:
- Change in appearance (e.g., periocular edema and ecchymosis, loss of hair on head if an area was shaved for surgery or to repair lacerations)
- Changes in motor and sensory function
- Dependence on others to meet basic needs
- Anticipated changes in lifestyle and roles associated with sensory and motor impairments and disturbed thought processes

INEFFECTIVE COPING NDx
Related to:
- Persistent headache
- Changes in motor and sensory function and thought processes
- Possibility of lengthy rehabilitation and changes in future lifestyle and roles

INTERRUPTED FAMILY PROCESSES NDx
Related to change in family roles and structure associated with a family member's motor and sensory impairments, disturbed thought processes, and possible need for lengthy rehabilitation

SPINAL CORD INJURY

Spinal cord injury (spinal cord trauma) is most often the result of sudden, external trauma (e.g., motor vehicle accident, fall, sports or recreational injury, act of violence), although it can be caused by a tumor or conditions affecting the vertebrae (e.g., stenosis, pathologic fractures). Spinal cord injuries are classified in general terms as being neurologically complete or incomplete based upon sacral sparing (presence of sensory or motor function in the most caudal sacral segments). A complete injury is defined as the absence of sacral sparing (sensory and motor function) in the lowest sacral segments, whereas an incomplete injury is defined as the presence of sacral sparing (some perseveration of sensory and motor function). A five-point scale is used to grade the degree of impairment in spinal cord injury: A = Complete; B = Sensory Incomplete; C = Motor Incomplete, D = Motor Incomplete; E = Normal. Additional incomplete syndromes, not part of the classification system, include central cord syndrome (incomplete injury with greater weakness in the upper limbs vs. lower limbs); Brown–Sequard syndrome (ipsilateral loss of proprioception, vibration, and motor control at and below the level of injury; sensory loss at level of injury; contralateral loss of pain and temperature sensation); anterior cord syndrome (loss of motor function, pain sensation and temperature at and below level of injury with preservation of light touch and joint position sense); and cauda equina syndrome (flaccid paralysis of lower extremities and motor/sensory function to the bladder).

Immediately after traumatic injury to the spinal cord, spinal shock (loss of motor, sensory, autonomic, and reflex activity below the level of the injury) occurs. Spinal shock usually lasts between 1 and 6 weeks but can persist for months. The neurological impairments that remain after the period of spinal shock depend upon the level of the cord injury (the higher the level, the greater the loss of body function) and the degree of cord involvement (complete/incomplete).

This care plan focuses on the adult client hospitalized with a complete injury of the spinal cord at the level of the fifth cervical vertebra (C5).

After the period of spinal shock, a client with a complete cord injury at the C5 level experiences loss of voluntary motor function below the clavicles; however, full neck, upper shoulder, and some bicep control and elbow flexion are retained. Sensory function is intact above the clavicles and in certain areas of the deltoids and forearms. The client can speak and use the diaphragm; however, breathing will be weakened. With rehabilitation, the client may be able to do things such as operate an electric wheelchair and a manual wheelchair with hand rim projections (quad pegs), feed self using assistive devices, use reflex activity to achieve an erection and stimulate bowel and bladder elimination, accomplish some change in body position, and operate some equipment (e.g., computer, telephone) using assistive devices.

Much of the information provided in this care plan is also applicable to spinal cord–injured clients in extended care, rehabilitation, and home settings.

Although the focus is on injury at the C5 level, the information can easily be individualized to plan nursing care for clients with injury to other segments of the spinal cord.

OUTCOME/DISCHARGE CRITERIA

The client will:
1. Have clear, audible breath sounds throughout lungs
2. Have no evidence of tissue irritation or breakdown
3. Have an adequate nutritional status
4. Experience optimal control of urinary and bowel elimination
5. Direct own care and perform or participate in self-care when possible
6. Have adequate tissue perfusion and thermoregulation
7. Have no signs and symptoms of complications resulting from the spinal cord injury and decreased mobility
8. Identify ways to prevent complications associated with spinal cord injury and decreased mobility
9. Demonstrate the ability to correctly use and maintain assistive devices
10. Identify ways to manage altered bowel and bladder function
11. State signs and symptoms to report to the health care provider
12. Identify resources that can assist with financial needs, home management, and adjustment to changes resulting from spinal cord injury
13. Share thoughts and feelings about the effects of spinal cord injury on self-concept, lifestyle, and roles
14. Develop a plan for adhering to recommended follow-up care including future appointments with health care provider and occupational and physical therapists and medications prescribed

Nursing Diagnosis   INEFFECTIVE BREATHING PATTERN NDx

Definition: Inspiration and/or expiration that does not provide adequate ventilation.

Related to:
• Neuromuscular impairment
• Decreased energy/fatigue
• Respiratory muscle fatigue
• Immobility
• Pain related to spinal cord injury/invasive procedures

CLINICAL MANIFESTATIONS

Subjective	Objective
Verbal self-report of difficulty breathing	Dyspnea; orthopnea; respiratory rate (adults [ages ≥14 years], <11 or >24 breaths/min; infants, <25 or >60 breaths/min; ages 1 to 4 years, <20 or >30 breaths/min; ages 5 to 14 years, <14 or >25 breaths/min); depth of breathing (tidal volume: adults, 500 mL at rest; infants, 6 to 8 mL/kg); decreased inspiratory/expiratory pressure; decreased minute ventilation; decreased vital capacity; nasal flaring; use of accessory muscles to breathe; altered chest excursion; pursed-lip breathing; prolonged expiration phases; increased anterior-posterior chest diameter; decreased pulse oximetry readings

RISK FACTOR

• Spinal cord injury at or above C-5 level

DESIRED OUTCOMES

The client will maintain effective breathing pattern as evidenced by:
a. Rate and depth of respirations within normal range for client
b. Symmetrical chest excursion
c. Oxygen saturation within normal ranges for client

NOC OUTCOMES

Respiratory status; ventilation; airway patency

NIC INTERVENTIONS

Airway management; respiratory monitoring; cough enhancement; ventilation assistance

NURSING ASSESSMENT	RATIONALE
Assess for signs and symptoms of an ineffective breathing pattern (e.g., shallow respirations, tachypnea, limited chest excursion, dyspnea, use of accessory muscles when breathing).	*Early recognition of signs and symptoms of an ineffective breathing pattern allows for prompt intervention.*
Monitor for and report a significant decrease in oximetry results.	*Oximetry is a noninvasive method of measuring arterial oxygen saturation. The results assist in evaluating respiratory status.*

THERAPEUTIC INTERVENTIONS	RATIONALE

Independent Actions

Implement measures to decrease fear and anxiety (e.g., assure client that breathing deeply will not dislodge tubes or cause incision to break open, interact with client in a confident manner).

Fear and anxiety may cause a client to breathe shallowly or to hyperventilate. Decreasing fear and anxiety allows the client to focus on breathing more slowly and taking deeper breaths.

Place client in a semi- to high-Fowler's positions unless contraindicated. Position with pillows to prevent slumping.
D ● ✦

A semi- to high-Fowler's positions allows for maximal diaphragmatic excursion and lung expansion. Prevention of slumping is essential because slumping causes the abdominal contents to be pushed up against the diaphragm and restricts lung expansion.

THERAPEUTIC INTERVENTIONS	RATIONALE
Implement measures to increase strength and activity tolerance if client is weak and fatigued (e.g., provide uninterrupted rest periods, maintain optimal nutrition). **D** ✦	*An increase in strength and activity tolerance enables the client to breathe more deeply and participate in activities to improve breathing pattern.*
If client must remain flat in bed, assist with position change at least every 2 hrs. **D** ● ✦	*Compression of the thorax and subsequent limited chest wall and lung expansion occur when the client lies in one position. Frequent repositioning promotes maximal chest wall and lung expansion.*
Instruct client to deep breathe or use incentive spirometer every 1 to 2 hrs. **D** ✦	*Deep breathing and use of an incentive spirometer promote maximal inhalation and lung expansion. Deep inhalation also stimulates surfactant production, which lowers alveolar surface tension and subsequently increases lung compliance and ease of inflation.*

Dependent/Collaborative Actions

Administer prescribed analgesics before planned activity. **D** ✦	*Pain reduction enables the client to breathe more deeply.*
Assist with positive airway pressure techniques (e.g., continuous positive airway pressure [CPAP], bilevel positive airway pressure [BiPAP], flutter/positive expiratory pressure [PEP] device), if ordered.	*Positive airway pressure techniques increase intrapulmonary (i.e., alveolar) pressure, which helps reexpand collapsed alveoli and prevent further alveolar collapse.*
Increase activity as allowed and tolerated. **D** ✦	*During activity, the client usually takes deeper breaths, thus increasing lung expansion.*
Consult appropriate health care provider (e.g., physician, respiratory therapist) if ineffective breathing pattern continues.	*Notifying the appropriate health care provider allows for modification of treatment plan.*

Nursing Diagnosis ## IMPAIRED PHYSICAL MOBILITY NDx

Definition: Limitation in independent, purposeful movement of the body or of one or more extremities.

Related to:
- Activity limitations associated with quadriplegia and immobilization of the spine
- Spasticity after the period of spinal shock associated with stimulation of the reflex arcs below the level of the injury
- Decreased motivation associated with fatigue and the physiological response to the extensive motor and sensory losses that have occurred
- Pain
- Loss of muscle mass, tone, and strength in areas of existing motor function (biceps, upper shoulders, and neck) associated with prolonged disuse (more likely to occur when client is in skeletal traction and must remain in bed)
- Contractures (if they develop)

CLINICAL MANIFESTATIONS

Subjective	Objective
Verbal self-report of pain; discomfort; fatigue	Difficulty moving; supporting the affected limb; exertional dyspnea; contractures; limited ability to perform gross and fine motor skills; limited range of motion (ROM); movement-induced tremor; postural instability; uncoordinated movements

RISK FACTORS

- Neuromuscular impairment related to spinal cord injury
- Sensory-perceptual impairment

DESIRED OUTCOMES

The client will improve mobility as evidenced by:
a. Increased physical activity
b. Movement of affected limb or limbs
c. Participation in activities of daily living (ADLs)
d. Demonstration of appropriate use of assistive devices to improve movement
e. Absence of contractures
f. Absence of redness/irritation to skin-no skin breakdown

NDx = NANDA Diagnosis   **D** = Delegatable Action   ● = UAP   ✦ = LVN/LPN   ⊜▶ = Go to ⊜volve for animation

NOC OUTCOMES	NIC INTERVENTIONS
Immobility consequences: physiological; neurological status: peripheral; spinal sensory/motor function	Positioning; exercise therapy: joint mobility; exercise therapy: muscle control

NURSING ASSESSMENT	RATIONALE
Assess client's movement ability and activity tolerance. Use a tool such as the Assessment Tool for Safe Patient Handling and Movement or the Functional Independence Measures (FIM).	Assessment of mobility is used to best determine how to facilitate movement. Assessment of activity tolerance provides a baseline for patient strength and endurance with movement.
Assess circulation, motion, and feeling in digits.	Circulation may be compromised by edema of extremities, which can lead to tissue necrosis and/or contractures.
Determine risk for skin breakdown using a risk assessment tool (e.g., Norton Scale, Braden Scale, Gosnell Scale).	Identification of clients at risk for skin breakdown allows for implementation of nursing interventions to prevent breakdown from occurring. Use of a scale provides for more accurate assessment.
Inspect the skin (especially bony prominences, dependent and/or edematous areas, perineum, area underneath halo vest, and areas of sensory loss) for pallor, redness, and breakdown.	Early recognition of signs and symptoms of skin impairment allows for prompt intervention.
Assess need for assistive devices.	Determine client's needs for assistive devices as well as proper use of wheelchairs, walkers, canes, and so on, to reduce incidence of falls.

THERAPEUTIC INTERVENTIONS	RATIONALE
Independent Actions Encourage and implement strength training activities: • Active and/or passive ROM • Ambulation • Use of trapeze for pull-ups • ADLs **D** ● ✦	Inactivity contributes to muscle weakening. Contractures can develop as early as 8 hrs of immobility. These activities maintain and increase the client's strength and ability to move.
Use assistive devices that are appropriate for the mobility level of the client. Assistive devices may include: • Crutches • Gait belt • Walker **D** ● ✦	Assistive devices help the caregivers decrease the potential for falls and/or injuries.
Cluster treatments and care activities to allow for uninterrupted periods of rest. **D** ● ✦	Increases client's tolerance and strength for activities.
Encourage patient with positive reinforcement during activities. **D** ● ✦	A positive approach to activities supports the client's accomplishment, engagement in new activities, and improves self-esteem.
Implement falls protocol.	Client safety is a priority.
Maintain the bed in low position and keep side rails up. **D** ● ✦	Reduces prolonged pressure on tissues, decreasing potential for tissue ischemia and pressure sores.

Implement measures to maintain healthy, intact skin:
• Keep skin lubricated, clean, and dry.
• Assist patient to turn and reposition every 2 hrs.
• Keep bed linens dry and wrinkle-free). **D** ● ✦
• Position client with appropriate devices (wedges, pillows, kinetic bed, air bed, gel mattress). **D** ●
• If client is wearing a halo vest:
  • Ensure the vest lining and skin beneath it are kept dry and intact
  • Make sure clothing worn under the vest is wrinkle free, and made of cotton
  • Cover all rough edges of vest with tape
	Healthy, intact skin reduces the risk of pressure sores and infection.
	
	Turning clients allows for appropriate circulation to tissues.
	
	Reduces prolonged pressure on tissues, decreasing potential for tissue ischemia and pressure sores
	Skin will become macerated from accumulation of moisture on the vest lining.
	Rough edges on the vest can cause lacerations of the skin.

THERAPEUTIC INTERVENTIONS	RATIONALE
Maintain an optimal nutritional status. Increase protein intake.	*Adequate nutrition is needed to maintain adequate energy level.*
Assist client with acceptance of immobility.	*Helps patient accept limitations and focus on a new quality of life.*

Dependent/Collaborative Actions

Consult appropriate health care provider: dietitian, physician, and occupational therapist.	*These individuals provide specific activities and exercise programs to improve strength and mobility.*
Administer pain medications before activities. **D** ✦	*Reduces muscle stiffness and tension, allowing the client to participate in activities.*
Notify appropriate health care provider (e.g., wound care specialist, physician).	*Wound care specialists can provide individualized treatment to improve healing of skin breakdown.*

Nursing Diagnosis   INEFFECTIVE THERMOREGULATION NDx

Definition: Temperature fluctuation between hypothermia and hyperthermia.

Related to:
- Interruption in the feedback system between the area below the level of cord injury and the hypothalamus, and loss of vasomotor tone below the level of the injury (these conditions result in the loss of compensatory responses to temperature changes [i.e., vasodilation, sweating, vasoconstriction, shivering, and piloerection])
- Reduction in heat generation associated with limited body movement (especially during period of spinal shock)

CLINICAL MANIFESTATIONS

Subjective	Objective
Verbal self-report of feeling too warm or too cold	Excessively warm or cool skin below the level of injury; temperature above or below normal range; tachycardia; hypotension/hypertension; shivering; skin cool to touch; pallor; slow capillary refill; cyanotic nail beds; piloerection; warm to touch; flushed skin; hypercapnia; seizures

RISK FACTORS
- Environmental temperature
- Edema
- Trauma

DESIRED OUTCOMES

The client will experience effective thermoregulation as evidenced by:
a. Verbalization of comfortable body temperature
b. Absence of excessively warm or cool skin below the level of the injury
c. Temperature within normal range

NOC OUTCOMES	NIC INTERVENTIONS
Thermoregulation	Temperature regulation: environmental management

NURSING ASSESSMENT	RATIONALE
Assess for signs and symptoms of ineffective thermoregulation (e.g., reports of feeling too warm or too cold, excessively warm or cool skin below the level of the injury, temperature above or below normal range).	*Early recognition of the signs and symptoms of inefficient thermoregulation allows for prompt intervention.*

THERAPEUTIC INTERVENTIONS	RATIONALE

Independent Actions

Implement measures to maintain effective thermoregulation:
- Perform actions to prevent hypothermia:
  - Maintain room temperature at 70°F.
  - Provide extra clothing and bedding as necessary. **D ● ✦**
  - Protect client from drafts. **D ● ✦**
  - Provide warm liquids for client to drink. **D ● ✦**
  - Avoid taking client outdoors when it is very cold. **D ● ✦**
- Perform actions to prevent hyperthermia:
  - Maintain room temperature at 70°F. **D ● ✦**
  - Avoid use of excessive clothing and bedding. **D ● ✦**
  - Remove extra clothing during physical and occupational therapy sessions.
  - Avoid taking client outdoors when it is very hot (especially if the humidity is high). **D ● ✦**

The client is not able to regulate body temperature due to loss of sympathetic control. These interventions focus on keeping the client's temperature as close to normal as possible.

Dependent/Collaborative Actions

Implement measures to maintain effective thermoregulation:
- Apply warming and cooling blanket as ordered. **D ● ✦**

Consult physician if above measures fail to maintain effective thermoregulation.

Notifying the physician allows for modification of the treatment plan.

Nursing Diagnosis | # RISK FOR AUTONOMIC DYSREFLEXIA NDx

Definition: Susceptible to life-threatening, uninhibited response of the sympathetic nervous system, post-spinal shock, in an individual with spinal cord injury or lesion at the 6th thoracic vertebra (T6) or above (has been demonstrated in patients with injuries at the 7th thoracic vertebra [T7] and the 8th thoracic vertebra [T8]), which may compromise health.

Related to:

Related to loss of autonomic nervous system control below the level of the cord injury (can occur once reflect activity returns after period of spinal shock):
- Cardiopulmonary stimuli—Deep vein thrombosis and pulmonary emboli
- GI stimuli—Bowel distention, constipation, digital stimulation, enemas, esophageal reflux, fecal impaction, gall stones, gastric ulcers, hemorrhoids, suppositories
- Musculoskeletal-integumentary stimuli—Cutaneous stimulation, pressure over bony prominences, pressure over genitalia, range-of-motion exercises, spasm, sunburns, wounds
- Neurological stimuli—Irritating stimuli below of injury, painful stimuli below level of injury
- Regulatory stimuli—Extreme environmental temperatures, temperature fluctuations
- Reproductive stimuli—Ejaculation, labor and delivery, menstruation, pregnancy
- Situational stimuli—Constrictive clothing, drug reactions, narcotic/opiate withdrawal, positioning, surgical procedures
- Urological stimuli—Bladder distension and spasm, calculi, catheterization, cystitis, epididymitis, surgery, urinary tract infection

CLINICAL MANIFESTATIONS

Subjective	**Objective**
Verbal self-report of a sudden pounding headache; blurred vision; nausea; feelings of apprehension	Sudden onset of severe hypertension; bradycardia; flushing above the lesion; pale extremities below the level of the lesion; profuse diaphoresis above level of injury; piloerection

RISK FACTORS
- Trauma
- Any stimulus that irritates or increases pressure below the level of injury

DESIRED OUTCOMES

The client will not experience autonomic dysreflexia as evidenced by:
a. Vital signs within normal range for client
b. Skin dry and usual color above the level of the injury
c. No reports of pounding headache, nasal congestion, and blurred vision

NOC OUTCOMES	NIC INTERVENTIONS
Symptom severity	Dysreflexia management

NURSING ASSESSMENT	**RATIONALE**
Assess for signs and symptoms of autonomic dysreflexia: • Sudden rise in B/P (systolic pressure may go as high as 300 mm Hg) • Bradycardia • Flushing and profuse diaphoresis above level of injury • Pounding headache • Nasal congestion • Blurred vision	*Autonomic dysreflexia is considered a medical emergency that may occur after the resolution of spinal shock. Early recognition of the signs and symptoms of autonomic dysreflexia allows for prompt intervention.*

THERAPEUTIC INTERVENTIONS	**RATIONALE**

Independent Actions

Implement measures to prevent stimulation of the sympathetic nervous system below the level of the cord injury to prevent autonomic dysreflexia.

- Perform actions to prevent distention of the bladder and bowel:

  Problems with the bladder and bowel are the two most frequent causes of autonomic dysreflexia.
  These interventions promote regular bladder and bowel emptying.

  - Attempt to initiate voiding periodically by stimulating the trigger zones of the reflex sacral arc (e.g., tap suprapubic area, stroke inner thigh, perform anal sphincter stretching, pull pubic hair); if voiding occurs, repeat stimulus as necessary to empty the bladder.

  - If possible, place client on bedside commode or toilet when triggering voiding reflex.

    Gravity promotes emptying of the bladder.

  - Instruct client to space fluid intake evenly throughout the day, rather than drinking a large quantity at one time.

    If the bladder fills rapidly and frequency of emptying is not increased, bladder distention occurs.

  - Instruct client to limit intake of alcohol and beverages containing caffeine such as colas, coffee, and tea.

    Alcohol and caffeine have a mild diuretic effect and act as irritants to the bladder; the increased urine production can result in bladder distention if the frequency of bladder emptying is not also increased, and the bladder irritation can trigger bladder spasms and subsequent incontinence.

  - Limit oral fluid intake in the evening. **D** ● ✦

    Limiting oral intake in the evening prevents the bladder from becoming overdistended during the night. As rehabilitation progresses, most clients do not perform intermittent catheterization or attempt to trigger voiding during the night.

  - Instruct client and others to avoid stimulating the voiding reflex trigger zones at times other than during bladder care.

    This reduces the risk of incontinence.

- Implement measures to prevent constipation:

  - Encourage client to drink hot liquids before scheduled bowel evacuation.

    Drinking hot liquids prior to a bowel evacuation helps stimulate peristalsis.

  - Assist client to eat at scheduled times and adhere to a routine time for defecation; follow client's preinjury pattern if possible. **D** ● ✦

    A scheduled eating and defection routine helps maintain continence.

  - Perform actions to prevent pressure on any area of the client's body below the level of the cord injury.

    Pressure below the level of injury may stimulate autonomic dysreflexia.

  - Instruct and assist client to change positions frequently.

    These actions decrease pressure on the non-innervated areas of the body.

  - Ensure that overbed tray is not resting on chest. **D** ● ✦
  - Ensure that clothing is not constrictive and shorts are not too tight.
  - Perform good nail care.

    Long fingernails may stimulate the sympathetic nervous system.

NDx = NANDA Diagnosis   **D** = Delegatable Action   ● = UAP   ✦ = LVN/LPN   ⊜▶ = Go to ⊖volve for animation

Continued...

THERAPEUTIC INTERVENTIONS	RATIONALE

Dependent/Collaborative Actions

- Perform actions that prevent pressure on any area of the client's body below the level of cord injury.
- Perform intermittent catheterization or insert indwelling catheter as ordered.
- Maintain patency of indwelling catheters. **D** ✦

These actions prevent the bladder from becoming distended and placing the client at increased risk for autonomic dysreflexia.

- Apply a topical anesthetic agent to any existing pressure ulcer.
- Apply a local anesthetic (e.g., Nupercainal ointment) if ordered before performing actions that can result in an exaggerated sympathetic response (e.g., urinary catheterization, removal of a fecal impaction, administration of an enema, care of any wound below the level of the injury).

Use anesthetic ointment to decrease the risk of aggravating the autonomic dysreflexia.

If signs and symptoms of autonomic dysreflexia occur:

- Immediately implement measures to promote venous pooling and subsequent decrease in B/P (e.g., raise head of bed and lower client's legs unless contraindicated; remove abdominal binder, antiembolism stockings, and intermittent pneumatic compression device if present).

Immediate treatment is important to prevent a hypertensive stroke. These actions decrease B/P.

- Administer antihypertensives (e.g., diazoxide, hydralazine, nitroprusside) as ordered.

Antihypertensive medications decrease blood pressure, which is important in stroke prevention.

- Monitor B/P and pulse frequently (usually every 3 to 5 minutes until treatments and/or medication take effect).
- Notify physician immediately if signs and symptoms persist or if complications resulting from severe hypertension occur (e.g., seizures, intraocular hemorrhage, cerebrovascular accident, myocardial infarction).

These complications can have a very deleterious impact on the body and should be treated immediately to prevent further insult to the body.

- Notify all persons participating in client's care of the episode of autonomic dysreflexia because such episodes can reoccur.

The client's treatment plan may need to be altered to address other effects of autonomic dysreflexia.

Nursing Diagnosis   ## SELF-CARE DEFICIT NDx (BATHING, DRESSING, FEEDING, AND TOILETING)

Definition: **Self-Care Deficit: Bathing NDx:** Inability to independently complete cleansing activities; **Self-Care Deficit: Dressing NDx:** Inability to independently put on or remove clothing; **Self-Care Deficit: Feeding NDx:** Inability to eat independently; **Self-Care Deficit: Toileting NDx:** Inability to independently perform tasks associated with bowel and bladder elimination.

Related to: Impaired physical mobility associated with quadriplegia, spasticity, decreased motivation, pain, weakness, and activity restrictions imposed by treatment plan

CLINICAL MANIFESTATIONS

Subjective	Objective
Verbal self-report of pain and/or weakness	Inability to move upper and/or lower extremies due to injury; muscle spasticity

DESIRED OUTCOME

The client will demonstrate increased participation in self-care activities within the limitations imposed by the treatment plan and effects of the spinal cord injury.

NOC OUTCOMES	NIC INTERVENTIONS
Self-care: activities of daily living; bathing; dressing; eating; self-care hygiene; toileting	Self-care assistance: dressing/grooming; self-care assistance: feeding; self-care assistance: toileting; self-care assistance: transfer

NURSING ASSESSMENT	RATIONALE
Assess readiness to engage in self-care activities. Determine level of motivation and family support.	*The level of client interest, motivation, and family support will determine when and how much self-care the client can assume.*

THERAPEUTIC INTERVENTIONS	RATIONALE

Independent Actions

- With client, develop a realistic plan for meeting daily physical needs. Inform client that with rehabilitation and use of assistive devices, he/she may be able to accomplish activities such as:
- Feeding self once meal has been set up
- Washing face and chest
- Combing front and sides of hair, brushing teeth, and shaving with an electric razor
- Participating in dressing upper body **D** ● ✦

Engaging client in self-care activities will demonstrate to client that he or she will be able to care for self after discharge.

Schedule care at a time when client is most likely to be able to participate (e.g., when analgesics are at peak effect, after rest periods, not immediately after physical therapy sessions or meals).

If the client is tired or experiencing pain, he/she will not be able to participate in activities of daily living, which may cause a decrease in morale if client has been previously successful in completing tasks.

Keep objects client can use independently within easy reach. **D** ● ✦

Provides the client a way to be independent will improve morale and decrease recovery time.

Allow adequate time for accomplishment of self-care activities. **D** ● ✦

Be sure not to rush the client. Learning new ways of caring for self may require additional time.

Encourage client to perform as much of self-care as possible within physical limitations and activity restrictions imposed by the treatment plan. **D** ● ✦

Allows client the ability to see that he/she can care for self and promotes self-confidence.

Perform for client the self-care activities that he/she is unable to accomplish. **D** ● ✦

Inform significant others of client's abilities to participate in own care.

Explain the importance to significant others of encouraging and allowing client to achieve an optimal level of independence.

Dependent/Collaborative Actions

When condition stabilizes and physician allows, implement measures to facilitate client's ability to perform self-care activities:

- Perform actions to increase mobility (e.g., tilt table, active and passive range of motion [ROM]).

These actions increase client's ability to become more mobile and to perform self-care activities.

- Consult occupational therapist regarding assistive devices available; reinforce use of these devices, which may include:

Consulting an occupational therapist allows for interdisciplinary care and use of tools and techniques to improve and enhance self-care abilities.

  - Rocker feeder, overhead sling, plate guard, sandwich holder, and broad-handled and/or swivel utensils for feeding self
  - Flexor-hinge splint or universal cuff to aid in brushing teeth, combing hair, and shaving with electric razor
  - Bath mitt for bathing face and chest
  - Velcro fasteners to facilitate dressing upper body

Nursing Diagnosis **RISK FOR INJURY** NDx

Definition: Susceptible to physical damage due to environmental conditions interacting with the individual's adaptive and defensive resources, which may compromise health.

Related to:
- Falls related to loss of motor function, use of kinetic bed, altered sitting balance if wearing a halo device (the structure and weight of the device alter the client's center of gravity), and unexpected body movements resulting from spasticity
- Burns related to loss of motor and sensory function and unexpected body movements resulting from spasticity

NDx = NANDA Diagnosis   **D** = Delegatable Action   ● = UAP   ✦ = LVN/LPN   ⊝▶ = Go to ⊝volve for animation

RISK FACTORS
- Changes in balance
- Weakness
- Loss of neuromuscular functioning

CLINICAL MANIFESTATIONS

Subjective	Objective
N/A	Inability to move upper and/or lower extremities due to injury; muscle spasticity

DESIRED OUTCOME

The client will not experience falls or burns.

NOC OUTCOMES	**NIC INTERVENTIONS**
Fall prevention behavior; falls occurrence	Fall prevention; environmental management; peripheral sensation management

NURSING ASSESSMENT	**RATIONALE**
Assess for signs and symptoms that client is at risk for injury.	*Early recognition of signs and symptoms that place the client at risk for injury allows for prompt intervention.*

THERAPEUTIC INTERVENTIONS	**RATIONALE**

Independent Actions

Implement measures to reduce the risk for injury:
- Perform actions to prevent falls:
  - If client is in a standard hospital bed, keep bed in low position with side rails up. **D ● ✦**
  - If client is in a kinetic bed, use safety measures such as safety straps and padded side pieces. **D ● ✦**
  - Keep safety belts securely fastened when client is on a stretcher or in a wheelchair. **D ● ✦**
  - Obtain adequate assistance when moving client; follow instructions from physical therapist on correct transfer techniques. **D ● ✦**
  - Implement measures to increase client's stability when in a wheelchair (e.g., use wheelchair equipped with an antitipping device, fasten safety belt around upper body and chair to stabilize trunk, use H-straps to keep legs positioned properly).
  - Do not rush client; allow adequate time for the accomplishment of transfers and position changes. **D ● ✦**
- Perform actions to prevent burns:
  - Let hot foods and fluids cool slightly before serving. **D ● ✦**
  - Supervise client while smoking; do not place ashtray on client's lap.
  - Assess temperature of bath water before and during use. **D ● ✦**
  - When client is in a wheelchair, instruct the client to avoid placing self next to sources of heat (e.g., heater, stove).
- Encourage client to request assistance whenever needed; have a specially adapted call signal available to client at all times.
- Perform actions to decrease spasticity (e.g., avoid stimulating extremities or muscle groups; assist client to change position and perform ROM activities).

These actions will decrease the client's risk for falls and potential injury.

Client may accidentally spill liquids; without ability to feel hot or cold, client may inadvertently cause a burn.

The cigarette could roll off the ashtray onto the client's clothing causing a fire and subsequent burns.

The client has lost sense of feeling and may not be aware that water is too hot and can cause burning.

This will cause the sides of the wheelchair to become hot and burn the client's skin.

Stretching to reach a call light may cause the client to lose balance and fall out of bed.

It is important to reduce the risk of unexpected body movements to prevent injury.

THERAPEUTIC INTERVENTIONS	RATIONALE
Include client and significance others in planning and implementing measures to prevent injury.	*Significant others should be informed on how to help prevent client injury.*
If injury does occur, initiate appropriate first aid and notify physician.	*Notification of the physician allows for modification of the treatment plan.*

Nursing Diagnosis ## RISK FOR VENOUS THROMBOEMBOLISM NDx

Definition: Susceptible to the development of a blood clot in a deep vein, commonly in the thigh, calf or upper extremity, which can break off and lodge in another vessel, which may compromise health.

Related to:
- Venous stasis associated with decreased mobility and decreased vasomotor tone below the level of the injury
- Hypercoagulability associated with increased blood viscosity (if fluid intake is inadequate) and increased levels of calcium in the blood from bone demineralization (can result from prolonged immobility)

CLINICAL MANIFESTATIONS

Subjective	Objective
Verbal self-report of pain or tenderness in an extremity	Increase in circumference of extremity; distention of superficial vessels in extremity; unusual warmth of extremity

RISK FACTORS	DESIRED OUTCOME
• Impaired mobility	Client will not develop a deep vein thrombosis.

NURSING ASSESSMENT	RATIONALE
Assess for and report signs and symptoms of a deep vein thrombus: • Pain or tenderness in extremity • Increase in circumference of extremity • Distention of superficial vessels in extremity • Unusual warmth of extremity	*Early recognition of signs and symptoms of deep vein thrombus allows for prompt intervention.*

NOC OUTCOMES	NIC INTERVENTIONS
Immobility consequences: physiological; tissue perfusion: peripheral	Embolus precautions; embolus care: peripheral

THERAPEUTIC INTERVENTIONS	RATIONALE
Independent Actions Implement measures to maintain adequate blood flow in legs to reduce the risk for thrombus formation and prevent a pulmonary embolism (e.g., maintain adequate fluid intake, use of thromboembolic disorder [TED] hose, position firm pillow between client's legs if spasms tend to cause legs to cross; instruct client to obtain assistance to reposition legs properly, if they do cross).	*Adequate blood flow in the legs reduces the risk for thrombus formation and prevents a thromboembolus from occurring.*
If signs and symptoms of a deep vein thrombus occur: • Maintain client on strict bed rest in a semi- to high-Fowler's positions. • Do not exercise, or massage any extremity known to have a thrombus.	*Avoid putting pressure on the posterior knees because this action will compress the leg veins, increasing turbulent blood flow, and increasing the risk of thrombus formation. If a thrombus is suspected, elevate the affected extremity and do not massage the area because of the danger of dislodging the thrombus.*
• Caution client to avoid activities that create a Valsalva response (e.g., holding breath while moving up in bed).	*Valsalva response changes pressure in the chest cavity, which may dislodge a venous thrombus.*

NDx = NANDA Diagnosis **D** = Delegatable Action ● = UAP ✦ = LVN/LPN ⊜▶ = Go to ⊜volve for animation

Continued...

THERAPEUTIC INTERVENTIONS	RATIONALE

• Perform actions to prevent autonomic dysreflexia:
   • Perform measures to decrease incidence of a distended bladder and/or bowel.
   • Prevent pressure on any area of the client's body below the level of cord injury because this may lead to autonomic dysreflexia.
	A full bladder or bowel is a major precipitator of autonomic dysreflexia.
	 Autonomic dysreflexia changes systemic B/P and may dislodge a clot from a vessel wall.

Collaborative/Dependent Actions
 Implement measures to prevent deep vein thrombus formation:
 • Apply mechanical devices designed to increase venous return in the immobile patient:
   • Sequential compression devices
   • Thromboembolic (TED) stockings **D** ✦
 • Maintain a minimum fluid intake of 2500 mL/day (unless contraindicated). **D** ✦
	These sequential compression devices and TED stockings decrease venous stasis in the lower extremities and increase venous return through the deep leg veins, which are prone to the formation of a thrombus.
	 Adequate hydration helps reduces blood viscosity and decreases the incidence of deep vein thrombus.

If signs and symptoms of a deep vein thrombus occur: • Administer anticoagulants: • Low- or adjusted-dose heparin • Fondaparinux • Warfarin • Low-molecular-weight heparin • Prepare client for diagnostic studies (e.g., d-dimer venography, duplex ultrasound, impedance plethysmography). • Maintain oxygen therapy as ordered. **D** ✦	*Anticoagulants, if indicated, help suppress the formation of clots.* *Additional studies may be indicated to confirm the presence of a deep vein thrombus, so the appropriate interventions can be implemented.* *Supplemental oxygen helps maintain adequate tissue oxygenation.*

Nursing Diagnosis SEXUAL DYSFUNCTION NDx

Definition: A state in which an individual experiences a change in sexual function during the sexual response phases of desire, excitation, and/or orgasm, which is viewed as unsatisfying, unrewarding, or inadequate.

Related to:
• Decreased libido associated with:
• Loss of sensory and voluntary motor function below the level of spinal cord injury
• Presence of a urinary catheter and/or fear of urinary and bowel incontinence
• Depression, disturbed self-concept
• Fear of rejection by partner
• Fear of autonomic dysreflexia (genital stimulation can cause dysreflexia)
• Decreased ability to control and maintain an erection associated with loss of ability to have a psychogenic erection (only reflexogenic erection is possible)
• Altered ejaculatory flow associated with impaired nerve function in the bladder neck (can result in retrograde ejaculation)

CLINICAL MANIFESTATIONS

Subjective	Objective
Verbal self-report of sexual dysfunction; stated inability to achieve sexual satisfaction or feelings of being sexually unattractive	Limitations imposed by quadriplegia specific to sexual dysfunction

RISK FACTORS
• Fear
• Trauma
• Loss of control of body

DESIRED OUTCOMES

The client will demonstrate beginning acceptance of changes in sexual functioning as evidenced by:
a. Verbalization of a perception of self as sexually acceptable and adequate
b. Statements reflecting beginning adjustment to the effects of the spinal cord injury on sexual functioning
c. Maintenance of relationship with significant other

NOC OUTCOMES	NIC INTERVENTIONS
Sexual identity; sexual functioning	Sexual counseling; support group

NURSING ASSESSMENT	RATIONALE
Assess for signs and symptoms of sexual dysfunction (e.g., verbalization of sexual concerns or inability to achieve sexual satisfaction, alteration in relationship with significant other, limitations imposed by paraplegia/quadraplegia).	*Recognition that the spinal cord injury patient will experience sexual dysfunction will alert the nurse to assess for both physical and mental alterations.*

THERAPEUTIC INTERVENTIONS	RATIONALE

Independent Actions

Implement measures to promote an optimal level of sexual functioning:

- Facilitate communication between client and partner; focus on the feelings the couple share and assist them to identify changes that affect their sexual relationship.

    Communication between partners about how the physical changes will affect their sexual relationship is important.

- Discuss ways to be creative in expressing sexuality (e.g., massage, fantasies, cuddling).

    Client will require education on ways that he or she can express sexuality.

- Suggest alternative methods of sexual gratification and use of assistive devices if appropriate; encourage partner to explore erogenous areas on the client's lips, neck, and ears.

    Learning different ways of maintaining a sexual relationship will take time.

- Arrange for uninterrupted privacy if desired by the couple. **D** ✦

    Arranging time for couples to explore their sexual relationship fosters closeness between partners.

- Inform male client and his partner of techniques for eliciting and maintaining reflexogenic erection (e.g., stimulate genitalia, stroke inner thigh, pull on pubic hairs, stimulate the rectum, manipulate the urinary catheter).

    Sexual activity in clients with spinal cord injury requires different approaches and the possible use of assistive devices.

- If client has difficulty maintaining an erection, encourage him to discuss various treatment options (e.g., vacuum erection aids, penile prosthesis) with physician if desired.

- If client experiences episodes of autonomic dysreflexia, instruct client to consult physician about ways to prevent it during sexual activity (e.g., have partner apply a local anesthetic to client's genitalia).

    To decrease the incidence of autonomic dysreflexia during sex, the client should be instructed to have the partner apply a local anesthetic to client's genitalia.

- Inform female client that vaginal lubrication can occur by local stimulation or can be enhanced by using a water-soluble lubricant.

    Female clients may need to use a water-soluble lubricant.

- If incontinence of urine is a concern, instruct client to:
    - Limit fluid intake 2 to 4 hrs before sexual activity.
    - Have bladder emptied immediately before sexual activity.

    These actions limit urinary incontinence during sexual activity.

- Instruct client to perform bowel care several hours before sexual activity.

    This action reduces the risk of bowel incontinence if anal or rectal stimulation occurs during sexual activity.

- If appropriate, involve partner in care of client.

    Involvement of partner of client helps the partner adjust to the changes in the client's appearance and body functioning and subsequently decreases the possibility of partner's rejection of the client.

- Encourage client to rest before sexual activity.

    The client needs to conserve energy before sexual activity to avoid fatigue.

- Instruct client and partner to establish a relaxed, unhurried atmosphere for sexual activity.

    Providing an unhurried atmosphere for sexual activity allows the client and partner to explore what activities will provide sexual gratification including varying positions, use of explicit films and assist devices.

- Discuss positions that may facilitate sexual activity (e.g., lying on side, client in supine position).

- Provide explicit films and literature if desired by client and/or partner.

- Include partner in above discussions and encourage continued support of the client.

    Changes in the client's functioning has a great impact on the partner, and to improve chances of a positive sexual relationship, the partner should be included in discussions on sexual activity.

NDx = NANDA Diagnosis   **D** = Delegatable Action   ● = UAP   ✦ = LVN/LPN   ⊜▶ = Go to ⊜volve for animation

Continued...

THERAPEUTIC INTERVENTIONS	RATIONALE
Dependent/Collaborative Actions Consult appropriate health care provider (e.g., sex counselor, physician) when client is ready for sexual counseling and/or sexual counseling appears indicated.	*The expertise of a sexual counselor will provide a multidisciplinary approach to a client's sexual activity.*

Nursing Diagnosis   INTERRUPTED FAMILY PROCESSES NDx

Definition: Break in the continuity of family functioning which fails to support the well-being of its members.
Related to:
* Change in family roles and structure associated with a family member's sudden, catastrophic injury, permanent disability, and need for extensive rehabilitation

CLINICAL MANIFESTATIONS

Subjective	Objective
Verbal self-report of being unable to accept client's quadriplegia or paraplegia	Disruptive family interactions; inability to use coping strategies; refusal to participate in client's care

RISK FACTORS
* Situational crisis
* Situational transition

DESIRED OUTCOMES

The family members/significant others, will demonstrate beginning adjustment to changes in functioning of a family member and family roles and structure as evidenced by:
a. Meeting client's needs
b. Verbalization of ways to adapt to required role and lifestyle changes
c. Active participation in decision-making and client's rehabilitation
d. Positive interactions with one another

NOC OUTCOMES	NIC INTERVENTIONS
Family coping; family functioning; family resiliency; family normalization	Family involvement promotion; family integrity promotion; family process maintenance; family support; family mobilization

NURSING ASSESSMENT	RATIONALE
Assess for signs and symptoms of interrupted family processes (e.g., inability to meet client's needs, statements of not being able to accept client's quadriplegia or make necessary role and lifestyle changes, inability to make decisions, inability or refusal to participate in client's rehabilitation, negative family interactions). Identify components of the family and the patterns of communication and role expectations.	*Early recognition of signs and symptoms of interrupted family processes allows for prompt intervention.*

THERAPEUTIC INTERVENTIONS	RATIONALE
Independent Actions Implement measures to facilitate family members' adjustment to client's diagnosis, changes in client's functioning within the family system, and altered family roles and structure: • Encourage verbalization of feelings about the client's quadriplegia and its effect on family structure; actively listen to each family member and maintain a nonjudgmental attitude about feelings shared.	*Verbalization of feelings promotes communication and support for family members and may positively impact coping.*

THERAPEUTIC INTERVENTIONS	RATIONALE
• Reinforce physician's explanations of the effects of the injury and planned treatment and rehabilitation.	*Information helps the client's family understand what is happening and keeps them informed of the management of care.*
• Assist family members to gain a realistic perspective of client's situation, conveying as much hope as appropriate.	*Keep the family informed concerning what is occurring, answer questions as needed, assist in their understanding of a spinal cord injury while maintaining hope for the future.*
• Provide privacy for the client and family and stress the importance of and facilitate the use of good communication techniques.	*It is important that the client and family share feelings as they deal with the client's body changes.*
• Assist family members to progress through their own grieving process; explain that they may encounter times when they need to focus on meeting their own needs rather than the client's needs.	*The client's injury has a major impact on the life of the family, and family members will go through a grieving process. They need to be reassured as they work through the changes that have occurred in the family processes.*
• Emphasize the need for family members to obtain adequate rest and nutrition and to identify and use stress management techniques.	*Family members need to take care of themselves so that they are better able to emotionally and physically deal with the changes and losses experienced.*
• Encourage and assist family members to identify coping strategies for dealing with the client's body changes and the effects on the family.	*Reinforce family members' regular coping mechanisms and implement new techniques as needed.*
• Assist family members to identify realistic goals and ways of reaching those goals.	*The setting of realistic goals will help the family feel that they have some control over the situation and their ability to care for the client once discharged.*
• Include family members in decision-making about the client and care; convey appreciation for their input and continued support of client.	*Including the family in the care of the client and decision-making helps improve family members' confidence in their ability to care for the client.*
• Encourage and allow family members to participate in client's care and rehabilitation.	
• Assist family members in identifying resources that can assist them in coping with their feelings and meeting their immediate and long-term needs (e.g., counseling and social services; caregiver assistance programs; pastoral care; service, church, and spinal cord injury groups); initiate a referral if indicated.	*Community resources can provide mental support, respite care, and information that can help the family reach rehabilitation goals.*

Dependent/Collaborative Actions

Consult appropriate health care provider (e.g., psychiatric nurse clinician, physician) if family members continue to demonstrate difficulty adapting to changes in client's functioning and family structure.	*Consultation with other health care providers may increase the family members' success in adapting to changes in the client's functioning and in the family structure.*

Collaborative Diagnosis **RISK FOR ASCENDING SPINAL CORD INJURY**

Definition: Extension of damage from the original spinal cord injury that ascends up the spinal cord.

Related to: Further damage to and/or ischemia of the cord above the C5 level associated with vasospasm of damaged vessels, progressive edema, bleeding, compression of cord by hematoma or bone fragments, and/or ineffective immobilization of an unstable cord injury

CLINICAL MANIFESTATIONS

Subjective	Objective
Verbal self-report of shortness of breath	Increased dyspnea; shallow respirations; dusky or cyanotic skin color; drowsiness; confusion; decreased B/P and heart rate; progressive loss of sensory and motor function

RISK FACTORS
- Trauma
- Changes in hemodynamic status

DESIRED OUTCOMES

The client will not experience spinal cord injury above the level of C5 as evidenced by:
a. Stable respiratory status
b. Stable B/P and pulse
c. No further loss of motor and sensory function

NURSING ASSESSMENT

Assess for and report signs and symptoms of ascending spinal cord injury:
- Respiratory failure (e.g., rapid, shallow respirations; dusky or cyanotic skin color; drowsiness; confusion)
- Significant decrease in B/P and pulse
- Further loss of motor and sensory function

RATIONALE

Early recognition of signs and symptoms of ascending spinal cord injury allows for prompt intervention.

THERAPEUTIC INTERVENTIONS

Independent Actions

Implement measures to prevent spinal cord injury above the level of C5:
- Perform actions to maintain immobilization of the spine until stabilization has been accomplished:
  - Do not release or adjust skeletal traction or halo device unless ordered.

  - If skeletal traction is present, keep traction rope and weights hanging freely.
  - Always use turn sheet and adequate assistance when repositioning client.
  - Never use the rods of the halo device as handles. **D** ● ✦

  - Check pin sites of halo or traction device every shift; notify physician if pins are loose. **D** ✦
  - If immobilization device fails (e.g., pins fall out, traction weights drop, rods on halo device disconnect):
    1. Stabilize client's head, neck, and shoulders with hands, sandbags, or cervical collar.
    2. Notify physician immediately.

- Use the jaw thrust method rather than hyperextending client's neck if respiratory distress occurs.

Collaborative/Dependent Actions
- Perform actions to prevent ascending spinal cord ischemia:
  - Implement measures to maintain adequate tissue perfusion.
  - Prepare client for decompression of the spinal cord (e.g., removal of hematoma or bone fragments) if planned.
  - Prepare client for surgical stabilization (e.g., fusion) if planned.

- Administer corticosteroids and calcium channel blockers if ordered.
If signs and symptoms of ascending spinal cord injury occur, be prepared to assist with intubation or tracheostomy and mechanical ventilation.

RATIONALE

Appropriate healing should occur before changes/adjustments in traction occur, because the changes may extend the area of spinal cord injury.
If weights are not hanging freely, the level of traction changes and may further the spinal cord injury.
Use of a turn sheet helps maintain the spine in proper alignment when repositioning the client.
Use of rods on the halo device to move a client places undue stress on the spinal cord and may further spinal cord injury.
Changes in the tightness of the halo pins or traction devices may extend the area of spinal cord injury.
Stabilize the client's head, neck, and shoulders with any means possible to prevent further injury.

The physician must be notified to reestablish traction as soon as possible, thus preventing further injury.
Hyperextending the client's neck may extend the spinal cord injury.

Anything that alters spinal cord tissue perfusion may cause spinal cord ischemia.
Decreases pressure on the spinal cord and improves circulation.

Administration of high doses of methylprednisolone within the first 8 hrs after spinal cord injury appears to be the most effective way of slowing the development of ischemia above the level of injury.
Calcium channel blockers decrease vasospasms.

Ascending spinal cord injuries may compromise the client's neurological stimulation to the lungs. Emergency care may be necessary to prevent death.

Collaborative Diagnosis **RISK FOR PARALYTIC ILEUS**

Definition: Paralysis of the intestines resulting in blockage of the intestines.

Related to: Absence of neural stimulation of the intestine associated with absence of autonomic nervous system and reflex activity below the level of the spinal cord injury during period of spinal shock

CLINICAL MANIFESTATIONS

Subjective	Objective
Verbal self-report of persistent abdominal pain and cramping	Firm, distended abdomen; absent bowel sounds; failure to pass flatus; abdominal x-ray showing distended bowel

RISK FACTORS
- Inability to follow treatment regimen
- Lack of fiber and food in diet

DESIRED OUTCOMES

The client will not develop a paralytic ileus as evidenced by:
a. Absence or resolution of abdominal pain and cramping
b. Soft, nondistended abdomen
c. Gradual return of bowel sounds
d. Passage of flatus

NURSING ASSESSMENT

Assess for and report signs and symptoms of paralytic ileus:
- Development of or persistent abdominal pain and cramping
- Firm, distended abdomen
- Absent bowel sounds
- Failure to pass flatus
Monitor results of abdominal x-ray.

RATIONALE

Early recognition of signs and symptoms of a paralytic ileus allows prompt intervention.

An abdominal x-ray that demonstrates distended bowel and may be indicative of a paralytic ileus.

THERAPEUTIC INTERVENTIONS

Collaborative/Dependent Actions
If signs and symptoms of paralytic ileus occur:
- Withhold all oral intake.
- Insert nasogastric tube and maintain suction as ordered. **D** ✦
Perform actions to maintain adequate tissue perfusion:
- Administer GI stimulants (e.g., metoclopramide) if ordered. **D** ✦

RATIONALE

Paralytic ileus results in cessation of normal peristalsis. The client should have nothing by mouth (NPO) and have a nasogastric tube in place to facilitate gastric decompression until the ileus is resolved.

GI stimulants help maintain adequate blood supply to the bowel.

Collaborative Diagnosis **RISK FOR GASTROINTESTINAL BLEEDING**

Definition: Bleeding that occurs in the gastrointestinal (GI) tract.

Related to:
- Erosions of the gastric and duodenal mucosa (can develop as a result of the increased output of hydrochloric acid that occurs with stress)
- Irritation of the gastric mucosa associated with side effect of certain medications (e.g., corticosteroids)

CLINICAL MANIFESTATIONS

Subjective	**Objective**
Verbal self-report of shoulder pain, abdominal pain	Frank/occult blood in stool or gastric contents; decreased B/P, increased heart rate; decreasing RBC count, Hgb and Hct levels

RISK FACTORS

- Stress
- Anxiety
- Medication regimen

DESIRED OUTCOMES

The client will not experience GI bleeding, as evidenced by:
a. No reports of shoulder pain
b. Absence of frank and occult blood in stool and gastric contents
c. B/P and pulse within normal range for client
d. RBC count, Hct and Hgb levels within normal range

NURSING ASSESSMENT	**RATIONALE**
Assess for and report signs and symptoms of GI bleeding (e.g., reports of shoulder pain [referred]; frank or occult blood in stool or gastric contents; decreased B/P; increased pulse rate; decreasing RBC count, Hct and Hgb levels).	*Early recognition of signs and symptoms of GI bleeding allows for prompt intervention.*

THERAPEUTIC INTERVENTIONS	**RATIONALE**

Independent Actions

Implement measures to prevent ulceration of the gastric and duodenal mucosa:

- Perform actions to decrease fear and anxiety (e.g., introduce client to staff, place call bell within client's hand, answer call promptly).

  These actions decrease fear, anxiety, and stress, thus decreasing the release of endogenous steroids.

- Instruct client to avoid acidic foods/fluids that stimulate hydrochloric acid secretions or irritate the gastric mucosa (e.g., coffee, caffeine-containing tea and colas; spices such as black pepper, chili powder, and nutmeg).

  Acidic foods/fluids increase acidity in the GI tract and risk for GI bleeding.

Dependent/Collaborative Actions

Implement measures to prevent ulceration of the gastric and duodenal mucosa:

- Administer histamine$_2$-receptor antagonists, proton-pump inhibitors, antacids, and/or cytoprotective agents, if ordered.

  Histamine receptor antagonists and proton-pump inhibitors suppress secretion of gastric acid. Antacids neutralize stomach acid and cytoprotective agents create a protective barrier against stomach acid and pepsin.

If signs and symptoms of GI bleeding occur:

- Insert nasogastric tube and maintain suction as ordered.

  Insertion of an NG tube to facilitate suction removes gastric acid and pressure on the gastric lining.

- Administer blood products and/or volume expanders if ordered.

  Hypotension may occur; administration of blood and/or volume expanders may be needed to maintain adequate blood pressure and tissue perfusion.

- Assist with measures to control bleeding (e.g., gastric lavage, endoscopic electrocoagulation) if planned.

  These interventions decrease or stops GI bleeding.

DISCHARGE TEACHING/CONTINUED CARE

Nursing Diagnosis # DEFICIENT KNOWLEDGE NDx; INEFFECTIVE FAMILY HEALTH MANAGEMENT NDx; OR INEFFECTIVE HEALTH MAINTENANCE*,†
NDx

Definition: **Deficient Knowledge NDx:** Absence of cognitive information related to a specific topic, or its acquisition; **Ineffective Family Health Management NDx:** A pattern of regulating and integrating into family processes a program for the treatment of illness and its sequelae that is unsatisfactory for meeting specific health goals of the family unit; **Ineffective Health Maintenance NDx:** Inability to identify, manage, and/or seek out help maintain well-being.

CLINICAL MANIFESTATIONS

Subjective	Objective
Verbal self-report of inability to manage illness; verbalizes inability to follow prescribed regimen	Inaccurate follow-through with instructions; inappropriate behaviors; experience of preventable complications of spinal cord injury

RISK FACTORS
- Cognitive deficit
- Financial concerns
- Failure to take action to reduce risk factors for complications of spinal cord injury

- Inability to care for oneself
- Difficulty in modifying personal habits and integrating treatments into lifestyle

NOC OUTCOMES

Knowledge: treatment regimen; health behavior; health resources; treatment procedure(s)

NIC INTERVENTIONS

Teaching: individual; teaching: prescribed exercise; teaching: psychomotor skills; health system guidance; financial resource assistance; support system enhancement

NURSING ASSESSMENT

Assess the client's ability to learn and readiness to learn. Assess the client's understanding of teaching.

RATIONALE

Learning is more effective when the client is motivated and understands the importance of what is to be learned. Readiness to learn changes based on situations, physical and emotional challenges.

THERAPEUTIC INTERVENTIONS

Desired Outcome: The client will identify ways to prevent complications associated with spinal cord injury and decreased mobility.

RATIONALE

Independent Actions
Instruct client in ways to prevent complications associated with spinal cord injury:
- Position firm pillow between legs if spasms tend to cause legs to cross.
- Wear an abdominal binder when changing from a reclining to a sitting position and take vasoconstrictor drugs if prescribed to prevent dizziness and fainting.
- Elevate legs periodically during the day.

Use of firm pillows between legs helps prevent thrombus formation and adduction contractures.
An abdominal binder supports the abdominal muscles and helps prevent injury.

Elevation of the legs prevents blood from pooling in the lower extremities and decreases the incidence of orthostatic hypotension.

*The nurse should select the diagnostic label that is most appropriate for the client's discharge teaching needs.
†Although the client will not be able to perform many of the following actions independently, he/she must be knowledgeable about them in order to provide proper instruction to significant others and attendant and maintain an active role in the rehabilitation process.

NDx = NANDA Diagnosis   **D** = Delegatable Action   ● = UAP   ✦ = LVN/LPN   ◉▶ = Go to ℮volve for animation

Continued...

THERAPEUTIC INTERVENTIONS	RATIONALE
• Implement measures to reduce severe spasticity (e.g., avoid fatigue and chills, change position at least every 2 hrs, take muscle relaxants as prescribed).	*These actions improve mobility and prevent contractures.*
• Use full-length and long-handled mirrors to examine all skin surfaces in the morning and the evening; increase pressure relief measures if any areas of redness or pallor develop.	*Daily skin assessment helps identify pressure areas to prevent skin breakdown.*
• Obtain a kinetic bed for home use if possible.	*Use of a kinetic bed helps prevent skin breakdown.*
• Wear shoes when in wheelchair.	*Wearing shoes helps prevents injury to feet.*
• Avoid putting items such as coins, keys, and wallet in skirt or pant pockets.	*These items can cause pressure on underlying skin areas when placed in skirt or pants pockets.*
• Avoid wearing tight-fitting belts, clothing, shoes, and jewelry; make sure that urine collection leg bag straps are not too tight.	*These actions assure that there is no unnecessary pressure on the skin that may lead to skin breakdown.*
• Replace wheelchair cushions when they become worn-out.	
• Implement measures to prevent hyperthermia (e.g., avoid excessive clothing and bedding, limit length of time in direct sunlight in hot weather, wear a wide-brimmed hat when in direct sun, park your car or van in the shade in hot weather and open the doors to let the vehicle cool down before getting inside).	*The client is unable to maintain body temperature. These interventions help prevent hyperthermia injuries.*
• Implement measures to prevent hypothermia (e.g., wear adequate amounts of clothing, wear a hat when in a cold environment, drink warm liquids).	*These actions help the client maintain appropriate body temperature.*
• Implement measures to prevent falls (e.g., always use safety belt during transfers and when in chair, be certain to have adequate assistance for transfer activity).	*These interventions help prevent client injuries.*
• Implement measures to prevent burns:	*These actions help prevent hyperthermia injuries.*
• Always check temperature of shower or bath water before use (can use bath water thermometer or have attendant check water temperature).	
• Never smoke when alone; do not place ashtray in lap.	
• Let hot foods/fluids cool slightly before attempting to feed self.	
• Never position self next to a stove, heater, or other major source of heat; be aware of where feet and legs are in relation to car heater when it is on.	
• Never use an electric heating pad or electric blanket.	
• Implement measures to prevent autonomic dysreflexia:	*Autonomic dysreflexia is a life-threatening emergency requiring immediate treatment. These actions help prevent autonomic dysreflexia. Bladder and bowel distention are the primary causes of dysreflexia and should be prevented.*
• Continue with effective bladder and bowel programs to prevent urinary retention and constipation/impaction.	
• Change position frequently.	
• Seek medical attention at first sign of infection, persistent pressure area, or ingrown toenail.	
• Apply a local anesthetic (e.g., Nupercainal ointment) to area being stimulated before procedures/activities that have previously resulted in episodes of autonomic dysreflexia (e.g., urinary catheterization, administration of an enema, sexual activity).	

THERAPEUTIC INTERVENTIONS	RATIONALE
Demonstrate the following procedures to client, significant others, and attendant: • Assisted coughing technique (quad-cough) • Heimlich maneuver • Skin care • Proper positioning and padding • Transfer techniques • Active and passive range-of-motion exercises • Application of elastic stockings, abdominal binder, and heel and elbow protectors • Emergency treatment of autonomic dysreflexia (e.g., elevate head of bed and lower client's legs, alleviate causative factor, administer an antihypertensive agent) Allow time for questions, clarification, and return demonstration.	*The client's family members should provide a return demonstration on client care and prevention of injuries so that they are able to perform these correctly and may help the client maintain functional status.*

THERAPEUTIC INTERVENTIONS	RATIONALE

Desired Outcome: The client will demonstrate the ability to correctly use and maintain assistive devices.

Independent Actions

Reinforce instructions from physical and occupational therapists regarding use of assistive devices. Allow time for questions, clarification, and return demonstration.	*Clarification of information and understanding of how to improve health status.*
Instruct and demonstrate for client proper maintenance of assistive devices (e.g., replace parts that are worn out or broken, clean wheel hubs and crossbars of wheelchairs per manufacturer's instructions, keep wheelchair tires properly inflated).	*Assist devices need to be kept in good working order to prevent client injury and help the client maintain independence and self-care.*

THERAPEUTIC INTERVENTIONS	RATIONALE

Desired Outcome: The client will identify ways to manage altered bowel and bladder function.

Independent Actions

Reinforce bladder and bowel training programs.	*Proper bladder and bowel elimination are important in preventing autonomic dysreflexia and other possible complications.*
Demonstrate bowel care (e.g., digital stimulation, insertion of suppositories, administration of enemas) and bladder care (e.g., stimulation techniques, intermittent catheterization, application of leg bag and bedside drainage bag, emptying of urinary collection bag). Allow time for questions, clarification, and return demonstration.	

THERAPEUTIC INTERVENTIONS	RATIONALE

Desired Outcome: The client will state signs and symptoms to report to the health care provider.

Independent Actions

• Instruct the client to report the following:
  • Cloudy or foul-smelling urine
  • Nausea and vomiting
  • Cough productive of purulent, green, or rust-colored sputum
	Client and significant others should be instructed on the clinical manifestations of infections and other changes in health status, and to inform their health care practitioner to prevent further injury or decline in health status.

Continued...

THERAPEUTIC INTERVENTIONS	**RATIONALE**

- Difficulty breathing or increased shortness of breath with activity
- Sudden or persistent shoulder pain (this can be a referred pain)
- Fever
- Chills or profuse sweating (can occur above the level of the injury)
- Increase in spasticity (could indicate an infection below the level of the injury)
- Unsuccessful bowel and/or bladder programs
- Redness in any extremity
- Swelling that appears suddenly, occurs only in one extremity, or does not subside overnight
- Increased restriction of any joint motion
- Persistent swelling over a joint
- Signs and symptoms of autonomic dysreflexia (e.g., pounding headache, sudden rise in B/P, blurred vision, slow pulse, flushing and sweating above level of injury, nasal congestion) that do not subside once the stimulus is removed
- Any area of persistent skin irritation or breakdown
- Indications of pregnancy (stress that appropriate prenatal care should be initiated as soon as possible)

THERAPEUTIC INTERVENTIONS	**RATIONALE**

Desired Outcome: The client will identify resources that can assist with financial needs, home management, and adjustment to changes resulting from spinal cord injury.

Independent Actions

Inform client and significant others about resources that can assist with financial needs, home management, and adjustment to changes resulting from spinal cord injury (e.g., spinal cord injury support and social groups; state and federally funded financial programs; home health agencies; community health agencies; local service groups; financial, individual, family, and vocational counselors).	*Community resources may provide the client and family with multiple levels of assistance (e.g., financial, social support, counseling).*
Initiate a social service referral if indicated.	*A referral may be required for the client and family to access community resources.*

THERAPEUTIC INTERVENTIONS	**RATIONALE**

Desired Outcome: The client, in collaboration with the nurse, will develop a plan for adhering to recommended follow-up care including future appointments with health care provider and occupational and physical therapists, and medications prescribed.

Independent Actions

Reinforce the importance of keeping scheduled follow-up visits with health care provider, occupational and physical therapists.	*The client requires life-long care and follow-up appointments help maintain health status.*
Explain the rationale for, side effects of, drug-to-drug and drug-to-food interactions, and importance of taking medications as prescribed.	*Knowledge of the medication regimen and the impact of these medications on the system, as well as how the medication regimen can be incorporated into the client's lifestyle, allows the client some mechanism of control of his/her disease and the ability to have an active part in treatment and care.*

THERAPEUTIC INTERVENTIONS	**RATIONALE**

Implement measures designed to improve client adherence:
- Include significant others and caregivers in teaching sessions.
- Encourage questions and allow time for reinforcement and clarification of information provided.

An informed client and family are better able to adhere to a treatment regimen.

- Provide written instructions on scheduled appointments with health care provider and occupational and physical therapists, medications prescribed, and signs and symptoms to report.

Understanding the impact of medications on the individual will allow the client to recognize changes and inform his/her health care practitioner as needed.

ADDITIONAL NURSING DIAGNOSES

FEAR AND ANXIETY NDx
Related to:
- Extensive loss of motor and sensory function
- Application of immobilization device to stabilize and align the cervical spine
- Lack of understanding of diagnostic tests, diagnosis, and treatment
- Unfamiliar environment
- Financial concerns
- Anticipated effects of the spinal cord injury on lifestyle and roles

ACUTE/CHRONIC PAIN NDx
- Headache related to contractures of the neck muscles (can occur in response to stress and/or neck pain)
- Neck pain related to nerve root irritation at the site of spinal cord injury, muscle stiffness while immobilization device is in place, and muscle strain associated with increased use of neck muscles after removal of immobilization device
- Upper arm and shoulder pain related to muscle strain associated with increased use of biceps and shoulders as activity progresses

IMBALANCED NUTRITION: LESS THAN BODY REQUIREMENTS NDx
Related to:
- Decreased oral intake associated with:
  - Dietary restrictions during period of spinal shock if paralytic ileus develops
  - Anorexia resulting from fatigue, depression and social isolation, the effect of negative nitrogen balance, and early satiety that occurs with decreased GI motility
  - Difficulty swallowing resulting from neck hyperextension and/or horizontal body position during the time that the cervical spine is immobilized
  - Difficulty feeding self
- Increased nutritional needs associated with an imbalance in the rate of catabolism and anabolism (Catabolic processes occur at a faster rate than anabolic processes in persons who have sustained a spinal cord injury and in those who are immobile.)

RISK FOR ASPIRATION NDx
Related to:
- Decreased ability to clear tracheobronchial passages associated with inability to cough forcefully resulting from weakness of the diaphragm and paralysis of the abdominal and intercostal muscles
- Difficulty swallowing associated with neck hyperextension and/or horizontal body positioning during the time that the cervical spine is immobilized

RISK FOR POWERLESSNESS NDx
Related to:
- Quadriplegia
- Dependence on others
- Changes in roles, relationships, and future plans

GRIEVING NDx
Related to extensive loss of motor and sensory function and the effects of this loss on future lifestyle and roles

RISK FOR LONELINESS NDx
Related to inability to participate in usual activities, decreased contact with significant others and friends while in the hospital and extended care or rehabilitation facility, depression, and withdrawal from others

IMPAIRED URINARY ELIMINATION NDx
Retention related to:
- Atony of bladder wall during period of spinal shock
- Spasticity of the external urinary sphincter and/or loss of ability to coordinate bladder contraction and relaxation of the external urinary sphincter after period of spinal shock
- Incomplete bladder emptying associated with horizontal positioning (in this position, the gravity needed for complete bladder emptying is lost)
Incontinence related to:
- Spasticity of the bladder after period of spinal shock and loss of ability to contract the external urinary sphincter voluntarily (incontinence can occur if the bladder contracts strongly when the external urinary sphincter is relaxed)
- Inadvertent stimulation of the voiding reflex

RISK FOR CONSTIPATION NDx
Related to:
- Decreased GI motility associated with:
  - Loss of autonomic nervous system function below the level of the injury during period of spinal shock
  - Decreased activity
- Lack of awareness of stool in rectum associated with sensory loss below the level of the injury
- Loss of central nervous system control over defecation reflex
- Decreased gravity filling of lower rectum associated with horizontal positioning
- Decreased intake of fluids and foods high in fiber

RISK FOR INFECTION NDx
- Pneumonia related to:
  - Stasis of secretions associated with decreased activity and decreased ability to clear tracheobronchial passages (Client is unable to cough forcefully as a result of weakness of the diaphragm and paralysis of the abdominal and intercostal muscles.)
  - Aspiration of foods/fluids (impaired swallowing can occur as a result of neck hyperextension and/or horizontal body positioning during the time that the cervical spine is immobilized)
- Urinary tract infection related to:
  - Growth and colonization of pathogens associated with urinary stasis
  - Introduction of pathogens associated with presence of an indwelling catheter and/or performance of intermittent catheterizations

- Skull pin site infection related to introduction of pathogens during or after insertion of skull pins

DISTURBED BODY IMAGE
Related to:
- Dependence on others to meet self-care needs
- Feelings of powerlessness
- Change in appearance associated with temporary presence of devices to immobilize the spine, necessity of wheelchair use, and spasticity after period of spinal shock
- Infertility (in males) associated with:
  - Possibility of retrograde ejaculation (can result from impaired nerve function in the bladder neck)
  - Decreased sperm formation and viability resulting from testicular atrophy and impaired temperature regulation in the testes
- Changes in body functioning, lifestyle, and roles

INEFFECTIVE COPING NDx
Related to:
- Depression, fear, anxiety, feelings of powerlessness, and ongoing grieving associated with spinal cord injury and its effects on body functioning, lifestyle, and roles
- Dependence on others to meet basic needs
- Lack of personal resources to deal with spinal cord injury and its effects
- Need for extensive rehabilitation

PARKINSON DISEASE

Parkinson disease (PD) is a neurodegenerative disease that leads to impairment of an individual's motor functioning. PD affects approximately 1 million individuals in the United States and 10 million worldwide. An estimated 4% of individuals with Parkinson disease are diagnosed before the age of 50 with the rate of newly diagnosed cases increasing with age. The prevalence of the disease ranges from 41 per 100,000 people in the 4th decade of life to more than 1,900 per 100,000 among those 80 years of age and older. PD is slightly more prevalent in whites than other ethnic groups, with men 1½ times more likely than women to have the disease. While the exact cause of PD is unknown, experts agree that the condition results from a combination of both genetic and environmental factors. Genetic risk factors include autosomal dominant genes (e.g., ANCA and LRRK2), autosomal recessive genes (e.g., PARK7, PINK1, PRKN), and risk factor modifier genes (e.g., GBA). Identified environmental risk factors include age (>60 years of age), gender (greater in men), chemicals from occupational exposure (e.g., farming, military), and head injury/traumatic brain injury.

The symptoms of PD develop from an imbalance of acetylcholine and dopamine in the brain. Injury to the dopamine-producing neurons in the substantia nigra and the basal ganglia lead to loss of dopamine. In normal movement, there is a balance between dopamine, an inhibitory neurotransmitter, and acetylcholine, an excitatory neurotransmitter. When this balance is lost, the individual with PD experiences the classic clinical manifestations of tremors, rigidity, akinesia or

bradykinesia, and postural changes. During the early stage of PD, these manifestations may develop alone or in combination; however, as the disease progresses, all of these manifestations are usually present. PD has an insidious onset that makes the diagnosis of the disease difficult until more pronounced symptoms appear. Other clinical manifestations seen as the disease progresses include shuffling gait; postural changes; loss of facial expressions; slurred speech; difficulty writing, eating, chewing, and swallowing; drooling; gastric retention; constipation; orthostatic hypotension; and urinary retention. Depression is often seen in individuals with PD.

While there is no definitive diagnostic test for PD, various symptoms and diagnostic tests can be used in combination. Researchers have identified lower levels of a protein-neurofilament light chain protein (NfL) in people with the disease and in healthy individuals versus people with other parkinsonian disorders. To consider a PD diagnosis, two of the four main symptoms must be present over a period of time: shaking or tremor, slowness of movement (bradykinesia), stiffness or rigidity of the arms or legs, and/or trouble with balance and possible falls (postural instability). Significant improvement in response to medication therapy confirms a diagnosis of PD.

There is no cure for PD. The standard treatment focuses on correcting the imbalance of neurotransmitters with medication. The medications approved for treatment of PD focus on improving the release of dopamine or blocking the effects of acetylcholine. The categories of medications used in PD are anticholinergics, dopamine precursors, dopamine agonists, monoamine oxidase B (MAO-B) inhibitors, and catechol-O-methyltransferase inhibitors. Additional treatment may include exercise to maintain the client's health status as long as possible. Specific exercises may be prescribed to maintain muscle tone, decrease rigidity, and improve the ability to swallow and speak. Clients with advanced PD or with unstable responses to medication, deep brain stimulation may be offered, which may stabilize medication fluctuations, reduce or halt involuntary movements, reduce tremor, reduce rigidity, and improve slowing of movements. Even with treatment, the disease is progressive, and ultimately clients will lose the ability to care for themselves.

This care plan focuses on the adult client hospitalized with signs and symptoms of PD. Much of the information is also applicable to clients receiving follow-up care in an extended care or rehabilitation facility or home setting.

OUTCOME/DISCHARGE CRITERIA

The client will:
1. Participate in activities of daily living
2. Engage in a regular exercise program to maintain strength
3. Maintain optimal nutritional status to meet caloric needs
4. Understand medication regimen
5. Develop a plan of care for adhering to recommended follow-up care

---

Nursing Diagnosis | **IMPAIRED PHYSICAL MOBILITY** NDx

Definition: Limitation in independent, purposeful physical movement of the body or of one or more extremities.

Related to: Physiological changes associated with Parkinson disease

CLINICAL MANIFESTATIONS

Subjective	Objective
Verbal self-report of pain; discomfort; fatigue	Decreased reaction time; rigidity of muscles with movement; tremors of upper extremities; limited ability to perform gross and fine motor skills; limited range of motion; intentional movement–induced tremor; postural instability; uncoordinated movements

RISK FACTORS

- Lack of motivation
- Weakness
- Depression

DESIRED OUTCOMES

The client will improve mobility as evidenced by:
a. Increased physical activity
b. Movement of affected limb or limbs
c. Participation in activities of daily living
d. Demonstration of appropriate use of assistive devices to improve movement

NOC OUTCOMES

Activity tolerance; fall prevention behavior; endurance

NIC INTERVENTIONS

Ambulation; joint mobility; fall precautions; exercise therapy

NURSING ASSESSMENT	**RATIONALE**
Assess client's movement ability and activity tolerance. Use a tool such as the Assessment Tool for Safe Patient Handling and Movement or the FIM.	*Assessment of mobility is used to best determine how to facilitate movement. Assessment of activity tolerance provides a baseline for patient strength and endurance with movement.*
Assess for hallmark signs of PD:	
• Tremors	*Tremors are more prominent at rest or during emotional stress. Tremors are due to a central nervous system imbalance between acetylcholine and dopamine.*
• Changes in handwriting, "pill-rolling," shaking of the head	
• Rigidity	
• Jerky quality of movement with passive range of motion	*May be observed unilaterally or bilaterally.*
• Bradykinesia	
• Decreased movement in blinking of eyelids, decreased movement of the arms while ambulating, difficulty with swallowing saliva, decreased facial expressions and movements of the hands, changes in posture	

Continued...

NURSING ASSESSMENT	RATIONALE
Assess emotional response to immobility.	Determine client's acceptance of limitations. This impacts implementation of therapeutic interventions.
Assess need for assistive devices.	Determine client's needs for assistive devices as well as proper use of wheelchairs, walkers, cane, and so on to reduce incidence of falls.

THERAPEUTIC INTERVENTIONS	RATIONALE

Independent Actions

Encourage and implement strength-training activities:
- Active and/or passive range of motion
- Ambulation
- Activities of daily living **D** ● ✦

Inactivity contributes to muscle weakening. Regular exercise decreases muscle rigidity and contractures while maintaining joint mobility and physical strength.

Use assistive devices to help client with movement:
- Crutches
- Gait belt
- Walker **D** ● ✦

Assistive devices help caregivers decrease the potential for falls and/or injuries.

Cluster treatments and care activities to allow for uninterrupted periods of rest. **D** ● ✦

Adequate rest increases client's tolerance and strength for activities.

Encourage patient with positive reinforcement during activities. **D** ● ✦

A positive approach to activities supports the client's accomplishment and engagement in new activities, and improves self-esteem.

Implement falls protocol.
- Maintain the bed in low position and keep side rails up. **D** ● ✦

These actions help prevent client falls.

Use sequential compression devices or antiembolic stockings. **D** ● ✦

These devices improve venous circulation and help prevent the development of thrombophlebitis in lower extremities.

Implement measures to maintain healthy, intact skin (e.g., keep skin lubricated, clean, and dry; instruct or assist client to turn every 2 hrs; keep bed linens dry and wrinkle-free). **D** ● ✦

These actions help client maintain healthy, intact skin and reduce the risk of pressure sores and infection.

Maintain an optimal nutritional status:
- Increase protein intake.
- Increase fluid intake to 2000 to 3000 mL/day unless contraindicated.

Adequate nutrition is needed to maintain adequate energy level.

Increased fluid intake maintains adequate hydration and helps prevent constipation and hardening of the stool.

Encourage coughing and deep breathing exercises and use of incentive spirometry.

Prevents buildup of secretions and promotes lung expansion.

Dependent/Collaborative Actions

Consult appropriate health care provider:
- Dietitian and physician and occupational therapists

These individuals provide specific activities and exercise programs to improve strength and mobility.

- Administer pain medications before activities.

Pain medications reduce muscle stiffness and tension, allowing the client to participate in activities.

Nursing Diagnosis **IMBALANCED NUTRITION: LESS THAN BODY REQUIREMENTS** NDx

Definition: Intake of nutrients insufficient to meet metabolic needs.

Related to:
- Decreased oral intake associated with anorexia and nausea
- Loss of nutrients associated with vomiting if present
- Difficulty in swallowing

CLINICAL MANIFESTATIONS

Subjective	objective
Verbal self-report of lack of appetite; fatigue; difficulty swallowing	Choking episodes; vomiting of food or fluids through the nares; loss of weight with adequate food intake; body weight 20% or more under ideal weight; capillary fragility; pale conjunctiva and mucous membranes; constipation; poor muscle tone; increased blood urea nitrogen (BUN) and serum creatinine levels; decreased serum albumin and preal-bumin levels; decreased Hct and Hgb levels, and WBC count

RISK FACTORS
* Lack of appetite
* Fatigue
* Depression

NOC OUTCOMES

Appetite; body image; bowel elimination; compliance behavior: prescribed diet; hydration; weight maintenance behavior

NIC INTERVENTIONS

Nutritional monitoring; nutritional counseling; nutritional management; aspiration precautions; weight management

NURSING ASSESSMENT	RATIONALE
Assess for and report signs and symptoms of malnutrition:	*Early recognition and reporting of signs and symptoms of malnutrition allows for prompt intervention.*
• Weight significantly below client's usual weight or below normal for client's age, height, and body frame	
• Decreased BUN and serum albumin, prealbumin, Hct, Hgb, and lymphocyte levels	
• Weakness and fatigue	
• Sore, inflamed oral mucous membrane	
• Pale conjunctiva	
Assess for physical difficulty with eating:	*Physical changes resulting from PD can lead to malnutrition.*
• Difficulty swallowing	
• Decreased gag reflex	
• Choking episodes	
• Vomiting from nares	
Monitor percentage of meals and snacks client consumes. Report a pattern of inadequate intake.	*An awareness of the amount of foods/fluids the client consumes alerts the nurse to deficits in nutritional intake. Reporting an inadequate intake allows for prompt intervention.*
Perform or assist with anthropometric measurements such as skinfold thickness, body circumferences (e.g., hip, waist, mid-upper arm), and bioelectrical impedance analysis if indicated. Report results that are lower than normal.	*Anthropometric measurements provide information about the amount of muscle mass, body fat, and protein reserves the client has. These assessments assist in evaluating the client's nutritional status.*

THERAPEUTIC INTERVENTIONS	RATIONALE
Independent Actions	
Implement measures to prevent choking and/or vomiting (e.g., eliminate noxious sites and odors). **D** ● ✦	*Choking and vomiting result in actual loss of nutrients.*
Implement measures to improve oral intake:	
• Perform actions to reduce nausea, pain, fear, and anxiety if present. **D** ● ✦	*Nausea, pain, fear, and anxiety all decrease client's appetite and oral intake.*
• Perform actions to relieve GI distention if present (e.g., encourage and assist client with frequent ambulation unless contraindicated). **D** ● ✦	*Distention of the GI tract (especially the stomach and duodenum) can result in stimulation of the satiety center and subsequent inhibition of the feeding center in the hypothalamus. This effect, along with the discomfort that occurs with distention, decreases appetite.*

Continued...

THERAPEUTIC INTERVENTIONS	RATIONALE
• Increase activity as allowed and tolerated. **D** ● ✦	*Activity usually promotes a general feeling of well-being, which can result in improved appetite.*
• Maintain a clean environment and a relaxed, pleasant atmosphere. **D** ● ✦	*Noxious sites and odors can inhibit the feeding center in the hypothalamus. Maintaining a clean environment helps prevent this from occurring. In addition, maintaining a relaxed, pleasant atmosphere can help reduce the client's stress and promote a feeling of well-being, which tends to improve appetite and oral intake.*
• Encourage a rest period before meals if indicated. **D** ● ✦ ✦	*The physical activity of eating requires some expenditure of energy. Fatigue can reduce the client's desire and ability to eat.*
• Provide oral hygiene before meals. **D** ●	*Oral hygiene moistens the oral mucous membrane, which may make it easier to chew and swallow. It freshens the mouth and removes unpleasant tastes. This can improve the taste of foods/fluids, which helps stimulate appetite and increase oral intake.*
• Serve foods/fluids that are appealing to the client and adhere to personal and cultural (e.g., religious, ethnic) preferences whenever possible. **D** ● ✦	*Foods/fluids that appeal to the client's senses (especially sight and smell) and are in accordance with personal and cultural preferences are most likely to stimulate appetite and promote interest in eating.*
• Serve frequent, small meals rather than large ones if client is weak, fatigues easily, and/or has a poor appetite. **D** ● ✦	*Providing small rather than large meals can enable a client who is weak or fatigues easily to finish a meal. A client who has a poor appetite is often more willing to attempt to eat smaller meals because they seem less overwhelming than larger ones. If smaller meals are served, the number of meals per day should be increased to help ensure adequate nutrition.*
• Encourage significant others to bring in client's favorite foods unless contraindicated and eat with him/her if client desires.	*A client's favorite foods/fluids tend to stimulate his/her appetite more than institutional foods/fluids. The presence of significant others during meals helps create a familiar social environment that can stimulate appetite and improve oral intake. In addition, relieving dyspnea decreases the client's anxiety about and preoccupation with breathing efforts and increases the ability to focus on eating and drinking.*
• Place client in a high-Fowler's positions for eating and drinking.	*Placing client in a high-Fowler's positions to eat reduces the risk for aspiration.*
• Provide foods that can be easily chewed and provide thickened liquids.	*These actions improve the client's ability to swallow foods and decrease incidence of choking and potential for aspiration.*
• Allow adequate time for meals; reheat foods/fluids if necessary. **D** ● ✦	*A client who feels rushed during meals tends to become anxious, lose his/her appetite, stop eating, and possibly choke.*
• Limit fluid intake with meals unless the fluid has a high nutritional value. **D** ● ✦	*When the stomach becomes distended, its volume receptors stimulate the satiety center in the hypothalamus and the clients reduces his/her oral intake. Drinking liquids with meals distends the stomach and may cause satiety before an adequate amount of food is consumed.*
• Ensure that meals are well balanced and high in essential nutrients.	*The client must consume a diet that is well balanced and high in essential nutrients in order to meet his/her nutritional needs. Dietary supplements are often needed to help accomplish this.*
• Allow the client to assist in the selection of foods/fluids that meet nutritional needs.	*The client who is actively involved in menu planning is more likely to adhere to the diet plan. Involvement in meal selection increases the client's sense of control, which promotes a feeling of well-being and can lead to an increased oral intake.*

Dependent/Collaborative Actions
Implement measures to improve oral intake and nutritional status:

• Administer medications that may be ordered to improve client's nutritional status (e.g., antiemetics, antidiarrheals, GI stimulants, and vitamins and minerals). **D** ✦	*Medications such as antiemetic, antidiarrheals, and GI stimulants may relieve vomiting, diarrhea, and distention of the GI tract, which decreases the discomfort that occurs with each of these signs and symptoms. Vitamins and minerals are needed to maintain metabolic functioning. If the client's dietary intake does not provide adequate amounts of them, oral and/or parenteral supplements may be necessary.*

THERAPEUTIC INTERVENTIONS	RATIONALE
• Obtain a dietary consult if necessary.	*A dietitian is best able to evaluate whether the foods/fluids selected will meet the client's nutritional needs.*
• Obtain a speech therapy consult.	*Speech therapists can work with the client to improve his/her ability to swallow.*
• Perform a calorie count if ordered. Report information to the dietitian and physician.	*A calorie count provides information about the caloric and nutritional value of the foods/fluids the client consumes. The information obtained helps the dietitian and physician determine whether an alternative method of nutritional support is needed.*
• Consult the physician about an alternative method of providing nutrition (e.g., parenteral nutrition, tube feeding) if client does not consume enough food or fluids to meet nutritional needs.	*If the client's oral intake is inadequate, an alternative method of providing nutrients needs to be implemented.*

Nursing Diagnosis RISK FOR ASPIRATION NDx

Definition: Susceptible to entry of gastrointestinal secretions, oropharyngeal secretions, solids, or fluids to the tracheobronchial passages, which may compromise health.

Related to:
• Impaired swallowing
• Decreased gag reflex
• Decreased facial muscle tone

CLINICAL MANIFESTATIONS

Subjective	Objective
N/A	Cough; tachypnea; dyspnea; tachycardia; dull percussion noted over affected lung area; presence of foods in aspirate

RISK FACTORS	DESIRED OUTCOMES
• Weakness • Eating too fast	The client will not aspirate secretions or foods/fluids as evidenced by: a. Clear breath sounds b. Resonant percussion over lungs c. Absence of cough, tachypnea, and dyspnea

NOC OUTCOMES	NIC INTERVENTIONS
Risk control: aspiration; body positioning: self-initiated; GI function; nausea and vomiting control; respiratory status; swallowing status	Aspiration precautions; respiratory monitoring; swallowing therapy; airway suctioning

NURSING ASSESSMENT	RATIONALE
Assess for and report signs and symptoms of aspiration of secretions or foods/fluids: • Rhonchi • Dull percussion note over affected lung area • Cough • Tachypnea • Dyspnea • Tachycardia • Presence of tube feeding in tracheal aspirate	*Early recognition of signs and symptoms of aspiration allows for prompt intervention.*
Assess for difficulty in swallowing and a decreased gag reflex.	*Allows for interventions to be implemented to decrease risk of aspiration.*

Continued...

NURSING ASSESSMENT	RATIONALE
Assist with diagnostic studies to determine whether aspiration is occurring during swallowing (e.g., videofluoroscopy).	*Aspiration of foods/fluids during swallowing process is evident on studies such as videofluoroscopy. Knowing when aspiration occurs during the swallowing process aids in the development of an individualized plan of care to prevent further aspiration.*
Monitor chest radiograph results. Report findings of pulmonary infiltrate.	*Evidence of pulmonary infiltrate on chest radiograph can indicate that aspiration has occurred.*

THERAPEUTIC INTERVENTIONS	RATIONALE

Independent Actions

Perform actions to decrease the risk of aspiration:

• Keep suction equipment readily available at bedside.	*This equipment is necessary to maintain patency of airway.*
• Position patient in high-Fowler's positions before initiating feeding.	*This position uses gravity to facilitate movement of food/fluids through the pharynx into the esophagus.*
• Maintain patient in an upright position 30 to 45 minutes after eating. **D** ● ✦	*Allows for observation of potential swallowing difficulty.*
• Supervise administration of oral intake.	
• Offer foods with a thicker consistency, which facilitates swallowing.	*Semisolid foods are more readily swallowed. Watery fluids are difficult for patients with dysphagia to manage.*
• Encourage client to chew each bite slowly and completely, and to eat slowly during meals. **D** ● ✦	*Complete mastication of food products improves the client's ability to swallow food.*
• Place foods/medications on unaffected side of the mouth. **D** ● ✦	*This action facilitates effective swallowing of food.*
• Provide oral care after feedings. **D** ● ✦	*Good oral hygiene after meals results in removal of any remaining food that could enter the pharynx and be aspirated into the lungs.*
• If client is receiving tube feedings, check tube placement before each feeding or on a routine basis if tube feeding is continuous.	*Verification of feeding tube placement ensures that the tube feeding solution goes into the alimentary tract rather than the lungs.*

Dependent/Collaborative Actions

Perform actions to decrease the risk of aspiration:

• Monitor chest radiograph results.	*Evidence of pulmonary infiltrates on chest radiograph can indicate that aspiration has occurred.*
• Administer antiemetics as ordered to prevent vomiting. **D** ✦	*Antiemetics reduce the risk of vomiting.*
• Consult appropriate speech therapist for swallowing difficulties.	*Dysphagia assessment can establish techniques to prevent aspiration in patients with impaired swallowing.*

Nursing Diagnosis   # CONSTIPATION NDx

Definition: Decrease in normal frequency of defecation accompanied by difficult or incomplete passage of stool and/or passage of excessively hard, dry stool.

Related to: Physiological changes that alter normal bowel functioning

CLINICAL MANIFESTATIONS

Subjective	Objective
Reports of straining with defecation; feeling of rectal fullness or pressure; inability to pass stool; headache; indigestion	Infrequent bowel movements; dry, hard, formed stool; hyperactive/hypoactive bowel sounds; distended abdomen; percussed abdominal dullness; severe flatus; hypoactive or hyperactive bowel sounds; palpable abdominal mass; oozing liquid stool

RISK FACTORS
- Lack of fiber in diet
- Abdominal muscle weakness
- Physical inactivity
- Decreased fluid intake
- Side effects of medications

DESIRED OUTCOMES

The client will maintain usual bowel elimination pattern as evidenced by:
a. Usual frequency of bowel movements
b. Passage of soft, formed stool
c. Absence of abdominal distention and pain, feeling of rectal fullness or pressure, and straining during defecation

NOC OUTCOMES

Bowel elimination; GI function; hydration; symptom control

NIC INTERVENTIONS

Constipation/impaction management

NURSING ASSESSMENT	RATIONALE
Ascertain client's usual bowel elimination habits.	Knowledge of the client's usual bowel elimination habits is essential in determining whether constipation is present because the frequency of defecation varies among individuals.
Assess for signs and symptoms of constipation: • Decrease in frequency of bowel movements • Passage of hard, formed stools • Anorexia • Abdominal distention and pain • Feeling of fullness or pressure in rectum • Straining during defecation	Early recognition of signs and symptoms of constipation allows for prompt intervention.
Assess bowel sounds. Report a pattern of decreasing bowel sounds.	Bowel sounds are produced by peristaltic activity. A pattern of decreasing bowel sounds indicates a decrease in bowel motility, which can lead to and be present with constipation.

THERAPEUTIC INTERVENTIONS	RATIONALE

Independent Actions
Implement measures to promote optimum bowel elimination:

• Encourage client to defecate whenever the urge is felt. **D** ● ✦	Repeated inhibition of the defecation reflex results in progressive weakening of the reflex. In addition, when the defecation reflex is inhibited, feces remain in the colon longer and water continues to be absorbed from the feces, making the stool drier, harder, and subsequently more difficult to evacuate.
• Assist client to toilet or bedside commode or place in high-Fowler's positions on bedpan for bowel movements unless contraindicated. **D** ● ✦	A sitting position aids in the expulsion of stool by taking advantage of gravity. This position also enhances the client's ability to perform the Valsalva maneuver, which increases intra-abdominal pressure and forces the fecal contents downward and into the rectum, where the defecation reflex is then elicited.
• Encourage client to relax, provide privacy, and have call signal within reach during attempts to defecate. **D** ● ✦	If the client is able to relax during attempts to defecate, he/she will be able to relax the levator ani muscle and external anal sphincter, thus facilitating the passage of stool.
• Encourage the client to establish a regular time for defecation, preferably within an hour after a meal. **D** ✦	Attempting to have a bowel movement within an hour after a meal, particularly breakfast, takes advantage of mass peristalsis, which occurs only a few times a day and is strongest after meals. Mass peristalsis is stimulated by the gastrocolic reflex, which is initiated by the presence of foods/fluids in the stomach and duodenum.
• Instruct client to increase intake of foods high in fiber (e.g., bran, whole grain breads and cereals, fresh fruits and vegetables) unless contraindicated.	Foods high in fiber provide bulk to the fecal mass and keep the stool soft because of the ability of fiber to absorb water. The increased bulkiness (mass) of the stools stimulates peristalsis, which promotes more rapid movement of stool through the colon. The shorter the time that feces remains in the intestine, the less water is absorbed from it, which helps prevent the formation of hard, dry stools that are difficult to expel.

Continued...

THERAPEUTIC INTERVENTIONS	RATIONALE
• Encourage client to drink hot liquids (e.g., coffee, tea) upon arising in the morning. • Encourage client to maintain regular exercise. • Encourage client to perform isometric abdominal strengthening exercises unless contraindicated.	*These interventions can stimulate peristalsis.*

Dependent/Collaborative Actions

Implement measures to promote optimum bowel elimination:

• Instruct client to maintain a minimal fluid intake of 2500 mL/day unless contraindicated.	*Inadequate fluid intake reduces the water content of feces, which results in hard, dry stool that is difficult to evacuate.*
• Increase activity as allowed and tolerated. **D** ● ✦	*Ambulation stimulates peristalsis, which promotes the passage of stool through the intestines.*
• When appropriate, encourage the use of nonnarcotic rather than opioid analgesics for pain management.	*Opioid analgesics slow peristalsis, which delays transit of intestinal contents. This delay also results in increased absorption of fluid from the fecal mass with the subsequent formation of hard, dry stool.*
• Administer laxatives as ordered. **D** ✦	*Laxatives/cathartics act in a variety of ways to soften the stool, increase stool bulk, stimulate bowel motility, and/or lubricate the fecal mass and thereby promote the evacuation of stool.*
• Administer cleansing and/or oil retention enemas if ordered. **D** ● ✦	*A cleansing enema stimulates peristalsis and evacuation of stool by distending the colon with a large volume of solution and/or by irritating the colonic mucosa. An oil retention enema facilitates the passage of stool by softening the fecal mass and lubricating the rectum and anal canal.*
• Consult physician about checking for an impaction and digitally removing stool if the client has not had a bowel movement in 3 days, if the client is passing liquid stool, or if other signs and symptoms of constipation are present.	*An impaction prohibits the normal passage of feces. Digital removal of an impacted fecal mass may be necessary before normal passage of stool can occur.*

Nursing Diagnosis **IMPAIRED VERBAL COMMUNICATION** NDx

Definition: Decreased, delayed, or absent ability to receive, process, transmit, and/or use a system of symbols.

Related to:
- Decreased tone in facial muscles
- Slow and/or slurred speech
- Decreased facial expression
- Decreased mobility of the tongue
- Decreased tone of voice

CLINICAL MANIFESTATIONS

Subjective	Objective
Verbal self-report of difficulty of expressing self	Unable to speak dominant language; speaks or verbalizes with difficulty; cannot speak; slurring/stuttering; difficulty forming words and sentences

RISK FACTORS	DESIRED OUTCOME
• Depression • Embarrassment • Change in muscle tone	The client will maintain positive interactions with others.

NOC OUTCOMES	NIC INTERVENTIONS
Communication: expressive	Communication enhancement: speech deficit; active listening

NURSING ASSESSMENT	RATIONALE
Assess for motor speech impairment or difficulty forming words.	*Provides a baseline assessment of client's status and allows for the implementation of appropriate interventions.*

THERAPEUTIC INTERVENTIONS	RATIONALE

Independent Actions
Implement measures to maintain positive communication:

• Approach communication with client as an adult. **D** ● ✦	*Inability to communicate can be frustrating. The client should be treated with dignity.*
• Ask questions that require short answers and allow time for the patient to respond. **D** ● ✦	*The client will need more time to express himself/herself. Short, simple answers will reduce client's frustration, allowing for easier communication.*
• Face client and maintain eye contact when client is speaking. **D** ● ✦	*In a calm, quiet environment the client can concentrate on communication efforts and can hear others more clearly.*
• Create a calm, quiet environment.	
• Provide rest periods before speech therapy. **D** ● ✦	
• Encourage client to routinely perform face and tongue exercises.	*These actions help the client maintain muscle tone, reduces rigidity and helps facilitate communication while decreasing frustration with the process.*
• Encourage client to sign or read out loud to self or family members.	
• Provide assistive communication aids such as pad/pencil, computer, word cards, or picture boards. **D** ● ✦	
• Encourage family to communicate with client. **D** ✦	*Family involvement will reinforce consistency of communication measures.*

Dependent/Collaborative Actions
Implement measures to maintain positive communication:

• Consult speech pathologist.	*Multidisciplinary plan of care can be developed.*

Nursing Diagnosis ## DISTURBED SELF-CONCEPT*

Definition
Disturbed Body Image NDx: Confusion in mental picture of one's physical self.
Situational Low Self-Esteem NDx: Development of a negative perception of self-worth in response to a current situation.
Ineffective Role Performance NDx: A pattern of behavior and self-expression that does not match the environmental context, norms, and expectations.

Related to:
• Loss of independent functioning
• Difficulty in communication

CLINICAL MANIFESTATIONS

Subjective	Objective
Verbal self-report of negative feelings about self	Lack of participation in activities of daily living; withdrawal from significant others; lack of planning to adapt to necessary changes in lifestyle

---

*This diagnostic label includes the nursing diagnoses of disturbed body image, low self-esteem, and ineffective role performance.

RISK FACTORS

- Changes in physical appearance
- Poor self-esteem

DESIRED OUTCOMES

The client will demonstrate beginning adaptation to changes in appearance, body functioning, and lifestyle as evidenced by:
a. Verbalization of feelings of self-worth
b. Maintenance of relationships with significant others
c. Active participation in activities of daily living
d. Verbalization of a beginning plan for integrating changes in appearance and body functioning into lifestyle

NOC OUTCOMES

Body image; personal autonomy; self-esteem; psychosocial adjustment: life change

NIC INTERVENTIONS

Body image enhancement; self-esteem enhancement; emotional support; support system enhancement; role enhancement; counseling

NURSING ASSESSMENT	RATIONALE
Assess for signs and symptoms of a disturbed self-concept (e.g., verbalization of negative feelings about self, withdrawal from significant others, lack of participation in activities of daily living, lack of plan for adapting to necessary changes in lifestyle).	*Early recognition of signs and symptoms of a disturbed self-concept allows for prompt treatment.*
Determine the meaning of changes in appearance, body functioning, and lifestyle to the client by encouraging verbalization of feelings and by noting nonverbal responses to the changes experienced.	*An understanding of what the change means to the client provides a basis for planning care.*

THERAPEUTIC INTERVENTIONS	RATIONALE
Independent Actions	
Be aware that client may grieve the loss of normal body functioning and change in appearance. Provide support during the grieving process.	*Allows client and significant others to grieve loss of normal body functioning; helps client work through changes that are occurring.*
Discuss client's feelings about disease symptoms.	*Discussion of feelings about the disease process helps the client in dealing with his/her physiological changes.*
Instruct client in ways to maintain health status as long as possible: • Maintain regular exercise program. • Maintain optimal diet. • Maintain performance of activities of daily living.	*These actions help the client maintain health status, decrease muscle rigidity, and improve muscle strength.*
Encourage significant others to allow client to do what he/she is able.	*This improves client's confidence in ability to care for self and enhances client's feelings of self-worth and assists with the development of a positive self-concept.*
Assist client's and significant others' adjustment by listening, facilitating communication, and providing information.	*These actions facilitate client and family acceptance of changes and changes in lifestyle.*
Encourage visits and support from significant others.	
Encourage client to pursue usual roles and interests and to continue involvement in social activities as much as possible.	*Pursuit of usual roles and activities helps the client maintain independence and social interaction as long as possible.*
Refer client and family to support groups	*Support groups may help client and family work through changes related to the disease process.*
Refer client and family to community organizations.	*Allows for continuity of care and support once discharged from an acute care facility.*

DISCHARGE TEACHING/CONTINUED CARE

Nursing Diagnosis **DEFICIENT KNOWLEDGE** NDx**; INEFFECTIVE FAMILY HEALTH MANAGEMENT** NDx**; OR INEFFECTIVE HEALTH MAINTENANCE** NDx*,†

Definition: **Deficient Knowledge NDx:** Absence of cognitive information related to a specific topic, or its acquisition; **Ineffective Family Health Management NDx:** A pattern of regulating and integrating into family processes a program for the treatment of illness and its sequelae that is unsatisfactory for meeting specific health goals of the family unit; **Ineffective Health Maintenance NDx:** Inability to identify, manage, and/or seek out help maintain well-being.

CLINICAL MANIFESTATIONS

Subjective	**Objective**
Verbal self-report of inability to manage illness; verbalizes inability to follow prescribed regimen	Inaccurate follow-through with instructions; inappropriate behaviors; experience of preventable complications of Parkinson disease

RISK FACTORS
- Cognitive deficit
- Financial concerns
- Failure to take action to reduce risk factors for complications of Parkinson disease

- Inability to care for oneself
- Difficulty in modifying personal habits and integrating treatments into lifestyle

NOC OUTCOMES

Knowledge: treatment regimen; health behavior; health resources; treatment procedure(s)

NIC INTERVENTIONS

Teaching: individual; teaching: prescribed activity/exercise; teaching: psychomotor skills; health system guidance; financial resource assistance; support system enhancement

NURSING ASSESSMENT

Assess the client's ability to learn and readiness to learn
Assess the client's understanding of teaching

RATIONALE

Learning is more effective when the client is motivated and understands the importance of what is to be learned. Readiness to learn changes based on situations, physical and emotional challenges.

THERAPEUTIC INTERVENTIONS

RATIONALE

Desired Outcome: The client will understand disease process and prognosis.

Independent Actions
Reinforce information concerning the disease and treatment modalities.

Knowledge of disease process and treatment helps the client and family understand the changes that are occurring and the importance of treatment in maintaining health status as long as possible. This improves the client's adherence to treatment regimen and allows the client to maintain a level of independence for as long as possible. Knowledge of the disease process may help with the client's ability to cope with physical changes.

*The nurse should select the diagnostic label that is most appropriate for the client's discharge teaching needs.
†Although the client will not be able to perform many of the following actions independently, he/she must be knowledgeable about them in order to provide proper instruction to significant others and attendant and maintain an active role in the rehabilitation process.

NDx = NANDA Diagnosis   **D** = Delegatable Action   ● = UAP   ✦ = LVN/LPN   ⊖▶ = Go to ⊖volve for animation

THERAPEUTIC INTERVENTIONS	RATIONALE

Desired Outcome: The client will verbalize an understanding of the rationale for and components of the recommended diet and the importance of maintaining optimal nutritional status.

Independent Actions
Provide instructions regarding ways to maintain an optimal nutritional status:
- Maintain an adequate diet with the appropriate mix of nutrients.

- Reinforce instructions related to taking small bites and chewing food thoroughly.
- Inform client that eating small, frequent meals rather than three large meals may help achieve the recommended calorie intake.
- Reinforce the benefits of eating when rested and in a relaxed atmosphere.

Adequate nutritional status is required for the body to work efficiently and maintain optimal muscle strength and energy to perform activities of daily living as long as possible. These actions improve the client's ability to swallow foods and decrease the risk of aspiration.

Eating in a relaxed environment improves the client's ability to maintain nutritional status and decreases risk of aspiration. When a client is anxious or rushed, there is an increased risk for aspiration.

THERAPEUTIC INTERVENTIONS	RATIONALE

Desired Outcome: The client will verbalize ways to maintain optimal muscle tone.

Independent Actions
Instruct client in ways that will maintain muscle strength for as long as possible:
- Maintain a regular exercise routine.
- Encourage client to maintain exercises that work the facial muscles (i.e., sing or read aloud, stick out tongue, move tongue from side to side).

Regular exercise including exercise of the facial muscles, improves balance, maintains muscle strength, and improves flexibility and mobility and the client's ability to verbally communicate.

THERAPEUTIC INTERVENTIONS	RATIONALE

Desired Outcome: The client will verbalize an understanding of medication regimen, including rationale, food and drug interactions, side effects, schedule for taking, and importance of taking as prescribed.

Independent Actions
Explain the rationale for, side effects of, food and drug interactions, and the importance of taking medications as prescribed. The client should understand which side effects require notification of the health care provider.

Reinforce importance of taking medications as prescribed.

Types of medications to treat PD include:
- Anticholinergics

Knowledge of medications and how they impact the system improves client adherence and helps enhance the client's understanding of the importance of adhering to the prescribed medication regimen. The client must be able to recognize alterations in functioning related to medication administration.

Missing doses of medications or not taking them as prescribed may adversely impact mobility.

Anticholinergics help control muscle activity.

THERAPEUTIC INTERVENTIONS	**RATIONALE**
• Dopamine agonists • Monoamine oxidase B inhibitor • Catechol-O-methyltransferase inhibitor	*Dopamine agonists, monoamine oxidase B inhibitors, and cate-chol-O-methyl-transferase inhibitors increase the amount of CNS dopamine available for use, which decreases muscle rigidity and tremors.*
Instruct client to inform physician before taking other prescription and nonprescription medications.	*Over-the-counter (OTC) medications may impact prescription medications and should not be taken without a health care provider's approval.*

THERAPEUTIC INTERVENTIONS	**RATIONALE**

Desired Outcome: The client will identify resources that can assist in the adjustment to changes resulting from PD and its treatment.

Independent Actions

Provide information about resources that can assist the client and significant others in adjusting to PD and its effects (e.g., local support groups, Parkinson disease foundations, counseling services).	*Client may need assistance from community organizations for both emotional and financial support, once discharged from the acute care facility.*

THERAPEUTIC INTERVENTIONS	**RATIONALE**

Desired Outcome: The client, in collaboration with the nurse, will develop a plan for adhering to recommended follow-up care including future appointments with health care provider and activity level.

Independent Actions

Reinforce importance of keeping follow-up appointments with health care provider.	*PD is a chronic illness and requires appropriate follow-up with health care providers.*
Implement measures to improve client's compliance:	
• Include significant others in teaching sessions if possible.	*Support from client's significant others is important in maintaining adherence to the therapeutic regimen.*
• Encourage questions and allow time for reinforcement and clarification of information provided.	*Improves client's and family's understanding of disease process and what to do to remain healthy.*
• Provide written instructions on future appointments with health care provider, medications prescribed, signs and symptoms to report, and future laboratory studies.	*Written instructions allow the client to refer to them after discharge as needed.*

ADDITIONAL NURSING DIAGNOSES

ACTIVITY INTOLERANCE NDx
Related to muscle weakness and fatigue

RISK FOR INJURY NDx
Related to altered gait and muscle weakness

CAREGIVER ROLE STRAIN NDx
Related to:
• Level of illness experienced by the client
• Duration of care required
• Complexity of care
• Caregiver isolation

BATHING SELF-CARE DEFICIT NDx; DRESSING SELF-CARE DEFICIT NDx; FEEDING SELF-CARE DEFICIT NDx; TOILETING SELF-CARE DEFICIT NDx
Related to:
• Muscle weakness
• Tremors
• Rigidity of movements

The Client With Alterations in Hematologic and Immune Function

HUMAN IMMUNODEFICIENCY VIRUS INFECTION AND ACQUIRED IMMUNE DEFICIENCY SYNDROME

Acquired immune deficiency syndrome (AIDS) is an infectious disease of the immune system and is considered the last phase of the clinical spectrum of infection by the human immunodeficiency virus (HIV). HIV is a retrovirus that affects the immune system cells in the body that have a CD4 receptor on their surface. The immune cells with the CD4 receptor include T helper cells, monocytes, macrophages, and dendritic cells. The CD4+ T lymphocytes (also called T4 or T-helper cells) have the greatest number of CD4 receptors and are consequently the major target of HIV. These lymphocytes are ultimately destroyed by HIV, which results in severely impaired cell-mediated immunity in the host. Humoral immune function is also impaired because the B lymphocytes are unable to respond appropriately to the presence of a new antigen without the help of normal CD4+ T lymphocytes. Macrophages and monocytes are the cells that are active in the immune response and are greatly impacted by HIV infection.

HIV has been isolated from all body fluids, but at this point, transmission has been associated only with blood, semen, amniotic fluid, vaginal secretions, and breast milk. The known routes of transmission are by intimate sexual contact, mucous membrane or percutaneous exposure to infected blood or blood products, and perinatal transmission from mother to child. In the United States, HIV is spread primarily through sexual contact with someone who has HIV without using a condom, as well as sharing intravenous drug equipment. Transmission to recipients of blood/blood products is rare. Occupational exposure and fetus exposure from women who are HIV positive have significantly decreased over the past several years.

Progression of HIV infection to a diagnosis of AIDS progresses in stages and is based on symptoms and CD4 cell levels.

Infection with HIV, and the subsequent clinical expression, is attributed to either the effects of the virus itself or the consequences of CD4+ T-lymphocyte depletion. Initial symptoms during the acute retroviral infection may occur as early as 2 to 4 weeks after exposure to HIV. During this phase, some individuals experience flu-like symptoms such as fever, headache, myalgias, lymphadenopathy, rash, fatigue, and a sore throat that may persist for a week or longer. The second phase of HIV infection is the chronic infection stage. In the early period of chronic infection, the person may be asymptomatic or continue to experience mild symptoms such as fatigue, headache, and lymphadenopathy. This early period often lasts as long as 10 years, depending on the rate of viral replication and the rapidity of CD4+ T-lymphocyte destruction. During this stage, the individual may not have any symptoms, but is still able to pass the HIV-related symptoms and spread the virus to others. AIDS is the last stage of HIV infection. In addition to the symptoms experienced in the previous stages, AIDS is diagnosed when immune suppression decreases to a CD4+ T-lymphocyte count <200 cells/mm^3 and the presence of one or more illnesses as specified by the Centers for Disease Control and Prevention (CDC). These AIDS-indicator conditions include a wide variety of immunosuppression-related illnesses.

There is no cure for HIV infection. Significant advances have been made in antiretroviral therapy and prevention of opportunistic infections. These have increased the long-term survival of individuals with HIV infection. Earlier treatment and the use of antiretroviral therapy, which consists of a combination of at least three or more antiretroviral agents, have made significant differences in sustaining viral suppression, slowing disease progression, and reducing drug resistance. Because of the side effects of the antiretroviral agents and lack of adherence to the drug regimen, current federal guidelines suggest that treatment be offered early following exposure.

This care plan focuses on the adult client with HIV infection hospitalized for treatment of a probable opportunistic infection and progression to an AIDS diagnosis. Much of the information is applicable to clients receiving follow-up care in an extended care facility or home setting.

OUTCOME/DISCHARGE CRITERIA

The client will:
1. Maintain adequate respiratory status
2. Maintain adequate nutritional status
3. Perform activities of daily living without undue fatigue or dyspnea
4. Demonstrate evidence that opportunistic infection, if present, is resolving
5. Manage signs and symptoms of neurological dysfunction

6. Maintain pain relief at an acceptable level
7. Show evidence that skin and oral mucous membranes are intact or healing appropriately
8. Have fewer episodes of diarrhea
9. Implement actions to prevent the spread of HIV
10. Implement actions to decrease the risk for developing opportunistic infections
11. Develop a plan to maintain an optimal nutritional status
12. State signs and symptoms to report to the health care provider
13. Discuss concerns and feelings about changes in mental and physical functioning and the social isolation and loneliness that may result from having AIDS
14. Identify resources that can assist with financial needs and adjustment to changes resulting from the diagnosis of AIDS
15. Develop a plan for adhering to recommended follow-up care including regular laboratory studies, future appointments with health care providers, and medications prescribed.

Nursing Diagnosis RISK-PRONE HEALTH BEHAVIOR NDx

Definition: Impaired ability to modify lifestyle and/or actions in a manner that improves the level of wellness.

CLINICAL MANIFESTATIONS

Subjective	Objective
Verbalization of inability to adhere to health care providers' recommendations; statements that imply non-acceptance of health status changes; continue unsafe sexual habits	Smoking, alcohol and IV drug abuse; Demonstrated hostility to health care providers; missing scheduled health care appointments

RISK FACTORS
• Economically disadvantaged
• History of health risk behaviors
• Lack of understanding of seriousness of disease
• Insufficient social support

DESIRED OUTCOMES
The client will experience improved health status as evidenced by:
1. Verbalization of acceptance of condition
2. Initiation of lifestyle changes consistent with disease process
3. Developing a plan for improved health status

NOC OUTCOME
Risk Identification; Health Education

NIC INTERVENTIONS
Self-Efficacy enhancement; self-acceptance
Health Education: Risk factor reduction; health care plan; identification of resources; mechanisms to reduce health risk behaviors

NURSING ASSESSMENT
Assess for and report signs and symptoms of risk-prone health behavior:
• Identify client's understanding of risky health behavior
• Identify client's understanding of barriers to positive health behavior
• Identify client's understanding of illness and sequelae if health behaviors are not improved

RATIONALE
Early recognition of client's risk-prone behavior allows for prompt intervention.

THERAPEUTIC INTERVENTIONS
Independent Actions
Evaluate client's understanding of disease diagnosis and of behaviors required to maintain optimal health.
Encourage client to discuss concerns and challenges to implementing behaviors to maintain optimal health.
Collaborate with client to identity support systems and available community resources.

RATIONALE
Provides a starting point to develop a plan of action.

Allows patient to express beliefs, fears, and potential challenges in adhering to health behaviors and required regimen.
Allows client to have input into plan of care and identification of available support and resources. By involving the client, it can also demonstrate to the nurse the level of involvement and interest in making behavioral changes.

Continued...

THERAPEUTIC INTERVENTIONS	RATIONALE
Encourage client to utilize known and practice new coping mechanisms.	*Provides reinforcement of what has worked in the past and helps the client to develop new mechanisms to support behavioral changes. Practicing coping mechanisms with the nurse will improve client self-confidence.*
Discuss high-risk behaviors including unsafe sexual practices, sharing of injection drug needles, and failure to follow prescribed medication regimen.	*Client may be uncomfortable discussing these issues with persons known to them. The nurse can discuss these issues in a non-judgmental manner and assist client's understanding of what behaviors need to change and how to implement required changes.*
Collaborative Actions	
Refer client to HIV specialists, social workers, and community resources	*Client may benefit from working with individuals specifically trained to deal with clients diagnosed with HIV.*

Nursing Diagnosis INEFFECTIVE HEALTH MANAGEMENT NDx (MEDICATION MANAGEMENT)

Definition: Pattern of regulating and integrating into daily living a therapeutic regimen for the treatment of illness and its sequelae that is unsatisfactory for meeting specific health goals.

CLINICAL MANIFESTATIONS

Subjective	Objective
Verbalization of not taking medications; confusion about medication regimen; lack of financial resources to pay for medication; complaint of experience of medication side effects	Continued decrease in serum CD4+T cell levels; experience of opportunistic diseases

RISK FACTORS

- Socioeconomic status
- Medication side effects
- Poor understanding of medication regimen
- Insufficient knowledge of therapeutic regimen
- Insufficient social support
- Difficulty navigating complex health care systems

DESIRED OUTCOMES

The client will demonstrate ability to adhere to medication regimen by:
1. Taking medications as prescribed
2. Set up a plan to assure refill and renewal of prescriptions
3. Improving CD4+T cell levels

NOC OUTCOMES

Medication administration; Self-care

NIC INTERVENTIONS

Self-Efficacy Enhancement; medication administration; Health Education: medication management; support system enhancement

NURSING ASSESSMENT	RATIONALE
Assess for and report signs and symptoms of lack of adherence to medication regimen: • Assess client's feelings about and understanding of medication regimen • Assess client's understanding of what can occur if not adhering to medication regimen • Assess for experienced side effects that may lead to non-adherence with medication regimen • Assess client's financial concerns related to medications prescribed	*Early recognition of client's lack of medication adherence allows for prompt intervention.*

THERAPEUTIC INTERVENTIONS	RATIONALE

Independent Actions

Discuss rationale for the prescribed medication regimen.

Understanding of the short- and long-term outcomes of the role of antiretroviral medications may help improve compliance. Missing medications or altering drug regimen may lead to increased viral load and/or cause the HIV to become resistant to the prescribed medications.

Collaborate with client to develop a schedule for medication administration.

Helps to decrease confusion related to polypharmacy and drug administration requirements.

Collaborate with client in developing a plan to find and access community financial and social support.

Involvement of the client in plan development may improve implementation.

Collaborative Actions

Discuss ways of decreasing specific antiretroviral side effects:

Inform the client that milder medication side effects may decrease over time.

- Encourage eating several small meals per day or drinking nutritional smoothies
- Decrease intake of greasy, fatty, spicy, and dairy food; decrease intake of vegetables, whole grains and nuts that are high in insoluble fiber

Helps to decrease impact of anorexia, nausea, and vomiting.

- Increase nutritious foods that provide energy; increase activity tolerance; avoid smoking and alcohol

These actions may decrease the incidence of diarrhea.

- Increase activity tolerance

These actions may decrease the incidence of fatigue.

- Moisturize skin daily, take cool/lukewarm showers; use laundry detergents that are non-irritating; wear clothing from natural fiber

Actions decrease the incidence of a rash.

- Avoid caffeine after 2:00 pm; avoid taking naps; exercise regularly

Actions decrease problems with sleeping.

- Decrease amount of fat and sugars in diet, eat foods high in omega-3 fatty acids; monitor blood glucose and cholesterol levels

Actions address increased cholesterol and blood glucose levels.

With approval from health care provider, explore alternative health care interventions (i.e., acupuncture, acupressure, relaxation techniques, etc.)

Consult the appropriate health care provider (i.e., dietitian, physical therapist, physician, etc.) for additional information and support in decreasing medication side effects

Consulting the appropriate health care provider allows for modification of the treatment regimen.

Nursing Diagnosis | ## IMBALANCED NUTRITION: LESS THAN BODY REQUIREMENTS NDx

Definition: Intake of nutrients insufficient to meet metabolic needs.

Related to:
- **Decreased oral intake** associated with:
  - Anorexia resulting from malaise, fatigue, fear, anxiety, pain, depression, increased levels of certain cytokines that depress appetite (e.g., tumor necrosis factor [TNF]), and some antiretroviral agents
  - Nausea, dyspnea, and cognitive impairment if present
  - Oral pain and/or dysphagia resulting from opportunistic lesions in the mouth, pharynx, and esophagus
- **Impaired utilization of nutrients** associated with:
  - Accelerated and inefficient metabolism of nutrients resulting from an increased resting energy expenditure that occurs with infection and increased levels of certain cytokines (e.g., TNF, interleukin-1)
  - Decreased absorption of nutrients if HIV and/or opportunistic infection involve the intestine
- **Loss of nutrients associated with persistent diarrhea and vomiting** if present

CLINICAL MANIFESTATIONS

Subjective	Objective
Verbalization of inadequate food intake; reported lack of food; aversion to eating; lack of interest in food	Body weight 20% or more under ideal body weight; loss of weight with adequate food intake; weakness of muscles required for swallowing or chewing; sore, inflamed buccal cavity; hyperactive bowel sounds; diarrhea; vomiting, excessive hair loss

RISK FACTORS

- Inability to digest food
- Inability to absorb nutrients
- Biological factors
- Disease progression
- Insufficient dietary intake

DESIRED OUTCOMES

The client will maintain an adequate nutritional status as evidenced by:
a. Weight within normal range for client
b. Normal blood urea nitrogen (BUN) and serum albumin, prealbumin, hematocrit (Hct), and hemoglobin (Hgb) levels and lymphocyte count
c. Usual strength and activity tolerance
d. Healthy oral mucous membranes

NOC OUTCOMES

Nutritional status; weight control

NIC INTERVENTIONS

Nutritional monitoring; nutritional management; nutrition therapy; exercise promotion: strength training

NURSING ASSESSMENT	RATIONALE

Assess for and report signs and symptoms of malnutrition:
- Weight significantly below client's usual weight or below normal for client's age, height, and body frame
- Weakness and fatigue
- Sore, inflamed oral mucous membrane
- Pale conjunctiva
- Lower-than-normal anthropometric measurements:
  - Skinfold thickness
  - Body circumferences (e.g., hip, waist, mid-upper arm)
  - Bioelectrical impedance analysis
Monitor percentage of meals and snacks client consumes. Report a pattern of inadequate intake.
	Early recognition of signs and symptoms of malnutrition allows for prompt intervention.

Monitor BUN, serum prealbumin, albumin, Hct, and Hgb levels	*Abnormal BUN, low serum prealbumin, albumin, Hct, and Hgb levels may indicate malnutrition. Because of the long (20-day) half-life of albumin, the value is a late indicator of malnutrition. Prealbumin has a half-life of 2 days and is a more timely, sensitive indicator of protein status.*

THERAPEUTIC INTERVENTIONS	RATIONALE

Independent Actions

Implement measures to maintain an adequate nutritional status:
- Perform actions to improve oral intake:
  - Implement measures to prevent breakdown of the oral mucous membrane and promote healing of existing lesions:

    Actions help to reduce oral/pharyngeal pain and improve swallowing.

    - Lubricate lips frequently. **D** ✦

      Maintains moisture and helps prevent breakdown.

    - Rinse mouth frequently with salt and warm water; baking soda and warm water; or a solution of salt, baking soda, and warm water. **D** ✦

      Alkalinizes the mouth and helps decrease bacteria count, soothes oral mucosa.

      Dry crackers and other foods help to soothe stomach and decrease nausea.

  - Implement measures to reduce nausea:

    The client may be oversensitive to strong odors and when exposed to them can cause nausea.

    - Encourage client to eat dry foods when nauseated. **D** ● ✦
    - Avoid serving foods with an overpowering aroma.

      Nausea is associated with the pain experience and relief of pain may decrease/eliminate nausea.

    - Implement measures to reduce pain.

THERAPEUTIC INTERVENTIONS	RATIONALE
• Increase activity as tolerated.	*Activity promotes a sense of well-being, which can improve appetite. Immobility is associated with negative nitrogen balance which increases anorexia.*
• If client is having difficulty swallowing, assist him/her to select nutritional foods/fluids that are easily chewed and swallowed (e.g., eggs, custard, macaroni and cheese, baby foods) and avoid serving foods that are sticky (e.g., peanut butter, soft bread).	*Fluids and soft foods may be less irritating to the GI mucosa and decrease incidence of nausea. High nutrient fluids will help to improve nutritional status.*
• Encourage a rest period before meals to minimize fatigue.	*Provides energy for client to eat meals.*
• Maintain a clean environment and a relaxed, pleasant atmosphere. **D** ●	*Decreases noxious odors and subsequent nausea.*
• Provide oral hygiene before meals. **D** ●	*Oral hygiene moistens the mouth, which may make it easier to chew and swallow; it also removes unpleasant tastes, which often improves the taste of foods/fluids.*
• Serve frequent, small meals rather than large ones if client is weak, fatigues easily, and/or has a poor appetite.	*Small frequent meals enhance nutritional status and help client to conserve energy.*
• If client is dyspneic, place in a high-Fowler's positions for meals and provide supplemental oxygen therapy during meals. **D** ● ✦	
• If client's sense of taste is altered, suggest adding extra sweeteners and flavorings/seasonings to foods.	*Implement only if the client is not experiencing nausea, as this may increase it.*
• Encourage significant others to bring in client's favorite foods and eat with him/her.	*Client may be more likely to eat when favorite foods are available and in the presence of supportive company.*
• Assist client with meals if indicated. **D** ●	*Support with eating and providing a calm, relaxed atmosphere may help the client to relax and enjoy meal time, thus increasing nutritional status.*
• Allow adequate time for meals; reheat foods/fluids as necessary. **D** ● ✦	
• Perform actions to control diarrhea:	*Collaborate with client to identify foods and fluids that can stimulate diarrhea. Avoiding these foods will decrease incidence.*
• Instruct client to avoid foods/fluids that may stimulate or irritate the bowel or cause the stool to be more liquid.	

Dependent/Collaborative Actions

Implement measures to maintain an adequate nutritional status:

• Perform actions to improve oral intake:	
• Administer prescribed antiemetics.	*Decreases incidence of nausea.*
• Obtain a dietary consult if necessary.	*Can provide for additional nutritional support and ideas for meal times and required caloric intake*
• Ensure that meals are well balanced and high in essential nutrients; offer high-protein, high-calorie dietary supplements:	*High-density foods will improve client's nutritional imbalance.*
• Elemental formulas	
• Nutrient-dense candy bars and soups if indicated	
• Administer the following if ordered:	*Helps to maintain nutritional status until client can maintain appropriate weight.*
• Vitamins and minerals	*Appetite stimulants and anabolic agents increase appetite and stimulate increased muscle mass.*
• Appetite stimulants	
• Anabolic agents	
Perform a calorie count if ordered. Report information to dietitian and physician.	*Provides baseline for collaboration in determining client's caloric needs and potential interventions to improve weight gain.*
Consult physician or physical therapist about a progressive exercise program.	*Exercise is necessary to promote the maintenance/buildup of lean body mass and help prevent wasting and improves blood nitrogen balance, thus decreasing anorexia.*
Consult physician about an alternative method of providing nutrition if client does not consume enough food or fluids to meet nutritional needs:	*Consulting the appropriate health care provider allows for modification of the treatment plan.*
• Parenteral nutrition	*These supplemental methods support client's nutritional needs until they are able to improve oral intake.*
• Tube feedings	

Nursing Diagnosis **RISK FOR INFECTION** NDx **(OPPORTUNISTIC INFECTION)**

Definition: Susceptible to invasive and multiplication of pathogenic organisms, which may compromise health.

Related to:
- Decreased resistance to infection associated with:
  - Cellular and humoral immune deficiencies associated with HIV infection
  - Inadequate nutritional status
  - Myelosuppression resulting from medications (e.g., zidovudine, antineoplastic agents, trimethoprim-sulfamethoxazole, ganciclovir, pyrimethamine)
- Stasis of respiratory secretions and/or urinary stasis if mobility is decreased
- Changes in integrity of skin associated with frequent invasive procedures

CLINICAL MANIFESTATIONS*

Subjective	Objective
Verbal self-reports of pain at areas of impaired skin integrity	Fever, chills, tachycardia, warm discharge over areas of impaired skin integrity

DESIRED OUTCOMES

The client will remain free of additional opportunistic infection as evidenced by:
1. Return of temperature toward client's normal range
2. Decrease in number of episodes of chills and diaphoresis
3. BP and heart rate within normal range for client
4. Normal or improved breath sounds
5. Absence or resolution of dyspnea
6. Stable or improved mental status
7. Voiding clear urine without reports of frequency, urgency, and burning
8. Maintenance of skin integrity
9. Stable or gradual increase in body weight
10. No reports of increased weakness and fatigue
11. White blood cell (WBC) and differential counts returning toward normal range
12. Negative results of cultured specimens

NOC OUTCOMES

Infection protection

NIC INTERVENTIONS

Infection control; monitoring

NURSING ASSESSMENT	RATIONALE
Assess for and report signs and symptoms of additional opportunistic infection (be alert to subtle changes in client, since the signs of infection may be minimal as a result of immunosuppression; also be aware that some signs and symptoms vary depending on the site of infection, the causative organism, and the age of the client): <ul><li>Increase in temperature above client's usual level</li><li>Increase in episodes of chills and diaphoresis</li><li>Hypotension (a symptom of sepsis)</li><li>Tachycardia development or worsening of abnormal breath sounds</li><li>Development or worsening of dyspnea</li><li>Development or worsening of cough</li><li>Changes in mental status</li><li>Cloudy urine</li><li>Reports of frequency, urgency, or burning when urinating</li><li>Urinalysis showing a WBC count greater than 5, positive leukocyte esterase or nitrites, or presence of bacteria</li><li>Vesicular lesions particularly on face, lips, and perianal area</li><li>New or increased reports of pain in and/or itching of skin lesions and surrounding tissue</li></ul>	*Early recognition of signs and symptoms of infection allows for prompt intervention.*

---

*Specific objective and subjective symptoms will depend on site of infection and causative organism.

NURSING ASSESSMENT	RATIONALE

- Further increase in weight loss, fatigue, or weakness
- Visual disturbances
- New or increased heat, pain, redness, swelling, or unusual drainage in any area
- New or increased irritation or ulceration of oral mucous membrane
- Dysphagia
- Significant change in WBC count and/or differential
- Positive results of cultured specimens (e.g., urine, vaginal drainage, stool, sputum, blood, drainage from lesions)

Assess results of complete blood cell count (CBC) with differential, and of all cultured specimens for positive results.

THERAPEUTIC INTERVENTIONS	RATIONALE

Independent Actions

Implement measures to prevent further infection:

- Use good hand hygiene and encourage client to do the same. **D** ● ✦
- Protect client from others with infection
- Maintain isolation precautions as indicated
- Maintain a clean, well-ventilated environment
- Encourage frequent deep breathing or use of incentive spirometry and ambulation
- Maintain aseptic and/or sterile technique during all invasive procedures:
  - Urinary catheterization
  - Venous and arterial punctures
  - Injections
- Anchor catheters/tubings:
  - Urinary
  - Intravenous
- Change equipment, tubings, and solutions used for treatments such as intravenous infusions, respiratory care, irrigations, and enteral feedings according to hospital policy.
- Maintain a closed system for drains (e.g., urinary catheter) and intravenous infusions whenever possible.
- Provide a low-microbe diet (e.g., thoroughly cooked foods, fruits and vegetables that have been washed thoroughly).
- Perform actions to prevent stasis of respiratory secretions:
  - Assist client to turn, cough, and deep breathe. **D** ● ✦
  - Increase activity as allowed and tolerated.
- Instruct and assist client to take a daily shower, perform good perineal care routinely and after each bowel movement.
- Perform actions identified in this care plan to reduce stressors, such as discomfort, dyspnea, and fear and anxiety.
- Perform actions to prevent breakdown of oral mucous membrane and promote healing of existing lesions:
  - Have client rinse mouth frequently with salt and warm water; baking soda and warm water; or a solution of salt, baking soda, and warm water.
  - Perform actions to prevent or treat skin breakdown.
  - Implement measures to relieve pruritus.

- Perform actions to prevent urinary retention:
  - Instruct client to urinate when the urge is first felt.
  - Promote relaxation during voiding attempts.

First line of defense in breaking the chain of infection and prevents cross-contamination.
Anyone with any illness should not engage with the client.
Reduces exposure to pathogens.
Decreases stasis of secretions and risk for a respiratory infection.

The use of aseptic/sterile technique reduces the risk of introduction of pathogens into the body.

Securing catheters and tubings reduces trauma to the tissues and risk for introduction of pathogens associated with the in-and-out movement of the tubing.
Decreases potential for organism growth.

Prevents contamination of a closed system.

Prevents exposure to pathogens from fresh fruits and vegetables.

Actions decrease stasis of secretions and potential for excretions of secretions.

Actions decrease potential for infection.

Reducing stress helps to prevent an increase in secretion of cortisol (cortisol interferes with some immune responses).
Salt water/baking soda mouth rinses help to alkalinize the mouth, which reduces bacteria, as bacteria thrive in acidic environments.

Healthy, intact skin reduces the risk of infection.
Decrease risk of tissue injury and potential for introduction of organisms.
Urinary retention increases risk for a urinary tract infection. Accumulation of urine creates an environment conducive to the growth and colonization of organisms.

NDx = NANDA Diagnosis   **D** = Delegatable Action   ● = UAP   ✦ = LVN/LPN   ●▶ = Go to ⊖volve for animation

Continued...

THERAPEUTIC INTERVENTIONS	RATIONALE

Dependent/Collaborative Actions

Implement measures to prevent further infection:

- Administer the following if ordered:
  - Antiretroviral agents
  - Immunomodulating agents (e.g., interleukin-2, colony-stimulating factors such as filgrastim and sargramostim)
  - Antimicrobial agents (prophylaxis for *Pneumocystis carinii* pneumonia, *Mycobacterium tuberculosis*, toxoplasmosis, and *Mycobacterium avium* complex is recommended for all clients with a CD4+ cell count below a critical level)
- Vaccines (e.g., hepatitis A, hepatitis B, pneumococcal pneumonia, influenza)
- Maintain a fluid intake of at least 2500 mL/day unless contraindicated.
- Perform actions to maintain an adequate nutritional status:
  - Obtain a dietary consult, if necessary, to assist client in selecting foods/fluids that meet nutritional needs.

Agents to reduce the rate of replication of HIV.
Agents to stimulate production/enhance activity of the WBCs.
Agents to treat current infection or prevent additional opportunistic infection.

Supports immune system.

Helps to prevent dehydration and stasis of secretions.

Supports immune system.

Nursing Diagnosis   DISTURBED BODY IMAGE NDx

Definition: Confusion in mental picture of one's physical self.

Related to: Diagnosis of HIV/AIDS:
- Alteration in self-perception
- Fear of reactions by others to diagnosis and chronic illness
- Alteration in body function

Treatment regimen

CLINICAL MANIFESTATIONS

Subjective	Objective
Verbal self-report of concerns about physiological functioning and changes; expression of fear of reaction by others; powerlessness; preoccupation with diagnosis	Lack of engagement in self-care

RISK FACTOR
- Diagnosis of HIV/AIDS
- Chronic illness

DESIRED OUTCOMES

The client will experience improvement in body image as evidenced by:
a. Verbalization and understanding of changes in health status
b. Identification of coping mechanisms to improve self-perception

NOC OUTCOMES

Body image enhancement

NIC INTERVENTIONS

Crisis Intervention: counseling; strengthening coping mechanisms

NURSING ASSESSMENT	RATIONALE

Assess client for disturbed body image:
- Expression of negative thoughts about self and self-functioning
- Lack of engagement in self-care

Early recognition and report of signs and symptoms of disturbed body image allows for prompt intervention.

THERAPEUTIC INTERVENTIONS	RATIONALE
Independent Actions	
Discuss and encourage verbalization of client's concerns	*Demonstrates acceptance of client and will help client discuss disease process and concerns related to potential lifestyle and social interaction changes.*
Acknowledge client's feelings common following diagnosis of chronic illness	*Demonstrates acceptance of the individual and normalcy of feelings/experiences.*
Perform care in a nonjudgmental, accepting manner	*Health care providers should not allow personal feelings about the client or client's diagnosis to impact the client's care or to support the client's negative thoughts of self.*
Discuss meaning of diagnosis, treatment, and potential body functioning changes	*Provides the nurse with a basis to develop a plan to support patient in psychological and physiological changes, and client teaching concerning disease process and self-care.*
	Reinforce coping mechanisms that have worked for the client in the past.
Identify coping mechanisms utilized in previous illnesses or with major life changes; collaborate with client to develop and practice new coping mechanisms	*Developing and practicing new coping mechanisms adds to the client's ability to deal with current changes being experienced.*
Involve significant other in discussion about illness, coping mechanisms, and plan of care (if client allows)	*Can strengthen client's relationship with significant others, can help to determine support that can be provided, and areas where more is needed. Allows client and significant others to develop realistic expectations related to the client's diagnosis and long-term support.*
Dependent and Collaborative Actions	
• Recommend participation in support groups and identification of community support services.	*Allows client and significant others to engage with others going through the same experience. Provides for sense of community with others. Supports continuum of care once client is discharged from a health care facility.*

Nursing Diagnosis RISK FOR DEFICIENT FLUID VOLUME NDx AND RISK FOR ELECTROLYTE IMBALANCE NDx

Definitions: **Risk for Deficient Fluid Volume NDx**: Susceptible to experiencing decreased intravascular, interstitial, and/or intracellular fluid volumes, which may compromise health; **Risk for Electrolyte Imbalance NDx**: Susceptible to changes in serum electrolyte levels, which may compromise health.

Related to
• **Risk for deficient fluid volume NDx:**
  • Excessive loss of fluid associated with diarrhea, diaphoresis, and vomiting if present
  • Decreased oral intake associated with anorexia, weakness, nausea, and oropharyngeal pain
• **Hypokalemia:**
  • Excessive loss of potassium associated with diarrhea and vomiting if present
  • Decreased oral intake
• **Hyponatremia:**
  • Excessive loss of sodium associated with diarrhea, profuse diaphoresis, and vomiting if present
  • Water retention associated with increased antidiuretic hormone (ADH) output resulting from opportunistic disease involvement of the lungs or central nervous system; potential alterations in renal function and adrenal insufficiency

CLINICAL MANIFESTATIONS

Subjective	Objective
Verbalization of weakness; confusion; complaints of dry mouth	Change in mental status; decreased skin turgor; postural hypotension; tachycardia; decreased urine output; cardiac dysrhythmias; nausea and vomiting; diarrhea

RISK FACTORS

- Abdominal ascites
- Sepsis
- Active fluid loss
- Pharmaceutical agent
- Compromised regulatory mechanism

DESIRED OUTCOMES

The client will maintain fluid and electrolyte balance as evidenced by:
a. Normal skin turgor
b. Moist mucous membranes
c. Stable weight
d. BP and pulse within normal range for client and stable with position change
e. Capillary refill time less than 2 to 3 seconds
f. Usual mental status
g. Balanced intake and output
h. Usual muscle strength
i. Soft, nondistended abdomen with normal bowel sounds
j. Absence of nausea, vomiting, diarrhea, abdominal cramps, and seizure activity
k. BUN, Hct, and serum potassium and sodium levels within normal range

NOC OUTCOMES

Fluid/electrolyte monitoring

NIC INTERVENTIONS

Fluid management; electrolyte management: hypokalemia; electrolyte management: hyponatremia

NURSING ASSESSMENT

Assess for and report signs and symptoms of:
- Deficient fluid volume
  - Decreased skin turgor, dry mucous membranes, thirst
  - Thirst
  - Weight loss of 2% or greater over a short period
  - Postural hypotension and/or low BP
  - Weak, rapid pulse
  - Capillary refill time greater than 2 to 3 seconds
  - Change in mental status
  - Decreased urine output (reflects an actual rather than potential fluid deficit)
- Hypokalemia
  - Cardiac dysrhythmias
  - Postural hypotension
  - Muscle weakness
  - Nausea and vomiting
  - Abdominal distention
  - Hypoactive or absent bowel sounds
- Hyponatremia
  - Nausea and vomiting
  - Malaise
  - Abdominal cramps
  - Lethargy
  - Confusion
  - Weakness
  - Seizures

Monitor serum electrolyte, BUN, creatinine levels

RATIONALE

Early recognition of signs and symptoms of fluid deficit and electrolyte imbalance allow for prompt intervention.
Thirst is an early symptom of dehydration.
Body weight changes of 1 kg (2.2 lbs) equal a fluid loss of 1 liter.
Cardiovascular changes of hypotension and tachycardia are signs of dehydration.
May not change in clients with fever.
Monitor I and O to provide for early identification of fluid loss.

Indications of hypokalemia are non-specific and primarily involve changes in muscle and cardiac function. Weakness and fatigue are the most common symptoms.

Indications of hyponatremia involve proper muscle and nerve function. Clinical manifestations range from nausea and malaise to obvious neurological changes.

Can identify changes over time and implement actions to prevent symptomology from occurring

THERAPEUTIC INTERVENTIONS

Independent Actions

Implement measures to prevent or treat imbalanced fluid and electrolytes:
- Perform actions to control diarrhea:
  - Instruct client to avoid foods/fluids that may stimulate or irritate the bowel or cause the stool to be more liquid.

RATIONALE

Persistent or severe diarrhea results in excessive loss of fluid and electrolytes.

THERAPEUTIC INTERVENTIONS	RATIONALE
• Perform actions to improve oral intake (e.g., prevent breakdown of oral mucous membrane). **D** ● ✦	*Foods or fluids that stimulate the bowel lead to increased intestinal motility and excessive mucus production that increases the liquidity of the intestinal contents.*
• Provide fresh water and other fluids at easy access, if oral fluids are allowed. **D** ● ✦	*Helps to maintain integrity of oral mucosa.* *Helps to maintain adequate intake of fluids. Weight gain is a sensitive indicator of fluid volume changes.*
• Perform actions to reduce fever (e.g., tepid sponge bath, cool cloths to groin and axillae).	*Decreases fluid loss.*
• Encourage intake of foods/fluids high in potassium: • Bananas, avocado, sweet potatoes, orange juice, raisins • Avocado • Potatoes • Raisins • Cantaloupe	*Helps to maintain adequate potassium levels.*
• Encourage intake of foods/fluids high in sodium • Processed cheese, canned soups, canned vegetables • Canned soups • Canned vegetables • Bouillon	*Helps maintain adequate sodium levels.*
Encourage intake of probiotics or live-culture yogurt or supplements with *lactobacillus acidophilus*	*Improves bowel bacteria that when out of balance due to disease processes or treatment may lead to diarrhea.*
Dependent/Collaborative Actions Implement measures to prevent or treat imbalanced fluid and electrolytes:	
• Administer antiemetics if ordered to control vomiting.	*Nausea can cause the client to decrease fluid intake. Treating vomiting helps to prevent loss of fluid and electrolytes.*
• Administer antidiarrheal agents if ordered	*Diarrhea leads to fluid and electrolyte loss.*
• Administer antipyretics if fever is present	*Helps to reduce body temperature and increased metabolic state associated with fever.*
• Maintain a fluid intake of at least 2500 mL/day unless contraindicated; if oral intake is inadequate or contraindicated, maintain intravenous and/or enteral therapy as ordered.	*Adequate fluid intake needs to be provided to ensure adequate hydration to support vascular fluid volume.*
• Administer electrolyte replacements if ordered.	*Serum electrolytes such as sodium and potassium have narrow therapeutic ranges, must be kept within normal limits for normal body functioning.*
Consult physician if signs and symptoms of imbalanced fluid and electrolytes persist or worsen.	*Consulting the appropriate health care provider allows for modification of the treatment plan.*

Nursing Diagnosis   IMPAIRED RESPIRATORY FUNCTION*

Definition: Ineffective Breathing Pattern NDx: Inspiration and/or expiration that does not provide adequate ventilation; **Ineffective Airway Clearance NDx:** Inability to clear secretions or obstruction from the respiratory tract to maintain a clear airway; **Impaired Gas Exchange NDx:** Excess or deficit in oxygenation and/or carbon dioxide elimination at the alveolar-capillary membrane.

Related to

Ineffective breathing pattern NDx: Changes in rate and depth of respirations associated with fear, anxiety, weakness, fatigue, infection, increased metabolic rate, and chest pain

Ineffective airway clearance NDx
• Increased production of secretions associated with some opportunistic infections of the lungs
• Stasis of secretions associated with decreased activity and poor cough effort resulting from fatigue and pain

Impaired gas exchange NDx
A decrease in effective lung surface associated with:
• Presence of infiltrates and/or cavities in the lung tissue resulting from opportunistic infection of the lungs (e.g., pneumococcal pneumonia [PCP], tuberculosis, histoplasmosis, etc.)
• Compression and/or replacement of lung tissue if an AIDS-related cancer such as Kaposi sarcoma or non-Hodgkin lymphoma is present

*This diagnostic label includes the following nursing diagnoses: ineffective breathing pattern, ineffective airway clearance, and impaired gas exchange.

NDx = NANDA Diagnosis   **D** = Delegatable Action   ● = UAP   ✦ = LVN/LPN   ⊖▶ = Go to ⊜volve for animation

CLINICAL MANIFESTATIONS

Subjective	Objective
Verbalization of difficulty vocalizing; verbal reports of restlessness	Dyspnea; tachypnea, orthopnea; diminished breath sounds; adventitious breath sounds; cough productive and non-productive; change in respiratory rate and rhythm

RISK FACTORS

- Pulmonary infection
- Immunosuppression
- Pneumocystis jiroveci pneumonia
- Mycobacterium tuberculosis
- Alveolocapillary membrane changes
- Respiratory muscle fatigue
- Retained secretions
- Excessive mucus

DESIRED OUTCOMES

The client will experience adequate respiratory function as evidenced by:
a. Normal rate and depth of respirations
b. Decreased dyspnea
c. Improved breath sounds
d. Symmetrical chest excursion
e. Usual mental status
f. Oximetry results within normal range
g. Arterial blood gas values within normal range

NOC OUTCOMES

Respiratory status: airway patency: ventilation; gas exchange

NIC INTERVENTIONS

Respiratory monitoring; airway management; chest physiotherapy; cough enhancement; ventilation assistance; oxygen therapy; medication administration

NURSING ASSESSMENT

Assess for and report signs and symptoms of impaired respiratory function:
- Rapid, shallow respirations
- Dyspnea, orthopnea
- Use of accessory muscles when breathing
- Abnormal breath sounds (e.g., diminished, bronchial, crackles [rales], wheezes)
- Asymmetrical chest excursion
- Cough (can be productive or dry and nonproductive depending on the opportunistic disease present)
Monitor SaO_2 levels, arterial blood gas values, chest x-ray results.

RATIONALE

Early recognition of signs and symptoms of impaired respiratory function allows for prompt intervention.

THERAPEUTIC INTERVENTIONS

Independent Actions
Implement measures to improve respiratory status:
- Place client in a semi- to high-Fowler's positions unless contraindicated; position with pillows to prevent slumping. **D** ● ✦

- Instruct client to breathe slowly if hyperventilating.
- If client must remain flat in bed, assist with position change at least every 2 hrs. **D** ● ✦
- Instruct client to deep breathe or use incentive spirometer every 1 to 2 hrs. **D** ● ✦

- Perform actions to promote removal of pulmonary secretions.
- Instruct and assist client to cough or "huff" every 1 to 2 hrs.

- Discourage smoking.

RATIONALE

High-Fowler's positions allow for maximum diaphragmatic excursion and lung expansion. Prevention of slumping is essential because slumping causes abdominal contents to be pushed up and decreases lung expansion.
Slowing the client's breathing will decrease incidence of lightheadedness
Repositioning helps to mobilize secretions.

Deep breathing and use of an incentive spirometer promote maximal inhalation, lung expansion, improve sputum expectoration, and decrease incidence of serious lung infections.
Coughing or "huffing" accelerates airflow through the airways, helps mobilize and clear mucus and foreign matter from the respiratory tract.
The irritants in smoke increase mucus production, impair ciliary function, and can cause damage to the bronchial and alveolar walls; the carbon monoxide decreases oxygen availability.

THERAPEUTIC INTERVENTIONS	RATIONALE

Dependent/Collaborative Actions

Implement measures to improve respiratory status:

- Maintain activity restrictions as ordered to reduce oxygen needs.

  Helps to prevent shortness of breath.

- Assist with positive airway pressure techniques (e.g., continuous positive airway pressure [CPAP], bilevel positive airway pressure [BiPAP], flutter/positive expiratory pressure [PEP] device) if ordered.

  Positive pressure airway techniques increase intrapulmonary (alveolar) pressure, which helps re-expand alveoli and prevent further alveolar collapse.

- Perform actions to promote removal of pulmonary secretions:
  - Implement measures to thin tenacious secretions and reduce dryness of the respiratory mucous membrane:
  - Maintain a fluid intake of at least 2500 mL/day unless contraindicated.
  - Humidify inspired air as ordered.

  Adequate hydration and humidified inspired air help thin secretions, thus facilitating mobilization and expectoration of secretions.

- Assist with administration of mucolytics (e.g., acetylcysteine) and diluent or hydrating agents (e.g., water, saline) via nebulizer if ordered.
- Assist with or perform postural drainage therapy (PDT) if ordered.
- Perform suctioning if ordered.
- Administer expectorants (e.g., guaifenesin) if ordered.

  Mucolytics and diluent or hydrating agents are mucokinetic substances that reduce the viscosity of mucus, thus making it easier for the client to mobilize and clear secretions from the respiratory tract. Postural drainage and suctioning help prevent stasis of secretions and their removal from the respiratory tract.

- Perform actions to reduce pain and fatigue:
  - Administer analgesics before activities and procedures that can cause pain and before pain becomes severe.

  Reducing pain enables the client to breathe more deeply and participate in activities to improve respiratory status.

- Maintain oxygen therapy as ordered. **D** ✦

  Supplemental oxygen helps to support tissue oxygenation requirements.

- Administer central nervous system depressants judiciously; hold medication and consult physician if respiratory rate is less than 12 breaths/min.

  Central nervous system depressants such as opioid narcotics cause depression of the respiratory center and cough reflex. This can result in stasis of secretions and hypoventilation with impaired gas exchange.

- Administer the following medications if ordered:
  - Bronchodilators

  Bronchodilators dilate terminal airways, improving oxygen delivery and ventilation.

  - Antimicrobials

  Antimicrobials may be given to prevent pneumonia.

  - Corticosteroids

  Corticosteroids decrease pulmonary inflammation and are usually reserved for moderate to severe cases of PCP due to risk of further immunosuppression.

Consult appropriate health care provider (e.g., respiratory therapist, physician) if signs and symptoms of impaired respiratory function persist or worsen.

Consulting the appropriate health care provider allows for modification of the treatment plan.

Nursing Diagnosis ## ACUTE/CHRONIC PAIN NDx

Definition: Acute Pain NDx: Unpleasant sensory and emotional experience associated with actual or potential tissue damage, or described in terms of such damage (International Association for the Study of Pain); sudden or slow onset of any intensity from mild to severe with an anticipated or predictable end, and with a duration of less than 3 months.

Chronic Pain NDx: Unpleasant sensory and emotional experience associated with actual or potential tissue damage, or described in terms of such damage (International Association for the Study of Pain); sudden or slow onset of any intensity from mild to severe, constant or recurring without an anticipated or predictable end, and a duration of greater than 3 months.

Oral, pharyngeal, and/or esophageal pain related to the presence of aphthous ulcers in the mouth and/or infections involving the oropharyngeal and esophageal mucosa (e.g., candidiasis, herpes simplex).

Abdominal pain related to nonspecific gastritis and opportunistic infection or neoplastic involvement of the intestine.

Neuropathic pain related to the effect of HIV, some opportunistic infections, and impact of medications (e.g., didanosine, zalcitabine, isoniazid) on the peripheral nerves.

Headache related to:

- Cranial inflammation/pressure associated with an opportunistic infection involving the sinuses or brain or the presence of a cerebral neoplasm
- Vasoactive cytokines that are present with HIV infection

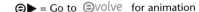
NDx = NANDA Diagnosis   **D** = Delegatable Action   ● = UAP   ✦ = LVN/LPN   ⊖▶ = Go to ⊖volve for animation

Chest pain related to:
- Inflammation of the parietal pleura associated with an opportunistic infection of the lungs
- Muscle strain associated with excessive coughing if present

Skin and local tissue pain related to:
- Skin lesions associated with opportunistic infection and/or Kaposi sarcoma
- Skin breakdown in perianal area associated with diarrhea

CLINICAL MANIFESTATIONS

Subjective	Objective
Verbal report of pain identifying changes in level of intensity using a pain rating scale; reported loss of appetite	Inability to breathe deeply, ambulate, sleep, or perform activities of daily living; crying; muscle rigidity; diaphoresis; blood pressure (BP) or pulse changes; increase in the rate and depth of breathing

RISK FACTORS
- Chronic physical disability
- Chronic psychosocial disability
- Medication side effects
- Disease processes fatigue

DESIRED OUTCOMES

The client will experience diminished pain as evidenced by:
a. Verbalization of a decrease in or absence of pain
b. Relaxed facial expression and body positioning
c. Increased participation in activities
d. Stable vital signs

NOC OUTCOMES

Comfort level; pain control; pain: disruptive effects

NIC INTERVENTIONS

Pain management; acute and chronic; environmental management: comfort; analgesic administration

NURSING ASSESSMENT	RATIONALE
Assess for and report signs and symptoms of pain: • Verbalization of pain • Grimacing • Reluctance to move or breathe deeply • Rubbing head • Reluctance to eat • Restlessness • Diaphoresis • Increased BP • Tachycardia	*Early recognition of signs and symptoms of acute or chronic pain allows for prompt intervention.*
Assess client's perception of the severity of pain using a pain intensity rating scale.	*Provides a more objective measure of pain experienced and a consistent standard for communication concerning pain.*
Assess the client's pain pattern: • Location • Quality • Onset • Duration • Precipitating factors • Aggravating factors • Alleviating factors	
Ask the client to describe previous pain experiences and methods used to manage pain effectively.	

THERAPEUTIC INTERVENTIONS	RATIONALE

Independent Actions

Implement measures to reduce pain: **D** ✦
* Perform actions to reduce fear and anxiety about the pain experience:
  * Assure client the need for pain relief is understood.
  * Plan methods for achieving pain control with client "including adjuvant methods of pain relief."
* Perform actions to reduce fear and anxiety:
  * Instruct client in relaxation techniques and encourage participation in diversional activities.
* Administer analgesics before activities and procedures that can cause pain and before pain becomes severe.

* Perform actions to reduce fatigue:
  * Organize nursing care to allow for uninterrupted periods of rest.

Collaborate with client to implement actions to achieve pain control
* Perform actions to prevent and treat oral mucous membrane and skin lesions:
  * Lubricate lips frequently. **D** ● ✦
  * Have client rinse mouth frequently with salt and warm water. **D** ● ✦

Actions help promote relaxation and subsequently increase the client's threshold and tolerance for pain.

Measures to promote relaxation and decrease anxiety (i.e., relaxation techniques, guided imagery), acupuncture, distraction, etc. can enhance relief of pain with or without drug interventions.

Pain relief improves client's ability to independently perform activities of daily living and increase activities, and will help to decrease difficulty in sleep.

Actions help to increase the client's threshold and tolerance for pain.

Collaborating with clients regarding pain control strategies provides the client a sense of control over the pain experience.

Provides additional moisture, removes bacteria, and improves oral mucosal integrity.

Dependent/Collaborative Actions

Implement measures to reduce pain:
* Administer the following if ordered:
  * Nonopioid (nonnarcotic) analgesics such as salicylates and other nonsteroidal anti-inflammatory agents
  * Opioid (narcotic) analgesics

* Tricyclic antidepressants (e.g., amitriptyline) and/or anticonvulsants (e.g., carbamazepine, gabapentin)
* Topical anesthetic/analgesic ointments (e.g., capsaicin)
* Oral anesthetic and/or protective agents (e.g., sucralfate, viscous xylocaine mixed with diphenhydramine elixir and a magnesium or aluminum antacid)
* Corticosteroids

* Antimicrobials and/or antineoplastic agents

Consult appropriate health care provider if adequate pain relief cannot be achieved with the above measures.

Nonopioid analgesics interfere with the transmission of pain impulses by inhibiting prostaglandin synthesis.

Opioid analgesics act by altering the client's perception of pain and emotional response to the pain experience.

Tricyclic antidepressants and anticonvulsant medications are used to treat painful neuropathies.

Topical anesthetics help alleviate skin and superficial neuropathic pain.

Anesthetic agents help control pain by inhibiting the initiation and conduction of pain impulses along sensory pathways.

Corticosteroids can decrease pain associated with some central nervous system lesions, sinusitis, and peripheral neuropathies.

These agents may be given to treat HIV infection and/or opportunistic disease(s) causing the pain.

Consulting the appropriate health care provider allows for modification of the treatment plan.

Nursing Diagnosis **SPIRITUAL DISTRESS** NDx

Definition: A state of suffering related to the impaired ability to experience meaning in life through connections with self, others, the world, or a superior being.

CLINICAL MANIFESTATIONS

Subjective	Objective
Self-reports of inability to forgive; ineffective relationships	

RISK FACTORS
- Stress
- Anxiety
- Chronic illness
- Fear of dying

DESIRED OUTCOMES

The client will maintain:
A sense of self-worth
Positive self-esteem
Connections with others
Connections with the world
Connections to a higher power than self

NOC OUTCOMES

Spiritual well-being

NIC INTERVENTIONS

Spiritual support; Spiritual Growth Facilitation

NURSING ASSESSMENT	**RATIONALE**
Assess for signs and symptoms of spiritual distress: Determine engagement in life activities that involve others Expressions of feelings of hopelessness, futility, and powerlessness Expressions of spiritual loss	*Early recognition of signs and symptoms of spiritual distress allows for prompt intervention.*

THERAPEUTIC INTERVENTIONS	**RATIONALE**

Independent Actions

Discuss client's engagement in spiritual religious activities.	*Allows nurse to determine what type of support client may require based on beliefs and level of engagement in spiritual/religious activities.*
Supports client's expression of anger, frustration, lack of spiritual connection, and feelings of loss, powerlessness, and fear.	*The nurse should reassure the client that these feelings are normal when diagnosed with a terminal illness. The nurse should provide non-judgmental care and allow the client to work through feelings.*
Collaborate with client in identify beliefs and values used to guide behavior.	*Helps client to clarify beliefs, values, and life goals.*

Collaborative Actions

Determine client's engagement with formalized religion and identity family and community resources including pastoral staff, grief and crisis counselors.	*Helps to engage others in supporting client. Provides post-discharge support for client and family.*
Identify and refer to community support groups with individuals of the same religious faith or spiritual convictions.	
Engage significant others in client's journey working through spiritual issues.	

DISCHARGE TEACHING/CONTINUED CARE

Nursing Diagnosis **INEFFECTIVE HEALTH MANAGEMENT NDx; INEFFECTIVE FAMILY HEALTH MANAGEMENT NDx**

Definition: Ineffective Health Management NDx: Pattern of regulating and integrating into daily living a therapeutic regimen for the treatment of illness and its sequelae that is unsatisfactory for meeting specific health goals; **Ineffective Family Health Management NDx:** A pattern of regulating and integrating into family processes a program for the treatment of illness and its sequelae that is unsatisfactory for meeting specific health goals of the family unit.

CLINICAL MANIFESTATIONS

Subjective	**Objective**
Self-report of the desire to manage illness; self-report of difficulty with prescribed regimen	Failure to include treatment regimen in daily routines; failure to take action to reduce risk factors; makes choices in daily living ineffective for meeting health goals; inadequate follow-through of instruction

RISK FACTORS

- Complex medication and treatment regimen
- Lack of recall
- Unfamiliarity with information, resources
- Economically disadvantaged
- Family conflict

NOC OUTCOMES	NIC INTERVENTIONS
Health Education	Health system guidance; teaching: disease process; teaching: prescribed diet; teaching: prescribed medication; communicable disease management; financial resource assistance

NURSING ASSESSMENT	RATIONALE
Assess the client's baseline understanding of: • Disease process • Therapeutic regimen • Health prevention measures	*Understanding the client's knowledge base allows for teaching appropriate information.*
Assess the client's access to resources to help with successful implementation of the treatment plan.	*Early identification of barriers to therapeutic regimen management allows for implementation of the appropriate interventions.*

THERAPEUTIC INTERVENTIONS	RATIONALE

Desired Outcome: The client will identify ways to prevent the spread of HIV.

Independent Actions

Instruct client in ways to prevent the spread of HIV to others:	*HIV is a fragile virus that is transmitted only under specified conditions. They include when client comes in contact with infected body fluids including blood, vaginal secretions, and breast milk. HIV is transmitted through sexual intercourse with an infected partner, exposure to infected body fluids, and perinatal transmission during pregnancy, at the time of delivery, or through breast-feeding.*
• If a spill of blood or other body fluids occurs, cleanse area with hot, soapy water or a household detergent and then disinfect with a solution of 1 part bleach to 10 parts water.	*HIV is rapidly destroyed after being exposed to chemical germicides such as household bleach.*
• Dispose of water used to clean up body fluid spills in the toilet.	*Prevents further contamination.*
• Do not share eating utensils, toothbrushes, razors, enema equipment, or sexual devices.	*Prevents transmission of HIV.*
• Avoid getting pregnant, but if pregnancy occurs, consult health care provider about antiretroviral therapy (e.g., zidovudine) to reduce the risk of perinatal transmission of HIV to infant.	*Consulting health care provider allows for early intervention.*
• Do not breast-feed infant.	
• Do not donate blood, sperm, or body organs.	
• If an intravenous drug user:	*Drug use in and of itself does not cause HIV.*
• Get involved in a needle and syringe exchange program.	*The major risk for HIV infection with drug use is the sharing of drug paraphernalia that may contain the blood of an infected individual. These interventions prevent exposure to other pathogens and transmission of HIV.*
• Do not share drug-injecting equipment (e.g., needles, syringes, cookers, cotton, rinse water).	
• Discard disposable needles and syringes after one use or clean them with household bleach and rinse thoroughly with water.	
• If sexually active with a partner:	*Safe sexual activity decreases the risk of exposure to HIV in semen and vaginal secretions. Abstinence is the most effective method.*
• Avoid multiple sexual partners and partners with risky sexual behaviors; be honest with desired partner about HIV infection.	
• Modify techniques so that both partners are protected from contact with body fluids.	
• Avoid unsafe sexual practices:	
• Sharing sex toys	
• Allowing ejaculate to come in contact with broken skin or mucous membranes	

Continued...

THERAPEUTIC INTERVENTIONS	RATIONALE
• Intercourse without a condom	
• Any activity that could cause tears in lining of vagina, rectum, or penis	
• Mouth contact with penis, vagina, or anal area	
• Avoid vaginal intercourse during menstruation (the contact with blood increases the risk of HIV transmission).	
• Instruct the client in effective use of condoms:	*Barriers should be used when engaging in insertive sexual activity. The effectiveness of male condoms is 80% to 90%.*
• Always use a barrier (male and/or female condom) during anal, vaginal, and oral penetration (condom should be applied before a body orifice is entered because HIV is found in preseminal fluid).	
• Use latex or polyurethane condoms (HIV can penetrate other types of materials).	
• Use condoms with a receptacle tip to reduce the risk of spillage of semen; if that type is unavailable, create a receptacle for ejaculate by pinching tip of condom as it is rolled on erect penis.	
• Lubricate outside of condom and area to be penetrated to minimize possibility of condom breakage.	
• Avoid lubricants made of mineral oil or petroleum distillates such as Vaseline or baby oil (these products weaken latex).	
• Hold condom at base of penis during withdrawal and use caution during removal of condom to prevent spillage of semen (penis should be withdrawn and condom removed before the penis has totally relaxed).	
• Dispose of condom immediately after use (a new one should be used for subsequent sexual activity).	
• Store condoms in a cool place to prevent them from drying out and breaking during use.	
• Do not use a condom if the expiration date on the package has passed, the package looks worn or punctured, or if the condom looks brittle or discolored or is sticky.	

THERAPEUTIC INTERVENTIONS	RATIONALE

Desired Outcome: The client will identify ways to decrease the risk for developing opportunistic infections.

Independent Actions

Instruct client in ways to decrease risk for developing an opportunistic infection:

• Cleanse kitchen and bathroom surfaces regularly with a disinfectant to prevent growth of pathogens.

• If respiratory equipment (e.g., inhalers, humidifier) is used at home, cleanse it as instructed and change water in humidifier daily.

• Wear gloves when gardening and when in contact with human or pet excreta (e.g., cleaning litter boxes, bird cages, and aquariums).

• Avoid exposure to body fluids during sexual activity and use latex or polyurethane condoms during sexual intercourse.

• Reduce the risk of food-borne illness.

  • Thoroughly wash hands and food preparation items and surfaces (e.g., knives, cutting board, countertop) before and after cooking, especially when working with raw meat, poultry, and fish.

HIV disease progression may be delayed by promoting a healthy immune system.

Actions that result in avoiding exposure to new infections are useful.

Prevents exposure to other pathogens.

THERAPEUTIC INTERVENTIONS	RATIONALE

- Avoid intake of foods/fluids with a high microorganism content (e.g., raw or undercooked poultry, seafood, meats, or eggs; unwashed fruits and vegetables; unpasteurized dairy products or fruit juices; raw seed sprouts; soft cheeses; anything that has passed its expiration date).
- Cook leftover foods or ready-to-eat foods (e.g., hot dogs) until steaming hot before eating.
- Avoid foods from delicatessen counters (e.g., prepared meats, salads, cheeses) and refrigerated pâtés and other meat spreads, or reheat these foods until steaming before eating.
- Do not drink water directly from lakes or rivers.
- Boil water for a full minute if a community "boil water" advisory is issued.

- Avoid activities such as cleaning, remodeling, or demolishing old buildings; exploring caves; disturbing soil beneath bird-roosting sites or cleaning chicken coops; being around disturbed native soil at building excavation sites or dust storms.
- Wash hands after handling pets and avoid contact with reptiles (e.g., snakes, lizards, turtles), baby chickens, and ducklings.
- Avoid swimming in lakes, rivers, and public pools.
- Keep living quarters well ventilated and change furnace filters regularly to reduce exposure to airborne disease.
- Avoid contact with persons who have an infection and those who have been recently vaccinated.
- Maintain an adequate balance between activity and rest.
- Drink at least 10 glasses of liquid each day unless contraindicated.
- Contact health care provider before undergoing vaccinations.

Old buildings, damp areas may be source of molds or environmental contaminants. Other areas may be considered to be endemic areas for histoplasmosis and coccidioidomycosis.

Action reduces the risk of exposure to environmental contaminants that may lead to viral or bacterial infection.

Supports immune system.

Many vaccines are composed of live viruses and create a health risk for those with compromised immune systems.

THERAPEUTIC INTERVENTIONS	RATIONALE

Desired Outcome: The client will verbalize ways to maintain optimal nutritional status.

Independent Actions

Provide instructions regarding ways to maintain an optimal nutritional status:

- Eat foods that are high in protein and calories.
- Try to eat a snack or a small meal or drink a nutritional supplement every 2 to 3 hrs.
- Take prescribed vitamins, appetite stimulants (e.g., megestrol acetate), and anabolic agents (e.g., oxandrolone).
- Participate in a progressive exercise program if possible.

Proper nutrition is essential to maintain body mass and ensure the necessary levels of vitamins and nutrients.

Each of these actions help to maintain nutritional status. Supplements may be required to stimulate appetite or provide additional nutritional support.

THERAPEUTIC INTERVENTIONS	RATIONALE

Desired Outcome: The client will state signs and symptoms to report to the health care provider.

Independent Actions

Stress importance of notifying the health care provider if the following signs and symptoms occur or if these existing signs and symptoms worsen:

- Persistent fever or chills
- Night sweats

Clients must notify the health care provider of signs and symptoms of disease progression and/or the development of opportunistic infections so the treatment plan can be modified.

Continued...

THERAPEUTIC INTERVENTIONS	RATIONALE

- Persistent headache or different type of headache
- Swollen glands
- Skin lesions or significant rash
- Reddish purple patches or nodules on any body area
- Ulcerations or white patches in the mouth
- Difficulty swallowing
- Persistent diarrhea or vomiting
- Perianal or vulvovaginal itching and/or pain
- Frequency, urgency, or burning on urination
- Cloudy or foul-smelling urine
- Dry cough or a cough productive of purulent, green, or rust-colored sputum
- Progressive shortness of breath
- Increasing weakness, fatigue, or weight loss
- Change in vision, spots that appear to drift in front of eye (floaters)
- Decline in mental function or level of consciousness
- Loss of strength and coordination in extremities
- Inability to maintain an adequate fluid intake
- Yellow discoloration of skin
- Bleeding from rectum that is not related to hemorrhoids
- Severe depression or anxiousness or feelings of being a danger to self or others
- Seizures

THERAPEUTIC INTERVENTIONS	RATIONALE

Desired Outcome: The client will identify resources that can assist with financial needs and adjustment to changes resulting from the diagnosis of HIV/AIDS.

Independent Actions

Provide information to client and significant others about private, local, state and federally funded financial programs and resources that can assist in adjustment to the diagnosis of AIDS (e.g., Ryan White HIV/AIDS Program, hospice programs, community support groups, HIV/AIDS Hotline, Project Inform).

Provides client and family with knowledge of resources to sustain therapeutic regimen if experiencing financial difficulties.

THERAPEUTIC INTERVENTIONS	RATIONALE

Desired Outcome: The client, in collaboration with the nurse, will develop a plan for adhering to recommended follow-up care including regular laboratory studies, future appointments with health care providers, and prescribed medication regimen.

Independent Actions

Stress the importance of adhering to the prescribed treatment regimen.

Reinforce the importance of keeping scheduled follow-up appointments for laboratory studies and with health care providers.

Explain the rationale for, side effects of, and importance of taking medications prescribed (e.g., antiretroviral agents, antimicrobial agents, hematopoietic agents, anabolic agents, appetite stimulants).

Inform client of techniques to decrease medication side effects.

Adherence to the prescribed regimen can reduce hospitalization, improve outcomes, and aid in maintaining optimal health status.

Helps health care professionals support client in maintenance of health and provides early recognition of disease process changes.

The medication regimen for clients with HIV/AIDS is very complex, has many side effects, and can be expensive. The more clients understand their medication regimen, the more successful they may be in adherence.

Experience of side effects is one reason for non-adherence. Knowing actions that can decrease incidence will help adherence to regimen.

THERAPEUTIC INTERVENTIONS	RATIONALE
Inform client of pertinent food and drug interactions and ways to decrease the experience of drug side effects.	*Providing this information allows the client to assume some control of their health care regimen and may improve adherence.*
Reinforce the importance of strictly adhering to the antiretroviral regimen prescribed (usually consists of a combination of at least three antiretroviral agents).	*Helps client understand the importance of taking medications as prescribed.*
Explain that not adhering to the prescribed regimen will limit the effectiveness of subsequent regimens.	*Full adherence to medication regimen prevents potential for resistance to retroviral medications.*
Explain the importance of taking the full dose of any antimicrobial agents prescribed. Reinforce the possibility that lifelong treatment with antimicrobials may be necessary.	*Antimicrobials such as trimethoprim-sulfamethoxazole [TMP-SMX]) may be necessary to prevent some opportunistic infections if the CD4+ cell count is critically low.*
Implement measures to improve client compliance: • Include significant others in teaching sessions if possible. • Encourage questions and allow time for reinforcement and clarification of information provided. • Provide written instructions regarding scheduled appointments with health care providers and laboratory, medications prescribed, signs and symptoms to report, and ways to prevent infection. • Collaborate with client and significant others to develop a plan for integration of health care regimen into activities of daily living.	*Including significant others in client teaching will help improve support for client and provides time for clarification of information.* *Written instructions provide informational resources for client and family to use once discharged from the acute care facility.* *Client engagement in developing the plan of care allows some control over the process, boosts confidence in their ability to manage health status, and improves adherence.*

ADDITIONAL NURSING DIAGNOSES

DIARRHEA NDx
Related to: A direct effect of HIV on the intestine or opportunistic disease involvement of the intestine
• Side effect of some antiretroviral agents (e.g., protease inhibitors, didanosine)

IMPAIRED COMFORT NDx (PRURITUS)
Related to:
• Dry skin associated with deficient fluid volume
• Pruritic folliculitis
• Dermatological disorders such as seborrheic dermatitis, photodermatitis, and psoriasis
• Side effects of some antimicrobials
• Oral and vulvovaginal candidiasis

IMPAIRED ORAL MUCOUS MEMBRANE NDx
Related to:
• Malnutrition and deficient fluid volume
• Infections such as candidiasis, herpes simplex, oral hairy leukoplakia, and bacterial gingivitis/periodontitis
• Kaposi sarcoma or lymphoma in the oral cavity

RISK FOR IMPAIRED SKIN INTEGRITY NDx
Related to:
Presence of cutaneous infections
  • Presence of skin disorders
  • Skin lesions associated with Kaposi sarcoma if present
Excessive scratching associated with pruritus
  • Increased skin fragility associated with malnutrition
  • Persistent contact with irritants associated with diarrhea
  • Damage to the skin and/or subcutaneous tissue associated with prolonged pressure on tissues, friction, or shearing if mobility is decreased

FEAR NDx/ANXIETY
Related to:
• Threat of permanent worsening of health status; possible disability and death
• Threat to self-concept associated with changes in physical and mental functioning (e.g., wasting syndrome, gait difficulty, poor coordination, dementia)
• Stigma associated with having AIDS
• Financial concerns
• Separation from support system
• Possibility of transmitting disease to others

INEFFECTIVE COPING NDx
Related to:
• Depression, fear, anxiety, and ongoing grieving associated with the diagnosis of HIV/AIDS and long-term illness
• Need for permanent change in lifestyle associated with impaired immune system functioning and potential for disease transmission to others
• Uncertainty of disease process and feelings of powerlessness over course of disease
• Need for disclosure of diagnosis with possibility of subsequent rejection and/or distancing by others and loss of employment and health benefits
• Guilt associated with past behavior and/or possibility of having transmitted HIV to others
• Lack of personal resources to deal with disability and premature death associated with youth
• Multiple losses (e.g., death of close friends with AIDS; loss of normal body functioning, family support, financial security, and/or usual lifestyle and roles)
• Chronic symptoms (e.g., pain, diarrhea, fatigue) if present

RISK FOR LONELINESS NDx
Related to:
- Fear of associating with others because of possibility of contracting an infection
- Stigma and discrimination associated with the diagnosis of HIV/AIDS and others' fear of contracting HIV
- Decreased participation in usual activities because of weakness, pain, fatigue, and fear of falls
- Withdrawal from others associated with fear of embarrassment resulting from decline in physical and mental functioning

INTERRUPTED FAMILY PROCESSES NDx
Related to:
- Diagnosis of terminal, communicable disease in family member
- Fear of disclosure of diagnosis with subsequent rejection of family unit
- Change in family roles and structure associated with progressive disability and eventual death of family member
- Financial burden associated with extended illness and progressive disability of client
- Fear of contracting disease from client
- Decisions made by client and his/her significant other about such issues as treatment plan, life support, and disposition of property that may conflict with the client's family of origin
- Anticipatory grief

DISTURBED SLEEP PATTERN NDx
Related to: Fear, anxiety, depression, frequent assessments and treatments, pain, diarrhea, pruritus, chills, night sweats, coughing and dyspnea (may occur if respiratory infection is present), unfamiliar environment, and the effect of some medications

INEFFECTIVE SEXUALITY PATTERN NDx
Related to:
- Rejection by desired partner associated with his/her fear of contracting HIV/AIDS
- Need to disclose to new partner(s) the diagnosis of HIV/AIDS
- Decreased sexual desire associated with fatigue, pain, weakness, anxiety, depression, and fear of transmitting or contracting disease

POWERLESSNESS NDx
Related to:
- The disabling and terminal nature of AIDS
- Increasing dependence on others to meet basic needs
- Changes in roles, relationships, and future plans

GRIEVING NDx
Related to:
- Having an incurable illness with an uncertain course and a high probability of premature death
- Changes in body functioning, appearance, lifestyle, and roles associated with the disease process

HYPERTHERMIA NDx
Related to: Stimulation of the thermoregulatory center in the hypothalamus by endogenous pyrogens that are released in an infectious process

FATIGUE NDx
Related to:
- Difficulty with sleep and rest patterns
- Increased energy utilization associated with the elevated metabolic rate that is present with infection
- Malnutrition

SEPSIS

Sepsis, as defined by the American College of Chest Physicians and Society of Critical Care Medicine, is a "life-threatening organ dysfunction caused by a dysregulated host response to infection" (Singer et.al., p. 804). The new criteria for a diagnosis of sepsis are altered mental status, rapid respiratory rate (>22 breaths/min), and low blood pressure (≤100 mm Hg systolic). Blood tests are no longer required for the diagnosis. Clients with two of the three criteria are considered to be septic.

The most common sites of infection that lead to sepsis are the lungs, blood, abdominal/pelvic cavity, and the urinary tract.

Once the causative organism enters the blood (referred to as septicemia or bacteremia), the toxins produced by the pathogens initiate a widespread inflammatory and immune response commonly referred to as the systemic inflammatory response syndrome. This inflammatory response is designed to be a protective process but if uncontrolled, triggers the release of many inflammatory mediators that subsequently cause widespread vasodilation, injury to the endothelium, and increased capillary permeability. This chain of events can lead to maldistribution of circulating blood with hypotension, hypoperfusion, and organ dysfunction. Septic shock, disseminated intravascular coagulation (DIC), and multiple organ dysfunction syndrome (MODS) can develop if this chain of events is not reversed.

According to the CDC, more than 1.5 million individuals will get sepsis each year in the United States. One in three patients who die in the hospital have sepsis. Individuals at highest risk for sepsis are infants, children, the elderly, and people who have serious injuries or medical problems such as diabetes, an impaired immune system, cancer, or liver disease. Sepsis occurs due to the failure of the body's defense mechanisms to an infection caused by bacteria, viruses, or fungi. However, bacterial infections are the most common cause.

The Quick Sepsis-related organ failure assessment (qSFOA) score is used to identify anyone who has an infection to identify clients at high risk for sepsis. The score utilizes the three criteria utilized to diagnose sepsis: altered mental status, rapid respiratory rate (>22 breaths/min), and low blood pressure (≤100 mm Hg systolic). Scores range from 0 to 3 points. The presence of two or more qSOFA indicators at onset of infection has been associated with a prolonged stay in the ICU or a greater risk of death. The qSOFA is a risk identification tool to help determine who may be at risk for the development of sepsis. The nurse should assess anyone who is suspected of having an infection using the qSOFA. Early recognition and prompt treatment are critical to decreasing the incidence of sepsis and improving client mortality.

This care plan focuses on care of the adult client hospitalized for treatment of sepsis.

OUTCOME/DISCHARGE CRITERIA

The client will:
1. Demonstrate evidence that infection is resolving
2. Maintain stable vital signs
3. Experience no signs and symptoms of complications
4. Verbalize understanding of ways to promote continued resolution of the existing infection
5. Discuss ways to reduce the risk for recurrent infections
6. List signs and symptoms to report to the health care provider
7. Develop a plan for adhering to recommended follow-up care including future appointments with health care provider, medications prescribed, and activity limitations

---

Nursing Diagnosis | # RISK FOR INEFFECTIVE PERIPHERAL TISSUE PERFUSION NDx
RISK FOR INEFFECTIVE CEREBRAL TISSUE PERFUSION NDx
RISK FOR DECREASED CARDIAC TISSUE PERFUSION NDx

Definition: **Risk for Ineffective Peripheral Tissue Perfusion NDx:** Susceptible to a decrease in blood circulation to the periphery, which may compromise health; **Risk for Ineffective Cerebral Tissue Perfusion NDx:** Susceptible to a decrease in cerebral circulation, which may compromise health; **Risk for Decreased Cardiac Tissue Perfusion NDx:** Susceptible to a decrease in cardiac (coronary) circulation, which may compromise health.

Related to:
- Maldistribution of circulating fluid volume associated with vasodilation, fluid shift that occurs with increased capillary permeability, and selective vasoconstriction occurring in response to inflammatory mediators (e.g., cytokines, complement, histamine, kinins)
- Hypovolemia associated with deficient fluid volume resulting from decreased fluid intake, excessive loss of fluid (e.g., diaphoresis, hyperventilation, vomiting, and/or diarrhea if present), and the fluid shift that occurs with increased capillary permeability
- Decreased cardiac output (occurs late in severe sepsis and shock) associated with the depressant effect of lactic acidosis, myocardial dysfunction related to inflammatory mediators (e.g., cytokines)

CLINICAL MANIFESTATIONS

Subjective	Objective
Restlessness	Decreased BP; confusion; cool extremities; pallor or cyanosis of extremities; diminished or absent peripheral pulses; slow capillary refill; edema; oliguria

RISK FACTORS

- Smoking
- Hyperlipidemia
- Sedentary lifestyle
- Underlying infection

DESIRED OUTCOMES

The client will maintain adequate tissue perfusion as evidenced by:
a. BP within normal range for client
b. Usual mental status
c. Extremities warm with absence of pallor and cyanosis
d. Palpable peripheral pulses
e. Capillary refill time less than 2 to 3 seconds
f. Absence of edema
g. Urine output at least 30 mL/h

NOC OUTCOMES

Circulation status; tissue perfusion: cardiac, cerebral and peripheral

NIC INTERVENTIONS

Circulatory care: arterial insufficiency; circulatory care: venous insufficiency; cerebral perfusion promotion; hypovolemia management; cardiac care: acute and rehabilitative

---

NDx = NANDA Diagnosis   **D** = Delegatable Action   ● = UAP   ✦ = LVN/LPN   ⊖▶ = Go to ⊖volve for animation

NURSING ASSESSMENT	RATIONALE
Assess for and report signs and symptoms of diminished tissue perfusion: • Decreased BP • Changes in heart rate and rhythm • Confusion • Cool, pale or cyanotic extremities • Diminished or absent peripheral pulses • Slow capillary refill >2 to 3 seconds • Edema • Oliguria <30 mL/h Monitor hemodynamic status: • Vital signs • Urine output • Central venous pressure (if applicable)	*Early recognition of signs and symptoms of ineffective tissue perfusion allows for prompt intervention.*

THERAPEUTIC INTERVENTIONS	RATIONALE

Dependent/Collaborative Actions
 	
• Perform actions to maintain adequate tissue perfusion:
  • Administer intravenous fluids (colloids/crystalloids) as ordered.
  • Administer vasopressors and positive inotropic agents if ordered to maintain adequate perfusion pressure and cardiac output.
• Perform actions to prevent or treat deficient fluid volume:
  • Control diarrhea if present.
  • Reduce nausea and vomiting if present.
  • Administer antimicrobial agents as ordered.
 	
Consult appropriate health care provider if signs and symptoms of diminished tissue perfusion persist or worsen.
	Maintaining adequate vascular volume helps to ensure adequate tissue perfusion. The massive vasodilation that occurs during sepsis results in a relative hypovolemia or distributive shock. Adequate volume replacement must occur first. If BP remains low after volume has been replaced, vasopressors and/or inotropes may be added to support circulation. Adequate tissue perfusion promotes delivery of oxygen at the tissue level.
	
	Antimicrobial agents help to resolve the infectious process and control the systemic inflammatory response.
	Allows for timely modification of the treatment plan

Nursing Diagnosis   RISK FOR IMBALANCED FLUID VOLUME NDx

Definition: Susceptible to a decrease, increase, or rapid fluid shift from one to the other of intravascular, interstitial, and/or intracellular fluid, which may compromise health. This refers to body fluid loss, gain, or both.

Related to:
• Decreased oral intake associated with anorexia, fatigue, and nausea if present
• Increased insensible fluid loss associated with diaphoresis and hyperventilation if present
• Excessive loss of fluid associated with vomiting and/or diarrhea if present with initial infection or as a side effect of antimicrobial therapy
• Fluid shift from the intravascular to interstitial space associated with the increased capillary permeability that occurs with a systemic inflammatory response

CLINICAL MANIFESTATIONS

Subjective	Objective
N/A	Decreased BP; decreased pulse pressure; decreased skin turgor; dry mucous membranes; tachycardia; elevated Hct; increased body temperature; decreased urine output; increased urine concentration; dependent edema; increased urine specific gravity

DESIRED OUTCOMES

The client will not experience deficient fluid volume as evidenced by:
a. Normal skin turgor
b. Moist mucous membranes
c. Stable weight
d. BP and heart rate within normal range for client and stable with position change
e. Usual mental status
f. BUN and Hct values within normal range
g. Balanced intake and output
h. Urine specific gravity within normal range

NOC OUTCOMES	NIC INTERVENTIONS
Fluid management: adequate hydration	Hypovolemia management; intravenous therapy; fever treatment; diarrhea management; nausea management

NURSING ASSESSMENT	RATIONALE
Assess for and report signs and symptoms of imbalanced fluid volume: • Decreased skin turgor • Dry mucous membranes, thirst • Weight loss of 2% or greater over a short period • Postural hypotension and/or low BP • Weak, rapid pulse • Neck veins flat when client is supine • Change in mental status • Decrease in urine output with increased specific gravity Monitor BUN and Hct values.	*Early recognition of signs and symptoms of imbalanced fluid volume allows for prompt intervention.*

THERAPEUTIC INTERVENTIONS	RATIONALE
Independent Actions Implement measures to prevent or treat imbalanced fluid volume Monitor blood pressure and heart rate.	*Decreased vascular fluid volume leads to decreased blood pressure and subsequent tachycardia. May demonstrate shift of fluid from intravascular to interstitial compartments.*
Monitor and document intake and output, correlating these findings with daily weight; measure urine specific gravity.	*Decreased urine output with increased specific gravity is indicative of hypovolemia. Correlation of changes in weight with I & O may indicate increased vascular permeability leading to edema.*
Monitor and document decreased peripheral pulses.	*May indicate changes in vascular fluid volume.*
Monitor and document incidence and level of edema.	*Indicates shift of vascular fluid volume into the interstitial tissues; increasing level of edema may indicate worsening fluid volume deficit.*
Dependent/Collaborative Actions Implement measures to prevent or treat imbalanced fluid volume: • Encourage oral intake of fluid if client is not on NPO; keep ice chips and water easily accessible to client.	*Helps to maintain fluid volume; helps to maintain oral cavity integrity; easy accessibility of water and ice chips provides clients a measure of control over care*

• Perform actions to reduce nausea and vomiting if present:
  • Administer antimicrobial agents with food unless contraindicated.
  • Administer prescribed antiemetics.
	Helps to prevent further loss of fluid.
	Helps client tolerate medications.
	Decreases incidence of nausea and vomiting.

• Perform actions to control diarrhea if present:
  • Consult physician about another antimicrobial agent if onset of diarrhea seems related to initiation of antimicrobial therapy.
  • Administer prescribed antidiarrheal agents.
	Prolonged diarrhea can lead to excessive fluid loss and exacerbate dehydration.

Continued...

THERAPEUTIC INTERVENTIONS	RATIONALE
• Perform actions to reduce fever.	*Actions help to reduce insensible fluid loss associated with diaphoresis and hyperventilation.*
• Administer antimicrobial agents as ordered to treat the infection and decrease the release of inflammatory mediators.	*Decreasing the release of inflammatory mediators associated with infection decreases capillary permeability and the resultant fluid shift.*
• Maintain a fluid intake of at least 2500 mL/day unless contraindicated; if oral intake is inadequate or contraindicated, maintain intravenous fluid therapy as ordered.	*Maintains adequate vascular volume to support cardiac functioning.*

Nursing Diagnosis   ## IMPAIRED GAS EXCHANGE NDx

Definition: Excess or deficit in oxygenation and/or carbon dioxide elimination at the alveolar-capillary membrane.

Related to: Decreased pulmonary blood flow associated with a reduction in systemic tissue perfusion resulting from inflammatory-mediated vasodilation, fluid shift with increased capillary permeability, and selective vasoconstriction
• Loss of effective lung surface associated with:
  • Hypoventilation-associated atelectasis and decrease in surfactant production with diminished blood flow to the lungs
  • Accumulation of secretions in the lungs subsequent to decreased mobility, poor cough effort, and increased production of secretions
  • Fluid accumulation in the lungs resulting from generalized endothelial damage and increase in capillary permeability that occur with a systemic inflammatory response

CLINICAL MANIFESTATIONS

Subjective	Objective
Verbal self-reports of shortness of breath; visual disturbances; headache upon awakening	Confusion; restlessness; dyspnea; irritability; somnolence; abnormal pulse oximetry and arterial blood gas values; abnormal skin color; abnormal breathing patterns; tachycardia; diaphoresis

RISK FACTORS
• Alveolocapillary membrane changes
• Ventilation perfusion abnormalities
• Smoking
• Respiratory infection

DESIRED OUTCOMES

The client will experience adequate oxygen/carbon dioxide exchange as evidenced by:
a. Usual mental status
b. Unlabored respirations at 12 to 20 breaths/min
c. Oximetry results within normal range
d. Arterial blood gas values within normal range
e. Maintain clear lung sounds

NOC OUTCOMES

Respiratory status: gas exchange
Acid-base balance

NIC INTERVENTIONS

Respiratory monitoring; cough enhancement; chest physiotherapy; oxygen therapy; airway management
Acid-base management: respiratory pattern; electrolyte imbalance; HCO_3 deficit

NURSING ASSESSMENT	RATIONALE
Assess for and report signs and symptoms of impaired gas exchange: • Restlessness, irritability • Confusion, somnolence • Tachypnea, dyspnea • Significant decrease in oximetry results • Decreased partial pressure of arterial oxygen (PaO_2) and/or increased partial pressure of arterial carbon dioxide ($PaCO_2$) Monitor pulse oximetry and arterial blood gas values	*Early recognition of signs and symptoms of impaired gas exchange allows for prompt intervention.*

THERAPEUTIC INTERVENTIONS	RATIONALE

Independent Actions

Implement measures to improve gas exchange: **D** ✦

- Place client in a semi- to high-Fowler's positions unless contraindicated.

Improves lung expansion, and decreases potential for aspiration.

- Instruct and assist client to change position, deep breathe, and cough at least every 2 hrs.

Provides for mobilization of secretions.

- If severely dyspneic and physically able, assist client to assume the tripod position (leaning forward, with elbows supported on the bedside table).

Decreases gastric pressure on the diaphragm and allows improved lung expansion.

- Discourage smoking.

The irritants in smoke increase mucus production, impair ciliary function, and can damage the bronchial and alveolar walls; the carbon monoxide decreases oxygen availability.

Dependent/Collaborative Actions

Implement measures to improve gas exchange:

- Perform actions to maintain adequate tissue perfusion:

Maintaining adequate tissue perfusion helps to ensure adequate pulmonary blood flow.

  - Administer intravenous fluids (colloids/crystalloids) as ordered.

  - Administer vasopressors and positive inotropic agents if ordered to maintain adequate perfusion pressure and cardiac output.

The massive vasodilation that occurs during sepsis results in a relative hypovolemia or distributive shock. Adequate volume replacement must occur first. If BP remains low after volume has been replaced, vasopressors and/or inotropes may be added to support circulation. Adequate tissue perfusion promotes delivery of oxygen at the tissue level.

  - Monitor intake and output.

Fluid balance is critical in sepsis. Intake and output must be measured to assure fluid balance. Fluid overload in the first 48–96 hrs is associated with increased mortality.

- Assist with positive airway pressure techniques (e.g., continuous positive airway pressure [CPAP], bilevel positive airway pressure [BiPAP], flutter/positive expiratory pressure [PEP] device) if ordered.

All actions help to open terminal airways/alveoli, increasing the surface area available for gas exchange to occur, resulting in improved oxygenation.

- Maintain activity restrictions as ordered; increase activity gradually as allowed and tolerated.

Restricting activity lowers the body's oxygen requirements and decreases cardiovascular energy requirement.

- Administer antimicrobial agents as ordered.

Antimicrobial agents help to resolve the infectious process and control the systemic inflammatory response.

Consult appropriate health care provider (respiratory therapist, physician) if signs and symptoms of impaired gas exchange persist or worsen.

Allows for modification of the treatment plan.

Nursing Diagnosis ## HYPERTHERMIA NDx

Definition: Core body temperature above the normal diurnal range due to failure of thermoregulation.

Related to: Stimulation of the thermoregulatory center in the hypothalamus by endogenous pyrogens that are released in an infectious process

CLINICAL MANIFESTATIONS

Subjective	Objective
Self-report of chills	Flushed skin; increase in body temperature; tachycardia; tachypnea; warm to touch

RISK FACTORS

- Illness or trauma
- Increased metabolic rate
- Dehydration
- Infection or Sepsis
- Burns

DESIRED OUTCOMES

The client will experience resolution of hyperthermia as evidenced by:
a. Skin usual temperature and color
b. Pulse rate between 60 and 100 beats/min
c. Respiratory rate 12 to 20 breaths/min
d. Normal body temperature

NOC OUTCOMES

Thermoregulation

NIC INTERVENTIONS

Hyperthermia treatment: fever treatment

NURSING ASSESSMENT

Assess for signs and symptoms of hyperthermia:
- Warm, flushed skin
- Tachycardia
- Tachypnea
- Elevated temperature

RATIONALE

Early recognition and reporting of signs and symptoms of hyperthermia allow for prompt intervention.

THERAPEUTIC INTERVENTIONS

Independent Actions

Implement measures to reduce fever:
- Perform actions to resolve the infectious process: **D** ✦
  - Implement measures to promote rest (assist client with activities of daily living, provide uninterrupted rest periods, limit visitors).
  - Encourage client to eat a well-balanced diet high in essential nutrients.
- Administer tepid sponge bath and/or apply cool cloths to groin and axillae if indicated. **D** ● ✦
- Use a room air conditioner and room fan to provide cool, circulating air.

RATIONALE

Preserves energy to focus on underlying condition causing an increased temperature.

Helps to fight off infection.

Decreases body temperature.

Cool, ambient temperature helps other measures to decrease body temperature. It is important to prevent shivering as this will increase oxygen consumption.

Dependent/Collaborative Actions

Implement measures to reduce fever:
- Perform actions to resolve the infectious process:
  - Maintain a fluid intake of at least 2500 mL/day unless contraindicated.
  - Administer antimicrobials as ordered.
- Apply cooling blanket if ordered
- Administer antipyretics if ordered.

Consult physician if temperature remains higher than 38.5°C.

Dehydration can lead to increased body temperature.

Treats/prevents infection.
Decreases core body temperature.

Allows for prompt alteration in interventions.

Nursing Diagnosis   # RISK FOR INFECTION NDx (SUPERINFECTION)

Definition: Susceptible to invasion and multiplication of pathogenic organisms, which may compromise health.

Related to:
- Decreased resistance to infection associated with depletion of immune mechanisms resulting from the current infection and treatment with antimicrobial agents
- Stasis of respiratory secretions and/or urinary stasis if mobility is decreased or with dehydration
- Break in skin integrity associated with frequent venipunctures or presence of invasive lines

CLINICAL MANIFESTATIONS

Subjective	**Objective**
Verbal self-reports of pain at areas of impaired skin integrity	Increased body temperature; redness, warmth; discharge over areas of impaired skin integrity

RISK FACTORS

- Prolonged hospitalization
- Trauma
- Smoking
- Aging
- Suppressed inflammatory response
- Invasive procedure
- Chronic illness
- Immunosuppression

DESIRED OUTCOMES

The client will have resolution of existing infection and remain free of superinfection as evidenced by:
a. Return of temperature toward normal range
b. Decrease in episodes of chills and diaphoresis
c. Pulse rate returning toward normal range
d. Normal or improved breath sounds
e. Absence or resolution of dyspnea and cough
f. Stable or improved mental status
g. Voiding clear urine without reports of frequency, urgency, and burning
h. No reports of increased weakness and fatigue
i. Absence or resolution of heat, pain, redness, swelling, and unusual drainage in any area
j. Absence of oral mucous membrane lesions and ulceration
k. WBC and differential counts returning toward normal range
l. Negative results of cultured specimens

NOC OUTCOMES

Risk identification: immune status; infection severity

NIC INTERVENTIONS

Infection control; infection protection

NURSING ASSESSMENT	**RATIONALE**
Assess for and report signs and symptoms of superinfection (be alert to subtle changes in client since the signs of infection may be minimal as a result of immunosuppression; signs and symptoms may vary depending on the site of the infection, the causative organism, and the age of the client): - Increase in body temperature - Increase in episodes of chills and diaphoresis - Increased pulse rate - Development or worsening of abnormal breath sounds - Development or worsening of dyspnea and/or cough - Decline in mental status - Cloudy urine; client reports of frequency, urgency, burning when urinating - Further increase in fatigue or weakness - New or increased heat, pain, redness, swelling, or unusual drainage in any area - Development or worsening of lesions or ulceration of oral mucous membrane - New or increased episodes of diarrhea and abdominal cramping or pain Monitor CBC with differential; culture results; urinalysis; chest x-ray results.	*Early recognition of signs and symptoms of an infection allows for prompt intervention.*

THERAPEUTIC INTERVENTIONS	**RATIONALE**
Independent Actions Implement measures to prevent superinfection: - Use good hand hygiene and encourage client to do the same. **D** ● ✦	*Prevents spread of infection and cross-contamination.*

NDx = NANDA Diagnosis   **D** = Delegatable Action   ● = UAP   ✦ = LVN/LPN   ⊖▶ = Go to ⊖volve for animation

Continued...

THERAPEUTIC INTERVENTIONS	RATIONALE
• Protect client from others with infection.	*Decreases client's potential for infection and decreases cross-contamination.*
• Encourage client to eat a well-balanced diet high in essential nutrients; provide dietary supplements if indicated.	*Necessary to produce cells that fight infection.*
• Maintain sterile technique during all invasive procedures.	*Prevents entrance of pathogens into the body.*
• Change intravenous insertion sites according to hospital policy.	*Decreases potential for infection.*
• Anchor catheter/tubings securely.	*Securely anchoring tubes/catheters reduces trauma to the tissues and the risk for introduction of pathogens associated with movement of the tubing. Intravenous devices are known to be a cause of hospital-acquired infections.*
• Change equipment, tubings, and solutions used for treatments such as intravenous infusions, respiratory care, irrigations, and enteral feedings according to hospital policy.	*Prevents introduction of pathogens into the body and reduces risk for nosocomial infections.*
• Maintain a closed system for drains (e.g., urinary catheter) and intravenous infusions whenever possible.	*Improves lung expansion and motility and potential excretion of secretions.*
• Perform actions to prevent stasis of respiratory secretions:	*Prevents cross-contamination.*
• Assist client to turn, cough, and deep breathe.	
• Instruct and encourage client to regularly use incentive spirometry	
• Increase activity as allowed and tolerated.	
• Use universal precautions if infection is present	
• Perform actions to prevent urinary retention/stasis:	
• Urinate when urge is felt.	
• Promote relaxation when voiding.	*Prevents stasis of urine, which increases the potential for infection. Urinary tract infections are a common cause of sepsis.*
• Instruct and assist client to perform good perineal care routinely and after each bowel movement.	*Prevents contamination from bacteria from the rectum and helps client to completely empty bladder.*
• If client has open lesions or wound drains, perform actions to prevent wound infection:	*Prevents cross-contamination.*
• Maintain sterile technique during wound care.	*Prevents cross-contamination and improves healing.*
• Instruct client to avoid touching wounds.	

Dependent/Collaborative Actions

Implement measures to prevent superinfection:

• Maintain a fluid intake of 2500 mL/day unless contraindicated.	*Helps to maintain adequate vascular fluid volume.*
• Consult physician about discontinuing urinary catheter if one is present.	*Decreases risk for hospital-acquired infection.*
• Consult physician about:	*Maintains nutritional status. TPN has a high glucose content, which provides a rich medium for bacterial growth. Monitor insertion site closely and change dressings using sterile technique and per facility policy for frequency. Specific antimicrobial therapy is determined by culture and sensitivity.*
• Enteral feeding rather than total parenteral nutrition (TPN) if nutritional replacement is necessary.	
Obtain cultures as ordered.	
• Use of sucralfate rather than antacids and histamine$_2$-receptor antagonists.	*These agents increase the pH of the stomach contents, which promotes bacterial overgrowth; aspiration of gastric contents with a high bacteria content increases the risk for pneumonia.*
• Administer antimicrobial agents as ordered.	*Until culture and sensitivity results are obtained, the client should be treated with a broad-spectrum antibiotic. Monitor and treat potential side effects from antibiotic therapy.*

POTENTIAL COMPLICATIONS OF SEPSIS

Collaborative Diagnosis   SEPTIC SHOCK

Definition: Sepsis-induced hypotension or the requirement for vasopressors or inotropes to maintain BP despite adequate fluid volume resuscitation combined with the presence of perfusion abnormalities that may include lactic acidosis, oliguria, and/or acute alteration in mental status.

Related to: Systemic hypoperfusion associated with maldistribution of circulating blood, deficient fluid volume, and/or decreased myocardial contractility resulting from an uncontrolled systemic inflammatory response to severe infection

CLINICAL MANIFESTATIONS

Subjective	Objective
Reports of confusion	Low arterial pressure; low systemic vascular resistance; systemic edema; tachycardia; temperature instability; oliguria; decreased SaO_2; changes in ABGs; cyanosis

DESIRED OUTCOMES

The client will not develop septic shock as evidenced by:
a. Systolic BP equal to or higher than 90 mm Hg
b. Usual mental status
c. Urine output at least 30 mL/h

d. Extremities warm and usual color
e. Capillary refill time less than 2 to 3 seconds
f. Palpable peripheral pulses

NURSING ASSESSMENT	RATIONALE

Assess for and report signs and symptoms of septic shock:
• Hyperdynamic or compensatory phase
  • Widened pulse pressure with the diastolic pressure dropping and little change in the systolic pressure
  • Restlessness
  • Tachycardia
  • Warm, flushed skin
• Hypodynamic or progressive phase
  • Systolic BP less than 90 mm Hg or a reduction of greater than 40 mm Hg from baseline
  • Cool, clammy skin
  • Change in level of consciousness
  • Decreased urine output
  • Rapid, shallow breathing
  • Rapid, thready pulse
	Early recognition of signs and symptoms of septic shock allows for prompt intervention.

Monitor serum lactate levels. Monitor acid-base status	*Indicates improving or declining client status.*

THERAPEUTIC INTERVENTIONS	RATIONALE
Dependent/Collaborative Actions Implement measures to maintain adequate tissue perfusion: • Administer intravenous fluids (crystalloids/colloids) as ordered.	*Supports intravascular volume and cardiovascular status.*
If signs and symptoms of septic shock occur: • Maintain intravenous fluid therapy as ordered.	*Treatment for septic shock focuses on the expansion of circulating volume to improve tissue perfusion. Fluid volume support is often not adequate to maintain blood pressure and cardiac output. Vasopressors and inotropic agents improve perfusion pressures and cardiac output.*
Administer vasopressors and positive inotropic agents • Maintain oxygen therapy as ordered.	*Oxygenation needs are increased, and supplemental support is required to decrease incidence of extreme lactic acidosis.*
• Administer antimicrobials as ordered.	*Antimicrobial agents are required to address infection. May start with a broad spectrum and change education based on culture and sensitivity results.*
• Prepare client for transfer to critical care unit.	*The patient often requires transfer to a critical care unit for invasive monitoring of hemodynamic status (Swan-Ganz catheter; central venous pressure; arterial line).*

⊖▶ | Collaborative Diagnosis | **RISK FOR DISSEMINATED INTRAVASCULAR COAGULATION**

Definition: A systemic blood clotting disorder most commonly associated with sepsis.

Related to: Widespread inflammation and the resulting endothelial damage associated with sepsis results in inappropriate triggering of the coagulation cascade due to the presence of tissue factor that is released by damaged or dead tissues

CLINICAL MANIFESTATIONS

Subjective	**Objective**
Reports of restlessness; agitation; confusion	Bleeding: rapid development of oozing from venipuncture sites, arterial lines, surgical wounds; ecchymotic lesions; bleeding in conjunctiva, nose, and gums Thrombosis: cyanosis of fingers/toes, nose, breast; symptoms of organ failure

DESIRED OUTCOMES

The client will not develop DIC as evidenced by:
a. Absence of petechiae, ecchymoses, and frank or occult bleeding
b. Usual color and temperature of extremities
c. Usual mental status
d. Fibrin degradation products (FDPs) and D-dimer results within normal range
e. Fibrinogen level, platelet count, activated partial thromboplastin time (APTT), prothrombin time (PT), and thrombin time within normal range

NURSING ASSESSMENT	**RATIONALE**
Assess for and report signs and symptoms of DIC: • Petechiae, ecchymoses • Frank or occult bleeding (e.g., oozing from venipuncture sites or surgical incisions, epistaxis, hematuria, gingival bleeding) • Cool, mottled extremities • Restlessness, agitation, confusion Monitor results of PT/PTT; FDP; fibrinogen level, D-dimer.	*Early recognition of signs and symptoms of DIC allows for prompt intervention.*

THERAPEUTIC INTERVENTIONS	**RATIONALE**

Independent Actions
If DIC occurs:
• Implement safety precautions to prevent further bleeding:
  • Avoid injections.
  • Avoid invasive procedures.
  • Discontinue any invasive lines with extreme caution.
  • Use electric rather than straight-edge razor for shaving.
	The body has depleted its clotting factors; thus, after any invasive procedure, excessive bleeding may occur. All these interventions will decrease or prevent increased bleeding.

Dependent/Collaborative Actions Implement measures to control infection and reduce the risk for an uncontrolled systemic inflammatory response in order to reduce the risk for DIC: • Administer antimicrobial agents as ordered. • Perform actions to reduce the risk for superinfection.	*Treat/prevent infections*
If DIC occurs: • Administer fresh frozen plasma, platelets, and/or cryoprecipitate if ordered.	*Blood clotting products replace deficit endogenous products and work to enhance clotting and decrease bleeding.*

• Administer medications to interrupt clotting:
  • Heparin
  • Antithrombin III
Heparin is contraindicated if platelet count is less than 50,000.
	Low-dose heparin can partially inhibit active coagulation in sepsis. Antithrombin III inhibits thrombin-mediated microvascular dysfunction and vascular injury associated with sepsis.

RISK FOR ORGAN ISCHEMIA/DYSFUNCTION (MULTIPLE ORGAN DYSFUNCTION SYNDROME)

Definition: The progressive and potentially reversible dysfunction of two or more organ or organ systems resulting from an uncontrolled inflammatory response to severe illness or injury. Mortality increases as the extent of organ failure increases.

Related to:
- Hypoperfusion of major organs associated with shock
- Microvascular thrombosis associated with DIC

CLINICAL MANIFESTATIONS

Subjective	Objective
N/A	Low-grade fever; tachycardia; dyspnea; altered mental status; individual organ failure; changes in acid-base balance

RISK FACTORS

- Bowel infarction
- Inadequate or delayed resuscitation
- Persistent infection
- Significant tissue injury
- Burns
- Trauma
- Acute pancreatitis
- Circulatory shock
- Adult respiratory distress syndrome
- Necrotic tissue

DESIRED OUTCOMES

The client will not develop organ ischemia/dysfunction as evidenced by:
a. Usual mental status
b. Urine output at least 30 mL/h
c. Unlabored respirations at 12 to 20 breaths/min
d. Audible breath sounds without an increase in adventitious sounds
e. Absence of new or increased abdominal pain, distention, nausea, vomiting, and diarrhea
f. BUN, creatinine, aspartate aminotransferase (AST), alanine aminotransferase (ALT), and lactate dehydrogenase (LDH) levels within normal range
g. Maintain acid-base balance
h. Maintain SaO_2 at >90

NURSING ASSESSMENT

Assess for and report signs and symptoms of:
- Cerebral ischemia (e.g., change in mental status)
- Urine output less than 30 mL/h (elevated BUN and creatinine levels)
- Acute respiratory distress syndrome (e.g., dyspnea, increase in respiratory rate, low arterial oxygen saturation [SaO_2], crackles)
- Gastrointestinal ischemia (e.g., hypoactive or absent bowel sounds, abdominal pain and distention, nausea, vomiting, diarrhea, hematemesis, blood in stool)
- Liver dysfunction (e.g., increased AST, ALT, and LDH levels; jaundice)

Monitor results of chest x-ray, complete metabolic panel, and ABGs.

RATIONALE

Early recognition of signs and symptoms of multiple organ dysfunction syndrome (MODS) allows for prompt intervention.

---

*The nurse should select the diagnostic label that is most appropriate for the client's discharge teaching needs.

THERAPEUTIC INTERVENTIONS	RATIONALE
Dependent/Collaborative Actions Implement measures to reduce the risk for organ ischemia/dysfunction: • Perform actions to maintain adequate tissue perfusion • Maintain fluid balance • Provide supplemental oxygenation • Maintain appropriate nutritional status • Monitor and document lab values and ABGs, noting significant trends over time • Monitor and document vital signs, noting significant trends over time • Perform actions to prevent and treat DIC Notify appropriate health care provider if client condition changes.	*Correction of vascular fluid volume with overload helps to decrease physiological impact of sepsis.* *Supplemental oxygen is required to address hypoxemia associated with sepsis and potential organ dysfunction.* *Nutritional support provides energy to fight infection and maintain body functions.* *Monitoring ABGs and lab values provides insight on changes in client's condition over time and should be correlated with other client assessment findings.* *Incidence of DIC is a contributing factor to MODS. Prevention and rapid treatment help to decrease the severity of organ dysfunction.* *Allows for prompt interventions.*

ADDITIONAL NURSING DIAGNOSES

FEAR NDx/ANXIRTY NDx
Related to:
• Unfamiliar environment
• Separation from significant others

• Severity of current condition
• Threat of death

SPLENECTOMY

Splenectomy is the surgical removal of the spleen. The most common indication for removal of the spleen is organ rupture. Causes of rupture include penetrating or blunt trauma to the spleen, operative trauma to the spleen during surgery on nearby organs, and damage to the spleen as a result of disease (e.g., mononucleosis, tuberculosis of the spleen). A splenectomy may also be indicated if the spleen is removing excessive quantities of platelets, erythrocytes, or leukocytes from the circulation (hypersplenism). Conditions associated with hypersplenism include infections such as mononucleosis, liver disease including hepatitis B, blood diseases characterized by abnormal blood cells, and problems with the lymphatic system. Additionally, splenectomy may be performed to treat splenic cysts and neoplasms. When feasible, a partial splenectomy is performed so that some of the spleen's immunological function is maintained.

This care plan focuses on the adult client hospitalized for a splenectomy. The care plan will need to be individualized according to the client's underlying disease process or the extensiveness of abdominal trauma necessitating the surgery.

OUTCOME/DISCHARGE CRITERIA

The client will:
1. Have surgical pain controlled
2. Have evidence of normal healing of surgical wound
3. Have no signs and symptoms of infection
4. Have no signs and symptoms of postoperative complications
5. Identify appropriate safety measures to follow because of increased risk for infection
6. State signs and symptoms to report to the health care provider
7. Develop a plan for adhering to recommended follow-up care including future appointments with health care provider, medications prescribed, wound care, and activity level

For a full, detailed care plan on this topic, go to http://evolve.elsevier.com/Haugen/careplanning/.
See Bibliography at the back of the book.

9

The Client With Alterations in Metabolic Function

DIABETES MELLITUS

Diabetes mellitus is a chronic, multisystem disease characterized by alterations in carbohydrate, fat, and protein metabolism resulting from abnormal insulin production, impaired insulin utilization, or both. The hallmark of this metabolic disorder is hyperglycemia.

Diabetes* is often complicated by structural and functional abnormalities in the blood vessels and nerves. The atherosclerotic changes that frequently occur in the large vessels (macroangiopathy) affect the cardiac, cerebral, and peripheral circulation. Thickening of the basement membrane of the capillaries (microangiopathy) can also occur and is especially significant when it involves the vessels in the eyes and kidneys. The neurological involvement can be manifested in a wide variety of ways and is referred to as diabetic neuropathy. Several different mechanisms are thought to contribute to the development of diabetic neuropathy. These include reduced blood flow to the nerves as a result of angiopathies and a metabolic defect in the polyol pathway resulting in accumulation of sorbitol in the nerves, which subsequently alters nerve function. The most common neuropathy is peripheral sensorimotor polyneuropathy, which has a gradual onset of sensory manifestations such as numbness and tingling, burning or shooting pain sensations, and/or hyperesthesia. Neuropathy of the autonomic nervous system is also common.

Parasympathetic involvement often occurs earlier and is more profound than sympathetic nervous system involvement, and manifestations vary depending on the system involved.

The two major types of diabetes are type 1 and type 2. Individuals with type 1 diabetes have an absolute insulin deficiency and are dependent on insulin replacement. The insulin deficiency is usually due to an immune-mediated destruction of the pancreatic beta-cells in a person with a genetic predisposition and a triggering environmental insult (e.g., viral infection). Individuals with type 2 diabetes have a relative deficiency of insulin caused by decreased tissue responsiveness to insulin (insulin resistance), a defect in insulin secretion, and inappropriate hepatic glucose production. Heredity plays a role in development of type 2 diabetes. Additional risk factors for type 2 diabetes include a history of gestational diabetes mellitus or impaired glucose tolerance, increasing age, obesity, and a sedentary lifestyle.

A sequence of pathophysiological events occurs in diabetes. When an insulin deficiency exists, glucose cannot be transported into the cells for energy metabolism. As a result, glucose accumulates in the blood and starts to spill into the urine once the level exceeds the renal threshold (>180 mg/dL). The high blood glucose acts as an osmotic diuretic, which leads to excessive diuresis and subsequent deficient fluid volume. Because the glucose cannot be used as an energy source by many cells, fat and protein are broken down to provide a source of energy for the starving cells. The free fatty acids that are mobilized from adipose tissue are converted by the liver to ketones to be used as an energy source. The ketones are strong acids and eventually deplete the body's buffer system and respiratory compensatory ability, leading to a state of metabolic acidosis. The simultaneous increase in glucagon and epinephrine release that occurs with an insulin deficiency exacerbates the hyperglycemia and ketogenesis. Continuation of these metabolic derangements leads to life-threatening imbalances.

This care plan focuses on the adult client who has had diabetes for many years and is being hospitalized because of difficulty stabilizing blood glucose levels. Many of the long-term vascular and neurological complications have been included in this care plan and should be individualized based on the client's current status. Much of the information in this care plan is applicable to clients receiving follow-up care in an extended care facility or home setting.

This care plan should be used in conjunction with the care plans on heart failure, myocardial infarction, cerebrovascular accident, hypertension, and/or chronic renal failure if the client is also being treated for one of these vascular complications of diabetes.

OUTCOME/DISCHARGE CRITERIA

The client will:
1. Have blood glucose stabilized within a desired range
2. Have signs and symptoms of vascular and neurological complications at a manageable level
3. Verbalize a basic understanding of diabetes mellitus

---

*Diabetes mellitus will be referred to as diabetes throughout the care plan.

NDx = NANDA Diagnosis   **D** = Delegatable Action   ● = UAP   ✦ = LVN/LPN   ⊜▶ = Go to ⊜volve for animation

4. Verbalize an understanding of medications ordered and demonstrate the ability to correctly draw up and administer insulin if prescribed
5. Verbalize an understanding of the principles of dietary management and be able to calculate and plan meals within the prescribed caloric distribution
6. Demonstrate the ability to perform blood glucose and urine tests correctly and interpret results accurately
7. Verbalize an understanding of the role of exercise in the management of diabetes
8. Identify health care and hygiene practices that should be integrated into lifestyle
9. Identify appropriate safety measures to follow because of the diagnosis of diabetes
10. State signs and symptoms of hypoglycemia and ketoacidosis and appropriate actions for prevention and treatment
11. State signs and symptoms to report to the health care provider
12. Share feelings and concerns about diabetes and its effect on lifestyle
13. Identify resources that can assist in the adjustment to and management of diabetes
14. Develop a plan for adhering to recommended follow-up care, including future appointments with health care provider and for laboratory studies

---

Nursing Diagnosis **RISK FOR UNSTABLE BLOOD GLUCOSE LEVEL** NDx

Definition: Susceptible to variation in serum levels of glucose from the normal range, which may compromise health.

Note: The following national definitions represent clinical conditions marked by variations in serum glucose levels:
- Hyperglycemia—blood glucose value >140 mg/dL
- Hypoglycemia—blood glucose value <70 mg/dL
- Diabetic ketoacidosis (DKA)—blood glucose value >250 mg/dL
- Hyperglycemic hyperosmolar nonketotic (HHNK)—blood glucose >600 mg/dL

Related to:
- Inadequate insulin production
- Ineffective action of insulin
- Inadequate insulin therapy/medication management
- Nonadherence to prescribed treatment plan (e.g., medication, diet, exercise)

CLINICAL MANIFESTATIONS

Subjective	Objective
Verbal self-report of fatigue, weakness, nausea, blurred vision, loss of appetite, and paresthesias	Objective findings depend upon the severity of variation of serum glucose from normal levels and can include but are not limited to polydipsia, polyuria, ketonuria, weight loss, dry mucous membranes, poor skin turgor, tachycardia, hypotension, Kussmaul respirations, acetone breath, nausea, vomiting, abdominal pain, altered level of consciousness.

RISK FACTORS

- Stress
- Obesity
- Excessive weight loss
- Infection
- Prescribed medications that release counter regulatory hormones (e.g., corticosteroids, thiazide diuretics, sympathomimetic agents, second generation antipsychotic agents)
- Drug use (e.g., cocaine)
- Alcohol abuse

DESIRED OUTCOMES

The client will experience normal or near-normal blood glucose levels as evidenced by:
a. Blood glucose levels <180 mg/dL at all times
b. Fasting blood glucose levels <110 mg/dL
c. Hemoglobin A1C <7%

NOC OUTCOMES

Hyperglycemia severity; hypoglycemia severity;

NIC INTERVENTIONS

Hyperglycemia management; hypoglycemia management

NURSING ASSESSMENT	RATIONALE
Assess for signs and symptoms of unstable glucose levels: • Altered neurological status (e.g., lethargy, headache, disorientation, seizures, decreased level of consciousness) • Excessive urine output • Excessive hunger	*Early recognition of signs and symptoms of variations in serum glucose levels allows for prompt intervention.*

Continued...

NURSING ASSESSMENT	RATIONALE
• Acetone breath • Nausea • Vomiting • Abdominal pain • Blurred vision Assess baseline/admission blood glucose levels: • Point-of-care finger stick (capillary specimen) • Serum hemoglobin A1C (if not performed within the last 3 months)	*Assessing the client's blood glucose levels determines effectiveness of glucose control and allows for adjustment to the treatment plan.*

THERAPEUTIC INTERVENTIONS	RATIONALE
Independent Actions Perform actions to maintain blood glucose at a near-normal level: • Monitor percentage of meals and snacks client consumes. • Provide meals and snack at regular intervals • Monitor fluid status (I & O), encourage oral intake as appropriate. • Report a pattern of inadequate or excessive intake. **D** ✦ • Minimize client's exposure to emotional and physiological stress • Restrict exercise when blood glucose levels are greater than 250 mg/dL, especially if ketones are present.	*Pattern of inadequate or excessive intakes will indicate need for further dietary teaching.* *Stress causes an increased output of epinephrine, glucagon, and cortisol all of which increase blood pressure.* *If blood sugar is >250, the client should not exercise until fast-acting insulin has been administered. In the presence of hyperglycemia, if the body does not produce enough insulin to use the glucose, body cells will continue to signal that they need glucose for fuel and will continue to signal the liver to produce more glucose elevating blood levels further.*

Dependent/Collaborative Actions
Implement measures to maintain blood glucose at a near-normal level, achieve ideal weight, and provide necessary nutrients:
Monitor blood glucose levels using point-of-care testing at intervals appropriate to dietary intake:
• Clients who are eating:
  • Blood glucose before meals (AC) and at bedtime (HS)
• Clients who are not eating:
  • Every 4 to 6 hrs
• Administer insulin and antihyperglycemic agents as ordered.
	
	Ongoing serial monitoring of blood glucose levels is necessary to evaluate effectiveness of treatment plan and allow for modification and evaluation of treatment plan.
	
	2017 American Diabetes Association guidelines for in-hospital care of diabetic clients identifies insulin as the preferred treatment for glycemic control. Basal insulin or basal insulin plus bolus correction is the preferred treatment for non-critically-ill clients with poor oral intake or those taking nothing by mouth.

Monitor for signs and symptoms of hypoglycemia (e.g., shakiness, tremor, sweating, weakness, dizziness).
• Implement hypoglycemic protocol:
  • Administer glucagon (if able to take PO).
  • Provide simple carbohydrate as indicated.
  • Provide complex carbohydrate/protein as indicated.
  • Administer IV glucose as indicated (if unable to take PO).
Maintain IV access as appropriate.
• Administer IV insulin as ordered for hyperglycemia.
• Administer IV glucose (D$_{50}$) for hypoglycemia.
• Consult dietitian to develop a diet/meal plan and/or reinforce dietary education.
• Perform a calorie count if ordered.
	Hypoglycemia in hospitalized clients is associated with adverse short-term and long-term outcomes including but not limited to macro–microvascular events and even death. Early identification and treatment can prevent further deterioration to a more severe episode with adverse outcomes.
	
	Depending on the blood glucose level, a functioning IV may be necessary for the administration of medications necessary to correct extreme blood glucose values.
	Improves clients' ability to care for themselves and maintain appropriate blood glucose levels.
	A calorie count helps determine appropriate volume of calories needed to maintain adequate nutrition and blood glucose levels.

NDx = NANDA Diagnosis   **D** = Delegatable Action   ● = UAP   ✦ = LVN/LPN   ⊝▶ = Go to ⊖volve for animation

Nursing Diagnosis   RISK FOR DEFICIENT FLUID VOLUME NDx

Definition: Susceptible to experiencing decreased intravascular, interstitial, and/or intracellular fluid volumes, which may compromise health.

Related to: Excessive loss of fluid associated with the osmotic diuresis resulting from uncontrolled blood glucose levels

CLINICAL MANIFESTATIONS

Subjective	Objective
Verbal self-report of thirst, weakness	Polyuria; weight loss; dry buccal mucosa; sunken eye balls; poor skin turgor; tachycardia; hypotension; shock

RISK FACTORS

- DKA
- HHNK syndrome
- Renal insufficiency associated with diabetes

DESIRED OUTCOMES

The client will maintain fluid balance as evidenced by:
- Vital signs within client's normal range
- Balanced intake/output
- Serum BUN/creatinine within client's normal range

NOC OUTCOMES

Fluid balance; shock severity: hypovolemic

NIC INTERVENTIONS

Fluid monitoring; fluid management; hypovolemia management; intravenous therapy

NURSING ASSESSMENT	RATIONALE
Assess vital signs for signs of excessive fluid loss: • BP—Hypotension • HR—Tachycardia • RR—Tachypnea	*Osmotic diuresis associated with uncontrolled glucose levels can lead to dehydration. Identification of signs of excessive fluid loss allows for prompt intervention.*
Assess for symptoms of excessive fluid loss: • Thirst • Dizziness • Changes in mentation • Dry mucous membranes • Orthostatic hypotension • Quality of peripheral pulses • Capillary refill >3 seconds • Dry skin turgor • Urine output—color, quantity	*Identification of symptoms of fluid loss allows for prompt intervention.*
Assess baseline laboratory values for evidence of excessive fluid loss: • Elevated BUN • Elevated creatinine • Urinalysis—elevated specific gravity • Elevated hematocrit • Osmolality—elevated urine and blood • Electrolytes for imbalance • Elevated glucose	*Baseline laboratory tests are valuable in cases of severe hydration. Baseline values allow for comparisons for monitoring the effectiveness of treatment.*

THERAPEUTIC INTERVENTIONS	RATIONALE

Independent Actions

Implement measures to restore optimum fluid balance.

Monitor vital signs as appropriate.   *Allows for monitoring effectiveness of treatment regimen.*

Continued...

THERAPEUTIC INTERVENTIONS	RATIONALE
Monitor hydration status as appropriate, including maintaining accurate intake and output records: • Weigh daily at consistent times. • Monitor color, quantity, and specific gravity of urine. Promote oral intake between meals as appropriate offering fluids every 1 to 2 hrs unless contraindicated.	*Helps restore circulating fluid volume.*
Dependent/Collaborative Actions Implement measures to restore optimum fluid balance. Establish and maintain patent IV access. Administer ordered IV fluids: • Monitor for fluid overload during administration (e.g., crackles, neck vein distention edema). Monitor additional laboratory results as ordered. Consult with physician if signs and symptoms of fluid volume deficit persist.	*Restores extracellular circulating fluid volume.* *Evaluates response to therapy and guides treatment regimen. Allows for modification of the treatment regimen.*

Nursing Diagnosis   RISK FOR ELECTROLYTE IMBALANCE NDx

Definition: Susceptible to changes in serum electrolyte levels, which may compromise health.

Related to: Increased serum osmolality and resulting movement of water out of the cells and associated metabolic acidosis associated with uncontrolled blood glucose levels.

CLINICAL MANIFESTATIONS

Subjective	Objective
Verbal self-report of weakness; nausea; abdominal pain	Lethargy; fatigue; agitation, restlessness, confusion, nausea, vomiting, dysrhythmias; diarrhea; constipation; convulsions; seizures; acetone (fruity) odor on breath

RISK FACTORS

- DKA
- HHNK
- Conditions associated with diabetes:
  - Impaired renal function
  - Malabsorption syndrome
  - Acid-base disorders
  - Multidrug regimens

DESIRED OUTCOMES

The client will maintain electrolyte balance as evidenced by:
- Vital signs within normal range for client
- Serum electrolyte values within normal range
- Blood glucose level <180 mg/dL
- Normal blood pH/acid-base balance (arterial blood gases [ABGs] and bicarbonate levels within normal range
- Normal serum osmolality
- Absence of serum and urine ketones

NOC OUTCOMES

Electrolyte balance; electrolyte and acid base balance

NIC INTERVENTIONS

Acid-base management; acid-base management: metabolic acidosis; electrolyte management; electrolyte management: electrolyte monitoring; fluid/electrolyte management

NURSING ASSESSMENT	RATIONALE
Assess vital signs for evidence of electrolyte imbalances: • Blood pressure • Hypotension—associated with hypermagnesemia; associated metabolic acidosis	*Early recognition of unstable vital signs allows for prompt intervention.*

NURSING ASSESSMENT	**RATIONALE**

• Heart rate
  • Irregularity/dysrhythmias associated with hyper/ hypokalemia; hypermagnesemia
• Respirations
  • Kussmaul respirations associated with metabolic acidosis; acetone (fruity) odor on breath	

Assess for signs and symptoms of electrolyte imbalances: • Neurological—lethargy, fatigue, agitation; confusion; restlessness; convulsion, seizures • Cardiac—dysrhythmias (irregular heart rate; tachycardia; life-threatening dysrhythmias)	*Early recognition of signs and symptoms of electrolyte imbalances allows for prompt intervention.*
Assess EKG tracings as indicated for changes related to electrolyte abnormalities (potassium). • Gastrointestinal—nausea; vomiting; abdominal pain; constipation; diarrhea • Musculoskeletal—muscle weakness; cramping; tetany; numbness; tingling	
Assess baseline laboratory values for additional abnormal electrolyte values. • Hyper/hypokalemia • Hyper/hyponatremia • Increase serum osmolality • Decreased serum bicarbonate • Elevated serum ketones • Elevated urine ketones • Anion gap metabolic acidosis (>30 mEq/L) • ABG/blood pH for metabolic acidosis	*Extreme variations in blood glucose levels can be accompanied by life-threatening alterations in electrolytes caused by hypertonicity induced movement of water out of the cells and related dilution of serum electrolytes; osmotic diuresis; shift of electrolytes into the cells related to administration of medications (e.g., insulin); associated metabolic acidosis.*

THERAPEUTIC INTERVENTIONS	**RATIONALE**
Independent Actions Perform actions to maintain electrolytes/acid-base balance at a near-normal levels: Monitor intake and output. **D** ● ✦	*Osmotic diuresis associated with uncontrolled glucose levels contributes to electrolyte abnormalities.*
Provide diet appropriate for client's electrolyte imbalance (e.g., potassium rich; low sodium; low carbohydrate)	*Adequate dietary intake of electrolytes can help maintain normal levels.*
Provide a safe environment for the client with neurological and/or neuromuscular manifestations of electrolyte imbalance. • Hourly rounding • Bed at lowest level • Side rails as appropriate for confusion	*Neuromuscular effects of electrolyte imbalances can increase the risk of injury (e.g., falls due to confusion).*
Dependent/Collaborative Actions Implement measures to maintain serum electrolytes/acid-base balance at a near-normal levels: Monitor serial serum electrolyte values for abnormalities.	*Ongoing monitoring of laboratory values allows for evaluation and adjustment of the treatment plan.*
Monitor for associated acid-base imbalances: • Decreased serum bicarbonate • Anion gap metabolic acidosis (>30 mEq/L) • Blood pH <7.35	*Extreme elevation of blood glucose levels can result in metabolic acidosis as the body breaks down fat and muscle for energy producing excessive ketones and fatty acids. Metabolic acidosis contributes to further electrolyte abnormalities, which may be life-threatening.*
Place on cardiac monitor as appropriate. Monitor EKG tracings as indicated for changes related to abnormal electrolyte levels (potassium, magnesium).	*Hypomagnesemia, hyperkalemia, and hypokalemia are associated with dysrhythmias that may be life-threatening.*

Continued...

THERAPEUTIC INTERVENTIONS	RATIONALE
Maintain patent IV access as appropriate.	*Intravenous administration of electrolyte replacements is the appropriate route to correct critical values. A patent IV must be obtained.*
• Administer IV solutions containing electrolytes as ordered.	
• Administer supplemental electrolytes as ordered.	
Administer electrolyte-binding or electrolyte-excreting resins (sodium polystyrene sulfonate (Kayexalate) as ordered.	*Renal insufficiency, often associated with diabetes, may interfere with the appropriate regulation of electrolyte abnormalities such as hyperkalemia. Administration of binding or excreting resins may be necessary to normalize critical values.*
Administer HCO_3 as indicated:	*Administration of HCO_3 corrects metabolic acidosis. Administration should be carefully guided by laboratory values.*
• Oral, if able to take PO	
• IV, if unable to take PO	
Consult dietitian to develop a diet/meal plan and/or reinforce dietary education.	*Improves clients' ability to care for themselves and maintain appropriate blood glucose levels*
Consult with physician on administration of electrolyte-sparing medications (e.g., spironolactone) as appropriate.	*Diuretic therapy contributes to electrolyte imbalances. Conversion to potassium-sparing medications may be warranted in the presence of hypokalemia.*
Consult physician if signs and symptoms of electrolyte imbalance persist or worsen.	*Allows for appropriate modification of the treatment plan.*

Nursing Diagnosis | INEFFECTIVE PERIPHERAL TISSUE PERFUSION NDx

Definition: Decreased blood circulation to the periphery, which may compromise health.

Related to:
• Peripheral polyneuropathy and/or peripheral vascular insufficiency associated with diabetes mellitus

CLINICAL MANIFESTATIONS

Subjective	Objective
Verbal self-report of burning, pain, numbness, tingling and/or increased sensitivity to sensory stimuli	Cool skin; decreased or absent lower extremity pulses; delayed capillary refill; edema; delayed in peripheral wound healing

RISK FACTORS
• Consistently high blood glucose levels
• Hypertension
• Sedentary lifestyle
• Smoking
• Wearing of tight shoes or constrictive clothing

DESIRED OUTCOMES

The client will sustain tissue perfusion to lower extremities as evidenced by:
a. Verbalization of decreased or absent extremity pain in lower extremities
b. Verbalization of decreased or absence of paresthesia (numbness/tingling) in lower extremities
c. Presence of peripheral pulses
d. Capillary refill time <3 seconds
e. Normal range for 6-minute walk test

NOC OUTCOMES

Comfort status: physical; pain control; tissue perfusion: peripheral; peripheral artery disease severity

NIC INTERVENTIONS

Pain management: chronic; environmental management: comfort; peripheral sensation management; circulatory care: venous insufficiency

---

NDx = NANDA Diagnosis   **D** = Delegatable Action   ● = UAP   ✦ = LVN/LPN   ⊖▶ = Go to ⊖volve for animation

NURSING ASSESSMENT	RATIONALE
Assess for: • Signs and symptoms of peripheral neuropathy (e.g., reports of persistent burning; sharp, shooting pain; numbness; tingling; or increased sensitivity to sensory stimuli [hyperesthesia]) • Signs and symptoms of peripheral vascular insufficiency (e.g., reports of cramping in calves precipitated by ambulation [intermittent claudication], delayed capillary refill, cold feet, dependent rubor, diminished or absent pulses; edema) • Stasis ulcers and tissue breakdown • Nonverbal signs of pain/discomfort (e.g., grimacing, guarding of affected area, reluctance to move, restlessness, diaphoresis, increased B/P, tachycardia) Assess client's perception of the severity of the pain/discomfort using an intensity rating scale.	*Early recognition of signs and symptoms of peripheral neuropathy and vascular insufficiency allows for prompt intervention.*
Assess the client's pattern of pain/discomfort (e.g., location, quality, onset, duration, precipitating factors, aggravating factors, alleviating factors). Ask the client to describe the methods used to manage the pain/discomfort effectively.	*Provides a baseline to measure changes in discomfort pattern. May indicate worsening of neuropathies.*

THERAPEUTIC INTERVENTIONS	RATIONALE
Independent Actions Implement measures to reduce discomfort: • Perform actions to reduce fear and anxiety about pain/discomfort (e.g., assure client that the need for relief of pain /discomfort is understood; plan methods for control of discomfort with client). • Perform actions to reduce stress (e.g., explain procedures, maintain a calm environment).	*These actions promote relaxation and subsequently increases client's threshold and tolerance for discomfort.*

• If client has hyperesthesia, implement measures to protect extremity from injury:
  • Provide a bed cradle **D** ● ✦
  • Sheepskin under feet/lower legs
  • Well-fitted shoes
  • Protect extremities from extremes in temperature
	Use of a bed cradle keeps bedding off affected extremities to decrease pressure on the skin. Sheepskin under feet/legs helps decrease pressure reducing the risk of pressure ulcers. Well-fitted shoes, made of soft materials with shock absorbing soles, help protect the feet from injury.

• Assist client with ambulation if walking relieves discomfort. **D** ● ✦ • If client is experiencing intermittent claudication, encourage short, more frequent walks.	*Walking often relieves lower extremity discomfort associated with neuropathies.* *Longer walks exacerbate pain associated with vascular insufficiency.*
• Provide or assist with additional nonpharmacologic measures for relief of pain/discomfort (e.g., position change, relaxation exercises, guided imagery, quiet conversation, restful environment).	*Use of nonpharmacologic measures provides relief of pain without sedation.*
Dependent/Collaborative Actions Implement measures to reduce pain/discomfort: • Perform actions to maintain blood glucose at a near-normal level (e.g., appropriate diet, exercise, blood glucose monitoring).	*Maintaining optimal glycemic control can actually alleviate or reduce neuropathic discomfort and the progression of neuropathy.*
• Administer the following medications if ordered to control discomfort: • Analgesics • Tricyclic antidepressants • Anticonvulsants (i.e., gabapentin or carbamazepine)	*Provides pain relief through a variety of mechanisms:* *Analgesics and tricyclic antidepressants work via the central nervous system (CNS).* *These anticonvulsants have been used to treat sharp or stabbing superficial burning pain.*

Continued...

THERAPEUTIC INTERVENTIONS	RATIONALE
• Capsaicin cream	*Capsaicin cream is useful in treatment of superficial pain.*
• Hemorrheologic agents (e.g., pentoxifylline)	*Hemorrheologic agents can improve peripheral blood flow and reduce discomfort associated with intermittent claudication.*
• Skeletal muscle relaxants or quinine sulfate	*Quinine sulfate can be used to treat leg cramps.*
• Consult appropriate health care provider (e.g., pharmacist, pain management specialist, physician) if above measures fail to provide adequate relief of discomfort	*If pain relief is inadequate, consultation with other member of the health care team provides a multidisciplinary approach to pain management*

Nursing Diagnosis RISK FOR DYSFUNCTIONAL GASTROINTESTINAL MOTILITY NDx

Definition: Susceptible to increased, decreased, ineffective, or lack of peristaltic activity within the gastrointestinal system, which may compromise health.

Related to: Delayed emptying of the stomach associated with autonomic neuropathy involving the gastrointestinal tract

CLINICAL MANIFESTATIONS

Subjective	Objective
Verbal self-report of abdominal gas, heart burn, fullness, bloating, and nausea	Palpable distended abdomen; decreased or absent bowel sounds

RISK FACTORS

- Stress
- Diabetes
- Lack of exercise

DESIRED OUTCOMES

The client will experience adequate gastric motility as evidenced by:
a. Verbalization decreased or absent abdominal pain/discomfort
b. Relaxed facial expression and body positioning

NOC OUTCOMES

Comfort level; symptom control

NIC INTERVENTIONS

Environmental management: comfort; nausea management; hyperglycemia management

NURSING ASSESSMENT	RATIONALE
Assess client for: • Verbal reports of gastric discomfort (e.g., gastric fullness, postprandial bloating, nausea) • Nonverbal signs of discomfort (e.g., grimacing, rubbing upper abdomen, restlessness, reluctance to move)	*Early recognition of signs and symptoms of gastric discomfort allows for prompt intervention.*

THERAPEUTIC INTERVENTIONS	RATIONALE
Independent Actions Implement measures to reduce gastric discomfort: • Perform actions to reduce the accumulation of gas and fluid in the stomach: • Encourage and assist client with frequent position changes and ambulation as tolerated. • Have client sit up during meals and for 1 to 2 hrs after meals. **D** ● ✦ • Provide small, frequent meals rather than three large ones; instruct client to ingest foods and fluids slowly. **D** ● ✦	*Activity stimulates gastrointestinal motility.* *Gravity promotes passage of food and fluid through the gastrointestinal tract.* *Small, frequent meals decrease abdominal fullness after meals.*

NDx = NANDA Diagnosis   **D** = Delegatable Action   ● = UAP   ✦ = LVN/LPN   ⊜▶ = Go to ⊜volve for animation

THERAPEUTIC INTERVENTIONS	RATIONALE
• Instruct client to avoid foods high in fat.	*Foods high in fat delay gastric emptying.*
• Instruct client to avoid activities such as chewing gum, drinking through a straw, and smoking.	*Avoiding these activities decreases air swallowing.*
• Instruct client to avoid intake of carbonated beverages and gas-producing foods (e.g., cabbage, onions, beans).	*Avoiding these foods/fluids reduces production of gas.*
• Encourage client to eructate whenever the urge is felt. **D ● ✦**	*Burping helps remove gas from the stomach.*
• Perform actions to reduce nausea if present:	
• Encourage client to take deep, slow breaths when nauseated.	*Slow, deep breaths help alleviate nausea.*
• Instruct client to avoid foods/fluids that irritate the gastric mucosa (e.g., spicy foods; caffeine-containing beverages such as coffee, tea, and colas).	*Foods that irritate the gastric mucosa increase the incidence of esophageal reflux and heartburn.*
• Eliminate noxious sights and odors from the environment. **D ● ✦**	*Noxious stimuli can cause stimulation of the vomiting center.*
• Instruct and assist client to change positions slowly. **D ● ✦**	*Rapid movement can result in stimulation of the chemoreceptor trigger zone and subsequent excitation of the vomiting center.*
• Avoid serving foods with an overpowering aroma; remove lids from hot foods before entering room. **D ● ✦**	*Powerful smells may stimulate the nausea center.*
• Instruct client to eat dry foods (e.g., toast, crackers) and avoid drinking liquids with meals when feeling nauseated.	*These actions help settle the client's stomach when nauseated.*
• Perform actions to maintain blood glucose at a near-normal level. (e.g., establishing an exercise routine, adhering to a diabetic diet).	*Maintaining optimal glycemic control seems to improve gastric emptying.*

Dependent/Collaborative Actions

Implement measures to reduce gastric discomfort:

• Perform actions to reduce the accumulation of gas and fluid in the stomach:	
• Administer medications that enhance gastric motility (e.g., metoclopramide) if ordered. **D ✦**	*Metoclopramide stimulates gastric motility, which improves gastric emptying.*
• Perform actions to reduce nausea if present:	
• Administer antiemetics as ordered. **D ✦**	*Antiemetics decrease nausea and emesis.*
Consult physician if gastric discomfort persists or worsens.	*Notification of the physician allows for modification of the treatment plan.*

Nursing Diagnosis   **INEFFECTIVE FAMILY HEALTH MANAGEMENT** NDx

Definition: A pattern of regulating and integrating into family processes a program for the treatment of illness and its sequelae that is unsatisfactory for meeting specific health goals of the family unit.

CLINICAL MANIFESTATIONS

Subjective	Objective
Verbal self-report of inability to manage care at home; lack of understanding of factors that contribute to acute and chronic complications; unwillingness or inability to modify personal habits and integrated treatments into lifestyle; statements reflecting a view that diabetes is curable or that the situation is hopeless and adherence will not improve health	Refusing medications; nonadherence to dietary restrictions

RISK FACTORS

- Lack of understanding of the implications of not following the prescribed treatment plan
- Feeling of lack of control over disease progression despite efforts to follow prescribed treatment plan
- Difficulty modifying personal habits and integrating necessary treatments and dietary regimen into lifestyle
- Insufficient financial resources

DESIRED OUTCOMES

The client will demonstrate the probability of effective therapeutic regimen management as evidenced by:
a. Willingness to learn about and participate in treatments and care
b. Statements reflecting ways to modify personal habits and integrate treatments into lifestyle
c. Statements reflecting an understanding of the implications of not following the prescribed treatment plan

NOC OUTCOMES

Adherence behavior; self-management: diabetes; knowledge: treatment regimen; health beliefs: perceived resources; health beliefs: perceived ability to perform

NIC INTERVENTIONS

Self-modification assistance; medication management; values clarification; teaching: disease process; teaching: prescribed diet; weight reduction assistance; financial resource assistance; support system enhancement

NURSING ASSESSMENT

Assess for indications that client may be unable to effectively manage the therapeutic regimen or may require further education:
- Statements reflecting inability to manage care at home
- Failure to adhere to treatment plan (e.g., refusing medications, not adhering to dietary restrictions)
- Statements reflecting a lack of understanding of factors that contribute to acute and chronic complications
- Statements reflecting an unwillingness or inability to modify personal habits and integrate necessary treatments into lifestyle
- Statements reflecting the view that diabetes is curable or that the situation is hopeless and that efforts to comply with treatments are useless

RATIONALE

Provides a baseline for client and family teaching and what specific concerns, lack of understanding, or level of acceptance is being experienced.

THERAPEUTIC INTERVENTIONS

Independent Actions
Implement measures to promote effective therapeutic management:
- Determine client's understanding of diabetes; clarify misconceptions and stress that diabetes is a chronic condition and adherence to the treatment plan may delay and/or prevent complications; caution the client that some complications may occur despite strict adherence to treatment plan.
- Encourage client to participate in assessment and treatments (e.g., blood glucose monitoring, selection of diet, insulin administration).
- Provide client with written instructions about future appointments with health care provider, diet, medications, exercise, signs and symptoms to report, and foot care.
- Discuss with client the difficulties of incorporating treatments into lifestyle; assist client in identifying ways to modify lifestyle rather than completely change it.

RATIONALE

Adherence to the treatment regimen will preserve the client's health for a longer period and may prevent some complications from occurring.

Through observation of the client's adherence to treatment regimen, the nurse can determine client's ability to care for self.

Written instructions provide the client an information resource once discharged.

Portrays a true picture of diabetes management and allows the client to determine what lifestyle modifications are feasible. This improves the client's ability to adhere to the treatment regimen.

THERAPEUTIC INTERVENTIONS	RATIONALE
• Encourage client to discuss concerns about the cost of medications, food, and supplies; obtain a social service consult to assist with financial planning and obtain financial aid if indicated.	*Diabetes can have a significant financial impact on clients and their families and should be discussed openly to assist clients with treatment management.*
• Encourage client to attend follow-up diabetic education classes.	*Continued education improves client's understanding about diabetes and interventions to improve health.*
• Provide information about and encourage utilization of resources that can assist client to make necessary lifestyle changes (e.g., diabetes support groups, counseling services, American Diabetes Association, diabetic cookbooks, and publications).	*Provides for continuum of care once discharged from the acute care facility.*
• Reinforce behaviors suggesting future compliance with the therapeutic regimen (e.g., participation in the treatment plan, statements reflecting plans for integrating treatments into lifestyle).	*Provides client feedback and can increase confidence in client's ability to care for self and adhere to treatment regimen.*
• Include significant others in explanations and teaching sessions and encourage their support; reinforce the need for client to assume responsibility for managing as much of care as possible.	*Informed family members can support the client in lifestyle changes and treatment regimen management.*

Nursing Diagnosis DEFICIENT KNOWLEDGE NDx OR INEFFECTIVE HEALTH MANAGEMENT* NDx

Definition: **Deficient Knowledge NDx:** Absence of cognitive information related to specific topic, or its acquisition; **Ineffective Health Management NDx:** Pattern of regulating and integrating into daily living a therapeutic regime for the treatment of illness and its sequelae that is unsatisfactory for meeting specific health goals.

CLINICAL MANIFESTATIONS

Subjective	Objective
Verbal self-report of inability to manage illness or inability to follow prescribed regimen	Inaccurate follow-through with instructions; inappropriate behaviors; experience of preventable complications of diabetes

RISK FACTORS
- Cognitive deficit
- Financial concerns
- Failure to take action to reduce modifiable risk factors
- Inability to care for oneself
- Difficulty in modifying personal habits and integrating treatments into lifestyle

NOC OUTCOMES	NIC INTERVENTIONS
Knowledge: treatment regimen; health behavior; health resources; treatment procedure(s)	Teaching: individual; teaching: prescribed exercise; teaching: psychomotor skills; health system guidance; financial resource assistance; support system enhancement

NURSING ASSESSMENT	RATIONALE
Assess client's ability to learn and readiness to learn. Assess client's understanding of teaching. Assess client's ability for self-care.	*Learning is more effective when client is motivated and understands the importance of what is to be learned. Readiness to learn changes based on situations and physical and emotional challenges.*

*The nurse should select the diagnostic label that is most appropriate for the client's discharge teaching needs.

THERAPEUTIC INTERVENTIONS	RATIONALE

Desired Outcome: The client will verbalize a basic understanding of diabetes and of medications ordered and demonstrate the ability to correctly administer insulin if prescribed.

Independent Actions

Determine client's understanding of diabetes mellitus.

Clarify misconceptions and reinforce teaching as necessary. Use available teaching aids (e.g., pamphlets, videotapes).

Explain the rationale for, side effects of, storage and care of, method of administration of, and importance of taking medications prescribed.

Provide instructions if client is to self-administer insulin.

If client is discharged with an insulin pump device, provide instructions regarding its management (e.g., changing the insertion site, filling syringes, changing batteries in pump).

Allow time for practice and return demonstration.

Instruct client to consult pharmacist or health care provider before taking other prescription and nonprescription medications (e.g., over-the-counter cold preparations).

Instruct client to inform all health care providers of medications being taken.

Baseline understanding is important in developing client teaching plan.

A variety of teaching methods are more effective, as individuals have varying styles of learning.

Knowledge of medications and how they impact the system improves client adherence. Help enhance the client's understanding of the importance of adhering to the prescribed medication regimen. The client must be able to recognize alterations in functioning related to medication administration.

Client and family members should be taught how to correctly administer insulin.

Client should not leave health care institution without an understanding of how to appropriately use the insulin pump to prevent or decrease the number of hyperglycemic and hypoglycemic events.

Demonstration provides the nurse time to provide client feedback and improves client's confidence in ability to care for self.

Over-the-counter medications may affect the hypoglycemic agent taken by the client.

This action prevents drug interactions when health care provider is prescribing new medications.

THERAPEUTIC INTERVENTIONS	RATIONALE

Desired Outcome: The client will verbalize an understanding of the principles of dietary management and be able to calculate and plan meals within the prescribed caloric distribution.

Independent Actions

Reinforce dietary instructions regarding the prescribed diabetic diet and methods of calculating the foods/fluids allowed (e.g., exchange list, consistent carbohydrate diet, Food Guide Pyramid).

Have client plan sample menus before discharge to ensure that he/she is able to calculate the diet correctly.

Explain the purpose of weight reduction if client has been placed on a caloric restriction to reduce weight. Reinforce need to avoid fasting and fad diets.

Instruct client on appropriate dietary adjustments that should be made if meal schedule or activity level has been significantly altered.

Reinforce the following principles of good dietary management:

* Eat three meals each day about 4 to 5 hrs apart and close to the same time each day; do not skip meals.
* Limit intake of concentrated sweets (e.g., sugar, candy, syrups, jams, jellies, cakes, pies, pastries, fruits packed in heavy syrup).
* Avoid foods high in saturated fat and cholesterol (e.g., butter, cheese, eggs, ice cream, red meat) and *trans* fats (e.g., stick margarine and shortening and foods such as commercial baked goods that are prepared with these products).

Knowledge of dietary instructions helps the client to determine appropriate foods to eat and to maintain proper blood glucose levels and nutritional status.

Planning sample menus provides client with an understanding of diet regulations and the ability to care for self.

Fasting or fad diets may impact client's ability to prevent hyperglycemic or hypoglycemic events.

Dietary adjustments help control blood glucose levels while maintaining adequate nutritional status.

Eating regularly timed meals helps prevent large variations in blood glucose levels.

An intake of concentrated sweets may precipitate a hyperglycemic event.

Foods high in saturated fat increase the development of atherosclerosis, hypertension, and coronary artery disease.

THERAPEUTIC INTERVENTIONS	RATIONALE
• Increase intake of foods high in soluble fiber (e.g., fruits, whole-grain cereals, green leafy vegetables).	*A high-fiber diet decreases blood glucose levels.*
• Read food/fluid labels and limit intake of those that contain significant amounts of sugar, honey, and nutritive sweeteners such as xylitol, sorbitol, and fructose (nutritive sweeteners are usually labeled as "sugar free" but are only "sucrose free," not carbohydrate free; however, they are not digested and absorbed as well as other carbohydrates and therefore contribute only 2 kcal/g as compared with 4 kcal/g of other carbohydrates).	*Client needs to understand what is in foods to prevent inadvertent increases in blood glucose levels.*
• Use artificial (nonnutritive or noncaloric) sweeteners such as saccharin (e.g., Sweet and Low), acesulfame (e.g., Sunett), and aspartame (e.g., Equal, NutraSweet) when possible.	*Client can use a sweetener without an increase in blood glucose levels.*
• Eat an afternoon carbohydrate snack (e.g., fresh fruit, ½ bagel, 1 cup skim milk) if taking an intermediate-acting insulin in the morning, and a snack at bedtime that includes protein and carbohydrate (e.g., milk and graham crackers, ½ meat sandwich, cheese and crackers) if taking an oral glucose-lowering agent or insulin in the evening.	*Appropriate snacks help maintain adequate blood glucose levels.*
• If alcoholic beverages are consumed:	
• Drink alcohol with food.	*Alcohol can decrease blood glucose levels shortly after drinking and for 8 to 12 hrs afterward. Alcohol can also block effects of diabetic medications.*
• Avoid liqueurs, sweet wines, wine coolers, and sweet mixes that contain large amounts of carbohydrates.	*Wines with high levels of carbohydrates will increase blood sugar levels without any nutritional value.*
• Do not substitute alcohol for anything in prescribed diet.	*Alcohol is not an adequate exchanger for any food type in a prescribed diet.*
	Alcohol may interfere with the liver's ability to produce glucose. If on a weight-control diet, client should avoid alcohol because it adds calories without any nutritional value.
• Limit alcohol intake to two drinks per day for men and one drink per day for women (a "drink" is considered to be 1½ oz of liquor, 12 oz of beer, or 5 oz of wine).	*If a client chooses to drink, he/she should drink only the recommended amount for clients with diabetes.*

THERAPEUTIC INTERVENTIONS	RATIONALE
Desired Outcome: The client will demonstrate the ability to perform blood glucose and urine tests correctly and interpret results accurately.	
Independent Actions	
Review with client how and when to perform a blood glucose measurement and calibrate and maintain a glucose monitoring device.	*Reinforces what client knows and provides an opportunity to expand client's understanding.*
Have client demonstrate blood glucose measurement. Reinforce teaching as necessary.	*Client demonstration of blood glucose measurement provides clients with confidence that they can appropriately monitor blood glucose levels and allows the nurse time to reinforce teaching.*
Instruct client to keep a record of test results and take the record of results to appointments with the health care provider.	*Maintenance of a test results record can provide the health care provider with a long-term view of client's adherence to therapeutic regimen and control of blood glucose level.*
Provide instructions on actions client should take when test results are abnormal. (Some clients are instructed to adjust insulin dose and dietary intake; others are instructed to notify appropriate health care provider).	*Written instructions provide an ongoing resource for client to use in controlling blood glucose level.*

THERAPEUTIC INTERVENTIONS	**RATIONALE**

Desired Outcome: The client will verbalize an understanding of the role of exercise in the management of diabetes.

Independent Actions

Explain how exercise affects blood sugar levels.

Exercise improves insulin's effectiveness, lowers hemoglobin A1c, promotes weight loss, and decreases cardiovascular risk factors.

Provide the following instructions about exercise and diabetes management:

- Maintain a regular exercise program, making sure to start exercise slowly and build up gradually.

  A regular program gives client an indication of how exercise affects blood glucose levels before increasing exercise intensity and length of time.

- Avoid exercising during insulin peak action time.

  This may precipitate a severe hypoglycemic episode.

- Try to exercise about 1 hr after a meal and about the same time of the day.

  Promotes better processing of glucose through increased insulin sensitivity.

- Avoid giving insulin in a site that will be heavily exercised.

  Increased circulation to the injection area will increase utilization of insulin, potentially causing a hypoglycemic event.

- Adjust insulin dosage before exercise according to physician's instructions.

  Adjusting the dosage helps decrease the potential for a hypoglycemic event during exercise.

- Consume extra carbohydrates before vigorous exercise and supplement carbohydrate intake (15–30 g) at 30- to 60-minute intervals during vigorous prolonged exercise.

  Extra carbohydrate before vigorous exercise helps prevent the potential for a hypoglycemic event.

- Maintain adequate hydration during periods of intense exercise.

  Adequate hydration is needed to prevent dehydration.

- Consume an extra bedtime snack on days that exercise has been prolonged or unusually vigorous.

  Doing so helps prevent hypoglycemic events.

- Do not exercise in extreme heat or cold.

  Hot and cold weather affect how the body uses insulin.

- Do not exercise at times when blood sugar is >250 mg/dL and ketones are present in urine or if blood sugar is >300 mg/dL.

  Strenuous exercise is perceived by the body as a stressor, leading to an increased output of counter regulatory hormones and a further increase in blood glucose.

- Perform blood glucose tests more frequently during periods of significant variation in activity level.

  More frequent blood glucose testing during exercise helps prevent large variations in blood glucose level.

- Carry a rapid-acting carbohydrate source (e.g., hard candy, glucose tablets) during exercise (especially if using insulin and if exercise is expected to be prolonged or vigorous).

  Doing so helps prevent hypoglycemic events.

- Stop any activity that causes extreme weakness, trembling, incoordination, or nausea.

  Client should be aware of clinical manifestations of hypoglycemia and stop exercising.

THERAPEUTIC INTERVENTIONS	**RATIONALE**

Desired Outcome: The client will identify health care and hygiene practices that should be integrated into lifestyle.

Independent Actions

Reinforce the importance of adhering to the following health care practices:

- Perform oral hygiene including brushing and flossing at least twice a day.
- Have regular dental appointments at least every 6 months.

  Individuals with diabetes are at higher risk for cavities, gum diseases, and oral infections. Good oral hygiene and regular dental appointments help prevent these from occurring.

- Have annual eye examinations (beginning 5 years after onset for type 1 and at onset for type 2 diabetes).

  Diabetes is the number one cause of blindness in the United States. Regular eye examinations allow for early recognition and treatment of changes and potentially decrease deleterious effects of diabetes.

- Avoid smoking.

  Smoking increases the risk for cardiovascular disease.

- Have feet examined by health care provider annually.

  Early identification of peripheral vascular changes helps prevent neuropathies, foot ulcers, and risk of infection.

Provide instructions about foot care:

- Inspect feet daily for cuts, redness, cracks, blisters, corns, and calluses; use a mirror to check bottoms of feet if necessary.

  Daily foot inspection allows for early identification of alterations that increase the risk of infections that may lead to amputation.

THERAPEUTIC INTERVENTIONS	RATIONALE
• Wash feet daily with a mild soap and warm water and dry gently but thoroughly.	*Doing so prevents breakdown of skin, particularly between toes.*
• Apply lanolin or other lubricating lotion to feet (except between toes) daily.	*Lubricants replace moisture lost from the skin. Lotion should have a low alcohol content to prevent skin dryness.*
• Keep feet dry by wearing cotton socks and avoiding shoes with rubber or plastic soles.	*Cotton socks absorb moisture from perspiration, decreasing risk of fungal infection. Shoes with rubber or plastic soles cause the feet to sweat.*
• Cut nails after a bath or shower; cut them straight across and smooth them with an emery board after cutting.	*The skin is softer after a shower, and proper cutting of nails helps prevent injury to the feet, decreasing the risk for infection.*
• See a podiatrist rather than using home remedies to treat corns, calluses, and ingrown nails or if help is needed with routine nail care.	*Professional foot care helps prevent injury and decrease the risk for infection.*
• Avoid wearing socks, stockings, or garters that are tight.	*These garments may further compromise peripheral blood flow.*
• Buy shoes that fit well and break them in gradually; it is best to buy shoes in the late afternoon when feet are at their largest.	*Peripheral neuropathy and loss of sensation increase the risk of foot injury from ill-fitting shoes.*
• Do not wear open-toed shoes, sandals, high heels, or thongs.	*These types of shoes increase the risk for trauma.*
• Do not walk barefoot; wear shoes or slippers when walking.	*Wearing shoes or slippers prevents foot injury.*
• Do not use a heating pad or hot water bottle on feet; test bath water with bath thermometer, wrist, or elbow before immersing feet (temperature should be 30°C–32°C [84°F–90°F]).	*Peripheral neuropathy and loss of pain and temperature sensation increase the risk for burns and other injuries.*
• Protect feet from extreme cold to prevent vasoconstriction and possible frostbite.	

THERAPEUTIC INTERVENTIONS	RATIONALE
Desired Outcome: The client will identify appropriate safety measures to follow because of the diagnosis of diabetes. **Independent Actions** Teach client the following safety precautions:	
• Always carry an identification card or wear a medical alert bracelet or tag identifying self as a diabetic patient; identification card should have the name of health care provider, the type and dose of insulin and/or oral agent(s), and measures to take if found behaving abnormally or unconscious.	*Carrying identification allows for prompt and appropriate treatment if client is alone and unable to speak.*
• Always carry a rapid-acting carbohydrate, such as glucose tablets or instant glucose gel.	*A rapid-acting carbohydrate is necessary to reverse hypoglycemic events.*
• If insulin-dependent, always have insulin readily available (carry in purse or briefcase).	*Insulin is necessary to reverse hyperglycemic events.*
• If traveling by plane, bus, or train:	
• Carry a letter from health care provider indicating the necessity of having syringes, blood glucose monitoring equipment, and medication.	*A letter from a health professional prevents problems with security when traveling with syringes and other supplies.*
• Keep snack items, a quick-acting source of carbohydrate, a full day's supply of food, blood glucose monitoring equipment, and an extra supply of insulin, injection equipment, and oral agents in carry-on luggage.	*These supplies are necessary to maintain adequate nutrition and appropriate blood glucose levels.*
• Consult physician about plans for pregnancy and maintain close prenatal supervision.	*Pregnancy impacts the way a client controls diabetes, and this should be monitored by a health care practitioner.*
• Keep a glucagon kit readily available and know how and when to use it; make sure significant other is also trained in how to use it.	*A glucagon kit can be used for severe hypoglycemic events.*

Continued...

THERAPEUTIC INTERVENTIONS	RATIONALE
• If ill but able to tolerate some foods/fluids:	
• Take usual dose of insulin or oral glucose-lowering agent unless blood glucose is low.	
• Check blood glucose every 4 hrs or a minimum of four times a day.	*Illness places an additional stress on blood glucose levels. To maintain adequate control, blood glucose levels need to be monitored more frequently.*
• If blood glucose is >240 mg/dL, test urine for ketones.	*Testing for ketones with a blood glucose >240 mg/dL provides early detection of DKA.*
• Drink 8 to 12 oz of caffeine- and alcohol-free fluid (e.g., broth, fruit juice, regular or diet soda, water, Gatorade) every hour.	*Caffeine and alcohol increase urine output and may increase risk for dehydration.*
• If not able to tolerate solid foods, substitute liquids and easily digested soft foods.	*Liquids and soft food can provide adequate nutrition.*
• Do not exercise.	*Exercise may cause hypoglycemia.*
• Notify physician if:	
• Unable to eat for >24 hrs	*Not eating or vomiting may significantly decrease blood glucose levels and increases client's risk for injury.*
• Vomiting or severe diarrhea persists for >4 hrs.	
• Blood glucose level is >300 mg/dL or ketones are present in urine.	*Increased blood glucose levels with presence of ketones in the urine may indicate DKA.*
• Having difficulty breathing or a change in mental status occurs	*These signs and symptoms are indicative of DKA and should be treated immediately.*
• Symptoms of dehydration, such as unusual thirst, dry mouth, or fever occur	
• Inform all health care providers of diabetic conditions.	*This helps the health care team provide the most appropriate care in a timely manner.*

THERAPEUTIC INTERVENTIONS	RATIONALE
Desired Outcome: The client will state signs and symptoms of hypoglycemia and ketoacidosis and appropriate actions for prevention and treatment.	
Independent Actions	
Reinforce the following information about hypoglycemia:	
• Factors that precipitate hypoglycemia (e.g., too much insulin or oral hypoglycemic agent, insufficient oral intake, excessive exercise, excessive alcohol intake)	*The client should be able to identify clinical manifestations of hyperglycemic or hypoglycemic events and the treatment necessary to regain appropriate blood glucose levels.*
• Signs and symptoms of hypoglycemia (e.g., shakiness, nervousness, weakness, hunger, sweating, nightmares, early-morning headache, incoordination, blood glucose <70 mg/dL)	
• Actions to take if signs and symptoms of hypoglycemia occur:	
• Test blood glucose if possible and if <70 mg/dL (or if symptoms are present but glucose testing is not possible), take 15 g of rapid-acting carbohydrate (e.g., half a glass of regular [sugar-containing] soft drink, three glucose tablets, half a tube of instant glucose); if taking acarbose (Precose) or miglitol (Glyset), only the glucose tablets or instant glucose will correct hypoglycemia quickly.	*The client needs to base interventions on blood glucose levels.*
• Retest glucose level in 15 minutes, and if still <70 mg/dL, take another 15 g of rapid-acting carbohydrate; if blood glucose level remains <70 mg/dL and/or symptoms persist for >30 minutes, consult health care provider.	*Retesting of glucose levels provides follow-up information, so client may determine next actions based on blood glucose levels.*

THERAPEUTIC INTERVENTIONS	**RATIONALE**

- After the hypoglycemic episode, consume a snack (e.g., graham crackers and a glass of milk, half a sandwich and half a glass of milk) if it will be longer than 30 minutes until the next meal.

Eating appropriate foods is important to maintain blood glucose level after the hypoglycemic event and prevent continued variations in blood glucose levels.

Teach significant others how to treat hypoglycemia:

- If client is awake but groggy, put corn syrup, honey, cake icing, or instant glucose in client's mouth between cheek and gum.
- If client loses consciousness, administer glucagon injection.

Family members should know what to do in a hypoglycemic event if client is unable to care for self.

Reinforce the following information about ketoacidosis:

- Factors that precipitate ketoacidosis (e.g., emotional stress, infection, failure to take insulin or oral glucose-lowering agent)

Helps client avoid situations in which client is at increased risk for ketoacidosis.

- Signs and symptoms of impending or actual ketoacidosis (e.g., unusual thirst; excessive urination; weakness; warm, flushed skin; blood glucose level >250 mg/dL; ketones in urine; abdominal pain; nausea and vomiting)
- Immediate actions to take if signs and symptoms of ketoacidosis occur:

If client and family are able to recognize signs and symptoms of ketoacidosis, they will be able to seek treatment early and prevent negative effects of ketoacidosis.

- Drink a cup or more of broth or sugar-free liquid if able to tolerate it.
- Administer insulin (if previously instructed in insulin coverage based on blood glucose results).
- Contact health care provider.

Immediate actions decrease the level of blood glucose and improve recovery time frame from ketoacidosis.

THERAPEUTIC INTERVENTIONS	**RATIONALE**

Desired Outcome: The client will state signs and symptoms to report to the health care provider.

Independent Actions

Instruct client to report the following:

- Unexplained episodes of hypoglycemia and ketoacidosis
- Unusual variations in blood glucose results
- A cut, scratch, or burn that becomes red, swollen, or tender or does not start to heal within 24 hrs
- Nausea and vomiting or severe diarrhea that lasts >4 hrs
- Temperature elevation that lasts >2 days
- Change in vision
- Development or worsening of symptoms that are indicative of long-term complications (e.g., burning or aching pain in extremity, decreased sensation in extremity, persistent gastric discomfort, frequent urination of small amounts, impotence, gait disturbances, chest pain, extreme fatigue, persistent dizziness, or lightheadedness)

These events should be reported to the client's health care practitioner to prevent further complications and for prompt implementation of therapeutic interventions.

THERAPEUTIC INTERVENTIONS	**RATIONALE**

Desired Outcome: The client will identify resources that can assist in the adjustment to and management of diabetes.

Independent Actions

Provide information about resources that can assist client and significant others in adjustment to and management of diabetes (e.g., American Diabetes Association, diabetic education classes, weight loss programs, diabetes support groups, counseling services, publications such as Diabetes Forecast, Internet sites [www.diabetes.org]). Initiate a referral if indicated.

Giving client resources provides for a continuum of care once client is discharged from the acute care facility.

THERAPEUTIC INTERVENTIONS	RATIONALE

Desired Outcome: The client, in collaboration with the nurse, will develop a plan for adhering to recommended follow-up care including future appointments with health care provider and for laboratory studies.

Independent Actions
Reinforce the importance of keeping follow-up appointments with health care provider and for laboratory studies.

Follow-up appointments allow for early recognition and treatment to help prevent or delay the macrovascular and microvascular complications of diabetes.

ADDITIONAL CARE PLANS

DIARRHEA NDx
Related to: Effects of autonomic neuropathy on intestinal motility

RISK FOR FALLS NDx
Related to:
- Gait abnormalities (may result from impaired proprioception and muscle weakness and loss of normal structure of the foot) and muscle weakness and diminished reflexes in one or more lower extremity associated with motor and sensory neuropathies that may be present
- Dizziness and syncope associated with postural hypotension that may be present as a result of autonomic neuropathy
- Diminished visual acuity

RISK FOR INJURY NDx
Burns related to:
- Decreased sensation in extremities (may be present as a result of peripheral polyneuropathy)

SEXUAL DYSFUNCTION NDx
Related to: Autonomic neuropathy and angiopathies that may occur (men may experience impotence and ejaculatory changes; women may experience changes in arousal pattern, vaginal lubrication, and orgasm)

INEFFECTIVE COPING NDx
Related to:
- Fear of complications and inability to manage them
- Discomfort
- Need to alter lifestyle
- Feeling of powerlessness
- Knowledge that condition is chronic and will require lifelong medical supervision, dietary regulation, and medication therapy

IMBALANCED NUTRITION: LESS THAN BODY REQUIREMENTS NDx
Related to:
- Decreased cellular uptake and utilization of glucose and a compensatory increase in metabolism of fat and protein stores associated with insulin deficiency
- Decreased oral intake associated with nausea and feeling of fullness resulting from delayed gastric emptying if diabetic gastroparesis is present

URINARY RETENTION NDx
Related to: Loss of bladder sensation and diminished contractility of the detrusor muscle associated with autonomic neuropathy involving the genitourinary system

CONSTIPATION NDx
Related to: Colonic atony or dilatation associated with autonomic neuropathy involving the large bowel

RISK FOR INFECTION NDx
Related to:
- Decreased efficiency of leukocyte function in a hyperglycemic environment
- Delayed healing of any break in skin integrity associated with decreased tissue perfusion and altered nutritional status (There is diminished protein synthesis and tissue repair when insulin is deficient.)

NDx = NANDA Diagnosis   **D** = Delegatable Action   ● = UAP   ✦ = LVN/LPN   ⊝▶ = Go to ⊝volve for animation

10

The Client With Alterations in the Gastrointestinal Tract

ABDOMINAL TRAUMA

Abdominal trauma involves injury to the body structures located between the diaphragm and the pelvis. Injury to abdominal contents occurs from a direct impact or movement of organs within the body as a result of rapid deceleration, causing rupture, lacerations, and/or tears in organs or blood vessels. Organs injured with abdominal trauma include the spleen, liver, stomach, large and small intestines, pancreas, kidneys, and urinary bladder. The large vessels in the abdomen, the aorta and vena cava, may also be injured.

Abdominal trauma occurs as the result of blunt or penetrating trauma. Blunt trauma is the result of motor vehicle accidents, assaults, sports injuries, or falls. In blunt trauma injury, the liver and spleen are the most commonly affected organs. Liver and splenic injuries can lead to profuse bleeding because these organs are highly vascular. The client with injuries to these organs may have upper right quadrant pain, abdominal rigidity and guarding with rebound tenderness, loss of bowel sounds, signs of hemorrhagic shock, and Kehr sign, which is seen with splenic rupture. Injury to the intestines leads to leakage of intestinal contents, leading to abdominal distention, pain, peritonitis, and sepsis, and may lead to multiple organ dysfunction syndrome (MODS). Other injuries that may be seen in individuals with abdominal trauma include pancreatic trauma, diaphragmatic rupture, urinary bladder rupture, tears in the great vessels, renal injury, and stomach and intestinal rupture.

Penetrating abdominal trauma can be caused by stabbing, gunshot, or impalement. In an individual with a penetrating injury it is important to determine the entry and exit point or the trajectory of a stab wound. The external injury may mask extensive internal injury.

A person admitted to the emergency department with an abdominal trauma is assessed using the "ABCDE" method: airway, breathing, circulation, and exposure disability.

Life-threatening injuries are identified and treated. Emergency care focuses on establishing or maintaining a patent airway, establishing or maintaining an effective breathing pattern, pain relief, fluid replacement, and prevention of shock and other potential complications. The initial resuscitation phase focuses on maintaining hemodynamic stability. In a hemodynamically unstable patient, rapid diagnostic evaluation can be accomplished by means of a diagnostic peritoneal lavage or the focused assessment with sonography for trauma (FAST). An exploratory laparotomy with repairs of injuries is required in hemodynamically unstable clients who have a penetrating abdominal injury. After stabilization of the client, care focuses on structural healing and prevention of complications.

This care plan focuses on the adult client hospitalized for treatment of abdominal trauma. Some of the information is applicable to clients receiving follow-up care at home.

OUTCOME/DISCHARGE CRITERIA

The client will:
1. Have evidence of normal healing of trauma and/or surgical wound
2. Have clear, audible breath sounds
3. Tolerate prescribed diet
4. Have surgical pain controlled
5. Have no signs and symptoms of complications
6. State signs and symptoms to report to the health care provider
7. Develop a plan for adhering to recommended follow-up care including future appointments with health care provider, medications prescribed, activity level, and wound care.

Nursing Diagnosis INEFFECTIVE BREATHING PATTERN NDx

Definition: Inspiration and/or expiration that does not provide adequate ventilation.

Related to:
- Increased rate of respirations associated with:
  - Fear and anxiety
  - Pressure on the diaphragm from abdominal distention

- Decreased rate of respirations associated with injury and/or the depressant effect of anesthesia and some medications (e.g., narcotic [opioid] analgesics, some antiemetics)
- Decreased depth of respirations associated with:
  - Reluctance to breathe deeply because of pain
  - Fear, anxiety, weakness, and fatigue
  - Restricted chest expansion resulting from positioning and elevation of the diaphragm if abdominal distention is present

CLINICAL MANIFESTATIONS

Subjective	Objective
Verbal self-report of shortness of breath	Dyspnea; orthopnea; increased respiratory rate; decreased depth of breathing; decreased minute ventilation; decreased vital capacity; nasal flaring; use of accessory muscles to breathe; altered chest excursion; pursed-lip breathing; decreased oxygen saturation; arterial blood gas (ABG) values: respiratory acidosis

RISK FACTOR

- Abdominal injury

DESIRED OUTCOMES

The client will maintain an effective breathing pattern as evidenced by:
a. Normal rate and depth of respirations
b. Absence of dyspnea

NOC OUTCOMES

Respiratory status: ventilation

NIC INTERVENTIONS

Ventilation assistance; respiratory monitoring

NURSING ASSESSMENT	RATIONALE
Assess for signs and symptoms of an ineffective breathing pattern: • Shallow or slow respirations • Limited chest excursion • Tachypnea or dyspnea • Use of accessory muscles when breathing	*Early recognition of signs and symptoms of an ineffective breathing pattern allows for prompt intervention.*
Assess/monitor pulse oximetry (arterial oxygen saturation [SaO₂]), ABG values as indicated.	*Monitoring continuous SaO₂ readings allows for the early detection of hypoxia.* *Assessment of ABG values allows for a more direct measurement of both the partial pressure of oxygen in arterial blood (PaO₂) and the partial pressure of carbon dioxide in arterial blood (PaCO₂), both of which reflect the adequacy of ventilation.*

THERAPEUTIC INTERVENTIONS	RATIONALE

Independent Actions
 Implement measures to improve breathing pattern:
• Perform actions to reduce fear and anxiety:
  • Promote a calm environment.
• Perform actions to reduce pain:
  • Reposition client for comfort.
  • Instruct client to support incision with hands or a pillow when moving or coughing.
• Instruct client to bend knees while coughing and deep breathing.
• Perform actions to reduce the accumulation of gas and fluid in the gastrointestinal (GI) tract:
  • Maintain patency of nasogastric (NG), gastric, or intestinal tubes if present.
	Reducing fear and anxiety helps to prevent shallow and/or rapid breathing.
	 Reducing pain helps to increase the client's willingness to move and breathe more deeply.
	
	 Relieves tension on abdominal muscles and incision.
	
	 Reducing the accumulation of gas in the GI tract decreases pressure on the diaphragm, facilitating more effective ventilation.

Continued...

THERAPEUTIC INTERVENTIONS	RATIONALE
• Have client deep breathe or use incentive spirometer every 1 to 2 hrs.	*Deep breathing and use of an incentive spirometer promote maximal inhalation and lung expansion.*
• Instruct client to breathe slowly if hyperventilating.	*Hyperventilation is an ineffective breathing pattern that can lead to respiratory alkalosis.*
	Clients can often slow breathing rate if they concentrate on doing so.
• Place client in a semi- to high-Fowler's position unless contraindicated.	*A semi- to high-Fowler's position allows for maximal diaphragmatic excursion and lung expansion.*
If client develops signs and symptoms of respiratory distress and impaired gas exchange (e.g., restlessness, confusion, significant decrease in oximetry results, decreased PaO_2 and increased $PaCO_2$ levels):	*Improves tissue oxygenation.*
• Prepare client for intubation and mechanical ventilation.	

Dependent/Collaborative Actions
Implement measures to improve breathing pattern:

• Maintain oxygen as ordered.	*Improves oxygen saturation if the client is unable to maintain normal oxygen saturation.*
• Assist with positive airway pressure techniques if ordered: • Continuous positive airway pressure (CPAP). • Bilevel positive airway pressure (BiPAP). • Flutter/positive expiratory pressure (PEP) device.	*Positive airway pressure techniques increase intrapulmonary (alveolar) pressure, which helps re-expand collapsed alveoli and prevent further alveoli collapse.*
• Administer central nervous system depressants judiciously: • Hold medication and consult physician if respiratory rate is less than 12 breaths/min.	*Central nervous system depressants cause depression of the respiratory center in the brainstem, which can result in a decreased rate and depth of respiration.*
• Perform actions to reduce pain: • Administer analgesics before activities and procedures that can cause pain and before pain becomes severe.	*Reducing pain helps to increase the client's willingness to move and breathe more deeply.*

Nursing Diagnosis **RISK FOR IMBALANCED FLUID VOLUME NDx;**
RISK FOR ELECTROLYTE IMBALANCE* NDx

Definition: **Risk for Imbalanced Fluid Volume NDx:** Susceptible to a decrease, increase, or rapid shift from one to the other of intravascular, interstitial, and/or intracellular fluid, which may compromise health. This refers to body fluid loss, gain, or both. **Risk for Electrolyte Imbalance NDx:** Susceptible to changes in serum electrolyte levels, which may compromise health.

Related to:
• **Deficient fluid volume NDx** related to excessive blood loss, loss of fluid associated with vomiting and NG tube drainage (if present)
• **Hypokalemia and metabolic alkalosis** related to loss of electrolytes and hydrochloric acid associated with blood loss, vomiting, and NG tube drainage

CLINICAL MANIFESTATIONS

Subjective	Objective
Verbal self-report of nausea; headache	Hypotension; tachycardia; prolonged capillary refill >2 to 3 seconds; decreased urine output; vomiting; abnormal serum electrolyte levels; flat neck veins when client is flat; increased urine specific gravity; increased blood urea nitrogen (BUN) and hematocrit (Hct) values

---

*The nurse should select the diagnostic label that is most appropriate based on the assessment of the client.

RISK FACTORS

* Injury
* Possible surgical procedure
* Ineffective fluid level and electrolyte replacement therapy

DESIRED OUTCOMES

The client will maintain fluid and electrolyte balance as evidenced by:

a. Blood pressure (BP) and pulse within normal range for client and stable with position change
b. Capillary refill time less than 2 to 3 seconds
c. Usual mental status
d. Balanced intake and output (I&O)
e. Urine specific gravity within normal range
f. Soft, nondistended abdomen with active bowel sounds
g. Absence of cardiac dysrhythmias, muscle weakness, paresthesias, twitching, spasms, and dizziness
h. BUN, Hct, serum electrolyte, and ABG values within normal range

NOC OUTCOMES

Fluid balance; electrolyte and acid-base balance

NIC INTERVENTIONS

Fluid management; electrolyte management: hypokalemia; electrolyte management: hypocalcemia; acid-base management: metabolic acidosis

NURSING ASSESSMENT

Assess for and report signs and symptoms of deficient fluid volume:

* Postural hypotension and/or low BP
* Weak, rapid pulse
* Capillary refill time longer than 2 to 3 seconds
* Neck veins flat when client is supine
* Change in mental status
* Decreased urine output with increased specific gravity (reflects an actual rather than potential fluid deficit)
* Significant increase in BUN and Hct above previous levels
* Hypokalemia (e.g., cardiac dysrhythmias, postural hypotension, muscle weakness, nausea and vomiting, abdominal distention, hypoactive or absent bowel sounds
* Metabolic acidosis (e.g., drowsiness; disorientation; stupor; rapid, deep respirations; headache; nausea and vomiting; cardiac dysrhythmias; low pH and carbon dioxide [CO_2] content)

RATIONALE

Early recognition of signs and symptoms of fluid and electrolyte imbalance allows for prompt treatment.

THERAPEUTIC INTERVENTIONS

Dependent/Collaborative Actions

Implement measures to treat fluid volume deficit:

* Perform actions to improve hypovolemia associated with recent abdominal injury:
  * Rapidly infuse warmed fluids.
* Administer blood and blood products as ordered.

* Perform actions to prevent nausea and vomiting (e.g., medicate as needed for pain relief).
* If a nasogastric (NG) tube is present and needs to be irrigated frequently and/or with large volumes of solution, irrigate it with normal saline rather than water.

* When oral intake is allowed and tolerated, assist client to choose foods/fluids high in potassium (e.g., bananas, orange juice, potatoes, raisins, cantaloupe, tomato juice).
* After initial fluid volume resuscitation, maintain a fluid intake of at least 2500 mL/day unless contraindicated.

RATIONALE

Clients who experience abdominal injuries often experience excessive bleeding. Replacement fluids are necessary to maintain vascular volume.
Replaces lost blood volume and improves oxygenation to the tissues.
Decreases loss of electrolytes.

Irrigation of an NG Tube with normal saline decreases the loss of electrolytes.

Maintains fluid volume and increases potassium intake.

Maintains vascular fluid volume status.

NDx = NANDA Diagnosis **D** = Delegatable Action ● = UAP ✦ = LVN/LPN ⓔ▶ = Go to ⓔvolve for animation

Continued...

THERAPEUTIC INTERVENTIONS	RATIONALE
• Monitor I&O and administer replacements as ordered.	*Maintains vascular fluid volume.*
• Administer electrolyte replacements (e.g., magnesium sulfate, sodium bicarbonate, potassium) if ordered.	*Helps prevent fluid volume deficit and maintains electrolyte levels.*
If signs and symptoms of hypovolemic shock occur:	
• Place the client flat in bed with legs elevated unless contra-indicated.	*Placing client flat on the bed and elevating the legs increases fluid return to the heart to maintain cardiac output.*
• Monitor vital signs frequently.	*Changes in vital signs indicate improvement or worsening of hypovolemic shock.*
• Administer oxygen as ordered.	*Improves tissue oxygenation.*
• Administer blood products and/or volume expanders as ordered.	*Replaces fluid and/or blood cells, which improves cardiac output and tissue oxygenation.*
• Prepare client for insertion of hemodynamic monitoring devices (e.g., central venous catheter, intra-arterial catheter) if planned.	*Improves ability to monitor hemodynamic changes.*
• Administer vasopressor medications as ordered.	*Improves BP and reduces heart rate.*

Nursing Diagnosis INEFFECTIVE PERIPHERAL TISSUE PERFUSION NDx

Definition: Decrease in blood circulation, which may compromise health.

Related to:
• Hypovolemia secondary to blood loss due to injury and/or subsequent surgical procedure

CLINICAL MANIFESTATIONS

Subjective	Objective
Verbal self-report of nausea, abdominal pain, or tenderness; dizziness and lightheadedness	Hypoactive or absent bowel sounds; nausea; abdominal distention; abdominal pain or tenderness; tachycardia; hypotension; cyanotic, pale skin; oliguria; capillary refill time greater than 2 to 3 seconds; elevated BUN and serum creatinine level; decreasing oxygen saturation

RISK FACTORS
• Decreased cardiac output
• Trauma
• Inadequate therapeutic regimen

DESIRED OUTCOMES

The client will maintain adequate tissue perfusion as evidenced by:
a. BP within normal range and stable with position change
b. Usual mental status
c. Extremities warm with absence of pallor and cyanosis
d. Palpable peripheral pulses
e. Capillary refill time less than 2 to 3 seconds
f. BUN and serum creatinine levels within normal limits
g. Urine output at least 30 mL/h

NOC OUTCOMES

Circulation status; tissue perfusion: abdominal organs; cardiac; cerebral; peripheral; pulmonary

NIC INTERVENTIONS

Circulatory care: arterial insufficiency; circulatory care: venous insufficiency; cerebral perfusion promotion; hypovolemia management

NURSING ASSESSMENT	RATIONALE
Assess for and report signs and symptoms of diminished tissue perfusion: • Significant decreased BP • Restlessness, confusion, or other change in mental status • Reports of dizziness or lightheadedness or occurrence of syncopal episodes • Cool, pale, or cyanotic skin • Diminished or absent peripheral pulses • Increasing abdominal girth • Capillary refill time greater than 2 to 3 seconds • Elevated BUN and serum creatinine levels • Oliguria	*Early recognition of signs and symptoms of diminished GI tissue perfusion allows for prompt intervention.*

THERAPEUTIC INTERVENTIONS	RATIONALE
Dependent/Collaborative Actions Implement measures to maintain adequate tissue perfusion: • Administer intravenous fluids and blood as ordered.	*Intravenous (IV) fluids and blood help to maintain adequate circulatory status and tissue perfusion.*
• Apply thromboembolism deterrent (TED) hose or a sequential compression device.	*Prevents pooling of blood in the extremities.*
• If the client is hypothermic, apply warming blankets to increase temperature.	*Hypothermia inhibits platelet function and decreases coagulation.*
• Administer coagulation factors as ordered.	*Coagulation factors improve body's ability to clot blood and decrease bleeding.*
• Administer supplemental oxygen.	*Helps to improve tissue oxygenation.*
• Prepare client for surgery to further control the bleeding.	

Nursing Diagnosis **ACUTE PAIN** NDx

Definition: Unpleasant sensory and emotional experience associated with actual or potential tissue damage, or described in terms of such damage (International Association for the Study of Pain); sudden or slow onset of any intensity from mild to severe with an anticipated or predictable end, and a duration of less than 3 months.

Related to:
• Injury
• Surgery

CLINICAL MANIFESTATIONS

Subjective Verbal self-report of pain	**Objective** Grimacing; diaphoresis; changes in BP; tachypnea; tachycardia; restlessness; grading behaviors

RISK FACTORS

• Abdominal trauma, bleeding into the abdomen, and surgical intervention

DESIRED OUTCOMES

The client will experience diminished pain as evidenced by:
a. Verbalization of decrease in or absence of pain
b. Relaxed facial expression and body positioning
c. Increased participation in activities
d. Stable vital signs

NOC OUTCOMES

Pain control: comfort level

NIC INTERVENTIONS

Analgesic administration; pain management acute; patient-controlled analgesia (PCA) assistance

---

NDx = NANDA Diagnosis   **D** = Delegatable Action   ● = UAP   ✦ = LVN/LPN   ⊜▶ = Go to ⊜volve for animation

NURSING ASSESSMENT	RATIONALE
Assess for signs and symptoms of pain (e.g., verbalization of pain, grimacing, reluctance to move, restlessness, diaphoresis, increased BP, tachycardia).	*Early recognition of signs and symptoms of pain allows for prompt intervention and improved pain control.*
Assess client's perception of the severity of pain using a pain intensity rating scale.	
Assess specific area of pain (e.g., location and quality); note that a finding of pain radiating to the left shoulder may indicate splenic bleeding (Kehr sign).	

THERAPEUTIC INTERVENTIONS	RATIONALE

Independent Actions

Implement measures to reduce fear and anxiety (e.g., assure client that the need for pain relief is understood; plan methods for achieving pain control with client; provide a calm environment).	*Fear and anxiety are experienced after a traumatic event. Reassurance that the client's issues are understood will help to control pain.*

Dependent/Collaborative Actions

Administer analgesics as ordered.	*Pharmacological therapy is an effective method of reducing or relieving pain. Use opioids with care because they decrease gastric motility.*
Postoperative pain: consult physician about an order for PCA if indicated.	*The use of PCA allows the client to self-administer analgesics within parameters established by the physician. This method facilitates pain management by ensuring prompt administration of the drug when needed, providing more continuous pain relief, and increasing the client's control over the pain.*
Consult appropriate health care provider (e.g., physician, pharmacist, pain management specialist) if above measures fail to provide adequate pain relief.	*Allows for alterations in treatment plan.*

Collaborative Diagnosis **RISK FOR PERITONITIS**

Definition: Inflammation of the peritoneum.

Related to:
- Release of intestinal contents into the peritoneal cavity resulting from abdominal trauma
- Exposure of abdominal contents to pathogens associated with a penetrating abdominal wound

CLINICAL MANIFESTATIONS

Subjective	Objective
Verbal self-report of increasing abdominal pain, rebound tenderness, and nausea	Temperature above 38°C; rigid abdomen; diminished or absent bowel sounds; tachycardia; hypotension; tachypnea; elevated white blood cell (WBC) count

RISK FACTOR
- Exposure to pathogens

DESIRED OUTCOMES

The client will not develop peritonitis as evidenced by:
a. Temperature stable and less than 38°C
b. Soft, nondistended abdomen
c. No increase in abdominal pain and tenderness, nausea, and vomiting
d. Normal bowel sounds
e. Stable vital signs

NURSING ASSESSMENT	RATIONALE
Assess for and report signs and symptoms of peritonitis (e.g., further increase in temperature or temperature above 38°C; distended, rigid abdomen; increase in severity of abdominal pain; rebound tenderness; increased nausea and vomiting; diminished or absent bowel sounds; tachycardia; tachypnea; hypotension; a WBC count greater than 15,000/mm^3).	*Early recognition of signs and symptoms of peritonitis allows for prompt intervention.*

THERAPEUTIC INTERVENTIONS	RATIONALE

Dependent/Collaborative Actions

Implement measures to prevent peritonitis:

- Administer antimicrobials as ordered.

  Prevents and/or treats infections.

- Perform actions to prevent inadvertent removal of wound drain if present:
  - Use caution when changing dressings surrounding drain. **D** ✦

    Prevents accidental dislodgment of a drain if present.

  - Provide extension tubing if necessary. **D** ✦

    Use of extension tubing enables client to move without placing tension on the drain.

  - Instruct client not to pull on drain and drainage tubing. **D** ✦

    Prevents accidental dislodgement of the drain.

- Maintain sterile technique during dressing changes and wound care. **D** ✦

  Prevents introduction of bacteria into the wound.

- Keep abdominal dressing clean and dry. **D** ✦

  Prevents stasis of drainage and decreases potential for infection.

If signs and symptoms of peritonitis occur:

- Withhold oral intake as ordered. **D** ✦

  Withholding oral intake decreases further increase in abdominal contents.

- Place client on bedrest in a semi-Fowler's position. **D** ✦

  Putting the client in a semi-Fowler's position assists in pooling or localizing GI contents and urine in the pelvis rather than under the diaphragm.

- Prepare client for diagnostic tests (e.g., abdominal radiograph, peritoneal aspiration, computed tomography, ultrasonography) if planned.

- Insert an NG tube and maintain suction as ordered. **D** ✦

  Decreases potential for GI distention.

- Administer intravenous fluids and/or blood volume expanders if ordered to prevent or treat shock.

  Maintains circulatory volume and prevents the increased capillary permeability that occurs with inflammation and the subsequent escape of protein, fluid, and electrolytes from the vascular space into the peritoneal cavity.

- Prepare client for surgical intervention (e.g., drainage and irrigation of peritoneum) if indicated.

  Decreases client's fear and anxiety and promotes understanding of what is to happen.

Collaborative Diagnosis | # RISK FOR SEPTIC SHOCK

Definition: A life-threatening medical condition that involves decreased tissue perfusion resulting from a systemic infection.

Related to:

- Systemic hypoperfusion associated with maldistribution of circulating blood, deficient fluid volume, and decreased myocardial contractility resulting from uncontrolled systemic inflammatory response to severe infection

CLINICAL MANIFESTATIONS

Subjective	Objective
N/A	Hypotension; tachycardia; widening pulse pressure; restlessness; warm, flushed skin; change in level of consciousness; capillary refill greater than 2 to 3 seconds; significant decrease in pulse oximetry values; changes in ABG values

RISK FACTORS

- Trauma
- Infection
- Decreased cardiac output
- Failure of regulatory mechanisms

DESIRED OUTCOMES

The client will not develop septic shock as evidenced by:
a. Systolic BP equal to or higher than 90 mm Hg
b. Usual mental status
c. Urine output at least 30 mL/h
d. Extremities warm and usual color
e. Capillary refill time less than 2 to 3 seconds
f. Palpable peripheral pulses

NURSING ASSESSMENT

Assess for and report signs and symptoms of septic shock:
- Hyperdynamic or compensatory phase (e.g., widened pulse pressure with the diastolic pressure dropping and little change in the systolic pressure; restlessness; tachycardia; warm, flushed skin)
- Hypodynamic or progressive phase (e.g., systolic BP less than 90 mm Hg or a reduction of greater than 40 mm Hg from baseline; cool, clammy skin; change in level of consciousness; decreased urine output; rapid, shallow breathing; rapid, thready pulse)

RATIONALE

Early recognition of signs and symptoms of septic shock allows for prompt intervention.

THERAPEUTIC INTERVENTIONS

Dependent/Collaborative Actions
Implement measures to maintain adequate tissue perfusion in order to reduce the risk for septic shock:
- Administer intravenous fluids and blood as ordered.

- Apply TED hose or a sequential compression device.
- If the client is hypothermic, apply warming blankets to increase temperature.
- Administer coagulation factors as ordered.

- Administer supplemental oxygen.
If signs and symptoms of septic shock occur:
- Maintain intravenous fluid therapy as ordered.
- Maintain oxygen therapy as ordered.
- Administer antimicrobials as ordered.

- Administer vasopressors and positive inotropic agents (dopamine, dobutamine, norepinephrine) as ordered.

RATIONALE

IV fluids and administration of blood help maintain adequate circulatory status and tissue perfusion.
Prevents pooling of blood in the extremities.
Hypothermia inhibits platelet function and decreases coagulation.

Coagulation factors improve the body's ability to clot blood and decrease bleeding.
Helps to improve tissue oxygenation.

Helps maintain adequate perfusion, blood pressure, and cardiac output.
Provides supplemental oxygen.
Treats infection, which helps decrease vasodilation caused by the systemic infection.
Vasopressors increase blood pressure and positive inotropic agents increase heart rate to maintain circulatory status.

Collaborative Diagnosis
RISK FOR ORGAN ISCHEMIA/DYSFUNCTION (MULTIPLE ORGAN DYSFUNCTION SYNDROME)

Definition: A life-threatening syndrome in which the body is unable to maintain homeostasis without intervention.

Related to:
- Hypoperfusion of major organs associated with septic shock
- Microvascular thrombosis associated with disseminated intravascular coagulation (DIC) if it occurs

CLINICAL MANIFESTATIONS

Subjective	Objective
N/A	Severe hypotension; tachycardia; urine output less than 30 mL/h; dyspnea, tachypnea; altered ABG values with low PaO_2; elevated BUN and serum creatinine levels; crackles throughout lungs; changes in mental status

RISK FACTORS

- Decreased cardiac output
- Infection
- Decreased vascular fluid volume
- Failure of regulatory mechanisms

DESIRED OUTCOMES

The client will not develop organ ischemia or dysfunction as evidenced by:
a. Usual mental status
b. Urine output at least 30 mL/h
c. Unlabored respirations at 12 to 20 breaths/min
d. Audible breath sounds without an increase in adventitious sounds
e. Absence of new or increased abdominal pain, distention, and diarrhea
f. BUN, creatinine, aspartate aminotransferase (AST), alanine aminotransferase (ALT), and lactate dehydrogenase (LDH) levels within normal range

NURSING ASSESSMENT

Assess for and report signs and symptoms of:
- Cerebral ischemia (e.g., change in mental status)
- Renal insufficiency (e.g., urine output <30 mL/h, elevated serum BUN and creatinine levels)
- Acute respiratory distress syndrome (ARDS) (e.g., dyspnea, increase in respiratory rate, low SaO_2, crackles)
- GI ischemia (e.g., hypoactive or absent bowel sounds, abdominal pain and distention, nausea, vomiting, diarrhea, hematemesis, blood in stool)
- Liver dysfunction (e.g., increased serum AST, ALT, and LDH levels; jaundice)

RATIONALE

Early recognition of signs and symptoms of MODS allows for prompt intervention.

THERAPEUTIC INTERVENTIONS

Dependent/Collaborative Actions

Implement measures to reduce the risk for organ ischemia/dysfunction:
- Administer antimicrobial agents as ordered.

- Maintain fluid intake of 2500 mL/day unless contraindicated.
- Use good hand hygiene.
- Maintain adequate nutritional status.
- Maintain sterile technique during all invasive procedures (e.g., urinary catheterization, venous and arterial punctures, injections).
- Consult physician about discontinuing urinary catheter if one is present.
- Anchor catheter/tubings securely.
- Change equipment, tubings, and solutions according to hospital policy.
- Maintain a closed system for drains (e.g., urinary catheter) and intravenous infusions whenever possible.
- Administer recombinant activated protein C (drotrecogin alfa) if ordered.

RATIONALE

Prevents/treats infections.

Maintains adequate vascular fluid volume.

Decreases transmission of infectious agents.
Required for healing and to fight off infections.
Decreases transmission of infectious agents.

A urinary catheter is another avenue by which the body's defenses can be breached and increases the risk for infection.
Prevents movement and accidental removal.
Decreases potential for infection.

Prevents introduction of infectious agents.

Drotrecogin alfa has antithrombotic, anti-inflammatory, and profibrinolytic activity and may reduce the risk of MODS.

DISCHARGE TEACHING/CONTINUED CARE

Nursing Diagnosis **DEFICIENT KNOWLEDGE** NDx**; INEFFECTIVE FAMILY HEALTH MANAGEMENT** NDx**; OR INEFFECTIVE HEALTH MAINTENANCE*** NDx

Definition: **Deficient Knowledge NDx:** Absence of cognitive information related to specific topic, or its acquisition. **Ineffective Family Health Management NDx:** A pattern of regulating and integrating into family processes a program for the treatment of illness and its sequelae that is unsatisfactory for meeting specific health goals of the family unit. **Ineffective Health Maintenance NDx:** Inability to identify, manage, and/or seek out help to maintain well-being.

CLINICAL MANIFESTATION

Subjective	Objective
Verbal requests for information; verbal statements indicating misunderstanding	Inadequate follow-through of instruction; inappropriate or exaggerated behaviors

RISK FACTORS

• Cognitive limitations or unfamiliarity of situation

NOC OUTCOMES	NIC INTERVENTIONS
Knowledge: treatment regimen; health behavior; health resources	Health system guidance; teaching: individual; teaching: prescribed activity/exercise; teaching: prescribed medications

NURSING ASSESSMENT	RATIONALE
Assess client's willingness to learn and knowledge related to the disease process. Assess for indications that the client may be unable to effectively manage the therapeutic regimen.	*The client's willingness to learn and knowledge base provides the basis for education.* *Early recognition of inability to understand disease process or self-care allows for change in the teaching plan.*

THERAPEUTIC INTERVENTIONS	RATIONALE

Desired Outcome: The client will identify ways to prevent postoperative infection.

Independent Actions
Instruct client in ways to prevent postoperative infection/injury:

• Continue with coughing and deep breathing every 2 hrs while awake.	*These activities improve lung expansion.*
• Continue to use incentive spirometer if activity is limited.	
• Increase activity as ordered.	
• Avoid contact with persons who have infections.	*Decreases potential for infection.*
• Avoid crowds during flu and cold seasons.	
• Decrease or stop smoking.	*Nicotine intake can increase cardiac workload and myocardial oxygen use, thereby decreasing the amount of oxygen necessary to fight infection.*
• Drink at least 10 glasses of liquid per day unless contraindicated.	*Adequate hydration is necessary to maintain fluid balance.*
• Maintain a balanced nutritional intake.	*Balanced nutritional intake is required for healing.*
• Maintain proper balance of rest and activity.	*Promotes healing.*
• Maintain good personal hygiene (especially oral care, hand washing, and perineal care).	*These activities decrease the potential for an infection.*
• Avoid touching any wound unless it is completely healed.	*Prevents introduction of pathogens and decreases potential for infection.*
• Maintain sterile or clean technique as ordered during wound care.	

*The nurse should select the diagnostic label that is most appropriate for the client's discharge teaching needs.

THERAPEUTIC INTERVENTIONS	**RATIONALE**

Desired Outcome: The client will state signs and symptoms to report to the health care provider.

Independent Actions
Instruct client to report the following signs and symptoms:

- Persistent low-grade fever or significantly elevated (≥38.3°C [101°F]) temperature.
- Difficulty breathing.
- Chest pain.
- Productive cough of purulent, green, or rust-colored sputum.
- Increasing weakness or inability to tolerate prescribed activity level.
- Increasing discomfort or discomfort not controlled by prescribed medications and treatments.
- Continued nausea or vomiting.
- Increasing abdominal distention and/or discomfort.
- Separation of wound edges.
- Increasing redness, warmth, pain, or swelling around wound.
- Unusual or excessive drainage from any wound site.
- Pain or swelling in calf of one or both legs.
- Urine retention.
- Frequency, urgency, or burning on urination.
- Cloudy or foul-smelling urine.

Signs and symptoms indicate the client may be experiencing complications from the abdominal injury and/or surgery. Signs and symptoms indicate possible infection of the surgical area or other body systems and possible thromboembolism.

THERAPEUTIC INTERVENTIONS	**RATIONALE**

Desired Outcome: The client, in collaboration with the nurse, will develop a plan for adhering to recommended follow-up care including future appointments with health care provider, medications prescribed, activity level, and wound care.

Independent Actions
Collaborate with client to develop a plan that includes:

Importance of keeping scheduled follow-up appointments with the health care provider.

How to follow physician's instructions on suggested activity level and treatment plan.

Explanation of rationale for, side effects of, and importance of taking medications as prescribed. Inform client of pertinent food and drug interactions.

Include significant others in teaching sessions if possible.

Encourage questions and allow time for reinforcement and clarification of information provided.

Provide written instructions on scheduled appointments with health care provider, dietary modification, activity level, treatment plan, medications prescribed, and signs and symptoms to report.

Reinforcing information improves understanding and adherence to treatment regimen and for follow-up care.

Maintenance of treatment plan is important for continued healing and maintenance of health.

Knowledge of medications and how they impact the system improves client adherence and helps enhance the client's understanding of the importance of adhering to the prescribed medication regimen. The client must be able to recognize alterations in functioning related to medication administration.

Involvement of the client's significant others improves the client's potential for success in maintaining the treatment regimen.

Helps improves client's understanding of discharge information.

Written instructions provide ongoing access to information once client is discharged from the acute care facility.

APPENDICITIS/APPENDECTOMY

Acute appendicitis is one of the most common indications for emergency abdominal surgery. The appendix is a small fingerlike pouch that extends from the inferior part of the cecum and is usually located in the right iliac region. The most common cause of appendicitis is obstruction of the lumen by a fecalith, a foreign body, an appendiceal calculus, a tumor, or intramural thickening caused by lymphoid hyperplasia. Obstruction of the appendix leads to increased luminal pressure, vascular congestion, bacterial invasion, and ultimately, necrosis and perforation of the appendix.

An appendectomy is the surgical removal of the appendix. It can be done via a laparotomy or laparoscopy. A laparoscopic appendectomy offers the advantage of shorter hospitalization and decreased morbidity and mortality but is contraindicated in persons with extensive intraperitoneal adhesions or other intestinal problems that would impede mobilization and dissection of the appendix.

This care plan focuses on the adult client with suspected appendicitis who is hospitalized for a possible appendectomy.

OUTCOME/DISCHARGE CRITERIA

The client will:
1. Have evidence of normal healing of surgical wound
2. Have clear, audible breath sounds
3. Tolerate prescribed diet
4. Have surgical pain controlled
5. Have no signs and symptoms of postoperative complications
6. State signs and symptoms to report to the health care provider
7. Develop a plan for adhering to recommended follow-up care including future appointments with health care provider, medications prescribed, activity level, and wound care

For a full, detailed care plan on this topic, go to http://evolve.elsevier.com/Haugen/careplanning/

BOWEL DIVERSION: ILEOSTOMY

An ileostomy is the diversion of the ileum from the abdominal cavity through an opening created in the abdominal wall. It may be performed after abdominal trauma or to treat conditions such as familial polyposis, intestinal cancer, and most commonly, inflammatory bowel disease that is refractory to conservative management. An ileostomy can be temporary or permanent.

A temporary ileostomy is usually created to allow the bowel to heal after traumatic abdominal injury or to permit healing of a newly constructed ileoanal reservoir (pouch). The ileoanal reservoir is a treatment option for some persons with inflammatory bowel disease or familial polyposis. In the initial surgery, the diseased portion of the intestine is removed, a temporary ileostomy is performed, and a reservoir is created in the rectal area using a portion of the ileum. After 2 to 4 months, the ileostomy is closed, and intestinal continuity is established between the remaining intestine and the ileoanal reservoir.

There are two types of permanent ileostomies. The standard (Brooke) ileostomy is the most common one. It is created by bringing a portion of the terminal ileum through the abdominal wall, usually in the right lower quadrant. The ileostomy drains intermittently but, because it cannot be regulated, a collection device must be worn over the stoma at all times. Another type of permanent ileostomy is the continent ileostomy (abdominal pouch). In this procedure, the terminal ileum is used to construct an intra-abdominal reservoir (Kock pouch). Initially, the reservoir drains via a catheter that is placed through the stoma and a surgically constructed one-way valve. After the surgical area heals, the catheter is removed, and the reservoir only needs to be drained periodically. If the system functions properly, the client does not need to wear a collection device over the stoma.

The type of permanent ileostomy constructed depends on the client's age, underlying disease process, and preference and expertise of the surgeon. A proctocolectomy (removal of the colon, rectum, and anus) is often done at the same time as a permanent ileostomy to treat the disease process or to prevent future bowel changes that could occur. If a proctocolectomy is not performed, the rectal stump is sutured across the top; the rectum stays intact and secretes mucus that is expelled via the anus.

This care plan focuses on the adult client with inflammatory bowel disease hospitalized for bowel diversion with creation of a permanent ileostomy. Much of the postoperative information is applicable to clients receiving follow-up care in an extended care facility or home setting.

OUTCOME/DISCHARGE CRITERIA

The client will:
1. Have surgical pain controlled
2. Have evidence of normal healing of the surgical wound
3. Have a medium pink to red, moist stoma and intact peristomal and perianal skin
4. Have no evidence of fluid and electrolyte imbalances
5. Maintain an adequate nutritional status
6. Have no signs and symptoms of postoperative complications
7. Verbalize a basic understanding of the anatomical changes that have occurred as a result of the bowel diversion
8. Identify ways to maintain fluid and electrolyte balance
9. Verbalize ways to maintain an optimal nutritional status
10. Identify methods of controlling odor and sound associated with ileostomy drainage and gas
11. Demonstrate the ability to change the pouch system, maintain integrity of the peristomal and perianal skin, and maintain adequate stomal integrity
12. Demonstrate the ability to properly use, clean, and store ostomy products
13. Demonstrate the ability to drain and irrigate a continent ileostomy if present
14. Identify ways to prevent and treat blockage of the stoma
15. State signs and symptoms to report to the health care provider

16. Share thoughts and feelings about the effect of altered bowel function on self-concept and lifestyle
17. Identify appropriate community resources that can assist with home management and adjustment to changes resulting from the bowel diversion
18. Develop a plan for adhering to recommended follow-up care including future appointments with health care provider, wound care, activity level, and medications prescribed

USE IN CONJUNCTION WITH STANDARDIZED PREOPERATIVE CARE PLAN

Nursing Diagnosis **DEFICIENT KNOWLEDGE** NDx

Definition: Absence of cognitive information related to a specific topic, or its acquisition.

RISK FACTORS
- Lack of knowledge regarding the surgical procedure, physical preparation for the bowel diversion, sensations that normally occur after surgery and anesthesia, expected appearance and function of the ileostomy, and postoperative care and management of the ileostomy

NOC OUTCOMES
Knowledge: treatment regimen; treatment procedure(s)

NIC INTERVENTIONS
Health system guidance; teaching: individual; teaching: procedure/treatment

NURSING ASSESSMENT	RATIONALE
Assess client's understanding of surgical procedure and outcome.	*Client's understanding of what may occur will decrease anxiety.*

THERAPEUTIC INTERVENTIONS	RATIONALE

Desired Outcome: The client will verbalize an understanding of the surgical procedure, preoperative care, and postoperative sensations and care of the ileostomy; verbalize an understanding of the appearance, function, and management of the ileostomy.

Independent Actions
Provide information regarding specific preoperative care and postoperative sensations and care for clients having a bowel diversion with ileostomy:
- Explain the preoperative bowel preparation (e.g., low-residue or clear liquid diet, cleansing enemas, laxatives, antimicrobial therapy).
- If proctocolectomy is planned, inform client that:
  - A perineal wound drain will be present after surgery.
- Occasional feelings of pressure in the perineal area are expected after surgery and that these will subside as edema decreases.
- If a continent ileostomy is planned, inform client that:
  - A catheter will be inserted into the reservoir during surgery and will extend from the stoma and drain into an external collection device; stress that this is a temporary measure (usually for 2–4 weeks).
  - The reservoir will need to be irrigated periodically (especially in the early postoperative period) to remove mucus that accumulates in the reservoir.
  - After removal of the stomal catheter, a catheter will be inserted into the stoma at regularly scheduled intervals.
Allow time for questions and clarification of information provided.
Arrange for a visit with an enterostomal therapy (ET) nurse if available.
Reinforce information provided by physician and/or ET nurse about the appearance and function of the ileostomy:
- The stoma will be medium pink to red and will be moist.

Improves client's understanding of what will occur during the operative procedure and what to expect during recovery. Information helps to decrease fear and anxiety and improve postoperative adherence to treatment regimen.

This keeps the reservoir from becoming distended while the suture lines are healing.

The bowel used to construct the reservoir initially secretes quite a bit of mucus.

This is to drain the reservoir so that an external collection device will not be needed.

The client should be well informed about what will occur before the procedure and what to expect in the postoperative period and subsequent changes that may occur following discharge.

NDx = NANDA Diagnosis   **D** = Delegatable Action   ● = UAP   ✦ = LVN/LPN   ⊝▶ = Go to ⊝volve for animation

Continued...

THERAPEUTIC INTERVENTIONS	RATIONALE
• The stoma will shrink in size as edema resolves during the first 6 weeks after surgery (final stoma height is usually 1.5–2.5 cm [about ½ to 1 inch] from the skin surface).	
• Slight bleeding of the stoma is expected when it is wiped with tissue.	
• For the first day or two after surgery, the stoma will drain a small amount of clear to white, blood-tinged fluid containing some mucus; after a few days, the color of the drainage will change to green and then light to medium brown as the diet progresses.	
• When the ileostomy begins to function (usually 2–3 days after surgery), the drainage will be watery and high volume (up to 1–2 L/day), but within a couple of weeks the amount will begin to decrease (expected amount of output after 2–3 months is 500–800 mL/day) and develop a thicker, paste-like consistency.	
Provide basic information about peristomal skin care, ways to control intestinal gas and odor of the effluent, products the client will be using after surgery, and irrigation and drainage of the reservoir (if a continent ileostomy is planned).	*Allows client more time to process information when given before surgery.*
Provide visual aids and allow client to handle ileostomy appliances that will be used in the immediate postoperative period. Provide a pouch clamp so that client can practice putting it on and taking it off an empty pouch.	*The client should become familiar with how to use the appliances to decrease stress postoperatively when using the appliances.*
Encourage client to try wearing a pouch system partially filled with water in order to experience how it feels and to determine whether the planned stoma site will be adequate for successful adhesion of the pouch.	*Allows the client to know what the pouch will feel like when working with a full pouch.*
Allow time for questions and clarification of information provided.	

USE IN CONJUNCTION WITH POSTOPERATIVE CARE PLAN

Nursing Diagnosis **RISK FOR IMBALANCED FLUID VOLUME** NDx**;**
RISK FOR ELECTROLYTE IMBALANCE* NDx

Definition: **Risk for Imbalanced Fluid Volume NDx:** Susceptible to a decrease, increase, or rapid shift from one to the other of intravascular, interstitial and/or intracellular fluid, which may compromise health. This refers to body fluid loss, gain, or both. **Risk for Electrolyte Imbalance NDx:** Susceptible to changes in serum electrolyte levels, which may compromise health.

Related to:
Risk for imbalanced fluid volume NDx:
• Restricted oral fluid intake before, during, and after surgery
• Blood loss
• Loss of fluid associated with vomiting, NG tube drainage, and/or high-volume ileostomy output

Risk for electrolyte imbalance NDx: Hypokalemia, hypomagnesemia, and hypochloremia related to loss of electrolytes associated with vomiting, NG tube drainage, decreased oral intake, and/or high-volume ileostomy output

Metabolic alkalosis related to:
• Loss of hydrochloric acid associated with vomiting and NG tube drainage
• Loss of bicarbonate ions associated with high-volume ileostomy output (effluent contains bicarbonate ions that would normally be absorbed throughout the large intestine)

---

*The nurse should determine the most appropriate nursing diagnoses based on client assessment.

CLINICAL MANIFESTATIONS

Subjective	Objective
Verbal self-report of weakness; confusion, nausea	Change in mental status; decreased skin turgor; postural hypotension; weak, rapid pulse; decreased urine output; cardiac dysrhythmias; nausea and vomiting; absent bowel sounds; decreased urine output; capillary refill ≤2 to 3 seconds; decreased electrolyte levels, decreased pH and CO_2 levels; positive Chvostek and Trousseau sign

RISK FACTORS

- Inadequate fluid replacement
- Surgery

DESIRED OUTCOMES

The client will not experience deficient fluid volume, hypokalemia, hypochloremia, hypomagnesemia, and acid-base imbalance as evidenced by:
a. Normal skin turgor
b. Moist mucous membranes
c. Stable weight
d. BP and pulse rate within normal range for client and stable with position change
e. Capillary refill time less than 2 to 3 seconds
f. Usual mental status
g. Balanced I&O within 48 hrs after surgery
h. Urine specific gravity within normal range
i. Return of peristalsis within expected time
j. Absence of cardiac dysrhythmias, twitching, muscle weakness, paresthesias, dizziness, headache, nausea, and vomiting
k. Negative Chvostek and Trousseau sign
l. BUN, serum electrolyte, and ABG values within normal range

NOC OUTCOMES

Fluid balance; electrolyte and acid-base balance

NIC INTERVENTIONS

Fluid monitoring; electrolyte management: hypokalemia; electrolyte management: hypomagnesemia; fluid/electrolyte management; acid-base monitoring; acid-base management: metabolic alkalosis; acid-base management: metabolic acidosis

NURSING ASSESSMENT

Assess for and report signs and symptoms of deficient fluid volume, hypokalemia, hypochloremia, hypomagnesemia, and metabolic alkalosis:
- Decreased skin turgor, dry mucous membranes, thirst
- Weight loss of 2% or greater over a short period
- Postural hypotension and/or low BP
- Capillary refill time greater than 2 to 3 seconds
- Neck veins flat when client is supine
- Change in mental status
- Continued low urine output 48 hrs after surgery with a change in specific gravity

RATIONALE

Early recognition of signs and symptoms of fluid volume deficit and electrolyte imbalance allow for prompt intervention.

Specific gravity will usually increase with an actual fluid volume deficit but may be decreased depending on the cause of the deficit.

Continued...

NURSING ASSESSMENT	RATIONALE
• Excessive ileostomy output (after bowel activity returns) • Elevated BUN • Changes in serum electrolyte levels • Drowsiness • Disorientation • Stupor • Rapid, deep respirations • Headache • Nausea and vomiting • Low pH and CO_2	*After bowel activity returns, expected output may be as high as 2000 mL/day, and then in 10 to 14 days it should begin to gradually decrease to 500 to 800 mL/day within 2 to 3 months.*

THERAPEUTIC INTERVENTIONS	RATIONALE

Independent Actions

Implement measures to prevent or treat fluid volume deficit:

• Perform actions to prevent nausea and vomiting (e.g., assist client to ingest food/fluid slowly, eliminate noxious sights and odors, medicate as needed for pain relief). **D** ✦	*Nausea often causes the client to have decreased fluid volume intake. Persistent vomiting results in excessive loss of fluid.*
• If an NG tube is present and needs to be irrigated frequently and/or with large volumes of solution, irrigate it with normal saline rather than water. **D** ✦	*Irrigation of the NG tube helps prevent fluid volume deficit and maintains electrolyte levels.*
• When oral intake is allowed and tolerated, assist client to choose foods/fluids high in potassium (e.g., bananas, orange juice, potatoes, raisins, cantaloupe, tomato juice).	*Helps to maintain electrolyte levels.*
• Encourage intake of foods that may thicken effluent (e.g., applesauce, bananas, boiled rice, tapioca, pretzels, creamy peanut butter, pasta).	*Foods that thicken fluid in the bowel help slow its progress through the bowel and allow for increased absorption of fluid and electrolytes.*
• Maintain a fluid intake of at least 2500 mL/day unless contraindicated. **D** ✦	*Maintains fluid volume.*
• Monitor I&O and administer fluid replacements as ordered.	*Monitoring I &O provides baseline for fluid volume replacement.*
• Perform actions to reduce fever if present (e.g., sponge client with tepid water, remove excessive clothing or bedcovers). **D** ● ✦	*Reduction of a fever prevents diaphoresis and subsequent loss of fluid.*
• Instruct client to avoid excessive intake of foods/fluids that may cause diarrhea (e.g., raw fruits and vegetables; prune juice; fatty, spicy, or extremely hot or cold items; coffee).	*Foods high in fiber, those that are spicy, very hot or cold, or with caffeine may induce diarrhea.*

Dependent/Collaborative Actions

Implement measures to prevent or treat fluid volume deficit:

• Administer antipyretics.	*Antipyretics are given to reduce fever.*
• Administer electrolyte replacements (e.g., magnesium sulfate, sodium bicarbonate, potassium) if ordered.	*Electrolyte replacements help to normalize fluid and electrolyte levels.*
• Administer antidiarrheal agents (e.g., loperamide, diphenoxylate hydrochloride) if ordered. **D** ✦	*Antidiarrheal medications prevent/treat diarrhea.*
Consult physician if signs and symptoms of deficient fluid volume and electrolyte imbalances persist or worsen.	*Notification of the physician allows for prompt alterations in the treatment plan.*

Nursing Diagnosis **RISK FOR IMPAIRED TISSUE INTEGRITY** NDx

Definition: Susceptible to damage to mucous membrane, cornea, integumentary system, muscular fascia, muscle, tendon, bone, cartilage, joint capsule, and/or ligament, which may compromise health.

Related to:
• Disruption of tissue associated with the surgical procedure
• Delayed wound healing associated with factors such as decreased nutritional status and inadequate blood supply to wound area

- Irritation of skin associated with:
  - Contact with wound drainage, ileostomy output (effluent is rich in proteolytic enzymes), soap residue and perspiration under the pouch, and/or mucus drainage from the anus (occurs if rectum was left intact)
  - Frequent or improper removal of tape, adhesives, or other substances used to secure pouch to the skin
  - Aggressive cleansing of peristomal area
  - Sensitivity to tape, pouch material, ostomy paste, and/or substances used to secure pouch to the skin (e.g., adhesive disk, skin barrier, adhesive spray)
  - Pressure from tubes, appliance belt, and/or pouch drainage valve or clamp

CLINICAL MANIFESTATIONS

Subjective	**Objective**
N/A	Redness of skin around suture line and stoma; redness of skin where tape or skin barrier had been removed; swelling of ileostomy stoma; drainage from wound

RISK FACTORS

- Surgical procedure
- Preoperative nutritional deficit
- Delayed nutritional therapy postoperatively

DESIRED OUTCOMES

The client will experience normal healing of surgical wounds as evidenced by:
a. Gradual reduction in periwound swelling and redness
b. Presence of granulation tissue if healing by secondary or tertiary intervention
c. Intact, approximated wound edges if healing is by primary intention

The client will maintain integrity of peristomal and perianal skin and skin in contact with wound drainage, tape, and tubings as evidenced by:
a. Absence of redness and irritation
b. No skin breakdown

NOC OUTCOMES

Wound healing: primary intention; ostomy self-care; tissue integrity: skin and mucous membranes

NIC INTERVENTIONS

Skin surveillance; pressure ulcer prevention; skin care: topical treatment; incision site care; ostomy care

NURSING ASSESSMENT

Assess for and report signs and symptoms of impaired wound healing (e.g., increasing periwound swelling and redness, pale or necrotic tissue in wounds healing by secondary or tertiary intention, separation of wound edges in wounds healing by primary intention).

Assess for signs and symptoms of:
- Peristomal irritation or breakdown (e.g., redness, inflammation, and/or excoriation of peristomal skin; reports of itching or burning under the pouch seal; inability to keep pouch on)
- Perianal irritation or breakdown (e.g., redness, inflammation, and/or excoriation of perianal skin; reports of itching or burning in perianal area).

RATIONALE

Early recognition of signs and symptoms of impaired wound healing allows for prompt treatment.

THERAPEUTIC INTERVENTIONS

Independent Actions
Implement measures to promote wound healing:

- Ensure that dressings are secure enough to keep them from rubbing and irritating wound.
- Carefully remove tape and dressings when performing wound care.

RATIONALE

Secure dressings help protect the wound from mechanical injury.

These actions decrease stress on the surgical area and support wound healing.

Continued...

THERAPEUTIC INTERVENTIONS	RATIONALE
• Remind client to keep hands away from the wound.	*Prevents cross contamination.*
• Instruct and assist client to support the surgical area when moving.	*Support surgical area. Helps to decrease discomfort and support incision area.*
• Instruct and assist client to splint wound when coughing.	*Helps to prevent infection.*
• Apply abdominal binder during periods of activity if ordered.	
• Encourage the client to eat a diet with adequate amounts of protein. **D** ✦	*Supports immune system and wound healing to prevent infection.*
Implement measures to prevent tissue irritation and breakdown in areas in contact with wound drainage, tape, and tubings:	
• Inspect dressings, wounds, and areas around drains; cleanse wound and change dressings when appropriate.	*These actions prevent wound drainage from contacting or remaining on the skin.*
• Maintain patency of drainage tubes.	
• Apply a collection device over drains that are draining copiously.	*Helps to decrease infections and supports wound healing.*
• Apply a protective barrier product to skin that is likely to be in frequent contact with drainage.	
• When positioning client, ensure that he/she is not lying on tubings. **D** ✦	*Pressure on the skin can compromise circulation to that area; if drainage tubing is occluded, there is an increased risk for leakage of drainage around the tubing.*
• Anchor all tubing securely. **D** ✦	*Anchoring tubing prevents excessive movement of tubes against tissues.*
• Apply a water-soluble lubricant to external nares every 2 to 4 hrs. **D** ✦	*Decreases irritation from NG tube and nasal airway or cannula.*
• Use Montgomery straps or tubular netting. **D** ✦	*Using Montgomery straps or netting helps avoid repeated application and removal of tape if frequent dressing changes are anticipated.*
• When removing tape, pull it in the direction of hair growth; use adhesive solvents if necessary. **D** ✦	*Prevents irritation to skin when removing tape.*
Implement measures to prevent peristomal irritation and breakdown:	
• Shave or clip hair from peristomal skin if necessary. **D** ✦	*Helps achieve an adequate pouch seal and reduce irritation when the pouch system is removed.*
• Patch test all products that will come in contact with the skin (e.g., sealant, ostomy paste, barrier, adhesive, and solvent) before initial use; do not use products that cause redness, rash, itching, or burning.	*The client may be allergic to products used against the skin. Patch testing them will prevent allergic reaction at the suture line or stoma site.*
• Change entire pouch system only when necessary (e.g., if pouch seal is leaking, if client reports burning or itching of the peristomal skin, when the stoma size changes); pouch system is usually changed every 3 days in early postoperative period and then should be able to remain in place for 5 to 7 days.	*Too frequent changes of the pouch system cause unnecessary irritation to the peristomal site.*
• Use a two-piece pouch system (e.g., faceplate and pouch, wafer with flange and pouch) during the initial postoperative period.	*This type of system allows the pouch to be removed to assess the stoma without having to remove the adhesive from the skin.*
• Perform actions to reduce peristomal irritation during removal of the pouch:	
• Place drops of warm water or solvent where the pouch system adheres to the skin; allow time for adhesive to loosen before removing pouch.	*These actions facilitate the removal of the pouch and decrease potential for drainage to contact the skin.*
• Remove pouch system gently and in direction of hair growth; hold skin adjacent to the skin barrier taut and push down slightly on skin.	

THERAPEUTIC INTERVENTIONS	RATIONALE

- Perform actions to prevent effluent from contacting the skin when changing the pouch system or pouch or when the pouch system is on:
  - Change the pouch or pouch system when the ileostomy is least active (e.g., upon awakening in the morning, before meals, 2–4 hrs after eating, before retiring at night).
  - Place a wick (rolled gauze pad or tampon) on the stoma opening when the pouch system or pouch is off.
  - Cleanse peristomal skin thoroughly with mild soap and water, rinse completely, and pat dry; use tepid rather than hot water. — *Prevents burning the skin.*
  - Apply skin sealant to the clean, dry peristomal skin before applying the skin barrier. — *Protects skin from the irritating effects of the adhesive.*
  - Always use a skin barrier (e.g., Reliaseal, Stomahesive). **D** ✦ — *Protects skin from the proteolytic enzymes in the effluent.*
  - Measure the diameter of the stoma; cut skin barrier the same size as stoma and select a pouch with an opening that is not more than 0.3 cm ($^1/_8$ inch) larger than the stoma (it may be necessary to create a pattern to use for cutting barrier and pouch openings if stoma has an irregular shape and cannot be measured using appliance manufacturer's standard measuring guide). — *Creates a barrier that is close to the size of the stoma, decreasing potential for contact between skin and proteolytic enzymes.*
  - Implement measures to achieve an adequate pouch seal:
    - (1) Avoid use of ointments or lotions on peristomal skin. — *Ointments and lotions can interfere with adequate adhesive bonding.*
    - (2) Follow manufacturer's instructions when applying skin products and pouch system. — *Prevents potential injury to skin and poor adhesive bonding.*
    - (3) Use products such as ostomy paste to skin in irregularities around stoma site before applying pouch system. — *Allows for an adequate seal in areas where there are body folds or scars.*
    - (4) Apply firm pressure and remove air pockets when applying pouch system; place client in a supine position. — *Increases tautness of skin surface during application and increases adequate pouch seal.*
  - Empty pouch when it is one third full of effluent or inflated with gas. **D** ✦ — *A heavy or inflated pouch can cause the pouch system to separate from the skin.*
  - Position pouch so gravity flow facilitates drainage away from stoma and peristomal skin. — *Prevents effluent stasis or backflow, which increases the chance of irritation to the skin.*
  - Rinse out bottom of drainable pouch after emptying it and then close pouch clamp securely. — *Prevents leakage of effluent*
  - Use a drainable pouch, 2-piece pouch system, and/or pouch with a release valve if gas is a problem; never puncture or cut the pouch to release gas. — *These actions prevent effluent from seeping out of the pouch and causing skin irritation.*
- If a belted pouch system is used, fasten the belt so that two fingers can slip easily between belt and skin. — *Use of a belted pouch system prevents excessive pressure on the skin and potential skin irritation.*
- Instruct and assist client to check pouch periodically to ensure that pouch clamp is not placing pressure on the skin. **D** ✦

Implement measures to prevent perianal irritation and breakdown:
- Keep perianal area dry and clean. — *Prevents irritation and potential breakdown.*
- Instruct client to regularly perform perineal exercises (e.g., relaxing and tightening perineal and gluteal muscles). — *Increases anal sphincter tone and reduces the risk of mucus leakage.*
- Place absorbent pads in client underwear if needed and change pads when they become damp. — *Prevents irritation of anal area and potential skin breakdown.*
- Apply moisture-barrier ointment to perianal area as ordered. **D** ● ✦

NDx = NANDA Diagnosis   **D** = Delegatable Action   ● = UAP   ✦ = LVN/LPN   ⊝▶ = Go to ⊝volve for animation

Continued...

THERAPEUTIC INTERVENTIONS	RATIONALE
If signs and symptoms of peristomal or perianal skin irritation or breakdown occur: • Cleanse areas gently with warm water. • Avoid use of any product that may have caused the irritation or breakdown. • Perform skin care as ordered or according to hospital procedure.	*Decreases further skin irritation.* *Prevents adverse skin reactions.* *Usual care may include exposing affected area to air for 20 to 30 minutes, applying an antifungal agent or corticosteroid preparation to affected skin, and/or covering all irritated skin with a solid skin barrier. This promotes skin healing.*
Consult appropriate health care provider (e.g., wound care specialist, ET nurse, physician) if area of irritation or breakdown does not improve within 48 hrs.	*Allows for prompt alteration in treatment plan.*

Collaborative Diagnosis **RISK FOR PERITONITIS**

Definition: Inflammation of the peritoneum.

Related to:
• Wound infection (a client with inflammatory bowel disease often has a decreased resistance to infection as a result of long-term preoperative corticosteroid use and decreased nutritional status)
• Leakage of intestinal contents into the peritoneum during surgery and/or postoperatively associated with loss of integrity of the sutures at sites of anastomoses or separation of the peristomal skin from the stoma (retraction of the stoma can occur as a result of slippage of sutures, impaired healing of surgical site, or shrinkage of the supporting tissues)
• Accumulation of wound drainage in the peritoneum

CLINICAL MANIFESTATIONS

Subjective	Objective
Verbal self-report of increasing abdominal pain; rebound tenderness	Hyperthermia, rigid abdomen, vomiting, tachycardia, tachypnea, hypotension, decreased or absent bowel sounds, increased WBC count or failure to decrease to normal levels

RISK FACTORS
• Surgery
• Exposure to pathogens
• Exposure of abdomen to intestinal fluids and content

DESIRED OUTCOMES

The client will not develop peritonitis as evidenced by:
a. Gradual resolution of abdominal pain
b. Soft, nondistended abdomen
c. Temperature declining toward normal
d. Stable vital signs
e. Absence of nausea and vomiting
f. Gradual return of normal bowel sounds
g. WBC count declining toward normal

NURSING ASSESSMENT	RATIONALE
Assess for and report signs and symptoms of peritonitis (e.g., increase in severity of abdominal pain; rebound tenderness; distended, rigid abdomen; increase in temperature; tachycardia; tachypnea; hypotension; nausea; vomiting; continued or diminished or absent bowel sounds; WBC counts that increase or fail to decline toward normal).	*Early recognition of signs and symptoms of peritonitis allows for prompt intervention.*

THERAPEUTIC INTERVENTIONS	RATIONALE

Independent Actions

Implement measures to prevent peritonitis:

- Implement measures to prevent wound infection:
  - Maintain an optimal nutritional status.

    Adequate nutrition is needed to maintain normal function of the immune system.
  - Do not apply dressing too tight.

    Dressings that are too tight decrease circulation to the surgical area and decrease healing.
  - Ensure dressings are secure enough to keep them from rubbing the wound.

    Prevents irritation to the wound.
  - Carefully remove tape from the wound.

    Decreases potential for injury to the stoma.
- Perform measures to maintain patency of wound drain if present:
  - Keep tubing free of kinks. **D** ✦

    Allows drainage to flow away from the wound and prevents distention of the conduit.
  - Empty collection device as often as necessary. **D** ✦

    Prevents stress on the wound and stasis of drainage and prevents distention of the conduit.
  - Maintain suction as ordered.

    Prevents stasis of secretions and prevents distention of conduit.
- Perform measures to prevent inadvertent removal of the tube:

    These actions prevent accidental dislodgement of a drain if present and enables the client to move without placing unnecessary tension on the drain.
  - Use caution when changing dressings surrounding drain. **D** ✦
  - Provide extension tubing if necessary. **D** ✦
  - Instruct client not to pull on drain and drainage tubing. **D** ✦

Dependent/Collaborative Actions

Implement measures to prevent peritonitis:

- Perform actions to prevent distention of the internal reservoir (if client has a continent ileostomy) or remaining segment of the ileum:

    Distention can cause strain on the suture lines and subsequent leakage of effluent into the peritoneal cavity.
  - Implement measures to prevent stomal obstruction:
    (1) Irrigate stoma if ordered.

    Removes excessive mucus that could block stoma.
    (2) Maintain a fluid intake of 2500 mL/day.

    Keeps effluent from becoming too thick and maintains fluid volume.
    (3) Administer oral medications crushed and mixed in water or in liquid or chewable form.

    Undigested pills can block stoma.
  - Instruct client to avoid activates such as drinking carbonated beverages, chewing gum, smoking, and eating gas-producing foods (e.g., cabbage, onions, broccoli, beans, cucumbers)

    Prevents accumulation of air and gas in the remaining intestine or internal reservoir.
  - Use only the prescribed amount of irrigating solution (e.g., 20–30 mL) when irrigating the stoma or internal reservoir.

    Prevents accumulation of fluid in the remaining intestine or internal reservoir.
  - Maintain patency of stomal catheter (e.g., keep stomal catheter and drainage bag below level of reservoir, keep catheter free of kinks, irrigate catheter as ordered).

    Promotes gravity drainage and prevents stasis or backflow of drainage.
  - Change pouch system carefully. **D** ✦

    Helps prevent unintentional dislodgement of the stomal catheter.
  - If client has a continent ileostomy and the stomal catheter is removed before discharge, assist client with drainage of the internal reservoir at scheduled intervals and when client feels increased abdominal pressure.

    Prevents accumulation of drainage in the internal reservoir.
- Do not reposition the stomal catheter.

    Repositioning could disrupt the suture line.
- If the peristomal skin separates from the stoma:

    Appropriate wound care facilitates the formation of granulation tissue in the affected area.
  - Perform wound care as ordered.
  - Prepare client for surgical reconstruction of the stoma if planned.
- Administer antimicrobials if ordered.

    Antimicrobials prevent and treat infections.

NDx = NANDA Diagnosis   **D** = Delegatable Action   ● = UAP   ✦ = LVN/LPN   ⊖▶ = Go to ⊖volve for animation

Continued...

THERAPEUTIC INTERVENTIONS	RATIONALE
• If signs and symptoms of peritonitis occur:	
• Withhold oral intake as ordered. **D** ✦	*Prevents increased pressure in the abdomen.*
• Place client on bedrest in a semi-Fowler's position. **D** ✦	*Positioning in a semi-Fowler's position assists in pooling or localizing GI contents in the pelvis rather than under the diaphragm.*
• Prepare client for diagnostic tests (e.g., abdominal radiograph, peritoneal aspiration, computed tomography, ultrasonography) if planned.	*Decreases client's fear and anxiety.*
• Insert an NG tube and maintain suction as ordered. **D** ✦	*Insertion of an NG tube to suction decreases potential for GI distention.*
• Administer intravenous fluids and/or blood volume expanders if ordered to prevent or treat shock.	*Administration of IV fluids maintains circulatory volume and prevents the increased capillary permeability that occurs with inflammation and the subsequent escape of protein, fluid, and electrolytes from the vascular space into the peritoneal cavity.*
• Prepare client for surgical intervention (e.g., drainage and irrigation of peritoneum, repair of sites of anastomoses) if indicated.	*Decreases client's fear and anxiety.*

Collaborative Diagnosis RISK FOR STOMAL CHANGES

Definition: Changes in the structure of the stoma.

Related to:

Necrosis related to intraoperative and/or postoperative interruption of blood supply to the stoma

Excessive bleeding related to irritation associated with aggressive cleansing of stoma and/or improper fit or application of pouch system

Prolapse related to loss of integrity of the sutures or pressure around the stoma

CLINICAL MANIFESTATIONS

Subjective	Objective
N/A	Changes in color of stoma to pale or dark blue, black, or purple; increased stoma height; increased stoma bleeding and/or edema

RISK FACTORS
- Surgery
- Preoperative poor skin integrity
- Inadequate or inappropriate stomal/skin therapy

DESIRED OUTCOMES

The client will maintain stomal integrity as evidenced by:
a. Medium pink to red stomal coloring
b. Expected stomal height
c. Absence of excessive bleeding and increasing edema of the stoma

NURSING ASSESSMENT	RATIONALE
Assess for and report signs and symptoms of impaired stomal integrity: • Pale, dark red, dusky blue, blue-black, or purple color of stoma • Increased height of stoma • Increased stomal edema or bleeding	*Early recognition of signs and symptoms of impaired stomal integrity allows for prompt treatment.*

THERAPEUTIC INTERVENTIONS	RATIONALE

Independent Actions
Use clear pouches during immediate postoperative period.
Implement measures to maintain integrity of stoma:
* Perform actions to maintain adequate stomal circulation:
  * Ensure that the openings of the skin barrier, faceplate, and pouch are not too small and that the stoma is centered in the openings.
* Instruct client to avoid wearing clothing that puts pressure on the stoma.
* Apply pouch system securely. **D** ✦
* Cleanse stoma gently using a soft cloth, gauze, or tissue. **D** ✦

If signs and symptoms of impaired stomal integrity occur:
* Perform stomal care as ordered.
* Prepare client for surgical revision of stoma if indicated.

Clear pouches allow for easy visibility and assessment of the stoma.
Prevents pressure on and around the stoma.

Prevents it from slipping and irritating or shearing stoma.
These actions prevent skin irritation and decrease risk for infection and injury.

Collaborative Diagnosis ## RISK FOR STOMAL OBSTRUCTION

Definition: Inability of fecal material to pass through the stoma.

Related to:
* Stomal edema and/or blockage of stoma

Subjective	**Objective**
Verbal self-report of abdominal cramping; nausea or increased feeling of fullness	Less than expected output; thin, watery effluent consistency

RISK FACTORS
* Surgery
* Inadequate flushing
* Lack of peristalsis
* Immobility

DESIRED OUTCOMES

The client will not develop stomal obstruction as evidenced by:
a. Expected amount and consistency of ileostomy output
b. No reports of abdominal cramping, nausea, or increased feeling of fullness
c. Absence of vomiting

NURSING ASSESSMENT	RATIONALE

Assess for and report signs and symptoms of stomal obstruction:

* Less than expected amount of ileostomy output

* Change in effluent consistency from a thicker consistency to a thin, watery liquid
* Reports of abdominal cramping, nausea, or increased feeling of fullness
* Vomiting

Early recognition of signs and symptoms of stomal obstruction allows for prompt intervention.
After return of peristalsis, output may be as high as 2000 mL/day and will gradually decrease to about 500 to 800 mL/day.
Postoperatively, effluent gradually becomes thicker; a return to thin, watery consistency may indicate blockage of stoma.

THERAPEUTIC INTERVENTIONS	RATIONALE

Independent Actions
Implement measures to prevent stomal obstruction:
* Irrigate stoma if ordered. **D** ✦
* Administer oral medications crushed and mixed in water or in liquid or chewable form. **D** ✦

Stomal irrigation removes excessive mucus that could block stoma.
Undigested pills can block stoma.

NDx = NANDA Diagnosis   **D** = Delegatable Action   ● = UAP   ✦ = LVN/LPN   ⊝▶ = Go to ⊝volve for animation

Continued...

THERAPEUTIC INTERVENTIONS	RATIONALE
• When oral intake is allowed, perform actions to prevent blockage of stoma by food:	
• Encourage client to eat small, frequent meals rather than three large ones.	*Small meals help keep effluent from becoming too thick and allow body time to more fully digest smaller amounts of food.*
• Instruct client to chew food thoroughly.	*Chewing thoroughly will increase absorption of food.*
• Instruct client to avoid or eat only small amounts of foods that are high in fiber.	*Fibrous foods absorb water in the intestinal tract.*
• Instruct client to avoid or eat only small amounts of foods that are hard to digest (e.g., popcorn, coconut, raw vegetables, fruits with seeds, celery, bean sprouts, bamboo shoots, whole kernel corn, potato skins, bran, nuts, fruit skins).	*Hard-to-digest foods increase abdominal distention.*
If food particles or mucus seem to be obstructing the stoma, implement measures to promote flow of effluent through the stoma:	
• Perform actions to relax the abdominal muscle that surrounds the stoma (e.g., apply warm compresses to the abdomen unless contraindicated, encourage participation in relaxing activities such as reading and listening to music).	*These actions decrease the stricture around the stoma from a contracted abdominal muscle.*
• Perform actions to break up or shift foods or mucus:	
• Encourage fluid intake unless contraindicated.	*Adequate fluid intake liquefies secretions, improving effluent flow out of the stoma.*
• Instruct and assist client to assume a knee-chest position.	*Positioning in the knee-chest position may break up or shift stomal blockage.*
• Gently massage peristomal area unless contraindicated.	*Gentle massage may stimulate peristalsis to move fecal material through the colon.*
• Assist with or gently perform digital dilation of stoma if ordered.	*Provides manual removal of blockage.*
• Irrigate ileostomy if ordered.	*Irrigation of the ileostomy may flush out blockage.*
Dependent/Collaborative Actions	
• Maintain fluid intake of 2500 mL/day unless contraindicated.	*Keeps effluent from becoming too thick.*
If stomal edema seems to be obstructing the stoma, consult physician about gently inserting a catheter through the stoma into the ileal segment.	
If signs and symptoms of stomal obstruction persist:	
• Withhold oral intake as ordered.	*Prevents food from further obstructing stoma.*
• Maintain intravenous fluid therapy.	*Prevents fluid volume deficit and increased viscosity of effluent.*
• Insert an NG tube and maintain suction as ordered.	*An NG tube to suction removes contents from stomach.*
• Prepare client for surgical intervention to remove obstruction if indicated.	*Decreases fear and anxiety.*

Nursing Diagnosis **INEFFECTIVE SEXUALITY PATTERNS** NDx

Definition: Expressions of concern regarding own sexuality.

Related to:
• Decreased libido associated with feelings of loss of femininity/masculinity and sexual attractiveness
• Fear of offensive odor or leakage of effluent and gas
• Fear of rejection by partner
• Discomfort resulting from surgical incision
• Depression

CLINICAL MANIFESTATIONS

Subjective	Objective
Verbal self-report of sexual concerns; expression of fear of rejection by partner	N/A

RISK FACTORS

- Changes in body
- Embarrassed by physical appearance

DESIRED OUTCOMES

The client will demonstrate beginning acceptance of changes in sexual functioning as evidenced by:
a. Verbalization of a perception of self as sexually acceptable and adequate
b. Statements reflecting beginning adjustment to the effects of the ileostomy on sexual functioning

NOC OUTCOMES

Body image; personal well-being; sexual functioning

NIC INTERVENTIONS

Body image enhancement; sexual counseling

NURSING ASSESSMENT	RATIONALE
Assess for signs and symptoms of sexual dysfunction (e.g., verbalization of sexual concerns, alteration in relationship with significant other, reports of anticipated changes in sexual activities or behaviors).	*Early recognition of signs and symptoms of changes in sexual functioning allows for prompt intervention.*

THERAPEUTIC INTERVENTIONS	RATIONALE

Independent Actions

Implement measures to promote optimal sexual functioning:

- Facilitate communication between client and partner; focus on the feelings the couple share and assist them to identify changes that may affect their sexual relationship.

Allows client and partner to explore concerns and work through issues related to changes that affect their sexual relationship.

- Perform actions to promote a positive self-concept (e.g., use odor-proof pouches, change appliance regularly).

Improves self-concept and self-esteem.

- Instruct client in ways to reduce risk of leakage of effluent during sexual activity:
  - Empty the pouch or drain internal reservoir (if present) before sexual activity.

These actions prevent leakage.

  - Secure appliance seal with tape for added security.

Prevents inadvertent dislodgement of the appliance and subsequent leakage.

- If client is concerned about odor, instruct client to:
  - Shower or bathe before sexual activity.
  - Use an odor-proof pouch or pouch deodorant.
  - Use cologne or perfume if desired.
  - Keep room well ventilated.

These actions prevent odor from effluent from being noticed during sexual activity, making the client less self-conscious.

- If client is concerned about the presence of the stoma and pouch system, discuss the possibility of:
  - Using opaque or patterned pouches or decorative pouch covers

Makes client less self-conscious about wearing the appliance.

  - Wearing underwear with the crotch removed (for females), boxer shorts (for males), or a cummerbund or stretch tube top around abdomen during sexual activity

Wearing crotchless underwear provides support for and covers the appliance during sexual activity.

- If client is concerned that operative site discomfort will interfere with usual sexual activity:
  - Assure client that discomfort is temporary and will diminish as the incision heals.
  - Encourage alternatives to intercourse or use of positions that decrease pressure on surgical site (e.g., side lying).

Decreases pressure on the surgical site or pressure from a partner on top of the client during sexual activity.

- If appropriate, involve partner in ileostomy care.

Facilitates partner's adjustment to the changes in client's appearance and body functioning and subsequently decreases the possibility of a partner's rejection of client.

- Encourage client to obtain written information regarding sexual activity from the United Ostomy Association and from manufacturers of ostomy products.

Provides for continuum of care and resources for the client once discharged from the acute care environment.

- Include partner in above discussion and encourage continued support of the client.

Allows client and partner to work through physical changes and emotional concerns together.

Continued...

THERAPEUTIC INTERVENTIONS	RATIONALE
Dependent/Collaborative Actions Consult appropriate health care provider (e.g., ET nurse, psychiatric nurse clinician, sex therapist, physician) if counseling is indicated.	*Provides for a multidisciplinary approach to client care.*

Nursing Diagnosis **DISTURBED SELF-CONCEPT***

Definition: **Disturbed Body Image: NDx** Confusion in mental picture of one's physical self.
Situational Low Self-Esteem: NDx Development of a negative perception of self-worth in response to a current situation.
Ineffective Role Performance: NDx A pattern of behavior and self-expression that do not match the environmental context, norms, and expectations.

Related to:
- Change in appearance associated with presence of stoma and pouch system
- Embarrassment associated with sounds and odor resulting from gas and effluent
- Dependence (usually temporary) on others for assistance with ileostomy management
- Loss of control over bowel elimination if client has conventional ileostomy
- Loss of ability to urinate normally
- Change in appearance associated with the presence of a stoma and appliance
- Changes in usual sexual functioning
- Possibility of impotence if nerve damage occurred during a proctocolectomy (use of nerve-sparing surgical techniques has greatly reduced the occurrence of nerve damage and subsequent impotence)

CLINICAL MANIFESTATIONS

Subjective Verbal self-report of negative feelings about self	**Objective** Lack of participation in activities of daily living; withdrawal from significant others; refusal to look at or touch stoma; lack of planning to adapt to necessary changes in lifestyle

RISK FACTORS
- Physical changes
- Depression
- Surgery
- Inability to perform perceived family role

DESIRED OUTCOMES

The client will demonstrate beginning adaptation to changes in appearance, body functioning, and lifestyle as evidenced by:
a. Verbalization of feelings of self-worth
b. Maintenance of relationships with significant others
c. Active participation in activities of daily living
d. Verbalization of a beginning plan for integrating changes in appearance and body functioning into lifestyle

NOC OUTCOMES

Body image; personal autonomy; self-esteem; psychosocial adjustment: life change

NIC INTERVENTIONS

Body image enhancement; self-esteem enhancement; emotional support; support system enhancement; role enhancement; counseling

NURSING ASSESSMENT	RATIONALE
Assess for signs and symptoms of a disturbed self-concept (e.g., verbalization of negative feelings about self, withdrawal from significant others, lack of participation in activities of daily living, refusal to look at or touch stoma, lack of plan for adapting to necessary changes in lifestyle).	*Early recognition of signs and symptoms of a disturbed self-concept allows for prompt treatment.*

---

*This diagnostic label includes the nursing diagnoses of disturbed body image, situational low self-esteem, and ineffective role performance.

NURSING ASSESSMENT	RATIONALE
Determine the meaning of changes in appearance, body functioning, and lifestyle to the client by encouraging verbalization of feelings and by noting nonverbal responses to the changes experienced.	*An understanding of what the change means to the client provides a basis for planning care.*

THERAPEUTIC INTERVENTIONS	RATIONALE

Independent Actions

Be aware that client may grieve the loss of usual bowel function and change in appearance. Provide support during the grieving process.	*Allow client and significant others to grieve loss of normal body functioning; helps to work through changes that are occurring.*
Emphasize the positive effects of the surgery on future lifestyle (e.g., the discomfort and frequent diarrhea associated with inflammatory bowel disease and the side effects of medications such as corticosteroids usually have had a disruptive effect on many aspects of the client's life).	*Unrealistic expectations may lead to difficulty in dealing with the physical changes that have occurred.*
Implement measures to promote optimal sexual functioning (e.g., ways to support stoma during sexual activity; proper positioning during sexual activity; ways to decrease odor from the stoma during sexual activity).	*Sexual activity may have a positive effect on self-esteem.*
Instruct and assist client in ways to reduce gas formation:	
• Avoid activities that can cause air swallowing (e.g., chewing gum, smoking).	*Prevents abdominal distention related to gas from air swallowing.*
• Limit intake of carbonated beverages and gas-producing foods (e.g., cabbage, onions, beans, radishes, broccoli, cucumbers).	*These foods cause gas production and abdominal distention.*
Instruct client in and assist with measures to reduce the odor of ileostomy drainage and/or gas:	*These interventions are effective in reducing noticeable pouch system odor.*
• Use odor-proof pouches and change appliance regularly.	
• Empty pouch regularly, rinse inside of pouch, and clean off any effluent before closing pouch.	
• Drain the reservoir of continent ileostomy at scheduled intervals and when it feels full to reduce possibility of leakage from stoma.	
• Use a disposable pouch and change it regularly, or clean reusable pouch thoroughly.	
• Perform actions to achieve an adequate pouch seal (e.g., patch test all products that come into contact with the skin, change/empty pouch when necessary, place a drop of warm water on the skin to increase adherence of the appliance, measure diameter of the stoma and cut skin barrier to prevent exposure to the effluent).	
• Limit intake of foods that cause effluent to have a strong odor (e.g., onions, fish, eggs, strong cheeses, asparagus).	
• Increase intake of foods/fluids that control odor (e.g., spinach, parsley, yogurt, buttermilk).	
• Change bed linens and clothing promptly if they become soiled.	
Inform client that pouch and clothing muffle sounds of bowel activity.	*Assures client that bowel sounds may not be noticed by others.*
Assure client that once stomal edema and discomfort associated with the surgery have resolved, the client will be able to dress as before with minor, if any, modifications.	*Realistic expectations about appearance and/or body functioning facilitate goal setting and are essential for positive adaptation to the changes experienced and integration of these changes into self-concept.*
Show client and significant others some of the attractive ileostomy products that are available (e.g., opaque or patterned pouches, pouch covers).	*Helps reduce client self-consciousness.*

Continued...

THERAPEUTIC INTERVENTIONS	RATIONALE
Encourage participation in activities that can assist client to integrate physical changes that have occurred (e.g., ileostomy care, bathing).	Supporting behaviors indicative of positive adaptation to changes encourages the client to repeat these behaviors. Repetition of positive adaptive behaviors facilitates the development of a positive self-concept.
Demonstrate acceptance of client using techniques such as touch and frequent visits.	Frequent visits and the use of touch convey a feeling of acceptance to the client. This enhances feelings of self-worth and assists with the development of a positive self-concept.
Support behaviors suggesting positive adaptation to changes that have occurred (e.g., willingness to care for ileostomy, compliance with the treatment plan, verbalization of feelings of self-worth, maintenance of relationships with significant others).	Improves client's confidence in ability to care for self. This enhances client's feelings of self-worth and assists with the development of a positive self-concept.
Encourage significant others to allow client to do what he/she is able.	Demonstrates to the client that independence can be re-established and/or self-esteem redeveloped.
Assist client's and significant others' adjustment by listening, facilitating communication, and providing information.	Demonstrates acceptance of physical changes by significant others and enhances self-worth.
Encourage visits and support from significant others.	
If acceptable to client, arrange for a visit with an ostomate of similar age and same sex who has successfully adjusted to an ileostomy.	Demonstrates that client is not alone in the changes experienced and ability to have a positive future.
Encourage client to pursue usual roles and interests and to continue involvement in social activities.	The ability to pursue usual roles and activities has a positive effect on the client's self-esteem.
Provide information about and encourage utilization of community agencies and support groups (e.g., ostomy groups; sexual, family, individual, and/or financial counseling).	Provides for continuum of care once the client has been discharged from the acute care setting.
If nerve damage that could result in impotence is believed to have occurred during a proctocolectomy, encourage client to discuss it and various treatment options (e.g., vacuum erection aids, penile prosthesis) with physician.	Helps client realize there are options if nerve damage has occurred.

Dependent/Collaborative Actions

Consult appropriate health care provider (e.g., psychologist, psychiatric nurse clinician, ET nurse, physician) if client seems unwilling or unable to adapt to changes resulting from the bowel diversion.	Allows for multidisciplinary interventions.

DISCHARGE TEACHING/CONTINUED CARE

Nursing Diagnosis ## DEFICIENT KNOWLEDGE NDx; INEFFECTIVE FAMILY HEALTH MANAGEMENT NDx; OR INEFFECTIVE HEALTH MAINTENANCE* NDx

Definition: **Deficient Knowledge NDx:** Absence of cognitive information related to specific topic, or its acquisition. **Ineffective Family Health Management NDx:** A attern of regulating and integrating into family processes a program for the treatment of illness and its sequelae that is unsatisfactory for meeting specific health goals of the family unit. **Ineffective Health Maintenance NDx:** Inability to identify, manage, and/or seek help to maintain well-being.

CLINICAL MANIFESTATIONS

Subjective	Objective
Verbal self-report of the problem	Inaccurate follow-through of instructions; inappropriate behaviors

*The nurse should select the diagnostic label that is most appropriate for the client's discharge teaching needs.

RISK FACTORS

- Denial of disease process and physical changes
- Cognitive deficiency
- Failure to participate in self-care while hospitalized

NOC OUTCOMES	NIC INTERVENTIONS
Knowledge: ostomy care; treatment regimen; diet	Health systems guidance; teaching: individual; teaching: disease process; teaching: prescribed diet; teaching: prescribed medication

NURSING ASSESSMENT	RATIONALE
Assess client's knowledge base related to the disease process. Assess for indications that the client may be unable to effectively manage the therapeutic regimen: • Statements reflecting inability to manage care at home • Failure to adhere to treatment plan	*The client's knowledge base provides the basis for education. Early recognition of inability to understand disease process or self-care allows for change in teaching modality.*

THERAPEUTIC INTERVENTIONS	RATIONALE
Desired Outcome: The client will verbalize a basic understanding of anatomical changes that have occurred as a result of the bowel diversion. **Independent Actions** Reinforce teaching regarding the anatomical changes that have occurred as a result of the bowel diversion. Use appropriate teaching aids (e.g., pictures, videotapes, anatomical models).	*Improves client's understanding of surgery and subsequent physical and lifestyle changes as a result of surgery.*

THERAPEUTIC INTERVENTIONS	RATIONALE
Desired Outcome: The client will identify ways to maintain fluid and electrolyte balance. Instruct client to drink at least 10 glasses of liquid per day unless contraindicated and to increase fluid intake during hot weather, during and after intense physical activity, when perspiring profusely, if urine is dark yellow, and during episodes of diarrhea; inform client that pale yellow urine is a good indicator of adequate fluid intake.	*These actions provide client with methods to maintain adequate fluid volume during weather and physical changes.*
Instruct client to perform the following actions to prevent excessive ileostomy output: • Avoid excessive intake of foods/liquids that may cause diarrhea (e.g., raw fruits and vegetables, prune juice, fatty foods, spicy foods, coffee). • Do not take laxatives or excessive amounts of magnesium-containing antacids (e.g., Milk of Magnesia, Mylanta, Maalox). • Take antidiarrheal agents (e.g., loperamide, diphenoxylate hydrochloride) as prescribed.	*Excessive ileostomy output may cause changes in fluid and electrolyte balance. These actions help prevent increased and excessive ileostomy output.*
If ileostomy output increases or becomes more watery, instruct client to: • Increase intake of foods that may thicken effluent (e.g., applesauce, bananas, boiled rice, tapioca, pretzels, creamy peanut butter, pasta).	*Foods that thicken fluid in the bowel help to slow its progress and allow for more fluid and electrolytes to be absorbed.*
• Increase intake of foods/liquids such as fruit juices, Gatorade, potatoes (without skins), bananas, and bouillon. • Drink a mixture of baking soda and water (usually ¼ to ½ teaspoon baking soda in 1 cup of water) if prescribed by physician.	*These actions help maintain electrolyte balance.*

NDx = NANDA Diagnosis   **D** = Delegatable Action   ● = UAP   ✦ = LVN/LPN   ⊝▶ = Go to ⊝*volve* for animation

THERAPEUTIC INTERVENTIONS	RATIONALE

Desired Outcome: The client will verbalize ways to maintain an optimal nutritional status.

Independent Actions
Provide instructions regarding ways to maintain an optimal nutritional status:

- Stress the importance of eating a well-balanced diet.

  Eating a well-balanced diet is necessary for postoperative healing and normal body functions.

- Stress the need to chew food thoroughly.

  Thoroughly chewing foods enhances digestion and subsequent absorption of nutrients.

- Stress the importance of taking vitamins and minerals as prescribed.

  Vitamin and mineral supplements enhance nutritional status.

THERAPEUTIC INTERVENTIONS	RATIONALE

Desired Outcome: The client will identify methods of controlling odor and sound associated with ileostomy drainage and gas.

Independent Actions
Reinforce instructions regarding ways to reduce gas formation and odor associated with ileostomy drainage and gas (e.g., avoid activities that can cause air swallowing, limit intake of carbonated beverages, use odor-proof pouches, change pouch regularly).

These actions prevent abdominal distention related to gas from air swallowing or intake of gas-producing foods. Reduction of odor and excessive bowel sounds help improve client's self-esteem.

Inform client that the ostomy pouch and clothing will muffle the sounds from the ileostomy.

THERAPEUTIC INTERVENTIONS	RATIONALE

Desired Outcome: The client will demonstrate the ability to change the pouch system, maintain integrity of the peristomal and perianal skin, and maintain adequate stomal integrity.

Independent Actions
Reinforce teaching regarding application of the pouch system, prevention of peristomal and perianal skin irritation and breakdown, and maintenance of adequate stomal integrity:

- Shave or clip hair from peristomal skin as necessary.

  Helps achieve an adequate pouch seal and reduces irritation when the pouch system is removed.

- Patch test all products to prevent irritation or allergic reaction when used.

  Helps prevent skin irritation surrounding the stoma.

- Change entire pouch system only when necessary.
- Place drops of warm water or solvent where the pouch system adheres to the skin.

  Facilitates removal of pouch system.

- Remove pouch system gently and in direction of hair growth; hold skin adjacent to the skin barrier taut and push down on skin slightly.

  Facilitates separation of pouch system and client's skin.

Support client's efforts to decrease odor of effluent and gas but discourage excessive changing and emptying of pouch or pouch system.

Excessive pouch system changing and emptying causes skin and stoma irritation.

Instruct and assist client to establish a routine for emptying and changing pouch or emptying ileostomy.

A routine for emptying and changing the pouch system reduces the risk of leakage of effluent and skin irritation.

Instruct client to follow special precautions for products used (e.g., skin sealants should be used only on healthy peristomal skin).

Skin sealants used on reddened and excoriated skin can cause further irritation.

THERAPEUTIC INTERVENTIONS	RATIONALE
Allow time for questions, clarification, practice, and return demonstration of emptying the pouch, changing the pouch system, and performing appropriate stoma and skin care.	*Improves client's self-confidence in ability to care for self.*

THERAPEUTIC INTERVENTIONS	RATIONALE

Desired Outcome: The client will demonstrate the ability to properly use, clean, and store ostomy products.

Independent Actions	
Instruct client regarding proper use of ostomy products that will be used after discharge.	*Improves client's self-confidence in ability to care for self.*
Demonstrate appropriate pouch system cleansing. Emphasize importance of:	*These actions in caring for the pouch system help decrease odors and prevent leakage of effluent onto the skin.*
• Rinsing inside of pouch each time it is emptied.	
• Soaking reusable pouch according to manufacturer's instruction and allowing it to dry thoroughly before reusing.	
Instruct client to avoid reusing disposable products and to discard a reusable pouch if it retains an odor after thorough cleansing or it becomes brittle.	
Discuss recommended methods of storing ostomy products based on manufacturer's recommendations.	

THERAPEUTIC INTERVENTIONS	RATIONALE

Desired Outcome: The client will demonstrate the ability to drain and irrigate a continent ileostomy if present.

Independent Actions	
Explain the gradual and progressive clamping routine if catheter will still be in the stoma of a continent ileostomy at time of discharge.	*Initially, the reservoir will need to be drained for 5 to 15 minutes every 3 to 4 hrs, but after about 6 months, it may need emptying only 2 to 3 times a day.*
If the stomal catheter has been removed, demonstrate the correct method of and explain the schedule for stomal catheter insertion.	
Demonstrate the correct technique for irrigating a continent ileostomy. Caution client to use only the prescribed amount of irrigant (usually 20–30 mL).	*Avoids overdistending and damaging the internal reservoir.*

THERAPEUTIC INTERVENTIONS	RATIONALE

Desired Outcome: The client will identify ways to prevent and treat blockage of the stoma.

Independent Actions	
Instruct client in ways to prevent blockage of the stoma:	
• Drink at least 10 glasses of liquid per day unless contraindicated.	*Adequate hydration helps liquefy stool.*
• Chew food thoroughly.	*Thoroughly chewing food prevents food particles from blocking stoma.*
	These foods can block the stoma.
• Avoid or eat only small amounts of foods that are high in fiber or hard to digest (e.g., popcorn, coconut, raw vegetables, bean sprouts, bamboo shoots, celery, caraway seeds, whole kernel corn, potato skins, fruit with seeds, nuts, fruit skins).	

Continued...

THERAPEUTIC INTERVENTIONS	RATIONALE
• Ensure that skin barrier and pouch openings are large enough to prevent mechanical constriction of the stoma.	*Appropriate sizing and placement of pouch system prevents the stoma from becoming blocked due to lack of appropriate drainage of effluent.*
Instruct client in ways to unblock the stoma:	
• Apply a warm compress to abdomen.	*These actions help relax abdominal muscles around the stoma and enhance removal of what is blocking the stoma.*
• Participate in relaxing activities (e.g., warm bath, reading).	
• Assume a knee-chest position.	
• Gently message the peristomal area.	
• Irrigate the stoma or gently perform digital dilation of the stoma if prescribed.	
Demonstrate techniques and have client provide a return demonstration of massage of the abdomen, irrigation of stoma, and digital dilation of stoma if appropriate.	*Enhances client's self-esteem and confidence in ability to care for self.*

THERAPEUTIC INTERVENTIONS	RATIONALE

Desired Outcome: The client will state signs and symptoms to report to the health care provider.

Independent Actions

Educate the client on signs and symptoms to report to the health care provider:

• Difficulty breathing.	*May indicate a thromboembolism.*
• Productive cough of discolored sputum.	*May indicate an infection.*
• Unusual or excessive drainage from the wound site.	
• Pain or swelling in the calf of one or both legs.	*May indicate a deep vein thrombus.*
• Unusual and continuous abdominal or pelvic pain.	*May indicate that pain has not been well controlled or possible injury to the client.*
• Temperature above 38°C (100.4°F).	*May indicate an infection or dehydration.*
• Absence of or reduction in urinary output despite an adequate fluid intake.	*May indicate a urinary tract infection.*
• Dark red, dusky blue, blue-black, purple, or pale stoma.	*May indicate strangulation of the stoma.*
• Change in color, consistency, or odor of effluent that is not readily identified as a response to food or fluid intake.	*May indicate a blockage in the bowel.*
• Unexplained change in shape, size, or height of stoma (use diagrams and descriptive terms so client does not confuse decreasing stoma size due to resolving edema with actual stomal retraction).	*May indicate injury, infection, or improper healing.*
• Excessive bleeding of stoma or bloody drainage from stoma.	*May indicate injury.*
• Difficulty accomplishing ileostomy care.	*May indicate lack of acceptance of physical changes or understanding of self-care.*
• Persistent skin irritation and breakdown.	*May lead to an infection.*
• Bright red, bumpy, itchy rash or white-coated area on skin around stoma.	*May indicate an allergic reaction or yeast infection.*
• Persistent thirst, dry mucous membranes, dizziness, or decreased urine output.	*May indicate dehydration/inadequate fluid volume.*
• Irregular pulse, muscle weakness and cramping, nausea, and vomiting.	*May indicate decreased serum potassium levels.*
• Headache, abdominal cramping, fatigue, and irritability.	*May indicate decreased serum sodium levels.*
• Thin, watery ileostomy output; absence of ileostomy output; unusual foul odor of gas; abdominal distention and/or nausea and vomiting that does not resolve within 2 hrs of implementing measures to relieve stomal blockage.	*These indicate a possible blockage of bowel above the stoma.*
• Persistent leakage of pouch systems.	*May indicate lack of understanding of self-care.*
• Persistent leakage of effluent from stoma if client has a continent ileostomy.	
• Fever; pain or cramping in reservoir area; pain when draining the reservoir; and/or persistent watery, high-volume ileostomy output.	*May indicate inflammation of the internal reservoir (pouchitis), which is a long-term complication that can develop in the client with a continent ileostomy.*

THERAPEUTIC INTERVENTIONS	RATIONALE
• Difficulty adjusting to changes in appearance and body functioning.	*May indicate depression and place the client at risk for poor self-care.*

THERAPEUTIC INTERVENTIONS	RATIONALE

Desired Outcome: The client will identify appropriate community resources that can assist with home management and adjustment to changes resulting from the bowel diversion.

Independent Actions

Provide information about community resources that can assist the client and significant others with home management and adjustment to changes resulting from the bowel diversion (e.g., local ostomy support groups; community health agencies; ET nurse; home health agencies; financial, individual, and family counseling services).	*Provides for continuum of care once client is discharged from the acute care facility.*

THERAPEUTIC INTERVENTIONS	RATIONALE

Desired Outcome: The client, in collaboration with the nurse, will develop a plan for adhering to recommended follow-up care including future appointments with health care provider, wound care, activity level, and medications prescribed.

Independent Actions

Collaborate with client to develop a plan to include:
How to adhere to instructions regarding activity limitations:

• Avoid strenuous exercise and lifting objects more than 10 lbs. for at least 6 weeks.	*Prevents potential injury to suture line and to stoma.*
• Avoid participating in contact sports.	
Provide client with a list of ostomy products he/she is using (including product name, size, and number) and where these supplies can be obtained.	*Provides for continuum of care once client is discharged from acute care facility.*
Explanation of the rationale for, side effects of, food and drug interactions, and the importance of taking medications as prescribed (e.g., electrolyte supplements, vitamins, antimicrobials).	*Knowledge of medications and how they impact the system improves client adherence to treatment regimen and understanding of the importance of adhering to the prescribed medication regimen. The client must be able to recognize alterations in functioning related to medication administration and what clinical manifestations that should be reported to the health care provider.*
Stress that oral medications should be crushed or in liquid, chewable, uncoated, or sugar-coated form rather than enteric-coated tablets or timed-release capsules.	*Medications should be in liquid, chewable, crushed, uncoated, or sugar-coated so absorption can take place before the medication is excreted. Unabsorbed medications may cause stomal blockage.*

ADDITIONAL NURSING DIAGNOSES

IMBALANCED NUTRITION: LESS THAN BODY REQUIREMENTS NDx
Related to:
- Decreased oral intake associated with prescribed dietary modifications; pain; weakness; fatigue; nausea; and fear of excessive ileostomy output, gas, and/or odor
- Inadequate nutrition replacement therapy
- Loss of nutrients associated with vomiting and excessive ileostomy output

- Decreased absorption of nutrients associated with loss of absorptive surface of the bowel resulting from surgical removal of a large portion of the intestine
- Increased nutritional needs associated with the increased metabolic rate that occurs during wound healing

INEFFECTIVE COPING NDx
Related to:
- Fear, anxiety, and depression associated with loss of control over bowel elimination (especially with a conventional ileostomy) and possibility of rejection by others

- Difficulty performing ileostomy care and incorporating the care into lifestyle
- Need for lifelong medical supervision

GRIEVING NDx
- Related to loss of usual manner of bowel elimination and change in appearance associated with the ileostomy

ENTERAL NUTRITION

Malnutrition, defined as an imbalance in the essential components of a healthy diet, is common in clients with acute and chronic illnesses cared for in both long-term and acute care settings. Left untreated, malnutrition can lead to compromise of the immune system, decreased respiratory ability, and muscle and adipose tissue wasting. Enteral nutrition, also known as tube feeding, is one method of providing nutritional support for malnourished clients who have a functioning GI tract but are unable to take any or enough oral nourishment.

Categories of malnutrition include protein-calorie malnutrition (PCM), marasmus, kwashiorkor, and micronutrient malnutrition, the less visible form of malnutrition resulting from deficiencies of vitamins and minerals. PCM can result from either primary or secondary factors. Primary PCM results from poor eating habits, whereas secondary PCM results from alterations in normal ingestion, digestion, absorption, or metabolism. Marasmus, which results from caloric and protein deficiencies, can lead to the loss of both muscle and body fat. Kwashiorkor results from a protein deficiency that occurs within the setting of a catabolic stress event such as surgery, burns, or infectious diseases. Micronutrient malnutrition results from deficiencies in vitamins A, B, C, D, and calcium, iron, and iodine, and other necessary nutrient components.

Several diagnostic studies can assist in assessment of a client's nutritional state. Serum albumin, the most frequently assessed value, with a half-life of 20 to 22 days, is not the best indicator of a client's current state of malnutrition because the value lags behind a client's current protein deficiency by as much as 14 days. Serum prealbumin, with a half-life of approximately 2 days, is a much better indicator of a client's current nutritional state. Serum transferrin, BUN, Hct, and hemoglobin (Hgb) levels and the lymphocyte count provide additional values that assist in understanding a client's current nutritional state. Anthropometric measurements such as skinfold thickness, body circumferences, and bioelectrical impedance analysis can provide information about the amount of muscle mass, body fat, and protein reserves the client has.

Enteral nutrition, or feeding through the GI tract, is the preferred route of nutrient delivery in hospitalized and critically ill clients. Enteral nutrition helps to prevent villous atrophy and promotes the local immune function of the gut. Enteral nutrition is delivered via an NG tube (short-term), or a tube placed in the duodenum or jejunum (long-term). Enteral nutrition can be delivered continuously or cyclically by pump, or intermittently by gravity or syringe bolus. The type of formula used for enteral nutrition varies depending upon the clinical diagnosis of the client.

This care plan focuses on the adult client undergoing enteral nutritional therapy in an acute care, extended care, or long-term care environment.

OUTCOME/DISCHARGE CRITERIA

The client will:
1. Progressively gain weight toward desired goal
2. Weigh within normal weight for height and age
3. Consume adequate nutrition to meet metabolic needs
4. Be free of signs of malnutrition
5. Maintain adequate fluid volume status
6. Recognize factors contributing to malnutrition/underweight
7. Be free of complications related to enteral feeding

Nursing Diagnosis **RISK FOR ASPIRATION** NDx

Definition: Susceptible to entry of gastrointestinal secretions, oropharyngeal secretions, solids, or fluids to the tracheobronchial passages, which may compromise health.

Related to:
- Decreased gastric motility
- Delayed gastric emptying
- Presence of a GI tube
- Residual gastric volumes
- Impaired swallowing
- Decreased level of consciousness

CLINICAL MANIFESTATIONS

Subjective	Objective
N/A	Rhonchi; cough; dyspnea; tachycardia; presence of tube feeding in aspirate; dull percussion note over affected lung area

RISK FACTORS
- Presence of endotracheal tube
- Depressed cough and gag reflex
- Tracheostomy

DESIRED OUTCOMES

The client will
- Swallow and digest oral, NG, or gastric feeding without aspiration
- Maintain patent airway and lung sounds

NOC OUTCOMES

Aspiration prevention

NIC INTERVENTIONS

Aspiration precautions; respiratory monitoring; swallowing therapy; airway suctioning

NURSING ASSESSMENT

RATIONALE

Assess client's level of consciousness, cough reflex, gag reflex, and swallowing ability.

Reduced level of consciousness, depressed gag or cough reflexes, and alterations in normal swallowing increase the risk for aspiration.

Assess for and report signs and symptoms of aspiration:
- Crackles
- Cough
- Tachycardia
- Presence of tube feeding aspirate
- Dyspnea
- Dull percussion note over affected area

Early recognition of signs and symptoms of aspiration allows for prompt intervention.

Assess client for signs of gastric retention:
- Feelings of fullness
- Nausea/vomiting
- Abdominal distention

Gastric retention can increase the risk for aspiration.

Monitor chest radiograph results. Report findings of pulmonary infiltrate.

Evidence of pulmonary infiltrate on chest radiograph can indicate that aspiration has occurred.

THERAPEUTIC INTERVENTIONS

RATIONALE

Independent Actions

Confirm tube placement before each feeding (for intermittent feedings) or at 4-hr intervals for continuous feedings (or per organizational policy):
- Aspirate stomach contents to verify tube placement.
- Check pH of gastric contents.
- After radiographic confirmation of placement, mark the feeding tube with indelible ink at the exit site from the lip or naris.
  - Observe for changes in the length of the external portion of the feeding tube.

The greatest risks associated with enteral nutrition are malposition of feeding tubes and aspiration. Secondary marking of the tube after initial radiographic confirmation of proper placement allows for additional visual confirmation of tube placement before administering medications or feeding.

Measuring the pH of feeding tube aspirate is of limited benefit with continuous tube feedings because the feedings buffer gastric secretions.

Implement measures during feeding to prevent aspiration: **D** ✦
- Elevate the head of the bed 30 degrees to 45 degrees at all times during feeding.
- Keep head of the bed elevated for 30 to 60 minutes after intermittent feeding.
- Discontinue feeding 30 to 60 minutes before placing the client in a supine position.

Head-of-bed elevation helps to prevent the regurgitation of gastric contents.

Check residual gastric volumes every 4 to 6 hrs: **D** ✦
- Holding of enteral nutrition should not occur for gastric residual volumes <500 mL in the absence of other signs of intolerance. Consult organizational policy.

Checking residual volumes helps to assess gastric emptying. Residual volumes increase with delayed gastric emptying. High gastric residual volumes increase the risk for aspiration of tube feeding formula. Clients are monitored closely for signs of intolerance.

Dependent/Collaborative Actions

Obtain a chest radiograph to confirm placement of an NG or orogastric feeding tube after insertion.

Radiography is the "gold standard" for ruling out respiratory placement of blindly inserted enteral feeding tubes.

NDx = NANDA Diagnosis   **D** = Delegatable Action   ● = UAP   ✦ = LVN/LPN   ⊝▶ = Go to ⊝volve for animation

Continued...

THERAPEUTIC INTERVENTIONS	RATIONALE
If client has an artificial airway (e.g., tracheostomy or endotracheal tube), maintain proper cuff inflation.	*Maintaining adequate cuff pressure helps to secure the airway and prevent aspiration.*
Notify the appropriate health care provider if signs and symptoms of aspiration develop.	*Notifying the appropriate health care provider allows for modification of the treatment plan.*

Nursing Diagnosis IMBALANCED NUTRITION: LESS THAN BODY REQUIREMENTS NDx

Definition: Intake of nutrients insufficient to meet metabolic needs.

Related to: The presence of biological, economical, or psychological factors that prevent the ingestion, digestion, or absorption of nutrients necessary to meet metabolic needs

CLINICAL MANIFESTATIONS

Subjective	Objective
Verbal self-report of abdominal cramping; abdominal pain; aversion to eating; lack of interest in food; perceived inability to eat food; altered taste sensation	Body weight 20% or more under ideal; diarrhea; hyperactive bowel sounds; weight loss with adequate food intake; poor muscle tone; pale mucous membranes; sore buccal cavity; capillary fragility; excessive hair loss

RISK FACTOR
Stress of illness

DESIRED OUTCOMES
The client will:
a. Progressively gain weight toward ideal body weight
b. Consume adequate nourishment
c. Be free of signs of malnutrition

NOC OUTCOMES

Nutritional status: biochemical measures; energy; food and fluid intake; nutrient intake

NIC INTERVENTIONS

Nutritional therapy; nutritional monitoring; nutritional management

NURSING ASSESSMENT	RATIONALE
Assess for and report signs and symptoms of intolerance of enteral feeding: • Vomiting • Diarrhea • Abdominal pain/distention • Constipation • Absence of bowel sounds	*Early recognition of signs and symptoms of problems with enteral feeding allows for prompt intervention.*
Perform or assist with anthropometric measurements such as skinfold thickness if indicated. Report lower than normal values.	*Anthropometric measurements provide information about a client's muscle mass, body fat, and protein reserves.*
Monitor albumin, prealbumin, transferrin, BUN, Hct, and Hgb levels and lymphocyte counts, reporting abnormal values.	*Laboratory values assist in determining the nutritional status of the client.*
Monitor bedside glucose values.	*After initiation of tube feeding, a client is at risk for hyperglycemia. Bedside glucose checks should be assessed. Elderly clients often have difficulty handling high glucose loads and should be monitored closely.*
Assess daily weights.	*Daily weight values will determine whether adjustments to caloric intake are necessary.*

THERAPEUTIC INTERVENTIONS	RATIONALE
Independent Actions Ensure patency of enteral tube: • Irrigate with water before and after intermittent feedings. **D** ✦ • Routinely flush tubes every 4 hrs with 20 to 100 mL sterile water. Monitor client tolerance of tube feeding: • If gastric residual volume greater than 200 to 250 mL, hold tube feeding for 1 hr and recheck residual. **D** ✦	*Feeding tube occlusions are often caused by coagulation of protein-based formulas.* *Routine water flushes with water are necessary to maintain tube patency.* *Tube feedings should not be automatically discontinued because of a single elevated residual volume. The feeding should be held for 1 hr and the client assessed for symptoms of gastric distress. Gastric residual volumes less than 200 mL can be replaced. Any amount greater than 200 mL should be discarded and documented as output. Refer to institutional policy as to current practice regarding residual volumes, as protocols may vary.*
Dependent/Collaborative Actions Consult dietician to determine the number of calories and type of nutrients needed. Administer enteral feedings as ordered. Continuous feedings should be administered via a pump. **D** ✦ Administer prokinetic agents. **D** ✦ Administer pancreatic enzyme solution if tube becomes clogged. Minimize interruptions to continuous tube feedings: • Maintain enteral feedings until the start of medical or diagnostic procedures. • Restart tube feeding within 1 hr unless contraindicated. If signs and symptoms of intolerance to tube feeding develop, consult appropriate health care provider.	*Enteral formulas may vary based on client diagnosis.* *Tube feedings are initiated slowly, increasing gradually during the first 24 to 48 hrs to minimize side effects (e.g., nausea/diarrhea).* *In the presence of high gastric volumes, prokinetic agents can be administered to promote gastric motility and prevent unnecessary cessation of tube feeding.* *Pancreatic enzyme solution with sodium bicarbonate has been successful in unblocking feeding tubes and in prolonging the time to occlusion. Other methods such as soft drinks and cranberry juice have not been consistently effective.* *Nutritional goals for enteral nutrition are often not met because of frequent interruption of feeding. Refer to institutional policy.* *Notifying the appropriate health care provider allows for modification of the treatment plan.*

Nursing Diagnosis RISK FOR DEFICIENT FLUID VOLUME NDx

Definition: Susceptible to experiencing decreased intravascular, interstitial, and/or intracellular fluid volumes, which may compromise health.

Related to: Diarrhea, vomiting, or inadequate fluid intake

CLINICAL MANIFESTATIONS

Subjective	**Objective**
Verbal self-report of weakness	Change in mental status; decreased urine output; increased urine concentration; decreased capillary refill; increased body temperature; elevated Hct; decreased skin turgor; dry skin/mucous membranes; increased pulse rate; decreased BP

RISK FACTORS

- Active fluid volume loss
- Failure of regulatory mechanisms

DESIRED OUTCOMES

The client will not experience a deficient fluid volume as evidenced by:
a. Normal skin turgor
b. Moist mucous membranes
c. Stable weight
d. BP and pulse rate within normal range for client
e. Capillary refill time less than 2 to 3 seconds
f. Usual mental status
g. BUN and Hct within normal limits
h. Balanced I&O

NOC OUTCOMES

Fluid balance

NIC INTERVENTIONS

Fluid monitoring; fluid management; hypovolemia management; intravenous therapy

NURSING ASSESSMENT

Assess for and report signs and symptoms of deficient fluid volume:
- Change in mental status
- Decreased urine output
- Increased urine concentration
- Hyperthermia
- Elevated Hct
- Decreased skin turgor
- Dry mucous membranes
- Increased pulse rate
- Decreased BP

RATIONALE

Early recognition of signs and symptoms of deficient fluid volume allows for prompt intervention.

THERAPEUTIC INTERVENTIONS

Independent Actions

Implement measures to decrease diarrhea:
- Check for medications that may contribute to diarrhea.
- Administer tube feeding at room temperature. **D** ✦
- Decrease the risk of contamination of tube feeding formula:
  - Wash hands with an antimicrobial soap or alcohol-based hand rub for 10 seconds before preparing, handling, and assembling any portion of the tube feeding system.
  - Discard feedings that have been infusing more than 8 to 12 hrs or follow manufacturer's guidelines. **D** ✦
  - Disinfect tube feeding container with 70% isopropyl alcohol, disinfecting the opening of the can and the rim before opening.
  - Refrigerate unused formula and record the date of opening.
  - Use closed systems when possible.
  - Change tubing every 24 hrs.

Dependent/Collaborative Actions

Implement measures to decrease diarrhea:
- Slow tube feeding rate or decrease the strength of the formula.

Implement measures to prevent dehydration:
- Increase supplemental fluids (water) via feeding tube or mouth as ordered.
- Monitor bedside glucose level upon initiation of feeding.

RATIONALE

Diarrhea is a common problem associated with enteral feeding. Feeding too fast, medications such as antibiotics, contamination of feeding formula, and type of formula can be contributing factors.

Contamination of tube feeding could introduce microbes, which could lead to development of diarrhea.

The more calorically dense the formula, the greater the need for supplemental fluids.

Protein content greater than 16% can lead to dehydration.

THERAPEUTIC INTERVENTIONS	RATIONALE
Consult the appropriate health care personnel (e.g., physician, dietician) if diarrhea persists, for a change in formula: • Formula with more fiber content Consult physician if signs and symptoms of deficient fluid volume persist or worsen.	*Notifying the appropriate health care provider allows for modification of the treatment plan.*

DISCHARGE TEACHING/CONTINUED CARE

Nursing Diagnosis ## DEFICIENT KNOWLEDGE NDx; INEFFECTIVE FAMILY HEALTH MANAGEMENT NDx; OR INEFFECTIVE HEALTH MAINTENANCE* NDx

Definition: **Deficient Knowledge NDx:** Absence of cognitive information related to specific topic, or its acquisition. **Ineffective Family Health Management NDx:** A pattern of regulating and integrating into family processes a program for the treatment of illness and its sequelae that is unsatisfactory for meeting specific health goals of the family unit. **Ineffective Health Maintenance NDx:** Inability to identify, manage, and/or seek help to maintain well-being.

CLINICAL MANIFESTATIONS

Subjective	Objective
Verbal self-report of inability to follow prescribed regimen	Inaccurate follow-through of instructions; inappropriate behaviors

RISK FACTORS

- Denial of disease process
- Cognitive deficiency
- Failure to reduce risk factors
- Lack of recall
- Information misinterpretation
- Unfamiliarity with information resources

NOC OUTCOMES	NIC INTERVENTIONS
Knowledge: treatment regimen; infection control	Teaching: individual; teaching: psychomotor skill

NURSING ASSESSMENT	RATIONALE
Assess client's readiness and ability to learn. Assess meaning of nutritional therapy to client.	*Early recognition of readiness to learn and meaning of nutritional therapy to client allows for implementation of the appropriate teaching interventions.*

THERAPEUTIC INTERVENTIONS	RATIONALE
Desired Outcome: The client will be able to demonstrate proper technique in mixing and handling of solutions and administration sets.	
Independent Actions Instruct client and family on the proper way to mix, handle, and store enteral feedings. • Allow time for return demonstration. Instruct client and family on proper care of enteral feeding administration sets: • Discard enteral feeding sets every 24 hrs. • Allow time for return demonstration.	*Enteral feeding should be refrigerated to prevent bacterial growth.* *Changing administration sets every 24 hrs helps prevent bacterial growth.*

*The nurse should select the nursing diagnostic label that is most appropriate for the client's discharge teaching needs

THERAPEUTIC INTERVENTIONS	RATIONALE

Desired Outcome: The client will be able to demonstrate proper care of gastrostomy or jejunostomy tube.

Independent Actions

Instruct the client and family to inspect the skin surrounding the feeding tube site on a daily basis.

The skin surrounding the feeding tube site may become irritated by gastric juices. The client should be instructed to report any redness or maceration.

Instruct client and family on protective skin care measures around the feeding tube site:
- Initially rinse with sterile water and dry.
- After healed, the client may wash with mild soap and water.
- A protective ointment may be used around the insertion site (zinc oxide, Karaya paste) until site is healed.
- Site should be kept clean and dry.

Actions help to protect the skin surrounding the feeding tube, preventing breakdown and infection.

Instruct client to report the following signs and symptoms to health care provider:
- Diarrhea
- Vomiting
- Constipation
- Redness or purulent drainage around gastrostomy or jejunostomy site
- Dislodgement of the tube

These signs and symptoms may be a result of infection, contaminated formula, inappropriate formula, or signs of an infection at the feeding tube insertion site. The appropriate health care provider must be notified to determine whether a change in formula is necessary or whether an infection has developed.

RELATED CARE PLANS

RISK FOR CONSTIPATION NDx
Related to:
- Poor fluid intake
- Formula components

RISK FOR INFECTION NDx
Related to:
- Bacterial contamination of tube feeding formula during preparation or administration
- Bacterial contamination of tube feeding delivery system
- Skin breakdown around jejunostomy or gastrostomy feeding tube site

GASTRECTOMY

Gastrectomy is the surgical removal of all or part of the stomach. There are two main types of gastrectomy; total or full gastrectomy and partial gastrectomy. A gastrectomy procedure is performed to treat numerous conditions including benign or cancerous tumors, bleeding, inflammation, perforations in the stomach wall, polyps or growths, and severe peptic or duodenal ulcers.

A total gastrectomy involves removal of the entire stomach and anastomosis of the esophagus to the jejunum (esophagojejunostomy). It may be considered as treatment for advanced stomach cancer or Zollinger-Ellison syndrome that is not controlled by more conservative measures. A total gastrectomy is performed infrequently because it is so difficult to maintain an adequate nutritional status postoperatively.

The more common type of gastrectomy performed is a partial gastrectomy. This less extensive surgery is most often done to treat cancers of the stomach, peptic ulcer disease that continues to be symptomatic despite conservative management, or to treat complications that develop as a result of the disease (e.g., perforation, gastric outlet obstruction, hemorrhage).

A partial gastrectomy usually involves excision of 40% to 75% of the distal stomach including the antrum (which contains the gastrin-secreting cells) and a portion of the body of the stomach that contains much of the parietal cell mass. GI continuity is re-established by anastomosis of the remaining stomach to the duodenum (gastroduodenostomy, or Billroth I) or jejunum (gastrojejunostomy, or Billroth II). In the latter procedure, the duodenal stump is left intact so that bile and pancreatic secretions can enter the jejunum. The decreased output of gastric secretions that results from a partial gastrectomy can be enhanced by a vagotomy (truncal, selective, or highly selective), which is often performed concurrently to further reduce stimulation of gastric secretions. A truncal vagotomy (resection of the vagal nerve trunks at the level of the esophageal hiatus) is the most effective in reducing gastric secretions; however, the extensive denervation also greatly suppresses gastric motility and impairs normal functioning of the pancreas, gallbladder, and small intestine. Because of this, a selective vagotomy (which preserves the hepatic and celiac branches of the vagus nerve) or highly selective vagotomy (which only affects the parietal cell mass) is performed more frequently.

This care plan focuses on the adult client who is hospitalized for a partial gastrectomy. Much of the postoperative information is applicable to clients receiving follow-up care in an extended care facility or home setting.

The client will:
1. Have surgical pain controlled
2. Have evidence of normal healing of the surgical wound
3. Have clear, audible breath sounds throughout lungs
4. Have no signs and symptoms of postoperative complications
5. Tolerate prescribed diet
6. Verbalize an understanding of ways to maintain an adequate nutritional status
7. Identify ways to control postvagotomy diarrhea if it occurs
8. Identify ways to manage dumping syndrome if it occurs
9. State signs and symptoms to report to the health care provider
10. Develop a plan for adhering to recommended follow-up care including future appointments with health care provider, medications prescribed, activity level, and wound care

For a full, detailed care plan on this topic, go to http://evolve.elsevier.com/Haugen/careplanning/.

BARIATRIC SURGERY

Bariatric surgery is performed to control obesity by restricting the amount of food that the stomach can hold, causing malabsorption of nutrients, or by a combination of both gastric restriction and malabsorption. The most common bariatric surgical procedures are gastric bypass, biliopancreatic diversion, sleeve gastrectomy, and adjustable gastric band. Most weight loss surgical procedures today are done using minimally invasive techniques.

The Roux-en-Y procedure, a gastric bypass procedure that produces 60% to 80% excess weight loss, is considered the gold standard of weight loss surgery. The procedure consists of two components. The first component involves the creation of a 30 mL stomach pouch by dividing the top of the stomach from the rest of the stomach. The second component involves the division of a small portion of the intestine with the bottom portion of the divided small intestine brought up to connect to the new stomach pouch and the top portion of the divided small intestine connected to a more distal portion of the small intestine. As a result, stomach acids and digestive enzymes from the bypassed stomach pass from the pouch directly into the jejunum, eventually mixing with food. The significantly smaller, newly created stomach pouch facilitates smaller meals, resulting in fewer consumed calories. In addition, the food stream is rerouted with less digestion of food in the smaller stomach pouch, resulting in less absorption of calories and nutrients.

The biliopancreatic diversion with duodenal switch also consists of two components: creation of a small tubular stomach pouch by removing a portion of the stomach and bypassing a large portion of the small intestine. Similar to other bariatric procedures, this procedure helps to reduce the volume of food consumed. Unlike other bariatric procedures, approximately ¾ of the small intestine is bypassed by the food stream. This surgery is considered the most effective procedure for the treatment of diabetes, resulting in great weight loss and the ability of clients to consume more normal meals. However, this procedure requires a longer hospitalization and carries the highest complication rate and risk for mortality than other bariatric procedures.

Sleeve gastrectomy,—performed via a laparoscopic approach, removes approximately 80% of the stomach, leaving a remaining pouch the size of a banana. This procedure does not involve the use of implantable foreign objects and induces a rapid, significant weight loss of >50%.

The adjustable gastric band, a minimally invasive procedure with a hospital stay usually less than 24 hrs, involves placement of an inflatable band around the upper portion of the stomach, creating a small pouch above the band and leaving the rest of the stomach below the band. The size of the stomach can be adjusted by filling the band with sterile saline injected through a port placed under the skin. Reducing the size of the opening is done gradually over time, reducing hunger and decreasing caloric consumption. In general, all bariatric surgical procedures cause favorable changes in gut hormones that suppress hunger, reduce appetite, and improve satiety.

Clients undergoing bariatric surgery are carefully screened physically and psychologically and must meet certain criteria before undergoing gastric reduction surgery. Qualifying criteria for bariatric surgery in most areas include body mass index (BMI) ≥ 4 m, or more than 100 lbs overweight, BMI ≥ 35 and at least one or more obesity-related co-morbidities such as type 2 diabetes, hypertension, sleep apnea, and other respiratory disorders, and/or an inability to achieve a healthy weight loss sustained for a period of time with prior weight loss efforts. The client must also be emotionally stable, have no uncontrolled or severe major illness, verbalize a willingness to adhere to lifelong dietary modifications, and have access to adequate follow-up medical care.

This care plan focuses on the adult client hospitalized for gastric reduction surgery. Much of the information is relevant to the client receiving continued care in the home setting.

The client will:
1. Have evidence of normal healing of surgical wounds
2. Have clear, audible breath sounds throughout lungs
3. Tolerate prescribed diet
4. Have no signs and symptoms of postoperative complications
5. Identify ways to prevent excessive stretching of the gastric pouch
6. Verbalize an understanding of ways to maintain an adequate nutritional status
7. Identify ways to reduce the risk of consuming excessive amounts of food, fluid, and calories
8. Demonstrate the ability to accurately calculate and measure the allotted amounts of food and fluid
9. State signs and symptoms to report to the health care provider
10. Identify community resources that can assist in the adjustment to prescribed dietary modifications and future changes in body image
11. Develop a plan for adhering to recommended follow-up care including future appointments with health care provider, activity level, medications prescribed, and wound care

NDx = NANDA Diagnosis   **D** = Delegatable Action   ● = UAP   ✦ = LVN/LPN   ⊜▶ = Go to ⊜volve for animation

PREOPERATIVE USE IN CONJUNCTION WITH PREOPERATIVE AND POSTOPERATIVE CARE PLANS FOR ADDITIONAL DIAGNOSES

Nursing Diagnosis   **DISTURBED SELF-CONCEPT***

Definition: **Disturbed Body Image NDx:** Confusion in mental picture of one's physical self.
Situational Low Self-Esteem NDx: Development of a negative perception of self-worth in response to a current situation.

Related to: Obesity and inability to lose weight by more conventional methods

CLINICAL MANIFESTATIONS

Subjective	Objective
Verbal self-report of feelings or perceptions that reflect an altered view of one's body in appearance, structure, or function; current challenges to self-worth; self-negating verbalizations; indecisive, nonassertive behavior	Lack of involvement in preoperative care or self-care

RISK FACTORS

- Obesity
- Poor self-esteem
- Ineffective dieting

DESIRED OUTCOMES

The client will demonstrate a positive self-concept as evidenced by:
a. Verbalization of feelings of self-worth
b. Positive statements regarding anticipated effects of surgical procedure
c. Maintenance of relationships with significant others
d. Active participation in preoperative care and self-care

NOC OUTCOMES

Body image; self-esteem

NIC INTERVENTIONS

Body image enhancement; self-esteem enhancement; emotional support; support system enhancement

NURSING ASSESSMENT	RATIONALE
Assess for signs and symptoms of a disturbed self-concept: • Verbalization of negative feeling about self • Withdrawal from significant others • Lack of participation in preoperative care or self-care	*Early recognition of signs and symptoms of a disturbed self-concept allows for prompt intervention.*

THERAPEUTIC INTERVENTIONS	RATIONALE
Independent Actions Implement measures to assist client to increase self-esteem (e.g., limit negative self-assessment, encourage positive comments about self, assist to identify strengths, give positive feedback about accomplishments, provide positive feedback about decision to have the surgery and lose weight).	*Self-esteem is a major component of one's view of self. An increase in self-esteem has a positive effect on the client's self-concept.*
Implement measures to reduce client's embarrassment about obesity:	
• Obtain information from physician regarding client's height and weight so that oversized equipment and supplies (e.g., bed, chair, commode, BP cuff, gowns, bathrobe) can be obtained before client is admitted.	*If the equipment is obtained ahead of time, it helps the client feel more comfortable in the health care environment.*
• Remove unnecessary furniture and equipment from room so client can move around easily. **D** ● ✦	*Improves client's mobility.*
• Provide privacy when weighing client. **D** ● ✦	*Privacy while weighing the client decreases client embarrassment.*

*This diagnostic label includes the nursing diagnoses of disturbed body image and chronic low self-esteem.

THERAPEUTIC INTERVENTIONS	RATIONALE
• Transfer client to and from operating room in own hospital bed rather than attempting to use a regular-sized stretcher.	*Prevents embarrassment when trying to transfer client to a regular-sized stretcher.*
Allow client to wear own clothes rather than hospital gown before and after surgery if desired.	*Provides client some control over the situation.*
Assure client that he/she will be assisted with usual grooming and makeup habits after surgery if necessary.	*Decreases anxiety concerning postoperative care.*
Arrange for a visit from an individual who has achieved weight loss after gastric reduction surgery if client desires.	*Provides client with an experiential perspective on postoperative care and lifestyle changes.*
If client is expressing concerns about the amount of excess skin that will be present after the majority of weight loss occurs (usually after 1–1½ years), provide information about various clothing styles that may be most flattering (e.g., long-sleeved shirts or blouses) and reconstructive surgery that is available to remove excess skin from abdomen, breasts, upper arms, and thighs.	*Decreases fear and anxiety concerning postoperative and lifestyle changes.*

Dependent/Collaborative Interventions

Consult physician if client has unrealistic expectations of postoperative weight loss and dietary management.	*Provides additional time for the physician to address client's concerns related to surgery and subsequent lifestyle changes.*

POSTOPERATIVE: USE IN CONJUNCTION WITH THE STANDARDIZED POSTOPERATIVE CARE PLAN

Nursing Diagnosis ## INEFFECTIVE BREATHING PATTERN NDx

Definition: Inspiration and/or expiration that does not provide adequate ventilation.

Related to:
• Increased rate of respirations associated with fear and anxiety
• Decreased rate of respirations associated with the depressant effect of anesthesia (effect lasts longer in the obese client because adipose tissue more readily absorbs and stores anesthetic agents) and some medications (e.g., narcotic [opioid] analgesics, some antiemetics)
• Decreased depth of respirations associated with:
  • Depressant effects of anesthesia and some medications (e.g., narcotic [opioid] analgesics, some antiemetics)
  • Reluctance to breathe deeply because of pain and fear of dislodging tubes
  • Fear, anxiety, weakness, and fatigue
  • Restricted chest expansion resulting from:
    (1) Limited diaphragmatic excursion (occurs because of the large amount of abdominal adipose tissue and postoperative abdominal distention)
    (2) Decreased activity (chest expansion is restricted by the bed surface when client is lying in bed)
    (3) Increased weight of the chest wall of an obese client (especially in women with large, pendulous breasts)

CLINICAL MANIFESTATIONS

Subjective	Objective
Verbal self-report of shortness of breath	Limited chest excursion; tachypnea; dyspnea; use of accessory muscles when breathing; decreased pulse oximetry less than 85%

RISK FACTORS
• Surgical procedure
• Obesity
• Immobility

DESIRED OUTCOMES

The client will maintain an effective breathing pattern as evidenced by:
a. Normal rate and depth of respirations
b. Absence of dyspnea

NDx = NANDA Diagnosis   **D** = Delegatable Action   ● = UAP   ✦ = LVN/LPN   ⊕▶ = Go to ⊖volve for animation

NOC OUTCOMES	NIC INTERVENTIONS
Respiratory status: ventilation	Respiratory monitoring; ventilation assistance

NURSING ASSESSMENT	RATIONALE
Assess for and report signs and symptoms of an ineffective breathing pattern: • Complaints of feeling short of breath • Shallow or slow respirations • Limited chest excursion • Tachypnea • Dyspnea • Use of accessory muscles when breathing	*Early recognition of signs and symptoms of an ineffective breathing pattern allows for prompt intervention.*
Monitor for and report a significant decrease in oximetry results.	*Oximetry is a noninvasive method of measuring SaO$_2$. The results assist in evaluating respiratory status.*

THERAPEUTIC INTERVENTIONS	RATIONALE
Independent Actions	
Implement measures to reduce chest or abdominal pain if present (e.g., splint incision with pillow during coughing and deep breathing). **D** ● ✦	*A client with upper abdominal pain often guards respiratory efforts and breathes shallowly to prevent additional discomfort.*
Implement measures to decrease fear and anxiety (e.g., assure client that breathing deeply will not dislodge tubes or cause incision to break open, interact with client in a confident manner). **D** ● ✦	*Fear and anxiety may cause a client to breathe shallowly or to hyperventilate.* *Decreasing fear and anxiety allows the client to focus on breathing more slowly and taking deeper breaths.*
Implement measures to increase strength and activity tolerance if client is weak and fatigued (e.g., provide uninterrupted rest periods, maintain optimal nutrition). **D** ● ✦	*An increase in strength and activity tolerance enables the client to breathe more deeply and participate in activities to improve breathing pattern.*
Assist client to deep breathe or use incentive spirometer every 1 to 2 hrs. **D** ● ✦	*Deep breathing and use of an incentive spirometer promote maximal inhalation and lung expansion.*
Instruct client to breathe slowly if hyperventilating.	*Hyperventilation is an ineffective breathing pattern that can eventually lead to respiratory alkalosis. The client can often slow breathing rate by concentrating on doing so.*
Position client with head of bed elevated at least 30 degrees at all times. **D** ● ✦	*This position allows for maximal diaphragmatic excursion and lung expansion.*
Instruct and assist client to use overhead trapeze and turn at least every 2 hrs.	*Repositioning promotes maximal chest wall and lung expansion.*
Add extensions to tubings if necessary.	*Enables client to turn and move without fear of dislodging tubes.*
Instruct client to bend knees while coughing and deep breathing.	*Relieves tension on abdominal muscles and incision.*
Instruct and assist client to splint incision with hands or pillow when coughing and deep breathing.	*Provides support to the abdomen and helps to decrease discomfort when coughing and deep breathing.*

Collaborative Diagnosis   RISK FOR OVERDISTENTION OF THE GASTRIC POUCH

Definition: Enlarged, expanded, or stretched.

Related to:
• Accumulation of gas and fluid in the pouch associated with:
  • Decreased peristalsis and/or impaired functioning of NG or gastrostomy tube
  • Obstruction of the pouch outlet (the channel between the pouch and distal stomach if gastroplasty performed or the opening between the pouch and jejunal loop if gastric bypass performed) resulting from edema and/or ingestion of medications or fluids that are too thick to pass through pouch outlet
• Excessive oral intake

CLINICAL MANIFESTATIONS

Subjective	Objective
Verbal self-report of frequent epigastric fullness and nausea	Vomiting

RISK FACTORS
- Physiological changes
- Inappropriate diet and intake

DESIRED OUTCOMES

The client will not experience overdistention of the gastric pouch as evidenced by:
a. Decreased reports of epigastric fullness
b. Absence of nausea and vomiting

NURSING ASSESSMENT	RATIONALE
Assess for and report signs and symptoms of overdistention of the gastric pouch (e.g., increasing reports of epigastric fullness, nausea, vomiting).	*Early recognition of signs and symptoms of overdistention of the gastric pouch allows for prompt intervention.*

THERAPEUTIC INTERVENTIONS	RATIONALE

Dependent/Collaborative Actions

Implement measures to prevent overdistention of the gastric pouch:

- Maintain patency of NG or gastric tube; irrigate the tube only if ordered and with no more than prescribed amount of solution. **D** ✦

    Reduces gas and fluid accumulation during period of decreased peristalsis.

- Encourage and assist client with frequent position changes and ambulation as soon as allowed and tolerated. **D** ● ✦

    Activity stimulates peristalsis, which promotes passage of food through the GI tract and decreases distention of the gastric pouch.

- Instruct the client to avoid activities such as chewing gum and smoking.

    Reduces air swallowing.

- Do not change position of NG or gastric tube unless ordered.

    The NG tube is usually positioned at the pouch outlet to help prevent obstruction of the opening into the distal stomach (if gastroplasty performed) or jejunal loop (if gastric bypass is performed).

- When oral intake is allowed:
    - Adhere strictly to prescribed oral intake schedule (clients usually begin with hourly liquid feedings of 30 mL and, over at least 6 weeks, progress to 5 or 6 small [1–2 oz] liquid meals per day with 1–2 oz of water allowed periodically between meals).

        The stomach size is reduced and the client will have to eat smaller meals to prevent overdistention of the stomach.

    - Provide client with allotted amounts of fluids at the proper times; discard skipped "meals." **D** ● ✦

        This is done so the client does not ingest feedings too close together, as this will cause overdistention of the stomach.

    - Instruct client to adhere to the liquid or blenderized diet as ordered.

        Oral intake that is too thick can block the pouch outlet, which may be narrower in the early postoperative period because of edema.

    - Administer oral medication in liquid or chewable form or crushed thoroughly. **D** ● ✦

        Prevents blockage of the pouch outlet.

- Encourage client to eructate whenever the urge is felt.

    Releases gas from the stomach

- Encourage use of nonnarcotic analgesics once severe pain has subsided.

    Opioid analgesics depress GI motility.

If signs and symptoms of overdistention occur:

Withhold all oral intake as ordered. **D** ● ✦

- Prepare client for upper abdominal radiographs to check placement of NG or gastric tube if present.

    Helps to reduce stomach distention.

    Determines appropriate placement of tubes and whether manipulation of them is required.

- Assist physician with adjustment or reinsertion of the NG or gastric tube if indicated.

Collaborative Diagnosis   ## RISK FOR PERITONITIS

Definition: Inflammation of the peritoneum.

Related to:
- Leakage of gastric contents into the peritoneum associated with disruption of the staple line (if gastroplasty performed) or proximal anastomosis (if gastric bypass performed)

NDx = NANDA Diagnosis   **D** = Delegatable Action   ● = UAP   ✦ = LVN/LPN   ⊖▶ = Go to ⊖volve for animation

CLINICAL MANIFESTATIONS

Subjective	Objective
Verbal self-report of abdominal pain	Nausea and vomiting; distended and rigid abdomen; diminished or absent bowel sounds; fever; tachypnea; increased WBC count

RISK FACTORS

- Surgery
- Exposure to pathogens
- Exposure of abdominal contents to irritating fluids

DESIRED OUTCOMES

The client will not develop peritonitis as evidenced by:
a. Gradual resolution of abdominal pain
b. Soft, nondistended abdomen
c. Temperature declining toward normal
d. Stable vital signs
e. Absence of nausea and vomiting
f. Gradual return of normal bowel sounds
g. WBC count declining toward normal

NURSING ASSESSMENT

Assess for and report signs and symptoms of peritonitis (e.g., increase in severity of abdominal pain; generalized abdominal pain; rebound tenderness; distended, rigid abdomen; increase in temperature; tachycardia; tachypnea; hypotension; nausea; vomiting; continued diminished or absent bowel sounds; WBC count that increases or fails to decline toward normal).

RATIONALE

Early recognition of signs and symptoms of peritonitis allows for prompt intervention.

THERAPEUTIC INTERVENTIONS

RATIONALE

Dependent/Collaborative Actions
Implement measures to prevent peritonitis:
- Implement measures to prevent wound infection:
  - Maintain an optimal nutritional status.
  - Administer vitamins and minerals as ordered. **D** ✦

  - Do not apply dressing too tight. **D** ✦
- Ensure dressings are secure enough to keep them from rubbing the wound.
  - Carefully remove tape from the wound. **D** ✦
  - Maintain adequate fluid volume of 2500 mL/day unless contraindicated. **D** ✦
- Perform measures to maintain patency of wound drain if present.
  - Keep tubing free of kinks. **D** ✦

  - Empty collection device as often as necessary. **D** ✦

  - Maintain suction as ordered. **D** ✦
- Perform measures to prevent inadvertent removal of the tube:
  - Use caution when changing dressings surrounding drain. **D** ✦
  - Provide extension tubing if necessary. **D** ✦
Instruct client not to pull on drain and drainage tubing. **D** ✦
- Perform actions to prevent stress on and subsequent leakage of gastric contents from the staple line or site of proximal anastomosis.
  - Implement measures to prevent overdistention of gastric pouch.

Adequate nutrition is needed to maintain normal function of the immune system. Vitamin and mineral supplements may be required to maintain nutritional status.
Tight dressings decrease circulation to the surgical site.
Applying secure dressings prevents wound irritation.

Prevents irritation of surgical site and damage to surrounding skin.
Maintains adequate circulatory volume.

Allows drainage to flow away from the wound and prevents distention of the conduit.
Prevents stress on the wound and stasis of drainage and prevents distention of the conduit.
Prevents stasis of secretions and prevents distention of conduit.

Prevents accidental dislodgement of a drain if present.

Enables client to move without placing tension on the drain.
Prevents accidental dislodgement of the drain.

Distention can cause strain on the suture lines, which may permit subsequent leakage of gastric contents into the peritoneal cavity.

THERAPEUTIC INTERVENTIONS	RATIONALE
• Implement measures to prevent nausea and vomiting (e.g., maintain patency of NG or gastric tube, eliminate noxious sights and odors from the environment, instruct client to change positions slowly, administer antiemetics and/or GI stimulants as ordered).	*Prevents pressure and strain on the abdominal wound and the proximal anastomosis.*
• Do not adjust position of NG or gastric tube unless ordered.	*Adjustment of the NG tube or gastric tube may cause disruption of staples or perforation at the site of proximal anastomosis.*

If signs and symptoms of peritonitis occur:
- Withhold oral intake and jejunostomy tube feedings as ordered.

  Prevents further leakage of food content into the abdominal cavity.
- Place client on bedrest in a semi-Fowler's position.

  Assists in pooling or localizing gastric contents in the pelvis rather than under the diaphragm.
- Prepare client for diagnostic tests (e.g., abdominal radiograph, computed tomography, ultrasound) if necessary.

  Decreases fear and anxiety.
- Assist physician with insertion of NG tube or gastric tube and maintain to suction as ordered.

  Removes secretions from the stomach.
- Administer antimicrobials as ordered.

  Treats infection.
- Administer intravenous fluids and/or blood volume expanders if ordered.

  IV fluids/blood volume expanders prevent or treat shock, which can result from the increased capillary permeability that occurs with inflammation and the subsequent escape of protein, fluid, and electrolytes from the vascular space into the peritoneal cavity.
- Prepare client for surgical intervention (e.g., repair of perforation) if planned.

  Decreases fear and anxiety.

Nursing Diagnosis **RISK FOR VENOUS THROMBOEMBOLISM** NDx

Definition: Susceptible to the development of a blood clot in a deep vein, commonly in the thigh, calf, or upper extremity, which can break off and lodge in another vessel, which may compromise health.

Related to:
- Venous stasis associated with decreased activity, increased blood viscosity (can result from deficient fluid volume), and pressure on abdominal vessels from excessive adipose tissue and abdominal distention
- Hypercoagulability associated with increased release of thromboplastin into the blood (occurs as a result of surgical trauma) and hemoconcentration and increased blood viscosity (can occur as a result of deficient fluid volume)
- Trauma to vein walls during surgery

CLINICAL MANIFESTATIONS

Subjective	Objective
Verbal self-report of pain or tenderness in an extremity	Increase in circumference of extremity; distention of superficial vessels in extremity; unusual warmth of extremity

RISK FACTORS
- Immobility
- Inadequate fluid intake
- Ineffective treatment regimen

DESIRED OUTCOMES

The client will not develop a deep vein thrombus as evidenced by:
a. Absence of pain, tenderness, swelling, and distended superficial vessels in extremities
b. Usual temperature of extremities

NOC OUTCOMES

Tissue perfusion: peripheral

NIC INTERVENTIONS

Embolus precautions; embolus care: peripheral

NDx = NANDA Diagnosis   **D** = Delegatable Action   ● = UAP   ✦ = LVN/LPN   ⊙▶ = Go to ⊜volve for animation

NURSING ASSESSMENT	**RATIONALE**
Assess for and report signs and symptoms of a deep vein thrombus: • Pain or tenderness in extremity • Increase in circumference of extremity • Distention of superficial vessels in extremity • Unusual warmth of extremity • Pain in area where thromboembolus lodged	*Early recognition of signs and symptoms of a deep vein thrombus allows for implementation of the appropriate interventions.*

THERAPEUTIC INTERVENTIONS	**RATIONALE**
Independent Actions Implement measures to prevent thrombus formation: **D** ✦ • Perform actions to prevent peripheral pooling of blood such as leg exercises: • Ankle rotation • Alternate dorsiflexion and plantar extension of both feet If signs and symptoms of a deep vein thrombus occur: **D** ✦ • Maintain client on bedrest until activity orders received. • Elevate foot of bed 15 to 20 degrees above heart level if ordered. • Discourage positions that compromise blood flow (e.g., pillows under knees, crossing legs, sitting for long periods).	*Leg and ankle exercises help promote venous return and reduce the risk of venous thromboembolism.* *These actions facilitate venous return to the heart.* *Avoid putting pressure on the posterior knees because this action will compress leg veins, increasing turbulent blood flow, and increase the risk of thromboembolism formation. If a thrombus is suspected, avoid activity, elevate the affected extremity, and do not massage the area because of the danger of dislodging the thrombus.*
Dependent/Collaborative Actions Implement measures to prevent thrombus formation: • Apply mechanical devices designed to increase venous return in the immobile patient: **D** ✦ • Sequential compression devices • Thromboembolic (elastic) stockings • Maintain a minimum fluid intake of 2500 mL/day (unless contraindicated). If signs and symptoms of a deep vein thrombus occur: • Administer anticoagulants: • Low- or adjusted-dose heparin • Fondaparinux • Warfarin • Low-molecular-weight heparin Prepare client for diagnostic studies (e.g., venography, duplex ultrasound, impedance plethysmography). If signs and symptoms of embolism occur: • Maintain client on strict bedrest in a semi- to high-Fowler's position. • Maintain oxygen therapy as ordered. • Prepare client for diagnostic tests (e.g. blood gases, D-dimer level, ventilation-perfusion lung scan; pulmonary angiography). • Prepare client for the following if planned: • Vena caval interruption • Embolectomy	*These devices decrease venous stasis in the lower extremities and increase venous return through the deep leg veins, which are prone to the formation of a thromboembolism. These devices should remain in place until the patient is ambulatory.* *Adequate hydration helps to reduce blood viscosity, which may contribute to the formation of a thrombus.* *Anticoagulants, if indicated, help to suppress the formation of clots.* *Additional studies may be indicated to confirm the presence of a thromboembolism, so the appropriate interventions can be implemented.* *Improves lung expansion and provides supplemental oxygen.* *Decreases client fear/anxiety to prevent further pulmonary emboli.* *Removal of emboli.*

DISCHARGE TEACHING/CONTINUED CARE

Nursing Diagnosis | **DEFICIENT KNOWLEDGE NDx; INEFFECTIVE FAMILY HEALTH MANAGEMENT NDx; OR INEFFECTIVE HEALTH MAINTENANCE* NDx**

Definition: Deficient Knowledge NDx: Absence of cognitive information related to specific topic, or its acquisition. **Ineffective Family Health Management NDx:** A pattern of regulating and integrating into family processes a program for the treatment of illness and its sequelae that is unsatisfactory for meeting specific health goals of the family unit. **Ineffective Health Maintenance NDx:** Inability to identify, manage, and/or seek help to maintain well-being.

RISK FACTORS
- Financial concerns related to lifestyle change
- Cognitive difficulty
- Inability to integrate exercise and diet into lifestyle

CLINICAL MANIFESTATIONS

> **Subjective**
> Verbal self-report of difficulty in implementing lifestyle changes; expressed financial concerns; refusal to participate in self-care

NOC OUTCOMES	NIC INTERVENTIONS
Compliance behavior; adherence behavior; health beliefs: perceived ability to perform; perceived control; knowledge: prescribed diet; treatment regimen	Weight reduction assistance; teaching: prescribed diet; behavior modification; support system enhancement; health system guidance; teaching: individual; teaching: prescribed diet; support system enhancement

NURSING ASSESSMENT	RATIONALE

Assess for indications that the client may be unable to effectively manage the therapeutic regimen:
  Failure to adhere to treatment plan while in the hospital (e.g., not adhering to dietary modifications and fluid restrictions, refusing to increase activity).
  Statements reflecting a lack of understanding of dietary modifications and factors that will cause stretching of the gastric pouch.
  Verbalization of an inability to integrate necessary dietary modifications and exercise program into lifestyle.
  Statements reflecting the belief that the surgical procedure will result in continued weight loss even without adherence to the prescribed dietary modifications.
	Early recognition of signs and symptoms of inability to effectively manage the therapeutic regimen allows for prompt intervention.

THERAPEUTIC INTERVENTIONS	RATIONALE
Desired Outcome: The client will verbalize an understanding of the lifestyle changes that need to be maintained as a result of gastric reduction surgery. Explain the surgical procedure and importance of dietary modifications and a balanced exercise program in terms the client can understand; emphasize that adherence to the treatment program is necessary if an optimal weight is to be attained.	*Understanding of surgical procedure will help client maintain diet and exercise program, as these will help client meet weight reduction goals.*

*The nurse should select the diagnostic label that is most appropriate for the client's discharge teaching needs.

Continued...

THERAPEUTIC INTERVENTIONS	RATIONALE
Inform the client that prescribed food and fluid modifications are not as strict after the surgical area has healed (usually 6–8 weeks).	After 6 to 8 weeks, the client has more dietary choices than those available in the early postoperative period.
Stress the positive effects of compliance with dietary modifications and exercise program (e.g., weight loss resulting in change in appearance; decreased risk of development or worsening of conditions such as diabetes mellitus, cardiovascular disease, respiratory problems, and arthritis).	Compliance with dietary modification and exercise program is important to continued weight reduction and subsequent maintenance.
Encourage activities other than eating to cope with stress (e.g., exercise).	Stress eating will interfere with dietary regimen.
Provide written instructions about future appointments with health care provider, dietary modifications, and signs and symptoms to report.	Provides an information resource for the client once discharged from the acute care facility.

THERAPEUTIC INTERVENTIONS	RATIONALE

Desired Outcome: The client will identify ways to prevent excessive stretching of the gastric pouch.

Independent Actions

Instruct client in ways to prevent excessive stretching of the gastric pouch:

	RATIONALE
• Decrease risk of blockage of the pouch outlet by:	
• Limiting oral intake to liquids and blenderized foods for about 6 to 8 weeks after surgery	Liquids and blenderized foods will exit the stomach quicker than solid food.
• Taking all prescription and nonprescription medications in liquid or chewable form or crushing them thoroughly	Unabsorbed pills may block output from the pouch.
• Chewing food thoroughly	Thoroughly chewing food breaks it down into small particles, which improves digestion and helps the bolus move more quickly out of the stomach.
• Do not exceed prescribed volume of food/fluid intake.	Limiting the volume of intake prevents overdistention of the stomach.
• Do not make up for skipped meals while on an hourly drinking/eating schedule.	Provides potential for overeating and stretching of the gastric pouch.
• Eat and drink slowly.	Eating and drinking slowly increases satiety, as this occurs approximately 20 minutes after beginning a meal.
• Avoid intake of carbonated beverages for 6 to 8 weeks after surgery and limit intake of these beverages after that time.	Carbonated beverages increase gas in the stomach and the potential for overdistention.
• When solid foods are allowed, consume fluids between rather than with meals.	Fluids will fill the stomach quickly and when combined with a meal can cause over distention of the stomach.

THERAPEUTIC INTERVENTIONS	RATIONALE

Desired Outcome: The client will verbalize an understanding of ways to maintain an adequate nutritional status.

Independent Actions

Instruct client regarding ways to maintain an adequate nutritional state:

	RATIONALE
• Do not skip meals.	Skipping meals will decrease caloric intake and can negatively affect nutritional status.
• Consume foods/fluids from each food group daily as diet advances.	Daily consumption from all the food groups provides for nutritional balance in the diet.
• Consume adequate amounts of protein (e.g., blenderized drinks containing peanut butter, pureed meats and fish, cottage cheese) as diet advances.	Prevents over distention of the stomach while maintaining nutritional status.
• Take vitamin and mineral supplements as prescribed.	Dietary supplements may be required to maintain nutritional status.
• Obtain dietary consult if indicated to assist client in planning meals.	Meal planning should include foods the client likes while providing the appropriate nutrition.

THERAPEUTIC INTERVENTIONS	**RATIONALE**

Desired Outcome: The client will identify ways to reduce the risk of consuming excessive amounts of food, fluid, and calories through accurately calculating and measuring the allotted amounts of foods and fluid.

Independent Actions

Instruct client in ways to reduce the risk of consuming excessive amounts of food, fluid, and calories:

- Limit food/fluid intake to prescribed volume.

  Consumption of excessive food/fluid and calories can lead to overdistention of the stomach and weight gain.

- Prepare food ahead of time, freeze in 1-oz portions using plastic ice cube trays or plastic bags, and then reheat only allowed amounts at mealtime.

  Helps with meal planning and for eating the appropriate amount of food.

- Have jars of prepared strained baby food products rather than high-calorie puddings and snacks on hand.

  These preparations are easily digested and won't overdistend the stomach.

- Have only low-calorie drinks available (other than the required high-protein supplements).

  Prevents increased caloric intake.

- Decrease the risk of hunger by adhering to a schedule of 5 or 6 meals per day as diet advances (each meal will usually consist of 2–4 tablespoons of food).

  Adhering to a schedule for meals provides for adequate nutrition without client becoming hungry between meals.

- Serve food on a small plate.

  Eating from a small plate provides an illusion that meals are larger than they really are.

- Eat and drink very slowly (use techniques such as putting fork down between bites of food and putting glass down between sips of fluid).

  Allows satiety center of the brain to register fullness before overeating.

- If going out to dinner, order an appetizer and have it served with everyone else's entrée.

  Allows the client to eat with party without feeling deprived.

- Avoid excessive intake of high-calorie foods/fluids.

  It is possible to maintain or gain weight if only high-calorie substances are consumed.

- Demonstrate ways to measure foods/fluids accurately using measuring spoons and a cup with 1-oz markings.

  These help the client understand the size of servings using common kitchen items.

- Allow time for questions, clarification, and return demonstration.

  Having a client do a return demonstration improves client's self-esteem and ability to be successful in lifestyle changes.

THERAPEUTIC INTERVENTIONS	**RATIONALE**

Desired Outcome: The client will state signs and symptoms to report to the health care provider.

Independent Actions

Educate the client on signs and symptoms to report to the health care provider:

- Difficulty breathing
- Productive cough of discolored sputum
- Unusual or excessive drainage from the wound site
- Pain or swelling in the calf of one or both legs
- Unusual and continuous abdominal or pelvic pain
- Temperature above 38°C (100.4°F)
- Absence of or reduction in urinary output despite an adequate fluid intake

  These clinical manifestations indicate a variety of complications from the surgery including deep vein thrombosis, thromboembolism, infection, and dehydration.

- Nausea and vomiting after consuming prescribed amount of foods/fluids

  Client may be experiencing dumping syndrome.

- Inability to adhere to dietary modifications
- Weight gain

  Increases potential weight gain.
  Indicates problems maintaining lifestyle changes.

- Inability to lose weight or excessive weight loss (expected weight loss is usually about 10 lbs. per month for the first year or 30% of preoperative body weight by the end of the first year)

NDx = NANDA Diagnosis   **D** = Delegatable Action   ● = UAP   ✦ = LVN/LPN   ⊜▶ = Go to ⊝volve for animation

Continued...

THERAPEUTIC INTERVENTIONS	RATIONALE
• Abdominal cramping, flushing, palpitations, weakness, and/or dizziness within 30 minutes after eating	*May indicate dumping syndrome, which sometimes occurs after bypass when the client begins to eat solid food; if dumping syndrome does occur, symptoms are usually mild and self-limiting or easily controlled with minor dietary modifications.*
Reinforce the physician's instructions regarding need to adhere to a schedule of moderate exercise (clients are usually instructed to begin a walking program and should be walking 1-2 miles/day by the fourth week after discharge).	*Regular moderate exercise improves activity tolerance and weight loss.*

THERAPEUTIC INTERVENTIONS	RATIONALE
Desired Outcome: The client will identify community resources that can assist in the adjustment to prescribed dietary modifications and future changes to body image.	
Independent Actions	
Provide information about community resources that can assist the client with adjustment to prescribed dietary modifications and future changes in body image (e.g., weight reduction groups, counseling services, support groups of persons who have had the same or similar surgery).	*Provides for continuum of care once client is discharged from the acute care facility.*
Initiate a referral if needed.	

THERAPEUTIC INTERVENTIONS	RATIONALE
Desired Outcome: The client, in collaboration with the nurse, will develop a plan for adhering to recommended follow-up care including future appointments with health care provider, activity level, medications prescribed, and wound care.	
Independent Actions	
Collaborate with the client to develop a plan for adherence that includes:	*Follow-up visits to the health care provider improve the potential for a client's adherence to treatment regimen and lifestyle changes.*
The importance of follow-up appointments with the health care provider.	
Including significant others in teaching sessions if possible.	*Knowledge of the required lifestyle changes improves the significant other's ability to support client's adherence to the treatment regimen.*
Encouraging questions and allow for reinforcement and clarification of information provided about treatment regimen.	
Providing written instructions on scheduled appointments with health care provider, dietary modifications, activity level, treatment plan, medications, and signs and symptoms to report.	*Provides an information resource for the client after discharge from the acute care facility.*

ADDITIONAL NURSING DIAGNOSES:

IMBALANCED NUTRITION: LESS THAN BODY REQUIREMENTS NDx
Related to:
- Decreased oral intake associated with nausea, pain, weakness, fatigue, prescribed dietary modifications, and early satiety resulting from small gastric pouch and delayed pouch emptying
- Inadequate nutritional replacement therapy
- Increased nutritional needs associated with the increased metabolic rate that occurs during wound healing

ACTUAL/RISK FOR IMPAIRED TISSUE INTEGRITY NDx
Related to:
- Disruption of tissue associated with the surgical procedure
- Delayed wound healing associated with factors such as decreased nutritional status and inadequate blood supply to wound area
- Irritation of skin associated with contact with wound drainage, pressure from tubes, and use of tape
- Difficulty keeping deep skinfold areas dry

- Damage to the skin and/or subcutaneous tissue associated with:
  - Friction or shearing when moving in bed
  - Pressure on tissue as a result of excessive body weight and decreased activity

GASTROINTESTINAL BLEED, ACUTE

GI bleeding, a symptom of a disorder in the digestive tract, accounts for a significant number of hospital admissions each year. The causes of GI bleeding are classified based on the location of the bleeding in the GI tract (upper vs. lower). Causes of bleeding in the upper GI tract include peptic ulcers (usually located in the stomach or duodenum), esophageal varices (swelling of the veins in the esophagus or stomach), Mallory-Weiss tear (tear in the esophagus or stomach most often due to severe vomiting or retching), and gastritis (general inflammation of the stomach lining usually from ingested materials). Additional risk factors that may contribute to the development of gastritis include regular use of NSAIDs or nonsteroidal anti-inflammatory drugs and/or steroids, chronic or excessive alcohol intake, burns, and trauma. Causes of lower GI bleeding include diverticulosis (small out-pockets that form in a weakened portion of the bowel wall), cancer, inflammatory bowel disease (e.g. Crohn disease, ulcerative colitis), infectious diarrhea, angiodysplasia (malformation of blood vessels in the wall of the GI tract), polyps, hemorrhoids, and fissures.

Acute GI bleeding first appears as vomiting of blood, bloody bowel movements, or black, tarry stools depending upon the location of the bleed. The severity of the bleeding ranges from slight oozing to frank, profuse hemorrhage and depends on whether the source is arterial, venous, or capillary. Significant bleeding is almost always arterial in nature. A GI bleed is considered massive if the bleed results in hemodynamic instability, acute anemia, and/or the need for blood transfusion. Hematemesis of bright red or "coffee ground" vomitus is often the initial symptom of an upper GI bleed. Melena (dark, tarry stools) can also indicate upper GI bleeding that is occurring at a slower rate. Additional symptoms associated with blood loss from a GI bleed include fatigue, weakness, shortness of breath, abdominal pain, and pale appearance.

Most people who experience a GI bleed spontaneously stop bleeding. However, treatment is initiated immediately in cases of massive bleeding and consists of endoscopic hemostasis of the bleeding vessel. Vasoactive medications such as epinephrine, octreotide, or vasopressin may also be administered to help stop the bleeding. Gastric lavage may be done before endoscopy to remove blood from the stomach and improve endoscopic visualization. If bleeding continues, surgery may be necessary. Subsequent treatment to prevent rebleeding depends on the cause of the bleeding.

This care plan focuses on the adult client hospitalized with a massive upper GI bleed. It should be used in conjunction with the care plans on peptic ulcer and cirrhosis if it is determined that the client's bleed is associated with either of these conditions.

OUTCOME/DISCHARGE CRITERIA

The client will:
1. Have adequate tissue perfusion
2. Tolerate prescribed activity without a significant change in vital signs, chest pain, dizziness, or extreme fatigue or weakness
3. Have no signs and symptoms of complications
4. Identify ways to reduce the risk for rebleeding
5. State signs and symptoms to report to the health care provider
6. Develop a plan for adhering to recommended follow-up care including future appointments with health care provider, medications prescribed, and dietary restrictions

| Nursing Diagnosis | **RISK FOR SHOCK** NDx |

Definition: Susceptible to an inadequate blood flow to the body's tissues that may lead to life-threatening cellular dysfunction, which may compromise health.

Related to: Hypovolemia/hypotension associated with GI bleeding

CLINICAL MANIFESTATIONS

Subjective	Objective
Verbal self-report of nausea, abdominal pain or tenderness; dizziness and lightheadedness	Hematemesis; bright red/maroon stool, hypoactive or absent bowel sounds; nausea; abdominal distention; abdominal pain or tenderness; tachycardia; hypotension; cyanotic, pale skin; oliguria; capillary refill time greater than 2 to 3 seconds; elevated BUN and serum creatinine levels

RISK FACTORS

- Active GI bleeding
- Inadequate fluid and/or blood volume replacement

DESIRED OUTCOMES

The client will maintain adequate tissue perfusion as evidenced by:
a. BP within normal range and stable with position change
b. Usual mental status
c. Extremities warm with absence of pallor and cyanosis
d. Palpable peripheral pulses
e. Capillary refill time less than 2 to 3 seconds
f. BUN and serum creatinine levels within normal limits
g. Urine output at least 30 mL/h

NOC OUTCOMES

Blood loss severity; circulation status; tissue perfusion: abdominal organs; cellular

NIC INTERVENTIONS

Bleeding reduction: GI; blood product administration; shock management; hypotension management; hypovolemia management

NURSING ASSESSMENT

Assess for and report signs of active or continued GI bleeding:
- Hematemesis
- Bright red or maroon stool

Assess for and report signs and symptoms of diminished tissue perfusion:
- Decreased BP
- Decline in systolic BP of more than 15 mm Hg when client changes from a lying to a sitting or standing position
- Restlessness, confusion, or other change in mental status
- Reports of dizziness or lightheadedness or occurrence of syncopal episodes
- Cool, pale, or cyanotic skin
- Diminished or absent peripheral pulses
- Capillary refill time greater than 2 to 3 seconds
- Elevated BUN and serum creatinine levels
- Oliguria

Assess baseline CBC, serum chemistry values.

RATIONALE

Early recognition of active or continued GI bleeding allows for prompt intervention.

Early recognition of signs and symptoms of diminished GI tissue perfusion allows for prompt intervention before shock develops.

Assessing baseline laboratory values allows for evaluation of effectiveness of interventions.

THERAPEUTIC INTERVENTIONS

Independent Actions

Implement measures to maintain adequate tissue perfusion:
- Maintain a minimum fluid intake of 2500 mL/day if able.
- Instruct client to change from a supine to an upright position slowly.
- Maintain a comfortable room temperature and provide client with adequate clothing and blankets. **D** ● ✦

Dependent/Collaborative Actions

Implement measures to maintain adequate tissue perfusion:
- Prepare client for measures that may be performed to control bleeding:
  - Endoscopic thermocoagulation, sclerotherapy, or banding of bleeding varices
  - Intra-arterial or intravenous administration of vasoactive medications (e.g., epinephrine, octreotide, vasopressin)
  - Surgery
- Administer intravenous fluids and/or blood products as ordered.

RATIONALE

Maintains adequate circulatory volume and tissue perfusion.
Allows time for autoregulatory mechanisms to adjust to the change in distribution of blood associated with an upright position
Exposure to cold causes generalized vasoconstriction.

Processes that will obliterate bleeding varices.

Maintains adequate circulatory status and tissue perfusion.

THERAPEUTIC INTERVENTIONS	RATIONALE

• Administer the following medications if ordered to reduce the risk of rebleeding:
  • Proton pump inhibitors (e.g., omeprazole, lansoprazole, pantoprazole, esomeprazole)
  • Histamine2-receptor antagonists (e.g., famotidine, ranitidine, nizatidine) **D** ✦
	These medications decrease acid production and irritation of the stomach lining.
	
	Histamine receptor antagonists and proton-pump inhibitors suppress secretion of gastric acid.

• Consult appropriate health care provider if signs and symptoms of diminished tissue perfusion persist or worsen.	*Allows for prompt alterations in interventions.*

Nursing Diagnosis | # RISK FOR ELECTROLYTE IMBALANCE NDx

Definition: Susceptible to changes in serum electrolyte levels, which may compromise health.

Related to:
• Hypokalemia, hypochloremia, and metabolic alkalosis related to loss of electrolytes and hydrochloric acid associated with vomiting and NG tube drainage

CLINICAL MANIFESTATIONS

Subjective	**Objective**
Verbal self-report of nausea; headache	Vomiting; positive Chvostek and Trousseau sign; abnormal serum electrolyte levels; metabolic alkalosis

RISK FACTORS
• Chronic illness
• Stress
• Infection
• Inadequate therapeutic regimen

DESIRED OUTCOMES

The client will maintain fluid and electrolyte balance as evidenced by:
a. Normal skin turgor
b. Moist mucous membranes
c. Stable weight
d. BP and pulse rate within normal range for client and stable with position change
e. Capillary refill time less than 2 to 3 seconds
f. Usual mental status
g. Balanced I&O
h. Urine specific gravity within normal range
i. Soft, nondistended abdomen with normal bowel sounds
j. Absence of cardiac dysrhythmias, muscle weakness, paresthesias, twitching, spasms, and dizziness
k. BUN, Hct, serum electrolyte, and ABG values within normal range

NOC OUTCOMES

Electrolyte and acid-base balance

NIC INTERVENTIONS

Electrolyte management: hypokalemia; electrolyte management: hypocalcemia; electrolyte management: hypomagnesemia; acid-base management: metabolic alkalosis; diarrhea management

*The nurse should select the diagnostic label that is most appropriate for the client's discharge teaching needs.

NDx = NANDA Diagnosis   **D** = Delegatable Action   ● = UAP   ✦ = LVN/LPN   ⊝▶ = Go to ⊝volve for animation

NURSING ASSESSMENT	RATIONALE
Assess for and report signs and symptoms of electrolyte imbalance: • Hypokalemia (e.g., cardiac dysrhythmias, postural hypotension, muscle weakness, nausea and vomiting, abdominal distention, hypoactive or absent bowel sounds) • Hypomagnesemia and/or hypocalcemia (e.g., anxiousness; irritability; cardiac dysrhythmias; positive Chvostek and Trousseau signs; numbness or tingling of fingers, toes, or circumoral area; hyperactive reflexes; tetany; seizures) • Metabolic alkalosis (e.g., confusion, hand tremor, lightheadedness, muscle twitching, nausea, vomiting, numbness or tingling in face, hands, or feet; prolonged muscle spasms)	Early recognition of signs and symptoms of electrolyte imbalance allows for prompt intervention.

THERAPEUTIC INTERVENTIONS	RATIONALE
Dependent/Collaborative Actions Implement measures to prevent or treat imbalanced fluid and electrolytes: • Perform actions to prevent nausea and vomiting: • Insert NG tube and maintain suction and/or perform gastric lavage if ordered. • Administer antiemetics if ordered. **D** ✦ • If gastric lavage is being done or NG tube is being irrigated frequently with large volumes of solution, consult physician about using saline rather than water. • Administer intravenous fluid and electrolytes as ordered. Consult physician if signs and symptoms of imbalanced fluid and electrolytes persist or worsen.	*Maintaining an NG tube to suction removes blood from the stomach, reducing the stimulus to vomit.* *Antiemetics decrease nausea and vomiting, which decreases fluid and electrolyte loss.* *Water is sometimes preferred because it breaks up clots better than saline, but irrigation with large volumes of water may create electrolyte imbalance.* *IV fluids maintain adequate circulatory balance.* *Notification of the physician allows for prompt alteration in interventions.*

Nursing Diagnosis RISK FOR ASPIRATION NDx

Definition: Susceptible to entry of gastrointestinal secretions, oropharyngeal secretions, solids, or fluids into the tracheobronchial passages, which may compromise health.

Related to: hematemesis and possible decreased level of consciousness

CLINICAL MANIFESTATIONS

Subjective N/A	Objective Rhonchi; dull percussion note over affected lung area; cough; tachypnea; dyspnea; tachycardia; chest radiograph results showing pulmonary infiltrate

RISK FACTORS
• Depressed gag reflex
• Increased gastric residual volume
• Increased intragastric pressure
• Impaired swallowing

DESIRED OUTCOMES
The client will not aspirate as evidenced by:
a. Clear breath sounds
b. Resonant percussion note over lungs
c. Absence of cough, tachypnea, and dyspnea

NOC OUTCOMES
Respiratory status: airway patency; gas exchange

NIC INTERVENTIONS
Respiratory monitoring; aspiration precautions; airway suctioning

NURSING ASSESSMENT	RATIONALE
Assess for and report signs and symptoms of aspiration (e.g., rhonchi, dull percussion note over affected lung area, cough, tachypnea, dyspnea, tachycardia, chest radiograph results showing pulmonary infiltrate).	*Early recognition of signs and symptoms of aspiration allows for prompt intervention.*

THERAPEUTIC INTERVENTIONS	RATIONALE

Independent Actions

Implement measures to reduce the risk for aspiration:

- Keep head of bed elevated at least 45 degrees if vital signs are stable, or position client on side (if client is hypotensive, elevating the head of bed is contraindicated).

This position uses gravity to facilitate movement of foods/fluids through the pharynx into the esophagus, where the risk of aspiration is greatly reduced.

Dependent/Collaborative Actions

Implement measures to reduce the risk for aspiration:

- Perform actions to prevent nausea and vomiting (e.g., insert NG tube, provide oral hygiene, eliminate noxious odors, administer antiemetics as needed). **D** ✦

These actions decrease incidence of nausea and vomiting, thus decreasing the risk of aspiration.

Withhold oral foods/fluids as ordered. **D** ● ✦

- Perform oropharyngeal suctioning and provide oral hygiene as often as needed. **D** ● ✦

Keeps the stomach empty, decreasing the chance of aspiration.
Suctioning and frequent oral hygiene remove any blood and vomitus and keeps oropharynx clean.

If signs and symptoms of aspiration occur:

- Perform tracheal suctioning.
- Withhold oral intake.
- Prepare client for chest radiograph.

Removes aspirate.
Keeps the stomach empty.
Shows where the aspirate has lodged and potential damage to the lungs.

Nursing Diagnosis RISK FOR ACTIVITY INTOLERANCE NDx

Definition: Susceptible to experiencing insufficient physiological or psychological energy to endure or complete required or desired daily activities, which may compromise health.

Related to:
- Anemia resulting from blood loss
- Hypoxia associated with anemia
- Difficulty resting and sleeping associated with assessment and treatments, fear, and anxiety

CLINICAL MANIFESTATIONS

Subjective	Objective
Verbal self-report of feeling tired; chest pain	Dyspnea on exertion; tachycardia with exertion; BP increase with exertion

RISK FACTORS

- Fatigue
- Shortness of breath
- Pain

DESIRED OUTCOMES

The client will not experience activity intolerance as evidenced by:
a. No reports of fatigue or weakness
b. Ability to perform activities of daily living without exertional dyspnea, chest pain, diaphoresis, dizziness, and a significant change in vital signs

NOC OUTCOMES

Activity tolerance; energy conservation; self-care activities of daily living

NIC INTERVENTIONS

Energy management; oxygen therapy; sleep enhancement

NDx = NANDA Diagnosis   **D** = Delegatable Action   ● = UAP   ✦ = LVN/LPN   ⊖▶ = Go to ⊖volve for animation

NURSING ASSESSMENT	RATIONALE
Assess for signs and symptoms of activity intolerance: • Statements of fatigue or weakness • Exertional dyspnea, chest pain, diaphoresis, or dizziness • Abnormal heart rate response to activity (e.g., increase in rate of 20 beats/min above resting rate, rate not returning to preactivity level within 3 minutes after stopping activity, change from regular to irregular rate) • Significant change (15-20 mm Hg) in BP with activity	*Early recognition of signs and symptoms of activity intolerance allows for prompt intervention.*

THERAPEUTIC INTERVENTIONS	RATIONALE

Independent Actions

Implement measures to prevent activity intolerance:
- Perform actions to promote rest and/or conserve energy:
  - Maintain prescribed activity restrictions.
  - Minimize environmental activity and noise. **D** ● ✦
  - Organize care to provide uninterrupted rest periods. **D** ● ✦
  - Assist with self-care activities. **D** ● ✦
  - Keep supplies and personal articles within easy reach. **D** ● ✦
  - Limit the number of visitors.
  - Instruct client in energy-saving techniques (e.g., using a shower chair when showering, sitting to brush teeth or comb hair).
  - Implement measures to promote sleep (e.g., allow client to continue usual sleep practices unless contraindicated, administer sedative-hypnotic as ordered).

Cells use oxygen and fat, protein, and carbohydrate to produce the energy needed for all body activities. Rest and activities that conserve energy result in a lower metabolic rate, which preserves nutrients and oxygen for necessary activities.

- Discourage smoking and excessive intake of beverages high in caffeine such as coffee, tea, and colas.

Both nicotine and excessive caffeine intake can increase cardiac workload and myocardial oxygen utilization, thereby decreasing the amount of oxygen necessary for energy production.

Instruct client to report a decreased tolerance for activity and to stop any activity that causes chest pain, shortness of breath, dizziness, or extreme fatigue or weakness.

These symptoms indicate that insufficient oxygen is reaching the tissues and that activity has been increased beyond a therapeutic level.

Dependent/Collaborative Actions

Implement measures to prevent activity intolerance:
- Administer the following if ordered to treat anemia if present:
  - Iron supplements
  - Packed red blood cells
- Maintain oxygen therapy as ordered. **D** ✦
- Implement measures to maintain an adequate nutritional status (e.g., provide a diet high in essential nutrients, provide dietary supplements as indicated, administer vitamins and minerals as ordered).

Anemia reduces the oxygen-carrying capacity of the blood. Resolution of anemia increases oxygen availability to the cells, which increases the efficiency of energy production and subsequently improves activity tolerance.
Provides supplemental oxygen.
Metabolism is the process by which nutrients are transformed into energy. If nutrition is inadequate, energy production is decreased, which subsequently reduces one's ability to tolerate activity.
Vitamins and minerals may be required to support nutritional status.

- Increase client's activity gradually as allowed and tolerated. **D** ● ✦

A gradual increase in activity helps prevent a sudden increase in cardiac workload and myocardial oxygen consumption and the subsequent imbalance between oxygen supply and demand.

Consult physician if signs and symptoms of activity intolerance persist.

Notifying the physician allows for modification of the treatment plan.

DISCHARGE TEACHING/CONTINUED CARE

Nursing Diagnosis **DEFICIENT KNOWLEDGE** NDx**; INEFFECTIVE FAMILY HEALTH MANAGEMENT** NDx**; or INEFFECTIVE HEALTH MAINTENANCE*** NDx

Definition: **Deficient Knowledge** NDx: Absence of cognitive information related to specific topic, or its acquisition. **Ineffective Family Health Management** NDx: A pattern of regulating and integrating into family processes a program for the treatment of illness and its sequelae that is unsatisfactory for meeting specific health goals of the family unit. **Ineffective Health Maintenance** NDx: Inability to identify, manage, and/or seek help to maintain well-being.

Subjective	Objective
Verbal self-report of inability to manage illness; inability to follow prescribed regimen	Inaccurate follow-through with instructions; inappropriate behaviors; unwillingness to participate in self-care

RISK FACTORS
* Cognitive deficit
* Financial concerns
* Inability to care for oneself
* Difficulty in modifying personal habits and integrating treatments into lifestyle

NOC OUTCOMES	NIC INTERVENTIONS
Knowledge: disease process; treatment regimen	Health system guidance; teaching: individual; teaching: disease process; teaching: prescribed diet; teaching: prescribed medication

NURSING ASSESSMENT	RATIONALE
Assess the client's ability to learn and readiness to learn. Assess the client's understanding of teaching.	*Learning is more effective when the client is motivated and understands the importance of what is to be learned. Readiness to learn changes based on situations and physical and emotional challenges.*

THERAPEUTIC INTERVENTIONS	RATIONALE

Desired Outcome: The client will identify ways to reduce the risk of bleeding.

Independent Actions
Instruct client on how to reduce the risk for rebleeding:
* Drink decaffeinated or caffeine-free tea and colas rather than those containing caffeine
* Avoid drinking coffee and alcohol or drink these beverages only in small amounts during or immediately following a meal
* Avoid ingestion of foods known to irritate gastric mucosa directly or increase gastric acid production (e.g., whole grains, chocolate, rich pastries, spicy foods, meat extracts, extremely hot foods)
* Avoid intake of any foods and fluids that cause gastric distress

These drinks/foods irritate GI lining, slow down healing, and/or may cause re-ulceration.

Neutralizes gastric acid.

*The nurse should select the diagnostic label that is most appropriate for the client's discharge teaching.

NDx = NANDA Diagnosis   **D** = Delegatable Action   ● = UAP   ✦ = LVN/LPN   ⊝▶ = Go to ⊝volve for animation

Continued...

THERAPEUTIC INTERVENTIONS	RATIONALE
• Eat three regularly scheduled meals (moderate-sized, rather than large) and snacks each day; do not skip meals • Eat slowly and chew food thoroughly • Maintain a calm, pleasant atmosphere at mealtime and whenever possible • Stop smoking • Maintain a balance of physical activity and rest • Avoid stressful situations whenever possible • Avoid ingestion of over-the-counter medications such as aspirin and ibuprofen; if it is necessary to take these or other ulcerogenic medications (e.g., corticosteroids), take them with antacids or food unless contraindicated and/or take enteric-coated or buffered preparations of the drugs if available • If it is necessary to take an NSAID, consult health care provider about taking it with a medication that helps protect the gastric mucosa (e.g., misoprostol, sucralfate) and/or switching to an NSAID known to be less irritating to the mucosa (e.g., a COX-2 inhibitor selective agent such as celecoxib, valdecoxib, and rofecoxib) • Take medications for ulcer treatment as prescribed	*A large bolus of food causes an increased output of hydrochloric acid and pepsin.* *Decreases stress and production of gastric acid.* *Smoking may cause ulcers, lowers healing, and contributes to reccurrence.* *Reduces stress and promotes healing.* *Physiological stress can lead to stress gastritis which results in inflammation of the stomach lining. In more serious cases, this can lead to the development of erosions and bleeding which may be further exacerbated with the ingestion of NSAIDS, aspirin and/or ibuprofen.* *Many medications cause gastric irritation and should be avoided or taken with antacids or food.* *Enhances ulcer healing and reduces recurrence.*

THERAPEUTIC INTERVENTIONS	RATIONALE
Desired Outcome: The client will state signs and symptoms to report to the health care provider. **Independent Actions** Instruct client to report: • Bloody or "coffee-ground" vomitus • Black or tarry stools • Persistent epigastric fullness or bloating, nausea and/or vomiting • Abdominal distention • Persistent or increased epigastric or abdominal pain • Persistent weakness and fatigue	*Indication of bleeding should be reported immediately to allow for prompt intervention.*

THERAPEUTIC INTERVENTIONS	RATIONALE
Desired Outcome: The client, in collaboration with the nurse, will develop a plan for adhering to recommended follow-up care including future appointments with health care provider, medications prescribed, and dietary restriction. **Independent Actions** Collaborate with client to develop a plan adherence that includes: The importance of keeping follow-up appointments with health care provider. Explanation of the rationale for, side effects of, and importance of taking prescriptions as prescribed. Inform client of pertinent food and drug interactions. Physician's instruction regarding dietary restrictions such as caffeinated beverages, alcohol, and spicy foods. Providing written instructions about future appointments with health care provider, prescribed medications, dietary restrictions, and signs and symptoms to report.	*The client should be monitored for a period of time to ensure adequate healing.* *Knowledge of the medication regimen and the impact of these medications on the system, as well as how the medication regimen can be incorporated into the client's lifestyle, allows the client some mechanism of control of his/her disease and the ability to have an active part in treatment and care.* *Irritants to the GI tract may increase potential for rebleeding.* *Provides a resource for information once the client has been discharged from the acute care facility.*

ADDITIONAL NURSING DIAGNOSIS

FEAR/ANXIETY NDx
Related to:
- Presence of large amount of blood in vomitus and NG tube drainage

- Concern that bleeding may not be controlled
- Lack of understanding of the cause of the bleeding, diagnostic tests, treatment plan, and prognosis
- Possible need to change lifestyle in order to prevent rebleeding

INFLAMMATORY BOWEL DISEASE: ULCERATIVE COLITIS AND CROHN DISEASE

Crohn disease and ulcerative colitis are idiopathic chronic inflammatory bowel diseases often jointly referred to as inflammatory bowel disease. Prolonged inflammation associated with these diseases results in damage to the GI tract. Crohn disease most often affects a portion of the small intestine, with damaged areas appearing as patches next to areas of healthy tissue, and inflammation that may reach through multiple layers of the GI tract wall, while ulcerative colitis occurs in the large intestine.

The exact cause of inflammatory bowel disease is unknown but is the result of a defective immune system. The classic clinical manifestations of inflammatory bowel disease include persistent diarrhea, abdominal pain and cramping, rectal bleeding/bloody stools, weight loss, and fatigue. The severity and pattern of signs and symptoms depend on the portion(s) of the bowel affected and depth of bowel wall involvement. Ulcerative colitis primarily involves the mucosa of the bowel wall, extending to the submucosa only in severe cases. It typically starts in the rectum and sigmoid colon and progresses in a continuous pattern through the colon. It rarely involves the small intestine. Crohn disease can occur anywhere in the GI tract. The most frequent sites of involvement are the terminal ileum and right colon. The entire thickness of the bowel wall is involved, and it has a segmental, discontinuous pattern of progression.

Clients with either condition may experience a number of the same complications; however, those with ulcerative colitis have a higher incidence of toxic megacolon and bowel perforation, whereas clients with Crohn disease have a higher incidence of perianal involvement and fistula formation. Some clients also experience extraintestinal manifestations such as liver and biliary involvement; kidney stones; arthritis; and skin, eye, and oral lesions. Clients with inflammatory bowel disease may require hospitalization during periods of exacerbation or if complications are suspected.

Cornerstones of medical treatment have traditionally included corticosteroids, sulfasalazine, nonsulfa-aminosalicylates, immunomodulator agents such as azathioprine and mercaptopurine, and the newest class of approved drugs—the biologics. Research indicates that there may be a defect in immunoregulation of inflammation in Crohn disease. This has led to the use of monoclonal antibodies that neutralize a cytokine (specifically, tumor necrosis factor-α) to treat persons with Crohn disease who have not been responsive to conventional therapy or who have draining enterocutaneous fistulas.

This care plan focuses on the adult client with severe abdominal pain and diarrhea who is hospitalized for medical management of inflammatory bowel disease. Much of the information is applicable to clients receiving follow-up care in an extended care facility or home setting.

OUTCOME/DISCHARGE CRITERIA

The client will:
1. Have decreased abdominal pain
2. Have fewer episodes of diarrhea
3. Tolerate prescribed diet and have an improved nutritional status
4. Be free of signs and symptoms of complications
5. Identify ways to reduce the incidence of disease exacerbation
6. Verbalize ways to maintain an optimal nutritional status
7. State ways to prevent perianal skin breakdown
8. Verbalize an understanding of medications ordered including rationale, food and drug interactions, side effects, schedule for taking, and importance of taking as prescribed
9. State signs and symptoms to report to the health care provider
10. Identify resources that can assist in the adjustment to changes resulting from inflammatory bowel disease and its treatment
11. Share feelings and thoughts about the effects of inflammatory bowel disease on lifestyle and self-concept
12. Develop a plan for adhering to recommended follow-up care including future appointments with health care provider and activity level

| Nursing/Collaborative Diagnosis | **RISK FOR IMBALANCED FLUID VOLUME** NDx **AND RISK FOR ELECTROLYTE IMBALANCE** NDx* |

Definition: Risk for Imbalanced Fluid Volume NDx: Susceptible to a decrease, increase, or rapid shift from one to the other of intravascular, interstitial and/or intracellular fluid, which may compromise health. This refers to body fluid loss, gain, or both. **Risk for Electrolyte Imbalance NDx:** Susceptible to changes in serum electrolyte levels, which may compromise health.

---

*The nurse should select the diagnostic label that is most appropriate for the client's discharge teaching needs.

NDx = NANDA Diagnosis   **D** = Delegatable Action   ● = UAP   ✦ = LVN/LPN   ⊝▶ = Go to ⊝volve for animation

Related to:
- **Risk for Imbalanced Fluid Volume NDx; Risk for Electrolyte Imbalance NDx: hypokalemia, hypomagnesemia,** and **hypocalcemia** related to:
  - Prolonged inadequate oral intake associated with pain, fatigue, prescribed dietary restrictions, and fear of precipitating an attack of abdominal cramping and diarrhea.
  - Impaired absorption of fluid and electrolytes associated with inflammation and scarring of the intestine
  - Excessive loss of fluid and electrolytes associated with persistent diarrhea (loss of potassium can occur as a result of treatment with corticosteroids)
- **Metabolic acidosis** related to excessive loss of bicarbonate associated with persistent diarrhea

CLINICAL MANIFESTATIONS

Subjective	**Objective**
Verbal self-report of nausea; headache	Poor skin turgor; dry, cracked mucous membranes; hypotension; weight loss; prolonged capillary refill greater than 2 to 3 seconds; decreased urine output; increased urine specific gravity; vomiting; positive Chvostek and Trousseau sign; abnormal electrolytes; metabolic acidosis

RISK FACTORS

- Chronic illness
- Failure of regulatory mechanisms
- Inadequate diet and fluid intake

DESIRED OUTCOMES

The client will maintain fluid and electrolyte balance as evidenced by:
a. Normal skin turgor
b. Moist mucous membranes
c. Stable weight
d. BP and pulse rate within normal range for client and stable with position change
e. Capillary refill time less than 2 to 3 seconds
f. Usual mental status
g. Balanced intake and output
h. Urine specific gravity within normal range
i. Soft, nondistended abdomen with active bowel sounds
j. Absence of cardiac dysrhythmias, muscle weakness, and seizure activity
k. Absence of headache, nausea, and vomiting
l. Negative Chvostek and Trousseau signs
m. Decreased serum electrolytes and ABGs within normal range

NOC OUTCOMES

Fluid balance; electrolyte and acid-base balance

NIC INTERVENTIONS

Fluid management; electrolyte management: hypokalemia; electrolyte management: hypocalcemia; electrolyte management: hypomagnesemia; acid-base management: metabolic acidosis; diarrhea management

NURSING ASSESSMENT

Assess for and report signs and symptoms of deficient fluid volume:
- Decreased skin turgor, dry mucous membranes, thirst
- Weight loss of 2% or greater over a short period
- Postural hypotension and/or low BP
- Weak, rapid pulse
- Capillary refill time longer than 2 to 3 seconds
- Neck veins flat when client is supine
- Change in mental status
- Decreased urine output with increased specific gravity (reflects an actual rather than potential fluid deficit)

RATIONALE

Early recognition of signs and symptoms of fluid and/or electrolyte imbalances allows for prompt treatment.

NURSING ASSESSMENT	RATIONALE
• Significant increase in BUN and Hct above previous levels • Hypokalemia (e.g., cardiac dysrhythmias, postural hypotension, muscle weakness, nausea and vomiting, abdominal distention, hypoactive or absent bowel sounds) • Hypomagnesemia and/or hypocalcemia (e.g., anxiousness; irritability; cardiac dysrhythmias; positive Chvostek and Trousseau signs; numbness or tingling of fingers, toes, or circumoral area; hyperactive reflexes; tetany; seizures) • Metabolic acidosis (e.g., drowsiness; disorientation; stupor; rapid, deep respirations; headache; nausea and vomiting; cardiac dysrhythmias; low pH and CO_2 content)	

THERAPEUTIC INTERVENTIONS	RATIONALE

Independent Actions
Implement measures to prevent or treat imbalanced fluid and electrolytes:
• Perform actions to control diarrhea (e.g., restrict intake as needed, reduce stress, avoid milk and milk products, foods high in fat, those high in fiber or residue, high in caffeine, spicy foods, extremely hot or cold fluids). **D** ● ✦
• When oral intake is allowed:
  • Assist client to select foods/fluids within the prescribed dietary regimen that would replenish electrolytes (be aware that many foods/fluids high in potassium and magnesium are contraindicated on a low-residue diet) **D** ● ✦
    (1) Foods high in potassium (e.g., bananas, avocado, raisins, potatoes, cantaloupe)
    (2) Foods high in magnesium (e.g., seafood)
 	
Dependent/Collaborative Actions
Implement measures to prevent or treat imbalanced fluid and electrolytes:
• Administer the following if ordered:
  • Maintain a fluid intake of at least 2500 mL/day unless contraindicated.
  • If oral intake is inadequate or contraindicated, maintain intravenous and/or enteral fluid therapy as ordered.
  • Electrolyte replacements (e.g., potassium chloride, magnesium sulfate, calcium gluconate, calcium carbonate)
• Vitamin D preparations **D** ✦
If signs and symptoms of hypomagnesemia or hypocalcemia occur, institute seizure precautions. **D** ● ✦
Consult physician if signs and symptoms of imbalanced fluid and electrolytes persist or worsen.
	Clients with Crohn disease may have an intolerance to lactose-rich foods because of a deficiency of lactase.
	The foods listed stimulate the bowel and increase the incidence of diarrhea.
	Oral intake of foods high in potassium are necessary to maintain adequate electrolyte balance.
	
	Required to prevent the client from becoming dehydrated.
	Replenishes electrolytes.
	
	Increases intestinal absorption of calcium.
	Low levels of magnesium and calcium have been associated with increased seizure activity.
	Notification of the physician allows for alterations in treatment plan.

Nursing Diagnosis   IMBALANCED NUTRITION: LESS THAN BODY REQUIREMENTS NDx

Definition: Intake of nutrients insufficient to meet metabolic needs.

Related to:
• Decreased oral intake associated with pain, fatigue, prescribed dietary restrictions, and the knowledge that eating often precipitates abdominal cramping and diarrhea
• Decreased absorption of nutrients associated with inflammation and scarring of the bowel
• Loss of nutrients associated with diarrhea and protein exudation from the inflamed bowel
• Impaired folate absorption associated with treatment with sulfasalazine
• Increased metabolism of nutrients associated with the increased metabolic rate that may be present during periods of exacerbation

---

CLINICAL MANIFESTATIONS

Subjective	Objective
Verbal self-report of weakness and fatigue; lack of appetite; irritability; poor self-esteem	Weight significantly below client's usual weight or below normal for client's age, height, and body frame; abnormal BUN and low serum prealbumin, albumin, Hct, Hgb, and folate levels and low lymphocyte count; pale conjunctiva

RISK FACTORS
- Treatment regimen
- Inadequate/inappropriate diet

DESIRED OUTCOMES
The client will have an improved nutritional status as evidenced by:
a. Weight approaching a normal range for client
b. Improved BUN and serum prealbumin, albumin, Hct, Hgb, and folate levels and lymphocyte count
c. Increased strength and activity tolerance
d. Healthy oral mucous membranes

NOC OUTCOMES
Nutritional status

NIC INTERVENTIONS
Nutritional monitoring; nutrition management; nutrition therapy; total parenteral nutrition (TPN) administration; enteral tube feeding

NURSING ASSESSMENT	RATIONALE
Assess for signs and symptoms of malnutrition: - Weight significantly below client's normal or below normal for client's age, height, and body frame - Abnormal BUN and low serum prealbumin, albumin, Hct, Hgb, and folate levels and low lymphocyte count - Weakness and fatigue - Sore, inflamed oral mucous membrane - Pale conjunctiva	*Early recognition of signs and symptoms of imbalanced nutrition allows for prompt intervention.*

THERAPEUTIC INTERVENTIONS	RATIONALE

Independent Actions

When oral intake is allowed, monitor the percentage of meals and snacks client consumes. **D ● ✦** Report a pattern of inadequate intake. **D ● ✦**	*The client's intake should be monitored to ensure adequate calories and nutrients.*

Dependent/Collaborative Actions

Implement measures to improve nutritional status:

- Administer TPN or enteral tube feeding if ordered. - Perform actions to reduce inflammation and hypermotility of the bowel (restrict intake; limit activity to bedrest as needed; limit milk and milk products, those high in fats, fiber, caffeine, spicy foods, extremely hot or cold foods/fluids).	*Provides adequate nutrition until oral intake may be resumed.* *These actions reduce episodes of diarrhea and increase absorption of nutrients.*
- Maintain activity restrictions as ordered (usually bedrest with bedside commode or bathroom privileges)	*Reduces caloric requirements.*

- When food or fluid is allowed:
  - Provide elemental formulas (e.g., Vivonex, Criticare HN) if ordered.
  - Progress diet as tolerated (usual progression is from elemental formulas to a low-residue, high-calorie, high-protein diet). **D ● ✦**
	Helps rest the bowel; these formulas are high in calories and nutrients, free of lactose and fiber, and absorbed in the proximal small bowel.

- Implement measures to reduce pain (e.g., encourage a rest period before meals). **D ● ✦**	*Minimizes fatigue.*

THERAPEUTIC INTERVENTIONS	RATIONALE
• Maintain a clean environment and a relaxed, pleasant atmosphere. **D** ● ✦	*Eliminates noxious odors, which may decrease appetite.*
• Provide oral hygiene before meals. **D** ● ✦	*Oral hygiene removes unpleasant tastes, which often improves the taste of foods/fluids.*
• Implement measures to improve the palatability of elemental formulas (e.g., offer a variety of flavors, serve chilled).	*A variety of measures help them to become more palatable.*
• Obtain a dietary consult if necessary to assist client in selecting foods/fluids that are appealing and adhere to personal and cultural preferences as well as the prescribed dietary modifications.	*Improves nutritional status while allowing individuals to eat foods they like.*
• Serve frequent, small meals rather than large ones if client is weak, fatigues easily, or has a poor appetite. **D** ● ✦	*Small, frequent meals promote better nutritional status for the client who tires easily.*
• Allow adequate time for meals; reheat foods/fluids if necessary. **D** ● ✦	*Clients who feel rushed during meals tend to become anxious, lose their appetite, and stop eating. Appetite is also suppressed if foods/fluids normally served hot or warm become cold and then do not appeal to the client.*
• Administer the following if ordered:	*Oral iron preparations may not be effective during an acute attack because they may be poorly absorbed from the inflamed bowel.*
• Iron	
• Vitamin preparations (e.g., fat-soluble vitamins, vitamin B₁₂, folic acid)	*Supplements of these vitamins may be required because they may not be adequately absorbed from the inflamed bowel.*
Perform a calorie count if ordered. Report information to dietitian and physician. **D** ✦	*Monitors client's nutritional status.*
Consult physician and/or dietitian if nutritional status continues to decline.	*Notification of the physician allows for alterations in treatment plan.*

Nursing Diagnosis   # ACUTE/CHRONIC PAIN NDx

Definition: **Acute Pain NDx:** Unpleasant sensory and emotional experience arising from actual or potential tissue damage, or described in terms of such damage (International Association for the Study of Pain); sudden or slow onset of any intensity from mild to severe with an anticipated or predictable end, and a duration of less than 3 months.

Chronic Pain NDx: Unpleasant sensory and emotional experience arising from actual or potential tissue damage, or described in terms of such damage (International Association for the Study of Pain); sudden or slow onset of any intensity from mild to severe, constant or recurring, without an anticipated or predictable end, and a duration of greater than 3 months.

Related to:
- **Abdominal pain and cramping** related to:
  - Inflammation and ulceration of the bowel
  - Interference with the flow of intestinal contents associated with narrowing of the intestinal lumen as a result of inflammation and hypertrophy and fibrosis of the bowel wall if present
- **Joint pain** related to extraintestinal involvement of the joints (peripheral arthritis, ankylosing spondylitis, and sacroiliitis are the most common joint disorders that occur)
- **Perianal pain** related to irritation and breakdown of the skin in the perianal area associated with persistent diarrhea and/or the presence of an anorectal abscess or fistula

CLINICAL MANIFESTATIONS

Subjective	Objective
Verbal self-report of reluctance to move; pain	Grimacing; rubbing abdomen, back, or joints; diaphoresis; increased BP; tachycardia; restlessness

RISK FACTOR

• Chronic illness

DESIRED OUTCOMES

The client will experience diminished pain as evidenced by:
a. Verbalization of same
b. Relaxed facial expression and body positioning
c. Increased participation in activities
d. Stable vital signs

NOC OUTCOMES

Comfort level: pain control

NIC INTERVENTIONS

Environmental management: comfort; analgesic administration

NURSING ASSESSMENT	**RATIONALE**
Assess for signs and symptoms of pain (e.g., verbalization of pain, grimacing, reluctance to move, restlessness, diaphoresis, increased BP, tachycardia).	*Early recognition of signs and symptoms of pain allows for prompt intervention and improved pain control.*
Assess client's perception of the severity of pain using a pain intensity rating scale.	*An awareness of the severity of pain being experienced helps determine the most appropriate interventions for pain management. Use of a pain intensity rating scale gives the nurse a clearer understanding of the pain being experienced and promotes consistency when communicating with others about the client's pain experience.*
Assess the client's pain pattern (e.g., location, quality, onset, duration, precipitating factors, aggravating factors, alleviating factors).	*Knowledge of the client's pain pattern assists in the identification of effective pain management interventions.*
Ask the client to describe previous pain experiences and methods used to manage pain effectively.	*Many variables affect a client's response to pain (e.g., age, sex, coping style, previous experience with pain, culture, cause of pain). Knowledge of the client's usual response to pain and methods previously used to manage pain effectively enables the nurse to evaluate the client's pain more accurately and facilitates the identification of effective strategies for pain management.*

THERAPEUTIC INTERVENTIONS	**RATIONALE**
Independent Actions	
Implement measures to reduce fear and anxiety (e.g., assure client that the need for pain relief is understood, plan methods for achieving pain control with client, provide a calm environment). **D** ● ✦	*Fear and anxiety can decrease the client's threshold and tolerance for pain and thereby heighten the perception of pain. In addition, pain management methods are not as effective if the client is tense and unable to relax.*
Implement measures to promote rest (e.g., minimize environmental activity and noise). **D** ● ✦	*Fatigue can decrease the client's threshold and tolerance for pain and thereby heighten the perception of pain. A well-rested client often experiences decreased pain and increased effectiveness of pain management measures.*
Perform actions to reduce inflammation and hypermotility of the bowel:	
• Perform actions to rest the bowel:	
• Restrict oral intake; maintain NPO during acute stage.	*Restricting intake and placing the client on NPO rests the bowel and conserves the individual's energy.*
• Maintain activity restrictions (initially may be limited to bedrest with bedside commode or bathroom privileges).	*Enhances healing of the bowel.*
When oral intake is allowed, diet usually progresses from elemental formulas to a low-residue diet. **D** ● ✦	*Elemental formulas are absorbed in the proximal small bowel and thereby minimize stimulation of the bowel.*
• Instruct the client to avoid the following foods/fluids that may be poorly digested or can act as irritants to the inflamed bowel:	*Clients with Crohn disease may have an intolerance to lactose-rich foods because of a deficiency of lactase.*
(1) Milk and milk products	
(2) Foods high in fat (e.g., fried foods, gravies)	*These foods cause an increase in the potential for diarrhea and irritation of the colon.*
(3) Foods high in fiber (e.g., whole-grain cereals, nuts, raw fruits and vegetables)	
(4) Foods high in caffeine (e.g., coffee, tea, colas)	
(5) Spicy foods	
(6) Extremely hot or cold foods/fluids	

THERAPEUTIC INTERVENTIONS	RATIONALE
Perform actions to relieve perianal pain if present: • Clean perianal area with medication wipes such as "Tucks" after each bowel movement. • Apply protective ointment or cream to perianal area after each bowel movement. **D** ● ✦	These actions help to decrease pain and irritation.
Instruct client to add new foods one at a time.	Adding one food at a time allows client to determine which foods cause more discomfort.
Provide small, frequent meals rather than three large ones.	Small, frequent meals are tolerated better than three large meals.

Dependent/Collaborative Actions

Perform actions to relieve perianal pain if present: • Consult physician about order for sitz baths. • Apply anesthetic preparation (e.g., Nupercainal, Tronolane) to perianal area or into rectum as ordered.	These actions decrease pain experienced in the perianal area.
Consult physician regarding measures to help relieve joint pain if present (e.g., application of brace/splint to affected joint, application of heat to affected joints).	Braces and splints support the joints and help to reduce pain.

Perform actions to reduce inflammation and hypermotility of the bowel:
• Administer anti-inflammatory medications:
  • Corticosteroids
  • Sulfasalazine or non-sulfa-aminosalicylates
  • Antidiarrheal agents **D** ✦
	Corticosteroids and sulfasalazine or non-sulfa-aminosalicylates reduce bowel inflammation.
	
	Antidiarrheal agents slow intestinal motility; however, these medications should be used with caution because of the risk of megacolon.

Administer analgesics before activities and procedures that can cause pain and before pain becomes severe. **D** ✦	The administration of analgesics before a pain-producing event helps minimize the pain that will be experienced. Analgesics are also more effective if given before pain becomes severe because mild to moderate pain is controlled more quickly and effectively than severe pain.
Provide or assist with nonpharmacological methods for pain relief. Examples include: • Cutaneous stimulation measures (e.g., pressure, massage, heat and cold applications, transcutaneous electrical nerve stimulation [TENS], acupuncture) • Relaxation techniques (e.g., progressive relaxation exercises, meditation, guided imagery) • Distraction measures (e.g., listening to music, conversing, watching television, playing cards, reading) • Position change	Nonpharmacological pain management includes a variety of interventions. It is believed that most of these are effective because they stimulate closure of the gating mechanism in the spinal cord and subsequently block the transmission of pain impulses. In addition, some interventions are thought to stimulate the release of endogenous analgesics (e.g., endorphins) that inhibit the transmission of pain impulses and/or alter the client's perception of pain. Many of the nonpharmacological interventions also help decrease pain by promoting relaxation.
Administer the following medications as ordered: • Opioid analgesics	Pharmacological therapy is an effective method of reducing or relieving pain. Opioid analgesics act mainly by altering the client's perception of pain and emotional response to the pain experience.
• Nonopioid analgesics such as acetaminophen and salicylates and other NSAIDs (e.g., ketorolac, ibuprofen, naproxen)	Nonopioid analgesics are thought to interfere with the transmission of pain impulses by inhibiting prostaglandin synthesis.
• Anesthetic agents (e.g., bupivacaine, etidocaine)	Anesthetics help control pain by inhibiting the initiation and conduction of pain impulses along the sensory pathways at and near the infusion site.
Consult physician about an order for PCA if indicated.	The use of PCA allows the client to self-administer analgesics within parameters established by the physician. This method facilitates pain management by ensuring prompt administration of the drug when needed, providing more continuous pain relief and increasing the client's control over the pain.
Consult appropriate health care provider (e.g., physician, pharmacist, pain management specialist) if above measures fail to provide adequate pain relief.	Notifying the appropriate health care provider allows for modification of the treatment plan.

NDx = NANDA Diagnosis   **D** = Delegatable Action   ● = UAP   ✦ = LVN/LPN   ⊝▶ = Go to ⊖volve for animation

| Nursing Diagnosis | **RISK FOR INFECTION** NDx |

Definition: Susceptible to invasion and multiplication of pathogenic organisms, which may compromise health.

Related to:
- Ulcerations in the bowel wall
- Lowered resistance to infection associated with malnutrition and treatment with corticosteroids and/or immunosuppressive agents
- Stasis of respiratory secretions and urine associated with decreased mobility if activity restrictions are prescribed

CLINICAL MANIFESTATIONS

Subjective	Objective
Verbal self-report of chills; malaise; lethargy; confusion; frequency, urgency, or burning with urination	Fever; tachycardia; loss of appetite; abnormal breath sounds; productive cough of purulent, green, or rust-colored sputum; cloudy urine; urinalysis showing a WBC count greater than 5 per high-power field, positive leukocyte esterase or nitrites, or presence of bacteria; elevated WBC count and/or significant change in differential

RISK FACTORS

- Exposure to pathogens
- Treatment regimen
- Lack of exercise
- Inadequate fluid intake

DESIRED OUTCOMES

The client will remain free of infection as evidenced by:
a. Temperature declining toward normal
b. Absence of chills
c. Pulse rate within normal limits
d. Normal breath sounds
e. Usual mental status
f. Cough productive of clear mucus only
g. Voiding clear urine without reports of frequency, urgency, and burning
h. No increase in episodes of diarrhea and abdominal cramping and pain
i. Absence of heat, pain, redness, swelling, and unusual drainage in any area
j. No reports of increased weakness and fatigue
k. WBC and differential counts returning toward normal
l. Negative results of cultured specimens

NOC OUTCOMES

Immune status; infection severity

NIC INTERVENTIONS

Infection control; infection protection

NURSING ASSESSMENT	RATIONALE

Assess for and report signs and symptoms of infection (be aware that some signs and symptoms vary depending on the site of infection, the causative agent, and the age and immune status of the client):
- Elevated temperature
- Chills
- Increased pulse rate
- Malaise, lethargy, acute confusion
- Loss of appetite
- Abnormal breath sounds
- Productive cough of purulent, green, or rust-colored sputum

Early recognition of signs and symptoms of infection allows for prompt intervention.

NURSING ASSESSMENT	RATIONALE

- Cloudy urine
- Reports of frequency, urgency, or burning when urinating
- Urinalysis showing a WBC count greater than 5 per high-power field, positive leukocyte esterase or nitrites, or presence of bacteria
- Heat, pain, redness, swelling, or unusual drainage in any area
- Elevated WBC count and/or significant change in differential

Obtain specimens (e.g., urine, wound drainage, vaginal drainage, sputum, blood) for culture as ordered. Report positive results.

Cultures are done to identify the specific organism(s) causing the infection. Culture results provide information that helps determine the most effective treatment.

THERAPEUTIC INTERVENTIONS	RATIONALE

Independent Actions

Maintain a fluid intake of at least 2500 mL/day unless contraindicated. **D** ● ✦

Adequate hydration helps prevent infection by:
- *Helping maintain adequate blood flow and nutrient supply to the tissues*
- *Promoting urine formation and subsequent voiding, which flushes pathogens from the bladder and urethra*
- *Thinning respiratory secretions so that they can more easily be removed by coughing or suctioning (respiratory secretions provide a good medium for growth and colonization of microorganisms)*

Use good hand hygiene and encourage client to do the same. **D** ● ✦

Good hand hygiene removes transient flora, which reduces the risk of transmission of pathogens. Use of products such as an antibacterial soap, a chlorhexidine solution, or an alcohol-based handrub agent can actually inhibit the growth of or kill microorganisms, which further reduces infection risk.

Adhere to the appropriate precautions established to prevent transmission of infection to the client (standard precautions, transmission-based precautions on other clients, neutropenic precautions). **D** ● ✦

Adhering to the appropriate precautions that have been established to help prevent the transmission of microorganisms reduces the client's risk of infection.

Use sterile technique during invasive procedures (e.g., urinary catheterizations, venous and arterial punctures, injections, tracheal suctioning, wound care) and dressing changes.

Use of sterile technique reduces the possibility of introducing pathogens into the body.

Anchor catheters/tubings (e.g., urinary, intravenous, wound drainage) securely. **D** ● ✦

Catheters/tubings that are not securely anchored have some degree of in-and-out movement. This movement increases the risk of infection because it allows for the introduction of pathogens into the body. It can also cause tissue trauma, which can result in colonization of microorganisms.

Change equipment, tubings, and solutions used for treatments such as intravenous infusions, respiratory care, irrigations, and enteral feedings according to hospital policy. **D** ✦

The longer that equipment, tubings, and solutions are in use, the greater the chance of colonization of microorganisms, which can then be introduced into the body.

Maintain a closed system for drains (e.g., wounds, chest tubes, urinary catheters) and intravenous infusions whenever possible.

Each time a drainage or infusion system is opened, pathogens from the environment have an opportunity to enter the body. Maintaining a closed system decreases this risk, which reduces the possibility of infection.

Change peripheral intravenous line sites according to hospital policy.

Peripheral intravenous line sites are changed routinely to reduce persistent irritation of one area of a vein wall and the resultant colonization of microorganisms at that site.

Provide appropriate wound care (e.g., use dressing materials that maintain a moist wound surface, assist with debridement of necrotic tissue, use dressing materials that absorb excess exudate, protect granulating tissue from trauma and contamination, maintain patency of wound drains). **D** ✦

Proper wound care facilitates wound healing and reduces the number of pathogens that enter or are present in the wound, which reduces the risk of the wound becoming infected.

Continued...

THERAPEUTIC INTERVENTIONS	RATIONALE
Protect client from others with infections. **D** ● ✦	*Protecting the client from others with infections reduces the client's risk of exposure to pathogens.*
Implement measures to maintain healthy, intact skin (e.g., keep skin lubricated, clean, and dry; instruct or assist client to turn every 2 hrs; keep bed linens dry and wrinkle-free). **D** ● ✦	*Healthy, intact skin reduces the risk for infection by:* • *Providing a physical barrier against the introduction of pathogens into the body* • *Removing many of the microorganisms on the surface of the skin by means of the constant shedding of the epidermis* • *Inhibiting the growth of some bacteria on the surface of the skin (sebum contains fatty acids, which create a slightly acidic environment that inhibits the growth of some bacteria)*
Implement measures to reduce stress (e.g., reduce fear, anxiety, and pain; help client identify and use effective coping mechanisms). **D** ● ✦	*Stress causes an increased secretion of cortisol. Cortisol interferes with some immune responses, which subsequently increases the client's susceptibility to infection.*
Instruct and assist client to perform good perineal care routinely and after each bowel movement. **D** ● ✦	*The perineal area contains a large number of organisms. Routine cleansing of the area reduces the risk of colonization of organisms and subsequent perineal, urinary tract, and/or vaginal infection.*
Instruct and assist client to perform good oral hygiene as often as needed. **D** ● ✦	*Frequent oral hygiene helps prevent infection by removing most of the food, debris, and many of the microorganisms that are present in the mouth. It also helps maintain the integrity of the oral mucosa, which provides a physical and chemical barrier to pathogens.*
Implement measures to prevent urinary retention (e.g., instruct client to urinate when the urge is felt, promote relaxation during voiding attempts). **D** ✦	*A client experiencing urinary retention is at increased risk for urinary tract infection because:* • *The urine that accumulates in the bladder creates an environment conducive to the growth and colonization of microorganisms.* • *Voiding does not occur, so microorganisms are not flushed from the mucous lining of the urethra; these microorganisms can colonize and ascend into the bladder.*
Implement measures to prevent stasis of respiratory secretions (e.g., assist client to turn, cough, and deep breathe; increase activity as allowed and tolerated; perform tracheal suctioning if indicated). **D** ✦	*Respiratory secretions provide a good medium for growth of microorganisms. By preventing stasis, there is less chance of colonization of microorganisms and a decreased risk for development of respiratory tract infection.*
Instruct client to receive immunizations (e.g., influenza vaccine, pneumococcal vaccine) if appropriate.	*Immunizations are often recommended to reduce the possibility of some infections in high-risk clients (e.g., those clients who are immunosuppressed, elderly, or have a chronic disease).*

Dependent/Collaborative Actions

Maintain an optimal nutritional status. Administer vitamins and minerals as ordered. **D** ✦	*Adequate nutrition is needed to maintain normal function of the immune system.*
Perform actions to reduce inflammation of the bowel: • Administer corticosteroids, aminosalicylates, and/or immunomodulating agents as ordered.	*These medications are given to prevent further ulceration of the bowel and subsequently reduce the risk of intestinal infection.*
Consult appropriate health care provider regarding initiation of antimicrobial therapy if indicated. Administer antimicrobials if ordered (antimicrobials are generally given only if surgery is planned or if the client has severe colitis and is at high risk for infection; however, metronidazole or ciprofloxacin may be prescribed by some practitioners for the relief of symptoms).	*Most antimicrobials disrupt cell wall synthesis, which halts the growth of or kills microorganisms. This can effectively reduce the client's risk for infection.*

Collaborative Diagnosis   # RISK FOR RENAL CALCULI

Definition: Crystallized stones in the urinary tract.

Related to:
• Crystalline deposits in the urine associated with:
  • Increased serum oxalate levels (dietary oxalate normally binds with calcium in the intestine and is excreted in the stool; in clients with inflammatory bowel disease, calcium is bound with the poorly absorbed fat and oxalate becomes available for absorption)

- Decreased flushing of solutes from the urinary tract if urine formation is reduced as a result of deficient fluid volume
- Treatment with sulfasalazine

CLINICAL MANIFESTATIONS

Subjective	Objective
Verbal self-report of flank pain; verbalization of nausea	Hematuria; vomiting

RISK FACTORS

- Chronic disease
- Treatment regimen

DESIRED OUTCOMES

The client will not develop renal calculi as evidenced by:
a. Absence of flank pain, hematuria, nausea, and vomiting
b. Clear urine without calculi

NURSING ASSESSMENT	RATIONALE
Assess for and report signs and symptoms of renal calculi (e.g., dull, aching or severe, colicky flank pain; hematuria; nausea; vomiting).	*Early recognition of signs and symptoms of renal calculi allows for prompt intervention.*

THERAPEUTIC INTERVENTIONS	RATIONALE

Independent Actions

Implement measures to prevent renal calculi:
- Maintain a minimum fluid intake of 2500 mL/day unless contraindicated. **D** ● ✦
- Encourage client to decrease intake of foods/fluids high in oxalate (e.g., tea, instant coffee, peanuts, chocolate, spinach).
- Encourage client to adhere to a low-fat diet.

Providing adequate hydration helps maintain adequate blood flow to the kidneys to maintain glomerular filtration rate.

Decreases absorption of oxalate from the intestine.

A low-fat diet reduces the amount of fat available to bind calcium, thereby freeing calcium to bind with oxalate.

Dependent/Collaborative Actions

If signs and symptoms of renal calculi occur:
- Strain all urine and save any calculi for analysis; report finding to physician.
- Maintain a minimum fluid intake of 2500 mL/day unless contraindicated.
- Administer analgesics and antispasmodic agents (e.g., oxybutynin) as ordered.
- Prepare client for removal of calculi (e.g., extracorporeal shock wave lithotripsy, percutaneous nephrolithotomy, ureteroscopy with lithotripsy and stone extraction) if planned.
- Implement measures to reduce inflammation of the bowel (e.g., administer corticosteroids, aminosalicylates, and/or immunomodulating agents as ordered).

Straining the urine helps to determine whether the client has passed a renal calculus.

Helps to flush out the urinary tract and helps to pass a renal calculi.

Analgesics and antispasmodic agents decrease/eliminate pain experienced with renal calculi.

Explain procedures to client and provide required preprocedure or preoperative interventions.

These agents decrease inflammation and are used to put the disease in remission.

Collaborative Diagnosis **RISK FOR PERIRECTAL, RECTOVAGINAL, ENTEROVESICAL, AND ENTEROENTERIC ABSCESSES AND FISTULAS**

Definition: Fistula, ulceration, or tear in the intestinal wall; abscess—an accumulation of pus in tissues or a body cavity.

Related to: Extension of a mucosal fissure or ulcer through the intestinal wall

---

NDx = NANDA Diagnosis   **D** = Delegatable Action   ● = UAP   ✦ = LVN/LPN   ⊖▶ = Go to ⊖volve for animation

CLINICAL MANIFESTATIONS

Subjective	Objective
Verbal self-report of increased or constant abdominal pain; verbalization of rectal pain	Fever; perianal redness, swelling, and bleeding; foul-smelling vaginal discharge; increased WBC count

RISK FACTOR

• Chronic illness

DESIRED OUTCOMES

The client will have resolution of any abscesses and fistulas that develop as evidenced by:
a. Temperature declining toward normal
b. Resolution of abdominal pain
c. Absence of perianal redness, swelling, and pain
d. No unusual vaginal drainage
e. Clear, yellow urine
f. WBC count declining toward normal

NURSING ASSESSMENT	RATIONALE
Assess for and report signs and symptoms of abscess and/or fistula formation (e.g., further increase in temperature; increased or more constant abdominal pain; perianal redness, swelling, and pain; foul-smelling vaginal discharge or passage of stool from vagina; dysuria; fecaluria; further increase in WBC count).	*Early recognition of signs and symptoms of abscess and/or fistula formation allows for prompt intervention.* *Corticosteroids, aminosalicylates, and/or immunomodulating agents reduce bowel inflammation.*

THERAPEUTIC INTERVENTIONS	RATIONALE

Dependent/Collaborative Actions
Implement measures to reduce inflammation of the bowel (e.g., administer corticosteroids, aminosalicylates, and/or immunomodulating agents as ordered).
If signs and symptoms of abscesses or fistulas occur:
• Prepare client for diagnostic studies (e.g., computed tomography, ultrasonography, barium enema).
• Administer the following medications if ordered:
  • Antimicrobial agents (e.g., metronidazole, ciprofloxacin)
  • Immunomodulator agents such as azathioprine, mercaptopurine, or a monoclonal antibody (e.g., infliximab)
• If a cutaneous fistula is present, perform wound care as ordered.
• Prepare client for surgical intervention (e.g., incision and drainage of abscess, resection of involved area) if planned.
	Promotes healing of the intestinal mucosa and subsequently decreases the risk for the development of abscesses and fistulas.
	
	Decreases client anxiety.
	
	Antimicrobials treat/prevent infection.
	Decreases inflammation and promotes healing.
	
	Explain procedures to client and provide required preoperative interventions.

Collaborative Diagnosis — RISK FOR TOXIC MEGACOLON

Definition: A life-threatening complication of inflammatory bowel diseases in which there is segmental or total dilation of the colon as a result of inflammation or infection.

Related to:
• Loss of colonic muscle tone associated with the effects of widespread inflammation in the bowel, use of some medications (e.g., opiates, anticholinergics), and hypokalemia

CLINICAL MANIFESTATIONS

Subjective	Objective
Verbal self-report of increasing abdominal pain and tenderness	Hypoactive or absent bowel sounds; abdominal percussion reveals tympany; sudden episodes of diarrhea; tachycardia; fever; increased WBC count

RISK FACTORS

- Chronic illness
- Treatment regimen

DESIRED OUTCOMES

The client will not develop toxic megacolon as evidenced by:
a. Absence of abdominal distention
b. Gradual resolution of abdominal pain
c. Active bowel sounds
d. Gradual resolution of diarrhea
e. Temperature and WBC count declining toward normal

NURSING ASSESSMENT

Assess for and report signs and symptoms of toxic megacolon:
- Abdominal distention and increased abdominal pain and tenderness
- Hypoactive or absent bowel sounds with tympanic percussion note over abdomen
- Sudden decrease in episodes of diarrhea
- Fever (usually >38.6°C) and tachycardia
- Increase in WBC count
- Abdominal radiograph showing colonic dilation

RATIONALE

Early recognition of signs and symptoms of toxic megacolon allows for prompt intervention.

THERAPEUTIC INTERVENTIONS

Dependent/Collaborative Actions

Implement measures to prevent development of toxic megacolon:
- Perform actions to reduce inflammation of the bowel (e.g., administer corticosteroids, aminosalicylates, and/or immunomodulating agents as ordered).
- Administer medications that slow GI motility (e.g., opioid analgesics, antidiarrheal agents, anticholinergics) judiciously.
- Perform actions to prevent or treat hypokalemia (e.g., eat foods high in potassium, take potassium supplements).

If signs and symptoms of toxic megacolon occur:
- Withhold oral intake as ordered.
- Consult physician about discontinuing any medications that slow GI motility (e.g., narcotic analgesics, antidiarrheal agents, anticholinergics).
- Insert NG tube and maintain suction as ordered.
- Administer the following if ordered:
  - Intravenous fluids

  - Corticosteroids
  - Antimicrobials (e.g., metronidazole)

- Prepare client for surgical intervention (e.g., colectomy) if planned.
- Implement measures to reduce inflammation of the bowel (e.g., administer corticosteroids, aminosalicylates, and/or immunomodulating agents as ordered).

RATIONALE

These medications reduce inflammation, which will help prevent toxic megacolon.

Opioid analgesics, anti-diarrheal agents and anticholinergics may cause constipation, thereby contributing to toxic megacolon.

Helps prevent megacolon.

Withholding oral intake helps decompress the colon.
Increasing motility helps to decompress the colon.

Insertion of an NG tube provides decompression of the GI tract.
IV fluids are given to maintain adequate vascular volume (third-space fluid shifting occurs as a result of increased capillary permeability associated with the inflammation and increased intraluminal pressure that are present with toxic megacolon).
Steroids reduce intestinal inflammation.
Antimicrobials help prevent infection, which is important because the risk of perforation is increased when toxic megacolon develops.
If above treatment is not effective in decompressing the colon, surgery is indicated.
These actions reduce intestinal narrowing and scar tissue formation.

NDx = NANDA Diagnosis   **D** = Delegatable Action   ● = UAP   ✦ = LVN/LPN   ⊖▶ = Go to ⊖volve for animation

| Collaborative Diagnosis | **RISK FOR PERITONITIS** |

Definition: Inflammation of the peritoneum.

Related to: Perforation of the bowel or leakage from an abscess or fistula

CLINICAL MANIFESTATIONS

Subjective	Objective
Verbal self-report of abdominal pain	Nausea and vomiting; distended and rigid abdomen; diminished or absent bowel sounds; fever; tachypnea; increased WBC count

RISK FACTORS

* Exposure to pathogens
* Treatment regimen

DESIRED OUTCOMES

The client will not develop peritonitis as evidenced by:
a. Temperature declining toward normal
b. Soft, nondistended abdomen
c. Gradual resolution of abdominal pain
d. Gradual return of normal bowel sounds
e. Absence of nausea and vomiting
f. Stable vital signs
g. WBC count declining toward normal

NURSING ASSESSMENT

Assess for and report signs and symptoms of peritonitis (e.g., increase in severity of abdominal pain; generalized abdominal pain; rebound tenderness; distended, rigid abdomen; increase in temperature; tachycardia; tachypnea; hypotension; nausea; vomiting; continued diminished or absent bowel sounds; WBC count that increases or fails to decline toward normal).

RATIONALE

Early recognition of signs and symptoms of peritonitis allows for prompt intervention.

THERAPEUTIC INTERVENTIONS

Dependent/Collaborative Actions
If signs and symptoms of peritonitis occur:
* Withhold oral intake as ordered.

* Place client on bedrest in a semi-Fowler's position.

* Prepare client for diagnostic tests (e.g., abdominal radiograph, computed tomography, ultrasonography) if planned.
* Insert NG tube and maintain suction as ordered.
* Administer antimicrobials (e.g., metronidazole) as ordered.
* Administer intravenous fluids and/or blood volume expanders if ordered.

* Prepare client for surgical intervention (e.g., repair of perforation, bowel resection) if planned.

RATIONALE

Oral intake irritates the colon and increases pain associated with peritonitis.
This position assists in pooling or localizing intestinal contents in the pelvis rather than under the diaphragm.
Provide preprocedure information as required by the client.

Decompresses the GI tract.
Helps decrease infection in the GI tract.
IV fluids and/or blood volume expanders prevent or treat shock that can result from the increased capillary permeability that occurs with inflammation and the subsequent escape of protein, fluid, and electrolytes from the vascular space into the peritoneal cavity.

DISCHARGE TEACHING/CONTINUED CARE

Nursing Diagnosis **DEFICIENT KNOWLEDGE** NDx**; INEFFECTIVE FAMILY HEALTH MANAGEMENT** NDx**; OR INEFFECTIVE HEALTH MAINTENANCE*** NDx

Definition: Deficient Knowledge NDx: Absence of cognitive information related to specific topic or its acquisition. **Ineffective Family Health Management:** A pattern of regulating and integrating into family processes a program for the treatment of illness and its sequelae that is unsatisfactory for meeting specific health goals of the family unit. **Ineffective Health Maintenance NDx:** Inability to identify, manage, and/or seek help to maintain well-being.

CLINICAL MANIFESTATIONS

Subjective	Objective
Verbal self-report of the problem	Inaccurate follow-through of instructions; inappropriate behaviors

RISK FACTORS

- Denial of disease process
- Cognitive deficiency
- Failure to reduce risk factors

NOC OUTCOMES	NIC INTERVENTIONS
Knowledge: diet; medication; treatment regimen	Health system guidance; teaching: individual; teaching: disease process; teaching: prescribed diet; teaching: prescribed medication

NURSING ASSESSMENT	RATIONALE
Assess client's ability and readiness to learn. Assess the client's understanding of teaching.	*Learning is more effective when the client is motivated and understands the importance of what is to be learned. Readiness to learn changes based on situations and physical and emotional challenges.*

THERAPEUTIC INTERVENTIONS	RATIONALE

Desired Outcome: The client will identify ways to reduce the incidence of disease exacerbation.

Independent Actions
Reinforce the importance of adhering to the prescribed treatment regimen.
Instruct the client regarding ways to reduce bowel irritation:

- Reduce intake of or avoid foods/fluids likely to be poorly digested or that may irritate the bowel (e.g., raw fruits and vegetables, whole-grain cereals, gravy, fried foods, spicy foods, milk and milk products, caffeine-containing beverages, extremely hot drinks, iced drinks, alcohol).
- Avoid use of laxatives.

Explain that stress can precipitate periods of exacerbation. Provide information about stress management classes and counseling services that may assist client to manage stress.

Irritation of the bowel may cause nausea and vomiting as well as an exacerbation of the disease.

Encourage client to find ways of reducing stress in his/her life, as this will decrease exacerbations of the disease.

THERAPEUTIC INTERVENTIONS	RATIONALE

Desired Outcome: The client will verbalize ways to maintain an optimal nutritional status.

*The nurse should select the diagnostic label that is most appropriate for the client's discharge teaching needs.

NDx = NANDA Diagnosis   **D** = Delegatable Action   ● = UAP   ✦ = LVN/LPN   ⊖▶ = Go to ⊖volve for animation

Continued...

THERAPEUTIC INTERVENTIONS	RATIONALE

Independent Actions

Provide instructions regarding ways to maintain an optimal nutritional status:

- Reinforce instructions regarding prescribed diet (a low-residue, high-calorie, high-protein diet is often recommended).
- Inform client that eating small, frequent meals rather than three large meals may help achieve the recommended high-calorie intake.
- Reinforce the benefits of eating when rested and in a relaxed atmosphere.
- Stress the importance of taking vitamins and minerals as prescribed.

Maintenance of nutritional status and the appropriate diet is important in decreasing exacerbations of the disease and maintaining nutritional status.

THERAPEUTIC INTERVENTIONS	RATIONALE

Desired Outcome: The client will state ways to prevent perianal skin breakdown.

Independent Actions

Provide the following instructions about ways to prevent perianal skin breakdown:

- Use soft toilet tissue for wiping after each bowel movement.
- Cleanse perianal area with a mild soap and warm water after each bowel movement; dry thoroughly.
- Apply a protective ointment or cream to perianal area after skin has been cleansed.

Each of these interventions prevents skin breakdown, which subsequently decreases the risk of infection and pain.

THERAPEUTIC INTERVENTIONS	RATIONALE

Desired Outcome: The client will verbalize an understanding of medications ordered including rationale, food, and drug interactions, side effects, schedule for taking, and importance of taking as prescribed.

Independent Actions

Explain rationale for, side effects of, and importance of taking medications prescribed. Inform client of pertinent food and drug interactions.
Examples:

- Sulfasalazine
- Corticosteroid

Instruct client to inform physician before taking other prescription and nonprescription medications.

Knowledge of the medication regimen and the impact of these medications on the system, as well as how the medication regimen can be incorporated into the client's lifestyle, allows the client some mechanism of control of his/her disease and the ability to have an active part in treatment and care.

Over-the-counter medications may impact prescription medications and should not be taken without a health care provider's approval.

THERAPEUTIC INTERVENTIONS	RATIONALE

Desired Outcome: The client will state signs and symptoms to report to the health care provider.

Independent Actions

Instruct client to report the following signs and symptoms:

- Recurrent episodes of diarrhea and abdominal pain and cramping
- Increasing abdominal distention
- Persistent vomiting
- Unusual rectal or vaginal drainage
- Burning on urination or brownish, foul-smelling urine
- Pain, swelling, or open sores in perianal area

The client and significant others should be aware of what symptoms are associated with exacerbations of the disease or infection and to report these to the health care provider.

THERAPEUTIC INTERVENTIONS	RATIONALE

- Continued weight loss
- Constipation
- Yellowing of skin, flank pain, change in vision, eye pain, or joint pain or swelling (can indicate extraintestinal involvement)

THERAPEUTIC INTERVENTIONS	RATIONALE

Desired Outcome: The client will identify resources that can assist in the adjustment to changes resulting from inflammatory bowel disease and its treatment.

Independent Actions

Provide information about resources that can assist the client and significant others in adjusting to inflammatory bowel disease and its effects (e.g., local support groups, Crohn's and Colitis Foundation of America, counseling services, stress management classes).

Client may require assistance from community organizations for both emotional and financial support once discharged from the acute care facility.

Reinforce importance of keeping follow-up appointments with health care provider.

Inflammatory bowel disease is a chronic illness and requires appropriate follow-up with health care providers.

THERAPEUTIC INTERVENTIONS	RATIONALE

Desired Outcome: The client, in collaboration with the nurse, will develop a plan for adhering to recommended follow-up care including future appointments with health care provider and activity level.

Independent Actions

Collaborate with the client to develop a plan for adherence that includes:

- Importance of frequent rest periods throughout the day.

Allows body to heal.

Implementing measures to improve client compliance:

- Include significant others in teaching sessions if possible
- Encouraging questions and allow time for reinforcement and clarification of information provided.
- Providing written instructions on future appointments with health care provider, medications prescribed, signs and symptoms to report, and future laboratory studies.

Support from client's significant others is important in maintaining compliance to the therapeutic regimen.
Improves client's and family's understanding of disease process and what to do to remain healthy.
Written instructions allow the client to refer to them after discharge as needed.

ADDITIONAL NURSING/COLLABORATIVE DIAGNOSIS

DISTURBED SLEEP PATTERN NDx
Related to frequent need to defecate, pain, fear, and anxiety

FEAR NDx
ANXIETY NDx
Related to:

- Symptoms being experienced (e.g., abdominal pain, persistent diarrhea, fever)
- Lack of understanding of diagnosis, diagnostic tests, and treatment
- Concern about need for surgery if disease condition cannot be medically controlled
- Anticipated changes in future lifestyle because of inability to control symptoms
- Concern about expense of hospitalization and treatment for a chronic disease

DISTURBED SELF-CONCEPT
Related to:

- Dependence on others to meet self-care needs
- Embarrassment associated with diarrhea
- Changes in sexual functioning associated with pain, fatigue, and weakness
- Changes in lifestyle associated with pain and chronic diarrhea

RISK FOR IMPAIRED TISSUE INTEGRITY NDx
Related to:

- Damage to the skin and/or subcutaneous tissue associated with prolonged pressure on the tissues, friction, and shearing that can occur when mobility decreased
- Frequent contact with irritants associated with persistent diarrhea
- Increased fragility of skin associated with malnutrition

NDx = NANDA Diagnosis   **D** = Delegatable Action   ● = UAP   ✦ = LVN/LPN   ⊜▶ = Go to ⊜volve   for animation

- Hyperthermia related to stimulation of the thermoregulatory center in the hypothalamus by endogenous pyrogens that are released in an inflammatory process

ACTIVITY INTOLERANCE NDx
Related to:
- Inadequate nutritional status
- Difficulty resting and sleeping associated with pain, frequent need to defecate, fear, and anxiety

- Tissue hypoxia associated with anemia resulting from:
  - Blood loss from the ulcerated bowel
  - Decreased oral intake and impaired absorption of iron, vitamin B_{12}, and folate
- Increased energy expenditure associated with the increased metabolic rate that may be present during period of exacerbation

INTESTINAL OBSTRUCTION AND BOWEL RESECTION

Intestinal (bowel) obstruction is a condition in which the intestinal contents fail to move through the bowel. The obstruction can be partial or complete and can develop slowly or rapidly. It can occur as a result of any factor that narrows the lumen of the intestine or interferes with peristalsis. Narrowing of the lumen results in a mechanical obstruction and can be caused by factors such as adhesions, tumors, inflammatory bowel disease, hernias, fecal impaction, intussusception, a volvulus, and strictures. In a nonmechanical obstruction, the bowel lumen remains open, but the intestinal contents are not propelled forward. Factors that can cause this paralytic (adynamic) ileus include abdominal surgery, effects of anesthesia and some medications (e.g., narcotic [opioid] analgesics, some antiemetics, anticholinergics, antidiarrheals), electrolyte imbalances such as hypokalemia, decreased blood flow to the intestine (can occur with conditions such as hypovolemia or blockage of mesenteric vessels as a result of an embolus, thrombus, or arteriosclerosis), spinal cord injury, and peritonitis.

Signs and symptoms of intestinal obstruction vary depending on the location, cause, and degree of the obstruction. Common clinical manifestations include abdominal pain and distention, nausea, and vomiting. Hyperactive, high-pitched bowel sounds are present early in the development of a mechanical obstruction. Bowel sounds are absent or hypoactive in nonmechanical obstruction and as mechanical obstruction worsens.

Treatment of intestinal obstruction is directed toward relieving symptoms, managing fluid and electrolyte imbalances, preventing complications, and determining and treating the cause of the obstruction. Most cases of nonmechanical obstruction do not necessitate surgery. Some mechanical obstructions can be treated nonsurgically (e.g., enemas and laxatives to remove fecal impaction, dilatation of obstructed portion of bowel via endoscopy, radiation, or chemotherapy to reduce tumor size, gentle instillation of barium to resolve an intussusception or reverse a sigmoid volvulus). Surgical intervention (intestinal resection with re-anastomosis or creation of an ileostomy or colostomy) is indicated when it is necessary to remove an obstruction that persists despite conservative management or to remove a segment of bowel that is strangulated or necrotic.

This care plan focuses on the adult client hospitalized with an intestinal obstruction and addresses what postoperative care is required if a bowel resection is required. Some of the information is applicable to clients receiving follow-up care in an extended care facility or home setting.

OUTCOME/DISCHARGE CRITERIA

The client who does not have surgery will:
1. Have absence of or minimal abdominal pain
2. Have gradual return of normal bowel function
3. Tolerate prescribed diet
4. Have no signs and symptoms of complications
5. Verbalize an understanding of ways to reduce the risk for recurrent intestinal obstruction
6. State signs and symptoms to report to the health care provider
7. Develop a plan for adhering to recommended diet, prescribed medications, ways to prevent recurrent intestinal obstruction, and future appointments with health care provider

POSTOPERATIVE

The client will:
1. Have absence of or minimal abdominal postoperative pain
2. Have gradual return of normal bowel function
3. Tolerate prescribed diet
4. Have no signs and symptoms of postoperative complications
5. Have clear, audible breath sounds throughout lungs
6. Have evidence of normal healing of surgical wound(s)
7. Verbalize an understanding of ways to reduce the risk for recurrent intestinal obstruction
8. State signs and symptoms to report to the health care provider
9. Develop a plan for adhering to recommended diet, prescribed medications, ways to prevent recurrent intestinal obstruction, and future appointments with health care provider

Nursing/Diagnosis RISK FOR IMBALANCED FLUID VOLUME NDx; RISK FOR ELECTROLYTE IMBALANCE*

Definition: Risk for Imbalanced Fluid Volume NDx: Susceptible to a decrease, increase, or rapid shift from one to the other of intravascular, interstitial, and/or intracellular fluid, which may compromise health. This refers to body fluid loss, gain, or both. **Risk for Electrolyte Imbalance NDx:** Susceptible to changes in serum electrolyte levels, which may compromise health.

Related to:

Risk for Imbalanced Fluid Volume NDx:
* Increased capillary permeability that results from increased intraluminal pressure in the distended bowel

Risk for Electrolyte Imbalance NDx; hypokalemia, hypochloremia, and **metabolic alkalosis** related to:
* Decreased absorption of intestinal fluid into the vascular space associated with inflammation and distention of the bowel (the sequestering of fluid in the intestine is a major factor with obstructions of the small intestine and proximal portion of the large intestine)
* Restricted oral intake
* Excessive loss of fluid and electrolytes associated with vomiting and NG tube drainage

CLINICAL MANIFESTATIONS

Subjective	Objective
Verbal self-report of nausea, headache, and abdominal pain	Poor skin turgor; dry, cracked mucous membranes; hypotension; weight loss; prolonged capillary refill greater than 2 to 3 seconds; decreased urine output; increased urine specific gravity; abdominal distention; vomiting; positive Chvostek and Trousseau signs; abnormal serum electrolyte levels; cardiac dysrhythmias, muscle weakness, paresthesias, twitching, spasms, and dizziness; increased BUN and Hct

RISK FACTORS

* Failure of regulatory mechanisms
* Inadequate fluid/food intake
* Immobility

DESIRED OUTCOMES

The client will maintain fluid and electrolyte balance as evidenced by:
a. Normal skin turgor
b. Moist mucous membranes
c. Stable weight
d. BP and pulse rate within normal range for client and stable with position change
e. Capillary refill time less than 2 to 3 seconds
f. Usual mental status
g. Balanced I&O
h. Urine specific gravity within normal range
i. Abdomen less distended and bowel sounds returning toward normal
j. Absence of cardiac dysrhythmias, muscle weakness, paresthesias, twitching, spasms, and dizziness
k. BUN, Hct, serum electrolyte, and ABG values within normal range

NOC OUTCOMES

Fluid balance; electrolyte and acid-base balance

NIC INTERVENTIONS

Fluid management; electrolyte management: hypokalemia; electrolyte management: hypocalcemia; electrolyte management: hypomagnesemia; acid-base management: metabolic acidosis; diarrhea management

*The nurse must determine the appropriate nursing diagnosis based on assessment of the client.

NURSING ASSESSMENT	RATIONALE
Assess for and report signs and symptoms of deficient fluid volume:	Early recognition of signs and symptoms of electrolyte imbalance allows for prompt treatment.

Assess for and report signs and symptoms of deficient fluid volume:

- Decreased skin turgor, dry mucous membranes, thirst
- Weight loss of 2% or greater over a short period
- Postural hypotension and/or low BP
- Weak, rapid pulse
- Capillary refill time longer than 2 to 3 seconds
- Neck veins flat when client is supine
- Change in mental status
- Decreased urine output with increased specific gravity (reflects an actual rather than potential fluid deficit)
- Significant increase in BUN and Hct above previous levels
- Hypokalemia (e.g., cardiac dysrhythmias, postural hypotension, muscle weakness, nausea and vomiting, abdominal distention, hypoactive or absent bowel sounds)
- Hypomagnesemia and/or hypocalcemia (e.g., anxiousness; irritability; cardiac dysrhythmias; positive Chvostek and Trousseau signs; numbness or tingling of fingers, toes, or circumoral area; hyperactive reflexes; tetany; seizures)
- Metabolic acidosis (e.g., drowsiness; disorientation; stupor; rapid, deep respirations; headache; nausea and vomiting; cardiac dysrhythmias; low pH and CO_2 content)
- Third-spacing
- Ascites
- Evidence of vascular depletion (e.g., postural hypotension, weak, rapid pulse; decreased urine output)

Early recognition of signs and symptoms of electrolyte imbalance allows for prompt treatment.

THERAPEUTIC INTERVENTIONS	RATIONALE

Independent Actions

Implement measures to prevent or treat imbalanced fluid and electrolytes:

- Perform actions to reduce nausea and vomiting (e.g., eliminate noxious stimuli, have patient change positions slowly, provide oral hygiene after each meal). **D** ● ✦

  These interventions decrease nausea and vomiting, helping to maintain positive fluid and electrolyte balance.

If an NG tube is present and needs to be irrigated frequently and/or with large volumes of solution, irrigate it with normal saline rather than water. **D** ✦

  Provides decompression of the stomach, and irrigation with normal saline causes less irritation of the gastric mucosa.

Dependent/Collaborative Actions

Implement measures to prevent or treat imbalanced fluid and electrolytes:

- Maintain intravenous fluid therapy as ordered.

  Prevents dehydration.
- Administer electrolyte replacement as ordered.

  Helps to maintain appropriate electrolyte balance.
- Administer albumin infusions if ordered.

  Increases colloid osmotic pressure and promotes mobilization of third-space fluid back into the vascular space.
- When oral intake is allowed, assist client to select foods/fluids within the prescribed dietary regimen that would replenish electrolytes. **D** ✦

  Oral intake of foods high in potassium is necessary to maintain adequate electrolyte balance.

Consult physician if signs and symptoms of imbalanced fluid and electrolytes persist or worsen.

  Notification of the physician allows for prompt alteration in the treatment plan.

Nursing Diagnosis **ACUTE PAIN** NDx **(ABDOMINAL)**

Definition: Unpleasant sensory and emotional experience arising from actual or potential tissue damage or described in terms of such damage (International Association for the Study of Pain); sudden or slow onset of any intensity from mild to severe with an anticipated or predictable end, and a duration of less than 3 months.

Related to:
- Distention of the intestinal lumen associated with the accumulation of gas and fluid
- Inflammation of the intestine (can occur as a result of the underlying cause of the obstruction [e.g., inflammatory bowel disease])

CLINICAL MANIFESTATIONS

Subjective	Objective
Verbal self-report of pain	Autonomic responses (e.g., diaphoresis; changes in BP, respiration, pulse rate; pupillary dilatation); expressive behavior (e.g., restlessness, moaning, crying, vigilance, irritability, sighing); changes in appetite and eating; protective gestures; guarding behavior; facial mask; sleep disturbance (eyes lack luster, fixed or scattered movement, beaten look, grimace); self-focus; narrowed focus (altered time perception, impaired thought processes, reduced interaction with people and environment); distraction behavior (e.g., pacing, seeking out other people and/or activities, repetitive activities)

RISK FACTOR
- Chronic illness

DESIRED OUTCOMES

The client will experience diminished pain as evidenced by:
a. Verbalization of same
b. Relaxed facial expression
c. Increased participation in activities
d. Stable vital signs

NOC OUTCOMES

Pain control; minimizing pain's disruptive effects

NIC INTERVENTIONS

Pain management; environmental management: comfort; analgesic administration

NURSING ASSESSMENT	RATIONALE
Assess for signs and symptoms of pain (e.g., verbalization of pain, grimacing, reluctance to move, restlessness, diaphoresis, increased BP, tachycardia).	*Early recognition of signs and symptoms of pain allows for prompt intervention and improved pain control.*
Assess client's perception of the severity of pain using a pain intensity rating scale.	*An awareness of the severity of pain being experienced helps determine the most appropriate interventions for pain management. Use of a pain intensity rating scale gives the nurse a clearer understanding of the pain being experienced and promotes consistency when communicating with others about the client's pain experience.*
Assess the client's pain pattern (e.g., location, quality, onset, duration, precipitating factors, aggravating factors, alleviating factors).	*Knowledge of the client's pain pattern assists in the identification of effective pain management interventions.*
Ask the client to describe previous pain experiences and methods used to manage pain effectively.	*Many variables affect a client's response to pain (e.g., age, sex, coping style, previous experience with pain, culture, cause of pain). Knowledge of the client's usual response to pain and methods previously used to manage pain effectively enables the nurse to evaluate the client's pain more accurately and facilitates the identification of effective strategies for pain management.*

THERAPEUTIC INTERVENTIONS	RATIONALE
Independent Actions	
Implement measures to reduce fear and anxiety (e.g., assure client that the need for pain relief is understood, plan methods for achieving pain control with client, provide a calm environment).	*Fear and anxiety can decrease the client's threshold and tolerance for pain and thereby heighten the perception of pain. In addition, pain management methods are not as effective if the client is tense and unable to relax.*
Prevent actions that will increase the accumulation of intestinal gas and fluid (e.g., using a straw, chewing gum). **D ● ✦**	*These actions can increase air swallowing and subsequent gas production.*
Implement measures to promote rest (e.g., minimize environmental activity and noise, provide care to allow for periods of uninterrupted rest). **D ● ✦**	*Fatigue can decrease the client's threshold and tolerance for pain and thereby heighten the perception of pain. A well-rested client often experiences decreased pain and increased effectiveness of pain management measures.*
When oral intake is allowed, advance diet slowly and instruct client to avoid intake of carbonated beverages and gas-producing foods (e.g., cabbage, onions, beans).	*Reduces gas in the GI tract.*
Dependent/Collaborative Actions	
Insert NG tube and maintain suction as ordered.	*Provides decompression and prevents gas accumulation in the stomach.*
Administer GI stimulants (e.g., metoclopramide) if ordered. **D ✦**	*Promotes intestinal motility (may be ordered if obstruction is not complete or is the result of a paralytic ileus).*
Administer analgesics as ordered (the use of opioid analgesics is often avoided until the cause of the obstruction is determined). **D ✦**	*The administration of analgesics before a pain-producing event helps minimize the pain that will be experienced. Analgesics are also more effective if given before pain becomes severe because mild to moderate pain is controlled more quickly and effectively than severe pain.*
Provide or assist with nonpharmacological methods for pain relief. Examples include: • Cutaneous stimulation measures (e.g., pressure, massage, heat and cold applications, TENS, acupuncture) • Relaxation techniques (e.g., progressive relaxation exercises, meditation, guided imagery) • Distraction measures (e.g., listening to music, conversing, watching television, playing cards, reading) • Position change	*Nonpharmacological pain management includes a variety of interventions. It is believed that most of these are effective because they stimulate closure of the gating mechanism in the spinal cord and subsequently block the transmission of pain impulses. In addition, some interventions are thought to stimulate the release of endogenous analgesics (e.g., endorphins) that inhibit the transmission of pain impulses and/or alter the client's perception of pain. Many of the nonpharmacological interventions also help decrease pain by promoting relaxation.*
Consult appropriate health care provider (e.g., physician, pharmacist, pain management specialist) if above measures fail to provide adequate pain relief.	*Notifying the appropriate health care provider allows for modification of the treatment plan.*

Nursing Diagnosis | **NAUSEA** NDx

Definition: A subjective phenomenon of an unpleasant feeling in the back of the throat and stomach, which may or may not result in vomiting.

Related to:
• Stimulation of the vomiting center associated with:
  • Stimulation of the visceral afferent pathways resulting from inflammation and distention of the intestine
  • Stimulation of the cerebral cortex resulting from pain and stress

CLINICAL MANIFESTATIONS

Subjective	**Objective**
Verbal self-report of nausea	Gagging; retching (dry heaving)

RISK FACTORS
- Chronic illness
- Gastric irritation

DESIRED OUTCOMES

The client will experience relief of nausea and vomiting as evidenced by:
a. Verbalization of relief of nausea
b. Absence of vomiting

NOC OUTCOMES

Nausea and vomiting severity

NIC INTERVENTIONS

Nausea management; vomiting management; environmental management: comfort

| **NURSING ASSESSMENT** | **RATIONALE** |

Assess for nausea and vomiting.
Determine:
- Duration
- Frequency
- Severity

Identification of the signs and symptoms of nausea and vomiting allows for prompt intervention.

| **THERAPEUTIC INTERVENTIONS** | **RATIONALE** |

Independent Actions
Implement measures to reduce nausea and vomiting:
- Maintain food and oral fluid restrictions as ordered.

Food/fluid restrictions and insertion of an NG tube decreases pressure within the abdomen.

Dependent/Collaborative Actions
- Insert NG tube and maintain suction as ordered.

- Eliminate noxious sights and odors from the environment.
- Instruct client to change positions slowly. **D** ● ✦

Provide oral hygiene after each emesis. **D** ● ✦

Reduce pain via medications, positioning, or distractions. **D** ✦
- Perform actions to reduce fear and anxiety (e.g., assure client that staff are nearby; provide a calm, restful environment; explain all tests and procedures).
Encourage client to take deep, slow breaths when nauseated. **D** ● ✦

Insertion of an NG tube will help to decompress the stomach and alleviate nausea and vomiting.
Noxious stimuli can cause stimulation of the vomiting center.
Rapid movements can result in chemoreceptor trigger zone stimulation and subsequent excitation of the vomiting center.
Oral hygiene removes the taste of emesis from the mouth and helps to decrease subsequent nausea.
Pain may stimulate chemoreceptor trigger zone and produce nausea.
Fear and anxiety may produce nausea.

Taking slow, deep breaths helps to relax the client and reduce stress.

Dependent/Collaborative Actions
Implement measures to reduce nausea and vomiting:
Administer antiemetics as ordered. **D** ✦

- When oral intake is allowed, advance diet slowly. Initially encourage bland floods such as Jello, rice, broth, toast, and dry crackers.
Consult a physician or a pharmacist if nausea continues.

Antiemetics raise the threshold of the chemoreceptor trigger zone, thus decreasing nausea.
Oral intake helps maintain nutritional status and should be advanced slowly to decrease the incidence of nausea.

Allows for continued intervention to decrease/eliminate nausea.

Collaborative/Nursing Diagnosis **RISK FOR PERITONITIS**

Definition: Inflammation of the peritoneum.

Related to: Release of intestinal contents into the peritoneal cavity associated with perforation of the bowel if it occurs

CLINICAL MANIFESTATIONS

Subjective	**Objective**
Verbal self-report of abdominal pain	Nausea and vomiting; distended and rigid abdomen; diminished or absent bowel sounds; fever; tachypnea; increased WBC count

---

RISK FACTORS
- Exposure to pathogens
- Chronic illness

DESIRED OUTCOMES

The client will not develop peritonitis as evidenced by:
a. Temperature stable and less than 36°C
b. Abdomen less distended and firm
c. No increase in abdominal pain and tenderness, nausea, and vomiting
d. Gradual return of normal bowel sounds
e. Stable vital signs
f. No increase in WBC count

NURSING ASSESSMENT	RATIONALE
Assess for and report signs and symptoms of peritonitis (e.g., further increase in temperature or temperature >38°C, abdomen more distended and firm, increase in severity of abdominal pain, rebound tenderness, increased nausea and vomiting, tachycardia, hypotension, increase in WBC count)	*Early recognition of signs and symptoms of peritonitis allows for prompt intervention.*

THERAPEUTIC INTERVENTIONS	RATIONALE
Dependent/Collaborative Actions	
• Implement measures to prevent peritonitis:	
• Perform actions to reduce the risk for perforation of the bowel:	
• Implement measures to decrease the accumulation of intestinal gas and fluid (e.g., insert an NG tube and attach to suction, avoid carbonated beverages, avoid gas-producing foods).	*These actions maintain decompression of the gut.*
• Continue with actions to treat the underlying cause of the obstruction (e.g., anti-inflammatory agents to treat inflammatory bowel disease, chemotherapeutic agents to reduce tumor size).	
• Administer antimicrobials if ordered.	*Antimicrobials reduce/prevent infection.*
If signs and symptoms of peritonitis occur:	
• Withhold oral food and fluids as ordered.	*Decreases pressure within the abdomen.*
Place client on bedrest in a semi-Fowler's position.	*Assists in pooling or localizing GI contents in the pelvis rather than the diaphragm.*
• Prepare client for diagnostic tests (e.g., abdominal radiograph, computed tomography) if planned.	*Decreases client's fear and anxiety.*
• Administer antimicrobials as ordered.	*Antimicrobials reduce infection.*
• Administer fluids and/or blood volume expanders if ordered.	*Fluid volume and/or blood expanders prevent or treat shock that can result from the increased capillary permeability that occurs with inflammation and the subsequent escape of protein, fluid, and electrolytes from the vascular space into the peritoneal cavity.*
• Prepare client for surgery (e.g., drainage and irrigation of the peritoneum, bowel resection) if planned.	*If infection is not controlled, a bowel resection may be required.*

Collaborative Diagnosis **RISK FOR INTESTINAL NECROSIS**

Definition: Death of intestinal tissue.

Related to:
- Obstruction of blood flow in the affected area associated with:
- Inflammation and distention of the bowel lumen
- Hypovolemia
- Mesenteric vessel thrombosis or embolus (can be a cause of nonmechanical obstruction)
- Strangulation of a portion of the intestine (especially if obstruction is a result of a hernia, strictures, adhesions, or a volvulus)

CLINICAL MANIFESTATIONS

Subjective	Objective
Verbal self-report of severe abdominal pain	Bloody diarrhea; increased WBC count

RISK FACTORS

- Exposure to pathogens
- Chronic illness
- Lack of exercise

DESIRED OUTCOMES

The client will not experience intestinal necrosis as evidenced by:
a. Decreased abdominal pain
b. Absence of bloody diarrhea
c. No increase in WBC count

NURSING ASSESSMENT

Assess for and report signs and symptoms of intestinal necrosis (e.g., severe, continuous abdominal pain; bloody diarrhea; WBC count that increases or fails to decline toward normal).

RATIONALE

Early recognition of signs and symptoms of complications of intestinal obstruction allows for prompt intervention.

THERAPEUTIC INTERVENTIONS

Dependent/Collaborative Interventions
Implement measures to improve blood flow to the intestine in order to prevent intestinal necrosis:

- Perform actions to prevent and treat deficient fluid volume (e.g., provide antiemetics for nausea and vomiting, insert NG tube as needed, maintain intravenous fluids as ordered, administer electrolytes as needed).

- Perform actions to reduce the accumulation of intestinal gas and fluid (e.g., instruct client not to chew gum, suck on ice or hard candy; insert NG tube as needed; avoid carbonated beverages).

- Prepare client for treatment of the underlying cause of vascular obstruction (e.g., mesenteric thrombectomy or embolectomy; surgery to repair hernia, release adhesions, or correct volvulus) if planned.

If signs and symptoms of intestinal necrosis occur:

- Administer antimicrobials if ordered.
- Prepare client for surgical resection of the affected bowel.

RATIONALE

Maintenance of fluid volume is necessary to maintain adequate circulation to the gut.

Decreases intestinal gas and fluid, which may decrease intestinal blood flow.

If obstruction is not resolved, surgery may be necessary. The type of surgical intervention depends upon the underlying cause of the obstruction.

Prevention of infection.
Usually performed if the client has extensive tissue necrosis or gangrenous patches have developed.

DISCHARGE INFORMATION IF CLIENT DOES NOT REQUIRE SURGERY

Nursing Diagnosis **DEFICIENT KNOWLEDGE** NDx**; INEFFECTIVE FAMILY HEALTH MANAGEMENT** NDx**; OR INEFFECTIVE HEALTH MAINTENANCE*** NDx

Definition: **Deficient Knowledge NDx**: Absence of cognitive information related to specific topic, or its acquisition; **Ineffective Family Health Management NDx**: A pattern of regulating and integrating into family processes a program for the treatment of illness and its sequelae that is unsatisfactory for meeting specific health goals of the family unit; **Ineffective Health Maintenance NDx**: Inability to identify, manage, and/or seek help to maintain well-being.

*The nurse must determine the appropriate diagnosis based on client assessment.

NDx = NANDA Diagnosis   **D** = Delegatable Action   ● = UAP   ✦ = LVN/LPN   ⊙▶ = Go to ⊖volve for animation

CLINICAL MANIFESTATIONS

Subjective	Objective
Verbal self-report of inability to manage illness; inability to follow prescribed regimen	Inaccurate follow-through with instructions; inappropriate behaviors; experience of preventable complications of abdominal trauma

RISK FACTORS

- Cognitive deficit
- Financial concerns
- Failure to reduce risk factors for complications of abdominal trauma
- Inability to care for oneself
- Difficulty in modifying personal habits and integrating treatments into lifestyle

NOC OUTCOMES	NIC INTERVENTIONS
Knowledge: disease process; treatment regimen	Health system guidance; teaching: individual; teaching: disease process; teaching: prescribed diet; teaching: prescribed medication

NURSING ASSESSMENT	RATIONALE
Assess the client's ability to learn and readiness to learn. Assess the client's understanding of teaching.	*Learning is more effective when the client is motivated and understands the importance of what is to be learned. Readiness to learn changes based on situations and physical and emotional challenges.*

THERAPEUTIC INTERVENTIONS	RATIONALE

Desired Outcome: The client will state signs and symptoms to report to health care providers.

Independent Actions
Instruct client to report the following signs and symptoms:

- Recurrent episodes of abdominal pain
- Increasing abdominal distention
- Nausea or vomiting
- Constipation
- Elevated temperature

Client awareness of what changes require health care intervention will improve timeliness of treatment for complications.

THERAPEUTIC INTERVENTIONS	RATIONALE

Desired Outcome: The client will verbalize an understanding of ways to minimize the risk of recurrence of intestinal obstruction.

Independent Actions
Collaborate with client to develop a plan for adherence that includes:
The physician's instructions regarding ways to prevent the risk for recurrent intestinal obstruction. For example:

- Follow-up radiation and/or chemotherapy if obstruction was caused by a tumor
- Dietary and medication management if obstruction was caused by inflammatory bowel disease
- Bowel care regimen if obstruction was caused by a fecal impaction.

Reinforcement of information provided by the physician allows for clients to ask questions and improve their understanding of the causes of recurrence of bowel obstruction, and the dietary interventions to help prevent further complications.

THERAPEUTIC INTERVENTIONS	**RATIONALE**

Desired Outcome: The client, in collaboration with the nurse, will develop a plan for adhering to recommended follow-up care including recommended diet, prescribed medications, ways to prevent recurrent intestinal obstruction, and future appointments with health care provider.

Independent Actions

Develop a plan for adherence that includes:

The importance of keeping follow-up appointments with health care provider.

Reinforcing physician's instructions regarding dietary restrictions and advancement of diet.

Reinforcing physician's instructions regarding prescribed medications.

Include significant others in teaching sessions if possible.

Encouraging questions and allow time for reinforcement and clarification of information provided.

Providing written instructions on future appointments with health care provider, dietary restrictions, medications prescribed, and signs and symptoms to report.

Allows for health care provider to monitor progress and alter interventions as needed.

Important to maintain nutritional status and to promote healing.

Adherence to the regimen is increased with education about prescribed medications.

Significant others may provide support to clients as they implement treatment regimen.

Allows client to internalize information and clarify any areas of confusion.

Allows quick reference once the client has been discharged.

POSTOPERATIVE INTERVENTIONS

Nursing Diagnosis **INEFFECTIVE BREATHING PATTERN** NDx

Definition: Inspiration and/or expiration that does not provide adequate ventilation.

Related to:
* Reluctance to breathe deeply due to pain, weakness, and a large abdominal incision
* Decreased rate and depth of respirations associated with the depressant effect of anesthesia

CLINICAL MANIFESTATIONS

Subjective	**Objective**
Verbal self-report of difficulty breathing	Alterations in depth of breathing; altered chest excursion; bradypnea; decreased minute ventilation; use of accessory muscles to breathe; dyspnea

RISK FACTOR
* Surgical procedure

DESIRED OUTCOMES

The client will maintain an effective breathing pattern as evidenced by:
a. Normal rate and depth of respirations
b. Absence of dyspnea

NOC OUTCOMES

Respiratory status: ventilation

NIC INTERVENTIONS

Ventilation assistance; respiratory monitoring

NDx = NANDA Diagnosis   **D** = Delegatable Action   ● = UAP   ✦ = LVN/LPN   ⊖▶ = Go to ℮volve for animation

NURSING ASSESSMENT	RATIONALE

Assess for signs and symptoms of an ineffective breathing pattern:
* Shallow or slow respirations
* Limited chest excursion
* Tachypnea or dyspnea
* Use of accessory muscles when breathing

Early recognition of signs and symptoms of an ineffective breathing pattern allows for prompt intervention.

Assess/monitor pulse oximetry (SaO$_2$) and ABG values as indicated.

Monitoring continuous SaO$_2$ readings allows for the early detection of hypoxia. Assessment of ABG values allows for a more direct measurement of both the PaO$_2$ and the PaCO$_2$, which reflect the adequacy of ventilation.

THERAPEUTIC INTERVENTIONS	RATIONALE

Independent Actions

Implement measures to improve breathing pattern:
* Perform actions to reduce fear and anxiety:
  * Promote a calm, restful environment.
* Perform actions to reduce pain:
  * Reposition client for comfort.
  * Instruct client to support incision when moving or coughing.
* Perform actions to reduce the accumulation of gas and fluid in the GI tract:
  * Maintain patency of NG, gastric, or intestinal tubes if present.
* Perform actions to increase strength and improve activity tolerance (e.g., increase activity as tolerated; provide for periods of rest; maintain adequate nutrition).
  * Implement measures to conserve energy.
* Have client deep breathe or use incentive spirometer every 1 to 2 hrs. **D** ✦
* Instruct client to breathe slowly if hyperventilating.

* Place client in a semi- to high-Fowler's position unless contraindicated. **D** ✦

Reducing the client's fear and anxiety helps to prevent shallow and/or rapid breathing.

Reducing pain helps to increase the client's willingness to move and breathe more deeply.

Reducing the accumulation of gas in the GI tract decreases pressure on the diaphragm, facilitating more effective ventilation.

Increasing activity tolerance enables the client to breathe more deeply and participate in activities to improve breathing pattern.

Deep breathing and use of an incentive spirometer promote maximal inhalation and lung expansion.

Hyperventilation is an ineffective breathing pattern that can lead to respiratory alkalosis.

A client can often slow breathing rate by concentrating on doing so.

A semi- to high-Fowler's position allows for maximal diaphragmatic excursion and lung expansion.

Dependent/Collaborative Actions

Implement measures to improve breathing pattern:
* Increase activity as allowed and tolerated.

* Assist with positive airway pressure techniques if ordered:
  * CPAP
  * BiPAP
  * Flutter/ PEP device
* Administer central nervous system depressants judiciously.
  * Hold medication and consult physician if respiratory rate is less than 12 breaths/min.
* Perform actions to reduce pain:
* Administer analgesics before activities and procedures that can cause pain and before pain becomes severe. **D** ✦

Consult appropriate health care provider if:
* Ineffective breathing pattern continues.
* Client develops signs and symptoms of impaired gas exchange such as restlessness, irritability, confusion, significant decrease in oximetry results, decreased PaO$_2$ and increased PaCO$_2$ levels.

During activity, especially ambulation, the client usually takes deeper breaths, thus increasing lung expansion.

Positive airway pressure techniques increase intrapulmonary (alveolar) pressure, which helps re-expand collapsed alveoli and prevent further alveoli collapse.

Central nervous system depressants cause depression of the respiratory center in the brainstem, which can result in a decreased rate and depth of respiration.

Reducing pain helps to increase the client's willingness to move and breathe more deeply.

Notifying the appropriate health care provider allows for modification of treatment plan.

Nursing Diagnosis   INEFFECTIVE AIRWAY CLEARANCE NDx

Definition: Inability to clear secretions or obstructions from the respiratory tract to maintain a clear airway.

Related to:
- Stasis of secretions associated with:
  - Decreased activity
  - Depressed ciliary function due to anesthesia
  - Inability to produce an effective cough effort due to abdominal incision and depressant effect of anesthesia and pain medications

CLINICAL MANIFESTATIONS

Subjective	Objective
Verbal self-report of difficulty breathing	Dyspnea, orthopnea; diminished breath sounds; adventitious breath sounds (crackles, rhonchi, wheezes); cough, ineffective or absent sputum production; difficulty vocalizing; wide-eyed; restlessness; changes in respiratory rate and rhythm; cyanosis

RISK FACTORS
- Surgical procedure
- Positioning inactivity

DESIRED OUTCOMES

The client will maintain clear, open airways as evidenced by:
- Normal breath sounds
- Normal rate and depth of respirations
- Absence of dyspnea

NOC OUTCOMES

Respiratory status: ventilation; airway patency

NIC INTERVENTIONS

Respiratory monitoring; airway management; cough enhancement

NURSING ASSESSMENT	RATIONALE
Assess for signs and symptoms of ineffective airway clearance: • Abnormal breath sounds • Rapid, shallow respirations • Dyspnea • Cough	*Early recognition of signs and symptoms of ineffective airway clearance allows for prompt intervention.*
Assess/monitor pulse oximetry (SaO₂) and ABG values as indicated.	*Monitoring continuous SaO$_2$ readings allows for the early detection of hypoxia.* *Assessment of ABG values allows for a more direct measurement of both PaO$_2$ and PaCO$_2$, which reflect the adequacy of ventilation.*

THERAPEUTIC INTERVENTIONS	RATIONALE
Independent Actions Implement measures to promote effective airway clearance: • Position client on side and/or insert an artificial airway if necessary.	*Positioning the client on the side will help open the airway by alleviating any obstruction causes by the tongue. An artificial airway helps prevent obstruction of airway by the tongue.*

• Perform actions to reduce pain:
  • Reposition client for comfort. **D** ● ✦
  • Instruct client to support incision when moving or coughing.
	Reducing pain helps to increase the client's willingness to move and breathe more deeply.

Instruct and assist client to change position at least every 2 hrs while in bed. **D** ● ✦	*Repositioning helps mobilize secretions.*

NDx = NANDA Diagnosis   **D** = Delegatable Action   ● = UAP   ✦ = LVN/LPN   ⊖▶ = Go to ⊖volve for animation

Continued...

THERAPEUTIC INTERVENTIONS	RATIONALE
• Perform actions to promote the removal of secretions:	
• Assist client to deep breathe and cough every 1 to 2 hrs.	*Deep breathing and coughing can help loosen secretions and enhance the effectiveness of coughing.*
• Support abdominal incision when coughing. **D** ✦	*Provides incisional support while coughing.*
• Discourage smoking.	*Irritants in smoke increase mucus production, impair ciliary function, and can cause inflammation and damage to the bronchial walls.*
• Perform suctioning if needed.	*Suctioning removes secretions from the large airways. It also stimulates coughing, which helps clear airways of mucus and foreign matter.*

Dependent/Collaborative Actions

Implement measures to promote effective airway clearance:

• Implement measures to thin tenacious secretions and reduce drying of the respiratory mucous membrane:	
• Maintain a fluid intake of at least 2500 mL/day unless contraindicated.	*Adequate hydration and humidified inspired air help thin secretions, which facilitates the mobilization and expectoration of secretions.*
• Humidify inspired air as ordered. **D** ✦	*These actions also reduce dryness of the respiratory mucous membrane, which helps enhance mucociliary clearance.*
• Assist with administration of mucolytics and diluent or hydrating agents via nebulizer if ordered: (1) Acetylcysteine (2) Water, saline	*Mucolytics and diluents or hydrating agents are mucokinetic substances that reduce the viscosity of mucus, thus making it easier for the client to mobilize and clear secretions from the respiratory tract.*
• Increase activity as allowed and tolerated. **D** ● ✦	*Activity helps to mobilize secretions and promotes deeper breathing.*
• Administer central nervous system depressants judiciously.	*Central nervous system depressants depress the cough reflex, which can result in stasis of secretions.*
Consult appropriate health care provider such as a physician or respiratory therapist if:	*Notifying the appropriate health care provider allows for modification of the treatment plan.*
• Signs and symptoms of ineffective airway clearance persist	
• Signs and symptoms of impaired gas exchange are present: • Restlessness • Irritability • Confusion • Significant decrease in oximetry results • Decreased PaO_2 and increased $PaCO_2$	

Nursing Diagnosis # IMBALANCED NUTRITION: LESS THAN BODY REQUIREMENTS NDx

Definition: Intake of nutrients insufficient to meet metabolic needs.

Related to:

• Inability to ingest food due to lack of bowel sounds
• Decreased oral intake associated with pain, weakness, fatigue, and nausea
• Increased nutritional needs associated with increased metabolic rate that occurs during wound healing

CLINICAL MANIFESTATIONS

Subjective	Objective
Verbal self-report of abdominal cramping or pain; aversion toward eating; lack of interest in food; altered taste sensation	Inadequate food intake; inability to ingest food; diarrhea; hypoactive or absent bowel sounds; weakness of muscles of mastication

RISK FACTORS

- Poor preoperative nutritional status
- Delayed postop nutritional therapy

DESIRED OUTCOMES

The client will maintain an adequate nutritional status as evidenced by:
a. Weight within normal range for client
b. Normal BUN and serum albumin, Hct and Hgb levels and lymphocyte count
c. Usual strength and activity tolerance
d. Healthy oral mucous membrane

NOC OUTCOMES

Nutritional status

NIC INTERVENTIONS

Nutritional monitoring; nutrition management; nutrition therapy; diet staging

NURSING ASSESSMENT	RATIONALE
Assess for and report signs and symptoms of malnutrition: - Weight significantly below client's usual weight or below normal for client's age, height, and body frame - Weakness and fatigue - Sore, inflamed oral mucous membrane - Pale conjunctiva	*Early recognition of signs and symptoms of malnutrition allows for prompt intervention.*
Assess for return of bowel function every 2 to 4 hrs.	*Once the client begins to expel flatus, the physician should be notified so oral intake can be resumed as soon as possible.*
Monitor serum albumin, prealbumin, total protein, ferritin, transferrin, Hgb, Hct, and electrolyte levels as indicated.	*Serum albumin levels less than 3.5 g/100 mL are considered a risk for poor nutritional status. Early recognition of abnormal lab values reflective of the client's overall nutritional state allows for prompt intervention.*
When oral intake is allowed, monitor percentage of meals and snacks client consumes. Report pattern of inadequate intake.	*An awareness of the amount of foods/fluids a client consumes alerts the nurse to deficits in nutritional intake. Reporting inadequate intake allows for prompt intervention.*

THERAPEUTIC INTERVENTIONS	RATIONALE

Independent Actions
When food or oral fluids are allowed, implement measures to maintain an adequate nutritional status:
- Implement measures to prevent nausea and vomiting: **D** ● ✦
  - Eliminate noxious sights and odors from the environment.
  - Encourage the client to take deep, slow breaths when nauseated.
  - Instruct client to change positions slowly.
  - Apply a cold washcloth to the client's forehead.
	The presence of nausea can decrease the appetite. Preventing nausea and vomiting can improve the client's appetite. These actions reduce nausea.

- Implement measures to reduce pain: - Instruct client to support incision with movement. **D** ✦	*The presence of pain decreases the appetite.*
Implement measures to reduce the accumulation of gas and fluid in the GI tract and prevent constipation. **D** ✦ - Encourage frequent position changes. - Encourage ambulation.	*The subsequent feeling of fullness that accompanies gas accumulation leads to an early feeling of satiety. These actions stimulate peristalsis and move gas and fluid through the bowel.*
- Encourage a rest period before meals.	*To conserve energy for consuming meals, rest periods before eating should be encouraged.*
- Provide nursing assistance during meals. **D** ● - Maintain a clean environment and a relaxed, pleasant atmosphere. **D** ●	*A pleasant environment helps to promote adequate intake.*
- Provide oral hygiene before meals. **D** ●	*Good oral hygiene enhances appetite. A moist oral mucosa makes chewing and swallowing easier. Oral hygiene can also remove unpleasant tastes, improving the taste of foods/fluids.*

NDx = NANDA Diagnosis   **D** = Delegatable Action   ● = UAP   ✦ = LVN/LPN   ⊜▶ = Go to ⊜volve for animation

Continued...

THERAPEUTIC INTERVENTIONS	RATIONALE
Serve frequent, small meals rather than large ones if client is weak, fatigues easily, and/or has a poor appetite. **D** ✦	*Small, frequent meals are better tolerated in clients with a poor appetite.*
• Encourage significant others to bring in client's favorite foods unless contraindicated. **D** ✦	*Allowing a client to eat foods they prefer enhances intake and nutritional status.*
• Allow adequate time for meals; reheat foods/fluids if necessary. **D** ●	*Research has demonstrated that it takes 35 minutes to feed the client who is willing to eat.*
• Limit fluid intake with meals (unless the fluid has high nutritional value). **D** ✦	*A high fluid intake with meals promotes a feeling of fullness and early satiety that may decrease actual food intake.*

Dependent/Collaborative Actions

When food or oral fluids are allowed, implement measures to maintain an adequate nutritional status:

• Implement measures to prevent nausea and vomiting:	
• Administer antiemetics as ordered. **D** ✦	*The presence of nausea can decrease the appetite. Preventing nausea and vomiting can improve the client's appetite.*
Implement measures to reduce pain:	
• Administer pain medications as ordered. **D** ✦	*The presence of pain decreases the appetite.*
• Increase activity as tolerated and allowed. **D** ●	*Activity promotes gastric emptying, which reduces the feeling of gastric fullness; it also usually promotes a sense of well-being, which can improve appetite.*
• Obtain a dietary consult if necessary to assist client in selecting foods/fluids that meet nutritional needs, are appealing, and adhere to personal and cultural preferences as well as the prescribed dietary modifications.	*A dietician or nutritional support team can help clients individualize their diet within prescribed dietary restrictions. Providing food in line with client's preferences can enhance adherence to prescribed diet.*
• Ensure that meals are well balanced and high in essential nutrients; offer dietary supplements if indicated.	*Dietary supplements have shown a positive relationship with weight gain, reduced mortality, and reduced length of hospitalization.*
• Administer vitamins and minerals if ordered. **D** ✦	*Vitamins and minerals are essential to many metabolic processes in the body.*
• Perform a calorie count if ordered. Report information to dietitian and physician. **D** ✦	*Information gathered from an accurate calorie count is used to determine the adequacy of a client's daily diet or the need for nutritional support.*
Consult physician about an alternative method of providing nutrition if client does not consume enough food or fluids to meet nutritional needs:	*Notifying the physician allows for modification of the treatment plan.*
• Enteral tube feedings	
• Parenteral nutrition	

POTENTIAL COMPLICATIONS AFTER SURGERY

Collaborative Diagnosis **RISK FOR ATELECTASIS**

Definition: Collapse of lung tissue caused by hypoventilated alveoli.

Related to:
• Shallow respirations
• Stasis of secretions in the alveoli and bronchioles

CLINICAL MANIFESTATIONS

Subjective	**Objective**
Verbal self-report of difficulty breathing	Diminished or absent breath sounds; dull percussion over affected area; increased respiratory rate; dyspnea; tachycardia; elevated temperature

RISK FACTORS

- Immobility
- Surgery
- Lack of adequate cough effort

DESIRED OUTCOMES

The client will not develop atelectasis as evidenced by:
a. Clear, audible breath sounds
b. Resonant percussion note over lungs
c. Unlabored respirations at 12 to 20 breaths/min
d. Pulse rate within normal range for client
e. Afebrile status

NURSING ASSESSMENT

Assess for and report signs and symptoms of atelectasis:
- Diminished or absent breath sounds
- Dull percussion note over affected area
- Increased respiratory rate
- Dyspnea
- Tachycardia
- Elevated temperature

Monitor pulse oximetry as indicated.

Monitor chest radiograph results.

RATIONALE

Early recognition of signs and symptoms of atelectasis allows for implementation of the appropriate interventions.

Pulse oximetry is an indirect measure of SaO$_2$. Monitoring pulse oximetry (SaO$_2$) allows for early detection of hypoxia and implementation of the appropriate interventions.
Chest radiograph provides confirmation of atelectasis.

THERAPEUTIC INTERVENTIONS

Independent Actions
Implement measures to prevent atelectasis: **D** ✦
- Perform actions to improve breathing pattern:
  - Encourage client to deep breathe.
  - Incentive spirometry
- Perform actions to promote effective airway clearance:
  - Turn, cough, and deep breathe.
If signs and symptoms of atelectasis occur:
- Increase frequency of position change, coughing or "huffing," deep breathing, and use of incentive spirometer.
Consult physician if signs and symptoms of atelectasis persist or worsen.

RATIONALE

Lack of movement places a client at risk for atelectasis. Changing positions frequently, coughing, and deep breathing help to expand the lungs, enhancing alveolar expansion.

Notifying the appropriate health care provider will allow for modification of the treatment plan.

Nursing Diagnosis **RISK FOR VENOUS THROMBOEMBOLISM** NDx

Definition: Susceptible to the development of a blood clot in a deep vein, commonly in the thigh, calf, or upper extremity, which can break off and lodge in another vessel, which may compromise health.

Related to:
- Venous stasis associated with decreased activity
- Positioning during and after surgery
- Abdominal distention that may put pressure on the abdominal vessels
- Increased blood viscosity from deficient fluid volume

CLINICAL MANIFESTATIONS

Subjective	Objective
Verbal self-report of pain or tenderness in an extremity	Increase in circumference of extremity; distention of superficial vessels in extremity; unusual warmth of extremity

RISK FACTORS

- Immobility
- Inadequate fluid replacement

DESIRED OUTCOMES

The client will not develop a deep vein thrombus as evidenced by:
a. Absence of pain, tenderness, swelling, and distended superficial vessels in extremities
b. Usual temperature of extremities
c. Pain in area where thromboembolism lodged

NURSING ASSESSMENT

Assess for and report signs and symptoms of a deep vein thrombus:
- Pain or tenderness in extremity
- Increase in circumference of extremity
- Distention of superficial vessels in extremity
- Unusual warmth of extremity

RATIONALE

Early recognition of signs and symptoms of thrombus allows for implementation of the appropriate interventions.

NOC OUTCOMES

Risk control: thrombus; tissue perfusion: peripheral

NIC INTERVENTIONS

Embolus precautions; embolus care: peripheral

THERAPEUTIC INTERVENTIONS

Independent Actions

Implement measures to prevent thrombus formation: **D** ✦
- Use of sequential compression device during and after surgery until ambulatory
- Perform actions to prevent peripheral pooling of blood such as leg exercises:
  - Ankle rotation
  - Alternate dorsiflexion and plantar flexion of both feet

If signs and symptoms of a deep vein thrombus occur: **D** ✦
- Maintain client on bedrest until activity orders received.
- Elevate foot of bed 15 to 20 degrees above heart level if ordered.
- Discourage positions that compromise blood flow (e.g., pillows under knees, crossing legs, sitting for long periods).

Dependent/Collaborative Actions

Implement measures to prevent thrombus formation:
- Apply mechanical devices designed to increase venous return in the immobile patient: **D** ✦
  - Sequential compression devices
  - Thromboembolic (elastic) stockings
- Maintain a minimum fluid intake of 2500 mL/day (unless contraindicated).

If signs and symptoms of a deep vein thrombus occur:
- Administer anticoagulants:
  - Low- or adjusted-dose heparin
  - Fondaparinux
  - Warfarin
  - Low-molecular-weight heparin
- Prepare client for diagnostic studies (e.g., venography, duplex ultrasound, impedance plethysmography).

RATIONALE

Sequential compression devices and leg and ankle exercises promote venous return and reduce the risk of venous thromboembolism.

Avoid putting pressure on the posterior knees, as this action will compress leg veins, increasing turbulent blood flow, and increase the risk of thromboembolism formation. If a thrombus is suspected, elevate the affected extremity and do not massage the area because of the danger of dislodging the thrombus.

These devices decrease venous stasis in the lower extremities and increase venous return through the deep leg veins, which are prone to the formation of a thromboembolism. These devices should remain in place until the patient is ambulatory.

Adequate hydration helps to reduce blood viscosity and decrease the incidence of a thromboembolism.

Anticoagulants, if indicated, help to suppress the formation of clots.

Additional studies may be indicated to confirm the presence of a thromboembolism, so the appropriate interventions can be implemented.

THERAPEUTIC INTERVENTIONS	RATIONALE
If signs and symptoms of embolism occur:	
• Maintain on strict bedrest in a semi- or high-Fowler's position	*Decreases pressure of the abdomen and help to increase lung expansion.*
• Maintain oxygen therapy as ordered	*Provides supplemental oxygenation.*
• Prepare client for diagnostic tests (e.g., blood gases, D-dimer level, ventilation, perfusion lung scan; pulmonary angiography)	*Identification of physiological changes due to embolism.*
• Prepare client for the following, if planned:	*Decreases client fear/anxiety.*
• Vena caval interruption	*Prevents further emboli.*
• Embolectomy	*Removal of emboli.*

Collaborative Diagnosis RISK FOR PARALYTIC ILEUS

Definition: Paralysis of the intestines resulting in blockage of the intestines.

Related to:
• Manipulation of intestines during abdominal surgery
• Depressant effect of anesthesia and some medications on bowel motility

CLINICAL MANIFESTATIONS

Subjective	Objective
Verbal self-report of persistent abdominal pain and cramping	Firm, distended abdomen; absent bowel sounds; failure to pass flatus; abdominal radiograph showing distended bowel

RISK FACTORS	DESIRED OUTCOMES
• Inadequate exercise • Surgery	The client will not develop a paralytic ileus as evidenced by: a. Absence or resolution of abdominal pain and cramping b. Soft, nondistended abdomen c. Gradual return of bowel sounds d. Passage of flatus

NURSING ASSESSMENT	RATIONALE
Assess for and report signs and symptoms of paralytic ileus: • Development of or persistent abdominal pain and cramping • Firm, distended abdomen • Absent bowel sounds • Failure to pass flatus	*Early recognition of signs and symptoms of a paralytic ileus allows for prompt intervention.*
Monitor results of abdominal radiograph.	*An abdominal radiograph that demonstrates distended bowel may be indicative of a paralytic ileus.*

THERAPEUTIC INTERVENTIONS	RATIONALE
Independent Actions	
Implement measures to prevent paralytic ileus:	*Early ambulation in a postoperative client promotes the return of peristalsis.*
• Increase activity as soon as allowed and tolerated.	
• Perform actions to prevent hypokalemia.	*Hypokalemia promotes atony of the intestinal wall, which results in a decrease in peristalsis.*
Dependent/Collaborative Actions	
If signs and symptoms of paralytic ileus occur:	*Paralytic ileus results in cessation of normal peristalsis. The client should have nothing by mouth (NPO) and have an NG tube in place to facilitate gastric decompression until the ileus is resolved.*
• Withhold all oral intake.	
• Insert NG tube and maintain suction as ordered.	

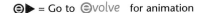

Continued...

THERAPEUTIC INTERVENTIONS	RATIONALE
If signs and symptoms of paralytic ileus occurs: • Administer GI stimulants (e.g., metoclopramide) if ordered.	*GI stimulants help to maintain adequate blood supply to the bowel.*

Collaborative Diagnosis RISK FOR DEHISCENCE

Definition: Pulling apart of a surgical wound at the suture line.

Related to:
• Inadequate wound closure
• Stress on incision line associated with persistent coughing
• Poor wound healing associated with decreased tissue perfusion of wound area and inadequate nutritional status

CLINICAL MANIFESTATIONS

Subjective	Objective
Verbal self-report of something "popping" or "giving way" at the incision site	Separation of edges of the wound

RISK FACTORS
• Poor preoperative nutritional status
• Surgery
• Delayed postoperative nutritional therapy

DESIRED OUTCOME
The client will not experience dehiscence as evidenced by intact, approximated wound edges.

NURSING ASSESSMENT	RATIONALE
Assess for and report evidence of wound dehiscence: • Separation of edges of the wound Assess for and immediately report signs and symptoms of evisceration: • Sudden profuse drainage of serosanguineous fluid from wound • Protrusion of intestinal contents	*Early recognition of evidence of wound dehiscence allows for implementation of the appropriate interventions.* *Total separation of wound layers sometimes results in dehiscence. This is an emergency situation that requires surgical intervention.*

THERAPEUTIC INTERVENTIONS	RATIONALE

Independent Actions
Implement measures to promote wound healing:
• Implement measures to reduce stress on the wound:
  • Limit movement of affected area.
  • If client has a chest or abdominal incision, instruct client to avoid coughing.
  • If client has an abdominal incision, place on bedrest in a semi-Fowler's position with knees slightly flexed.
	Proper wound healing decreases the risk of dehiscence.
	Decreasing stress on the incision reduces the risk of wound dehiscence.

Dependent/Collaborative Actions If dehiscence occurs: • Cover wound with a sterile, nonadherent dressing. • Apply skin closures (e.g., butterfly tape, Steri-Strips) to the incision line if appropriate. • Assist with re-suturing the wound if indicated.	*A wound that has dehisced requires a sterile, nonadherent dressing. The choice of a dry dressing or wet dressing will depend upon the presence of evisceration.*

DISCHARGE TEACHING

Nursing Diagnosis **DEFICIENT KNOWLEDGE** NDx**; INEFFECTIVE FAMILY HEALTH MANAGEMENT** NDx**; OR INEFFECTIVE HEALTH MAINTENANCE*** NDx

Definition: **Deficient Knowledge NDx:** Absence of cognitive information related to specific topic or its acquisition. **Ineffective Family Health Management NDx:** A pattern of regulating and integrating into family processes a program for the treatment of illness and its sequelae that is unsatisfactory for meeting specific health goals of the family unit. **Ineffective Health Maintenance NDx:** Inability to identify, manage, and/or seek help to maintain well-being.

CLINICAL MANIFESTATIONS

Subjective	Objective
Verbal self-report of inability to manage illness; inability to follow prescribed regimen	Inaccurate follow-through with instructions; inappropriate behaviors; experience of preventable complications of wound dehiscence

RISK FACTORS

- Cognitive deficit
- Financial concerns
- Inability to care for oneself
- Difficulty in modifying personal habits and integrating treatments into lifestyle

NOC OUTCOMES	NIC INTERVENTIONS
Knowledge: treatment regimen	Teaching: individual; teaching: prescribed activity/exercise; teaching: prescribed medication; health system guidance

NURSING ASSESSMENT	RATIONALE
Assess the client's ability to learn and readiness to learn. Assess the client's understanding of teaching.	*Learning is more effective when the client is motivated and understands the importance of what is to be learned. Readiness to learn changes based on situations and physical and emotional challenges.*

THERAPEUTIC INTERVENTIONS	RATIONALE

Desired Outcome: The client will identify ways to prevent postoperative infection.

Independent Actions
Instruct client in ways to prevent postoperative infection:	
• Continue with coughing (unless contraindicated) and deep breathing every 2 hrs while awake.	*These actions work to expand the lungs, mobilize secretions, and provide adequate oxygenation for healing.*
• Continue to use incentive spirometer if activity is limited.	
• Increase activity as ordered.	
• Avoid contact with persons who have infections.	*Decreases client's exposure to infectious agents.*
• Avoid crowds during flu and cold seasons.	
• Decrease or stop smoking.	*The irritants in smoke increase mucus production, impair ciliary function, and can cause inflammation and damage to the bronchial and alveolar walls; the carbon monoxide decreases oxygen availability.*
• Drink at least 10 glasses of liquid per day unless contraindicated.	*Maintains adequate fluid for circulation.*
• Maintain a balanced nutritional intake.	*Protein is required for appropriate wound healing.*

*The nurse should select the nursing diagnostic label that is most appropriate for the client's discharge teaching needs.

NDx = NANDA Diagnosis   **D** = Delegatable Action   ● = UAP   ✦ = LVN/LPN   ⊖▶ = Go to ⊖volve for animation

Continued...

THERAPEUTIC INTERVENTIONS	RATIONALE
• Maintain proper balance of rest and activity.	*Supports wound healing and recovery from surgery.*
• Maintain good personal hygiene (especially oral care, hand washing, and perineal care).	*Prevents cross contamination, contamination of the surgical wound, and potential for infection.*
• Avoid touching any wound unless it is completely healed.	
• Maintain sterile or clean technique as ordered during wound care.	

THERAPEUTIC INTERVENTIONS	RATIONALE

Desired Outcome: The client will demonstrate the ability to perform wound care.

Independent Actions

Discuss the rationale for, frequency of, and equipment necessary for the prescribed wound care.

Client adherence is improved if client understands what to do and how to use equipment as needed.

Provide client with the necessary supplies (e.g., dressings, irrigating solution, tape) for wound care and with names and addresses of places where additional supplies can be obtained.

Improves adherence to wound care.

Demonstrate wound care and proper cleansing of any reusable equipment. Allow time for questions, clarification, and return demonstration.

Improves client's confidence in ability to care for self.

THERAPEUTIC INTERVENTIONS	RATIONALE

Desired Outcome: The client will state signs and symptoms to report to the health care provider.

Independent Actions

Instruct the client to report the following signs and symptoms:

- Persistent low-grade fever or significantly elevated (≥38.3°C [101°F]) temperature
- Difficulty breathing
- Chest pain
- Cough productive of purulent, green, or rust-colored sputum
- Increasing weakness or inability to tolerate prescribed activity level

These clinical manifestations indicate complications that include infection, thromboembolism, and poor nutritional status.

- Increasing discomfort or discomfort not controlled by prescribed medications and treatments

May indicate increasing problems or tolerance to medication.

- Continued nausea or vomiting
- Increasing abdominal distention and/or discomfort

May indicate a recurrence of the bowel obstruction.

- Separation of wound edges
- Increasing redness, warmth, pain, or swelling around wound
- Unusual or excessive drainage from any wound site
- Pain or swelling in calf of one or both legs
- Urine retention
- Frequency, urgency, or burning on urination

May indicate dehydration or urinary tract infection.

- Cloudy or foul-smelling urine

THERAPEUTIC INTERVENTIONS	RATIONALE

Desired Outcome: The client, in collaboration with the nurse, will develop a plan for adhering to recommended follow-up care including future appointments with health care provider, dietary modifications, activity level, treatments, and medications prescribed.

THERAPEUTIC INTERVENTIONS	RATIONALE

Independent Actions

Collaborate with client in developing a plan for adherence that includes:

The importance of keeping scheduled follow-up appointments with the health care provider.

Physician's instructions about dietary modifications. Obtain a dietary consult for client if needed.

The physician's instructions on suggested activity level and treatment plan.

The rationale for, side effects of, and importance of taking medications prescribed.

Inform client of pertinent food and drug interactions.

Implement measures to improve client compliance:

- Include significant others in teaching sessions if possible.

- Encourage questions and allow time for reinforcement and clarification of information provided.

- Provide written instructions on scheduled appointments with health care provider, dietary modifications, activity level, treatment plan, medications prescribed, and signs and symptoms to report.

Improves adherence to treatment regimen and for follow-up care.

Important for continued healing and maintenance of health.

Improves adherence if client understands what to do for self-care.

Knowledge of medications and how they impact the system improves client adherence to treatment regimen and understanding of the importance of adhering to the prescribed medication regimen. The client must be able to recognize alterations in functioning related to medication administration and what clinical manifestations should be reported to the health care provider.

Improves the ability of significant others to support client adherence to the treatment regimen.

Improves client understanding of discharge information.

Provides an information resource for the client after discharge from the acute care facility.

ADDITIONAL NURSING DIAGNOSES

IMPAIRED ORAL MUCOUS MEMBRANE NDx
Related to:
- Deficient fluid volume associated with restricted oral intake and fluid loss resulting from vomiting and NG tube drainage
- Decreased salivation associated with deficient fluid volume, restricted oral intake, and the effect of some medications (e.g., narcotic [opioid] analgesics, some antiemetics)
- Mouth breathing when NG tube is in place

RISK FOR CONSTIPATION NDx
Related to decreased GI motility associated with manipulation of bowel during abdominal surgery, depressant effect of anesthesia and narcotic (opioid) analgesics, and decreased activity

DISTURBED SLEEP PATTERN NDx
Related to fear, anxiety, discomfort, inability to assume usual sleeping position, and frequent assessments and treatments

RISK FOR INFECTION NDx
Pneumonia related to stasis of pulmonary secretions and aspiration (if it occurs)

Wound infection related to:
- Contamination associated with introduction of pathogens during or after surgery
- Decreased resistance to infection associated with factors such as diminished tissue perfusion of wound area and inadequate nutritional status

Urinary tract infection related to:
- Increased growth and colonization of microorganisms associated with urinary stasis

- Introduction of pathogens associated with an indwelling catheter if present

RISK FOR FALLS NDx
Related to:
- Weakness and fatigue
- Dizziness or syncope associated with postural hypotension resulting from peripheral pooling of blood and blood loss during surgery
- Central nervous system depressant effect of some medications (narcotic [opioid] analgesics, some antiemetics)
- Presence of tubing or equipment

RISK FOR ASPIRATION NDx
Related to:
- Decreased level of consciousness and absent or diminished gag reflex associated with depressant effect of anesthesia and narcotic (opioid) analgesics
- Supine positioning
- Increased risk for gastroesophageal reflux associated with increased gastric pressure resulting from decreased GI motility

FEAR/ANXIETY NDx
Related to:
- Unfamiliar environment
- Pain
- Lack of understanding of surgical procedure performed, diagnosis, and postoperative treatment plan
- Possible change to body image and roles
- Financial concerns

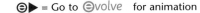

PARENTERAL NUTRITION

Early nutritional therapy, implemented within 48 hrs of either hospital admission or surgery, is supported by various consensus statements and professional guidelines as critical to reducing patient morbidity and mortality. Early enteral nutrition, advocated for the preservation of the mucosal barrier of the gut, is associated with both lower hospital costs and shorter hospital lengths of stay. However, certain clinical conditions may interfere with the client's ability to ingest, digest, or absorb nutrients, resulting in the need for parenteral nutrition.

Parenteral nutrition is defined as the delivery of nutrients by a route other than the GI system (e.g., bloodstream). The primary goal of parenteral nutrition is to provide the nutrients necessary to meet the metabolic needs of the client and allow for growth of new tissue. Clinical conditions that necessitate the use of parenteral nutrition include chronic, severe diarrhea and/or vomiting, complicated surgery or trauma, GI obstruction, GI tract anomalies, severe anorexia, severe malabsorption, and short bowel syndrome.

Parenteral nutrition is composed of both a base solution of dextrose and protein in the form of amino acids and prescribed levels of electrolytes, vitamins, and trace elements. The caloric intake requirement of clients in need of parenteral nutrition therapy far exceeds the 1200 to 1500 cal/day necessary to maintain normal physiological function. Carbohydrates in the form of dextrose and fat emulsions supply the calories that compose parenteral nutrition. While exact parenteral nutrition formulations are based upon individual client nutritional requirements, disease states, metabolic conditions, and medication use, there are accepted standard ranges of parenteral nutrition elements based on age and normal physiological requirements.

To minimize complications associated with nonfeeding, total caloric recommendations include 20 to 30 kcal/kg/day, daily protein of 1.5 to 2 g/kg/day, and fluid requirements of 30 to 40 mL/kg/day in clients who are stressed. Standard distribution of nonprotein calories includes 70% to 85% from carbohydrates and 15% to 30% supplied by fats. Fat content of parenteral solutions is not to exceed Food and Drug Administration recommendations of 2.5 g/kg/day. Fats are administered slowly over 12 to 24 hrs using concentrations of 10%, 20%, or 30% fat emulsion solutions. Standard electrolyte requirements include 10 to 15 mEq calcium, 8 to 20 mEq magnesium, 20 to 40 mmol phosphorous, 1 to 2 mEq/kg sodium, 1 to 2 mEq/kg potassium, and chloride as needed to maintain acid-base balance.

A common metabolic complication associated with the administration of parenteral nutrition is hyperglycemia. Both hyperglycemia and insulin resistance can occur in clients receiving parenteral nutrition. Parenteral nutrition solutions have high glucose concentrations that range between 20% and 50%. As a result, clients receiving parenteral nutrition should have blood glucose levels checked every 4 to 6 hrs, maintaining target blood glucose levels between 100 and 150 mg/dL or as indicated by institutional protocol. To avoid hypoglycemic episodes, parenteral infusions should not be abruptly discontinued for any reason.

Parenteral nutrition, prepared using strict aseptic techniques by a pharmacist, can be administered through a peripherally inserted catheter or centrally inserted device. Central administration is indicated for long-term support, or when the client has high protein and caloric requirements necessitating the administration of hypertonic solutions (>20% glucose concentration) that are caustic to peripheral veins. Parenteral nutrition administered through peripheral veins can be safely accomplished with minimal vein irritation using solutions with an osmolarity of up to 900 mOsm/L.

Safe, effective preparation, administration, and storage of parenteral solutions require a multidisciplinary health care team. Prescribing, preparing, and administering parenteral therapy require the expertise of physicians, pharmacists, dieticians, and nurses. ***This care plan focuses on the adult client undergoing parenteral nutritional therapy in an acute care, extended care, or long-term care environment.***

OUTCOME/DISCHARGE CRITERIA

The client will:
1. Progressively gain weight toward desired goal
2. Weigh within normal weight for height and age
3. Consume adequate nutrition to meet metabolic needs
4. Be free of signs of malnutrition
5. Maintain adequate fluid volume status
6. Recognize factors contributing to malnutrition/underweight
7. Be free of complications related to parenteral feeding

Nursing Diagnosis   **RISK FOR UNSTABLE BLOOD GLUCOSE LEVEL** NDx

Definition: Susceptible to variation in serum levels of glucose from the normal range, which may compromise health.

Related to:
- Insulin resistance associated with the stress of illness and/or diabetes
- Administration of hypertonic parenteral solutions
- Interruption in administration of parenteral nutritional therapy
- Inadequate blood glucose monitoring

CLINICAL MANIFESTATIONS

Subjective	Objective
Verbal self-report of hyperglycemia: thirst; dizziness; blurred vision; nausea	Hyperglycemia: polyuria; elevated serum glucose level; vomiting; dehydration
Verbal reports of hypoglycemia: hunger	Hypoglycemia: sweating; weakness; tremors

RISK FACTORS

* Physical health status
* Weight loss

DESIRED OUTCOME

The client will maintain blood glucose level between 90 and 130 mg/dL or close to 110 mg/dL in the critically ill client.

NOC OUTCOMES

Blood glucose levels; electrolyte and acid-base balance; hyperglycemia severity; hypoglycemia severity

NIC INTERVENTIONS

Hyperglycemia management; hypoglycemia management

NURSING ASSESSMENT	RATIONALE
Assess client for signs and symptoms of hyper/hypoglycemia: • Hyperglycemia: thirst, dizziness, blurred vision, polyuria, increased serum glucose level, nausea/vomiting, dehydration • Hypoglycemia: hunger, weakness, sweating, tremors	*Early recognition of signs and symptoms of hyper/hypoglycemia allows for prompt intervention.*
Assess serum blood glucose every 4 to 6 hrs during administration of parenteral nutrition.	*Because of the high dextrose concentration of most parenteral nutritional solutions, and possible insulin resistance in diabetic clients, blood glucose monitoring is warranted during therapy. Hypoglycemia may occur with abrupt cessation of parenteral nutrition because of the steady production of insulin by the pancreas in response to the high glucose concentration of parenteral solutions.* *Assessment determines the patient's tolerance of the infusion.*
Assess serum electrolyte levels for imbalances and report any deviations from normal.	*The exact amount of electrolytes needed in a parenteral solution will vary by client condition. Blood testing of serum electrolyte levels should occur several times a week to ensure electrolyte values remain therapeutic.* *Refeeding syndrome, characterized by electrolyte imbalances and fluid retention, can be associated with long-standing malnutrition.*

THERAPEUTIC INTERVENTIONS	RATIONALE
Independent Actions Implement interventions to reduce the risk of hypoglycemia: • Administer infusion using an infusion pump. • Ensure patency of infusion site (e.g., peripheral or central catheter). • Monitor bedside serum glucose levels every 4 to 6 hrs.	*The pancreas becomes accustomed to producing insulin at a level necessary to keep blood glucose levels within a normal range.* *Any abrupt cessation of an infusion of TPN places the client at risk for hypoglycemia.* *Administration of parenteral nutrition using an infusion pump allows for appropriate hourly rate regulation and detection of interruption of infusion when/if infusion site becomes occluded or obstructed.*

Continued...

THERAPEUTIC INTERVENTIONS	RATIONALE
Dependent/Collaborative Actions	
Infuse a 10% or 20% dextrose solution (based on the amount in the parenteral solution) if the formula bag is empty before the next solution is available.	*Administration of dextrose-containing solutions helps to prevent hypoglycemia in a client whose system has adjusted to the high levels of glucose in parenteral solutions.*
Administer insulin as prescribed.	*Supplemental insulin in accordance with a sliding scale may be necessary, as an increase in serum blood glucose level is expected after initiation of parenteral nutritional therapy.*
Implement hypoglycemic protocol for blood glucose level less than 70 mg/dL:	*The brain requires a constant supply of glucose to properly function. Untreated hypoglycemia can lead to loss of consciousness, seizures, coma, and/or death.*
• For the conscious patient, ingestion of 15 to 20 g of simple carbohydrate (e.g., 4–6 oz fruit juice)	
• In acute care settings, or with patients who are unconscious, administer 20 to 50 mL of 50% dextrose IV push.	
• Recheck blood glucose level 15 minutes after intervention and repeat treatment if client's blood glucose level remains less than 70 mg/dL.	
Notify the appropriate health care provider if signs and symptoms of hyperglycemia or hypoglycemia, or other electrolyte imbalances develop:	*Notifying the appropriate health care provider allows for modification of the treatment plan.*
• Physician provider	
• Dietician/nutritional consultant	

Nursing Diagnosis RISK FOR INFECTION NDx

Definition: Susceptible to invasion and multiplication of pathogenic organism, which may compromise health.

Related to:
• Administration of fluids that support bacterial growth
• Placement of central venous catheter (invasive procedure)
• Malnutrition
• Decreased defense mechanisms

CLINICAL MANIFESTATIONS

Subjective	Objective
Verbal self-report of nausea; malaise; chills	Erythema, tenderness, and exudate at venous access site; increased temperature; increased WBC count, abnormal differential count; positive blood and/or wound cultures

RISK FACTORS
• Chronic illness
• Inadequate immune response
• Exposure to pathogens

DESIRED OUTCOMES

The client will:
a. Remain free from symptoms of infection
b. Maintain WBC and differential count within normal range
c. Demonstrate appropriate care of infection-prone site
d. State signs and symptoms of infection of which to be aware

NOC OUTCOMES

Infection severity

NIC INTERVENTIONS

Infection control; infection protection

NURSING ASSESSMENT	RATIONALE
Assess client's venous access site for signs and symptoms of infection: • Nausea • Malaise • Erythema • Tenderness and exudate at venous access site • Chills • Fever • Increased WBCs • Abnormal differential count • Positive blood/wound cultures Monitor complete blood count, blood and wound culture results for abnormalities.	*Early recognition of signs and symptoms of infection allows for prompt intervention.*

THERAPEUTIC INTERVENTIONS	RATIONALE

Independent Actions

Wash hands before and after each patient encounter. Maintain aseptic technique when administering solution: • Administer parenteral solutions not containing fat emulsion through a 0.22-micron Millipore filter. • Administer parenteral solutions containing fat emulsions through a 1.2-micron filter. • Change filters and tubing in accordance with institutional policy, marking the date and time of initiation of use: • Change every 24 hrs if lipid emulsions are used. • Change every 72 hrs if amino acids and dextrose is used.	*Parenteral nutritional therapy, because of the high glucose concentrations, provides an excellent environment for microbial growth.* *The use of in-line filters helps reduce or eliminate the infusion of particulates, microprecipitates, microorganisms, pyrogens, and air.*
Visually inspect solution before administration for any visual indication of precipitates, color changes (turbidity), or leaks.	*If any abnormalities are suspected, the solution should be returned to the pharmacy promptly for replacement.*
Change peripheral IV sites and dressings in accordance with institutional policy/Centers for Disease Control and Prevention (CDC) guidelines for infection prevention. Complete all parenteral solution infusions at the ordered rate within 24 hrs of initiation.	*Catheter-related infection and septicemia can occur in patients receiving parenteral nutrition through both central and peripheral access devices.* *At room temperature, parenteral solutions and fat emulsions provide a medium for bacterial growth.*

Dependent/Collaborative Actions

Obtain blood cultures as indicated. Obtain culture of venous access device catheter tip if discontinued. Notify physician provider if signs and symptoms of systemic or site infection develop.	*Notifying the appropriate health care provider allows for modification of the treatment plan.*

DISCHARGE TEACHING/CONTINUED CARE

Nursing Diagnosis DEFICIENT KNOWLEDGE NDx; INEFFECTIVE FAMILY HEALTH MANAGEMENT NDx; OR INEFFECTIVE HEALTH MAINTENANCE* NDx

Definition: Deficient Knowledge NDx: Absence of cognitive information related to specific topic or its acquisition. **Ineffective Family Health Management NDx:** A pattern of regulating and integrating into family processes a program for the treatment of illness and its sequelae that is unsatisfactory for meeting specific health goals of the family unit. **Ineffective Health Maintenance NDx:** Inability to identify, manage, and/or seek help to maintain well-being.

*The nurse should select the nursing diagnostic label that is most appropriate for the client's discharge teaching needs.

CLINICAL MANIFESTATIONS

Subjective	Objective
Verbal self-report of inability to manage illness; verbalizes inability to follow prescribed regimen	Inaccurate follow-through with instructions; inappropriate behaviors

RISK FACTORS

- Cognitive deficit
- Financial concerns
- Inability to care for oneself

NIC OUTCOMES

Knowledge: treatment regimen; knowledge: infection management

NOC INTERVENTIONS

Teaching: individual; teaching: psychomotor skill

NURSING ASSESSMENT	RATIONALE
Assess client's readiness and ability to learn. Assess meaning of nutritional therapy to client.	*Early recognition of readiness to learn and meaning of nutritional therapy to client allows for implementation of the appropriate teaching interventions.*

THERAPEUTIC INTERVENTIONS	RATIONALE

Desired Outcome: The client will demonstrate the proper technique when changing infusion tubing and parenteral solution bags.

Independent Actions

Instruct client and family on the proper way to mix, handle, and store parenteral feedings.

- Allow time for return demonstration.

Instruct client and family on proper care of parenteral solution administration sets:

- Administer solution using appropriate filter.
- Discard administration sets every 72 hrs for solutions with amino acids/dextrose.
- Discard administration sets every 72 hrs for solutions containing lipid emulsions.

Instruct client and family on the proper handling and storage of solutions:

- Solutions must be infused within 24 hrs.
- Mixed solutions must be refrigerated until ½ hr before use.

Proper care of parenteral feedings is necessary to prevent contamination.

Given the high glucose concentration found in parenteral solutions, proper filtration and line maintenance is necessary to prevent bloodstream infections.

Parenteral nutritional therapy, because of the high glucose concentrations, provides an excellent environment for microbial growth.

The use of in-line filters helps reduce or eliminate the infusion of particulates, microprecipitates, microorganisms, pyrogens, and air. At room temperature, parenteral solutions and fat emulsions provide a medium for bacterial growth.

THERAPEUTIC INTERVENTIONS	RATIONALE

Desired Outcome: The client will demonstrate proper care of venous access device.

Independent Actions

Instruct client and family on the proper method of changing central line or venous access dressings.
Allow time for return demonstration.

Sterile dressing care of long-term venous access devices is necessary to prevent the development of catheter line sepsis.

THERAPEUTIC INTERVENTIONS	RATIONALE

Desired Outcome: The client will verbalize signs and symptoms of infection to report to health care provider.

Independent Actions

Instruct client and family to report any signs and symptoms of systemic or localized (catheter site) infection to the health care provider immediately.

Notifying the appropriate health care provider allows for modification of the treatment plan.

RELATED CARE PLAN

PEPTIC ULCER

A peptic ulcer is a break in the continuity of the GI mucosa that is exposed to acidic digestive secretions. The areas most often involved are the stomach and duodenum. Erosion of these areas can result from direct damage to the mucosa or from an increase in mucosal permeability, which allows gastric acids to diffuse through the mucosal barrier into the underlying tissue. The two most common causes of peptic ulcers are infection with *Helicobacter pylori (H. pylori)* and use of aspirin or other NSAIDs. Other factors believed to have a role in ulcer development, exacerbation, and/or recurrence include ingestion of alcohol, coffee, certain foods and spices, and caffeine; medications such as corticosteroids and some chemotherapeutic agents; smoking; stress; hypovolemia (can result in ischemia of the GI mucosa and subsequent alteration in mucosal permeability); certain disease conditions (e.g., Zollinger-Ellison syndrome, chronic obstructive pulmonary disease, pancreatitis, chronic renal failure); and genetic predisposition.

Peptic ulcers are usually classified by location (e.g., gastric, duodenal) and by the extensiveness of erosion (e.g., acute [superficial erosion with minimal inflammation], chronic [erosion of mucosa and submucosa with scar tissue formation]). Causative factors and the relationship between eating and occurrence of pain vary depending on the location and extensiveness of the ulcer. The characteristic symptom of a peptic ulcer is chronic, intermittent epigastric pain that is described as burning, aching, gnawing, or cramping.

Medical treatment of a peptic ulcer focuses on eradicating *H. pylori* infection if present, decreasing the degree of gastric acidity, and promoting mucosal integrity and regeneration. Surgical intervention (e.g., vagotomy, pyloroplasty, partial gastrectomy) may be indicated if symptoms cannot be medically controlled; if ulcers recur frequently; or if complications such as hemorrhage, perforation, or obstruction occur in the ulcerated area(s).

This care plan focuses on the adult client hospitalized for evaluation and medical treatment of a peptic ulcer that has become increasingly symptomatic. Much of the information presented here is applicable to clients receiving care in an extended care facility or home setting.

OUTCOME/DISCHARGE CRITERIA

The client will:
1. Have pain controlled
2. Have no signs and symptoms of complications
3. Verbalize a basic understanding of peptic ulcer disease and the importance of adhering to the prescribed treatment plan
4. Identify ways to promote healing of the existing ulcer and prevent recurrence of peptic ulcer
5. Verbalize an understanding of medications ordered including rationale, food and drug interactions, side effects, schedule for taking, and importance of taking as prescribed
6. State signs and symptoms to report to the health care provider
7. Develop a plan for adhering to recommended follow-up care including future appointments with health care provider

For a full, detailed care plan on this topic, go to http://evolve.elsevier.com/Haugen/careplanning/.

Nursing Care of the Client With Disturbances of the Liver, Biliary Tract, and Pancreas

CHOLECYSTECTOMY

⊖▶ A laparoscopic cholecystectomy is the standard surgical approach for removal of the gallbladder. It is performed to treat symptomatic cholecystitis or cholelithiasis, or both. A cholecystectomy can be done via laparoscopy or through a right subcostal incision (i.e., open cholecystectomy). A laparoscopic cholecystectomy is the procedure of choice because of the short hospitalization (<2 days), reduced postoperative pain, and a more rapid return to usual activities. An open cholecystectomy is indicated when the client is in the last trimester of pregnancy or has a gangrenous or perforated gallbladder, a suspected gallbladder malignancy, a history of multiple abdominal surgeries, severe inflammation that obscures the structures of the hepatobiliary triangle, or large stones in the biliary ducts or is morbidly obese. An open cholecystectomy may also be performed when problems are encountered during a laparoscopic cholecystectomy. If common bile duct stones are present, they can often be extracted endoscopically, but a choledocholithotomy may be necessary if the stones are large. After a choledocholithotomy, a T-tube is placed in the common bile duct to maintain adequate flow or drainage of bile until ductal edema subsides.

This care plan focuses on the adult client hospitalized for an open cholecystectomy with common bile duct exploration.

OUTCOME/DISCHARGE CRITERIA

The client will be able to:
1. Have pain controlled at a level that ensures client's comfort while not interfering with activities of daily living.
2. Tolerate prescribed diet
3. Have evidence of normal healing of surgical wound(s) and normal skin integrity around T-tube site
4. Maintain clear, audible breath sounds throughout the lungs
5. Have no signs and symptoms of postoperative complications
6. Demonstrate the ability to appropriately care for T-tube and surrounding skin if T-tube is present
7. Verbalize understanding of the rationale for and components of a low- to moderate-fat diet if prescribed
8. State signs and symptoms to report to the health care provider
9. Develop a plan for adhering to recommended follow-up care including future appointments with health care provider, wound care, medications prescribed, and activity level

See Care Plan on Cholelithiasis/Cholecystitis and the Standardized Preoperative and Postoperative Care Plans for additional diagnoses.

Nursing Diagnosis **INEFFECTIVE BREATHING PATTERN** NDx

Definition: Inspiration and/or expiration that does not provide adequate ventilation.

Related to:
- Increased rate of respirations associated with:
  - Decreased rate of respirations associated with depressant effect of anesthesia and other medications (e.g., opioid analgesics)
- Decreased depth of respirations associated with:
  - Depressant effect of anesthesia and other medications (e.g., opioid analgesics)
  - Reluctance to breathe deeply because of pain
  - Fear, anxiety, weakness, and fatigue
  - Restricted chest expansion resulting from positioning and elevation of the diaphragm if abdominal distention is present

CLINICAL MANIFESTATIONS

Subjective	Objective
Verbal reports of shortness of breath	Dyspnea; bradypnea, tachypnea; decreased depth of breathing; decreased inspiratory/expiratory pressure; decreased minute ventilation; use of accessory muscles; altered chest excursion

RISK FACTORS

- Surgery
- Immobility
- Fatigue
- Pain
- Anxiety

DESIRED OUTCOMES

The client will maintain an effective breathing pattern, as evidenced by:
a. Normal rate and depth of respirations
b. Absence of dyspnea
c. Oxygenation adequate for client needs

NOC OUTCOMES

Respiratory status: ventilation

NIC INTERVENTIONS

Respiratory monitoring

NURSING ASSESSMENT

Assess for signs and symptoms of an ineffective breathing pattern:
- Shallow or slow respirations
- Limited chest excursion
- Tachypnea or dyspnea
- Use of accessory muscles when breathing

Assess/monitor pulse oximetry (arterial oxygen saturation [SaO_2]),

RATIONALE

Early recognition of signs and symptoms of an ineffective breathing pattern allows for prompt intervention.

Shallow, rapid respirations, lack of chest excursion, and holding one's breath may lead to inadequate oxygenation and atelectasis.

Monitoring continuous SaO_2 readings allows for the early detection of hypoxia.

THERAPEUTIC INTERVENTIONS

Independent Actions

Implement measures to improve breathing pattern:
- Perform actions to reduce fear and anxiety:
  - Promote a calm, restful environment. **D** ● ✦
- Perform actions to reduce pain:
  - Reposition client for comfort.
  - Instruct client to support incision with hands or a pillow when moving or coughing. **D** ● ✦
- Assist client to bend knees while coughing and deep breathing. **D** ● ✦
- Perform actions to increase strength and improve activity tolerance:
  - Implement measures to conserve energy. **D** ● ✦
  - Have client deep breathe or use incentive spirometer every 1 to 2 hrs. **D** ✦
- Instruct client to breathe slowly if hyperventilating. **D** ✦

  - Place client in a semi- to high-Fowler's position unless contraindicated.
  - If client must remain flat in bed, assist with position change at least every 2 hrs. **D** ✦

RATIONALE

Reducing fear and anxiety helps to minimize shallow and/or rapid breathing.

Pain reduction increases the client's willingness to move and breathe deeply.

Supporting abdominal incision will decrease muscle tension and potential pain and discomfort when moving or coughing.

Relieves tension on abdominal muscles and incision allowing for better chest expansion.

Increasing activity tolerance enables the client to breathe deeply and participate in activities to improve breathing pattern.

Deep breathing and use of an incentive spirometer promote maximal inhalation and lung expansion.

Hyperventilation is an ineffective breathing pattern that can lead to respiratory alkalosis. A client can often slow breathing rate through focused concentration.

A semi- to high-Fowler's position allows for maximal diaphragmatic excursion and lung expansion.

Compression of the thorax and subsequent limited chest wall expansion occur when the client lies in one position. Frequent repositioning promotes maximal chest wall and lung expansion.

Dependent/Collaborative Actions

Implement measures to improve breathing pattern:
- Increase activity as allowed and tolerated.

During activity, especially ambulation, encourage the client to takes deep breaths, thus increasing lung expansion.

NDx = NANDA Diagnosis   **D** = Delegatable Action   ● = UAP   ✦ = LVN/LPN   ⊖▶ = Go to ⊖volve for animation

Continued...

THERAPEUTIC INTERVENTIONS	RATIONALE

• Administer central nervous system depressants judiciously:
  • Hold medication and consult physician if respiratory rate is less than 12 breaths/min.
• Perform actions to reduce pain:
  • Administer analgesics before activities and procedures than can cause pain and before pain becomes severe. **D** ✦
Consult appropriate health care provider if:
• Ineffective breathing pattern continues.
• Client develops signs and symptoms of impaired gas exchange such as restlessness, irritability, confusion, significant decrease in oximetry results, decreased partial pressure of oxygen in arterial blood (PaO_2) and increased partial pressure of carbon dioxide in arterial blood ($PaCO_2$) levels.
	Central nervous system depressants cause depression of the respiratory center in the brainstem, resulting in decreased rate and depth of respiration.
	Reducing pain helps to increase the client's willingness to move and breathe more deeply.
	
	Notifying the appropriate health care provider allows for modification of treatment plan.

Collaborative Diagnosis **RISK FOR ABSCESS FORMATION**

Definition: An accumulation of pus in any area of the body.

Related to:
• Accumulation of drainage in the surgical area and subsequent invasion area by microorganisms and neutrophils

CLINICAL MANIFESTATIONS

Subjective	Objective
Verbalization of pain in the surgical area	Redness, swelling, and/or warmth in the surgical area; fever; tachycardia; increased white blood cell (WBC) count

RISK FACTORS	DESIRED OUTCOMES
• Surgery • Exposure to pathogens	The client will not develop an abscess, as evidenced by: a. Lack of redness, warmth, or swelling of the surgical site b. Temperature declining toward normal c. WBC count declining toward normal

NURSING ASSESSMENT	RATIONALE
Assess for and report signs and symptoms of infection or abscess (e.g., increased or more constant abdominal pain, increase in temperature and pulse rate, further increase in WBC count).	*Early recognition of signs and symptoms of infection or abscess allows for prompt intervention.*

THERAPEUTIC INTERVENTIONS	RATIONALE
Independent Actions Implement measures to prevent infection and or accumulation of drainage in the surgical area: • Keep surgical site and puncture wounds clean and dry. • Monitor surgical wound or puncture sites for any drainage • Change dressings as ordered	*Prevents development of infection.* *The surgical wounds may initially drain serous-sanguineous fluid, but this should decrease in the hours following surgery.* *Dressing changes allow for assessment of the wound, help to provide protection from bile fluids that can cause skin breakdown.*

THERAPEUTIC INTERVENTIONS	RATIONALE

• Perform actions to maintain patency of wound drain and/or T-tube, if present:
  • Implement measures to prevent stasis and reflux of drainage: **D** ✦
  • Monitor color and characteristics of NG and T-tube drainage, if present:
    (1) Keep drainage tubing free of dependent loops and kinks (prevent kinking by placing a gauze roll under the drain tube and anchoring it to the skin or dressing with tape).
    (2) Keep collection device(s) below drain insertion site(s) unless ordered otherwise (physician may order T-tube collection device to be positioned just slightly below, level with, or above drain insertion site).
    (3) Empty collection device(s) as often as necessary and at least every shift. **D** ● ✦
	Promotes drainage of fluids from the wound, preventing stasis of fluids and reducing the risk for abscess formation and skin breakdown.
	Drainage may initially contain blood; this should change to greenish brown in the first few hours following surgery.
	
	Maintains appropriate drainage and prevents it from leaking into the abdomen.
	
	Reduces loss of bile.
	
	Prevents stasis of fluids.

Implement measures to prevent inadvertent removal of wound drain and/or T-tube: • Instruct client not to pull on drain(s) and drainage tubing. • Use caution when changing dressings surrounding drain(s). • Attach collection device(s) securely to abdominal dressing. • Maintain client in a semi- to high-Fowler's position as much as possible when in bed. **D** ✦	 *These actions prevent the T-tube from becoming dislodged, which can introduce bacteria into the body.* *Removes drainage from site and contact with skin—helps to maintain skin integrity* *Improves lung expansion and promotes drainage of respiratory secretions.*
Dependent/Collaborative Actions If signs and symptoms of an abscess occur: • Prepare client for diagnostic tests (e.g., ultrasonography, computed tomography, culture and sensitivity of wound). • Administer antimicrobials if ordered. • Prepare client for surgical intervention (e.g., incision and drainage of abscess) if planned.	 *Alleviates fear and anxiety.* *Alleviate infections.* *Alleviates fear and anxiety.*

DISCHARGE TEACHING/CONTINUED CARE

Nursing Diagnosis **DEFICIENT KNOWLEDGE** NDx; **OR INEFFECTIVE HEALTH MANAGEMENT*** NDx

Definition: Deficient Knowledge NDx: Absence of cognitive information related to a specific topic, or its acquisition: **Ineffective Health Management NDx:** Pattern of regulating and integrating into daily living a therapeutic regimen for the treatment of illness and its sequelae that is unsatisfactory for meeting specific health goals.

Related to:
• Insufficient interest in learning
• Misinformation provided by others
• Difficulty managing complex treatment regimen
• Difficulty navigating complex health care systems
• Insufficient social support

CLINICAL MANIFESTATIONS

Subjective	Objective
Verbalizes inability to manage illness; verbalizes inability to follow prescribed regimen	Inaccurate follow-through with instructions; inappropriate behaviors; experience of preventable complications of surgery

*The nurse should select the diagnostic label that is most appropriate for the client's discharge teaching needs.

NDx = NANDA Diagnosis   **D** = Delegatable Action   ● = UAP   ✦ = LVN/LPN   ⊖▶ = Go to ⊖volve for animation

RISK FACTORS
- Cognitive deficit
- Financial concerns
- Failure to take action to reduce risk factors for complications of surgery (if performed)
- Inability to care for oneself
- Difficulty in modifying personal habits and integrating treatments into lifestyle

NOC OUTCOMES	NIC INTERVENTIONS
Knowledge: Treatment regimen; health behaviors; health resources; Treatment procedures.	Teaching individualized prescribed medication, diet, activities; teaching: health system guidance; teaching: support systems.

NURSING ASSESSMENT	RATIONALE
Assess the client's ability to learn and readiness to learn. Assess the client's understanding of teaching.	*Learning is more effective when the client is motivated and understands the importance of what is to be learned. Readiness to learn changes based on situations, physical, and emotional challenges.*

THERAPEUTIC INTERVENTIONS	RATIONALE

Desired Outcome: The client will demonstrate the ability to appropriately care for T-tube and surrounding skin if T-tube is present.

The client demonstration is important to ensure that the client understands how to care for the T-tube and prevent complications following surgery and hospital discharge.

Independent Actions
If the client is to be discharged with a T-tube in place, instruct regarding care of the T-tube and surrounding skin:
- Cleanse the skin around the T-tube insertion site daily, and cover the site with a dry sterile dressing; apply zinc oxide cream to skin around insertion site if skin is irritated.

These actions help to prevent infection and skin breakdown.

- Keep the T-tube drainage collection device in the position prescribed (usually slightly below the insertion site).

Helps to maintain drainage patency and promote drainage.

- Keep the tubing pinned to the dressing and avoid any kinks or tension on the tubing.

Prevents unnecessary pressure or pulling on the T-tube.

- Empty the drainage collection device at least twice daily or more often if needed; keep a record of the amount of drainage.

Monitors output, noting changes in volume.

- When emptying the drainage collection device, check to see that the tube has not become dislodged (this can be easily monitored if the tube is marked at the skin line before discharge).

If tube becomes dislodged, client should contact the health care provider.

- Clamp T-tube only as instructed.

Clamping the T-tube helps prevent bile leakage.

Allow time for questions, clarification, and return demonstration of care of T-tube and surrounding skin.

Improves client's confidence in ability to care for self.

THERAPEUTIC INTERVENTIONS	RATIONALE

Desired Outcome: The client will verbalize an understanding of the rationale for and components of a low- to moderate-fat diet if prescribed

If the client understands the rationale for diet requirements and what may occur when they are not followed. This may improve client adherence.

Independent Actions
Explain the rationale for avoiding excessive fat intake for the first 4 to 6 weeks after surgery (many physicians instruct client to just avoid foods that cause epigastric discomfort).

Initially large amounts of fat can cause gastric upset and gastric discomfort. Over time, the client will learn the amount of fat that causes gastric discomfort.

Instruct client to increase fat intake gradually and introduce foods/fluids high in fat (e.g., butter, cream, whole milk, ice cream, fried foods, gravies, nuts) one at a time.

Gradual increase in fat intake allows the body to become used to absorbing fats, without severe epigastric discomfort.

THERAPEUTIC INTERVENTIONS	RATIONALE

Desired Outcome: The client will state signs and symptoms to report to the health care provider.

When the client understands what needs to be monitored and reported, it may improve client adherence with contacting their health care provider.

Independent Actions
Instruct the client to report the following signs and symptoms to health care provider:

- Persistent low-grade fever or significantly elevated temperature (≥38.8°C [101°F])
- Difficulty breathing
- Chest pain
- Cough productive of purulent, green, or rust-colored sputum
- Increased weakness or inability to tolerate prescribed activity level
- Increasing discomfort or discomfort not controlled by prescribed medications and treatments
- Nausea and vomiting

- Decreased urine output
- Frequency, urgency, or burning on urination
- Cloudy or foul-smelling urine
- Urine retention
- Clay-colored stools or dark amber urine
- Development of increased itchiness or yellowing of skin
- When the T-tube drainage subsides or after the T-tube has been removed, purulent drainage from the T-tube or green-brown drainage around T-tube or from wound site
- A significant increase in or more than 500 mL/day of drainage from T-tube
- A sudden marked decrease in T-tube drainage or increase in length of the T-tube (may indicate that the T-tube has become dislodged)
- Abdominal distention or rigidity

- Persistent heartburn, feeling of bloating, or nausea
- Loose stools that continue for longer than 2 to 3 months
Instruct client in ways to prevent postoperative infection:

- Continue with coughing unless contraindicated and deep breathing every 2 hrs while awake.
- Continue to use incentive spirometer if activity is limited.
- Increase activity as ordered.

- Avoid contact with persons who have infections.
- Avoid crowds during flu and cold seasons.
- Drink at least 10 glasses of liquid per day, unless contraindicated.
- Maintain a balanced nutritional intake.
- Maintain proper balance of bedrest and activity.
- Maintain good personal hygiene (e.g., oral care, handwashing, and perineal care).
- Maintain sterile or clean technique as ordered during wound care.
- Provide client with supplies necessary for wound care.

Instruct client to avoid heavy lifting for 4 to 6 weeks.

These clinical manifestations indicate that the client may be experiencing complications from surgery, if performed. They indicate possible infection of the surgical area or other body systems and possible thromboembolism.
Indication of a respiratory infection.

Could indicate a poor diet, as well as an infection.

May indicate something has changed in the client's condition and should be reported to the health care provider.
May indicate increased consumption of fatty foods or potential blockage of T-tube, if present.
Indicates a possible urinary tract infection or decrease fluid intake.

These changes indicate bile leaking into the abdomen and onto the client's skin.
May indicate a blockage or an infection.

This change may indicate increased bile production or infection.

These changes may indicate T-tube has become dislodged or is blocked.

May indicate consumption of too many fatty foods or potential abdominal abscess.
May indicate consumption of a high level of fat in the diet.

Understanding rationale may improve adherence to treatment regimen.
Coughing and deep breathing exercises help to improve oxygenation to the tissues, expand the lungs, and prevent stasis of secretions.
These actions prevent thromboembolism and improve ability to resume normal activities.
Prevents exposure of client to others who are ill and decreases the risk for an infection.
Maintains adequate hydration and vascular fluid volume.

An appropriate diet with adequate protein improves the body's ability to heal.
These actions help prevent infection.

Improves client's adherence to treatment regimen and decreases potential for infection.
The client should not do any heavy lifting until approved by the health care provider. Lifting may cause a rupture of suture line.

Continued...

THERAPEUTIC INTERVENTIONS	RATIONALE
Desired Outcome: The client, in collaboration with the nurse, will develop a plan for adhering to recommended follow-up care including future appointments with health care provider, wound care, medications prescribed, and activity level	*Important so the nurse knows that the client understands what is expected postoperatively.*
Independent Actions	
Explain the rationale for, side effects of, schedule for taking, and importance of taking medications prescribed. Inform client of pertinent food and drug interactions.	*Knowledge of disease process and treatment helps the client and family understand the changes that are occurring and the importance of treatment in maintaining health status. This improves client's adherence to treatment regimen and allows client to maintain a level of independence.*
If the client has had a laparoscopic cholecystectomy, mild shoulder pain may persist for a week after surgery until the carbon dioxide used during surgery is completely absorbed. Inform client that lying on his/her left side with the right knee flexed may help relieve this pain.	*Appropriate positioning postoperatively helps relieve pain.*

CIRRHOSIS

Cirrhosis is a chronic liver disease that is caused by extensive destruction of the parenchymal cells in the liver. These cells are eventually replaced by fibrous scar tissue with subsequent change in liver structure and functioning. These structural changes impair portal blood flow that results in venous congestion in other organs and systems such as the spleen and gastrointestinal tract.

The most common causes of cirrhosis include chronic infection with hepatitis B and C viruses and alcohol use. Laennec cirrhosis, alcohol-induced, is the second most common form of the disease. Other causes include exposure to toxic chemicals or drugs, genetic causes of cirrhosis (including alpha1-antitrypsin deficiency, Wilson disease, and hemochromatosis), heart failure, and conditions that cause persistent bile flow obstruction (e.g., primary biliary cirrhosis, primary sclerosing cholangitis).

All types of cirrhosis have similar signs and symptoms. Clinical manifestations are reflective of the degree of impaired liver function and portal hypertension–induced venous congestion. Alcohol-related cirrhosis may have additional manifestations such as cerebral degeneration and demyelinating neuropathies thought to be a direct result of the toxic effects of alcohol and/or associated vitamin deficiencies. Treatment of cirrhosis is supportive and directed at slowing the progression of liver scar tissue and decreasing the incidence and/or severity of complications. The primary goals of treatment are to eliminate or manage the factors/conditions that contributed to the development of cirrhosis, provide a high nutrient diet, reduction of further liver damage, and rest to reduce the metabolic demands on the liver. A liver transplant may be indicated to treat end-stage liver disease.

***This care plan focuses on the adult client with alcoholic (Laennec) cirrhosis hospitalized for management** of increasing ascites and peripheral edema. Much of the information is applicable to clients receiving follow-up care in an extended care facility or home setting.*

OUTCOME/DISCHARGE CRITERIA

The client will:
1. Maintain adequate nutritional intake
2. Perform activities of daily living without extreme fatigue or dyspnea
3. Maintain reduced or resolution of ascites and edema
4. Have no evidence of life-threatening complications
5. Discuss ways to prevent further liver damage
6. Discuss the for and components of the recommended diet
7. Reduce stress or trauma to the esophageal blood vessels
8. Describe ways to prevent bleeding
9. Implement ways to reduce the risk of infection
10. Describe methods to relieve pruritus
11. State signs and symptoms to report to the health care provider
12. List community resources that can assist with home management and adjustment to lifestyle changes necessary for effective management of cirrhosis
13. Discuss concerns and feelings about the diagnosis of cirrhosis; prognosis; and effects of the disease process and its treatment on self-concept, lifestyle, and roles
14. Develop plan for adhering to recommended follow-up care including future appointments with health care provider, medications prescribed, and activity level

Nursing Diagnosis INEFFECTIVE BREATHING PATTERN NDx

Definition: Inspiration and/or expiration that does not provide adequate ventilation.

Related to:
- Increased rate of respirations associated with fear and anxiety
- Decreased depth of respirations associated with:
  - Weakness and fatigue
  - Decreased lung compliance (distensibility) resulting from pleural effusion (hepatic hydrothorax) that occurs due to excess fluid volume and passage of ascetic fluid into the pleural space
  - Restricted chest expansion resulting from positioning and pressure on the diaphragm as a result of ascites

CLINICAL MANIFESTATIONS

Subjective	Objective
Complaints of shortness of breath	Dyspnea; orthopnea; bradypnea, tachypnea; decreased depth of breathing; decreased inspiratory/expiratory pressure; decreased minute ventilation; decreased vital capacity; nasal flaring; use of accessory muscles; use of three-point position; altered chest excursion; pursed-lip breathing; prolonged expiration phases

RISK FACTORS
- Chronic illness
- Failure of body's regulatory mechanisms
- Respiratory muscle fatigue

DESIRED OUTCOMES

The client will have an improved breathing pattern, as evidenced by:
  a. Regular rate and depth of respirations
  b. Decreased dyspnea
  c. Symmetric chest excursion
  d. Arterial blood gas (ABG) and vital capacity within acceptable range

NOC OUTCOMES

Respiratory status: ventilation

NIC INTERVENTIONS

Ventilation assistance; respiratory monitoring

NURSING ASSESSMENT	RATIONALE
Assess for signs and symptoms of an ineffective breathing pattern: • Shallow or slow respirations • Limited chest excursion • Tachypnea or dyspnea • Use of accessory muscles when breathing Assess/monitor pulse oximetry (arterial oxygen saturation [SaO_2]), ABG values as indicated.	*Early recognition of signs and symptoms of an ineffective breathing pattern allows for prompt intervention.* *Change in breathing rate and depth may be due to presence of fluid accumulation in the abdomen causing pressure on the lungs and decreased diaphragmatic excursion. This leads to increased respiratory rate and possible use of accessory muscles.* *Monitoring continuous SaO_2 readings allows for the early detection of hypoxia.* *Assessment of ABG values provides a more direct measurement of both the partial pressure of oxygen in arterial blood (PaO_2) and the partial pressure of carbon dioxide in arterial blood ($PaCO_2$), which reflect the adequacy of ventilation.*

THERAPEUTIC INTERVENTIONS	RATIONALE
Independent Actions Implement measures to improve breathing pattern: • Perform actions to increase strength and activity tolerance (e.g., maintain activity restrictions, maintain a calm environment, organize nursing care to provide for periods of rest, limit number of visitors and their length of stay). **D** ● ✦	*These actions provide longer rest periods and may increase a client's willingness and ability to move, deep breathe, and use incentive spirometer.*

NDx = NANDA Diagnosis   **D** = Delegatable Action   ● = UAP   ✦ = LVN/LPN   ⊖▶ = Go to ⊖volve for animation

Continued...

THERAPEUTIC INTERVENTIONS	RATIONALE

• Perform actions to restore fluid balance:
  • Restrict sodium intake as ordered.
  • Maintain fluid restriction.
	Reduces fluid accumulation in the peritoneal cavity and pleural space, thus decreasing pressure on the diaphragm.

• Encourage client to periodically rest in a recumbent position.	*Lying down reduces peripheral pooling of blood, which increases effective circulating volume and renal blood flow and subsequently promotes diuresis.*
• Place client in a semi-Fowler's position (a high-Fowler's position is uncomfortable if ascites is severe). **D** ● ✦	*Decreases less compression on the diaphragm from an extended abdomen.*
• Instruct client to deep breathe or use incentive spirometer every 1 to 2 hrs.	*Deep breathing and use of an incentive spirometer promote maximal inhalation and lung expansion, which reduces incidence of atelectasis and enhances mobilization of secretions*
• Instruct client to avoid intake of gas-forming foods (e.g., beans, cauliflower, cabbage, onions), carbonated beverages, and large meals.	*Avoidance of gas-forming foods prevents gastric distention and additional pressure on the diaphragm.*
Dependent/Collaborative Actions Implement measures to improve breathing pattern:	
• Assist with positive airway pressure techniques (e.g., continuous positive airway pressure [CPAP], bilevel positive airway pressure [BiPAP], flutter/positive expiratory pressure [PEP] device), if ordered.	*Positive airway pressure techniques increase intrapulmonary (alveolar) pressure, which helps expand collapsed alveoli and prevent further alveoli collapse.*
• Administer central nervous system depressants judiciously; hold medication and consult physician if respiratory rate is less than 12 breaths/min.	*Reducing pain helps to increase the client's willingness to move and breathe more deeply.*
• Assist with thoracentesis and/or paracentesis if performed.	*Removal of pleural and/or peritoneal fluid allows for increased chest and lung expansion.*
Consult appropriate health care provider (e.g., respiratory therapist, physician) if: • Ineffective breathing pattern continues. • Signs and symptoms of impaired gas exchange (e.g., restlessness, irritability, confusion, significant decrease in oximetry results, decreased PaO_2 and increased $PaCO_2$ levels) are present.	*Notifying the appropriate health care provider allows for prompt modification of treatment plan.*

Nursing/Collaborative Diagnosis: **RISK FOR IMBALANCED FLUID VOLUME** NDx **RISK FOR ELECTROLYTE IMBALANCE** NDx **AND THIRD-SPACING**

Definition: **Risk for Imbalanced fluid volume NDx:** Susceptible to a decrease, increase, or rapid shift from one to the other of intravascular, interstitial and/or intracellular fluid, which may compromise health. This refers to body fluid loss, gain, or both; **Risk for electrolyte imbalance NDx:** Susceptible to changes in serum electrolyte levels, which may compromise health.

Related to:
• Sodium and water retention associated with an increased serum aldosterone level resulting from:
  • Inability of the liver to metabolize aldosterone
  • Activation of the renin-angiotensin-aldosterone mechanism as a result of decreased renal blood flow (occurs because of a decrease in intravascular volume that results from vasodilation and from third-spacing and sequestration of fluid in the splanchnic system)
• Low plasma colloid osmotic pressure associated with hypoalbuminemia (a result of decreased hepatic synthesis of albumin and prolonged inadequate nutrition)
• Compromised regulator mechanisms
  Increased pressure in the portal system and hepatic lymph system associated with blood flow backup resulting from structural changes in the liver

CLINICAL MANIFESTATIONS

Subjective	**Objective**
Verbalization of shortness of breath	Jugular venous distention; decreased hemoglobin (Hgb) and hematocrit (Hct); weight gain over short period of time; dyspnea; intake exceeds output; pleural effusion; orthopnea; S_3 heart sound; pulmonary congestion; change in respiratory pattern; change in mental status; blood pressure changes; pulmonary artery pressure changes; oliguria; specific gravity changes; azotemia; electrolyte imbalance; restlessness; anxiety; adventitious breath sounds (crackles); edema, may progress to anasarca; increased central venous pressure; positive hepatojugular reflex; paroxysmal nocturnal dyspnea

RISK FACTORS

- Hyperaldosteronism
- Poor nutritional status
- Portal hypertension
- Hepatomegaly
- Compromised regulatory mechanism
- Ascites

DESIRED OUTCOMES

The client will experience resolution of fluid and electrolyte imbalance fluid, as evidenced by:
a. Decline in weight toward client's normal weight
b. B/P and pulse rate within normal range for client and stable with position change
c. Absence or resolution of S_3 heart sound or Electrocardiogram (ECG) changes
d. Balanced intake and output
e. Usual mental status
f. Electrolyte (e.g., sodium and potassium) levels returning toward normal range
g. Decreased dyspnea, peripheral edema, and neck vein distention
h. Improved breath sounds
i. Resolution of ascites
j. Usual muscle tone and strength
k. Absence of nausea and vomiting

NOC OUTCOMES

Fluid balance; fluid overload severity; electrolyte and acid-base balance

NIC INTERVENTIONS

Fluid/electrolyte management

NURSING ASSESSMENT	**RATIONALE**
Assess for and report:	*Early recognition of signs and symptoms of fluid and electrolyte imbalance allows for prompt treatment.*
• Signs and symptoms of excess fluid volume:	
• Weight gain of 2% or greater in a short period	*Rapid fluid gain may be noted in changes in daily weight.*
Signs and symptoms of abnormal potassium and sodium levels	*Change in potassium and sodium impacts cardiac functioning and fluid volume.*
• Elevated blood pressure	*B/P elevates with increase in vascular fluid volume and decreases if fluid has shifted out of the vascular space.*
• Development or worsening of S_3 heart sound; ECG changes	*S_3 heart sounds indicate vascular fluid overload ECG changes indicate decreased potassium levels.*
• Intake greater than output	*Indicates increased fluid retention.*
• Change in mental status	*May reflect impending hepatic encephalopathy.*
• Low serum sodium level	*May result from diuretic therapy and a low-sodium diet.*
• Dyspnea, orthopnea, crackles (rales), diminished or absent breath sounds	*Indicates increased pulmonary congestion.*
• Peripheral edema	*Indicates changes in capillary status.*
• Distended neck veins	*Increased vascular fluid volume.*

NDx = NANDA Diagnosis   **D** = Delegatable Action   ● = UAP   ✦ = LVN/LPN   ⊖▶ = Go to ⊖volve for animation

Continued...

NURSING ASSESSMENT	RATIONALE
• Signs and symptoms of third-spacing: • Ascites • Dyspnea and diminished or absent breath sounds	*Early recognition of signs and symptoms of third-spacing allows for prompt treatment.*
• Evidence of vascular depletion (e.g., postural hypotension; weak, rapid pulse; decreased urine output)	*Indications of potential changes in vascular fluid status and/or loss of vascular integrity.*
• Chest radiograph results showing pulmonary vascular congestion, pleural effusion, or pulmonary edema	*Confirmation of increased vascular fluid retention.*
• Low serum albumin levels	*Results in fluid shifting out of the vascular space because albumin is required to maintain plasma colloid osmotic pressure.*

THERAPEUTIC INTERVENTIONS	RATIONALE
Dependent/Collaborative Actions Implement measures to restore fluid balance: • Perform actions to reduce excess fluid volume: • Restrict sodium intake as ordered. • Maintain fluid restrictions if ordered.	*Sodium and fluid restriction helps to minimize fluid retention in extravascular tissues.*
• Encourage client to rest periodically in a recumbent position. **D** ● ✦	*Lying down reduces peripheral pooling of blood, which increases effective circulating volume and renal blood flow and subsequently promotes diuresis.*
• Administer diuretics if ordered (e.g., potassium-sparing diuretics such as spironolactone and amiloride). **D** ✦	*Potassium-sparing diuretics reduce fluid volume by increasing urinary output and decrease retention of sodium.*
• Perform actions to promote mobilization of fluid back into the vascular space and to prevent further third-spacing:	*Improves renal blood flow, which increases water excretion and reduces activation of the renin-angiotensin-aldosterone mechanism.*
• Administer albumin infusions, if ordered.	*Albumin infusions increase vascular colloid osmotic pressure and pulls fluid back into the vascular system.*
Monitor serum Na⁺ and K⁺ levels. Administer electrolyte replacements as ordered.	*Maintenance of Na and K levels is important to maintain adequate cardiac functioning. When administering potassium replacements, it is important to monitor the infusion carefully to prevent further complication.*
Consult physician if signs and symptoms of imbalanced fluid and electrolytes persist or worsen.	*Notifying the appropriate health care provider allows for prompt modification of treatment plan.*

Nursing Diagnosis IMBALANCED NUTRITION: LESS THAN BODY REQUIREMENTS NDx

Definition: Intake of nutrients insufficient to meet metabolic needs.

Related to:
• Reduced oral intake associated with dyspepsia, fatigue, dyspnea, dislike of the prescribed diet, and feeling of fullness from ascites
• Reduced metabolism and storage of nutrients by the liver associated with a reduction of functional liver tissue
• Malabsorption of fats and fat-soluble vitamins associated with impaired bile production and flow.

CLINICAL MANIFESTATIONS

Subjective	Objective
Verbalization of lack of appetite; fatigue; sore buccal membrane irritability; abdominal cramping/pain	Loss of weight with adequate food intake; body weight 20% or more under ideal weight; inflamed buccal cavity; capillary fragility; pale conjunctiva and mucous membranes; poor muscle tone; excessive hair loss; amenorrhea

RISK FACTORS

- Chronic illness
- Anorexia
- Poor nutritional status
- Poor dietary habits
- Economically disadvantages
- Inability to absorb nutrients

DESIRED OUTCOMES

The client will maintain an adequate nutritional status, as evidenced by:
a. Dry weight approaching normal for the client (dry weight achieved after fluid volume excess has been resolved)
b. Normal blood urea nitrogen (BUN) and serum albumin, prealbumin, hematocrit (Hct), and hemoglobin (Hgb) levels, and normal lymphocyte count
c. Improved strength and activity tolerance
d. Healthy oral mucous membrane

NOC OUTCOMES

Nutritional status

NIC INTERVENTIONS

Nutritional monitoring; nutritional counseling; nutritional management; nutritional therapy

NURSING ASSESSMENT

Assess for and report signs and symptoms of malnutrition:
- Weight significantly below client's usual weight or below normal for client's age, height, and body frame
- Decreased serum prealbumin, BUN, a albumin, Hct and Hgb levels and decreased lymphocyte count
- Weakness and fatigue
- Sore, inflamed oral mucous membrane
- Pale conjunctiva

Monitor percentage of meals and snacks client consumes. Report a pattern of inadequate intake.

RATIONALE

Early recognition and reporting of signs and symptoms of malnutrition allows for prompt intervention.

An awareness of the amount of food/fluid the client consumes alerts the nurse to deficits in nutritional intake. Reporting an inadequate intake allows for prompt intervention.

THERAPEUTIC INTERVENTIONS

Independent Actions
Implement measures to improve nutritional status:
- Implement measures to reduce dyspepsia (e.g., keep head of bed elevated for 2–3 hrs after eating; provide small, frequent meals; encourage client to ingest foods slowly; avoid carbonated beverages; do not use a straw). **D** ● ✦

Encourages a rest period before meals. **D** ● ✦
- Provide a clean environment and a relaxed, pleasant atmosphere. **D** ● ✦

- Serve frequent, small meals if client is weak, fatigues easily, and/or has a poor appetite. **D** ● ✦

- Elevate the head of bed as tolerated for meals. **D** ● ✦

- Provide adequate time for meals; reheat foods/fluids if necessary. **D** ● ✦
- Reduce fluid intake with meals unless the fluid has a high nutritional value. **D** ✦
- Increase activity as allowed and tolerated. **D** ● ✦

- Assist and instruct client to adhere to the following dietary recommendations:

RATIONALE

Elevation of the head of the bed after eating decreases pressure on abdomen, which may improve appetite. Small frequent meals and refraining from the use of carbonated beverages or a straw decrease pressure in the abdomen.
Minimizes fatigue.
A clean environment and a relaxed, pleasant atmosphere can help to reduce the client's stress and promote a feeling of well-being, which tends to improve appetite and oral intake.
Providing small rather than large meals can enable a client who is weak or fatigues easily to finish a meal. In addition, a client who has a poor appetite is often more willing to attempt to eat smaller meals because they seem less overwhelming than larger ones. If smaller meals are served, the number of meals per day should be increased to help ensure adequate nutrition.
Helps reduce dyspnea and feeling of fullness (a high-Fowler's position may be too uncomfortable if ascites is severe).
Appetite is also suppressed if foods/fluids normally served hot or warm become cold and do not appeal to the client.
Drinking liquids with meals distends the stomach and may cause satiety before an adequate amount of food is consumed.
Activity usually promotes a sense of well-being, which can improve appetite.
The client should understand what foods and fluids will improve nutritional status.

NDx = NANDA Diagnosis   **D** = Delegatable Action   ● = UAP   ✦ = LVN/LPN   ⊖▶ = Go to ⊖volve for animation

Continued...

THERAPEUTIC INTERVENTIONS	RATIONALE
• Avoid skipping meals.	*Skipping meals reduces caloric intake.*
• Consume a diet high in calories (2000–3000 calories/day) and carbohydrates.	*A high-calorie and high-carbohydrate diet will improve the client's nutritional status.*
• Limit protein intake with hepatic encephalopathy.	*Changes in the client's metabolism due to liver failure can cause hepatic encephalopathy, because ammonia is not metabolized and passes through the liver unchanged and can become a cerebral toxin.*
• Consume meals that are well balanced and high in essential nutrients.	*The client must consume a diet that is well balanced and high in essential nutrients to meet nutritional needs.*

Dependent/Collaborative Actions

Implement measures to improve nutritional status:

• Implement measures to restore fluid volume (e.g., restrict sodium intake; maintain fluid restrictions as ordered; administer diuretics as ordered).	*Reduces fluid in the peritoneal cavity and subsequently reduces the feeling of fullness*
• Administer vitamins and minerals (e.g., fat-soluble vitamins, thiamine, folic acid, iron), if ordered.	*Vitamins and minerals are needed to maintain metabolic functioning. If the client's dietary intake does not provide adequate amounts of them, oral and/or parenteral supplements may be necessary.*
• Instruct client to use herbs, spices, and salt substitutes (if approved by a physician).	*Use of spices makes low-sodium diet more palatable.*
• Obtain a dietary consult if necessary.	*A dietitian is best able to evaluate whether the foods/fluids selected will meet the client's nutritional needs.*
• Perform a calorie count if ordered. Report information to the dietitian and physician.	*A calorie count provides information about the caloric and nutritional value of the foods/fluids the client consumes. This information helps the dietitian and physician determine whether an alternative method of nutritional support is needed.*
• Consult physician about an alternative method of providing nutrition (e.g., parenteral nutrition, tube feeding) if client does not consume enough food or fluids to meet nutritional needs.	*If the client's oral intake is inadequate, an alternative method of providing nutrients needs to be implemented.*

Nursing Diagnosis | # IMPAIRED COMFORT NDx (PRURITUS)

Definition: Perceived lack of ease, relief, and transcendence in physical, psychospiritual, environmental, cultural, and/or social dimensions.

Related to: Stimulation of itch receptors in the skin by bile acid metabolites that accumulate in the blood as a result of bile flow obstruction

CLINICAL MANIFESTATIONS

Subjective	Objective
Self-report of skin itching	Persistent scratching or rubbing of skin

RISK FACTOR	DESIRED OUTCOMES
• Illness-related symptoms	The client will experience relief of pruritus, as evidenced by: a. Verbalization of same b. No scratching or rubbing of skin

NOC OUTCOMES	NIC INTERVENTIONS
Comfort status: symptom control	Pruritus management

NURSING ASSESSMENT	RATIONALE
Assess for the following: • Reports of itchiness • Persistent scratching or rubbing of skin	*Early recognition of signs and symptoms of pruritus allows for prompt intervention.*

THERAPEUTIC INTERVENTIONS	RATIONALE

Independent Actions

Instruct client in and/or implement measures to relieve pruritus:

• Apply cool, moist compresses to pruritic areas. **D** ● ✦	*Cold/cool compresses provide a counter sensation that decreases the urge to rub or scratch the area.*
• Apply emollient creams or ointments frequently. **D** ● ✦	*Creams and ointments prevent dryness.*
• Add emollients, cornstarch, or baking soda to bath water. **D** ● ✦	*Use of these products in bath water reduces skin dryness and provides a protective barrier.*
• Use tepid water and mild soaps for bathing. **D** ● ✦	*Use of tepid water and mild soaps decreases skin dryness.*
• Pat skin dry after bathing, making sure to dry thoroughly. **D** ● ✦	*Rubbing of the skin with a towel after a bath can stimulate itching.*
• Maintain a cool environment. **D** ● ✦	*A cool environment provides a counter sensation that decreases urge to rub or scratch.*
• Encourage participation in diversional activity including watching TV, listening to music, mindfulness-based relaxation.	*Distracts client from focusing on the itch.*
• Implement cutaneous stimulation techniques (e.g., massage, pressure, vibration, stroking with soft brush) at sites of itching or acupressure points.	*Cutaneous stimulation blocks the neurotransmission of the itch sensation.*
• Encourage client to wear loose cotton garments and avoid clothes or blankets made from wool.	*Wearing loose clothing and non-wool blankets decreases skin irritation.*

Dependent/Collaborative Actions

Instruct client in and/or implement measures to relieve pruritus:

• Administer the following medications if ordered: • Antihistamines (e.g., diphenhydramine, hydroxyzine [Atarax])	*Antihistamines block histamine, which stimulates itchy sensations.*
• Bile acid–sequestering agents (e.g., cholestyramine).	*Bile acid–sequestering agents bind with the bile acids in the intestines, prevent absorption, and enhance elimination, thereby decreasing itch sensations.*
Consult appropriate health care provider (e.g., clinical nurse specialist, physician) if aforementioned measures fail to alleviate pruritus or if the skin becomes excoriated.	*Notification of the appropriate health care provider allows for prompt modification in treatment plan.*

Nursing Diagnosis ## ACTIVITY INTOLERANCE NDx

Definition: Insufficient physiologic or psychological energy to endure or complete required or desired daily activities.

Related to:

• Tissue hypoxia associated with anemia resulting from:
  • Decreased production of red blood cells (RBCs), resulting from a decreased intake and absorption of vitamins and minerals and an inability of the liver to store vitamins and minerals
  • Excessive RBC destruction resulting from hypersplenism (if venous congestion has resulted in splenomegaly, the spleen will destroy RBCs faster than usual)
  • Blood loss if bleeding has occurred
• Loss of muscle mass, tone, and strength associated with malnutrition and disuse if mobility has been limited for an extended period
• Decrease in available energy associated with inability of the liver to metabolize glucose, fats, and proteins properly
• Difficulty resting and sleeping associated with dyspnea, discomfort, frequent assessments and treatments, fear, anxiety, and unfamiliar environment

---

NDx = NANDA Diagnosis   **D** = Delegatable Action   ● = UAP   ✦ = LVN/LPN   ⊖▶ = Go to ⊖volve for animation

CLINICAL MANIFESTATIONS

Subjective	Objective
Self-report of fatigue or weakness	Abnormal heart rate or B/P response to activity; exertional discomfort or dyspnea; ECG changes reflecting dysrhythmias or ischemia; unable to speak during physical activity

RISK FACTORS

- Chronic illness
- Poor nutritional status
- Immobility
- Impaired digestive processes

DESIRED OUTCOMES

The client will demonstrate an increased tolerance for activity, as evidenced by:
a. Verbalization of feeling less fatigued and weak
b. Ability to perform activities of daily living without exertional dyspnea, chest pain, diaphoresis, dizziness, and significant changes in vital signs

NOC OUTCOMES

Rest; energy conservation; activity tolerance

NIC INTERVENTIONS

Energy management; oxygen therapy; nutrition management; sleep enhancement

NURSING ASSESSMENT

Assess for signs and symptoms of activity intolerance:
- Statements of fatigue or weakness
- Exertional dyspnea, chest pain
- Diaphoresis or dizziness
- Abnormal heart rate response to activity (e.g., increase in rate of 20 beats/min above resting rate, rate not returning to preactivity level within 3 minutes after stopping activity, change from regular to irregular rate)
- Significant change (15-20 mm Hg) in B/P with change in activity level.

RATIONALE

Early recognition of signs and symptoms of activity intolerance allows for prompt intervention.

THERAPEUTIC INTERVENTIONS

Independent Actions
Implement measures to improve activity tolerance:
- Perform actions to promote rest and/or conserve energy
- Maintain prescribed activity restrictions.
- Minimize environmental activity and noise. **D** ● ✦
- Provide uninterrupted rest periods. **D** ● ✦
- Assist with care. **D** ● ✦
- Keep supplies and personal articles within easy reach. **D** ● ✦
- Limit the number of visitors.
- Instruct client in energy-saving techniques (e.g., using a shower chair when showering, sitting to brush teeth or comb hair).

- Implement measures to reduce fear and anxiety (e.g., assure client that staff are nearby, explain all tests and procedures, encourage verbalization of fear and anxiety).
- Implement measures to promote sleep (e.g., elevate head of bed and support arms on pillows to facilitate breathing; discourage intake of fluids high in caffeine, especially in the evening; encourage relaxing diversional activities in the evening).

- Implement measures to reduce discomfort (e.g., proper positioning). **D** ✦

RATIONALE

Cells use oxygen and fat, protein, and carbohydrate to produce the energy needed for all body activities. Rest and activities that conserve energy result in a lower metabolic rate, which preserves nutrients and oxygen for necessary activities. These actions promote energy conservation and rest.
Avoids stress due to inability to obtain desired objects and prevents potential for client injury.
Allows for rest and decreases exposure to potential infectious organism.
These techniques help client to maintain activities of daily living while decreasing fatigue.
Fear and anxiety interfere with a client's ability to rest.

Increased hours of sleep improve the client's ability to increase level of activity.

Decreasing discomfort improves the client's ability to perform activities and to rest.

THERAPEUTIC INTERVENTIONS	RATIONALE
• Discourage smoking and excessive intake of beverages high in caffeine such as coffee, tea, and colas.	*Both nicotine and excessive caffeine intake can increase cardiac workload and myocardial oxygen utilization, thereby decreasing the amount of oxygen necessary for energy production.*
• Implement measures to improve respiratory status (e.g., encourage use of incentive spirometer; elevate head of bed; assist with turning, coughing, and deep breathing) if ineffective breathing pattern, ineffective airway clearance, or impaired gas exchange is contributing to client's activity intolerance.	*Altered respiratory function can lead to inadequate tissue oxygenation, which results in less efficient energy production and a reduced ability to tolerate activity. Improving respiratory status increases the amount of oxygen available for energy production. It also eases the work of breathing, which reduces energy expenditure.*

Dependent/Collaborative Actions

Implement measures to improve activity tolerance:

• Implement measures to maintain an adequate nutritional status (e.g., provide a diet high in essential nutrients, provide dietary supplements as indicated, administer vitamins and minerals as ordered).	*Metabolism is the process by which nutrients are transformed into energy. If nutrition is inadequate, energy production is decreased, which subsequently reduces one's ability to tolerate activity.*
• Implement measures to treat anemia, if present (e.g., administer prescribed iron, folic acid, and/or vitamin B$_{12}$; administer packed RBCs as ordered).	*Anemia reduces the oxygen-carrying capacity of the blood. Resolution of anemia increases oxygen availability to the cells, which increases the efficiency of energy production and subsequently improves activity tolerance.*
• Implement measures to promote sleep (e.g., maintain oxygen therapy during sleep, administer sleep aids and analgesics).	*Improves tissue oxygenation.* *Improves client's ability to rest/sleep.*
• Increase client's activity gradually as allowed and tolerated.	
Instruct client to report a decreased tolerance for activity and to stop any activity that causes chest pain, a marked increase in shortness of breath, dizziness, or extreme fatigue or weakness.	*Progressive activity helps strengthen the myocardium, which enhances cardiac output and improves activity tolerance.* *Changes in a client's activity tolerance may indicate worsening disease process or inadequate treatment regimen.*
Consult physician if signs and symptoms of activity intolerance persist or worsen.	*Notification of the physician allows for prompt modification of the treatment plan.*

Collaborative/Nursing Diagnosis **ACUTE CONFUSION** NDx **AND CHRONIC CONFUSION** NDx

Definition: **Acute Confusion NDx:** Reversible disturbances of consciousness, attention, cognition and perception that develop over a short period of time, and which last less than 3 months; **Chronic Confusion NDx:** Irreversible, progressive, insidious, and long-term alteration of intellect, behavior and personality, manifested by impairment in cognitive functions (memory, speech, language, decisionmaking, and executive function), and dependency in execution of daily activities

Related to: Disturbances in central nervous system functioning associated with accumulation of toxic substances (e.g., ammonia) in the brain, toxic effects of long-term alcohol use, deficiencies of certain vitamins (e.g., thiamine), and hypoxia if anemia is moderate to severe

CLINICAL MANIFESTATIONS

Subjective	Objective
N/A	Alteration in behavior, personality, short- and long-term memory, social functioning, inability to perform at least one daily activity; and cognitive impairment

RISK FACTORS

- Alcohol use
- Inability of body to remove toxins
- Poor nutritional status
- Impaired metabolic functioning
- Functional impairment
- Age > 60 years old
- Infection

DESIRED OUTCOMES

The client will demonstrate decreased confusion, as evidenced by:
a. Improved ability to grasp ideas
b. Improved short- and long-term memory
c. Longer attention span
d. Absence or resolution of inappropriate behavior
e. Oriented to person, place, and time

NOC OUTCOMES

Cognitive orientation

NIC INTERVENTIONS

Environmental management; environmental management: safety behavioral management

NURSING ASSESSMENT

Assess for episodes of disorientation to person, place, and time; episodes of inappropriate behavior; impaired decision-making ability; impaired attention span, inability to perform one or more daily activities

RATIONALE

Early recognition of signs and symptoms of confusion allows for prompt intervention.

THERAPEUTIC INTERVENTIONS

RATIONALE

Dependent/Collaborative Actions
Implement measures to maintain optimal thought processes:

- Perform actions to improve nutritional status (e.g., provide a diet high in essential nutrients, provide dietary supplements as indicated, administer vitamins and minerals as ordered). **D** ✦

- Perform actions to prevent or manage hepatic coma (e.g., prevent constipation, decrease potential for gastrointestinal hemorrhage, maintain fluid and electrolytes).

- Administer central nervous system depressants such as opioids, sedative-hypnotics, and antianxiety agents with extreme caution; question any order for a normal adult dose of these medications. **D** ✦

- Administer thiamine if ordered. **D** ✦

- Maintain oxygen therapy as ordered.

If client shows evidence of confusion or disorientation:
- Speak to the client by name. **D** ● ✦

- Reorient client to person, place, and time as necessary **D** ● ✦
- Place familiar objects, clock, and calendar within client's view. **D** ● ✦
- Approach client in a slow, calm manner; allow adequate time for communication. **D** ● ✦
- Repeat instructions as necessary using clear, simple language and short sentences.
- Maintain a consistent and fairly structured routine, and write out a schedule of activities for client to refer to if desired.
- Have client perform only one activity at a time, and allow adequate time for performance of activities. **D** ● ✦
- Encourage client to make lists of planned activities, questions, and concerns.
- Assist client to problem solve if necessary.

Provides vitamins and minerals that are essential for normal neurologic functioning and treatment of anemia which improves oxygenation.

These actions eliminate or control levels of ammonia and other nitrogenous substances which impair cognitive functioning.

Liver damage associated with cirrhosis reduces normal drug metabolism and may lead to increased serum blood levels/toxicity of these medications. Medications may also cause cognitive impairment.
Thiamine is essential for appropriate neurologic functioning and binds with iron which helps to decrease the iron load on the liver.
Helps maintain appropriate tissue oxygenation.

The client may respond to name even when unable to recognize others.
Frequent reorientation may provide the client with a sense of security.
Placing familiar objects helps to orient client and provides a sense of security.
These actions help the client remain calm and increase appropriate communication.
Repetition of information increases potential for client understanding.

Structure provides a sense of security and ability to cope with cognitive changes.

Decreases client's risk of becoming confused and subsequently frustrated in performing multiple activities.
Structure provides the client with a sense of security.

Provides client some control over the situation.

THERAPEUTIC INTERVENTIONS	RATIONALE
• Maintain realistic expectations of client's ability to learn, comprehend, and remember information provided; provide client with a written copy of instructions.	*Decreases frustration of client, significant others, and nurses.*
• Encourage significant others to be supportive of client. Instruct them in methods of dealing with client's confusion.	*Decreases client and family frustration and agitation. Allows client's significant others to be involved in care and improves their understanding of the situation,*
• Inform client and significant others that cognitive and emotional functioning may to improve with treatment.	*Provides hope to client and significant others for the client's future cognitive abilities.*
Consult physician if disturbed thought processes worsen.	*Notification of the physician allows for prompt modification of the treatment plan.*

Nursing Diagnosis | **RISK FOR BLEEDING** NDx

Definition: Susceptible to a decrease in blood volume, which may compromise health.

Related to:
• Decreased production of clotting factors associated with impaired liver function and decreased available vitamin K (can occur from malnutrition, antimicrobials that suppress activity of intestinal flora, and impaired absorption of vitamin K as a result of bile flow obstruction)
• Thrombocytopenia associated with hypersplenism (if venous congestion has resulted in splenomegaly, the spleen will destroy platelets faster than usual)

NOC OUTCOMES	NIC INTERVENTIONS
Blood coagulation	Bleeding precautions; blood products administration

CLINICAL MANIFESTATIONS

Subjective	**Objective**
Verbalization of unusual joint pain and fatigue	Petechiae, purpura, and ecchymoses; gingival bleeding; prolonged bleeding from puncture sites; epistaxis, hemoptysis; further increase in abdominal girth; frank or occult blood in the stool, urine, or vomitus; menorrhagia; restlessness, confusion; hypotension and tachycardia; decrease in Hct and Hgb levels

RISK FACTORS
• Poor nutritional status
• Lack of clotting factors
• Early destruction of blood cells
• Gastrointestinal condition
• Impaired liver function

DESIRED OUTCOMES

The client will not experience unusual bleeding, as evidenced by:
a. Skin and mucous membranes free of petechiae, purpura, ecchymoses, and active bleeding
b. Absence of unusual joint pain
c. No further increase in abdominal girth
d. Absence of frank and occult blood in stool, urine, and vomitus
e. Usual menstrual flow
f. Vital signs within normal range for client
g. Stable or improved Hct and Hgb levels
h. No change in client's energy status

NDx = NANDA Diagnosis   **D** = Delegatable Action   ● = UAP   ✦ = LVN/LPN   ⊖▶ = Go to ⊖volve for animation

NURSING ASSESSMENT	RATIONALE
Assess client for and report signs and symptoms of unusual bleeding: • Petechiae, purpura, ecchymoses • Gingival bleeding • Prolonged bleeding from puncture sites • Epistaxis, hemoptysis • Unusual joint pain • Further increase in abdominal girth • Frank or occult blood in the stool, urine, or vomitus • Menorrhagia • Restlessness, confusion • Decreasing B/P and increased pulse rate • Decrease in Hct and Hgb levels Monitor platelet count and coagulation test results (e.g., prothrombin time or international normalized ratio [INR], activated partial thromboplastin time, bleeding time). Report abnormal values.	*Early recognition of signs and symptoms of bleeding allows for prompt intervention.*

THERAPEUTIC INTERVENTIONS	RATIONALE
Dependent/Collaborative Actions Implement measures to reduce bleeding: • Perform actions to reduce risk of bleeding from esophageal varices (e.g., reduce excess fluid volume; avoid straining to have a bowel movement, coughing, sneezing, lifting heavy objects; avoid spicy foods or ones that may cause trauma to the esophagus).	*These actions reduce pressure or irritation on esophageal vessels.*
• Avoid giving injections whenever possible; consult physician about prescribing an alternative route for medications ordered to be given intramuscularly or subcutaneously.	*May cause increased and unnecessary bleeding.*
• When giving injections or performing venous or arterial punctures, use the smallest-gauge needle possible and apply gentle, prolonged pressure to the site after the needle is removed.	*Helps to decrease bleeding from puncture sites.*
• Caution client to avoid activities that increase the risk for trauma (e.g., shaving with a straight-edge razor, using stiff bristle toothbrush or dental floss).	*Cuts or mucous membrane irritation, even minor ones, may cause excessive bleeding.*
• Whenever possible, avoid intubations (e.g., nasogastric) and procedures that can cause injury to the rectal mucosa (e.g., taking temperature rectally, inserting a rectal suppository, administering an enema).	*Decreases bleeding associated with trauma.*
• Pad side rails if client is confused or restless.	*Decreases risk for client injury.*
• Perform actions to prevent injury (e.g., keep bed in low position; keep needed items within easy reach; assist with ambulation; keep floor clear of clutter; provide ambulatory aids).	
• Instruct client to avoid blowing nose forcefully or straining to have a bowel movement; consult physician about an order for a decongestant and/or laxative if indicated.	*Reduces pressure in esophageal vessels.*

• Administer the following if ordered:
  • Vitamin K injections
  • Platelets
  • Fresh frozen plasma (FFP)
  • Cryoprecipitate
	Administration of these medications improves clotting ability.

If bleeding occurs and does not subside spontaneously: • Apply firm, prolonged pressure to bleeding area(s) if possible.	*Each action enhances the body's clotting ability.*

THERAPEUTIC INTERVENTIONS	RATIONALE
• If epistaxis occurs, place client in a high-Fowler's position and apply pressure and ice pack to nasal area.	*Application of pressure and ice packs to the nose increases potential for clotting.*
• Maintain oxygen therapy as ordered.	*Improves oxygenation.*
• Administer vitamin K (e.g., phytonadione) injections, whole blood, or blood products (e.g., FFP, platelets) as ordered.	*Enhances or replaces clotting factors.*
• Assess for and report signs and symptoms of hypovolemic shock (e.g., restlessness; confusion; significant decrease in B/P; rapid, weak pulse; rapid respirations; cool skin; urine output <30 mL/h).	*Notifying the physician allows for prompt modification of the treatment plan.*

Collaborative Diagnosis **RISK FOR ASCITES**

Definition: An abnormal accumulation of fluid in the peritoneal cavity.

Related to:
• Low plasma colloid osmotic pressure associated with hypoalbuminemia (a result of decreased hepatic synthesis of albumin and prolonged inadequate nutrition)
• Increased pressure in the portal system and hepatic lymph system associated with blood flow backup resulting from structural changes in the liver
• A generalized increase in hydrostatic pressure associated with excess fluid volume

CLINICAL MANIFESTATIONS

Subjective	**Objective**
Verbalization of abdominal pressure and discomfort	Increasing abdominal girth; dull percussion note over the abdomen; abdominal fluid wave; protruding umbilicus; bulging flanks; dyspnea

RISK FACTORS
• Poor nutritional status
• Chronic illness
• Impaired synthesis of proteins
• Hyperaldosteronism
• Alcoholism

DESIRED OUTCOMES

The client will have decreased ascites, if present, as evidenced by:
a. Decrease in abdominal girth
b. Abdominal percussion note more tympanic

NURSING ASSESSMENT	RATIONALE
Assess for signs and symptoms of ascites: • Increase in abdominal girth (daily measurement of abdominal girth should be done at the same time and in the same location on the abdomen with client in the same position) • Dull percussion note over abdomen with finding of shifting dullness • Presence of abdominal fluid wave • Protruding umbilicus and bulging flanks	*Early recognition of the signs and symptoms of ascites allows for prompt treatment.*

THERAPEUTIC INTERVENTIONS	RATIONALE
Dependent/Collaborative Actions Perform actions to reduce excess fluid volume, promote mobilization of fluid back into the vascular space, and prevent further third-spacing by: • Restrict sodium intake as ordered. • Maintain fluid restrictions if ordered.	*These actions decrease fluid retention.*

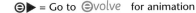

NDx = NANDA Diagnosis   **D** = Delegatable Action   ● = UAP   ✦ = LVN/LPN   ⊜▶ = Go to ⊜volve for animation

Continued...

THERAPEUTIC INTERVENTIONS	RATIONALE
• Encourage client to rest periodically in a recumbent position. **D** ✦	*Lying down reduces peripheral pooling of blood, which increases effective circulating volume and renal blood flow and subsequently promotes diuresis.*
• Administer diuretics if ordered (e.g., potassium-sparing diuretics such as spironolactone and amiloride are often used initially). **D** ✦	*Diuretics reduce fluid volume by increasing urinary output, and improve renal blood flow, which increases water excretion and reduces activation of the renin-angiotensin-aldosterone mechanism.*
If signs and symptoms of ascites are present and persist or worsen:	
• Consult physician.	*Notification of the physician allows for prompt modification of treatment plan.*
• Assist with paracentesis.	*Paracentesis removes fluid from abdomen.*
• Administer albumin infusions if ordered.	*Albumin increases colloid osmotic pressure and pulls fluid back into the vascular system.*
• Prepare client for a portal systemic shunt procedure (e.g., transjugular intrahepatic portosystemic shunt [TIPS]), if planned.	*Informing clients about the procedure helps to reduce anxiety.* *This procedure decreases portal hypertension and subsequently reduces ascites.*
• Administer vitamin K and blood products, if ordered.	*Vitamin K and blood products improve the body's clotting ability.*
If signs and symptoms of bleeding esophageal varices occur:	
• Turn client on side and suction as necessary.	*Reduces risk of aspiration.*
• Maintain oxygen therapy as ordered.	*Improves cellular oxygenation.*
• Assist with administration of octreotide (Sandostatin) or vasopressin, if ordered (nitroglycerin is often given with vasopressin).	*Octreotide and vasopressin cause constriction of the splanchnic vessels and reduce blood flow to the portal vein.* *Nitroglycerin lowers portal pressure and reduces vasoconstrictor side effects of vasopressin.*
• Prepare client for endoscopic sclerotherapy or ligation of varices, if planned.	*Knowing what may happen during a procedure may reduce fear and anxiety.*
• Assist with insertion of a gastroesophageal balloon tube (e.g., Sengstaken-Blakemore tube); maintain balloon pressure and suction and perform lavage as ordered.	*A gastroesophageal balloon tube places pressure on the esophageal varices to decrease bleeding and increase clotting.*
• Administer vitamin K (e.g., phytonadione) injections, whole blood, or blood products (e.g., FFP, platelets) as ordered.	*Vitamin K, blood, and blood products increase the body's clotting ability.*
• Prepare client for a TIPS or surgery (e.g., esophageal transection with reanastomosis, distal splenorenal shunt), if planned.	*Reduces client's fear and anxiety.*

Collaborative Diagnosis   RISK FOR HEPATIC (PORTAL-SYSTEMIC) ENCEPHALOPATHY (HEPATIC COMA)

Definition: Central nervous system damage associated with liver disease.

Related to:
- Altered brain function associated with:
  - The effect of toxic end products of intestinal protein digestion (e.g., ammonia) on the brain
  - Replacement of true neurotransmitters by false neurotransmitters
  - Increased brain sensitivity to certain substances (e.g., benzodiazepines, γ-aminobutyric acid [GABA])
- Decreased activity of urea cycle enzymes if zinc deficiency is present

CLINICAL MANIFESTATIONS

Subjective	Objective
Verbalization of weakness and lethargy	Changes in fine motor movements such as handwriting and drawing; asterixis; slowed or slurred speech; emotional liability; agitation; belligerence; disorientation; fetor hepaticus; unresponsiveness; increased serum ammonia level

RISK FACTORS
- Inability of body to remove toxins
- Hypokalemia
- Medication regimen

DESIRED OUTCOMES

The client will not develop hepatic encephalopathy, as evidenced by:
a. Usual speech and handwriting
b. Usual mental status
c. Absence of asterixis and fetor hepaticus
d. Serum ammonia level within normal range

NURSING ASSESSMENT

Assess for and report signs and symptoms of hepatic encephalopathy (e.g., change in handwriting, inability to draw simple figures or numbers, asterixis, slow or slurred speech, inability to concentrate, emotional lability, disordered sleep, agitation, belligerence, disorientation, lethargy, fetor hepaticus [musty or fruity odor on breath], unresponsiveness).

Monitor serum ammonia levels; report elevated values.

RATIONALE

Early recognition of signs and symptoms of hepatic encephalopathy allows for prompt intervention.

Increased serum ammonia levels are an indication of declining liver function, and it is no longer able to change ammonia to urea.

THERAPEUTIC INTERVENTIONS

Dependent/Collaborative Actions
Implement measures to reduce the risk for hepatic coma:
- Perform actions to eliminate or control the following conditions that increase levels of ammonia and other nitrogenous substances:
  - Constipation

  - Gastrointestinal hemorrhage

  - Hypokalemia and/or metabolic alkalosis
  - Renal failure
  - Excessive protein intake
  - Eat small frequent meals

  - Infection
  - Dehydration/hypovolemia

  - If client is to receive blood transfusions, request fresh rather than stored blood.
- Consult physician about discontinuation of prescribed medications that are potential hepatotoxins (e.g., isoniazid, amiodarone, 6-mercaptopurine, erythromycin, phenytoin).
- Administer central nervous system depressants such as opioids, sedative-hypnotics, and antianxiety agents with extreme caution.

If signs and symptoms of hepatic encephalopathy occur:
- Maintain client on strict bedrest.
- Maintain dietary protein restrictions as ordered; increase protein intake slowly as encephalopathy resolves
- Encourage intake of vegetable proteins rather than animal proteins.
- Ensure a high carbohydrate (CHO) intake or administer intravenous (IV) glucose or tube feedings as ordered.
- Administer enemas and/or cathartics as ordered.

RATIONALE

Results in increased formation and absorption of ammonia and mercaptans from the gut.
Intestinal bacteria convert the protein in blood to ammonia and other nitrogenous substances.
These conditions contribute to increased levels of ammonia.
Decreases excretion of ammonia.
Intestinal bacteria convert protein to ammonia and other nitrogenous substances. Ammonia levels increase when the liver is unable to change ammonia to urea.
Small meals prevent protein loading.
Bacteria that produce urease break urea into ammonia.
Reduced blood flow to the liver results in decreased detoxification of ammonia and other toxins.
Stored blood contains more ammonia and citrate.

Discontinuation of hepatotoxic medications prevent further liver damage.

Many of these agents are metabolized in the liver and may precipitate nonnitrogenous coma.

Rest reduces metabolic demands on the liver.
Vegetable proteins are less ammonia genic.
Protein loading increases production of ammonia.

A high CHO intake or IV glucose provides a rapid energy source and decreases metabolism of endogenous proteins.
Enemas and/or cathartics hasten expulsion of intestinal contents so that bacteria have less time to convert proteins to ammonia and other nitrogenous substances.

Continued...

THERAPEUTIC INTERVENTIONS	RATIONALE
• Administer the following medications if ordered:	
• Antimicrobials that suppress activity of the intestinal flora (e.g., neomycin, metronidazole)	*Antimicrobials suppress activity of intestinal flora, which decreases protein breakdown in the intestine and thus reducing the production of ammonia.*
• Lactulose	*Promotes excretion of ammonia in the stool, decreases the pH value of colon to less than 6, thereby decreasing absorption of ammonia, promotes growth of healthy bacteria, decreases ammonia production, and increases assimilation of nitrogenous products by bacteria.*
• Probiotics	*Probiotics may enhance tolerance the protein load, lower ammonia levels, and improve neurologic symptoms*
• Zinc supplements	*Stimulates ureagenesis (several enzymes in the urea cycle are zinc dependent) and improves psychometric performance in patients with hepatic encephalopathy.* *Zinc supplementation might play an important role in the prevention of hepatic encephalopathy by activating glutamine synthetase.*
• Institute general safety precautions	*Prevents client injury.*

Nursing Diagnosis   **RISK FOR SPIRITUAL DISTRESS** NDx

Definition: Susceptible to an impaired ability to experience and integrate meaning and purpose in life through connectedness within self, literature, nature, and/or a power greater than oneself, which may compromise health.

Related to:
• Chronic illness
• Increased dependence upon others
• Increased risk of death
• Loss of normal body function

CLINICAL MANIFESTATIONS

Subjective	Objective
Self-report of hopelessness; despair, spiritual distress	Disengagement in activities that used to bring client joy; change in client's routine activities; depression, inability to forgive; changes in relationships

RISK FACTORS
• Chronic illness	• Increased risk of death
• Loss of independence	• Failure of body's regulatory mechanisms

NOC OUTCOMES	NIC INTERVENTIONS
Spiritual Health	Spiritual Support

NURSING ASSESSMENT	RATIONALE
Observe client for actions that indicate difficulties in finding meaning and purpose in life	*Early recognition of signs and symptoms of spiritual distress allows for prompt interventions.*

THERAPEUTIC INTERVENTIONS	RATIONALE
Independent Actions	
Identify client's religious or spiritual beliefs.	*Provides a baseline for understanding client's preferences and planning of care.*
Provide a calm, peaceful environment.	*May allow client and family to express feelings.*
Be actively present and listen to client's concerns related to loss of independence, hopelessness, and helplessness.	*It is important to understand client and family perspective.*

THERAPEUTIC INTERVENTIONS	RATIONALE
Use therapeutic communication skills of nonjudgmental active listening.	*May help client to verbalize concerns and determine solutions.*
Provide opportunities for client and family to participate in mediation, prayer, and spiritual activities.	*Provides for healing of past and present client concerns.*
Dependent/Collaborative Actions	
Consult client's spiritual advisor (if present), pastoral care, or crisis counseling.	*Provides others to help support client and family in dealing with illness and its impact on the individual and family.*
Encourage client and family to participate in support groups.	*Allows client and family members to interact and communicate with others experiencing same or similar situations.*

Nursing Diagnosis INEFFECTIVE FAMILY HEALTH MANAGEMENT NDx

Definition: A pattern of regulating and integrating into family processes a program for the treatment of illness and its sequelae of illness that is unsatisfactory for meeting specific health goals of the family unit.

CLINICAL MANIFESTATIONS

Subjective	**Objective**
Self-report of inability to manage illness; verbalizes inability to follow prescribed regimen	Inaccurate follow-through with instructions; inappropriate behaviors

RISK FACTORS

- Ineffective family process
- Change in lifestyle
- Chronic illness
- Economically disadvantaged

DESIRED OUTCOMES

The client and significant other will demonstrate the probability of effective therapeutic regimen management, as evidenced by:
a. Willingness to learn about and participate in treatment plan and care
b. Statements reflecting ways to modify personal habits and integrate treatments into lifestyle
c. Statements reflecting an understanding of the implications of not following the prescribed treatment plan

NOC OUTCOMES

Compliance behavior; treatment behavior: illness or injury; knowledge: treatment regimen; health beliefs: perceived resources; perceived ability to perform

NIC INTERVENTIONS

Self-modification assistance; values clarification; substance use treatment; teaching: prescribed diet; financial resource assistance; support system enhancement

NURSING ASSESSMENT	RATIONALE
Assess for indications that the client and significant others may be unable to manage the therapeutic regimen effectively:	*Allows the nurse to tailor the client's education based on client's and significant others' abilities and concerns.*
• Statements reflecting inability to manage care at home	
• Failure to adhere to treatment plan (e.g., not adhering to dietary modifications and fluid restrictions, refusing medications)	
• Statements reflecting a lack of understanding of the factors that will cause further progression of liver failure	
• Statements reflecting an unwillingness or inability to modify personal habits and integrate necessary treatments into lifestyle	
• Statements reflecting the view that cirrhosis has resolved once he/she is feeling better or that there is no way to control the disease and efforts to comply with treatments are useless	

NDx = NANDA Diagnosis   **D** = Delegatable Action   ● = UAP   ✦ = LVN/LPN   ⊝▶ = Go to ⊝volve for animation

THERAPEUTIC INTERVENTIONS	RATIONALE
Independent Actions Implement measures to promote effective therapeutic regimen management:	
• Explain cirrhosis in terms the client and significant others can understand; stress that cirrhosis is a chronic disease and adherence to the treatment plan is necessary to delay and/or prevent complications.	*Increased knowledge about the disease process and self-care will improve adherence.*
• Encourage questions and clarify misconceptions about cirrhosis and its effects.	
• Encourage participation in the treatment plan.	*Improves sense of control and ability to care for self once discharged*
• Provide instructions on weighing self and calculating dietary sodium and protein content; allow time for return demonstration.	*Important to know whether a significant weight gain is occurring, which can represent increased fluid retention.*
• Determine areas of difficulty and misunderstanding and reinforce teaching as necessary.	*Increasing knowledge about the disease process and self-care will improve adherence.*
• Provide written instructions about scheduled appointments with health care provider, medications, signs and symptoms to report, weighing self, and dietary modifications.	*Provides information resource for client and significant others to refer to as needed after discharge.*
• Assist client and significant others to identify ways treatments can be incorporated into lifestyle; focus on modifications of lifestyle rather than complete change.	*Improves adherence to treatment regimen if client and significant others determines how lifestyle can be modified.*
• Encourage client and significant others to discuss concerns about the cost of hospitalization, medications, and lifelong follow-up care; obtain a social service consult to assist with financial planning and to obtain financial aid if indicated.	*Allows for clarification of issues and support in dealing with chronic illness.*
• Provide information about and encourage utilization of community resources that can assist client to make necessary lifestyle changes (e.g., drug and alcohol rehabilitation programs).	*Provides ongoing assistance following discharged.*
• Reinforce behaviors suggesting future compliance with the therapeutic regimen (e.g., statements reflecting plans for integrating treatments into lifestyle, participation in diet planning, statements reflecting an understanding of the importance of eliminating alcohol intake).	*Enhances client's and significant others' self-confidence for self-care and adherence to treatment regimen.*
• Include significant others in explanations and teaching sessions and encourage their support; reinforce the need for client to assume responsibility for managing as much of care as possible.	*Enhances potential for adherence to the treatment regimen.*
Consult appropriate health care provider (e.g., social worker, physician) about referrals to community agencies if continued instruction, support, or supervision is needed.	*Provides a multidisciplinary approach to care following discharge.*

DISCHARGE TEACHING/CONTINUED CARE

Nursing Diagnosis   **DEFICIENT KNOWLEDGE** NDx; **INEFFECTIVE HEALTH MANAGEMENT*** NDx

Definition: **Deficient Knowledge NDx:** Absence of cognitive information related to a specific topic, or its acquisition.
Ineffective Health Management NDx: Pattern of regulating and integrating into daily living a therapeutic regimen for the treatment of illness and its sequelae that is unsatisfactory for meeting specific health goals.

---

*The nurse should select the diagnostic label that is most appropriate for the client's discharge teaching needs.

CLINICAL MANIFESTATIONS

Subjective	Objective
Self-report of inability to manage illness; verbalizes inability to follow prescribed regimen	Inaccurate follow-through with instructions; inappropriate behaviors; experience of manageable complications of cirrhosis

RISK FACTORS

- Cognitive deficit
- Financial concerns
- Failure to take action to reduce risk factors for complications of cirrhosis
- Inability to care for oneself
- Difficulty in modifying personal habits and integrating treatments into lifestyle
- Difficulty navigate complex health care systems

NOC OUTCOMES	NIC INTERVENTIONS
Knowledge: diet; disease process; treatment regimen	Health system guidance; teaching: individual; teaching: disease process; teaching: prescribed diet; teaching: prescribed activity/exercise substance abuse treatment

NURSING ASSESSMENT	RATIONALE
Assess the client's ability to learn and readiness to learn. Assess the client's understanding of teaching.	*Learning is more effective when the client is motivated and understands the importance of what is to be learned. Readiness to learn changes based on situations and physical and emotional challenges.*

THERAPEUTIC INTERVENTIONS	RATIONALE

Desired Outcome: The client will identify ways to prevent further liver damage.

Independent Actions

Provide the following instructions regarding ways to prevent further liver damage:

- Avoid the following hepatotoxic agents:
  - Alcohol
  - Cleaning agents containing carbon tetrachloride and solvents (these are toxic even when inhaled)
  - Industrial chemicals such as nitrobenzene, disulfide, and tetrachloroethane
- Take acetaminophen (e.g., Tylenol) only when necessary and do not exceed the recommended dose.
- Adhere to the following precautions to prevent hepatitis:
  - Eat only in restaurants that have been inspected and approved by health authorities.
  - If blood transfusions are anticipated, arrange to donate and receive autologous blood rather than commercially obtained blood, if possible.
  - Avoid sharing food or eating utensils and handling toiletry items of others.
  - Practice safe sex (e.g., condom use for intercourse).
  - Avoid anal sex.
  - Do not share drug paraphernalia (e.g., needles, syringes, cookers, rinse water, straws for intranasal inhalation).

Hepatotoxic substances increase liver problems in processing proteins and medications.

Acetaminophen is processed through the liver and can impact liver functioning.

Foods must be appropriately prepared and under appropriate hygienic conditions.
Prevents exposure to blood products that may carry hepatitis.

These actions prevent sharing of body fluids, which increases potential for exposure to hepatitis A and/or B, which can further compromise liver functioning.

Continued...

THERAPEUTIC INTERVENTIONS	RATIONALE
• Get vaccinations for hepatitis A and B if recommended by health care provider.	*Decreases risk if exposed to hepatitis A and/or B.*
• If traveling to a developing country:	
(1) Receive immune globulin and vaccines for hepatitis (e.g., hepatitis B vaccine, hepatitis A vaccine) as recommended by health care provider.	
(2) Drink only bottled water, and avoid eating raw fruits and vegetables washed or prepared with local water when in the country.	

THERAPEUTIC INTERVENTIONS	RATIONALE

Desired Outcome: The client will verbalize an understanding of the rationale for and components of the recommended diet.

Independent Actions

Explain the rationale for a diet low in sodium, and teach the client how to identify sodium in the diet and decrease sodium intake:	*Increased sodium intake leads to retention of fluid, which may increase the incidence of ascites and lower extremity edema.*
• Read food labels and calculate sodium content of items; avoid those products that tend to have high sodium content (e.g., canned soups and vegetables, tomato juice, commercial baked goods, commercially prepared frozen or canned entrees and sauces).	
• Do not add salt when cooking foods or to prepared foods; use low-sodium herbs and spices, if desired.	
• Avoid cured and smoked foods, salty snacks, and commercially prepared foods.	
• Avoid routine use of over-the-counter medications with a high sodium content (e.g., some antacids, Alka-Seltzer).	
Obtain a dietary consult to assist client in planning meals that will meet prescribed dietary modifications.	*Provides multidisciplinary approach to client care.*

THERAPEUTIC INTERVENTIONS	RATIONALE

Desired Outcome: The client will identify ways to reduce stress on or trauma to the esophageal blood vessels.

Independent Actions

Provide the following instructions about ways to reduce stress on or trauma to the esophageal blood vessels:

Adhere to prescribed measures to reduce fluid retention (e.g., fluid restriction, low-sodium diet, diuretics).	*Prevents increased fluid volume that puts increased pressure on the esophageal vessels.*
Avoid activities that increase intra-abdominal pressure (e.g., straining to have a bowel movement, coughing, sneezing, lifting heavy objects).	*These activities increase intrathoracic pressure, which places additional pressure on the esophageal vessels.*
Avoid eating foods that might cause mechanical trauma to the esophageal varices (e.g., chips).	*May cause tearing of the esophageal vessels.*

THERAPEUTIC INTERVENTIONS	RATIONALE

Desired Outcome: The client will identify ways to prevent bleeding.

Independent Actions

Instruct client about ways to minimize risk of bleeding:	
• Avoid taking aspirin and other nonsteroidal antiinflammatory agents (e.g., ibuprofen) on a regular basis.	*Aspirin blocks platelet adherence, which is necessary for clotting, and will increase bleeding.*

THERAPEUTIC INTERVENTIONS	RATIONALE
• Use an electric rather than a straight-edge razor. • Floss and brush teeth gently. • Cut nails carefully. • Avoid situations that could result in injury (e.g., contact sports). • Avoid putting sharp objects (e.g., toothpicks) in mouth. • Do not walk barefoot. • Avoid blowing nose forcefully. • Avoid straining to have a bowel movement. Instruct client to control any bleeding by applying firm, prolonged pressure to the area, if possible.	*These actions decrease the risk of injury.* *Avoiding these actions decreases pressure on esophageal vessels.* *Improves body's blood clotting ability.*

THERAPEUTIC INTERVENTIONS	RATIONALE

Desired Outcome: The client will identify ways to reduce the risk of infection

Independent Actions

Instruct client in ways to reduce risk of infection:

• Maintain coughing and deep breathing exercises or use of incentive spirometer every 2 hrs while awake as long as activity is limited.	*Improves lung expansion and decreases stasis of secretions.*
• Increase activity as tolerated. • Avoid contact with persons who have an infection. • Avoid crowds, especially during flu and cold seasons. • Decrease or stop smoking.	*Decreases risk for exposure to infection.* *Smoking decreases ciliary activity and the ability to expel infectious agents with coughing.*
• Drink at least 10 glasses of liquid per day unless on a fluid restriction. • Adhere to recommended diet. • Take supplemental vitamins and minerals as prescribed. • Maintain good personal hygiene. • Receive immunizations (e.g., influenza vaccine, pneumococcal vaccine, hepatitis vaccines) if approved by health care provider.	*Maintains adequate hydration and vascular fluid volume.* *Malnutrition decreases the client's ability to fight off infection.* *Prevents cross-contamination.* *Enhances body's immune system and resistance to infection.*

THERAPEUTIC INTERVENTIONS	RATIONALE

Desired Outcome: The client will identify ways to relieve pruritus.

Independent Actions

Instruct client in and/or implement measures to relieve pruritus:

• Apply cool, moist compresses to pruritic areas.	*Cool/cold compresses provide a counter sensation that decreases the urge to rub or scratch the area.*
• Apply emollient creams or ointments frequently.	*Creams and ointments prevent dryness and subsequent itchy skin.*
• Add emollients, cornstarch, or baking soda to bath water.	*Adding these products to bath water decreases skin dryness and provides a protective barrier.*
• Use tepid water and mild soaps for bathing.	*Use of tepid water and mild soaps decreases skin dryness.*
• Pat skin dry after bathing, making sure to dry thoroughly.	*Rubbing of the skin with a towel after a bath can stimulate itching.*
• Maintain a cool environment.	*A cool environment provides a counter sensation that decreases urge to rub or scratch.*
• Encourage participation in diversional activity.	*Distracts client from focusing on the itch.*
• Use relaxation techniques—progressive muscle relaxation; mindfulness-based relaxation.	*Helps to decrease stress and anxiety.*
• Use cutaneous stimulation techniques (e.g., massage, pressure, vibration, stroking with soft brush) at sites of itching or acupressure points.	*Cutaneous stimulation decreases itching sensations by blocking neurotransmission of the sensation.*
• Encourage client to wear loose cotton garments and avoid clothes or blankets made from wool.	*Decreases skin irritation.*

NDx = NANDA Diagnosis   **D** = Delegatable Action   ● = UAP   ✦ = LVN/LPN   ⊝▶ = Go to ⊝volve for animation

Continued...

THERAPEUTIC INTERVENTIONS	RATIONALE
• Take medications as prescribed:	
• Antihistamines (e.g., diphenhydramine, hydroxyzine [Atarax])	*Antihistamines block histamine, which stimulates itchy sensations.*
• Bile acid–sequestering agents (e.g., cholestyramine)	*Bile acid–sequestering agents bind with the bile acids in the intestines, prevent absorption, and enhance elimination, thereby decreasing itch sensations.*

THERAPEUTIC INTERVENTIONS	RATIONALE

Desired Outcome: The client will state signs and symptoms to report to the health care provider.

Independent Actions

Stress the importance of reporting the following signs and symptoms:

• Rapid weight gain or loss	*Indicates changes in protein levels and retention of fluid volume.*
• Increasing size of abdomen	*May indicate ascites.*
• Increased swelling of lower extremities	*Indicates potential changes in vascular status.*
• Increasing shortness of breath	*May indicate heart failure.*
• Increased itchiness or yellowing of skin	*Indicates jaundice or increasing retention of bile acids.*
• Temperature elevation lasting more than 2 days	*Indicates infection.*
• Red, rust-colored, or smoky urine; bloody or tarry stools; blood in sputum or vomitus; persistent bleeding from nose, mouth, or skin; prolonged or excessive menses; excessive bruising; severe or persistent headache; or sudden abdominal or back pain	*Indicates inability of the body's clotting factors to control bleeding.*
• Tremors or changes in behavior, speech, or handwriting	*Indicates changes in neurologic status.*

THERAPEUTIC INTERVENTIONS	RATIONALE

Desired Outcome: The client will identify community resources to support lifestyle changes and support home management for effective management of cirrhosis

Independent Actions

Provide information regarding community resources that can assist client and significant others with lifestyle changes and home management of chronic disease (e.g., Meals on Wheels, home health agencies, transportation services, drug and alcohol rehabilitation programs, counseling services).	*Provides for continuation of care after discharge from the acute care facility.*

THERAPEUTIC INTERVENTIONS	RATIONALE

Desired Outcome: The client, in collaboration with the nurse, will develop a plan to adhere for recommended follow-up care including future appointment with health care provider, medications prescribed, and activity level.

Independent Actions

Reinforce the importance of keeping follow-up appointments with health care provider.	*Cirrhosis is a chronic illness, and follow-up appointments are important to maintain health status.*
Explain the rationale for, side effects of, and food and drug interactions and importance of taking medications prescribed.	*Knowledge of medications and how they impact the system improves client adherence to treatment regimen and understanding of the importance of adhering to the prescribed medication regimen. The client must be able to recognize alterations in functioning related to medication administration and what clinical manifestations that should be reported to the health care provider.*
Reinforce physician's instructions regarding activity level. Stress the importance of rest.	*Important in maintaining health status and ability to maintain activities of daily living.*

ADDITIONAL NURSING DIAGNOSES

RISK FOR INFECTION NDx
Related to:
- Lowered resistance to infection associated with:
  - Diminished function of the Kupffer cells in the liver (these cells normally phagocytize bacteria)
  - Malnutrition
  - Leukopenia resulting from hypersplenism (if venous congestion has resulted in splenomegaly, the spleen will destroy leukocytes faster than usual)
  - Serum complement deficiency resulting from decreased production of complement proteins by the liver
- Colonization of bacteria in the ascetic fluid (spontaneous bacterial peritonitis)
- Stasis of secretions in the lungs and urinary stasis if mobility is decreased

RISK FOR INJURY NDx
Falls related to:
- Weakness
- Dizziness (can result from anemia and the postural hypotension that occurs with third-spacing)
- Balance and gait disturbances that can occur with deficiencies of thiamine and/or vitamin B_{12}
- Disturbed thought processes (e.g., agitation, confusion)

Burns and lacerations related to:
- Paresthesias that can occur with deficiencies of thiamine and vitamin B_{12}
- Tremors and jerky, restless movements associated with delirium tremens ("DTs"), if present

INEFFECTIVE COPING NDx
Related to:
- Changes in appearance (e.g., edema, ascites, jaundice, spider angiomas, gynecomastia)
- Alterations in sexual functioning (e.g., impotence, decreased libido)
- Dependence on others to meet self-care needs
- Disturbed thought processes
- Stigma of having a chronic illness
- Possible changes in lifestyle and roles

DISTURBED SLEEP PATTERN NDx
Related to: Unfamiliar environment, frequent assessments and treatments, decreased physical activity, discomfort, fear, anxiety, and inability to assume usual sleep position because of orthopnea

FEAR AND ANXIETY NDx
Related to:
- Difficulty breathing
- Unfamiliar environment and separation from significant others
- Lack of understanding of the diagnosis, diagnostic tests, and treatments
- Uncertainty of prognosis
- Financial concerns
- Possibility of changes in lifestyle and roles

HEPATITIS

Hepatitis is the inflammation of the liver and remains a worldwide concern. Inflammation of the liver impacts its ability to detoxify substances, metabolize medications, produce clotting factor, synthesize plasma protein, metabolize proteins, fats, and carbohydrates, activate enzymes, and store glycogen.

Hepatitis is most commonly caused by a virus. Other causes of hepatitis include alcohol abuse, exposure to some prescriptions, over-the-counter medications, toxins, or autoimmune diseases. The five major causative viruses are hepatitis A virus (HAV), hepatitis B virus (HBV), hepatitis C virus (HCV), hepatitis E virus (HEV), and the delta virus or hepatitis D virus (HDV). Other viruses that can also cause liver inflammation include cytomegalovirus (CMV), Epstein-Barr virus (EBV), and yellow fever. Less common causes of viral hepatitis include adenovirus, CMV, EBV, and, rarely, herpes simplex virus (HSV).

Hepatitis A and E are both spread by the fecal-oral route. Hepatitis B is transmitted sexually, perinatally, and parenterally (primarily in IV drug users who share needles). In the United States, hepatitis A, B, and C are responsible for more than 90% of US cases of acute viral hepatitis. Hepatitis A and B are the most common cases of acute hepatitis in the United States. Hepatitis C is the most common cause of chronic hepatitis.

The various forms of hepatitis have similar clinical manifestations. Signs and symptoms vary in severity and are based on the level of liver involvement. Many cases go undetected because the person has very mild symptoms or is asymptomatic. Elevated serum aminotransferases (alanine aminotransferase [ALT] and aspartate aminotransferase [AST]) are hallmarks of acute hepatitis. Other signs and symptoms include flulike symptoms, nausea, fatigue, mild-to-moderate right upper quadrant pain, and symptoms of bile flow obstruction (e.g., jaundice, pruritus, dark amber urine, light-colored stools). The only definitive way to distinguish the various forms of viral hepatitis is by the presence of antigens and antigenic subtypes and the subsequent development of antibodies to these antigens.

Hospitalization of persons with hepatitis is usually not indicated except for some high-risk individuals (e.g., the elderly, immunocompromised persons, persons with other disease conditions that are complicated by the treatment of hepatitis) and persons with severe disease. Signs and symptoms of severe disease include a marked prolongation of prothrombin time, a serum bilirubin level more than 10 times normal, symptoms of encephalopathy, the presence of edema and/or ascites, or an inability to maintain adequate hydration. Chronic hepatitis may result in cirrhosis with portal hypertension and subsequent liver failure.

The treatment of acute hepatitis is primarily supportive and directed toward reducing the metabolic demands on the liver and promoting cell regeneration. If the client has hepatitis B, C, or D, close follow-up should be encouraged to determine whether medication therapy is indicated to prevent and treat chronic hepatitis.

This care plan focuses on the adult client with acute viral hepatitis hospitalized because of persistent nausea, worsening of liver function test results, and a prolonged prothrombin time. Much of the information is applicable to clients receiving follow-up care in an extended care facility or home setting.

OUTCOME/DISCHARGE CRITERIA

The client will:
1. Remain free of nausea
2. Have no evidence of bleeding or progressive liver degeneration

3. Maintain adequate nutritional intake
4. Perform activities of daily living without fatigue
5. Describe ways to prevent the spread of hepatitis to others
6. Identify ways to prevent further liver damage
7. Develop a plan to adhere to the recommended diet
8. State signs and symptoms to report to the health care provider
9. Develop a plan for adhering to recommended follow-up care including activity level, medications prescribed, and future appointments with health care provider and for laboratory studies

---

Nursing Diagnosis # RISK FOR DEFICIENT FLUID VOLUME NDx

Definition: Susceptible to experiencing decreased intravascular, interstitial, and/or intracellular fluid volumes, which may compromise health.

Related to:
- Decreased oral intake associated with anorexia and nausea
- Excessive loss of fluid if diaphoresis and/or persistent vomiting is present

CLINICAL MANIFESTATIONS

Subjective	Objective
Self-report of thirst; dry mouth, feeling weak	Decreased urine output; increased urine concentration; weight loss; decreased venous filling; increased body temperature; decreased pulse volume/pressure; change in mental status; elevated Hct; decreased skin/tongue turgor; dry skin/mucus membranes; tachycardia; decreased B/P

RISK FACTORS	DESIRED OUTCOMES
• Inadequate fluid intake • Exposure to pathogens • Medication regimen • Nausea and vomiting	The client will not experience a deficient fluid volume, as evidenced by: a. Normal skin turgor b. Moist mucous membrane c. Stable weight d. B/P and heart rate within normal range for client and stable with position change e. Capillary refill time less than 2 to 3 seconds f. Usual mental status g. BUN and Hct within appropriate range for the client h. Balanced intake and output

NOC OUTCOMES	NIC INTERVENTIONS
Fluid balance; hydration	Fluid management; IV therapy

NURSING ASSESSMENT	RATIONALE
Assess for and report signs and symptoms of deficient fluid volume: • Decreased skin turgor, dry mucous membranes, thirst • Weight loss of 2% or greater over a short period • Postural hypotension and/or low B/P • Weak, rapid pulse	*Early recognition of signs and symptoms of fluid volume deficit allows for prompt intervention.*

NURSING ASSESSMENT

RATIONALE

- Capillary refill time greater than 2 to 3 seconds
- Flat neck veins when supine
- Decreased urine output with increased specific gravity (reflects an actual rather than potential fluid deficit)
- Change in mental status
- Increased BUN and Hct values

THERAPEUTIC INTERVENTIONS

RATIONALE

Independent Actions

Implement measures to prevent deficient fluid volume:
- Perform actions to reduce nausea and prevent vomiting:
  - Instruct client to ingest food/fluid slowly.
  - Eliminate noxious sights and odors. **D** ● ✦
- Perform actions to improve oral intake:
  - Encourage rest before meals.
  - Provide oral hygiene before meals. **D** ● ✦

  - Allow adequate time for meals; reheat foods and fluids as needed. **D** ● ✦
- Perform actions to reduce fever, if present (administer tepid sponge bath, administer antipyretics, if ordered).
- Maintain fluid intake of at least 2300 mL/day unless contraindicated; if oral intake is inadequate or contraindicated, maintain IV and/or enteral fluid therapy as ordered.

Nausea often causes the client to have decreased fluid intake. Persistent vomiting results in excessive loss of fluid. These actions help prevent the experience of nausea.

Minimizes fatigue.
Removes unpleasant tastes, which often improves the taste of foods/fluids.
Improves client's ability to enhance oral fluid intake.

Reduction of fever decreases fluid loss from diaphoresis.

Adequate fluid intake needs to be provided to ensure adequate hydration.

Nursing Diagnosis **IMBALANCED NUTRITION: LESS THAN BODY REQUIREMENTS** NDx

Definition: Intake of nutrients insufficient to meet metabolic needs.

Related to:
- Decreased oral intake associated with anorexia and nausea
- Loss of nutrients associated with persistent vomiting, if present
- Reduced metabolism and storage of nutrients by the liver associated with an alteration in normal liver function as a result of inflammation
- Malabsorption of fats and fat-soluble vitamins associated with impaired bile flow resulting from inflammation of the liver
- Increased utilization of nutrients associated with the increased metabolic rate that is present with infection
- Insufficient interest in food
- Inability to absorb nutrients

CLINICAL MANIFESTATIONS

Subjective	Objective
Self-report lack of appetite; fatigue; irritability; poor self-esteem	Loss of weight with adequate food intake; body weight 20% or more under ideal weight; sore, inflamed buccal cavity; capillary fragility; pale conjunctiva and mucous membranes; poor muscle tone; excessive hair loss; amenorrhea

RISK FACTORS

- Chronic illness
- Change in normal digestive process
- Treatment regimen
- Anorexia, nausea, vomiting, diarrhea

DESIRED OUTCOMES

The client will maintain an adequate nutritional status, as evidenced by:
a. Weight within normal range for the client
b. Normal BUN and serum albumin, prealbumin, Hct and Hgb levels, and normal lymphocyte count
c. Improved strength and activity tolerance
d. Healthy oral mucous membrane

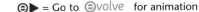

NDx = NANDA Diagnosis   **D** = Delegatable Action   ● = UAP   ✦ = LVN/LPN   ⊜▶ = Go to ℮volve for animation

NOC OUTCOMES	NIC INTERVENTIONS
Nutritional status	Nutritional monitoring; nutrition management; nutrition therapy; nutritional counseling; nausea management

NURSING ASSESSMENT	RATIONALE
Assess for and report signs and symptoms of malnutrition: • Weight significantly below client's usual weight or below normal for client's age, height, and body frame • Abnormal BUN and low serum albumin, prealbumin, Hct, Hgb, and ammonia levels and low lymphocyte count • Weakness and fatigue • Sore, inflamed oral mucous membrane • Pale conjunctiva	*Early recognition and reporting of signs and symptoms of malnutrition allow for prompt intervention.*
Monitor percentage of meals and snacks client consumes. Report a pattern of inadequate intake.	*An awareness of the amount of food/fluid the client consumes alerts the nurse to deficits in nutritional intake. Reporting an inadequate intake allows for prompt intervention.*

THERAPEUTIC INTERVENTIONS	RATIONALE

Independent Actions

Implement measures to maintain an adequate nutritional status:
- Perform actions to improve oral intake:
  - Implement measures to prevent nausea and vomiting if indicated (e.g., eliminate noxious sights and odors). **D** ● ✦

    Nausea may prevent a client from eating. Vomiting results in actual loss of nutrients and fluid volume.
  - Implement measures to control diarrhea, if present (e.g., discourage intake of spicy foods and foods high in fiber or lactose).

    Increased intestinal motility that occurs with or causes diarrhea results in a decreased absorption of nutrients in the bowel.
  - Maintain a clean environment and a relaxed, pleasant atmosphere. **D** ● ✦

    Noxious sights and odors can inhibit the feeding center in the hypothalamus. Maintaining a clean environment helps prevent this from occurring, which may improve appetite and oral intake.
  - Encourage a rest period before meals.

    Minimizes fatigue, which decreases client's ability to complete a meal.
  - Provide oral hygiene before meals. **D** ● ✦

    Removes unpleasant tastes, which often improves the taste of foods/fluids.
  - Serve foods/fluids that are appealing to the client and adhere to personal and cultural (e.g., religious, ethnic) preferences whenever possible.

    Foods/fluids that appeal to the client's senses (especially sight and smell) and are in accordance with personal and cultural preferences are most likely to stimulate appetite and promote interest in eating.
  - Serve frequent, small meals rather than large ones if client is weak, fatigues easily, and/or has a poor appetite.

    Providing small rather than large meals can enable a client who is weak or fatigues easily to finish a meal.
  - Provide adequate time for meals; reheat foods and fluids as needed. **D** ● ✦

    Clients who feel rushed during meals tend to become anxious, lose their appetite, and stop eating. Appetite is also suppressed if foods/fluids normally served hot or warm become cold and do not appeal to the client.
  - Limit fluid intake with meals unless the fluid has high nutritional value.

    Limiting fluid intake with meals reduces early satiety and subsequent decreased food intake.
  - Increase activity as allowed and tolerated. **D** ● ✦

    Activity promotes a sense of well-being, which can improve appetite.
- Encourage client to consume meals that are well balanced and high in essential nutrients; offer dietary supplements if client's caloric intake is inadequate.

  The client must consume a diet that is well balanced and high in essential nutrients to meet nutritional needs. Dietary supplements are often needed to help accomplish this.
- Assist and instruct client to adhere to the following dietary recommendations:
  - Avoid skipping meals.

    Skipping meals may decrease caloric and nutritional intake.
  - Consume a diet high in calories (2000–3000 calories/day) and carbohydrates; if unable to tolerate food, suck on hard candy and drink fruit juices and regular soft drinks.

    Consumption of adequate calories is required to maintain nutritional status.
  - Maintain a moderate to high protein intake (unless serum ammonia level is high or clinical evidence of encephalopathy is present).

    Adequate protein intake promotes healing of the liver.

THERAPEUTIC INTERVENTIONS	RATIONALE

Dependent/Collaborative Actions

Implement measures to maintain an adequate nutritional status:

- Administer medications that may be ordered to improve client's nutritional status (e.g., antiemetics, antidiarrheals, vitamins and minerals). **D** ✦

- Obtain a dietary consult if necessary.

- Perform a calorie count if ordered. Report information to the dietitian and physician.

Consult the physician about an alternative method of providing nutrition (e.g., parenteral nutrition, tube feeding) if client does not consume enough food or fluids to meet nutritional needs.

These medications decrease incidence of nausea, vomiting, and diarrhea. Vitamin and minerals may be required to maintain adequate nutritional status

A dietitian is best able to evaluate whether the foods/fluids selected will meet the client's nutritional needs.

A calorie count provides information about the caloric and nutritional value of the foods/fluids the client consumes. The information obtained helps the dietitian and physician to determine whether an alternative method of nutritional support is needed.

If the client's oral intake is inadequate, an alternative method of providing nutrients needs to be implemented.

Nursing Diagnosis ## NAUSEA NDx

Definition: A subjective phenomenon of an unpleasant feeling in the back of the throat and stomach, which may or may not result in vomiting.

Related to: Stimulation of the vomiting center associated with stimulation of the visceral afferent pathways as a result of:
- Inflammation of the gastrointestinal tract resulting from immune complex–mediated tissue responses to the viral infection
- Gaseous distention resulting from impaired fat digestion if bile flow is obstructed
- Sour taste
- Anxiety
- Noxious tastes

CLINICAL MANIFESTATIONS

Subjective	Objective
Verbalization of nausea	N/A

RISK FACTORS
- Chronic illness
- Treatment regimen
- Liver capsule stretch

DESIRED OUTCOME

The client will experience relief of nausea as evidenced by verbalization of same.

NOC OUTCOMES

Nausea and vomiting control

NIC INTERVENTIONS

Nausea management; environmental management

NURSING ASSESSMENT	RATIONALE
Assess for complaints of nausea.	*Early recognition of nausea allows for prompt treatment.*

THERAPEUTIC INTERVENTIONS	RATIONALE

Independent Actions

Implement measures to reduce nausea and prevent vomiting:
- Eliminate noxious sights and odors from the environment. **D** ● ✦
- Instruct client to change positions slowly.

- Encourage client to take deep, slow breaths when nauseated. **D** ✦

Noxious stimuli can cause stimulation of the vomiting center.

Rapid movement can result in stimulation of the chemoreceptor trigger zone and subsequent excitation of the vomiting center.
Provides relaxation and helps to decrease nausea.

Continued...

THERAPEUTIC INTERVENTIONS	RATIONALE
• Encourage client to avoid intake of foods/fluids high in fat (e.g., butter, cream, whole milk, ice cream, fried foods, gravies, nuts).	*Avoiding foods/fluids high in fat prevents a delay in gastric emptying and reduces nausea associated with impaired fat digestion.*
• Avoid serving foods with an overpowering aroma; remove lids from hot foods before entering room. **D ● ✦**	*Noxious stimuli can cause stimulation of the vomiting center.*
• Instruct client to eat dry foods (e.g., toast, crackers) and avoid drinking liquids with meals if nauseated.	*Eating dry foods and avoidance of drinking liquids with meals decrease the incidence of nausea.*
• Provide small, frequent meals; instruct client to ingest foods and fluids slowly.	*Eating small frequent meals and eating slowly prevent overdistention of the stomach and stimulation of the chemoreceptor trigger zone and subsequent excitation of the vomiting center.*
• Instruct client to avoid foods/fluids that irritate the gastric mucosa (e.g., spicy foods; caffeine-containing beverages such as tea, coffee, and colas).	*Avoidance of foods that irritate the gastric mucosa decreases the incidence of nausea.*
Dependent/Collaborative Actions	
Implement measures to reduce nausea and prevent vomiting:	
• Administer antiemetics, if ordered (phenothiazines are contraindicated because of their potential cholestatic effects).	*Antiemetics decrease nausea and/or vomiting.*
Consult physician if aforementioned measures fail to control nausea.	*Notification of the physician allows for prompt alterations in treatment plan.*

Nursing Diagnosis **RISK FOR BLEEDING** NDx

Definition: Susceptible to a decrease in blood volume, which may compromise health.

Related to:
• Decreased production of clotting factors associated with impaired liver function
• Impaired vitamin K absorption if bile flow is obstructed (normal bile flow is necessary for absorption of vitamin K)

DESIRED OUTCOMES

The client will not experience unusual bleeding, as evidenced by:
a. Skin and mucous membranes free of petechiae, purpura, ecchymoses, and active bleeding
b. Absence of unusual joint pain
c. No increase in abdominal girth
d. Absence of frank and occult blood in stool, urine, and vomitus
e. Usual menstrual flow
f. Vital signs within normal range for client
g. Stable or improved Hct and Hgb values

NURSING ASSESSMENT	RATIONALE
Assess client for and report signs and symptoms of unusual bleeding:	*Early recognition of signs and symptoms of bleeding and progressive liver degeneration allows for prompt intervention.*
• Petechiae, purpura, ecchymoses	
• Gingival bleeding	
• Prolonged bleeding from puncture sites, epistaxis, hemoptysis	
• Unusual joint pain	
• Increase in abdominal girth	
• Frank or occult blood in stool, urine, or vomitus	
• Menorrhagia	
• Restlessness, confusion	

THERAPEUTIC INTERVENTIONS	RATIONALE

Dependent/Collaborative Actions
Implement measures to prevent bleeding:

- Avoid giving injections whenever possible; consult health care provider for alternative routes for medication administration

  Giving the client injections increases risk of bleeding when clotting factors are diminished.

- When giving injections or performing venous or arterial punctures, use the smallest-gauge needle possible and apply gentle, prolonged pressure to the site after the needle is removed.

  These actions help to decrease bruising and improve clotting at the injection site.

- Encourage client to avoid activities that increase the risk for trauma (e.g., shaving with a straight-edge razor, using stiff bristle toothbrush or dental floss).

  Trauma increases the risk of bleeding when clotting factors are diminished.

- Pad side rails if client is confused or restless. **D** ● ✦

  Decreases potential for client injury.

- Whenever possible, avoid intubations (e.g., nasogastric) and procedures that can cause injury to the rectal mucosa (e.g., inserting a rectal suppository or tube, administering an enema).

  Trauma during procedures increases the risk of bleeding when clotting factors are diminished.

- Perform actions to reduce the risk for falls (e.g., avoid unnecessary clutter in room, instruct client to wear shoes/slippers with nonslip soles when ambulating). **D** ● ✦

  Placing client on risk for falls protocol decreases risk for injury.

- Instruct client to avoid blowing nose forcefully or straining to have a bowel movement; consult physician about an order for a decongestant and/or laxative if indicated.

  These actions may rupture small blood vessels and increase the incidence of bleeding.

- Administer the following if ordered to improve clotting ability:
  - Vitamin K injections **D** ✦
  - Platelets
  - FFP

  Administration of vitamin K, platelets, and FFP replaces deficient clotting factors.

If bleeding occurs and does not subside spontaneously:

- Apply firm, prolonged pressure to bleeding area(s) if possible.

  Application of pressure to the bleeding site improves clotting ability.

- If epistasis occurs, place client in a high-Fowler's position, have client lean forward and apply pressure and/or ice pack to nasal area. **D** ● ✦

  Proper positioning helps to prevent aspiration of blood from the nasal cavity. Application of pressure or ice to the nasal area improves clotting.

- Maintain oxygen therapy as ordered. **D** ✦

  Provides supplemental oxygenation to the tissues.

- If esophageal bleeding occurs:
  - Turn client on side and suction as necessary. **D** ✦

    These actions reduce the risk for aspiration.

  - Assist with administration of octreotide (Sandostatin) or vasopressin, if ordered.

    Octreotide/vasopressin constricts splanchnic vessels and reduces blood flow to the portal vein, decreasing pressure on esophageal varices.

  - Prepare client for endoscopic sclerotherapy or ligation of varices if planned.

    Decreases client's fear and anxiety.

  - Assist with insertion of a gastroesophageal balloon tube (e.g., Sengstaken-Blakemore tube,); maintain balloon pressure, suction client, and perform lavage, if ordered.

    The gastroesophageal balloon tube places pressure on bleeding varices, which improves clotting.

- Administer vitamin K injections, whole blood, or blood products (e.g., FFP, platelets) as ordered.

  Administration of vitamin K, blood, FFP, and platelets replaces deficient clotting factors.

- Assess for and report signs and symptoms of hypovolemic shock (e.g., restlessness; confusion; significant decrease in B/P; rapid, weak pulse; rapid respirations; cool skin; urine output <30 mL/h).

  Allows for prompt alteration in treatment plan.

Collaborative Diagnosis | **RISK FOR PROGRESSIVE LIVER DEGENERATION (E.G., FULMINANT HEPATITIS, CHRONIC ACTIVE HEPATITIS**

Definition: Degradation of liver cells.

Related to: Viral infection

CLINICAL MANIFESTATIONS

Subjective	Objective
Reports of weakness, itching	Increased jaundice, weakness, and pruritus
	Edema, ascites, bleeding
	Encephalopathy (e.g., change in handwriting, slow or slurred speech, emotional lability, agitation, asterixis, disorientation, lethargy)
	Further increase in prothrombin time
	Further elevation of serum AST, ALT, alkaline phosphatase, and bilirubin; low serum albumin

RISK FACTORS

- Chronic illness
- Inadequate/ineffective treatment regimen
- Nonadherence to treatment regimen

DESIRED OUTCOMES

The client will not experience progressive liver degeneration, as evidenced by:
a. Remaining free of signs and symptoms of hepatitis disease progression
b. Absence of edema, ascites, and bleeding
c. Usual mental status
d. Coagulation test results and serum AST, ALT, alkaline phosphatase, bilirubin, and albumin levels within or returning toward normal limits

NURSING ASSESSMENT

Assess for signs and symptoms of progressive liver degeneration:
- Worsening of signs and symptoms (e.g., increased jaundice, weakness, and pruritus)
- Edema, ascites
- Bleeding
- Encephalopathy (e.g., change in handwriting, slow or slurred speech, emotional lability, agitation, asterixis, disorientation, lethargy)
- Further increase in prothrombin time
- Further elevation of serum AST, ALT, alkaline phosphatase, and bilirubin levels
- Low serum albumin level

RATIONALE

Early recognition of signs and symptoms of progressive liver degeneration allows for prompt intervention.

THERAPEUTIC INTERVENTIONS

Dependent/Collaborative Actions
If signs and symptoms of progressive liver degeneration occur:
- Implement measures to decrease levels of ammonia and other nitrogenous substances (e.g., administer neomycin if ordered, administer lactulose if ordered, maintain prescribed dietary protein restriction). **D** ✦
- Implement measures to reduce the risk for injury (e.g., keep side rails up, maintain seizure precautions). **D** ● ✦
- Prepare client for liver transplant if planned.

RATIONALE

Neomycin attacks the ammonia-forming bacteria in the gastrointestinal tract. Lactulose draws ammonia from the blood stream into the colon for excretion. A low-protein diet reduces the buildup of nitrogen metabolites and ammonia in the blood stream.
Implement hospital protocols to reduce risk for injury.

Decreases client's fear and anxiety and improves client understanding of procedure.

DISCHARGE TEACHING/CONTINUED CARE

Nursing Diagnosis   **DEFICIENT KNOWLEDGE NDx; INEFFECTIVE HEALTH MANAGEMENT; INEFFECTIVE FAMILY HEALTH MANAGEMENT* NDx**

Definition: Deficient Knowledge NDx: Absence of cognitive information related to a specific topic or its acquisition.
Ineffective Health Management NDx: Pattern of regulating and integrating into daily living a therapeutic regimen for the treatment of illness and its sequelae that is unsatisfactory for meeting specific health goals.
Ineffective Family Health Management NDx: A pattern of regulating and integrating into family processes a program for the treatment of illness and the sequelae that is unsatisfactory for meeting specific health goals of the family unit.

CLINICAL MANIFESTATIONS

Subjective	Objective
Self-report of inability to manage illness; verbalizes inability to follow prescribed regimen	Inaccurate follow-through with instructions; inappropriate behaviors; experience of preventable complications of hepatitis

RISK FACTORS
- Cognitive deficit
- Economically disadvantaged
- Failure to take action to reduce risk factors for complications of hepatitis
- Inability to care for oneself
- Difficulty in modifying personal habits and integrating treatments into lifestyle
- Complex treatment regimen

NOC OUTCOMES

Knowledge: disease process; treatment regimen; health behavior; infection control and prevention

NIC INTERVENTIONS

Health education; teaching: disease process; teaching: prescribed diet; teaching: prescribed medication; teaching: individual

NURSING ASSESSMENT	**RATIONALE**
Assess client's knowledge base related to the disease process.	*The client's knowledge base provides the basis for education.*
Assess for indications that the client may be unable to effectively manage the therapeutic regimen:	*Early recognition of inability to understand disease process or self-care allows for change in teaching modality.*
• Statements reflecting inability to manage care at home	
• Failure to adhere to treatment plan (e.g., refusing medications)	
• Statements reflecting a lack of understanding of factors that may cause further progression hepatitis	
• Statements reflecting an unwillingness or inability to modify personal habits and integrate necessary treatments into lifestyle	
• Statements reflecting view that there is not a cure for most forms of hepatitis or that the situation is hopeless, and efforts to comply with the treatment plan are useless	

---

*The nurse should select the diagnostic label that is most appropriate for the client's discharge teaching needs.

NDx = NANDA Diagnosis   **D** = Delegatable Action   ● = UAP   ✦ = LVN/LPN   ⊝▶ = Go to ⊝volve for animation

THERAPEUTIC INTERVENTIONS	RATIONALE

Desired Outcome: The client will identify ways to prevent the spread of hepatitis to others.

Independent Actions

Provide the following instructions on ways to prevent the spread of hepatitis to others:

- If client has hepatitis A, provide instructions on how to adhere to the following precautions for 1 to 2 weeks after the onset of jaundice:
  - Wash hands thoroughly after having a bowel movement.
  - Use separate toilet facilities if possible; if separate toilet facilities are not available, clean toilet seat with a chlorine solution after use.
  - Wash bedding, towels, and underwear in hot, soapy water; wash them separately from other articles.
  - Do not donate blood or work in food services until approved by physician.
- If client has hepatitis B, C, or D, instruct him/her to adhere to the following precautions until health care provider states that transmitting hepatitis to others is no longer a risk:
  - Wash hands thoroughly after urinating and having a bowel movement.
  - Do not share personal articles (e.g., toothbrush, straight-edge razor, thermometer, washcloth).
  - Do not share food, cigarettes, or eating utensils.
  - If any injections (e.g., insulin, vitamin B_{12}) are given at home, use disposable equipment and dispose of it properly to reduce the risk of others coming in contact with contaminated needles.
  - Do not share drug paraphernalia (e.g., needles, straws for intranasal inhalation).
  - Use disposable eating utensils or wash utensils separately in hot, soapy water.
  - Avoid intimate sexual contact; once sexual activity is resumed, avoid intercourse during menstruation and intermenstrual bleeding and make sure that a condom is used during intercourse.
  - Do not donate blood.
- Instruct client to inform household and sexual contacts to see health care provider for appropriate immunization and testing for early detection of hepatitis.

These actions by the client prevent exposure of others to the client's blood and/or body fluids.

Prevents cross-contamination and decreases disease exposure to others.

Prevents personal injury.

Reduces the risk of others exposure to contaminated needles.

Prevents spread of disease.

Allows for testing and appropriate treatment of individuals who have been exposed to the individual with hepatitis.

THERAPEUTIC INTERVENTIONS	RATIONALE

Desired Outcome: The client will describe methods of preventing further liver damage

Independent Actions

Provide the following instructions regarding ways to prevent further liver damage:

- Avoid alcohol intake for a minimum of 6 months.

- Avoid contact with known liver toxins (e.g., cleaning agents containing carbon tetrachloride, solvents, industrial chemicals such as nitrobenzene, disulfide, and tetrachloroethane).

Alcohol is hepatotoxic and will exacerbate the clinical manifestations of hepatitis.
These agents are hepatotoxic and should be avoided.

THERAPEUTIC INTERVENTIONS	RATIONALE

• Take acetaminophen (e.g., Tylenol) only when necessary, and do not exceed the recommended dose or take it after drinking alcohol because of its potential toxic effect.
• Take precautions to prevent recurrent hepatitis:
  • Avoid unnecessary transfusions; if transfusions are necessary, arrange to donate and receive autologous blood rather than commercially obtained blood if possible.
  • Practice safe sex (e.g., condom use during intercourse); if sexual partner is a carrier, consult health care provider about receiving a hepatitis B vaccination.
  • Avoid sharing food, eating utensils, and toiletry items.
  • Avoid sharing drug paraphernalia (e.g., needles, syringes, cookers, rinse water, straws for intranasal inhalation).
  • Eat only in restaurants that have been inspected and approved by health authorities.
  • Get vaccinations for hepatitis A and B if recommended by health care provider.
  • Avoid anal sex.
• Inform all health care providers of history of hepatitis because a number of medications (e.g., chlorpromazine, acetaminophen, allopurinol, amiodarone, erythromycin, 6-mercaptopurine, phenytoin) can be hepatotoxic and should not be prescribed if alternatives are available.
	Acetaminophen at high doses is hepatotoxic, and, when combined with alcohol, the two substances compete for the substrates of metabolism.
	These actions decrease the client's exposure to other viral types of hepatitis or individuals with other viral infections.
	
	Informing all health care providers of history of hepatitis prevents unintended prescription of medications that may be hepatotoxic.

THERAPEUTIC INTERVENTIONS	RATIONALE

Desired Outcome: The client will develop a plan to adhere to the prescribed diet

Independent Actions

Collaborate with the client to develop a plan to adhere to the prescribed diet.	*Developing a plan that includes foods on a required diet and the impact of this diet on the system gives the client tools to have more control of the disease process and maintain an active role in treatment and care.*

THERAPEUTIC INTERVENTIONS	RATIONALE

Desired Outcome: The client will state signs and symptoms to report to the health care provider

Independent Actions

Stress the importance of reporting the following signs and symptoms: • Persistent or recurrent loss of appetite, nausea, fatigue, or weight loss. • Vomiting. • Increased itchiness or yellowing of skin. • Swelling of lower extremities, rapid weight gain, or increased size of abdomen. • Red, rust-colored, or smoky urine; bloody or tarry stools; blood in sputum or vomitus; prolonged or excessive bleeding from nose, mouth, or skin; prolonged or excessive menses; excessive bruising; severe or persistent headache; or sudden abdominal or back pain. • Changes in behavior, speech, or handwriting.	*These are signs and symptoms of progression of liver disease, and the client's health care professional should be notified to initiate prompt interventions.*

NDx = NANDA Diagnosis   **D** = Delegatable Action   ● = UAP   ✦ = LVN/LPN   ⊝▶ = Go to ⊝volve for animation

THERAPEUTIC INTERVENTIONS	RATIONALE

Desired Outcome: The client, in collaboration with the nurse, will develop plan for adhering to recommended follow-up care including activity level, medications prescribed, and future appointments with health care provider and for laboratory studies

Independent Actions

Collaborate with the client in developing a plan for progressive increased activity based on a physician's instructions regarding activity level. Stress the importance of rest during convalescent phase (from 6 weeks to 6 months).

Collaborate with the client to develop a schedule for follow-up appointments with health care provider and for laboratory studies

Collaborate with the client to develop a schedule for medication administration.

Educate the client on the rationale for prescribed medications and what side effects to monitor for and which ones should be reported to the health care provider.

Schedule time for the client to demonstrate the ability to perform subcutaneous injections, if required.

Provide client with information about and encourage participation in drug and alcohol rehabilitation programs if indicated.

Implement measures to improve client's adherence:
- Include significant others in teaching if possible.

- Encourage questions, and allow time for reinforcement and clarification of information provided.
- Provide written instructions regarding scheduled appointments with health care provider and for laboratory studies, medications prescribed, activity restrictions, and signs and symptoms to report.

Rest is critical for client healing and prevention of further liver damage.

Follow-up is critical because this is a long-term illness that requires various tests and evaluations to be treated properly.

Knowledge of the medication regimen and the impact of these medications on the system, as well as how the medication regimen can be incorporated into the client's lifestyle, allows the client some mechanism of control of his/her disease and the ability to have an active part in treatment and care.

Encourages adherence with treatment regimen.

Reduces further liver damage and potential infections.

Involvement of the client's significant others helps them to support the client and improves client's adherence to the treatment regimen.

Improves client understanding of treatment regimen and reinforces self-reliance and confidence in ability to care for self.

Provides the client and significant others a resource of information following discharge from the acute care facility.

ADDITIONAL NURSING DIAGNOSES

ACUTE PAIN NDx
- **Right upper quadrant** related to inflammation of the liver
- **Myalgias/arthralgias** related to the presence of circulating immune complexes and activation of the complement system associated with viral infection

RISK FOR ACTIVITY INTOLERANCE NDx
Related to:
- Inadequate nutritional status
- Increased energy utilization associated with the increased metabolic rate present in an infectious process
- Difficulty resting and sleeping associated with frequent assessments and treatments, discomfort, anxiety, and unfamiliar environment

FEAR AND ANXIETY NDx
Related to:
- Unfamiliar environment and lack of understanding of diagnosis and diagnostic tests
- Lack of definitive treatment for hepatitis and the possibility of serious complications
- Possible transmission of disease to others and rejection by others because of their fear of contracting hepatitis
- Temporary restrictions of some usual activities (e.g., vigorous exercise, contact sports, sexual activity, alcohol consumption)

PANCREATITIS, ACUTE

Acute pancreatitis is an inflammation of the pancreas with premature activation of enzymes that cause local damage to the organ, autodigestion, and fibrosis. These changes can lead to life-threatening complications including shock, diabetes, acute respiratory distress syndrome (ARDS), and end-organ dysfunction and failure.

After an episode of mild to moderate acute pancreatitis, the structure and function of the pancreas often return to normal. However, with more severe and/or recurrent episodes of acute pancreatitis, irreversible changes can occur and chronic pancreatitis can develop.

The most common causes of acute pancreatitis are biliary tract obstruction caused by gallstones and long-term alcohol abuse.

Some less frequent causes include external trauma to the abdomen, trauma to the pancreas during pancreatic endoscopy or abdominal surgery, bacterial and viral infections, some antibiotics, and metabolic disorders such as chronic hypercalcemia and genetic hyperlipidemia.

Often the presenting symptom of acute pancreatitis is sudden onset of epigastric in the upper left quadrant or abdomen, radiating to the back or shoulder. Pain increases with coughing, movement, and deep breathing, and pain may be associated with nausea, vomiting, and anorexia. As the disease progresses, shock, renal failure, and end-organ dysfunction/failure may occur. Patients with alcohol-induced pancreatitis may not experience any pain and generally present with abdominal fullness, indigestion, hiccups, fever, hypotension, and tachycardia.

The goal of treatment is to prevent further autodigestion of the pancreas and prevent systemic complications. If the cause of pancreatitis is gallstones, surgery is performed after pancreatic inflammation has subsided and the patient is stable.

This care plan focuses on the adult client hospitalized with acute pancreatitis. Some of the information is applicable to clients receiving follow-up care in an extended care facility or home setting.

OUTCOME/DISCHARGE CRITERIA

The client will:
1. Have no clinical manifestations of complications
2. Maintain relief of severe pain
3. Maintain adequate nutritional and fluid intake
4. Describe methods to prevent overstimulation and further trauma to the pancreas
5. Develop a plan to implement dietary modifications
6. State signs and symptoms to report to the health care provider
7. Develop a plan for adhering to recommended follow-up care including future appointments with health care provider and medications prescribed.

Nursing Diagnosis ## ACUTE PAIN NDx (EPIGASTRIC WITH RADIATION TO THE BACK)

Definition: Unpleasant sensory and emotional experience associated with actual or potential tissue damage, or described in terms of such damage (International Association for the Study of Pain); sudden or slow onset of any intensity from mild to severe with an anticipated or predictable end, and a duration of less than 3 months.

Related to:
- Distention of the pancreas associated with inflammation and obstruction of pancreatic ducts
- Peritoneal irritation associated with escape of activated pancreatic enzymes into the peritoneum

CLINICAL MANIFESTATIONS

Subjective	Objective
Verbal or coded report of pain; difficulty sleeping due to experience of pain;	Autonomic responses (e.g., diaphoresis; changes in B/P, respiration, pulse; pupillary dilatation); expressive behavior (e.g., restlessness, moaning, crying, vigilance, irritability, sighing); changes in appetite and eating; protective gestures; guarding behavior; facial mask; evidence of sleep disturbance (eyes lack luster, fixed or scattered movement, beaten look, grimace)

RISK FACTORS
Inflammation of the pancreas

DESIRED OUTCOMES

The client will experience diminished pain, as evidenced by:
a. Verbalization of a decrease in or absence of pain
b. Relaxed facial expression and body positioning
c. Increased participation in activities
d. Stable vital signs

NOC OUTCOMES

Pain Level; pain control

NIC INTERVENTIONS

Pain management; analgesic administration; patient-controlled analgesia (PCA) assistance; nonpharmacologic interventions

NURSING ASSESSMENT

Assess for signs and symptoms of pain (e.g., verbalization of pain, grimacing, reluctance to move, restlessness, diaphoresis, increased B/P, tachycardia).

Assess client's perception of the severity of pain using a pain intensity rating scale.

Assess the client's pain pattern (e.g., location, quality, onset, duration, precipitating factors, aggravating factors, alleviating factors).

Ask the client to describe previous pain experiences and methods used to manage pain effectively.

RATIONALE

Early recognition of signs and symptoms of pain allows for prompt intervention and improved pain control.

An awareness of the severity of pain being experienced helps determine the most appropriate interventions for pain management. Use of a pain intensity rating scale gives the nurse a clearer understanding of the client's pain experience, changes in pain over time, and promotes consistency when communicating with others.

Knowledge of the client's pain pattern assists in the identification of effective pain management interventions.

Many variables affect a client's response to pain (e.g., age, sex, coping style, previous experience with pain, culture, cause of pain). Understanding of the client's usual response to pain and methods previously used to manage pain effectively enables the nurse to evaluate the client's pain more accurately and facilitates the identification of effective strategies for pain management.

THERAPEUTIC INTERVENTIONS

Independent Actions

Implement measures to reduce pain:

- Implement measures to reduce fear and anxiety (e.g., assure client that the need for pain relief is understood, collaborate with client on methods for achieving pain control, provide a calm, restful environment). **D** ✦
- Perform actions to promote rest (e.g., minimize environmental activity and noise). **D** ● ✦

Collaborate with client on nonpharmacologic measure to decrease pain (e.g., Mindfulness based stress reduction (MBSR), distraction, guided imagery).

Allow client to sit or lie with knees and trunk flexed.

Dependent/Collaborative Actions

Implement measures to reduce pain:

- Administer analgesics before activities and procedures that can cause pain and before pain becomes severe.
- Administer IV analgesics before pain becomes too severe.
- Consider PCA pain administration.

- Perform actions to reduce pancreatic stimulation:
  - Withhold all food and oral fluid as ordered. **D** ✦

  - Implement measures to reduce the amount of hydrochloric acid in the stomach:
    (1) Insert a nasogastric tube and maintain suction, if ordered.
    (2) Administer histamine$_2$-receptor antagonists, if ordered.
  - Minimize client's exposure to odor and sight of food until oral intake is allowed.

RATIONALE

Promotes relaxation and subsequently increases the client's threshold and tolerance for pain.

These actions reduce fatigue and subsequently increase the client's threshold and tolerance for pain.

Decreases pancreatic stimulation, thus reducing client's pain experience.

Enhances patient's coping skills

This position relieves pressure on the inflamed pancreas

Improves ability to perform activities of daily living without discomfort and promotes rest.

Severe, prolonged pain is more difficult to relieve and increases anxiety and fear.

Provides client more control over pain relief and promotes client involvement in care.

Food and fluid cause the release of secretin and/or cholecystokinin, which stimulate the output of pancreatic secretions.

When hydrochloric acid enters the duodenum, it stimulates the release of pancreatic enzymes.

Removes fluid and hydrochloric acid from the stomach.

Histamine receptor antagonists and proton pump inhibitors suppress secretion of gastric acid.

Prevents stimulation of gastric secretions and the subsequent output of pancreatic secretions.

THERAPEUTIC INTERVENTIONS	RATIONALE
• When oral intake is allowed:	
(1) Advance diet slowly.	*Slow advancement increases tolerance to oral intake.*
(2) Provide small, frequent meals rather than three large ones. **D** ✦	*Small, frequent meals decrease stretch of the stomach and subsequent discomfort.*
(3) Avoid foods/fluids high in fat (e.g., butter, cream, whole milk, ice cream, fried foods, gravies, nuts), spicy foods, and caffeine-containing beverages (e.g., coffee, tea, colas), if ordered.	*These foods cause release of pancreatic enzymes, which cause pain.*
• Provide or assist with additional nonpharmacologic measures for pain relief (e.g., massage; position change; progressive relaxation exercises; restful environment; diversional activities such as watching television, reading, or conversing).	*Nonpharmacologic pain management includes a variety of interventions. It is believed that most of these are effective because they stimulate closure of the gating mechanism in the spinal cord and subsequently block the transmission of pain impulses. In addition, some interventions are thought to stimulate the release of endogenous analgesics (e.g., endorphins) that inhibit the transmission of pain impulses and/or alter the client's perception of pain. Many of the nonpharmacologic interventions also help to decrease pain by promoting relaxation.*
• If client is receiving epidural analgesia, perform actions to maintain patency of the system (e.g., keep tubing free of kinks, tape catheter securely, use caution when moving client to avoid dislodging catheter).	*Use of epidural analgesia helps to decrease pain without causing increased sedation.*
• Assist with peritoneal lavage if performed.	*Removes activated pancreatic enzymes and debris that cause peritoneal irritation and subsequent pain*
Consult appropriate health care provider (e.g., pharmacist, pain management specialist, physician) if aforementioned measures fail to provide adequate pain relief.	*Allows for prompt alterations in the treatment plan.*

Nursing Diagnosis IMBALANCED NUTRITION: LESS THAN BODY REQUIREMENTS NDx

Definition: Intake of nutrients insufficient to meet metabolic needs.

Related to:
• Decreased oral intake associated with nausea, pain, prescribed dietary restrictions, and feeling of fullness resulting from abdominal distention
• Loss of nutrients associated with vomiting
• Decreased utilization of nutrients associated with impaired digestion of fats, proteins, and carbohydrates resulting from loss of normal outflow of pancreatic enzymes
• Increased nutritional needs associated with the increased metabolic rate that occurs with pancreatitis

CLINICAL MANIFESTATIONS

Subjective	Objective
Verbalization of lack of appetite; fatigue; irritability; poor self-esteem	Weight loss; body weight 20% or more under ideal weight; pale conjunctiva and mucous membranes; excessive hair loss; amenorrhea

RISK FACTORS
• Impaired digestion
• Insufficient dietary intake
• Treatment regimen
• Inability to absorb nutrients

DESIRED OUTCOMES

The client will maintain an adequate nutritional status, as evidenced by:
a. Weight within normal range for the client
b. Normal BUN and serum albumin, prealbumin, Hct and Hgb levels, and normal lymphocyte count
c. Usual strength and activity tolerance
d. Healthy oral mucous membrane

NDx = NANDA Diagnosis   **D** = Delegatable Action   ● = UAP   ✦ = LVN/LPN   ⊝▶ = Go to ⊝volve for animation

NOC OUTCOMES	NIC INTERVENTIONS
Nutritional status	Nutritional monitoring; nutrition management; nutrition therapy; nausea management; pain management; total parenteral nutrition (TPN) administration

NURSING ASSESSMENT	RATIONALE
Assess for and report signs and symptoms of malnutrition: • Weight significantly below client's usual weight or below normal for client's age, height, and body frame • Abnormal BUN and low serum albumin, prealbumin, Hct, and Hgb levels and low lymphocyte count • Weakness and fatigue • Sore, inflamed oral mucous membrane • Pale conjunctiva	*Early recognition and reporting of signs and symptoms of malnutrition allows for prompt intervention.*
Monitor and report changes in percentage of meals and snacks client consumes.	*An awareness of the amount of foods/fluids the client consumes alerts the nurse to deficits in nutritional intake. Reporting an inadequate intake allows for prompt intervention.*

THERAPEUTIC INTERVENTIONS	RATIONALE

Independent Actions

Implement measures to maintain an adequate nutritional status:

- Limit activity as ordered. — *Limiting activity decreases energy utilization and metabolic rate.*
- When food or oral fluids are allowed perform actions to improve oral intake:
  - Implement measures to reduce ascites and accumulation of gas and fluid in the gastrointestinal tract (e.g., proper positioning, encourage client not to eat or drink foods that cause gas production [caffeine, beans, drinking with a straw, chewing gum]). — *These actions reduce abdominal distention and the subsequent feeling of fullness and early satiety.*
  - Implement measures to reduce nausea and vomiting:
    - maintain fluid and food restrictions as ordered,
    - provide oral hygiene at regular intervals
    - reduce pain,

    Decreasing nausea and vomiting will prevent fluid and electrolyte loss. Providing oral hygiene may decrease nausea and enhance appetite.
    Reduction of pain decreases potential for nausea and vomiting.

  Maintain a clean environment and relaxed, pleasant atmosphere. — *Noxious sites and odors can inhibit the feeding center in the hypothalamus. Maintaining a clean environment helps prevent this from occurring. In addition, maintaining a relaxed, pleasant atmosphere can help reduce the client's stress and promote a feeling of well-being, which tends to improve appetite and oral intake*

- Increase activity as allowed and tolerated. **D** ● ✦ — *Activity usually promotes a sense of well-being, which can improve appetite.*
- Allow adequate time for meals; reheat foods/fluids if necessary. **D** ● ✦ — *Clients who feels rushed during meals tend to become anxious, lose their appetite, and stop eating. Appetite is also suppressed if foods/fluids normally served hot or warm become cold and do not appeal to the client.*
- Limit fluid intake with meals (unless the fluids have high nutritional value). **D** ✦ — *Intake of oral fluids with meals causes stomach distention and can cause satiety before an adequate amount of food is consumed.*
- Ensure that meals are well balanced and high in essential nutrients. — *Maintenance of nutritional status.*

Dependent/Collaborative Actions

Implement measures to maintain an adequate nutritional status:

- Administer nasogastric feeding or TPN, if ordered. — *Provides nutrition if client is unable to tolerate oral intake.*
- Administer vitamins and minerals. — *Vitamins, minerals, and supplements are needed to maintain metabolic functioning.*

THERAPEUTIC INTERVENTIONS	RATIONALE
• Administer pancreatic enzymes	*Supplemental pancreatic enzymes aid in the digestion of foods.*
• Administer albumin	*Albumin increases osmotic pressure and pulls fluid into the vascular compartment.*
Implement measures to reduce pain (position properly, administer pain meds as ordered). **D** ✦	*Pain reduction increases a client's appetite and ability to tolerate diet.*
• Perform a calorie count, if ordered. Report information to dietitian and physician.	*A dietitian is best able to evaluate whether the foods/fluids selected will meet the client's nutritional needs.*
Reassess nutritional status on a regular basis and report decline.	*Allows for prompt alterations in treatment plan.*

Nursing/Collaborative Diagnosis **RISK FOR IMBALANCED FLUID VOLUME NDx RISK FOR ELECTROLYTE IMBALANCE NDx**

Definition: Risk for Imbalance Fluid Volume NDx: Susceptible to a decrease, increase, or rapid shift from one to the other of intravascular, interstitial, and/or intracellular fluid, which may compromise health. This refers to body fluid loss, gain, or both; **Risk for Electrolyte Imbalance NDx:** Susceptible to changes in serum electrolyte balance, which may compromise health.

Related to:
• **Risk for imbalanced fluid volume NDx** related to:
  • Disease process
  • Decreased oral intake
  • Excessive loss of fluid associated with vomiting and nasogastric tube drainage
• Third-spacing related to increased vascular permeability associated with the inflammatory response and activation of kinin peptides such as bradykinin and kallidin (occurs when the pancreatic enzyme trypsin enters systemic circulation)

Related to:
Risk for electrolyte imbalance NDx
• **Hypokalemia, hypochloremia, and metabolic alkalosis** related to loss of electrolytes and hydrochloric acid associated with vomiting and nasogastric tube drainage
• **Hypocalcemia** related to:
  • Binding of calcium to the undigested fats in the intestine (enzymes such as lipase and phospholipase A are not released into the intestinal tract to digest fats so calcium binds with the free fats and is excreted in the stool)
Hypoalbuminemia associated with increased vascular permeability that occurs with inflammation

CLINICAL MANIFESTATIONS

Subjective	Objective
Self-report of fatigue and weakness; complaints of dizziness; anxiousness; irritability; complaints of numbness and tingling of fingers, toes, or circumoral area	Decreased skin turgor; dry mucous membranes; weight loss of 2% or greater over a short period; postural hypotension; weak rapid pulse; flat neck veins when supine; changes in mental status; capillary refill greater than 2 to 3 seconds; decreased urine output with increased specific gravity; cardiac dysrhythmias; vomiting; hypoactive or absent bowel sounds; muscle twitching; positive Chvostek and Trousseau sign; hyperactive reflex

RISK FACTORS

- Failure of regulatory mechanisms
- Chronic illness
- Inadequate intake
- Exposure to pathogens
- Mechanical loss of electrolytes

DESIRED OUTCOMES

The client will not experience an imbalance in fluid volume or electrolytes, as evidenced by:
a. Normal skin turgor
b. Moist mucous membranes
c. Stable weight
d. B/P and pulse rate within normal range for client and stable with position change
e. Capillary refill time less than 2 to 3 seconds
f. Usual mental status
g. Balanced intake and output
h. Urine specific gravity within normal range
i. Soft, nondistended abdomen with normal bowel sounds
j. Absence of cardiac dysrhythmias, muscle weakness, paresthesias, muscle twitching or spasms, dizziness, tetany, and seizure activity
k. Negative Chvostek and Trousseau signs
l. BUN, Hct, serum electrolyte, and ABG values within normal range

NOC OUTCOMES

Maintain fluid/electrolyte balance

NIC INTERVENTIONS

Fluid/electrolyte management: hypokalemia; electrolyte management: hypocalcemia; acid-base monitoring; acid-base management: metabolic alkalosis

NURSING ASSESSMENT

Assess for and report signs and symptoms of fluid and electrolyte imbalance:
- Monitor cardiovascular status (i.e., changes in blood pressure and for postural hypotension, heart rate, rhythm, capillary refill time, flat or distended neck veins, changes in urine output)
- Monitor respiratory status (i.e., changes in breath sounds with the development of adventitious sounds).
- Changes in mental status
- Decreased skin turgor, dry mucous membranes, thirst
- Weight loss or gain of 2% over a short period
- Monitory I&O
- Monitor serum electrolytes (i.e., potassium, calcium)
- Monitor intake and output (I & O), BUN, and creatinine and Hct levels and changes in blood pressure from client's normal

RATIONALE

Early recognition of signs and symptoms of imbalanced fluid and electrolytes allows for prompt intervention.

THERAPEUTIC INTERVENTIONS

Dependent/Collaborative Actions
Implement measures to prevent or treat fluid volume and electrolyte imbalance:
- Perform actions to reduce nausea and vomiting (maintain fluid and food restrictions as ordered; reduce pain, eliminate noxious sights and odors from the environment). **D** ● ✦
- If a nasogastric tube is present and needs to be irrigated frequently and/or with large volumes of solution, irrigate it with normal saline rather than water.

RATIONALE

These actions prevent loss of fluid and electrolytes and alterations in metabolic status.

Maintains patency of nasogastric tube.

THERAPEUTIC INTERVENTIONS	RATIONALE
• Administer fluid and electrolyte replacements as ordered.	*Replaces lost fluid and electrolytes to normalize values.*
• Maintain a fluid intake of at least 2500 mL/day unless contraindicated. **D** ● ✦	*Adequate fluid intake is required to maintain adequate circulatory volume.*
• When oral intake is allowed:	
• Assist client to select the following foods/fluids:	
(1) For potassium deficits teach client about foods that are high in potassium (e.g., bananas, potatoes, cantaloupe, avocados, raisins)	*Maintains adequate level of potassium.*
(2) For calcium deficit, teach client about foods that are high in calcium such as milk and milk products (if client is on a low-fat diet, items such as ice cream, whole milk, butter, and cream should be omitted)	*Maintains adequate level of calcium.*
• Administer pancreatic enzymes (e.g., pancreatin, pancrelipase) if ordered.	*Promotes fat digestion so that there is less fat available to bind with calcium.*
Consult physician if signs and symptoms of fluid volume and electrolyte imbalances persist or worsen.	*Notification of the physician allows for prompt alterations in treatment plan.*
Monitor serum albumin levels. Report below-normal levels.	*Low serum albumin levels result in fluid shifting out of the vascular space because albumin normally maintains plasma colloid osmotic pressure.*
Implement measures to prevent further third-spacing and/or promote mobilization of fluid back into vascular space:	
• Administer albumin infusions if ordered.	*Albumin increases colloid osmotic pressure which pulls fluid into the vascular compartment.*
• Perform actions to decrease pancreatic stimulation; withhold all food and oral fluid as ordered. **D** ✦	*Food and fluid, especially those that are acidic or have a high protein or fat content, upon entering the duodenum cause the release of secretin and/or cholecystokinin, which stimulate the output of pancreatic secretions.*
Implement measures to reduce hydrochloric acid in the stomach.	*As hydrochloric acid enters the duodenum, it stimulates the release of secretin, which may stimulate significant output of pancreatic secretions.*
• Insert a nasogastric tube and maintain suction as ordered.	*Placing a nasogastric tube to suction removes the acid from the stomach.*
• Administer histamine receptor antagonists if ordered.	*Histamine receptor antagonists inhibit the action of histamine on the parietal cells, which blocks gastric acid secretion.*
• Minimize client's exposure to odor and sight of food until oral intake is allowed.	*Decreasing the client's exposure to the sight and odor of food prevents stimulation of gastric secretions and the subsequent output of pancreatic secretions.*
Consult physician if signs and symptoms of third-spacing persist or worsen.	*Notification of the physician allows for prompt alterations in treatment plan.*

Nursing Diagnosis ## RISK FOR INFECTION NDx **(SEPSIS)**

Definition: Susceptible to invasion and multiplication of pathogenic organisms, which may compromise health.

Related to:
- Release of bacteria into the blood associated with:
  - Presence of infected necrotic areas or leakage of infected pseudocysts or abscesses into the blood stream (necrotic areas, pseudocysts, and abscesses can develop as a result of destruction of pancreatic and surrounding tissue by the activated proteolytic enzymes)
  - Peritonitis (if it occurs)
- Decreased resistance to infection associated with decreased nutritional status
- Break in skin integrity associated with frequent venipunctures or presence of invasive lines

---

NDx = NANDA Diagnosis   **D** = Delegatable Action   ● = UAP   ✦ = LVN/LPN   ⊖▶ = Go to ⊖volve for animation

CLINICAL MANIFESTATIONS

Subjective	**Objective**
Self-report of chills/lethargy; loss of appetite	Elevated temperature; diaphoresis; tachypnea; tachycardia; confusion increase in WBC count above previous levels and/or significant change in differential; positive blood cultures

RISK FACTORS

- Exposure to pathogens
- Failure of immune response
- Poor nutritional status

DESIRED OUTCOMES

The client will not experience sepsis, as evidenced by:
a. No further increase in temperature
b. Absence of chills and diaphoresis
c. Pulse and respiratory rate within normal range for client
d. WBC and differential counts returning to normal
e. Negative blood culture results

NOC OUTCOMES

Immune status; infection severity

NIC INTERVENTIONS

Infection protection; infection control

NURSING ASSESSMENT	**RATIONALE**
Assess for and report signs and symptoms of sepsis (e.g., increase in temperature, chills, diaphoresis, tachypnea, tachycardia, increase in WBC count above previous levels and/or significant change in differential, positive cultures).	*Early recognition of signs and symptoms of sepsis allows for prompt intervention.*

THERAPEUTIC INTERVENTIONS	**RATIONALE**

Dependent/Collaborative Actions
Implement measures to prevent sepsis:

- Perform actions to decrease pancreatic stimulation (e.g., keep client NPO; maintain nasogastric tube to suction, remove noxious sights and smells).

  These actions reduce pancreatic enzyme stimulation which decrease destruction of pancreatic and peripancreatic tissue, thus preventing subsequent development of necrotic areas, pseudocysts, and abscesses.

- Perform actions to prevent and treat peritonitis (e.g., keep client NPO, place client in a semi-Fowler's position, administer antimicrobials).

  Prevents and decreases incidence of peritonitis.

- Prepare client for drainage of an abscess or pseudocyst or surgical resection of necrotic tissue if planned.

  Prevents spread of infection and decreases incidence of sepsis.

- Maintain strict aseptic and sterile technique during all invasive procedures (e.g., venous and arterial punctures, prompt dressing changes).

  Limits external bacteria being introduced in the system.

- Maintain an adequate nutritional status (e.g., provide frequent small, highly nutritious meals; maintain a clean environment and a relaxed, pleasant atmosphere)

  Adequate nutrition is necessary for cellular development and a robust immune response to pathogens.

- Perform actions to reduce pain and anxiety (e.g., administer pain medication as needed and before pain becomes severe; provide a calm, restful environment; explain diagnostic tests and treatment plan).

  Pain and anxiety reduction prevents an increase in secretion of cortisol, which interferes with some immune responses.

- Change IV line sites, tubing, and solutions using aseptic technique according to hospital policy and maintain a closed system for IV infusions, whenever possible.

  Decreases potential for the introduction of foreign bacteria into the system.

- Anchor catheters/tubings (e.g., IV) securely.

  Reduces trauma to the tissues and the risk for introduction of pathogens associated with in-and-out movement of the tubing.

THERAPEUTIC INTERVENTIONS	RATIONALE
• Administer antimicrobials as ordered.	*Antimicrobials prevent and/or treat infections.*
If signs and symptoms of sepsis occur, assess for and immediately report signs and symptoms of septic shock (e.g., systolic B/P < 90 mm Hg; rapid, weak pulse; restlessness; agitation; confusion; urine output < 30 mL/h; cool, pale, mottled, and/or cyanotic extremities; capillary refill time >3 seconds; diminished or absent peripheral pulses).	*Allows for prompt alterations in treatment plan.*

Nursing Diagnosis INEFFECTIVE BREATHING PATTERN NDx

Definition: Inspiration and/or expiration that does not provide adequate ventilation.

Related to:
• Increased rate of respirations associated with fear and anxiety
• Decreased depth of respirations associated with:
  • Depressant effects of some medications (e.g., narcotic [opioid] analgesics, some antiemetics)
  • Reluctance to breathe deeply due to abdominal pain
  • Restricted chest expansion resulting from positioning and abdominal pressure on the diaphragm

CLINICAL MANIFESTATIONS

Subjective	Objective
Verbalization of shortness of breath; inability to breathe deeply	Dyspnea; increased respiratory rate; decreased depth of breathing; use of accessory muscles to breathe; altered chest excursion; prolonged expiration phases; decreased SaO_2

RISK FACTORS
• Abdominal distention and pain

DESIRED OUTCOMES

The client will have an improved breathing pattern, as evidenced by:
a. Normal rate and depth of respirations
b. Decreased dyspnea
c. Symmetric chest excursion
d. Oxygenation saturation >90%

NOC OUTCOMES

Respiratory status: ventilation, vital signs

NIC INTERVENTIONS

Ventilation assistance; respiratory monitoring; breathing patterns

NURSING ASSESSMENT	RATIONALE
Assess for signs and symptoms of an ineffective breathing pattern: • Shallow or slow respirations • Limited chest excursion • Tachypnea or dyspnea • Use of accessory muscles when breathing	*Early recognition of signs and symptoms of an ineffective breathing pattern allows for prompt intervention.*

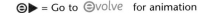

Continued...

NURSING ASSESSMENT	RATIONALE
Assess/monitor pulse oximetry (arterial oxygen saturation [SaO₂]), ABG values as indicated.	*Monitoring continuous SaO$_2$ readings allows for the early detection of hypoxia.* *Assessment of ABG values provides a more direct measurement of both the partial pressure of oxygen in arterial blood (PaO$_2$) and the partial pressure of carbon dioxide in arterial blood (PaCO$_2$), which reflect the adequacy of ventilation.*

THERAPEUTIC INTERVENTIONS	RATIONALE

Independent Actions

Implement measures to improve breathing pattern:

- Perform actions to reduce fear and anxiety (e.g., assure client that staff is nearby; provide a calm, restful environment; explain all tests and procedures). **D** ✦

- Perform actions to reduce pressure on the diaphragm:
  - Implement measures to reduce gas and fluid accumulation in the gastrointestinal tract (avoid carbonated beverages and chewing gum; avoid gas-producing foods). **D** ✦

- Position client in a semi- to high-Fowler's position unless contraindicated; support with pillows. **D** ✦
- If client must remain flat in bed, assist with position change at least every 2 hrs. **D** ● ✦
- Instruct and assist client to deep breathe or use incentive spirometer every 1 to 2 hrs.

- Reinforce splinting of abdomen with deep breathing and coughing

Prevents the shallow and/or rapid breathing that can occur with fear and anxiety.

These actions decrease incidence of abdominal distention and pressure on the diaphragm.

Prevents slumping and decreases pressure on the diaphragm which prevents adequate lung expansion.

Changing position while on bed rest prevents stasis of lung secretion and skin breakdown

Deep breathing and use of incentive spirometry improve lung expansion. Presence of the nurse may be helpful in decreasing client anxiety and assures appropriate use of the incentive spirometer.

Abdominal splinting may enhance client's deep breathing and cough effort.

Dependent/Collaborative Actions

- Implement measures to prevent diaphragmatic pressure from abdominal distention-insertion of nasogastric tube and maintain to suction, if ordered.

- Increase activity as allowed and tolerated. **D** ✦

- Schedule rest periods around times of increased activity.

- Administer central nervous system depressants judiciously; hold medication and consult physician if respiratory rate is less than 12 breaths/min.
- Administer supplemental oxygen as ordered.

Consult appropriate health care provider (e.g., respiratory therapist, physician) if:
- Ineffective breathing pattern continues.
- Signs and symptoms of atelectasis (e.g., diminished or absent breath sounds, dull percussion note over affected area, increased respiratory rate, dyspnea, tachycardia, elevated temperature) develop.
- Signs and symptoms of impaired gas exchange (e.g., restlessness, irritability, confusion, significant decrease in oximetry results, decreased PaO₂ and increased PaCO₂ levels) are present.

Decreasing pressure on the diaphragm will allow for improved lung expansion.

Insertion of a nasogastric tube will reduce stimulation of the pancreas and removes hydrochloric acid from the stomach.

Movement enhances circulation and lung expansion, decreases dyspnea, and increases activity tolerance.

Helps to conserve client's energy and ability to participate in desired activities.

Central nervous system depressants can significantly reduce respiratory rate and subsequently cause a significant decrease in oxygenation.

Improves ability to maintain adequate oxygenation to body tissues

Notifying the appropriate health care provider allows for prompt modification of treatment plan.

Each of these clinical manifestations may indicate worsening condition

Nursing Diagnosis	**RISK FOR SHOCK** NDx

Definition: Susceptible to an inadequate blood flow to the body's tissues that may lead to life-threatening cellular dysfunction, which may compromise health.

Related to:
- Deficient fluid volume associated with restricted oral intake and fluid loss resulting from vomiting and nasogastric tube drainage
- Peripheral vasodilation and increased vascular permeability with subsequent third-spacing subsequent to activation of kinin peptides such as bradykinin and kallidin (occurs when the pancreatic enzyme trypsin enters systemic circulation)

CLINICAL MANIFESTATIONS

Subjective	Objective
Self-report of feeling agitated; anxiety; thirst	Changes in mental status; agitation; confusion; hypotension; tachycardia; cool skin; restlessness; rapid respirations; pallor and cyanosis; oliguria, dry mucous membranes

RISK FACTORS

- Inadequate fluid intake
- Increased toxins in the blood
- Failure of regulatory mechanisms

DESIRED OUTCOMES

The client will not develop hypovolemic shock, as evidenced by:
a. Usual mental status
b. Stable vital signs
c. Skin warm and usual color
d. Palpable peripheral pulses
e. Urine output at least 30 mL/h
f. Moist mucous membranes

NOC OUTCOMES

Shock prevention

NIC INTERVENTIONS

Shock management: cardiac; vasogenic; volume

NURSING ASSESSMENT	RATIONALE

Assess for and report signs and symptoms of:
- Deficient fluid volume and third-spacing:
  - Decreased skin turgor, dry mucous membranes, thirst
  - Weight loss of 2% or greater over a short period
  - Postural hypotension and/or low B/P
  - Weak, rapid pulse
  - Capillary refill time greater than 2 to 3 seconds
  - Flat neck veins when supine
  - Change in mental status
  - Decreased urine output with increased specific gravity (reflects an actual rather than potential fluid volume deficit)
  - Increased BUN and Hct
- Bleeding (e.g., gray-blue discoloration around umbilicus [Cullen sign], green-blue or purple-blue discoloration of flanks [Grey Turner sign], increased abdominal or back pain, increased abdominal girth, decreasing B/P and increased pulse rate, decreased Hct and Hgb levels)

Early recognition of signs and symptoms of hypovolemic shock allows for prompt intervention.

Continued...

NURSING ASSESSMENT	RATIONALE

• Hypovolemic shock:
  • Restlessness, agitation, confusion, or other change in mental status
  • Significant decrease in B/P
  • Postural hypotension
  • Rapid, weak pulse
  • Rapid respirations
  • Cold, clammy skin
  • Pallor, cyanosis, decreasing SaO_2
  • Diminished or absent peripheral pulses
  • Urine output less than 30 mL/h
	Indicate deteriorating client condition and could be life threatening.

THERAPEUTIC INTERVENTIONS	RATIONALE

Dependent/Collaborative Actions
Implement measures to prevent hypovolemic shock:
• Monitor fluid volume and electrolytes:
  • Measure I & O
  • Monitor IV or oral fluid intake
  • Monitor serum electrolytes as ordered
	Maintenance of vascular fluid volume and treatment of changes as required decrease potential for hypovolemic shock.

• Perform actions to reduce pancreatic stimulation (e.g., withhold all food and oral fluid intake as ordered; insert a nasogastric tube and maintain to suction as ordered; administer histamine receptor antagonists).	*Actions that decrease the amount of elastase that is activated and released into the tissue and systemic circulation. This decreases the risk for bleeding and loss of vascular fluid volume.*
If signs and symptoms of hypovolemic shock occur: • Place client flat in bed with legs elevated, unless contraindicated.	*Placing the client in this position increases B/P and helps to maintain blood flow to the vital organs.*
• Monitor blood pressure, heart rate, and SaO_2.	*Monitors changes in client's status.*
• Administer oxygen as ordered.	*Maintains tissue oxygenation.*
• Administer whole blood, blood products, and/or volume expanders, if ordered.	*Administration of blood and blood products increases vascular fluid volume and B/P.*
• Prepare client for transfer to the critical care unit and insertion of hemodynamic monitoring devices (e.g., central venous catheter, intra-arterial catheter), if indicated.	*Central monitoring of central hemodynamic status allows for more rapid intervention and should done in the critical care unit.*

Collaborative Diagnosis | **RISK FOR PERITONITIS**

Definition: Inflammation of the peritoneum.

Related to:
• Escape of activated pancreatic enzymes from the pancreas into the peritoneum
• Leakage of necrotic substances into the peritoneum associated with rupture of an infected pancreatic or peripancreatic abscess or pseudocyst
• Suppuration in areas of pancreatic and peripancreatic necrosis

CLINICAL MANIFESTATIONS

Subjective	Objective
Verbalization of increasing abdominal pain; rebound tenderness; nausea	Temperature greater than 38°C; rigid abdomen; diminished or absent bowel sounds; tachycardia; hypotension; tachypnea; elevated WBC count

RISK FACTOR

- Exposure to pathogens

DESIRED OUTCOMES

The client will not develop peritonitis, as evidenced by:
a. Gradual resolution of abdominal pain
b. Soft, nondistended abdomen
c. Temperature declining toward normal
d. Stable vital signs
e. Decreased nausea and vomiting
f. Gradual return of normal bowel sounds
g. WBC count declining toward normal

NURSING ASSESSMENT

Assess for and report signs and symptoms of peritonitis (e.g., increase in severity of abdominal pain; generalized abdominal pain; rebound tenderness; distended, rigid abdomen; further increase in temperature; tachycardia; tachypnea; hypotension; increased nausea and vomiting; diminished or absent bowel sounds; WBC count that increases or fails to decline toward normal).

RATIONALE

Early recognition of signs and symptoms of peritonitis allows for prompt intervention.

THERAPEUTIC INTERVENTIONS

Dependent/Collaborative Actions

Implement measures to prevent peritonitis:
- Perform actions to reduce pancreatic stimulation (e.g., maintain food and oral fluid restrictions, if ordered; place client in a semi-Fowler's position). **D** ✦
- Administer antimicrobials, if ordered.
- Prepare client for drainage or removal of infected pseudocysts and abscesses and resection of necrotic tissue if planned.

If signs and symptoms of peritonitis occur:
- Withhold oral intake as ordered.
- Place client on bedrest in a semi-Fowler's position.

- Prepare client for diagnostic tests (e.g., abdominal radiograph, computed tomography, ultrasonography) if planned.
- Insert a nasogastric tube and maintain suction as ordered.

- Administer antimicrobials as ordered.
- Administer IV fluids and/or blood volume expanders if ordered, to prevent or treat shock.
- Prepare client for and assist with peritoneal lavage if performed.

RATIONALE

These actions decrease activation of the pancreatic enzymes within the pancreas and reduce the risk for their escape into the peritoneum.
Antimicrobials treat and/or prevent infections.
Decreases client's fear and anxiety.

Decrease activation of the pancreatic enzymes within the pancreas.

Proper positioning assists in pooling or localizing gastrointestinal contents in the pelvis rather than under the diaphragm.
Decreases client's fear and anxiety.

Removal of the gastric contents decreases activation of the pancreatic enzymes within the pancreas and reduces the risk for further leakage into the peritoneum.
Antimicrobials treat infection.
Administration of IV fluids or blood expanders increase vascular fluid volume.
Peritoneal lavage removes toxins from the peritoneal cavity.

Collaborative Diagnosis | **RISK FOR UNSTABLE BLOOD GLUCOSE LEVEL** NDx

Definition: Susceptible to variation in serum levels of glucose from the normal range, which may compromise health.

Related to:
- Increased glucagon and decreased insulin output associated with pancreatic enzyme damage to the islet cells
- The increased glucagon, cortisol, and catecholamine output associated with stress

CLINICAL MANIFESTATIONS

Subjective	Objective
Verbalization of feeling hungry and tired	Polydipsia; polyuria; polyphagia; change in mental status; blood glucose level greater than 200 mg/dL

RISK FACTORS

- Decreased dietary intake
- Failure of regulatory mechanisms
- Inadequate treatment regimen

NOC OUTCOMES	NIC INTERVENTIONS
Hyperglycemia severity; hypoglycemia severity; blood glucose monitoring	Hyperglycemia management; hypoglycemia management; blood glucose monitoring

DESIRED OUTCOMES

The client will maintain a safe blood glucose level, as evidenced by:
a. Absence of polydipsia, polyuria, and polyphagia
b. Usual mental status
c. Serum glucose between 60 and 200 mg/dL

NURSING ASSESSMENT	RATIONALE
Assess for and report signs and symptoms of hyperglycemia (e.g., polydipsia, polyuria, polyphagia, change in mental status, blood glucose levels >200 mg/dL the parameter specified by the health care provider).	*Early recognition of signs and symptoms of hyperglycemia allows for prompt intervention.*

THERAPEUTIC INTERVENTIONS	RATIONALE

Dependent/Collaborative Actions

Implement measures to prevent hyperglycemia:

- Perform actions to reduce pancreatic stimulation (e.g., maintain food and oral fluid restrictions if ordered, place client in a semi-Fowler's position, administer antimicrobials).

  Decreases activation of the pancreatic enzymes within the pancreas and prevents further damage to the pancreatic islet cells.

- Perform actions such as relieving discomfort, explaining all tests and procedures, and providing a restful environment to reduce stress.

  Stress causes an increased output of epinephrine, norepinephrine, glucagon, and cortisol that result in a further increase in blood glucose levels.

If signs and symptoms of hyperglycemia occur:

- Administer insulin or oral hypoglycemic agents, if ordered.

  Insulin and oral hypoglycemic agents decrease blood glucose levels. Appropriate insulin administration may prevent development of ketoacidosis.

- Assess for and report signs and symptoms of ketoacidosis (e.g., warm, flushed skin; thirst; weakness; lethargy; hypotension; increased abdominal pain; fruity odor on breath; Kussmaul respirations; blood glucose >250 mg/dL; ketones in blood and urine; low serum pH and CO_2 content).

  Notification of the physician of signs and symptoms of ketoacidosis allows a for modification of the treatment plan.

- If client does not have a history of diabetes or chronic pancreatitis, offer assurance that the hyperglycemia is expected to resolve as the pancreatitis does.

  When pancreatitis is resolved, the extent of pancreatic destruction will determine which medications the client will need upon discharge from the hospital.

Collaborative Diagnosis ## RISK FOR ORGAN ISCHEMIA/DYSFUNCTION

Definition: A life-threatening syndrome in which the body is unable to maintain homeostasis without intervention.

Related to:

- Hypoperfusion of major organs associated with hypovolemic and/or septic shock, if present, and decreased myocardial contractility (can occur as a result of the release of myocardial depressant factor in response to the inflammatory process that occurs in pancreatitis)
- Microvascular thrombosis associated with disseminated intravascular coagulation (DIC) if it occurs (activation of clotting mechanisms can occur in response to the presence of activated proteolytic enzymes in the blood vessels and/or the procoagulant effects of some inflammatory mediators)

CLINICAL MANIFESTATIONS

Subjective	Objective
N/A	Severe hypotension; tachycardia; urine output less than 30 mL/h; dyspnea, tachypnea; decreasing SaO_2; altered ABG values with low PaO_2; elevated serum BUN and creatinine levels; crackles throughout lungs; changes in mental status

RISK FACTORS

- Failure of regulatory mechanisms

DESIRED OUTCOMES

The client will not develop organ ischemia/dysfunction, as evidenced by:
a. Usual mental status
b. Urine output at least 30 mL/h
c. Unlabored respirations at 12 to 20 breaths/min
d. Audible breath sounds without an increase in adventitious sounds
e. Absence of new or increased abdominal pain, distention, nausea, vomiting, and diarrhea
f. BUN and serum creatinine, AST, ALT, and lactate dehydrogenase (LDH) levels within normal range
g. $SaO_2 > 90$

NURSING ASSESSMENT

Assess for and report signs and symptoms of organ ischemia/dysfunction:
- Cerebral ischemia (e.g., change in mental status)
- Renal insufficiency (e.g., urine output <30 mL/h, elevated BUN and serum creatinine levels)
- Acute respiratory distress syndrome (e.g., dyspnea, increase in respiratory rate, low SaO_2, crackles)
- Gastrointestinal ischemia (e.g., increasing and severe abdominal pain, nausea, and abdominal distention; continued hypoactive or absent bowel sounds; development of or increased episodes of vomiting; diarrhea; hematemesis; blood in stool)
- Liver dysfunction (e.g., increased serum AST, ALT, and LDH levels)

RATIONALE

Early recognition of organ ischemia/dysfunction allows for prompt intervention.

THERAPEUTIC INTERVENTIONS

Dependent/Collaborative Actions

Implement measures to reduce the risk for organ ischemia/dysfunction:
- Perform actions to prevent hypovolemic shock (administer fluids and electrolytes as ordered; maintain fluid intake of at least 2500 mL/day).
- Perform actions to prevent sepsis (administer antimicrobials as ordered; maintain aseptic or sterile technique on all procedures; maintain adequate nutrition status).
- Perform actions to treat DIC if it occurs (e.g., implement safety precautions to prevent further bleeding; administer FFP, platelets, and/or cryoprecipitate, if ordered; administer medications such as heparin and antithrombin III if ordered, to interrupt clotting).
- Maintain IV therapy as ordered.

RATIONALE

When pancreatic tissue dies, pancreatic enzymes and blood may escape into the abdomen, causing sepsis, which subsequently leads to systemic hypoperfusion. Prompt identification and intervention may prevent patient from progressing to organ ischemia/dysfunction.

These actions prevent introduction of bacteria into the system; nutrition is important for the body's ability to fight off infections.

Actions maintain fluid volume, replace used clotting factors, and prevent injury to client.

Maintains adequate vascular fluid volume.

Continued...

THERAPEUTIC INTERVENTIONS	RATIONALE
• Maintain oxygen therapy as ordered. • Administer vasopressors (e.g., dopamine, norepinephrine) and/or positive inotropic agents (e.g., dobutamine) as ordered. If signs and symptoms of organ ischemia/MODS occur, prepare client for transfer to critical care unit.	*Maintains adequate oxygenation of tissues.* *Vasopressors and positive inotropic agents cause vasoconstriction and increase the force of cardiac contractions to maintain adequate tissue perfusion and cardiac output.* *Client requires intensive monitoring and care that will be received in the intensive care unit.*

DISCHARGE CARE/CONTINUED CARE

Nursing Diagnosis

DEFICIENT KNOWLEDGE NDx; INEFFECTIVE HEALTH MANAGEMENT NDx; OR INEFFECTIVE FAMILY HEALTH MANAGEMENT* NDx

Definition: **Deficient Knowledge NDx:** Absence of cognitive information related to a specific topic or its acquisition; **Ineffective Health Management NDx:** Pattern of regulating and integrating into daily living a therapeutic regimen for the treatment of illness and its sequelae that is unsatisfactory for meeting specific health goals; **Ineffective Family Health Management NDx:** A pattern of regulating and integrating into family processes a program for the treatment of illness and its sequelae that is unsatisfactory for meeting specific health goals of the family unit.

Related to:
• Specific topic (lack of specific information necessary for clients/significant others) to make informed choices regarding condition/treatment/lifestyle changes
• Pattern of regulating and integrating into daily living and family processes a therapeutic treatment regimen.

CLINICAL MANIFESTATIONS

Subjective	Objective
Verbalizes inability to manage illness; verbalizes inability to follow prescribed regimen	Inaccurate follow-through with instructions; inappropriate behaviors; experience of preventable complications of pancreatitis

RISK FACTORS
• Cognitive deficit
• Financial concerns
• Failure to take action to reduce risk factors for complications of pancreatitis
• Inability to care for oneself
• Difficulty in modifying personal habits and integrating treatments into lifestyle and family processes

DESIRED OUTCOMES

The client will:
a. Identify ways to prevent overstimulation of and further trauma to the pancreas
b. Develop a plan to implement recommended dietary modifications
c. State signs and symptoms to report to the health care provider
d. Develop a plan for adhering in recommended follow-up care

NOC OUTCOMES

Knowledge: treatment regimen; diet; disease process

NIC INTERVENTIONS

Health Education
Health system guidance; teaching: individual; teaching: disease process; teaching: prescribed diet; teaching: prescribed medication

*The nurse should select the diagnostic label that is most appropriate for the client's discharge teaching needs.

NURSING ASSESSMENT	RATIONALE
Assess client's and family's knowledge base related to the disease process.	*The client's and family's knowledge base provides the basis for education.*
Assess for indications that the client and family may be unable to effectively manage the therapeutic regimen:	*Early recognition of inability to understand disease process or self-care allows for change in teaching modality.*
• Statements reflecting inability to manage care at home	
• Failure to adhere to treatment plan (e.g., refusing medications)	
• Statements reflecting a lack of understanding of factors that may cause further progression of pancreatitis	
• Statements reflecting an unwillingness or inability to modify personal habits and integrate necessary treatments into lifestyle	

THERAPEUTIC INTERVENTIONS	RATIONALE

Desired Outcome: The client and family will identify actions to prevent overstimulation of and further trauma to the pancreas

Independent Actions

Instruct client and family on actions that prevent overstimulation of and further trauma to the pancreas:

• Maintain a balanced program of rest and exercise.	*Decreases stimulation of the pancreas.*
• Avoid drinking alcohol.	*Alcohol can cause blockage of pancreatic ducts that drain into the pancreatic duct.*
• Adhere to recommended dietary modifications.	*Prevents overstimulation of the pancreas.*
If indicated, provide information about and encourage use of community resources that can assist client to make necessary lifestyle changes (e.g., alcohol rehabilitation program).	*Provides continuum of care post discharge from the acute care facility.*

THERAPEUTIC INTERVENTIONS	RATIONALE

Desired Outcome: The client and family will develop a plan to implement recommended dietary modifications

Independent Actions

Instruct client and family regarding dietary modifications necessary to prevent overstimulation of the pancreas during the recovery period:	*Enhances client's knowledge of recommended foods that the client can eat and tolerate. Client and family need to identify food preferences and ones that are allowed on the recommended diet.*
• Eat small, frequent meals rather than three large ones.	*Smaller meals require less pancreatic enzymes and energy by the patient to consume.*
• Avoid foods/fluids high in fat (e.g., butter, cream, whole milk, ice cream, fried foods, gravies, nuts).	*Foods/fluids high in fat increase the release of pancreatic enzymes.*
• Avoid spicy foods and caffeine-containing beverages (e.g., coffee, tea, colas).	*Spicy foods can simulate increased release of pancreatic enzymes.*
Obtain a dietary consult if client needs assistance in planning meals that incorporate dietary modifications.	*A dietitian can work with the client and family to integrate into meals plans foods that the client likes and are part of the recommended diet.*

THERAPEUTIC INTERVENTIONS	RATIONALE

Desired Outcome: The client and family will state signs and symptoms to report to the health care provider

Independent Actions

Instruct client to report:

• Stools that float and are grayish, greasy, and foul-smelling	*Indicates a very high fat content resulting from impaired flow of the pancreatic enzyme lipase into the intestinal tract.*
• Persistent or recurrent abdominal or back pain	*May indicated continued disease processes.*

Continued...

THERAPEUTIC INTERVENTIONS	RATIONALE
• Nausea or vomiting	*May indicate recurrence of pancreatitis, as well as the complications of bleeding and infection.*
• Abdominal distention or increasing feeling of fullness	
• Excessive thirst or excessive urination	*These symptoms may indicate decreased insulin production and increased serum glucose levels.*
• Irritability or confusion	
• Continued or unexplained weight loss	
• Bluish areas on the back or abdomen	*May indicate bleeding within the abdomen.*
• Persistent or recurrent temperature elevation	*These symptoms may indicate an infection or progression of disease processes.*
• Fever, chills	
• Difficulty breathing	

THERAPEUTIC INTERVENTIONS	RATIONALE

Desired Outcome: The client and family, in collaboration with the nurse, will develop a plan for adhering in recommended follow-up care including future appointments with heath care provider and medications prescribed

Independent Actions

Reinforce the importance of keeping follow-up appointments with health care provider. Client should develop and post in a prominent site a calendar of follow-up appointments.

Allows the health care provider to monitor client's health status.

Explain the rationale for, side effects of, and importance of taking medications prescribed (e.g., vitamins, antimicrobials, pancreatic enzymes). Inform client of pertinent food and drug interactions.

Client should develop a schedule for medication administration.

Knowledge of medications and how they impact the system improves client adherence to treatment regimen and understanding of the importance of adhering to the prescribed medication regimen. The client and family should be able to recognize alterations in functioning related to medication administration and know what clinical manifestations should be reported to the health care provider.

Implement measures to improve client's compliance:
• Include significant others in teaching sessions if possible.

Allows for others to support client as needed.

• Encourage questions and allow time for reinforcement and clarification of information provided.

Allows for a more complete understanding of the client's condition by client and significant others and for the nurse to evaluate client's knowledge of the treatment regimen.

• Provide written instructions on scheduled appointments with health care provider, medications prescribed, and signs and symptoms to report.

Written instructions provide an information resource following discharge from the acute care facility.

ADDITIONAL DIAGNOSES

IMPAIRED ORAL MUCOUS MEMBRANE INTEGRITY NDx

Related to:
• Fluid volume deficit associated with restricted oral intake and fluid loss resulting from vomiting and nasogastric tube drainage
• Decreased salivation associated with deficient fluid volume, restricted oral intake, and the side effect of some medications (e.g., narcotic [opioid] analgesics, some antiemetics)
• Mouth breathing if nasogastric tube is in place

FEAR NDx AND ANXIETY NDx
Definition:

Related to:
• Severe pain
• Unfamiliar environment
• Lack of understanding of diagnostic tests, treatment plan, and prognosis

NAUSEA NDx

Definition: A subjective phenomenon of an unpleasant feeling in the back of the throat and stomach, which may or may not result in vomiting.

Related to:
• Stimulation of the vomiting center associated with:
  • Stimulation of the visceral afferent pathways from abdominal distention and inflammation of the pancreas
  • Stimulation of the cerebral cortex resulting from pain and stress

12

The Client With Alterations in the Kidney and Urinary Tract

UROLITHIASIS (RENAL STONES)

Urolithiasis is the development of stones from crystalized solute in the urinary tract. Nephrolithiasis refers to stones that form in the kidney and ureterolithiasis refers to stones in the ureters. Renal stones occur more frequently in men than in women, and in Caucasians than in Blacks. In the United States, these stones occur more frequently in the southeastern area of the country and during the summer months. This area-specific incidence is thought to be associated with dehydration associated with humidity, sweating, and decreased consumption of water.

There are four main types of kidney stones. Calcium stones, which are the most common type, are composed of calcium and/or oxalate and phosphorus. Uric acid stones form when the urine is too acidic and can be composed of just uric acid or combined with calcium. Struvite stones are associated with urinary tract infections where the bacteria produce ammonia, and are made up of magnesium, ammonium, and phosphate. The rarest type of stone is a cysteine stone and occurs in individuals with a genetic disorder that allows cysteine to leak from the kidney into the urine. Regardless of the type of stone, it may lodge anywhere within the kidneys, ureters, bladder, or urethra. Kidney stones may form anywhere in the urinary tract. They may be asymptomatic until the stone lodges in the ureter or if there is urinary obstruction. The most common area for stones to obstruct urine flow and elimination from the body is in the ureteropelvic junction, where the urine exits the kidney and the lower third of the ureter. Unless the stone is passed or removed, blockage of urine elimination can cause severe complications including pyelonephritis, urosepsis, and irreversible renal damage. Surgical removal of the stone is required if the stone is large and causing severe urine obstruction. The type of procedure performed depends on the stone's size, location, and critical nature of the blockage. A ureteroscopy is used for large stones in the lower end of the ureter. The extracorporeal shock-wave lithotripsy (ESWL) is used for smaller stones (between 2 and 4 mm) in the kidney or ureter. In the ESWL procedure, the client is placed on a water-filled cushion. The surgeon uses x-rays to identify the precise location of the stone. High-energy sound waves are used to break the stone

into smaller, passible fragments. Conscious sedation or general anesthesia is used during the procedure. The client is typically discharged a few hours following the procedure. The client will be required to drink lots of fluid, and to strain or filter the urine to obtain stone fragments for testing.

For large (>2 cm), odd shaped, or stones not resolved by ESWL, the client may undergo a percutaneous nephrolithotomy and percutaneous nephrolithotripsy. These procedures involve percutaneous access to the kidney. In the nephrolithotomy, the stone is removed directly from the kidney. If a percutaneous nephrolithotripsy is done, the stone can be broken up using high-frequency sound waves and then the fragments are removed. Both procedures are conducted using general anesthesia and may require a short hospital stay. Although these procedures are minimally invasive, there is a risk for infection, bleeding, and complications associated with general anesthesia.

Discharge teaching should focus on action that will prevent recurrence of kidney stones. The client should be taught about adequate hydration, dietary restrictions (depending on the type of stone), and follow-up care.

This care plan focuses on the adult client having a kidney stone and surgical removal.

OUTCOME/DISCHARGE CRITERIA

The client will:
1. Maintain pain-free status
2. Maintain adequate urine output
3. Have no evidence of wound or urinary tract infection
4. Have no signs and symptoms of postoperative complications
5. Demonstrate the ability to strain/filter urine if ordered
6. State signs and symptoms to report to the health care provider
7. Develop a plan for adhering to recommended follow-up care including prevention recurrence of kidney stones, follow-up care with the heath care provider, medication regimen, and measures to prevent complications

Preoperative—Refer to Standardized Preoperative Care Plan
Postoperative—Refer to Standardized Postoperative Care Plan

ACUTE PAIN NDx

Definition: Unpleasant sensory and emotional experience associated with actual or potential tissue damage, or described in terms of such damage (International Association for the Study of Pain); sudden or slow onset of any intensity from mild to severe with an anticipated or predictable end, and with a duration of less than 3 months.

Related to:
- Partial or complete obstruction within the urinary tract
- Fear and anxiety specific to inability to pass stone
- Stone removal procedure if performed

CLINICAL MANIFESTATIONS

Subjective	Objective
Verbal self-report of pain, expression of fear and anxiety	Facial expressions of grimacing, restlessness, increased blood pressure (BP) and heart rate

RISK FACTORS

- Kidney stone
- Surgery

DESIRED OUTCOMES

The client will experience decreased pain as evidenced by:
a. Verbalization of decrease or absence of pain
b. Stable vital signs
c. Decreased or absent restlessness and grimacing

NOC OUTCOMES

Pain level

NIC INTERVENTIONS

Acute pain management: patient-controlled analgesia (PCA) assistance, analgesic administration

NURSING ASSESSMENT

Assess for signs and symptoms of pain
- Verbalization of pain
- Grimacing
- Restlessness
- Increased BP
- Tachycardia
- Assess client's perception of the severity of pain using a pain intensity rating scale
- Assess client's pain pattern (e.g., location, onset, quality, duration, aggravating factors)
- Ask client to describe previous pain experience and methods that were effective in relieving pain

RATIONALE

Early recognition of signs and symptoms of pain allows for prompt intervention and improved pain control.

Assessment of the severity of pain being experienced helps determine the most appropriate intervention. Use of a pain intensity rating scale provides the nurse a clear understanding of the pain being experienced and promotes consistency when communicating with others.

Knowledge of client's pain pattern assists in the identification of effective pain management intervention.

Knowledge of client's usual pain response and effective methods to alleviate pain supports the identification of effective pain management.

THERAPEUTIC INTERVENTIONS

Independent Actions
Implement measures to reduce fear and anxiety.
- Provide a calm environment.
- Answer call light quickly when notified of experience of pain. **D** ● ✦
- Assure client pain experience is understood and will be addressed.
- Implement measures to promote rest. **D** ● ✦
- Minimize environmental activity, light, and noise.

RATIONALE

Fear and anxiety can increase the clients experience of pain and interventions may not be as effective if the patient is unable to relax.

Fatigue can decrease client tolerance for pain. Rest often helps decrease the experience of pain and enhance effectiveness of pain interventions.

THERAPEUTIC INTERVENTIONS	RATIONALE
Provide or assist with adjuvant nonpharmacological methods of pain relief. **D** ● ✦ • Relaxation techniques (e.g., progressive relaxation exercises, mindfulness-based stress reduction (MBSR), meditation, focused breathing, guided imagery). • Distraction measures (e.g., music, conversing, watching TV, reading). **D** ● ✦ • Position changes. **D** ● ✦ • Provide warm blankets or heating pad to pain location.	*These nonpharmacological interventions are thought to be effective as they stimulate the closure of the gating mechanism in the spinal cord, thus blocking pain transmission. Other interventions may increase endorphin levels and promote relaxation.*
Encourage 2 to 3 L/day of fluid unless contraindicated. Document episodes of increased or persistent pain.	*Pain from kidney stones is colicky in nature and may worsen when lying in the supine position.* *Hydration increases urine production and output, preventing urinary stasis and promoting passing of the stone* *This may indicate increasing or complete obstruction of urine flow and may require immediate surgical intervention.*

Dependent/Collaborative Actions

Administer analgesics as indicated (e.g., opioids, oxycodone, acetaminophen, ibuprofen, ketorolac). Administer on a routine schedule to prevent pain from becoming too severe.	*Kidney stone pain is acute and colicky in nature. Parenteral narcotics are best to address this type of pain. Nonsteroidal anti-inflammatory drugs (NSAIDs) can also be effective when used alone or in combination with other medications for mild to moderate pain.*
Request PCA device.	*Allows client to maintain control of pain medication.*
Administer antispasmodics; calcium channel blockers, and alpha-adrenergic blockers.	*These medications help decrease spasms of the urinary tract and may facilitate stone passage.*
Notify the health care provider of increased episodes of pain or persistent pain.	*May indicate passing of stone or possible blockage. Notification of health care provider allows for prompt intervention.*

Nursing Diagnosis ## IMPAIRED URINARY ELIMINATION NDx

Definition: Dysfunction in urine elimination.

Related to: Obstruction to urine flow and output caused by renal calculus
Postoperative edema of the urinary tract

CLINICAL MANIFESTATIONS

Subjective	Objective
Verbal self-report of continued or persistent pain and difficulty in voiding, bladder fullness, increased frequency of attempting to void	Changes in urine output volume, color, and consistency; increased frequency in voiding pattern; distended bladder; changes in blood urea nitrogen (BUN) and creatinine levels

RISK FACTORS

- Age
- Surgery
- Kidney stone
- Poor bladder tone

DESIRED OUTCOMES

The client will maintain adequate urine output and elimination pattern as evidenced by:
a. Usual frequency of urination
b. Output >30 mL/h
c. Voiding clear urine
d. Absence of pain or burning upon urination
e. BUN and creatinine clearance levels within client's normal range

NOC OUTCOMES

Urinary elimination

NIC INTERVENTIONS

Urinary management, urinary retention care

NDx = NANDA Diagnosis   **D** = Delegatable Action   ● = UAP   ✦ = LVN/LPN   ⊖▶ = Go to ⊖volve for animation

NURSING ASSESSMENT	RATIONALE

Assess for and report the following:
  Normal urinary elimination patterns
  Possible urinary retention:
  • Reports of frequent urgency to empty bladder
  • Bladder distention
  • Post-void residual bladder fullness
  • Urine output <30 mL/h
Note color, clarity, and consistency of urine
	Early recognition of signs and symptoms of urinary retention allows for prompt intervention.
	Knowledge of client's voiding pattern may help to identify subtle changes that indicate urinary retention.
	A palpable bladder provides evidence of urinary retention.
	A post-void residual bladder scan can indicate if client is able to fully empty bladder.
	Changes in the color, clarity, and consistency of the urine may indicate stasis or possible urinary tract infection.

THERAPEUTIC INTERVENTIONS	RATIONALE

Independent Actions

Encourage increased fluid intake, if not contraindicated.	*Increased hydration dilutes the urine and may support passage of the stone or other debris.*
Instruct client to urinate when the urge is felt.	*Helps to prevent stasis.*
Implement measures to promote relaxation during voiding attempts (e.g., provide privacy, hold a warm blanket against abdomen, place client's hands in warm water).	*A client who is relaxed when trying to urinate is better able to relax the pelvic floor muscles and external urinary sphincter and allow voiding to occur.*
Assist client to assume a normal position for voiding (usually sitting for females and standing for males) unless contraindicated. **D** ● ✦	*A sitting or standing position uses gravity to facilitate bladder emptying. Allowing client to assume their routine voiding position also promotes relaxation and facilitates voiding.*
Strain urine and document any passage of stones and send to the laboratory for analysis. **D** ● ✦	*Helps to determine client's ability to pass the stone or stone fragments. Analysis of the type of stone is important in determining choice of therapy.*

Dependent/Collaborative Actions

Administer medications as ordered:
  α-Adrenergic blockers (i.e., tamsulosin, terazosin, doxazosin)
  Calcium channel blockers (i.e., nifedipine).
	For small distal ureteral stones, α-adrenergic blockers and calcium channel blockers have been shown to relax the smooth muscles of the ureter and decrease colic events, thus facilitating stone passage. Decreasing colicky events may decrease need for analgesic medications.

Corticosteroids (i.e., deltasone).	*Steroids reduce inflammation and neutrophil-induced damage to the ureter. When used in combination with α-adrenergic blockers and/or calcium channel blockers, steroids improve stone passage and decrease expulsion time.*
Monitor, document, and report any changes in lab values: BUN and creatinine.	*Changes in BUN and creatinine indicate kidney dysfunction.* *Determines presence of infection and causative agents. Sensitivity determines appropriate antibiotic therapy.*
Culture and sensitivity results.	*Provides client information on what to expect and helps to alleviate fear and anxiety.*

Prepare client for surgical procedures to remove the stone including:
  Ureteroscopy for stone removal and potential stent placement.
  Extracorporeal shockwave lithotripsy (ESWL)
  Percutaneous nephrolithotomy.	

Nursing Diagnosis ▎ **RISK FOR INFECTION** NDx **(URINARY TRACT)**

Definition: Susceptible to invasion and multiplication of pathogenic organisms, which may compromise health.

Related to: Increased growth and colonization of microorganisms associated with urinary stasis

CLINICAL MANIFESTATIONS

Subjective	Objective
Verbalization of frequency, urgency, and burning upon urination	Elevated temperature: urinalysis showing increased white blood cells (WBCs) and presence of bacteria; positive urine cultures

RISK FACTORS

- Poor hygiene
- Stasis of urine from inability to pass kidney stone
- Gender
- Suppressed immune system

DESIRED OUTCOMES

The client will remain free of urinary tract infection as evidenced by:
a. Clear urine
b. Absence of frequency, urgency, and burning on urination
c. Absence of chills and fever
d. Urinalysis slowing <5 WBCs, negative leukocyte esterase and nitrates and presence of bacteria
e. Negative urine culture

NOC OUTCOMES

Infection Protection

NIC INTERVENTIONS

Infection Control

NURSING ASSESSMENT

Assess for and report signs and symptoms of urinary tract infection:
- Presence of cloudy urine
- Self-reports of frequency, urgency, or burning upon urination
- Chills
- Elevated temperature
- Urinalysis showing >5 WBCs; positive leukocyte esters or nitrates or presence of bacteria
- Positive urine culture

RATIONALE

Early recognition of signs and symptoms of urinary tract infection allows for prompt intervention.

THERAPEUTIC INTERVENTIONS

Independent Actions

Encourage client to increase fluid intake if not contraindicated. **D** ● ✦

Encourage client to urinate when urge is first felt. **D** ● ✦

Teach female client to wipe from front to back after urinating or defecating. **D** ✦
Encourage client to wash hands before and after urinating and defecating. **D** ✦
Avoid use of irritating feminine products.
Monitor and document urine output, color, clarity, and verbalization of frequency, urgency, or burning. **D** ● ✦

Dependent/Collaborative Actions
Administer intravenous fluids if ordered.

Obtain lab studies:
   Urine culture and sensitivity.
   Serum complete blood count (CBC).
Notify health care provider if signs and symptoms occur.

RATIONALE

Increased hydration dilutes urine and stimulates more frequent urination, which allows for bacteria to be flushed from the system.
Helps to prevent urinary stasis.
Perineal hygiene performed in this manner reduces risk for urinary tract infection.
Prevents exposure to new bacteria and prevents cross-contamination.

Vaginal deodorant sprays, douches, and powders in the genital area can irritate the urethra.

Changes in volume of urine output, color, clarity and verbalization of frequency, urgency, or burning may indicate urinary tract infection. Decreased urine output may also indicate dehydration.

Increased hydration will increase frequency of voiding and help to flush out debris and bacteria.
Positive cultures indicate a urinary infection.

Elevated WBCs may indicate an infection and need for antibiotics.
Allows for timely modification of treatment regimen.

NDx = NANDA Diagnosis   **D** = Delegatable Action   ● = UAP   ✦ = LVN/LPN   ⊖▶ = Go to ⊖volve for animation

| Nursing Diagnosis | **RISK FOR DEFICIENT FLUID VOLUME** NDx |

Definition: Susceptible to experiencing decreased intravascular, interstitial, and or/intracellular fluid volumes, which may compromise health.

Related to:
- Fluid loss due to vomiting
- Decreased intake due to nausea
- Post-procedure and/or post-stone passage diuresis

CLINICAL MANIFESTATIONS

Subjective	Objective
Verbalization of thirst and dry mouth	Weight loss, increased body temperature, increased hematocrit (Hct), decreased skin turgor, increased heart rate, decreased BP; capillary refill >3 seconds

RISK FACTORS
- Active fluid loss
- Failure of regulatory mechanisms
- Aging-loss of thirst and fluid volume reserve

DESIRED OUTCOMES

The client will not experience a deficient fluid volume as evidenced by:
a. Normal skin turgor
b. Moist mucous membranes
c. Stable weight
d. BP and heart rate within normal range for client and stable with position change
e. Capillary refill time <2 to 3 seconds
f. Hct within normal limits
g. Balanced intake and output (I&O)

NOC OUTCOMES

Fluid management; hydration

NIC INTERVENTIONS

Fluid monitoring; fluid support

NURSING ASSESSMENT	RATIONALE
Assess for signs and symptoms of fluid volume deficit: - Decreased skin turgor - Dry mucous membranes, verbalization of thirst - Weight loss of 2% or greater over a short period of time - Postural hypotension and/or decreased blood pressure - Weak rapid pulse - Capillary refill time >2 to 3 seconds - Increased Hct levels	*Early recognition of signs and symptoms of deficit in fluid volume allows for prompt intervention.*

THERAPEUTIC INTERVENTIONS	RATIONALE
Independent Actions	
Monitor and document I & O and correlate with daily weight.	*A change in body weight of 1 kg (2.2 lbs) equals 1 L fluid loss. Decreased urine output may indicate dehydration.*
Monitor color, clarity, and consistency of urine output and urine osmolality.	*As urine output decreases, urine becomes darker and specific gravity and osmolality increase. A specific gravity of >1.030 indicates hypovolemia.*
Document incidence of nausea, vomiting, and diarrhea.	*Clients who have a kidney stone and have not passed it may experience nausea, vomiting, and diarrhea associated with pain, as the celiac ganglion innervates both the stomach and kidneys.*
Encourage increased fluid intake up to 3–4 L/day if not contraindicated. **D** ● ✦	*Maintains vascular fluid volume and may help to flush out renal stones and any bacteria or debris present.*
Monitor and document changes in heart rate, blood pressure, skin turgor, and capillary refill.	*All are indicators of fluid volume status.*
Dependent/Collaborative Actions	
Administer antiemetic and antidiarrheal medications.	*Decreases fluid volume loss.*
Administer IV fluids as ordered.	*Supports hemodynamic status and fluid volume replacement, and improves renal perfusion.*

THERAPEUTIC INTERVENTIONS	RATIONALE
Monitor and document trends in Hct levels.	*Provides feedback on status of hydration and effectiveness of hydration interventions.*
Encourage appropriate dietary intake including liquids and avoid spicy foods.	*Provides fluid and nutrients to maintain balance. Spicy foods irritate the gastrointestinal (GI) tract and may increase incidence of nausea and vomiting.*

Nursing Diagnosis ## DEFICIENT KNOWLEDGE NDx; INEFFECTIVE HEALTH MANAGEMENT NDx; INEFFECTIVE FAMILY HEALTH MANAGEMENT* NDx

Definition: Deficient Knowledge NDx: Absence of cognitive information related to a specific topic, or its acquisition; **Ineffective Health Management NDx:** Pattern of regulating and integrating into daily living a therapeutic regimen for the treatment of illness and its sequelae that is unsatisfactory for meeting specific health goals; **Ineffective Family Health Management NDx:** A pattern of regulating and integrating into family processes a program for the treatment of illness and its sequelae that is unsatisfactory for meeting specific health goals of the family unit.

CLINICAL MANIFESTATIONS

Subjective	Objective
Verbalization of concerns about potential recurrence of illness and inability to follow prescribed regimen	Inconsistent follow-through with treatment regimen; lack of engagement in self-care or inclusion of family in client education; frequent questioning about therapeutic regimen

RISK FACTORS

- Cognitive deficit
- Multifaceted health care regimen
- Difficulty modifying personal habits and integration of treatment regimen into lifestyle
- Lack of family support
- Lack of financial resources

NOC OUTCOMES	NIC INTERVENTIONS
Knowledge: disease process; treatment regimen	Discharge planning, health education: teaching: disease process; teaching; diet; teaching: prescribed medication; teaching: prescribed exercise

NURSING ASSESSMENT	RATIONALE
Assess client's ability to learn and readiness to learn Assess client's understanding of teaching Assess client's psychomotor skills to assure ability to perform required actions	*Learning is more effective when the client is motivated and understands the importance of what is to be learned. Readiness to learn changes based on situations and physical and emotional challenges.*

THERAPEUTIC INTERVENTIONS	RATIONALE
Desired Outcome: The client will demonstrate ability to strain urine as part of treatment regimen.	*Knowledge of the purpose for treatment regimen is the starting point for patient education and knowledge enhancement.*
Independent Action Assess client's knowledge of the purpose for voided urine straining. Discuss with client the importance of straining all voided urine specimens, and to notify the health care provider when stone has passed.	*The client should strain all voided urine to determine when the stone has passed out of the urinary tract.*

*The nurse should select the diagnostic label that is most appropriate for the client's discharge teaching needs.

NDx = NANDA Diagnosis   **D** = Delegatable Action   ● = UAP   ✦ = LVN/LPN   ⊖▶ = Go to ⊖volve for animation

Continued...

THERAPEUTIC INTERVENTIONS	RATIONALE
Demonstrate and request a return demonstration of how to strain voided urine and how to clean strainer.	*Demonstration of what is required of client supports learning of a new skill. The return demonstration provides the nurse with information on how well the client understands what is required and time for feedback to improve skills. Cleaning of strainer prevents cross-contamination.*
Provide the client with written instructions on how to strain voided urine.	*Provision of written instructions provides a resource for client to use post discharge from acute care setting.*

THERAPEUTIC INTERVENTIONS	RATIONALE
Desired Outcome: The client and significant other will develop a plan to implement required lifestyle changes to prevent recurrence of kidney stone development.	*Provides baseline understanding of disease process and what can be done to prevent kidney stone recurrence.*

Independent Actions

Assess client understanding of the correlation between lifestyle and stone formation.

Assist the client in developing a plan to implement life style changes:

- Maintain adequate fluid intake to assure urine output of 2 to 3 L/day

- Increase intake of water-filled fruits and vegetables

- Have client develop a plan to increase fluid intake throughout the day, particularly with meals and following increased physical activity

- Review dietary recommendations as appropriate:

- To decrease the incidence of uric acid stones:
  - Limit intake or cut down on high-purine foods such as red meat, organ meats, and shellfish and follow a healthy diet that contains mostly vegetables and fruits, whole grains, and low-fat dairy products.

- For oxalate stones:
  - Eat and drink calcium and oxalate-rich foods together during a meal or limit oxalate-rich foods (e.g., peanuts, rhubarb, spinach, beets, sesame seeds, chocolate, and sweet potatoes).

- For calcium stones:
  - No diet limitations at present; take calcium citrate supplements as needed
  - Encourage client to decrease sodium intake

Increase intake of vitamin B$_6$ and magnesium-rich foods.

Request consultation with the dietitian to assist client in developing appropriate menus for an appropriate intake.

Have the client put together 3 days of menus.

Encourage regular physical activity and development of an exercise program.

Have the client write out a plan on how to increase physical activity and to maintain an exercise routine.

Encourage client to avoid all over-the-counter medications and discuss use of herbal supplements with physician.

Encourage client to quit smoking if applicable; assist in plan development or referral to community resources.

Adequate hydration is required to maintain renal perfusion and development of urine output to a level that reduces stone formation.

Increasing hydration during these times is important, as urine solute load is highest following meals and increased physical activity.

Dietary recommendation changes depend on the type of kidney stone.

Decrease intake of uric acid precursors.

Foods that are high in purines predispose the client for uric acid stones.

Research indicates that eating and drinking calcium and oxalate-rich foods together is better than entirely limiting oxalate and calcium intake. When eaten together, oxalate and calcium bind to one another in the stomach and intestines before they can reach the kidneys, thus making it less likely that kidney stones will form.

There are no studies that support calcium limitations in reducing stone formation. Calcium citrate binds with oxalates and improves calcium absorption

Sodium in the diet may lead to dehydration and a high-sodium diet increases the amount of calcium in the urine.

Supplemental intake of magnesium (~200–400 mg/day) and vitamin B6 (~100 mg/day) reduce kidney stone development.

Provides client time with a nutritional expert who can help in choosing appropriate foods and menu development.

Provides for assessment of client's understanding of dietary recommendations and ability to implement appropriate dietary changes.

With decreased activity, the bones increase calcium release; additionally, exercise can help maintain appropriate weight for height and decrease incidence of high blood pressure, a condition that increases the risk for kidney stones.

Decreases incidence of drug interactions.

Smoking may contribute to the development of kidney stones, as it increases levels of calcium in the body.

THERAPEUTIC INTERVENTIONS	RATIONALE
Allow client to ask questions and express concerns related to therapeutic regimen and lifestyle changes.	*Lifestyle changes can be stressful and anxiety producing. Providing an accepting and open environment helps client work through feelings concerning changes without fear of judgment. It also enhances client's sense of confidence in ability to make changes and control over changes.*

THERAPEUTIC INTERVENTIONS	RATIONALE

Desired Outcome: This client will verbalize signs and symptoms to be reported to the health care provider.

Client should understand the incidence of stone recurrence is 15% at 1 year and 50% at 10 years. Knowledge of signs and symptoms and notification of the health care provider allows for prompt intervention.

Independent Actions

Review with client and provide a written list of what signs and symptoms should be reported to the health care provider.
- Increased temperature
- Chills
- Decreased urine output
- Presence of cloudy, dark urine
- Recurrent pain
- Presence of blood in urine
- Weight gain or loss over a short period of time

Indicates potential dehydration and/or infection.

Indicates potential stone blockage of urine flow. If not resolved, can lead to kidney damage.
Indicates trauma or kidney damage.
Indicates fluid imbalance.

THERAPEUTIC INTERVENTIONS	RATIONALE

Desired outcome: The client, in collaboration with the nurse, will a develop plan for adhering to recommended follow-up care including future appointments with health care provider, medications prescribed, activity level, wound care.

Independent Actions

Reinforce physician's instructions regarding
Post-procedure care:
- Increase activity as tolerated
- Avoid lifting objects over 7 lbs. or strenuous exercise until approved by health care provider.

Maintain adequate hydration
Develop schedule for administration of medications if ordered
Collaborate with family members for follow-up Appointments

Reinforcing information improves client understanding of requirements following discharge.

Decreases potential for re-occurrence of stones.
Improves potential for adherence to medication regimen.
Improves potential for attendance at follow-up appointments.

CYSTECTOMY WITH URINARY DIVERSION

Cystectomy is the surgical removal of the bladder to treat a malignancy of the bladder, congenital bladder anomalies, neurogenic bladder, and irreparable bladder trauma. A cystectomy may also be performed to prevent further deterioration of renal function associated with chronic bladder infection. A cystectomy may involve removal of just the bladder (simple cystectomy); however, when there is an invasive malignancy, a more radical procedure is performed. In men, the procedure is called a radical cystoprostatectomy and involves removal of the bladder, prostate, seminal vesicles, lower ureters and, in some cases, the urethra and some or all the pelvic lymph nodes. In women, the procedure is called radical cystectomy or anterior exenteration and usually includes removal of the bladder, urethra, uterus, fallopian tubes, ovaries, anterior vaginal wall, lower ureters, and often some or all the pelvic lymph nodes.

Removal of the bladder requires reconstruction of the lower urinary tract.

Removal of the bladder requires reconstruction of the urinary tract. All three available methods involve using segments of the GI tract for reconstruction of the removed areas of the urinary tract. There are three main types of urinary diversions. They include ileal conduit, creation of a pouch reservoir, and neobladder-to-urethra diversion.

In the first method, the ileal conduit method, the ureters are implanted in a segment of the intestine. The end of the segment is then brought through the abdominal wall, creating a stoma. The second method involves the creation of an internal reservoir (e.g., Kock pouch, Mainz pouch, Indiana pouch). In this method, the ureters are implanted in a resected portion of intestine that has been remodeled to create a reservoir. Another segment of the reservoir is used to create the stoma that is brought out through the abdominal wall. Urinary reflux from the reservoir back through the ureters and the uncontrolled flow of urine from the reservoir through the stoma are prevented by the surgical positioning of the ureters, reservoir, and stoma or by the construction of one-way valves at these sites. After healing occurs, a catheter is inserted into the stoma at regularly scheduled intervals (usually every 4–6 hrs once the reservoir stretches to its full capacity) to drain the reservoir. If the system functions properly, the client does not need to wear a urinary collection appliance over the stoma. The last type of urinary diversion involves reconstruction of a segment of the intestine into a "new" bladder. The ureters are connected to the "new" bladder and voiding requires contraction of the abdominal muscles.

The type of urinary diversion selected depends on many factors including the client's preference, age, body build, ability to learn about and participate in care of the urinary diversion, prognosis, and ability to tolerate lengthy surgery; the integrity of the client's ureters, kidneys, and intestinal tract; the advice of the enterostomal therapy nurse; and the expertise of the surgeon.

This care plan focuses on the adult client hospitalized for a cystectomy with urinary diversion by means of a conventional conduit. Some additional nursing interventions are also included for the client with a continent internal reservoir. Much of the postoperative information is applicable to clients receiving follow-up care in an extended care facility or home setting.

OUTCOME/DISCHARGE CRITERIA

The client will:
1. Maintain an adequate urine output via the urinary diversion

2. Maintain surgical pain control
3. Have evidence of normal healing of surgical wound
4. Have a medium pink to red, moist stoma and intact peristomal skin
5. Have no signs and symptoms of postoperative complications
6. Verbalize a basic understanding of the anatomical changes that occurred as a result of surgery
7. Demonstrate the ability to change the urostomy appliance and maintain stomal and peristomal skin integrity if present
8. Demonstrate the ability to properly clean reusable urostomy equipment, if ostomy is present
9. Demonstrate the ability to drain and irrigate a continent internal reservoir if present
10. Identify ways to control odor of the urostomy drainage and appliance if present
11. Discuss ways to prevent urinary tract infection
12. State signs and symptoms to report to the health care provider
13. Share thoughts and feelings about altered urinary elimination and its effect on body image and lifestyle
14. Identify and connect with appropriate community resources that can assist with home management and adjustment to changes resulting from the urinary diversion
15. Develop plan for adhering to recommended follow-up care including future appointments with health care provider, wound care, activity level, and medications prescribed

For a full, detailed care plan on this topic, go to http://evolve.elsevier.com/Haugen/careplanning/.

NEPHRECTOMY

Nephrectomy is the surgical removal of all or part of a kidney. Indications for a nephrectomy include renal carcinoma, massive traumatic injury to the kidney, polycystic kidney disease (especially if the kidney is bleeding or severely infected), calculi, pyelonephritis, glomerulonephritis, and renal sclerosis resulting from hypertension. The kidney may also be removed for the purpose of donation.

The surgical approach used to perform a nephrectomy depends on the extensiveness of the planned surgery; the client's age, body build, and physiological status; the underlying pathology; and prior surgical incisions. The approach commonly used for a simple nephrectomy (removal of just the kidney) is the flank approach. Other open procedure approaches (e.g., thoracoabdominal, transabdominal, dorsolumbar) may be necessary when greater visualization, improved access, or a radical nephrectomy (removal of the kidney, renal artery and vein, adrenal gland, proximal ureter, regional lymph nodes, and surrounding fat and fascia) is necessary. Although it is most often necessary to remove the entire kidney, advances in renal imaging, earlier diagnosis of renal disease, and improved surgical techniques have provided surgeons with an option of performing a partial nephrectomy (nephron-sparing nephrectomy) in some instances. In these situations, a laparoscopic rather than an open approach is often feasible.

This care plan focuses on the adult client hospitalized for a simple unilateral nephrectomy. Much of the postoperative information is applicable to clients receiving follow-up care in an extended care facility or home setting. The care plan will need to be individualized according to the client's diagnosis, prognosis, and plans for subsequent treatment.

OUTCOME/DISCHARGE CRITERIA

The client will:
1. Have evidence of normal healing of the surgical wound
2. Have adequate functioning of the remaining kidney
3. Have clear, audible breath sounds throughout lungs
4. Have no signs and symptoms of postoperative complications
5. Verbalize ways to maintain health of the remaining kidney
6. State signs and symptoms to report to the health care provider
7. Share thoughts and feelings about the loss of the kidney
8. Develop plan for adhering to recommended follow-up care including future appointments with health care provider, medications prescribed, activity level, wound care, and plans for subsequent treatment of the underlying disorder.

See Standardized Preoperative and Postoperative Care Plans for additional diagnoses.

Nursing Diagnosis   INEFFECTIVE BREATHING PATTERN NDx

Definition: Inspiration and/or expiration that does not provide adequate ventilation.

Related to:
- Increased rate of respirations associated with fear and anxiety
- Decreased rate of respirations associated with the depressant effect of anesthesia and some medications (e.g., narcotic [opioid] analgesics, some antiemetics)
- Decreased depth of respirations associated with:
  - Depressant effect of anesthesia and some medications (e.g., narcotic [opioid] analgesics, some antiemetics)
  - Reluctance to breathe deeply resulting from incisional pain and fear of dislodging chest tube if present
  - Positioning, weakness, fatigue, and elevation of the diaphragm (can occur if abdominal distention is present)

CLINICAL MANIFESTATIONS

Subjective	Objective
Verbal report of shortness of breath and difficulty breathing	Alterations in rate and depth of breathing; altered chest excursion; bradypnea; decreased minute ventilation; use of accessory muscles to breathe; decreased SaO_2 and changes in arterial oxygenation measured via arterial blood gases (ABGs)

RISK FACTORS
- Surgery
- Obesity
- Immobility

DESIRED OUTCOMES

The client will maintain an effective breathing pattern as evidenced by:
a. Normal rate and depth of respirations
b. Absence of dyspnea
c. $SaO_2 > 92\%$

NOC OUTCOMES

Respiratory status: ventilation

NIC INTERVENTIONS

Respiratory monitoring; ventilation assistance

NURSING ASSESSMENT	RATIONALE
Assess for signs and symptoms of the following: • Ineffective breathing pattern • Shallow or slow respirations • Limited chest excursion • Tachypnea or dyspnea • Use of accessory muscles when breathing	*Early recognition of signs and symptoms of an ineffective breathing pattern allows for prompt intervention.*
Assess/monitor pulse oximetry (arterial oxygen saturation [SaO_2]), ABG values as indicated.	*Monitoring continuous SaO_2 readings allows for the early detection and treatment of hypoxia.* *Assessment of ABG values allows for a more direct measurement of both the partial pressure of oxygen in arterial blood (PaO_2) and the partial pressure of carbon dioxide in arterial blood ($PaCO_2$), which reflect the adequacy of ventilation.*

THERAPEUTIC INTERVENTIONS	RATIONALE

Independent Actions
Implement measures to improve breathing pattern:
• Perform actions to reduce fear and anxiety:
  • Promote a calm, restful environment. **D** ● ✦
  • Assure client that deep breathing will not dislodge chest tube if present. **D** ✦
	Reducing fear and anxiety helps prevent shallow and/or rapid breathing.

Continued...

THERAPEUTIC INTERVENTIONS	RATIONALE

• Perform actions to reduce pain:
  • Reposition client for comfort. **D** ● ✦
  • Instruct and assist client to support incision when moving or coughing.
  • Provide adjuvant methods of pain control including relaxation techniques, guided imagery, distraction.
	Reducing pain helps increase the client's willingness to move and breathe more deeply.

• Perform actions to reduce the accumulation of gas and fluid in the GI tract: • Maintain patency of nasogastric (NG), gastric, or intestinal tubes if present. **D** ✦	*Reducing the accumulation of gas in the GI tract decreases pressure on the diaphragm, facilitating more effective ventilation.*

• Perform actions to increase strength and improve activity tolerance:
  • Implement measures to conserve energy. **D** ● ✦
  • Ambulate as able following surgery.
	Increasing activity tolerance enables the client to breathe more deeply and participate in activities to improve breathing pattern.

• Assist client to deep breathe or use incentive spirometer every 1 to 2 hrs. **D** ✦	*Deep breathing and use of an incentive spirometer promote maximal inhalation and lung expansion.*
• Instruct client to breathe slowly if hyperventilating. • Provide with a paper bag if lightheadedness occurs.	*Hyperventilation is an ineffective breathing pattern that can lead to respiratory alkalosis. A client can often slow breathing rate by concentrating on doing so. Lightheadedness with hyperventilation indicates decreased blood carbon dioxide levels*
• Place client in a semi- to high-Fowler's position unless contraindicated. **D** ● ✦	*A semi- to high-Fowler's position allows for maximal diaphragmatic excursion and lung expansion.*
• If client must remain flat in bed, assist with position change at least every 2 hrs. **D** ● ✦	*Compression of the thorax and subsequent limited chest wall expansion occur when the client lies in one position. Frequent repositioning promotes maximal chest wall and lung expansion.*
• Provide pillow support between lower costal margin and iliac crest when client is lying on operative side. **D** ● ✦	*Decreases strain on flank incision and subsequently increases the ease of deep breathing.*

Dependent/Collaborative Actions

Implement measures to improve breathing pattern:

• Increase activity as allowed and tolerated. **D** ● ✦ • Assist with ambulation.	*During activity, especially ambulation, the client usually takes deeper breaths, thus increasing lung expansion.*

• Assist with positive airway pressure techniques if ordered:
  • Continuous positive airway pressure (CPAP)
  • Bilevel positive airway pressure (BiPAP)
  • Flutter/positive expiratory pressure (PEP) device
  • Oscillating Positive Expiratory Pressure (OPEP) device.
	Positive airway pressure devices increase intrapulmonary (alveolar) pressure, which helps re-expand collapsed alveoli and prevent further alveoli collapse.

• Administer central nervous system (CNS) depressants judiciously: • Hold medication and consult physician if respiratory rate is less than 12 breaths/min. **D** ✦	*CNS depressants cause depression of the respiratory center in the brainstem, which can result in a decreased rate and depth of respiration.*
• Perform actions to reduce pain: • Administer analgesics before activities and procedures that can cause pain and before pain becomes severe. **D** ✦	*Reducing pain increase the client's willingness to move and breathe more deeply.*
• May require round-the-clock routine medication administration in early postoperative period.	*Prevents pain from becoming uncontrollable.*
• Request PCA.	*PCA is a method of pain control and provides some control over situation*

Consult appropriate health care provider if:

• Ineffective breathing pattern continues. • Client develops signs and symptoms of impaired gas exchange such as restlessness, irritability, confusion, significant decrease in oximetry results, decreased PaO_2 and increased $PaCO_2$ levels.	*Notifying the appropriate health care provider (e.g., physician, respiratory therapist) allows for modification of treatment plan.*

Nursing Diagnosis **RISK FOR SHOCK** NDx

Definition: Susceptible to an inadequate blood flow to the body's tissues that may lead to life-threatening cellular dysfunction, which may compromise health.

Related to: Excessive blood loss during surgery (the renal area is highly vascular) and hemorrhage after surgery

CLINICAL MANIFESTATIONS

Subjective	Objective
Self-report of feeling lightheaded or dizzy; weakness	Confusion; agitation; restlessness; hypotension; tachycardia; urine output <30 mL/h; cool, clammy skin; diminished or absent peripheral pulses; pallor; cyanosis

RISK FACTORS

- Failure of regulatory mechanisms
- Inadequate fluid volume replacement

DESIRED OUTCOMES

The client will not develop hypovolemic shock as evidenced by:
a. Usual mental status
b. Stable vital signs
c. Skin warm and usual color
d. Palpable peripheral pulses
e. Warm, dry skin
f. Urine output at least 30 mL/h
g. Stable weight at client's normal range

NOC OUTCOMES

Fluid balance; fluid management

NIC INTERVENTIONS

Fluid monitoring; fluid management: fluid administration

NURSING ASSESSMENT	RATIONALE
Assess for and report signs and symptoms of hypovolemic shock: • Restlessness, agitation, confusion, or other change in mental status • Significant decrease in blood pressure (BP) • Postural hypotension • Rapid, weak pulse • Rapid respirations • Cool, clammy skin • Pallor, cyanosis • Diminished or absent peripheral pulses • Urine output less than 30 mL/h • Change in weight greater than 2 lbs	*Early recognition of signs and symptoms of hypovolemic shock allows for prompt of intervention.*
Monitor hemoglobin (Hgb), Hct, and prothrombin time (PT)/ partial thromboplastin time (PTT) values	*Elevated clotting times may contribute to postoperative hemorrhage and hypovolemic shock. Monitoring Hgb/Hct and PT/PTT will allow for implementation of the appropriate interventions.*
Monitory hemodynamic values if present: • Central venous pressure (CVP)	*If present, hemodynamic values are beneficial in guiding fluid resuscitation and preventing fluid volume overload.*

THERAPEUTIC INTERVENTIONS	RATIONALE
Independent Actions Monitor I&O and correlate findings with daily weight. Encourage fluid intake if not contraindicated. Keep fluids easily accessible to client. Monitor vital signs. Assess and document indications of hypovolemia (e.g., dry mucous membranes, verbalization of thirst).	*Helps to determine fluid preplacement needs. Body weight changes of 1 kg (2.2 lbs) represent a fluid loss of 1 L.* *Provides support for vascular fluid volume.* *Maintenance of oral intake keeps oral mucosa moist and improves gastric functioning while supporting vascular fluid volume.* *Increased heart rate, decreased blood pressure, and dry mucous membranes are indicative of dehydration.*

NDx = NANDA Diagnosis **D** = Delegatable Action ● = UAP ✦ = LVN/LPN ⊜▶ = Go to ⊜volve for animation

Continued...

THERAPEUTIC INTERVENTIONS	RATIONALE
Dependent/Collaborative Actions Implement measures to prevent hypovolemic shock:	These actions prevent further loss of blood or vascular fluid volume, which may contribute to hypovolemic shock.
• If bleeding occurs, apply firm, prolonged pressure to area if possible.	Promotes clotting.
• Perform actions to prevent deficient fluid volume.	
• Maintain intravenous access and administration of fluid; may require large-bore access or a peripherally inserted central (PIC) line.	Provides vascular fluid volume replacement which may include volume expanders.
• Instruct client to splint incisional area with hands or pillow when turning and coughing.	Splinting the incision area when turning and coughing reduces stress on the surgical wound to reduce risk for hemorrhage.
• Implement measures to reduce pain, nausea and vomiting (e.g., administer medications for pain, eliminate noxious sights and odors, reduce fear and anxiety, instruct to change position slowly).	Retching action with vomiting places stress on the surgical wound. Preventing nausea and vomiting reduces this stress on the incision.
If signs and symptoms of hypovolemic shock occur:	
• Place client flat in bed with legs elevated unless contraindicated.	Elevation of legs facilitates the return of blood pooled in the extremities to the central circulation, improving blood flow to the vital organs.
• Monitor vital signs frequently.	
If signs and symptoms of hypovolemic shock occur:	
• Administer oxygen as ordered.	Supplemental oxygen is beneficial because oxygen delivery to the tissues is compromised in shock states.
• Administer blood and/or volume expanders if ordered.	Blood and/or fluid volume expanders will help restore circulating volume. The agent of choice is driven by laboratory values and oxygen levels.

• If not already present, prepare client for insertion of hemodynamic monitoring devices:
   • Central venous catheter.
   • Intra-arterial catheter.
	Hemodynamic monitoring devices can measure preload/filling pressures, which are low in hypovolemic shock states.

Collaborative Diagnosis RISK FOR PARALYTIC ILEUS

Definition: Paralysis of the intestines resulting in blockage of the intestines.

Related to:
• Manipulation of the bowel during surgery
• Depressant effect of anesthesia and some medications (e.g., narcotic [opioid] analgesics, some antiemetics) on bowel motility
• Hypovolemia if it occurs can cause decreased blood supply to the intestine

CLINICAL MANIFESTATIONS

Subjective	Objective
Verbal reports of persistent abdominal pain and cramping, loss of appetite; nausea	Firm, distended abdomen; absent bowel sounds; failure to pass flatus; abdominal radiograph showing distended bowel; nausea and vomiting

RISK FACTORS
• Surgery
• Inadequate fluid volume replacement
• Immobility

DESIRED OUTCOMES
The client will not develop a paralytic ileus as evidenced by:
a. Absence or resolution of abdominal pain and cramping
b. Soft, nondistended abdomen
c. Gradual return of bowel sounds
d. Passage of flatus

NURSING ASSESSMENT	RATIONALE
Assess for and report signs and symptoms of paralytic ileus: • Development of or persistent abdominal pain and cramping • Firm, distended abdomen • Absent bowel sounds • Failure to pass flatus • Abdominal radiograph showing distended bowel • Lack of appetite • Nausea and vomiting	*Early recognition of signs and symptoms of paralytic ileus allows for prompt intervention.*

THERAPEUTIC INTERVENTIONS	RATIONALE
Dependent/Collaborative Actions Implement measures to prevent paralytic ileus: • Increase activity as soon as allowed and tolerated following surgery.	*Activity increases peristalsis.*
• Perform actions to prevent hypokalemia if present (e.g., prevent nausea and vomiting, administer fluid and electrolytes as ordered, when oral intake is allowed help client to select foods high in potassium).	*Prevention of hypokalemia is important because it prevents resultant decrease in peristalsis.*
• Perform actions to maintain adequate tissue perfusion (e.g., maintain fluid intake of 2500 mL/day unless contraindicated, administer blood and blood products as ordered, instruct and assist client to perform active foot and leg exercises every 1–2 hrs while awake).	*Maintains adequate vascular fluid volume that supports blood supply to the bowel.* *Increased activity promotes peristalsis.*
• Administer GI stimulants (e.g., metoclopramide) if ordered. • Administer medications to decrease experience of nausea and vomiting.	*GI stimulants stimulate peristalsis.* *Decreases fluid and electrolyte loss.*
If signs and symptoms of paralytic ileus occur: • Withhold all oral intake. • Insert NG tube and maintain suction as ordered.	*Decreases potential for a bowel obstruction.* *Placement of an NG tube to facilitate suction helps remove fluid and gastric secretions from the stomach and decreases potential for a bowel obstruction.*

Collaborative Diagnosis **RISK FOR PNEUMOTHORAX**

Definition: An accumulation of air space between the lung and chest wall which causes the lung to collapse.

Related to: An accumulation of air in the pleural space associated with surgical opening of the pleura (occurs most frequently with thoraco-abdominal and flank approaches) and/or malfunction of chest tube if present

CLINICAL MANIFESTATIONS

Subjective	**Objective**
Verbalization of shortness of breath	Absent breath sounds; hyperresonant percussion; rapid, shallow, and/or labored respirations; restlessness; agitation; confusion; ABG values that have worsened; decreasing SaO_2 levels, chest radiograph showing a lung collapse

RISK FACTORS
• Surgery
• Central line placement
• Immobility
• Ineffective cough effort
• Obesity

DESIRED OUTCOMES
The client will experience normal lung re-expansion if pneumothorax occurs as evidenced by:
a. Audible breath sounds and resonant percussion note by the third to fourth postoperative day
b. Unlabored respirations at 12 to 20 breaths/min
c. ABG values returning toward normal
d. $SaO_2 > 90\%$
e. Chest radiograph showing lung re-expansion

NDx = NANDA Diagnosis **D** = Delegatable Action ● = UAP ✦ = LVN/LPN ⊖▶ = Go to ⊖volve for animation

NURSING ASSESSMENT	RATIONALE

Assess for and immediately report signs and symptoms of:
- Malfunction of the chest drainage system, if present (e.g., respiratory distress, lack of fluctuation in water seal chamber without evidence of lung re-expansion, excessive bubbling in water seal chamber, significant increase in subcutaneous emphysema)
- Further lung collapse (e.g., extended area of absent breath sounds with hyperresonant percussion note; rapid, shallow, and/or labored respirations; tachycardia; increased chest pain; restlessness; confusion; ABG results that have worsened; significant decrease in oximetry results)
- Monitor ABGs and SaO_2 levels

Monitor chest radiograph results. Report findings of delayed lung re-expansion or further lung collapse

Early recognition of the signs and symptoms of pneumothorax allows for prompt intervention.

THERAPEUTIC INTERVENTIONS	RATIONALE

Independent Actions

Implement measures to promote lung re-expansion and prevent further lung collapse:
- Perform actions to maintain patency and integrity of chest drainage system:
  - Maintain fluid levels in the water seal and suction chambers as ordered.

    Maintains negative pressure within the lungs.
  - Maintain occlusive dressing over chest tube insertion site.

    An occlusive dressing over the chest tube insertion site maintains negative pressure seal.
  - Tape all connections securely.

    Securely taping the tubings/connections prevents tubing from being disconnected and maintains a closed drainage system.
  - Tape the tubing to the chest wall close to insertion site.

    Taping the tubing to the chest wall reduces the risk of inadvertent removal of the chest tube.
  - Position tubing to promote optimum drainage (e.g., coil excess tubing on bed rather than allowing it to hang down below the collection device, keep tubing free of kinks).

    These actions promote chest tube drainage.
  - Drain fluid that accumulates in tubing into the collection chamber.

    Maintains patency of the drainage system.
  - Avoid clamping, stripping, or milking of chest tubes. If ordered with visible clots, manipulate the tubing using a hand-over-hand method while moving along the drainage tube.

    Clamping chest tubing prevents the escape of air or fluid increasing risk of tension pneumothorax.

    Chest tube stripping or milking causes extreme negative pressures in the tube and pleural space and may damage lung tissues.
  - Keep drainage collection device below level of client's chest at all times.

    Maintaining the drainage device below the level of the client's chest prevents backflow of drainage into the lungs.
  - Perform actions to facilitate the escape of air from the pleural space (e.g., maintain suction as ordered, ensure that the air vent is open on the drainage collection device if system is set to water seal only).

    Helps to maintain expansion or re-expand lung tissue following a pneumothorax.
  - Perform actions to improve breathing pattern and facilitate airway clearance (e.g., encourage client to cough and deep breathe every 1–2 hrs; use incentive spirometry every 2 hrs; ambulate as ordered and as tolerated).

    These actions improve lung expansion and removal of secretions.

If signs and symptoms of further lung collapse occur:
- Maintain client on bedrest in a semi- to high-Fowler's position.

  Positioning the client in a semi- to high-Fowler's position improves the client's ability to expand the lungs and decreases abdominal pressure on the diaphragm.
- Maintain oxygen therapy as ordered.

  Supplemental oxygen helps maintain tissue oxygenation.

THERAPEUTIC INTERVENTIONS	RATIONALE
• Assess for and immediately report signs and symptoms of tension pneumothorax (e.g., severe dyspnea, increased restlessness and agitation, rapid and/or irregular pulse rate, hypotension, neck vein distention, shift in trachea from midline).	*Emergency treatment is required to prevent further respiratory difficulty and prevent further complications.*
• Assist with clearing of existing chest tube and/or insertion of a new tube.	*Reestablishes a closed drainage system.*

DISCHARGE TEACHING/CONTINUED CARE

Nursing Diagnosis **DEFICIENT KNOWLEDGE NDx; INEFFECTIVE HEALTH MANAGEMENT NDx; INEFFECTIVE FAMILY HEALTH MANAGEMENT* NDx**

Definition: **Deficient Knowledge NDx:** Absence of cognitive information related to a specific topic, or its acquisition; **Ineffective Health Management NDx:** Pattern of regulating and integrating into daily living a therapeutic regimen for the treatment of illness and its sequelae that is unsatisfactory for meeting specific health goals; **Ineffective Family Health Management NDx:** A pattern of regulating and integrating into family processes a program for the treatment of illness and its sequelae that is unsatisfactory for meeting specific health goals of the family unit.

CLINICAL MANIFESTATIONS

Subjective	Objective
Verbalizes inability to manage illness; verbalizes inability to follow prescribed regimen	Inaccurate follow-through with instructions; inappropriate behaviors; experience of preventable complications of surgery and living with one kidney.

RISK FACTORS

- Cognitive deficit
- Financial concerns
- Failure to reduce risk factors for complications of surgery
- Inability to care for oneself
- Difficulty in modifying personal habits and integrating treatments into lifestyle

NOC OUTCOMES	NIC INTERVENTIONS
Knowledge: treatment regimen; disease management	Teaching: individual; teaching: disease process; teaching: prescribed activity/exercise; teaching: prescribed medication; health system guidance

NURSING ASSESSMENT	RATIONALE
Assess client's readiness and ability to learn. Assess meaning of illness to client.	*Early recognition of readiness to learn and meaning of illness to client allows for implementation of the appropriate teaching interventions.*

THERAPEUTIC INTERVENTIONS	RATIONALE

Desired Outcome: The client will verbalize ways to maintain health of the remaining kidney.

*The nurse should select the diagnostic label that is most appropriate for the client's discharge teaching needs.

NDx = NANDA Diagnosis   **D** = Delegatable Action   ● = UAP   ✦ = LVN/LPN   ⊝▶ = Go to ⊝volve for animation

Continued...

THERAPEUTIC INTERVENTIONS	RATIONALE

Independent Actions

Instruct client regarding ways to maintain health of the remaining kidney:

- Adhere to precautions to prevent a urinary tract infection:
  - Perform actions to prevent urinary stasis:
    - (1) Drink at least 10 glasses of liquid per day unless contraindicated.
    - (2) Urinate whenever the urge is felt.
    - (3) Avoid long periods of inactivity (if unable to maintain a program of moderate activity, be sure to change positions frequently).
  - Wipe from front to back after urinating and defecating (if female).
  - Keep perineal area clean and dry.
- Immediately report signs and symptoms of a urinary tract infection (e.g., chills; fever; urgency, frequency, or burning on urination; cloudy or foul-smelling urine).
- Notify physician if a cold or other infection persists for more than 2 to 3 days or if unable to maintain an adequate fluid intake.
- Inform other health care providers about the nephrectomy so that prophylactic antimicrobials may be initiated before dental work and invasive procedures such as cystoscopy and minor surgeries.
- Avoid activities that might cause trauma to the remaining kidney (e.g., contact sports, horseback riding).
- Inform physician of all prescription and nonprescription medications being taken and before taking any new medications since they might cause damage to the remaining kidney (e.g., ibuprofen, ciprofloxacin, captopril, quinine, naproxen, lithium, neomycin, gentamicin, pentamidine, vancomycin, cyclosporine).
- Consult health care provider before undergoing any diagnostic test involving the use of contrast media.
- If nephrectomy was performed because of renal calculi, reinforce physician's instructions about diet, drug therapy, and daily fluid requirements.
- If surgery was necessary because of renal hypertension, reinforce the physician's instructions about methods of controlling BP (e.g., dietary modification, medication, physical exercise on regular basis, weight loss if overweight).

Rationale column:

Hydration is required to maintain vascular fluid volume and adequate blood flow to the kidneys.
Prevents stasis of urine in the bladder.
Activity improves circulation and helps to prevent urine stasis.

Appropriate perineal hygiene prevents urinary tract exposure to vaginal or rectal bacteria. Moisture provides a medium for growth of bacteria.
Urinary tract infections require prompt intervention.

Hydration is important to maintain fluid volume and adequate blood flow to the kidneys.

Helps prevent infections.

Prevents injury.

Many medications are nephrotoxic and should not be taken. Knowledge of medications and supplements helps to prevent drug-to-drug interactions

Some agents used during these procedures can damage the remaining kidney.
Prevents formation of stones in the remaining kidney, and provides adequate hydration. Dietary recommendations help to decrease incidence and recurrence of kidney stones.
Client needs to control BP to prevent destruction of the nephrons on the remaining kidney.

THERAPEUTIC INTERVENTIONS	RATIONALE

Desired Outcome: The client will state signs and symptoms to report to the health care provider.

Independent Actions

Instruct client to report signs and symptoms to their health care provider:

- Difficulty breathing
- Productive cough of discolored sputum
- Unusual or excessive drainage from the wound site
- Pain or swelling in the calf of one or both legs
- Unusual and continuous abdominal or pelvic pain
- Temperature above 38°C (100.4°F)

These clinical manifestations should be reported to the health care provider because they require prompt intervention.
May indicate a pulmonary embolism.
May indicate dehydration or respiratory infection.
May indicate an infection.
May indicate a deep vein thrombosis.
May indicate an infection.

THERAPEUTIC INTERVENTIONS	RATIONALE
• Unexplained weight gain • Decreased urine output • Flank pain on the nonoperative side • Blood in the urine	*May indicate loss of or changes in kidney function, dehydration, or development of a kidney stone.*

THERAPEUTIC INTERVENTIONS	RATIONALE

Desired Outcome: The client, in collaboration with the nurse, will a develop plan for adhering to recommended follow-up care including future appointments with health care provider, medications prescribed, activity level, wound care, and plans for subsequent treatment of the underlying disorder.

Independent Actions
Reinforce physician's instructions regarding activity:
- Gauge activity according to tolerance and allow adequate rest periods.
- Avoid lifting objects over 7 to 10 lbs, pushing heavy objects, and exercising strenuously for specified length of time (usually 4–8 weeks).

Clarify plans for follow-up visits and subsequent treatment of the underlying disorder (e.g., chemotherapy, radiation therapy) if appropriate.

Collaborate with client to develop a schedule of appointments for follow-up care.

Refer client to community support groups

These actions prevent unnecessary stress on the suture line. Helps to conserve energy.
Prevents stress/injury to suture line and abdominal tissues.

Clarity of information improves client's understanding of long-term care and adherence to treatment regimen.
Provides for continuum of care following discharge from acute care facilities.

ACUTE KIDNEY INJURY AND CHRONIC KIDNEY DISEASE

Acute kidney injury (AKI) is an abrupt decline in kidney function. Symptoms range from very subtle changes in renal function to complete renal failure. The majority of cases of AKI are reversible with early diagnosis and treatment. The causes of AKI may be classified as prerenal, intrarenal, and postrenal failure. Prerenal AKI is the most common type of AKI. It occurs when blood flow to the kidneys has been significantly decreased so the kidneys are no longer able to concentrate urine. The loss of renal blood flow can be caused by conditions such as hypovolemia due to blood loss from trauma, severe hypotension from sepsis, cardiac failure, massive pulmonary embolism, and renal artery clamping or stenosis. Intrarenal AKI results from an injury to the kidney itself. Potential causes of intrarenal failure include acute tubular necrosis, acute glomerulonephritis, malignant hypertension, and injury to the glomerulus from nephron-toxic medications and/or dye used during procedures. Postrenal AKI results from a blockage of urine outflow from the kidneys. Causes of postrenal failure include kidney stones, tumors, injury, and/or edema that block the ureters.

Diagnosis and treatment of AKI focuses on the cause of the failure. A thorough client history will help identify the underlying cause of renal failure. Diagnostic studies used to diagnose AKI include urinalysis, serum BUN and creatinine levels and ratio, and the fractional excretion of sodium. The results of these studies vary depending upon the type of AKI present.

AKI and recovery of renal function progress in phases: initiation, oliguric, diuresis, and recovery. The initiation phase begins with the insult to the kidneys and continues until signs and symptoms begin. This phase can last from hours to days. Prevention of permanent injury may be possible within this phase. The maintenance or oliguric phase begins when the urine output is decreased to less than 400 mL/day. The decline in urine output indicates renal damage that does not respond to compensatory mechanisms.

The diuretic phase begins with a gradual increase in daily urine output of at least 1 to 3 L/day. In this phase, the kidneys are beginning to recover waste excretion processes but cannot concentrate urine.

In the recovery phase, the BUN and serum creatinine levels begin to decline and glomerular filtration rates (GFRs) increase. Recovery is gradual and can take up to 1 year for renal function to stabilize. In many cases, there is some permanent loss of renal function. AKI is reversible in most cases, but it can lead to chronic kidney disease (CKD). This is a progressive, irreversible loss of kidney function that usually develops gradually over many years. The leading causes of CKD are diabetes mellitus and hypertension. CKD can also develop after acute renal failure (ARF) that has resulted in irreversible renal damage.

There are five stages in CKD that are delineated by the GFR. Normal GFR is 125 mL/min. Stage 1 may maintain a normal or high GFR (GFR > 90 mL/min). Although kidney dysfunction is occurring, it may be undiagnosed due to lack of symptoms. In stage 2, there is a mild reduction of GFR to 60 to 89 mL/min. Symptoms that may occur during this stage are hypertension, polyuria, or nocturia. Otherwise, the individual remains asymptomatic. GFR in stage 3 is reduced to 30 to 59 mL/min. The individual remains asymptomatic; however, fluid and electrolyte changes are occurring. In stage 4, the GFR decreases to 15 to 29 mL/min. The client experiences symptoms related to metabolic acidosis, hyperphosphatemia, anemia, elevated triglycerides, and fluid and electrolyte imbalances.

In stage 5, the last stage of CKD, the GRF will decrease to less than 15% of normal. This stage is also known as end stage renal disease (EDSR).

There is a buildup of nitrogenous substances (e.g., urea, creatinine) to levels high enough to cause toxic effects on other body systems. Typical signs and symptoms can include lethargy, irritability, extreme fatigue and weakness, pruritus, nausea and vomiting, muscle cramping, and stomatitis. Fluid, electrolyte, and acid-base imbalances also worsen, and dialysis or kidney transplantation is necessary for survival.

This care plan focuses on the adult client with AKI who has progressed to the oliguric phase and is hospitalized for treatment and further evaluation of renal function. Much of the information is also applicable to clients in an extended care facility or home setting.

OUTCOME/DISCHARGE CRITERIA

The client will:
1. Not exhibit signs and symptoms of uremic syndrome
2. Maintain BP within a safe range

3. Maintain fluid, electrolyte, and acid-base balance within a safe range for the client
4. Tolerate expected level of activity
5. Have no evidence of infection
6. Maintain adequate nutritional status
7. Verbalize a basic understanding of AKI and CKD
8. Identify ways to slow the progression of kidney damage
9. Develop a plan to maintain fluid restrictions and dietary modifications
10. Demonstrate the ability to accurately weigh self, measure fluid I&O, and monitor own BP
11. List ways to reduce the risk of infection
12. Identify ways to manage signs and symptoms that often occur as a result of CKD
13. Share feelings and concerns about the effects of renal failure on lifestyle and roles
14. State signs and symptoms to report to the health care provider
15. Identify community resources that can assist with adjustment to changes resulting from CRF
16. Develop a plan for adhering to recommended follow-up care including future appointments with health care provider and medications prescribed

Nursing Diagnosis **EXCESS FLUID VOLUME** NDx

Definition: Surplus intake and/or retention of fluid.

Related to:
• Compromised regulatory mechanisms
• Fluid intake in excess of prescribed restrictions

CLINICAL MANIFESTATIONS

Subjective	Objective
Verbalization of shortness of breath	Weight gain of 2% or greater over a short period; hypertension; presence of an S3 heart sound; tachycardia; intake greater than output; changes in mental status; crackles (rales) and diminished or absent breath sounds; dyspnea, orthopnea; peripheral edema; distended neck veins; chest radiograph showing pulmonary vascular congestion, pleural effusion, or pulmonary edema

RISK FACTOR
• Compromised regulatory mechanisms
• Acute renal injury
• CKD

DESIRED OUTCOMES

The client will experience resolution of excess fluid volume as evidenced by:
a. Decline in weight toward client's normal
b. BP within normal range for client
c. Absence of an S3 heart sound
d. Balanced I&O
e. Usual mental status
f. Normal breath sounds
g. Absence of dyspnea, orthopnea, peripheral edema, and distended neck veins

NOC OUTCOMES	NIC INTERVENTIONS
Fluid balance; electrolyte and acid-base balance; fluid overload severity	Fluid/electrolyte monitoring; fluid management

NURSING ASSESSMENT	RATIONALE
Assess for and report signs and symptoms of excess fluid volume: • Weight gain of 2% or greater over a short period • Elevated BP (BP may not be elevated if fluid has shifted out of vascular space) • Presence of an S3 heart sound • Bounding pulse • Intake greater than output • Changes in mental status • Crackles (rales) and diminished or absent breath sounds • Dyspnea, orthopnea • Peripheral edema • Distended neck veins • Chest radiograph showing pulmonary vascular congestion, pleural effusion, or pulmonary edema	*Early recognition of signs and symptoms of excess fluid volume allows for prompt intervention.*

THERAPEUTIC INTERVENTIONS	RATIONALE
Independent Actions Weigh client daily at the same time of day using the same scale and with similar weight of clothing. **D** ✦ Monitor I&O and correlate with daily weight I&O should include all oral and parenteral intake of fluid. Output should include an estimate all insensible losses temperature will have increased. Monitor and document urine specific gravity, noting trends over time. Instruct client in ways to decrease thirst and keep oral mucous membranes moist (e.g., space fluid intake evenly throughout the hours client is awake, rinse mouth frequently with water, breathe through nose rather than mouth). Monitor lab and diagnostic studies values and analyze trends over time: Potassium, sodium, BUN and creatinine, H&H; serial chest x-rays; arterial pH.	*Daily weights are important for comparisons. A sudden weight gain may be an indication of fluid volume excess.* *A change in body weight of 1 kg (2.2 lbs) equals 1 L of fluid. Increased weight over a short period of time may indicate declining kidney function. Insensible water loss is estimated to be between 40 and 600 mL in an adult under normal circumstances.* *Urine specific gravity is used to measure kidney function. Findings less than 1.010 indicate declining kidney function.* *Ability to alleviate thirst and keep oral mucous membranes moist promotes compliance with oral fluid restrictions. Allows client to have fluid intake throughout a 24-hrs period and to maintain a sense of control.* *Monitoring trends over time helps to identify level of declining kidney function.*
Dependent/Collaborative Actions Implement measures to reduce excess fluid volume: • Maintain fluid restrictions as ordered (intake allowed is usually 500–700 mL plus the amount of urine output in the previous 24 hrs). **D** ✦ • If client is receiving numerous and/or a large volume of intravenous medications, consult the pharmacist to prevent excessive fluid administration (e.g., stop primary infusion during administration of intravenous medications, dilute medication in the minimum amount of solution).	*Reduction of excess fluid volume reduces stress on the heart and vascular system.* *Ability to alleviate thirst and keep oral mucous membranes moist promotes compliance with oral fluid restrictions.* *Prevents fluid volume excess.*

Continued...

THERAPEUTIC INTERVENTIONS	RATIONALE
• Restrict sodium intake as ordered. **D** ✦	*Reducing sodium intake decreases fluid retention.*
• Administer diuretic if ordered. **D** ✦	*Diuretics increase excretion of water and some solutes.*
• Administer vasodilators and antihypertensive agents as ordered.	*These agents may be ordered to decrease systemic vascular resistance (SVR) and maintain or increase renal perfusion.*
• Prepare client and assist with dialysis, if ordered (e.g., hemodialysis, peritoneal dialysis, or continuous renal replacement therapy).	*Dialysis is done to decrease fluid volume while correcting electrolyte and acid-base balance. Determination of the type of dialysis utilized depends on degree of kidney functioning and client's ability to tolerate the procedure.*
Consult physician if signs and symptoms of excess fluid volume persist or worsen.	*Notification of the physician allows for prompt alterations in treatment plan.*

Nursing Diagnosis RISK FOR DECREASED CARDIAC OUTPUT NDx

Definition: Susceptible to inadequate blood pumped by the heart to meet metabolic demands of the body, which may compromise health.

Related to:
• Fluid volume changes from declining kidney functioning
• Electrolyte imbalances and metabolic acidosis
• Changes in afterload and preload
• Impaired cardiac contractility
• Alteration in preload and stroke volume

CLINICAL MANIFESTATIONS

Subjective	Objective
Verbalization of fatigue, restlessness	Changes in blood pressure and heart rate; changes in electrocardiogram (ECG); development of S3 & S4 heart sounds; changes in fluid, electrolytes and metabolic status; changes in ECG patterns

RISK FACTORS
• AKI
• CKD

DESIRED OUTCOMES

The client will maintain adequate cardiac output as evidenced by:
a. Blood pressure and heart rate with normal range for client
b. Strong and palpable peripheral pulses
c. Maintained mental status appropriate for client
d. Maintained preload and stroke volume
e. Absence of adventitious lung sounds
f. Capillary refill <2 to 3 seconds

NOC
Cardiopulmonary status: Hemodynamic status: fluid volume

NIC
Hemodynamic regulation; fluid regulation; electrolyte management

NURSING ASSESSMENT	RATIONALE
Assess for and report signs and symptoms of decreased cardiac output: • Changes in blood pressure and heart rate • Presence of S3 & S4 heart sounds • ECG rhythm changes • Intake greater than output • Changes in mental status • Crackles (rales) and diminished or absent breath sounds • Dyspnea, orthopnea • Peripheral edema • Distended neck veins • Capillary refill >3 seconds • Changes in serum electrolyte levels	*Early recognition of signs and symptoms of decreased cardiac output will allow for prompt treatment.*

NURSING INTERVENTIONS	RATIONALE
Independent Actions	
Monitor BP and heart rate.	*Increased fluid volume associated with hypertension and renal failure, subsequent uremia, and increased SVR decrease cardiac output. In clients with AKI, heart failure may be reversible.*
Monitor and document ECG changes.	*A client with declining renal filtration may experience multiple electrolyte changes.* *Hypokalemia—ECG-flattened T-wave, peaked P wave, development of U waves* *Hyperkalemia—ECG-peaked T wave, widened QRS complex, prolonged R-R interval, flattened T wave* *Hypokalemia—prolonged QT interval* *Client may development additional heart sounds associated with excess fluid volume.*
Auscultate heart sounds. Assess skin color and nail beds and capillary refill time, and SaO₂ levels.	*Declining kidney function also impacts the production of erythropoietin. With decreased erythropoietin, there is a decrease in circulating red blood cells (RBCs). Additionally, decreased SaO₂ levels may occur with fluid volume excess.* *Early identification of respiratory congestion and heart enlargement is associated with declining kidney function.*
Monitor serial chest x-rays and/or reports. Encourage bedrest and appropriate rest periods. Schedule nursing interventions and procedures to allow for prolonged periods of rest.	*Decreases oxygen consumption and cardiac workload.*
Dependent/Collaborative Action	
Administer medications are ordered: Sodium bicarbonate	*Hyperkalemia of 6.5 mEq or higher constitutes a medical emergency. Administration of sodium bicarbonate will temporarily decrease potassium levels by shifting potassium back into the cell.*
Inotropic agents	*Increases myocardial contractility and stroke volume.*
Calcium Gluconate	*Given for hypocalcemia and to stabilize the cell membrane from depolarization in a hyperkalemic state.*
Monitor serum electrolyte levels, noting trends over time: Potassium	*A potassium level of >6.5 mEq is considered a medical emergency and requires prompt intervention.*
Calcium	*Calcium is involved in maintenance of heart rate and rhythm. Calcium deficit increases toxic effects of potassium.*
Administer and restrict fluid as indicated.	*Adequate cardiac functioning requires the appropriate level of vascular fluid volume.*
Provide supplemental oxygen as ordered.	*Provides supplemental oxygen to support appropriate cardiac functioning.*

NDx = NANDA Diagnosis   **D** = Delegatable Action   ● = UAP   ✦ = LVN/LPN   ⊖▶ = Go to ⊖volve for animation

Nursing Diagnosis **RISK FOR ELECTROLYTE IMBALANCE** NDx

Definition: Susceptible to changes in serum electrolyte levels, which may compromise health.

Related to:
- **Hyponatremia**
  - Excessive fluid intake in relation to output that causes a delusional hyponatremia
  - Loss of sodium associated with diuretic therapy
- **Hypernatremia**
  - Decreased ability of the kidneys to excrete sodium
  - Increased aldosterone output associated with activation of the renin-angiotensin-aldosterone mechanism if decreased renal blood flor has occurred as a result of the underlying disease process
  - Dietary sodium intake in excess of prescribed restrictions.
- **Hyperkalemia**
  - Decreased ability of the kidneys to excrete potassium
  - Increased cellular release of potassium associated with progressive renal tissue damage and metabolic acidosis
  - Dietary intake of potassium in excess of prescribed restrictions
  - Use of potassium-sparing diuretics or medications
  - Use of salt substitutes containing potassium
- **Hypocalcemia**
  - Decreased intestinal absorption of calcium associated with inability of the kidneys to activate vitamin D to its active metabolite that is required t0 stimulate calcium absorption from the small intestines
  - Hypophosphatemia that causes a reciprocal drop in calcium
- **Hypermagnesemia**
  - Decreased ability of the kidneys to excrete magnesium
  - Excessive intake of magnesium-containing antacids, laxatives or both
- **Hyperphosphatemia**
  - Hypocalcemia causes an increase in phosphorus
  - Decreased ability of the kidneys to excrete phosphorus

CLINICAL MANIFESTATIONS

Subjective	Objective
Hyponatremia: Self-report of nausea, abdominal cramps and weakness	**Hyponatremia:** Vomiting, confusion, seizures, low serum sodium level
Hypernatremia: Self-report of thirst, weakness	**Hypernatremia:** Dry, sticky mucous membranes; restlessness, elevated temperature; seizures; elevated serum sodium level
Hyperkalemia: Self-report of muscle weakness	**Hyperkalemia:** Bradycardia with irregular pulse; diarrhea and intestinal colic,; Electrocardiogram (ECG) showing peaked T wave, prolonged PR interval, and/or widened QRS; elevated potassium level
Hypocalcemia: Self-report of feeling anxious, numbness or tingling in fingers, toes, or circumoral area	**Hypocalcemia:** Irritability; Chovstek's and Trousseau's sign; hyperactive reflexes; tetany; seizures; serum calcium level lower than normal
Hypermagnesemia: Self-report of nausea and weakness	**Hypermagnesemia:** Flushed, warm skin, vomiting; drowsiness; hypotension; bradycardia; bradypnea; higher than normal serum magnesium level
Hyperphosphatemia: Self-report of numbness or tingling in hands and feet	**Hyperphosphatemia:** Tetany; seizures; elevated serum phosphorus level

RISK FACTORS

- Disease process that effects the kidney's ability to excrete electrolytes
- Prescribed drugs – diuretics and laxatives
- Decreased level of vitamin D
- Failure of physiological regulatory mechanisms
- Excessive potassium salt substitutes
- Poor adherence to dietary regimen
- Use of OTC medications

DESIRED OUTCOMES

The client will not experience an electrolyte imbalance as evidenced by:
a. Serum electrolyte values within normal limits
b. Absence of seizure activity, vomiting, abdominal cramps, diarrhea, and thirst
c. Normal ECG with a regular pulse 60 to 80 beats/min.
d. Usual muscle tone and strength
e. Negative Chvostek's and Trousseau's sign
f. Absence of numbness and tingling in fingers, toes and circumoral area,; hyperreflexia, and tetany

NOC OUTCOMES

Electrolyte balance; Fluid balance

NIC INTERVENTIONS

Fluid/electrolyte monitoring; Fluid/electrolyte management

NURSING ASSESSMENT

Assess for and report signs and symptoms of:
- **Hyponatremia:** Nausea. Vomiting, abdominal cramps, lethargy, confusion, weakness, seizures, and low serum sodium level
- **Hypernatremia:** Thirst, drug stick mucous membranes, restlessness; lethargy; weakness; elevated temperature, seizures, elevated serum sodium level
- **Hyperkalemia:** Slow or irregular pulse, paresthesias; muscle weakness and flaccidity; diarrhea and intestinal colic ECG showing peaked T waves, prolonger PR interval, and/or widened QRS, elevated serum potassium levels
- **Hypocalcemia:** Anxiousness; irritability; positive Chvostek's and Trousseau's sign; numbness or tingling of fingers, toes or circumoral area; hyperactive reflexes; tetany; seizures; serum calcium level that is lower than normal
- **Hypermagnesemia:** Flushed, warm skin; nausea; vomiting; muscle weakness; drowsiness; lethargy; hypotension; bradypnea; bradycardia; higher than normal serum magnesium level
- **Hyperphosphatemia:** Paresthesia; tetany; seizures; seizures, higher than normal serum phosphorus level

RATIONALE

Early recognition of signs and symptoms of electrolyte imbalance allows for prompt intervention.

THERAPEUTIC INTERVENTIONS

Dependent/Collaborative Actions
Implement measures to prevent or treat **hyponatremia**:
- Maintain fluid restriction as ordered.
- Increase dietary allotment of sodium if ordered. **D** ● ✦

- Administer loop diuretics.
Implement measures to prevent or treat **hypernatremia**:
- Maintain maximum fluid intake allowed. **D**
- Maintain dietary sodium restriction if ordered.
- Administer thiazide diuretics if ordered.

RATIONALE

Maintenance of fluid restrictions prevents dilutional hyponatremia.
Increased intake of sodium decrease the dilutional effects of vascular fluid retention.
Loop diuretics promote excretion of water.

Maintain appropriate balance between vascular fluid volume and sodium volume.
Thiazide diuretics increase excretion of sodium and water.
Notification of the health care provider allows for prompt alternation in treatment plan.

Continued...

THERAPEUTIC INTERVENTIONS	RATIONALE
Consult health care provider if high serum sodium levels persist.	
Implement measures to prevent or treat **hyperkalemia**:	
• Maintain dietary restrictions of potassium by limiting intake of foods/ fluids such as bananas, potatoes, raisings avocados and orange juice, and use of salt substitutes.	*Restricting intake of potassium-rich foods helps maintain a normal level of serum potassium.*
• Instruct client to consult health care provider or a dietitian about which salt substitutes can be safely used.	*Most salt substitutes contain potassium. The client would be taught which ones are safe for them to use.*
• Perform actions to reduce the cellular release of potassium:	
(1) Encourage client to consume the amount of dietary protein allowed.	*During the breakdown of proteins, potassium is released.*
(2) Provide allotted amount of carbohydrates.	*Ingestion of carbohydrates spares protein by providing a quick energy source.*
(3) Perform actions to prevent infection:	*Prevention of an infection prevents an increase in the metabolic rate and a subsequent increase in protein catabolism.*
• use sterile technique when doing invasive procedures,	
• use good handwashing and encourage client do to the same	
• rotate intravenous line sites according to hospital policy	
• Implement measure to prevent or treat metabolic acidosis (e.g., administer sodium bicarbonate).	*In metabolic acidosis, potassium is moved out of the cell in exchange for hydrogen, thus increasing the extracellular potassium level.*
• If signs and symptoms of hyperkalemia are present, consult health care provider before administering prescribed potassium supplements and other medications that can increase potassium levels (e.g., potassium penicillin G, potassium-sparing diuretics, some beta-blockers, and angiotensin-converting enzyme (ACE) inhibitors, and Angiotensin II receptor ARBS blocker).	*Prevents increased potassium levels.*
Administer the following mediations if ordered:	
• Loop diuretics	*Increases renal excretion of potassium.*
• Cation-exchange resins (e.g., sodium polystyrene sulfonate [Kayexalate])	*Administration of sodium polystyrene sulfonate increases potassium excretion via the intestines (action exchanging sodium for potassium).*
• Intravenous insulin and hypertonic glucose solutions.	*Infusion of hypertonic glucose solutions and insulin enhances transport of potassium back into the cells.*
If signs and symptoms of hyperkalemia persist or worsen:	*Notification of the healthcare provider allows for prompt alterations in the treatment plan.*
• Consult health provider.	
• Have intravenous calcium preparation (e.g., calcium gluconate) readily available.	*Administration of calcium gluconate counteracts the effect of a high potassium level on the heart.*
Implement measure to prevent or treat **hypercalcemia**:	
• Provide dietary sources of calcium (e.g., mile and milk products). **D** ● ✦	*Ensures calcium is present in the client's diet.*
• Administration of vitamin D (e.g., paricalcitol, calcitriol) and calcium supplements if ordered. **D** ● ✦	*Vitamin D is required for the absorption of calcium.*
• Perform measures to prevent or treat hyperphosphatemia (e.g., restrict phosphorus intake).	*Calcium and phosphate have an inverse relationship, and a high phosphate level leads to hypocalcemia.*
• Avoid rapid or aggressive treatment of acidosis.	*Rapidly reversing acidosis can results in decreased ionization of calcium.*
If signs and symptoms of hypocalcemia occur:	
• Institute seizure precautions.	*Prevents client injury*
• Administer calcium preparations (e.g. calcium gluconate, calcium carbonate) as ordered.	*Increases calcium levels.*

THERAPEUTIC INTERVENTIONS	RATIONALE
Implement measure to prevent or treat **hypermagnesemia:**	*Magnesium is absorbed from these agents.*
• Avoid giving laxatives and antacids that contain magnesium (e.g., Milk of Magnesia, Gelusil, Mylanta, Maalox).	
• Maintain dietary restrictions if ordered by limiting intake of foods/fluids such as seafood, green leafy vegetables and legumes.	*Because the kidneys are unable to regular the electrolytes, decreasing intake of magnesium is the most appropriate way to maintain decreased magnesium levels.*
Consult health care provider if signs and symptoms of hypermagnesemia persist or worsen.	*Notification of the health care provider allows for prompt alteration in the treatment plan.*
Implement measures to prevent or treat **hyperphosphatemia:**	
• Restrict dietary intake of phosphorus if ordered by limiting intake of foods/fluids such as poultry, nuts, mile, mile products, eggs, legumes, and some cola beverages.	*Administration of phosphate-binding medications binds with phosphate and decreases the free phosphate levels available in the body.*
• Administer phosphate-binding medication such as sevelamar (Renagel), aluminum-containing agents (e.g., Amphojel, Basaljel), calcium acetate (e.g., PhosLo), and calcium carbonate (e.g., Tums), if ordered.	*These foods and fluids contain phosphate and will increase blood phosphate levels.*
• Consult that health care provider if signs and symptoms of hyperphosphatemia persist or worsen.	*Notification of the health care provider allows for prompt alteration in treatment plan.*

Nursing Diagnosis IMBALANCED NUTRITION: LESS THAN BODY REQUIREMENTS NDx

Definition: Intake of nutrients insufficient to meet metabolic needs.

Related to:
• Decreased oral intake associated with fatigue and dislike of prescribed diet
• Prescribed dietary modifications (especially protein restrictions that are necessary in order to control the serum levels of nitrogenous substances)

CLINICAL MANIFESTATIONS

Subjective	Objective
Verbalization of lack of appetite, fatigue, poor self-esteem	Loss of weight with adequate food intake; sore, inflamed buccal cavity; capillary fragility; irritability; pale conjunctiva and mucous membranes; poor muscle tone; excessive hair loss; amenorrhea

RISK FACTORS
• Poor adherence to dietary regimen
• AKI
• CKD

DESIRED OUTCOMES

The client will maintain an adequate nutritional status as evidenced by:
a. Weight within normal range for the client
b. Serum albumin, prealbumin, Hct, and Hgb levels and lymphocyte count within normal range
c. Usual or improved strength and activity tolerance
d. Healthy oral mucous membrane

NOC OUTCOMES	NIC INTERVENTIONS
Nutritional status: weight maintenance	Nutritional monitoring; nutritional counseling; nutritional management; nutrition therapy; weight gain assistance; weight management

NURSING ASSESSMENT	RATIONALE
Assess for and report signs and symptoms of malnutrition: • Weight significantly below client's usual weight or below normal for client's age, height, and body frame • Low serum albumin, prealbumin, Hct, and Hgb levels and low lymphocyte count • Weakness and fatigue (may also reflect decreasing renal function) • Sore, inflamed oral mucous membranes • Pale conjunctiva	*Early recognition and reporting of signs and symptoms of malnutrition allows for prompt intervention.*
Monitor percentage of meals and snacks client consumes. Document and report a pattern or inadequate intake	*An awareness of the amount of foods/fluids the client consumes alerts the nurse to deficits in nutritional intake. Reporting an inadequate intake allows for prompt intervention.*

THERAPEUTIC INTERVENTIONS	RATIONALE

Independent Actions

Implement measures to improve oral intake: • Increase activity as allowed and tolerated. **D** ● ✦	*Activity usually promotes a general feeling of well-being, which can result in improved appetite.*
• Maintain a clean environment and a relaxed, pleasant atmosphere. **D** ● ✦	*Noxious sites and odors can inhibit the feeding center in the hypothalamus. Maintaining a clean environment helps prevent this from occurring. In addition, maintaining a relaxed, pleasant atmosphere can help reduce the client's stress and promote a feeling of well-being, which tends to improve appetite and oral intake.*
• Encourage a rest period before meals if indicated.	*The physical activity of eating requires some expenditure of energy. Fatigue can reduce the client's desire and ability to eat.*
• Provide oral hygiene between and before meals. **D** ● ✦ • Offer frequent mouth care. • Allow client to chew gum, use of breath mints, sugarless hard candy.	*Oral hygiene moistens the oral mucous membrane and stimulates saliva production, which may make it easier to chew and swallow. It also freshens the mouth and removes unpleasant tastes. This can improve the taste of foods/fluids, which helps stimulate appetite and increase oral intake.*
• Serve foods/fluids that are appealing to the client and adhere to personal and cultural preferences whenever possible.	*Foods/fluids that appeal to the client's senses (especially sight and smell) and are in accordance with personal and cultural preferences are most likely to stimulate appetite and promote interest in eating.*
• Serve frequent, small meals rather than large ones if client is weak, fatigues easily, and/or has a poor appetite. **D** ✦	*Providing small rather than large meals can enable a client who is weak or fatigues easily to finish a meal.*
• Allow adequate time for meals; reheat foods/fluids if necessary. **D** ● ✦	*Clients who feel rushed during meals tend to become anxious, lose their appetite, and stop eating.*
• Encourage client to eat the maximum amount of protein allowed; instruct client to satisfy protein requirements with foods/fluids that are complete proteins and contain essential amino acids (e.g., eggs, milk, meat, poultry) if serum phosphorus level is not too high.	*Client needs to have protein to maintain normal body functions.*
• Weigh daily at same time with same clothing. Analyze trends over time	*Allows for a more accurate weight to be obtained.*

THERAPEUTIC INTERVENTIONS	RATIONALE
Dependent/Collaborative Actions	
Consult dietitian.	*Assist client to identify highly nutritious foods within prescribed diet.*
Perform a calorie count if ordered. Report information to the dietitian and physician.	*The client must consume a diet that is well balanced and high in essential nutrients in order to meet nutritional needs. Dietary supplements are often needed to help accomplish this.*
Consult the physician about an alternative method of providing nutrition (e.g., parenteral nutrition, tube feeding) if client does not consume enough food or fluids to meet nutritional needs.	*Notification of the physician allows for prompt alteration in the treatment plan.*

Nursing Diagnosis **RISK FOR INFECTION** NDx

Definition: Susceptible to invasion and multiplication of pathogenic organisms, which may compromise health.

Related to:
- Lowered resistance to infection associated with:
  - Immunosuppression secondary to uremia
- Malnutrition
- Stasis of secretions in the lungs and urinary stasis if mobility is decreased
  - Invasive procedures and insertion of IV lines and urinary catheter

CLINICAL MANIFESTATIONS

Subjective	**Objective**
Self-report of chills/lethargy; loss of appetite	Elevated temperature; diaphoresis; tachypnea; tachycardia; confusion; increase in WBC count above previous levels and/or significant change in differential; positive blood cultures

RISK FACTORS

- Exposure to pathogens
- Failure of immune response
- Poor nutritional status
- AKI
- CKD

DESIRED OUTCOMES

The client will not experience an infection as evidenced by:
a. Temperature with normal limits
b. Absence of chills and diaphoresis
c. Pulse and respiratory rate within normal range for client
d. WBC and differential within normal limits
e. Negative blood culture results

NOC OUTCOMES

Immune status; infection severity

NIC INTERVENTIONS

Infection protection; infection control

NURSING ASSESSMENT	RATIONALE
Assess for and report signs and symptoms of infection: increase in temperature, chills, diaphoresis, tachypnea, tachycardia, increase in WBC and differential count and/or significant change in differential, positive blood cultures.	*Early recognition of signs and symptoms of an infection allows for prompt intervention.*

THERAPEUTIC INTERVENTIONS	RATIONALE

Independent Actions

Implement measures to prevent the development of an infection:

Maintain good handwashing technique. Teach client appropriate handwashing technique: — *Reduces risk of exposure and cross-contamination.*

- Minimize the use of invasive procedures when possible. — *Prevents induction of bacteria into the system.*
- Change dressings, IV tubing, and invasive lines using aseptic technique and as directed by facility policy.
- Anchor catheters/tubings (e.g., intravenous) securely. — *Reduces trauma to the tissues and the risk for introduction of pathogens associated with in-and-out movement of the tubing.*
- Encourage deep breathing exercises, coughing and/or use of incentive spirometry, frequent position changes, and ambulation if able. — *Enhances mobilization and excretion of respiratory secretions, thereby reducing the risk of respiratory infection.*
- Perform actions to maintain an adequate nutritional status (e.g., increase activity as tolerated; maintain a clean environment and a relaxed, pleasant atmosphere; serve several small meals rather than three large ones). — *Adequate nutrition is necessary for cellular development and to fight off infection.*
- Perform actions to reduce stress (e.g., reduce pain and nausea; provide a calm, restful environment; explain diagnostic tests and treatment plan). — *Stress reduction prevents an increase in secretion of cortisol, which interferes with some immune responses.*
- Monitor vital signs. **D** ● ✦ — *Elevated temperature, BP, and heart rate may indicate an infection.*

Dependent/Collaborative Actions

- Monitor WBC with differential. — *Leukocytosis is associated with AKI and kidney injury. In the differential, a high number of immature WBCs are indicative of an infection (i.e., shift to the left).*
- Administer antimicrobials as ordered. — *Antimicrobials prevent and/or treat infections. Dosage may need to be adjusted due to impaired renal clearance.*

Obtain culture and sensitivity as ordered. — *Allows for prompt and appropriate treatment for an infection.*

Nursing Diagnosis   **RISK FOR DEFICIENT FLUID VOLUME** NDx

Definition: Susceptible to experiencing decreased intravascular, interstitial, and or/intracellular fluid volumes, which may compromise health.

Related to:
- Excessive diuresis in diuretic phase of AKI
- Inadequate fluid intake

CLINICAL MANIFESTATIONS

Subjective	Objective
Verbalization of thirst and dry mouth	Weight loss, increased body temperature, increased Hct, decreased skin turgor, increased heart rate, decreased blood pressure; capillary refill >3 seconds

RISK FACTORS

- Acute kidney failure
- Aging-loss of thirst and fluid volume reserve

DESIRED OUTCOMES

The client will not experience a deficient fluid volume as evidenced by:
a. Normal skin turgor
b. Moist mucous membranes
c. Stable weight
d. BP and hear rate within normal range for client and stable with position change
e. Capillary refill time <2 to 3 seconds
f. Hct within normal limits
g. Balanced I&O

NOC OUTCOMES

Fluid management; hydration status

NIC INTERVENTIONS

Fluid monitoring; fluid support

NURSING ASSESSMENT

Assess for signs and symptoms of fluid volume deficit:
- Decreased skin turgor
- Dry mucous membranes, verbalization of thirst
- Weight loss of 2% or greater over a short period of time
- Postural hypotension and/or decreased blood pressure
- Weak rapid pulse
- Capillary refill time >2 to 3 seconds
- Increased Hct levels

RATIONALE

Early recognition of signs and symptoms of deficit fluid volume allows for prompt intervention.

THERAPEUTIC INTERVENTIONS

Independent Actions

Monitor and document I&O and correlate with daily weight. Calculate insensible fluid loss.

Encourage and monitor fluid intake. Provide client easy access to fluids to support increased fluid needs. **D** ● ✦

Monitor and document changes in heart rate, BP, dry mucous membranes, skin turgor, and capillary refill.

Dependent/Collaborative Actions

Monitor and document trends in Hct levels.
Monitor serum sodium levels.

RATIONALE

A change in body weight of 1 kg (2.2 lbs) equals 1 L fluid loss. Decreased urine output may indicate dehydration. Insensible fluid loss is approximately 400 to 660 mL in a normal adult.

During the diuresis stage of AKI, close monitoring of fluid intake and output (I/O) helps to prevent fluid volume overload.

Orthostatic hypotension and tachycardia are indicative of hypovolemia. Dry mucous membranes, poor skin turgor, and delayed capillary refill indicate dehydration and may indicate inadequate fluid volume replacement.

Elevation may indicate dehydration.
Increased sodium loss occurs in the diuretic phase of AKI. Increased sodium in the kidneys increases fluid loss. Sodium restrictions may be indicted to decrease the volume of ongoing fluid loss.

⊖▶ **Collaborative Diagnosis** ## RISK FOR METABOLIC ACIDOSIS

Definition: Elevated level of serum acidity (pH < 7.35).

Related to:
- Decreased ability of the kidneys to excrete hydrogen ions and reabsorb bicarbonate
- Hyperkalemia (the body attempts to compensate for high serum potassium levels by shifting hydrogen ions into the vascular space in exchange for potassium ions)

CLINICAL MANIFESTATIONS

Subjective	Objective
Verbalization of fatigue, headache, and nausea	Drowsiness; disorientation; stupor; rapid, deep respirations; vomiting; cardiac dysrhythmias; pH <7.35; increased anion gap (>12 mEq/L)

RISK FACTORS

- Changes in regulatory mechanisms
- AKI
- CKD

DESIRED OUTCOMES

The client will not experience metabolic acidosis as evidenced by:
a. Usual mental status
b. Unlabored respirations at 12 to 20 breaths/min
c. Absence of headache, nausea, vomiting, and cardiac dysrhythmias
d. ABG values within a safe range for client (pH 7.35–7.45)
e. Serum anion gap within a normal range (3–11 mEq/L)

NURSING ASSESSMENT	RATIONALE
Assess for and report signs and symptoms of metabolic acidosis (e.g., drowsiness; disorientation; stupor; rapid, deep respirations; headache; nausea; vomiting; cardiac dysrhythmias; pH <7.35 and CO_2 content; increased anion gap [>12 mEq/L]).	*Early recognition of signs and symptoms of metabolic acidosis allows for prompt intervention.*

THERAPEUTIC INTERVENTIONS	RATIONALE
Dependent/Collaborative Actions	
Implement measures to prevent or treat metabolic acidosis:	
• Perform actions to prevent or treat hyperkalemia (e.g., maintain dietary restrictions of potassium, limit use of salt substitutes, limit intake of dietary protein). **D** ✦	*Decreases potassium levels in the system or prevents elevated potassium levels from occurring.*
• Administer sodium bicarbonate if ordered.	*Administration of bicarbonate decreases acidosis of the blood.*
Consult physician if signs and symptoms of acidosis persist or worsen.	*Notification of the physician allows for prompt alterations in treatment plan.*

Collaborative Diagnosis ## RISK FOR UREMIC SYNDROME

Definition: A syndrome associated with progressive renal failure.

Related to: Accumulations of serum nitrogenous substances (e.g., creatinine, urea) associated with extensive loss of renal function (signs and symptoms usually occur when the GFR falls to <10% of normal)

CLINICAL MANIFESTATIONS

Subjective	Objective
Self-reports of inability to concentrate; increasing weakness and fatigue; hallucinations; nausea; itching; muscle cramps; restless feelings in the legs during rest; joint pain; metallic or bitter taste in mouth	Increasing serum BUN and creatinine levels; cardiac dysrhythmias; confusion; sallow or grayish bronze skin; stomatitis; vomiting; unusual bleeding; pericarditis; fever; asterixis; seizures

RISK FACTOR
- Failure of regulatory mechanisms

DESIRED OUTCOMES

The client will not experience uremic syndrome as evidenced by:
a. Pulse regular at 60 to 100 beats/min
b. Usual mental status
c. Usual skin color
d. Improved strength and activity tolerance
e. No reports of nausea, insomnia, itching, muscle cramping, joint pain, paresthesia, and/or taste alterations
f. Intact oral mucous membrane
g. Absence of vomiting, unusual bleeding, pericarditis, asterixis, and seizure activity

NURSING ASSESSMENT

Assess for and report the following:
- Increasing BUN and serum creatinine levels
- Decreasing creatinine clearance levels
- Signs and symptoms of uremic syndrome:
  - Cardiac dysrhythmias
  - Difficulty concentrating, lethargy, confusion, or hallucinations
  - Sallow or grayish bronze skin
  - Increased weakness or fatigue
- Reports of nausea, insomnia, itching, muscle cramps, joint pain, paresthesias, restless feeling in legs during periods of inactivity, or metallic or bitter taste in mouth
- Stomatitis
- Vomiting
- Unusual bleeding (e.g., ecchymoses; prolonged bleeding from puncture sites; gingival bleeding; frank or occult blood in stool, urine, or vomitus)
- Pericarditis (e.g., chest pain that frequently radiates to shoulder, neck, back, and arm [usually left]; pericardial friction rub; elevated temperature)
- Asterixis, seizures

RATIONALE

Early recognition of signs and symptoms of uremic syndrome allows for prompt intervention.

THERAPEUTIC INTERVENTIONS

Independent Actions
Implement measures to reduce the levels of serum nitrogenous substances to prevent uremic syndrome:
- Perform actions to maintain an adequate nutritional status (e.g., serve small, frequent meals; allow adequate time to complete meals; eat the appropriate amount of proteins; take dietary supplements if indicated). **D** ● ✦
- Consult a dietitian.
- Perform actions to prevent infection (e.g., maintain adequate fluid intake, use sterile technique during all invasive procedures, promote good handwashing, change peripheral intravenous line sites according to hospital policy).
- Implement measures as ordered to control disease conditions such as diabetes that have caused or contributed to renal failure.

Dependent/Collaborative Actions
- Consult the physician before administering medications that are known to be nephrotoxic (e.g., NSAIDs, aminoglycosides).

RATIONALE

These actions assist the client in maintenance of an adequate nutritional status while reducing catabolism of body proteins, which contribute to uremic syndrome.

Assists client to identify foods appropriate for a protein-restricted diet.
Prevention of infection prevents an increase in the metabolic rate and subsequent cellular catabolism.

Prevents further renal damage.

Client should be informed of medications that are nephrotoxic and should not take any over-the-counter medications without consulting his/her health care provider.

Continued...

THERAPEUTIC INTERVENTIONS	RATIONALE
If signs and symptoms of uremic syndrome occur:	
• Prepare client for dialysis if planned.	*Dialysis removes toxins from the blood.*
• Maintain a safe environment for client (e.g., side rails up while in bed, assistance with ambulation as needed, constant supervision if indicated, seizure precautions).	*Implementation of hospital policy related to falls and other precautions decreases potential for client injury.*
• Administer antidysrhythmics as ordered; restrict activity if indicated. **D** ✦	*Treats cardiac dysrhythmias.*
• Administer antiemetics as ordered. **D** ✦	*Antiemetics decrease the incidence of nausea.*
• Provide small, frequent meals; instruct client to ingest foods/fluids slowly.	
• Use tepid water and mild soap for bathing; apply emollient creams or ointments frequently. **D** ● ✦	*Use of tepid water for bathing and creams and ointments reduce the incidence of pruritus.*
• Administer antihistamines if ordered. **D** ✦	*Antihistamines block the release of histamines, which stimulate itchy sensations.*
• Instruct client to push feet against a hard surface when leg cramps occur; apply warm packs to affected areas.	*Actions help control muscle cramps.*
• Instruct client to avoid substances such as extremely hot, spicy, or acidic foods/fluids; assist with frequent oral hygiene; apply oral protective pastes as ordered.	*Avoidance of hot, spicy, and/or acidic foods reduces the severity of stomatitis.*
• Apply gentle, prolonged pressure after injections and venous and arterial punctures; instruct client to use an electric rather than a straight-edge razor and to use a soft bristle toothbrush for oral hygiene.	*These actions prevent and/or decrease incidence of bleeding.*
• Apply firm, prolonged pressure to bleeding area if possible; administer clotting factors or vitamin K if ordered.	*Administration of clotting factors and/or vitamin K helps improve body's clotting ability and control bleeding.*
• Maintain activity restrictions as ordered; administer an anti-inflammatory agent and analgesics if ordered. **D** ✦	*Anti-inflammatory agents treat pericarditis. Analgesics decrease sensation of pain.*

DISCHARGE TEACHING/CONTINUED CARE

Nursing Diagnosis **DEFICIENT KNOWLEDGE** NDx**; INEFFECTIVE FAMILY HEALTH MANAGEMENT** NDx **INEFFECTIVE HEALTH MANAGEMENT*** NDx

Definition: Deficient knowledge NDx: Absence of cognitive information related to a specific topic, or its acquisition; **Ineffective Family Health Management NDx:** A pattern of regulating into family processes a program for the treatment of illness and its sequelae that is unsatisfactory for meeting specific health goal of the family unit; **Ineffective Health Management NDx:** Pattern of regulating and integrating into daily living a therapeutic regimen for the treatment of illness and its sequelae that is unsatisfactory for meeting specific health goals.

Related to:
• Specific topic (lack of specific information necessary for clients/significant others) to make informed choices regarding condition/treatment/lifestyle changes

CLINICAL MANIFESTATIONS

Subjective	Objective
Verbalizes inability to manage illness; verbalizes inability to follow prescribed regimen	Inaccurate follow-through with instructions; inappropriate behaviors; experience of preventable complications of renal failure

---

*The nurse should select the diagnostic label that is most appropriate for the client's discharge

RISK FACTORS
- Cognitive deficit
- Financial concerns
- Failure to reduce risk factors for complications of renal failure
- Inability to care for oneself
- Difficulty in modifying personal habits and integrating treatments into lifestyle
- Insufficient knowledge of therapeutic regimen

NOC OUTCOMES	NIC INTERVENTIONS
Knowledge: treatment regimen; diet; infection control; cardiac medication	Health system guidance; teaching: individual; teaching: disease process; teaching: prescribed activity/exercise; teaching: prescribed medication

NURSING ASSESSMENT	RATIONALE
Assess client's readiness and ability to learn Assess meaning of illness to client	*Early recognition of readiness to learn and meaning of illness to client allows for implementation of the appropriate teaching interventions.*

THERAPEUTIC INTERVENTIONS	RATIONALE

Desired Outcome: The client will verbalize understanding of AKI and CKD.

Independent Actions

Explain renal failure in terms that client can understand. Use appropriate teaching aids (e.g., pictures, videotapes, kidney models).	*Client's understanding of the disease process will increase adherence with treatment regimen.*

THERAPEUTIC INTERVENTIONS	RATIONALE

Desired Outcome: The client will identify ways to slow the progression of kidney damage.

Independent Actions

Provide instructions regarding ways to slow the progression of kidney damage:

• Control hypertension by adhering to dietary modifications and taking medications as prescribed.	*Prevents further damage to the kidneys and decreases impact of vascular fluid volume changes on the heart.*

• Reduce the risk of urinary tract infection by:
  • Cleaning perineal area thoroughly after each bowel movement
  • Wiping from front to back after urination and defecation (if female)
	Proper perineal hygiene prevents urinary tract exposure to vaginal or rectal bacteria.

• Consuming the maximum amount of fluids allowed.	*Maintenance of appropriate fluid intake maintains vascular fluid volume.*

• Reduce the risk of nephrotoxic reactions by:
  • Consulting the appropriate health care provider before:
  (1) Taking any additional prescription and nonprescription drugs
	Many over-the-counter and prescription medications are nephrotoxic.

(2) Undergoing diagnostic testing that requires use of a contrast medium	*Inform health care provider of renal failure, as dyes used in diagnostic testing can be nephrotoxic.*
(3) Resuming any occupation or hobby involving exposure to chemicals or fumes.	*Fumes may be nephrotoxic and can cause further kidney injury.*
• Avoid contact with products such as antifreeze, pesticides, carbon tetrachloride, mercuric chloride, lead, arsenic, and creosote.	*Free radicals associated with these materials increase destruction of renal tissue.*
Assist client and significant others to identify ways in which the above-described health care measures can be incorporated into lifestyle.	*Allows client control of how he/she will be able to care for self postdischarge. It will also provide confidence in his/her ability to care for self.*

THERAPEUTIC INTERVENTIONS	RATIONALE

Desired Outcome: The client will develop a plan to adhere to fluid restrictions and dietary modifications.

Independent Actions

Reinforce the importance of adhering to and following physician's instructions about fluid restrictions and dietary modifications.

The client should understand the impact of following prescribed fluid restrictions and dietary modification as well as the impact on the system when the restrictions and modifications are not followed.

Reinforce dietitian's instructions on how to calculate and measure dietary allotments. Have client develop sample menus.

Allows client to determine appropriate meals based on treatment regimen.

If client is on a protein- and sodium-restricted diet, inform him/her that numerous salt-free and protein-free products are available. Provide names of local stores that carry these products.

Provides client with options for diet and flavoring of foods. Developing a list and a plan to adhere to diet restrictions provides client some level of control.

Collaborate with client to develop a list of foods they like that meet the diet restriction requirements.

If client is on a fluid restriction, instruct to:

- Take oral medications with soft foods (e.g., applesauce, pudding).

This allows client to take medications without using liquids.

- Reduce thirst by:
  - Sucking on sugar-free hard candy, popsicles, or ice cubes made with favorite juices. Rinse oral cavity with non-alcoholic rinses.

Maintains moist oral mucous membranes without fluid volume excess and decreases thirst. Caution client that the fluid volume of the popsicle and ice cubes must be considered as oral fluid intake.

  - Spacing fluids evenly throughout the hours client is awake.

Spacing fluid intake throughout the day helps maintain moist oral mucous membranes and improves client adherence to fluid restrictions.

- Set out the 24-hrs allotment of liquids in the morning in order to visualize the amount allowed for the day.

Helps client determine when are the best times to drink fluid allotment.

THERAPEUTIC INTERVENTIONS	RATIONALE

Desired Outcome: The client will demonstrate the ability to accurately weigh self, measure fluid I&O, and monitor own BP.

Independent Actions

If client needs to monitor weight, instruct client to weigh at the same time, on the same scale, and with similar amounts of clothing on.

Weight measurements should be performed daily at the same time and under the same conditions for more precise measurements.

Demonstrate how to measure and record fluid intake and urinary output if indicated. Stress that any substance that is liquid at room temperature is counted as fluid intake.

Accurate documentation and monitoring are important to determine appropriate amount of fluid intake.

If client needs to monitor BP, provide instructions on how to take, read, and record it.

Regular monitoring of blood pressure helps prevent hypertension and its deleterious effects on the kidneys.

Allow time for questions, clarification, practice, and return demonstration. Instruct client to take record of weights, fluid intake, urinary output, and BP readings to appointments with health care provider.

Allowing time for questions, clarification, and return demonstrations allows the nurse to evaluate the effectiveness of teaching and make the appropriate adjustments to the teaching plan. It also improves client's self-confidence in his/her ability to care for self and manage disease process.

THERAPEUTIC INTERVENTIONS	RATIONALE

Desired Outcome: The client will identify ways to reduce the risk of infection.

THERAPEUTIC INTERVENTIONS	RATIONALE

Independent Actions

Instruct client in ways to reduce the risk of infection:

- Avoid contact with persons who have an infection.
- Avoid crowds during the flu or cold season.
- Decrease or stop smoking.
- Drink allotted amounts of liquids.
- Maintain good personal hygiene.
- Maintain a good nutritional status.
- Maintain an adequate balance between activity and rest.

- Take antimicrobials as prescribed before scheduled dental work, invasive diagnostic procedures, or surgery.

These actions prevent exposure to individuals who may have an infection or improve the client's ability to fight infections.
Smoking weakens the immune system and causes irritation of the mouth and respiratory system.
Oral hygiene moistens mucous membranes and promotes the production of saliva. These help to maintain good oral health.
Required to maintain an adequate functioning immune system.
Sleep deprivation may decrease the production of cytokines in the immune system.
Prevents infection from normal body flora.
Dosages may require adjustment based on level of renal injury

THERAPEUTIC INTERVENTIONS	RATIONALE

Desired Outcome: The client will identify ways to manage signs and symptoms that often occur as a result of chronic renal failure.

Independent Actions

Provide instructions regarding ways to manage the following signs and symptoms that often occur as a result of chronic renal failure:

- Weakness and fatigue
  - Schedule frequent rest periods throughout the day.

  - Maintain a good nutritional status.
- Dry mouth
  - Space fluid allotments evenly throughout waking hours.
  - Perform oral hygiene frequently.
- Decreased libido (can occur as a result of weakness, fatigue, depression, and side effects of some medications)
  - Schedule rest periods before and after sexual activity.
  - Explore creative ways of expressing sexuality (e.g., massage, fantasies, cuddling).

Knowledge of disease process and how to decrease the impact of risk factors and disease progression helps the client and family understand why lifestyle changes are required to maintain health status. This improves client's adherence to treatment regimen and allows client to maintain a level of independence for as long as possible.
Important to conserve energy.
Provides energy for desired activities.

Dry mouth increases the client's risk for infection.

May need to plan activities to assure appropriate rest prior to activity.

THERAPEUTIC INTERVENTIONS	RATIONALE

Desired Outcome: The client will state signs and symptoms to report to the health care provider.

Independent Actions

Instruct client to report the following:

- Weight gain of more than 0.5 kg (1 lb) per day or a continued weight loss.
- Persistent nausea or vomiting.

- Increasing fatigue or weakness.
- Difficulty concentrating and making decisions.
- Confusion.

- Persistent or severe headache.
- Palpitations or chest pain.

These clinical manifestations should be reported to the health care provider and require prompt attention.
This level of weight gain indicates fluid volume excess.

Persistent nausea and vomiting may indicate changes in serum electrolyte levels.
These clinical manifestations indicate a decreased ability of the kidneys to remove toxins from the body.
Increasing confusion may reflect declining kidney functioning and reflect increased uremia.
Indicates increased B/P or vascular fluid volume.

Continued...

THERAPEUTIC INTERVENTIONS	RATIONALE
• Red, rust-colored, or smoky urine; bloody or tarry stools; blood in sputum or vomitus; persistent bleeding from nose, mouth, or any cut; prolonged or excessive menses; excessive bruising; or sudden abdominal or back pain.	*May indicate infection, anemia, or decreased level of clotting factors.*
• Fever or chills.	*Indicates an infection.*
• Numbness or tingling in extremities, persistent restless feeling in legs during periods of inactivity.	*May indicate anemia and/or changes in electrolyte levels.*
• Change in skin color (e.g., bronze, yellow-gray, brownish gray, increased pallor).	*May indicate anemia or dialysis-related hemochromatosis.*
• Impotence, infertility, or amenorrhea.	*Could indicate hormonal imbalances caused by increasing serum levels of nitrogenous substances.*
• Increasing BP.	*Increasing blood pressure may indicate excess vascular fluid volume and/or increased sodium levels.*
• Swelling of feet, ankles, or hands.	*Reflects declining ability of the kidneys.*
• Shortness of breath.	
• Diarrhea or constipation.	*Diarrhea and/or constipation can occur as a side effect of antacid therapy; physicians generally recommend alternating antacids containing magnesium with those containing aluminum or calcium to prevent these bowel problems.*
• Persistent itching.	*May indicate high plasma calcium levels.*
• Oral pain or breakdown of oral mucous membrane.	*Indicates increased uremia.*
• Muscle pain or cramping.	*Decreased serum potassium/magnesium.*
• Twitching or seizures.	*May indicate uremic encephalopathy.*
• Joint or bone pain.	*Could indicate renal osteodystrophy resulting from effects of hypocalcemia and hyperphosphatemia.*

THERAPEUTIC INTERVENTIONS	RATIONALE

Desired Outcome: The client will identify community resources that can assist with adjustment to changes resulting from chronic renal failure.

Independent Actions

Provide information about community resources that can assist the client and significant others to adjust to changes resulting from chronic renal failure (e.g., local chapter of the American Kidney Association, vocational rehabilitation, social services, counseling services).	*Provides for continuum of care and support of the client after discharge from the acute care facility.*
Initiate a referral if indicated.	*May be required for client to receive service or coverage by health care insurance/Medicare/Medicaid.*

THERAPEUTIC INTERVENTIONS	RATIONALE

Desired Outcome: The client, in collaboration with the nurse, will develop a plan for adhering to recommended follow-up care including future appointments with health care provider and medications prescribed.

Independent Actions

Reinforce the importance of keeping follow-up appointments with health care provider. Collaborate with the client to develop a plan for attendance at follow-up appointments.	*Client should understand that he/she has a chronic illness and should be monitored by a health care professional to maintain level of health as long as possible.*

THERAPEUTIC INTERVENTIONS	RATIONALE
Explain the rationale for, side effects of, and importance of taking prescribed medications. Inform client of pertinent food and drug interactions.	*Knowledge of medications and how they impact the system improves client adherence to treatment regimen and understanding of the importance of adhering to the prescribed medication regimen. The client must be able to recognize alterations in functioning related to medication administration and what clinical manifestations should be reported to the health care provider.*
Reinforce the importance of consulting the appropriate health care provider (e.g., pharmacist, nurse practitioner, physician) before taking any prescription and nonprescription drugs. Explain that:	
• Some drugs such as ibuprofen, neomycin, and naproxen are nephrotoxic and can hasten the progression of renal failure.	*Nephrotoxic medications hasten the progression of renal failure.*
• Some drugs such as aspirin and digoxin are excreted by the kidneys and can rapidly build to toxic levels in the body (usual dosages may need to be reduced or a different medication may need to be taken).	*Some drugs quickly build up to toxic levels because they are excreted by the kidneys.*
• Some drugs contain ingredients that affect electrolyte balance and elevate BP (e.g., many cold remedies).	
Include significant others in explanations and teaching sessions and encourage their involvement in plan development.	*Including significant others in teaching helps them understand how to appropriately support the client and improves adherence to the treatment regimen.*
Reinforce the need to the client to assume responsibility for managing as much of care as possible.	*Improves client's confidence in ability to care for self and maintain independence as long as possible.*

ADDITIONAL NURSING DIAGNOSES

ACTIVITY INTOLERANCE NDx
Related to:
- Inadequate tissue oxygenation associated with anemia resulting from:
  - Decreased secretion of erythropoietin as a result of impaired renal function (erythropoietin stimulates the bone marrow to produce RBCs)
  - Shortened survival time of RBCs (as renal failure progresses, the nitrogenous substances in the blood increase and cause increased hemolysis of RBCs)
- Inadequate nutritional status

RISK FOR CONSTIPATION NDx
Related to:
- Decreased intake of foods high in fiber and fluids associated with prescribed restrictions
- Decreased GI motility associated with decreased activity and the effect of some medications (e.g., those containing aluminum or calcium, iron preparations)

IMPAIRED ORAL MUCOUS MEMBRANE NDx
Related to:
- Injury to lips and oral mucosa
- Bad taste in mouth
- Stomatitis
- Lack of saliva

FEAR AND ANXIETY NDx
Related to:
- Prescribed fluid restriction
- Lack of understanding of diagnosis, diagnostic tests, and treatment plan
- Uncertainty as to extensiveness of loss of renal function
- Anticipated change in health status, lifestyle, and roles as a result of progressive loss of renal function
- Awareness of probable future need for dialysis or renal transplantation
- Financial concerns

GRIEVING NDx
Related to: Progressive loss of kidney function and the effects of this on lifestyle and roles

---

NDx = NANDA Diagnosis **D** = Delegatable Action ● = UAP ✦ = LVN/LPN ⊖▶ = Go to ⊖volve for animation

The Client With Alterations in Musculoskeletal Function

AMPUTATION

An amputation is the surgical removal of all or part of a limb. Amputation of an upper or lower extremity may be performed to treat conditions such as tumors, uncontrollable infection, or gangrene and may be indicated in situations involving tissue destruction resulting from trauma or thermal injury (e.g., frostbite, electrocution, burns). The majority of amputations are performed on the lower extremities of persons with severe peripheral vascular disease. In these instances, the ischemic limb is removed to prevent life-threatening infection and/or relieve severe, persistent discomfort. The location of a limb amputation (e.g., above the knee, below the knee) is determined by factors such as the adequacy of circulation in the involved extremity; the client's age, general health, anticipated mobility; and the requirements for proper fit and optimal function of the prosthetic device.

There are two types of surgical amputations performed: open and closed. The open type is performed if the client has an infected limb. The wound is left open with wound treatments applied until the infection resolves. The wound is then closed during a second surgical procedure. An open amputation may also be done if the client has a high risk for developing a wound or bone infection postoperatively. A closed amputation, which consists of soft tissue flaps sutured over the bone, is the type of amputation most frequently performed. The basic techniques for postoperative management of the residual limb after a closed amputation include use of a soft compression or rigid dressing. The technique selected depends on the client's underlying disease process and physiological status and whether the prosthetic fitting will be immediate, early (usually within 10 to 30 days), or delayed or is not expected to occur (unplanned).

OUTCOME/DISCHARGE CRITERIA

The client will:
1. Maintain pain relief
2. Have evidence of normal healing of the surgical wound
3. Achieve expected level of mobility
4. Not exhibit signs and symptoms of postoperative complications
5. Demonstrate ways to prevent contractures, increase strength, and improve mobility
6. Demonstrate correct transfer and ambulation techniques and proper use of ambulatory aids
7. Identify ways to maintain health of the remaining lower extremity
8. Demonstrate the ability to care for the residual limb
9. Identify ways to manage phantom limb pain if it occurs
10. State signs and symptoms to report to the health care provider
11. Share feelings and thoughts about the change in body image and effects of the amputation on lifestyle and roles
12. Identify community resources that can assist with home management and adjustment to changes resulting from the amputation
13. Develop a plan for adhering to recommended follow-up care including future appointments with health care provider, prosthetist, and physical therapist; medications prescribed; and activity level

This care plan focuses on the adult client hospitalized for a planned below-the-knee, closed amputation. Refer to the preoperative care plan for information for preparation for surgery. Much of the postoperative information is applicable to clients receiving follow-up care in an extended care facility or home setting.

Nursing Diagnosis **DEFICIENT KNOWLEDGE** NDx

Definition: Absence of cognitive information related to a specific topic, or its acquisition.

Related to:
- Surgical procedure
- Hospital routines associated with surgery
- Physical preparation for the amputation

- Sensations that may occur after surgery and anesthesia
- Postoperative care and management of the residual limb
- Postoperative activity and exercises

CLINICAL MANIFESTATIONS

Subjective	Objective
Verbalization of concerns about loss of lower limb Questioning about how to live in the future	Inaccurate follow-through of instructions, exaggerated behaviors

RISK FACTORS

- Cognitive limitations
- Unfamiliar with surgical procedure
- Grieving
- Age
- Chronic illness
- Fear of unknown

DESIRED OUTCOMES

NOC OUTCOMES

Knowledge: treatment regimen; prescribed activity

NIC INTERVENTIONS

Amputation care; teaching: individual;
teaching: preoperative; teaching: prescribed exercise

NURSING ASSESSMENT	RATIONALE
Assess client's readiness and ability to learn. Assess client's understanding of scheduled procedure. Assess meaning of current illness and future changes to client.	*Early recognition of readiness to learn, meaning of illness to client, and understanding of schedule procedure allows for implementation of the appropriate teaching interventions.*

NURSING INTERVENTIONS	RATIONALE

Independent Actions

Allow time for client to express fear, anxiety, and grief over loss of limb and subsequent lifestyle changes.

Assess for understanding of procedure and postoperative plan of care.

Explain that after surgery, the client will experience actual limb pain and may experience phantom limb sensation. This type of pain may be described as:

- Tingling.
- Throbbing.
- Feeling of pins/needles in the amputated limb.

Provide the following information about postoperative phantom limb pain, including:

- It does not occur in all clients.
- The type of pain experienced varies from client to client and can be similar to pain experienced before the amputation
- It may be triggered by pressure on other body areas.
- Measures will be implemented to provide effective control of the pain if it occurs.

Provide instructions on ways to prevent residual limb contractures that will be implemented following surgery:

- Avoid sitting for long periods.
- Avoid placing pillows under residual limb.
- Maintain residual limb in proper alignment.

Allowing client to express concerns and grieve over loss prior to teaching concerning postoperative care can improve client's ability to understand and engage in care and surgical preparation.
Provides baseline for patient education.

Residual limb pain is pain originating from the site of the amputated limb. It is felt during the early post-amputation period and may decrease with wound healing.

Phantom limb is a sensation that pain felt in the amputated area of the limb. This pain may reduce in frequency and intensity over time but may persist for several years.

The client needs to be assured that the nurse understands about phantom limb pain, and that all pain will be appropriately treated.
Information about phantom limb pain provides client with a basis for the pain and increases the potential that the client will be able to recognize pain and what may cause it and possible treatments.

Continued...

NURSING INTERVENTIONS	RATIONALE
Inform the client of the need to lie prone several times during the day	*Limb contractures can result from prolonged flexion of the knee or prolonged flexion, hyperextension, abduction, adduction, or external rotation of the hip.*
• Perform range-of-motion exercises as instructed • Assure client that support will be provided to do range-of-motion exercises	*Lying prone several times a day promotes hip flexion and decreases incidence of hip contractures.* *Range of motion exercises helps to maintain muscle strength and flexibility as well as improving circulation.*
Provide the client time for return demonstration in the following exercises: • Range-of-motion exercises • Strengthening exercises for the upper extremities, chest, residual limb, unaffected lower extremity, and abdominal muscles. Assure client that support will be provided to do range-of-motion exercises.	*Stressing importance of and demonstrating exercises prior to surgery will decrease anxiety following surgery when client will be expected to move and complete range-of-motion exercises which help to reduce incidence of contractures.*
Provide instructions regarding: • Use of overhead trapeze. • Transfer techniques. • Use of mobility aids (e.g., crutches, cane, walker).	*Proper instruction regarding the use of assistive devices reduces the risk of further injury. Ability to use supportive devices will allow client some measure of self-care.*
Reinforce the physician's explanation about the type of prosthesis and dressings planned. If an immediate prosthetic fitting (immediate postoperative prosthesis [IPOP]) is planned, inform client that: • A rigid dressing (plastic or plaster) will be placed on the residual stump during surgery, and the pylon (temporary artificial limb) will attach to the socket on the end of this dressing. • In addition to providing a means of securing the pylon, the rigid dressing will help shape the residual limb, reduce edema and support tissue in the surgical area, minimize pain during activity, and promote maturation of the residual limb. • Ambulation using the temporary prosthesis usually begins 24–48 hrs after surgery and progresses from walking between parallel bars to using ambulatory aids such as a walker, cane, or crutches if needed.	*Adequate education regarding immediate or delayed prosthetic fitting enables the client to know what to expect in the postoperative period, reducing the fear of the unknown.*
If there are no plans for an immediate prosthetic fitting, inform client that: • A soft compression dressing (soft dressing covered by an elastic bandage or sock) will be placed on the residual limb during surgery. • The elastic bandage or sock will be reapplied if it slips, wrinkles, or loosens. • Mobility will be accomplished using a wheelchair, walker, and/or crutches. • Fitting for a temporary prosthesis (if planned) will not occur until after the surgical site has healed (usually 3 to 6 weeks after surgery).	*Ambulatory aids may be needed if client's gait is not steady or only partial weight-bearing is allowed as the surgical area heals.* *The dressing will help reduce edema and support tissue in the surgical area and shape the stump for future prosthetic fitting if planned.*
Allow adequate time for client questions and return demonstrations.	*Helps client to understand although the prosthesis is not immediately available, it is expected that the client will be out of bed and moving following surgery. Client may need time to learn techniques to perform return demonstrations. Allowing client time to do this helps to decrease anxiety and confidence in ability to perform required actions following surgery.*

Nursing Diagnosis **ACUTE/CHRONIC PAIN** NDx

Definition: Acute Pain NDx: Unpleasant sensory and emotional experience associated with actual or potential tissue damage, or described in terms of such damage (International Association for the Study of Pain); sudden or slow onset of any intensity from mild to severe with anticipated or predictable end, and with a duration of less than 3 months.

Chronic Pain NDx: Unpleasant sensory and emotional experience associated with actual or potential tissue damage, or described in terms of such damage (International Association for the Study of Pain); sudden or slow onset of any intensity from mild to severe, constant or recurring without an anticipated or predictable end, and with a duration of greater than 3 months.

Related to:
- Incisional pain related to tissue trauma and reflex muscle spasms associated with the amputation, irritation from drainage tube, and stress on surgical area associated with movement
- Phantom limb pain related to altered neural transmission associated with interruption in usual nervous system pathways resulting from the amputation

CLINICAL MANIFESTATIONS

Subjective	Objective
Verbalization of pain in affected limb; verbalization of phantom pain with and/or reluctance to move or participate in self-care	Restlessness; diaphoresis; increased BP; tachycardia, tachypnea, grimacing with movement and guarding behaviors

RISK FACTORS
- Inadequate pain relief
- Altered mobility/limited mobility
- Muscle spasms
- Chronic illness
- Fear/anxiety

DESIRED OUTCOMES

The client will experience diminished pain as evidenced by:
a. Self-report of decreased pain
b. Vital signs within normal range for client
c. No guarding actions or grimacing with movement, or restlessness

NOC OUTCOMES

Pain control; comfort status

NIC INTERVENTIONS

Pain management; analgesic administration

NURSING ASSESSMENT

Assess for and report signs and symptoms of acute/chronic pain:
- Verbal reports of pain
- Restlessness
- Diaphoresis
- Increased BP
- Increased heart rate
- Grimacing with movement

RATIONALE

Early recognition of signs and symptoms of acute/chronic pain allows for prompt intervention.

Continued...

NURSING ASSESSMENT	RATIONALE

• Guarding actions
  • Assess client's perception of the severity of pain using a pain intensity rating scale
  • Assess client's pain pattern (e.g., location, onset, quality, duration, aggravating factors)
  • Ask client to describe previous pain experience and methods that were effective in relieving pain
	Assessment of the severity of pain experienced helps determine most appropriate interventions. Use of a pain intensity rating scale provides the nurse a clear understanding of the pain being experienced and promotes consistency when communicating with others.
	
	Knowledge of client's usual pain response and effective methods to alleviate pain supports the identification of effective pain management.

THERAPEUTIC INTERVENTIONS	RATIONALE

Independent Actions

Assess pain using a pain scale including severity, quality, intensity, radiation, and onset of new and different pain.

Provides baseline for pain experience and use of a standard tool improves communication among health care team. Change in type of pain experienced may indicate developing complications (e.g., compartment syndrome).

Provide adjuvant methods of acute pain relief:
• Relaxation techniques (e.g., mindfulness-based stress reduction [MBSR]).
• Guided imagery.
• Music/watching TV.
• Support client's preferred coping mechanisms.

Adjuvant pain relief refocuses attention, and relaxation techniques help to relax muscles. Use of known coping mechanisms reinforces effectiveness and client self-confidence in using them.

Implement measures to reduce phantom limb pain if it occurs:
• Instruct client to apply pressure on residual limb by walking on pylon or pressing limb against a firm surface unless contraindicated.
• Encourage participation in diversional activities. **D** ✦
• Reposition limb to decrease excessive pressure on any part of the body. **D** ✦

Phantom limb pain occurs in approximately 80% of individuals and may occur early in the postoperative period. The client taught about the syndrome and methods to reduce and cope with the pain.

For chronic phantom limb pain, consider alternative methods of pain control:
• Acupuncture
• Massage
• Virtual reality therapy
• Mirror box therapy
• Transcutaneous electrical nerve stimulation (TENS)

Phantom pain is a common complication following limb amputation. It is thought that phantom pain results from a combination of peripheral, spinal, central and psychological factors. Alternative therapies for this type of pain have been shown to be effective including acupuncture and area massage. The client should be encouraged to explore what alternative treatments will help to control pain.

Dependent/Collaborative Actions

Administer medication to decrease pain and phantom pain:
Opioids; NSAIDs, topical, oral, and IV methods of administration; prevent pain from becoming so severe that it takes a long time to provide relief; consider scheduling pain medication administration at set hours for the first 24 hrs following surgery.

Multiple types of pain medication may be used to provide pain relief. The goal is to maintain pain control and preventing the pain to become too severe.

Tricyclic antidepressants

Tricyclic antidepressants help to alter the transmission of pain impulses and/or the client's perception of pain.

Anticonvulsants

Anticonvulsants help to inhibit neurotransmission of pain sensation.

Request order for patient-controlled pain analgesia (PCA)

Allows client control over administration of pain medication.

Consult appropriate health care provider (e.g., physician, pain management specialist) about use of TENS, biofeedback, acupuncture, hypnosis, and/or other methods of pain control

Consultation with the appropriate health care provided can assist client improving both short-term and long-term pain control and relief.

Nursing Diagnosis IMPAIRED TISSUE INTEGRITY/RISK FOR IMPAIRED TISSUE INTEGRITY NDx

Definition: Impaired Tissue Integrity NDx: Damage to the mucous membrane, cornea, integumentary system, muscular fascia, muscle, tendon, bone, cartilage, joint capsule, and/or ligament: **Risk for Impaired Tissue Integrity NDx:** Susceptible to damage to the mucous membrane, cornea, integumentary system, muscular fascia, muscle, tendon, bone, cartilage, joint capsule, and/or ligament, which may compromise health.

Related to:
- Disruption of tissue associated with the amputation
- Delayed wound healing associated with factors such as:
  - Decreased nutritional status
    Decreased blood supply to wound area resulting from the underlying disease process, edema of the residual limb, and/or excessive or prolonged pressure on operative site (may occur as a result of noncompliance with weight-bearing limitations, improper residual limb wrapping, and/or slippage of the residual limb dressing)
- Irritation of skin associated with contact with wound drainage, pressure from tubings, and use of tape
- Damage to the skin and/or subcutaneous tissue associated with prolonged pressure on tissues, friction, and/or shearing while mobility is decreased

CLINICAL MANIFESTATIONS

Subjective	Objective
N/A	Increased periwound swelling and redness; pale or necrotic tissue in wound healing by secondary intention; separation of wound edges in wounds healing by primary intention

RISK FACTORS
- Altered mobility
- Decreased tissue perfusion
- Altered nutritional status
- Smoking

DESIRED OUTCOMES
The client will:
a. Experience normal healing of the surgical wound
b. Maintain tissue integrity as evidenced by absence of redness and irritation, and no skin breakdown

NOC OUTCOMES
Wound healing: primary intention; wound secondary intention

NIC INTERVENTIONS
Wound care; skin surveillance; pressure ulcer care; pressure ulcer prevention; positioning

NURSING ASSESSMENT	RATIONALE
Assess for and report signs and symptoms of impaired skin integrity: • Increased periwound swelling and redness • Pale or necrotic tissue in wounds healing by secondary or tertiary intention • Separation of wound edges in wounds healing by primary intention Assess the following for pallor, redness, irritation, and breakdown: • Skin areas in contact with wound drainage, tape, and tubings • Back, coccyx, and buttocks • Elbows and remaining heel	*Early recognition of signs and symptoms of impaired skin integrity allows for prompt intervention.*

THERAPEUTIC INTERVENTIONS	RATIONALE
Independent Actions • Elevate limb for the first 24–48 hrs. • Monitor vital signs, palpate pulses, capillary refill.	*Stable vital signs and no changes in strength and intensity of pulses are indications of perfusion.*

NDx = NANDA Diagnosis   **D** = Delegatable Action   ● = UAP   ✦ = LVN/LPN   ⊝▶ = Go to ⊝volve for animation

Continued...

THERAPEUTIC INTERVENTIONS	RATIONALE
• Assess neurovascular status of extremities—movement, sensations, color, temperature.	*Changes in skin color, temperature, sensation, and movement may indicate any of the following: tissue edema or hematoma at suture line that may lead to tissue necrosis; circulation to wound may be decreased if a pressure dressing is applied.*
• Monitor dressing (soft pressure wrap or rigid), noting amount and color of drainage.	*Clients on anticoagulants may have increased bleeding and be at risk for a hematoma. Increased drainage from the wound may also require increased fluid intake to maintain cardiovascular status.*
• Monitor pain status, noting any increase or inability to obtain pain relief or sudden changes.	*Hematoma or deep venous thrombosis (DVT) formation may lead to increased pain or sudden changes in pain characteristics.*
Implement measures to prevent tissue irritation and breakdown resulting from decreased mobility:	
• Assist client to turn at least every 2 hrs unless contraindicated. **D** ● ✦	*Prolonged and/or excessive pressure on the skin obstructs capillary blood flow to that area. The resultant hypoxia, impaired flow of nutrients, and accumulation of waste products in the area of obstructed flow make that tissue more susceptible to breakdown.*
• Position client properly; use pressure-reducing or pressure-relieving devices (e.g., pillows, gel or foam cushions, alternating pressure mattress, kinetic bed, air-fluidized bed) if indicated. **D** ● ✦	
• Instruct client to use overhead trapeze to lift self and shift weight at least every 30 minutes.	*Measures that prevent excessive pressure or ensure that pressure is relieved often enough to avoid obstruction of capillary blood flow help maintain skin integrity.*
• Lift and move client carefully using a turn sheet and adequate assistance.	
Keep bed linens dry and wrinkle-free. **D** ● ✦	
• Apply a protective covering such as a hydrocolloid or transparent membrane dressing to areas of the skin susceptible to breakdown (e.g., coccyx, heel, elbows).	*Prevents maceration and decreases potential breakdown when client is on bedrest.* *Reduces the risk of pressure ulcers over bony prominences or dependent areas.*
• Encourage early range-of-motion exercises and ambulation.	*Improves circulation and complications associated with prolonged bedrest. Improves client's self-confidence in ability to ambulate post amputation.*
• Monitor client's nutritional status. **D** ● ✦	*Adequate nutritional status promotes wound healing.*
• Encourage fluid intake. **D** ● ✦	*Maintenance of vascular fluid volume is required to provide adequate circulation.*
Dependent/Collaborative Actions	
• Maintain intravenous fluid or blood products as ordered.	*Supports vascular fluid volume to maintain adequate circulatory status.*
• Apply antiembolic hose or sequential compression device on nonoperative limb.	*Supports venous return to the heart and prevention of DVT.*
• Administer anticoagulants if ordered.	*Prevention of DVT and hematoma formation.*
Monitor laboratory values:	
• Hemoglobin and hematocrit.	*An increased H & H may indicate dehydration, which impairs tissue perfusion.*
If tissue integrity changes:	
• Notify appropriate health care provider (e.g., wound care specialist, physician).	*Allows for prompt revision in treatment regimen.*

<hr>

Nursing Diagnosis   **IMPAIRED PHYSICAL MOBILITY** NDx

Definition: Limitation in independent, purposeful movement of the body or of one or more extremities.

Related to:
- Surgical procedure - below-knee amputation
- Insufficient muscle strength and/or nutritional status
- Insufficient understanding of how to use adaptive equipment
- Changes in sense of balance
- Sedentary lifestyle
- Pain
- Reluctance to initiate movement

CLINICAL MANIFESTATIONS

Subjective	**Objective**
Verbalization of inability to perform range-of-motion exercises; fear of falling	Lack of engagement in activities of daily living (ADLs), refusal to participate in range-of-motion activities or ambulation with or without support

RISK FACTORS

- Trauma
- Surgery
- Nutritional status
- Lack of interest

DESIRED OUTCOMES

The client will demonstrate adequate status as evidenced by:
a. Participation in ADLs as able
b. Begin ambulation with assistance as ordered
c. Perform range-of-motion and/or resistance exercises
d. Demonstration and use of adaptive equipment (e.g., wheelchair, prosthesis, crutches, walker)

NOC OUTCOMES

Ambulation; exercise participation; knowledge of body mechanics: performance; self-care: ADLs

NIC INTERVENTIONS

Exercise therapy: ambulation, balance, muscle control; self-care: ADLs; body mechanics: positioning and strengthening

NURSING ASSESSMENT

- Assess client's ability and activity tolerance
- Assess client's understanding on how to do range-of-motion and resistance exercises
- Assess client's desire and motivation to maintain physical mobility
- Assess client's muscle strength and ability to use adaptive equipment

RATIONALE

Provides understanding of client's ability and desire to participate in self-care and to enhance mobility.

Determine client's acceptance of permanent physical changes and subsequent limitations.

Determine client's ability to use assistive devices; provides a baseline for further education.

THERAPEUTIC INTERVENTIONS

RATIONALE

Independent Actions

- Demonstrate and encourage client to participate in range-of-motion, resistance, and isometric exercises for affected and unaffected limb. **D** ● ✦

- Assist client in prone positioning at least 2 to 3 times/day, providing support for affected limb. **D** ● ✦
- Assist client in ADLs, allowing client to do as much self-care as possible. **D** ● ✦

- Teach client transfer techniques from bed to wheel chair, bed to chair, and how to support affected limb; use of crutches, walker, and other assistive devices.

- Provide appropriate nutrition and calorie intake. **D** ● ✦

Dependent/Collaborative Actions

Collaborate with and consult appropriate health care provider to support client learning, abilities, and level of independence (rehabilitation, prosthesis fitting, physical therapy, etc.).

Inactivity contributes to muscle weakness and positional skin breakdown. If mobility is impaired, contractures can develop and will limit client's ability to maintain self-care, mobility, and independence. Resistance and isometric exercises maintain and enhance muscle strength.

Helps to prevent hip contractures and skin injury if client is on bedrest.

Improves client self-confidence in ability to care for self. Provides the nurse time to assess if more support or teaching of appropriate techniques is required.

Ambulation and moving out of bed improve circulation and muscle strength. Improves client self-confidence in ability to maintain independence. Appropriate use of assistive devices prevents contractures and improves confidence in ability to care for self.

Required to maintain muscle strength and wound healing.

Provides a collaborative approach to client care.

Nursing Diagnosis RISK FOR SURGICAL SITE INFECTION NDx

Definition: Susceptible to invasion of pathogenic organisms at surgical site, which may compromise health.

Related to:
- Surgical procedure
- Inadequate primary defenses
- Environmental exposure to pathogens—hospitalization
- General anesthesia

CLINICAL MANIFESTATIONS

Subjective	Objective
Verbal self-report of chills, loss of energy, fatigue	Elevated temperature; increased heart rate; adventitious lung sounds, positive cultures; Increased WBC and differential; heat, swelling, and/or drainage from wound

RISK FACTORS
- Surgery
- Chronic illness
- Malnutrition
- Obesity

DESIRED OUTCOMES

The client will remain free of infection as evidenced by:
a. Absence of fever and chills
b. Pulse rate within normal limits for client
c. Usual mental status
d. Normal breath sounds
e. Free of productive cough
f. Absence of heat, pain, redness, or swelling from surgical wound or any other area
g. WBC within normal limits
h. Negative results of culture specimens

NOC OUTCOMES

Wound healing: primary intention; secondary intention; infection status: infection severity

NIC INTERVENTIONS

Infection control; wound care nutrition management

NURSING ASSESSMENT	RATIONALE
Assess and report signs and symptoms of infection: • Elevated temperature • Chills and fever • Increased heart rate • Malaise, lethargy, confusion • Loss of appetite • Adventitious breath sounds • Productive cough with purulent sputum • Cloudy urine • Elevated WBC count with changes in differential • Obtain culture specimens; report positive results	*Early recognition of signs and symptoms of infection allows for prompt intervention.* *Changes in WBC's may indicate an infection.* *Culture results identify the specific organism(s) causing the infection. Culture and sensitivity results provide information that helps determine the most effective intervention.*

THERAPEUTIC INTERVENTIONS	RATIONALE
Independent Actions • Monitor vital signs. • Maintain good hand hygiene and teach client to do the same. • Monitor surgical site.	 *Monitor changes over time that may indicate infection.* *Hand hygiene is important in preventing infections.* *Note wound healing and any changes that indicate an infection—redness, swelling, increased temperature and drainage.*

THERAPEUTIC INTERVENTIONS	RATIONALE
• Change dressings using aseptic techniques.	*Prevents cross-contamination and prevents introduction of new bacteria.*
• Encourage fluid intake and provide adequate nutrition. **D** ● ✦	*Hydration maintains adequate tissue perfusion. Supports maintenance of immune system and supports wound healing.*
• Use sterile techniques during invasive procedures.	*Reduces the possibly of introducing pathogens into the body.*
• Change dressings, IV sites, and line tubing as ordered and per hospital policy.	*The longer equipment, tubing, and solutions are in use, the greater the chance of colonization of microorganisms, which can be introduced into the body.*
• Protect client from others with infection.	*Reduces exposure to new pathogens.*
• Encourage client to turn, cough, deep breath, and use incentive spirometry at regular intervals.	*Prevents skin breakdown, promotes movement and excretion of secretions.*

Dependent/Collaborative Actions

• Obtain culture and sensitivity of wound, drainage, urine, or sputum as ordered.	*Allows for prompt and appropriate intervention for infection.*
• Administer/increase IV fluids as ordered.	*Hydration supports vascular fluid volume and nutrient supply to tissues; promotes urine formation and voiding, flushing out system.*
• Administer antibiotics as ordered.	*Sensitivity obtained with specimen culture identifies the most effective antibiotic to use. A broad-spectrum antibiotic may be ordered until sensitivity results are obtained.*

Nursing Diagnosis **DISTURBED BODY IMAGE** NDx

Definition: Confusion in mental picture of one's physical self.

Related to:
• Alteration in body function
• Surgical procedure
• Alteration in self-perception

CLINICAL MANIFESTATIONS

Subjective	Objective
Verbal self-report of loss; negative self concept; fear of others' reactions	Uninvolved in care; not looking at or touching residual limb; refusal to discuss loss

RISK FACTORS
• Culture
• Surgery
• Lack of social support
• Depression

DESIRED OUTCOMES

The client will have improving body image as evidenced by:
a. Verbalization of acceptance of self with change in physical body
b. Verbalization of feelings of self-worth
c. Maintenance of relationship with others
d. Involvement in self-care activities
e. Engagement and understanding of lifestyle changes required due to amputation
f. Appropriate use adaptive devices or prostheses

NOC OUTCOMES

Body image; health status; amputation care

NIC INTERVENTIONS

Body image enhancement; amputation care: engagement; health status: acceptance; self-esteem: enhancement

NURSING ASSESSMENT	RATIONALE
Assess for and report signs and symptoms of disturbed body image: • Verbalization of negative feelings about self • Withdrawal from significant others • Lack of participation in ADLs • Refusal to look at or touch the residual limb • Lack of plan for adapting to necessary changes in lifestyle	*Early recognition of signs and symptoms of disturbed body image allows for prompt intervention.*

THERAPEUTIC INTERVENTIONS	RATIONALE
Independent Actions • Allow client to express feelings of loss and change in self-image. • Stay with client during the first dressing change to provide support as the client views the residual limb for the first time. • Discuss with client the availability of a natural-looking prosthesis. • Clarify misconceptions about future limitations on physical activity. Emphasize that a high level of mobility can be achieved with a prosthesis in place and/or use of crutches, walker, or cane. • Encourage client's participation in activities that can assist in the integration of the physical changes that have occurred (e.g., exercise, bathing, wrapping residual limb). Provide assistance as needed. • Demonstrate acceptance of client using techniques such as touch and frequent visits. • Encourage significant others to do the same. • Avoid referring to the residual limb as a "stump" unless that is a term the client prefers. • Support behaviors suggesting positive adaptation to the amputation (e.g., willingness to care for residual limb, compliance with treatment plan, verbalization of feelings of self-worth, maintenance of relationships with significant others). • Encourage significant others to allow client to do what he/she is able so that independence can be re-established and/or self-esteem redeveloped. • Encourage client to have contact with others so that client can test and establish a new self-image. • Assist client's and significant others' adjustment by listening, facilitating communication, and providing information. • Assist client and significant others to have similar expectations and understanding of future lifestyle and to identify ways that personal and family goals can be adjusted rather than abandoned. • Encourage visits and support from significant others. • Encourage client to continue involvement in social activities and to pursue usual roles and interests. If previous roles, interests, and hobbies cannot be pursued, encourage development of new ones. • If acceptable to client, arrange for a visit with an individual who has successfully adjusted to the loss of a limb.	*Demonstrates acceptance of client and their physical changes. Helps in developing a trusting therapeutic relationship.* *Provides support to client, shows acceptance, and gives the client an opportunity to ask questions while viewing the residual limb.* *A change in appearance can initiate a grieving response and change in self-image. Successful resolution of grief assists the client to accept changes and experience and integrate the changes into self-image.* *Activities that help clients acknowledge and deal with the changes that have occurred in their body facilitate the incorporation of changes into the brain's schemata of the body.* *Frequent visits and the use of touch convey a feeling of acceptance to the client. This enhances feelings of self-worth and assists in the development of a positive self-esteem and body image.* *Supporting behaviors indicative of positive adaptation to change encourages the client to repeat these behaviors. Repetition of positive adaptive behaviors facilitates the development of a positive self-esteem and body image.* *Allowing clients to do as much as they are able facilitates the re-establishment of independence, which enhances feelings of self-esteem.* *Allows client to see how others react to them and helps to develop new self-image.* *Enhances relationships and provides emotional support.* *Assures client and significant others have the same understanding and are working toward the same goals. Helps to decrease future conflict and frustration.* *Enhances relationships and provides emotional support.* *Shows that some aspects of life will remain the same. Enhances self-esteem in that not all aspects of life have changed.* *Helps client understand that they are not alone. Allows for client to ask questions and what mechanisms/adaptive techniques are effective.*

THERAPEUTIC INTERVENTIONS	RATIONALE
• Provide information about and encourage utilization of community agencies and support groups (e.g., National Amputation Foundation; vocational rehabilitation; family, individual, and/or financial counseling).	*Community agencies and support groups provide the opportunity for clients to see that they are not experiencing a unique problem, to share feelings and concerns, to profit from the experience of others with similar difficulties, and to learn new skills necessary to rebuild self-esteem. All these factors help the client to establish a positive self-concept, body image, and self-esteem.*
Dependent/Collaborative Actions Consult appropriate health care provider (e.g., psychiatric nurse clinician, social worker, physical therapist physician) if client seems unwilling or unable to adapt to changes resulting from the amputation.	*Consulting the appropriate health care provider allows for modification of the treatment plan.*

DISCHARGE TEACHING/CONTINUED CARE

Nursing Diagnosis · **DEFICIENT KNOWLEDGE** NDx; **INEFFECTIVE HEALTH MANAGEMENT** NDx; **INEFFECTIVE FAMILY HEALTH MANAGEMENT** NDx*

Definition: **Deficit Knowledge NDx:** Absence of cognitive information related to a specific topic, or its acquisition; **Ineffective Health Management NDx:** Pattern of regulating and integrating into daily living a therapeutic regimen for the treatment of illness and its sequelae that is unsatisfactory for meeting specific health goals; **Ineffective Family Health Management NDX:** A pattern of regulating and integrating into family processes a program for the treatment of illness and its sequelae that is unsatisfactory for meeting specific health goals of the family unit.

Related to:
- Insufficient knowledge of therapeutic regimen
- Changes in health status
- Loss of limb
- Inability to manage treatment regimen
- Family conflict

CLINICAL MANIFESTATIONS

Subjective	**Objective**
Verbalizes inability to manage illness, verbalizes inability to follow prescribed treatment regimen	Inaccurate follow-through of instructions, inappropriate/exaggerated behaviors

RISK FACTORS
- Grieving
- Loss of self-esteem
- Lack of desire to improve health status
- Cognitive deficit
- Inability to care for oneself
- Difficulty integrating treatment into lifestyle and family processes
- Economically disadvantaged

DESIRED OUTCOME

The client will demonstrate appropriate wound care and ways to prevent contractures, increase strength, and improve mobility.

NOC OUTCOMES

Knowledge: fall prevention; prescribed activity; treatment regimen

NIC INTERVENTIONS

Health system guidance; teaching: individual; teaching: prescribed activity/exercise

*The nurse should select the nursing diagnostic label that is most appropriate for the client's discharge teaching needs.

NURSING ASSESSMENT	RATIONALE
Assess client's readiness and ability to learn. Assess meaning of illness to client.	*Early recognition of readiness to learn and meaning of illness to client allows for implementation of the appropriate teaching interventions.*

THERAPEUTIC INTERVENTIONS	RATIONALE

Independent Actions

Instruct client in the following ways to prevent contractures, increase strength, and/or improve mobility:

• Performing range-of-motion exercises of residual limb and other extremities. • Require client to provide return demonstration range-of-motion exercises of residual limb and other extremities.	*Inactivity contributes to muscle weakening. Contractures can develop as early as 8 hrs of immobility. Actions help to maintain and increase client's strength and ability to move.*
• Lying prone several times a day with pillow under abdomen and residual limb.	*Lying prone several times a day promotes hip flexion and decreases incidence of hip contractures. Improves lower body muscle tone and promotes improved balance when using prosthesis.*
• Performing knee bends, standing on toes, balancing on the unaffected leg without support, and performing quadriceps- and gluteal-setting exercises. • Performing pushups, flexion and extension of arms holding weights, and arm pulley exercises.	*Facilitates use of ambulatory aids and increases upper body strength to support movement.*

THERAPEUTIC INTERVENTIONS	RATIONALE

Desired Outcome: The client will demonstrate correct transfer and ambulation techniques and proper use of ambulatory aids.

Independent Actions

• Reinforce instructions about correct transfer and ambulation techniques, amount of weight-bearing allowed, and proper use of ambulatory aids (e.g., crutches, walker, cane). • Allow time for client to demonstrate ability to use ambulatory aids.	*Ensuring the client's understanding of the use of assistive devices reduces the risk of additional injury. Allow time for questions and return demonstration to assess the need for further instruction.*

THERAPEUTIC INTERVENTIONS	RATIONALE

Desired Outcome: The client will identify ways to maintain health of the remaining lower extremity.

Independent Actions

Instruct client in ways to maintain health of the remaining lower extremity:

• Wear a well-fitting shoe to protect foot from pressure and trauma.	*Shoes should be modified by an orthopedist to ensure that body weight is evenly distributed when prosthesis is used.*
• Perform foot and nail care using appropriate technique.	*Helps to prevent infection and skin breakdown.*
• Avoid breaks in the skin to reduce risk of infection.	*Client should be taught to monitor feet skin and nails to note when skin changes occur and notify the appropriate health care individul.*
• Stop smoking.	*Smoking causes vasoconstriction, which reduces blood flow, compromising oxygen and nutrient delivery to tissues.*
• Avoid sitting with legs crossed and wearing socks, stockings, or garters that are tight.	*Helps to reduce the risk of compromising peripheral blood flow.*
• Adhere to regular follow-up care if diabetes or peripheral vascular disease was a factor leading to the need for amputation.	*Helps prevent further loss of viable tissue and potential further loss of extremity.*

THERAPEUTIC INTERVENTIONS	RATIONALE

Desired Outcome: The client will demonstrate the ability to care for the residual limb.

THERAPEUTIC INTERVENTIONS	**RATIONALE**

Independent Actions

Instruct client in ways to care for the residual limb while dressing is in place:

If client has a soft compression dressing (soft dressing covered by an elastic bandage or sock) over the residual limb:

- Demonstrate the technique for rewrapping or changing the elastic bandage or sock.

  Action should be performed routinely during the day and if the dressing slips or the elastic bandage or sock becomes soiled or wrinkled.

- Demonstrate and allow for return demonstration of the technique for changing the dressing if client is expected to do this after discharge.

  Improves client's self-confidence in self-care and allows nurse to make any corrections to technique prior to discharge.

If client has a rigid dressing over the residual limb:

- Stress the importance of removing the pylon when in bed.
- Explain that the dressing should be positioned securely before applying the pylon (a belt may be needed to maintain the proper position of the rigid dressing during ambulation).

  Reduces the risk of twisting the residual limb.

- Caution client to adhere to weight-bearing restrictions until the surgical area heals completely.

  Careful positioning prevents injury to residual limb and prevents irritation or discomfort when ambulating.

- Require return demonstration of technique.

  Allows complete healing of the surgical site and decreases potential for injury.

Inform client about expected care of the residual limb once the dressings are no longer needed:

  Improves client's self-confidence in self-care and allows nurse to make any corrections to technique prior to discharge.

- The limb will need to be inspected daily using a hand mirror if necessary.

  It is important to monitor suture line for changes and surrounding skin for injury or infection.

- The residual limb will need to be washed and patted dry daily.

  Prevents irritation when bathing and potential for skin injury. Moist skin provides potential for infection and skin breakdown.

- Emollients and powders should not be applied to the residual limb.

  Prevents potential for infection or irritation.

THERAPEUTIC INTERVENTIONS	**RATIONALE**

Desired Outcome: The client will verbalize how to care for the prosthesis and residual limb if a permanent prosthesis is planned.

Independent Actions

Provide the client with information about anticipated care of the prosthesis and residual limb if a permanent prosthesis is planned:

- After the incision heals, the residual limb should be toughened by massaging it, pushing it against a firm surface, and/or pulling on it with a hand-held towel.

  A toughened limb is more resistant to irritation and breakdown from the constant pressure exerted on it by the prosthesis

- A residual limb sock should be worn next to the skin.

  Helps to reduce friction between residual limb and the socket.

- Only residual limb socks recommended by the prosthetist should be used; socks should be changed daily, laundered gently in cool water with a mild soap, and laid flat to dry.

  Actions help to prevent skin injury, irritation, and infection.

Replace worn or damaged residual limb socks. They should not be mended.

  Area of mending will cause irritation, breakdown and potential for infection.

- A prosthetist should examine the prosthesis on a regular basis and monitor the fit of the socket so that repairs and adjustments can be made when necessary (e.g., as the residual limb continues to shrink, if a weight loss or gain of 5 to 10 lbs occurs).

  Assures appropriate fit and decreases potential for further injury or falls.

- The socket should be cleansed daily with a damp cloth and dried thoroughly.
- Care should be taken to keep the leather or metal components of the prosthesis dry.

Continued...

THERAPEUTIC INTERVENTIONS	RATIONALE
• Shoes worn with the prosthesis should be kept in good repair.	*Helps to prevent skin breakdown and potential for infection.*
• If skin breakdown occurs, the prosthesis should not be worn until the area has been checked by the physician and/or prosthetist.	*Shoes should remain in good repair help to maintain a steady, even gait, prevent injury from a fall, and to avoid damage to the prosthesis.*
• The prosthesis should be applied on arising and worn for the prescribed length of time.	*Pressure from prosthesis prevents residual limb edema.*
• An elastic sock may need to be worn over the residual limb whenever the prosthesis is removed.	*The sock helps prevent development of edema in the residual limb and subsequent difficulty in reapplication of the prosthesis.*

THERAPEUTIC INTERVENTIONS	RATIONALE

Desired Outcome: The client will identify ways to manage phantom limb pain if it occurs.

Independent Actions

Instruct client in ways to manage phantom limb pain if it occurs:	*Educating the client regarding varying pain management modalities provides the client with options for a choice of treatment that best meets individualized pain management needs.*
• Apply intermittent pressure to residual limb by walking on pylon or pressing the limb against a firm surface.	
• Participate in diversional activities, watching TV, listening to music	*Diversional activities help to refocus client's attention.*
• Take medications as prescribed.	*Many of these interventions decrease muscle tension and can be used independent or as adjuvant to medications for pain relief.*
• Encourage client to consult appropriate health care provider about the use of therapies such as TENS, biofeedback, acupuncture, guided imagery mindfulness-based stress reduction (MBSR), and hypnosis to assist in pain control if indicated.	
• Reassure client that phantom limb pain usually disappears, but caution that it may take months to years.	*Client should be made aware that phantom limb pain can change over time. Pain is a subjective experience and the time frame for phantom pain to disappear is very individualized.*

THERAPEUTIC INTERVENTIONS	RATIONALE

Desired Outcome: The client will state signs and symptoms to report to the health care provider.

Independent Actions

Instruct client to report these additional signs and symptoms:	*Educating the client regarding signs and symptoms to report to the health care provider allows for implementing appropriate interventions, altering the plan of care, and reducing the risk of potential complications.*
• Development of and/or persistent phantom limb pain	
• Persistent or increased residual limb swelling	
• Difficulty with full extension of residual limb	*May require more physical therapy for muscle strengthening.*
• Inability to maintain balance	*May indicate a clot causing decreased circulation.*
• Change in color of residual limb (e.g., pallor, cyanosis, duskiness)	
• Persistent slippage or increased tightness of elastic bandage or sock	*Requires further evaluation to assure proper prosthesis fit.*
• Loosening of rigid dressing	
• Drainage from the wound	*Should be reported immediately, as these symptoms may indicate an infection.*
• Experience of chills, fever	

THERAPEUTIC INTERVENTIONS	RATIONALE

Desired Outcome: The client will identify community resources that can assist with home management and adjustment to changes resulting from the amputation.

THERAPEUTIC INTERVENTIONS	RATIONALE

Independent Actions

Provide information about community resources that can assist the client and significant others with home management and adjustment to changes resulting from the amputation (e.g., home health agency; social services; individual, family, and occupational counseling; amputee support groups; National Amputation Foundation).

Social support can aid the client in obtaining necessary resources to adapt to physical changes and obtain the necessary long-term assistance to maintain independence.

THERAPEUTIC INTERVENTIONS	RATIONALE

Desired Outcome: The client, in collaboration with the nurse, will develop a plan for adhering to recommended follow-up care including future appointments with health care provider, prosthetist, and physical therapist; medications prescribed; and activity level.

Independent Actions

Emphasize the importance of adhering to prescribed weight-bearing restrictions and exercise program.

Adherence to a plan of care reduces the risk of complications. Attendance at follow-up appointments allows health care providers ongoing assessment and evaluation, and allows for modification of treatment regimen as required.

Collaborate with client in developing a plan for follow-up appointments, schedule for exercises, list of medications, exercises, and side effects to monitor.

Provides the client a sense of control in relation to their life and how they can assure adherence with treatment regimen.

ADDITIONAL NURSING DIAGNOSIS

RISK FOR FALLS NDx
Related to:
- Weakness and fatigue
- Dizziness or syncope associated with postural hypotension resulting from peripheral pooling of blood and blood loss during surgery
- Central nervous system (CNS) depressant effect of some medications (e.g., narcotic [opioid] analgesics)
- Difficulty with balance, prosthesis control, and transfer and ambulation techniques

GRIEVING NDx
Related to:
- Loss of a limb
- Changes in body image and usual lifestyle and roles

FRACTURE (HIP) WITH INTERNAL FIXATION OR PROSTHESIS INSERTION

A fractured hip is the term used to describe a fracture of femur close to the hip bone. Hip fractures are classified according to the specific location of the fracture. A common classification system divides hip fractures into three types: femoral neck fractures (also referred to as proximal or intracapsular fractures), intertrochanteric fractures, and subtrochanteric fractures (the latter two types are sometimes referred to as extracapsular fractures).

A fractured hip is one of the most common orthopedic injuries in the elderly related to the increased incidence of osteoporosis and falls in the elderly population. Although a fractured hip can be treated by traction, the preferred treatment is surgery because it allows earlier mobility.

Surgery involves insertion of a femoral head prosthesis or reduction and internal fixation of the fracture with an intramedullary fixation device, cannulated screws, or a dynamic compression hip screw with a plate assembly. Internal fixation with preservation of the femoral head is the preferred treatment for hip fractures, but the femoral head and neck can be replaced with a prosthetic device (e.g., Austin Moore prosthesis) if an intracapsular fracture has occurred and factors are present that increase the risk for avascular necrosis and/or nonunion. Ideally, surgery is performed within 12 to 24 hrs after the injury, especially if the client has a displaced femoral neck. During the preoperative period, traction is usually applied to stabilize and reduce the fracture and reduce muscle spasms and pain.

This care plan focuses on the elderly adult client who is hospitalized for surgical repair of a hip fracture. Much of the postoperative information is applicable to clients receiving follow-up care in an extended care facility or home.

OUTCOME/DISCHARGE CRITERIA

The client will:
1. Show evidence of normal healing of the surgical wound
2. Maintain clear, audible breath sounds throughout lungs
3. Maintain expected level of mobility
4. Have adequate fracture reduction and healing
5. Maintain hip pain controlled
6. Have no signs and symptoms of infection or postoperative complications
7. Demonstrate correct transfer and ambulation techniques and proper use of ambulatory aids
8. Demonstrate the ability to correctly perform the prescribed exercises
9. Verbalize an understanding of activity and position restrictions necessary to prevent dislocation of the prosthesis or internal fixation device
10. Identify ways to reduce the risk of falls in the home environment
11. State signs and symptoms to report to the health care provider
12. Identify community resources that can assist with home management and provide transportation
13. Develop a plan for adhering to recommended follow-up care including future appointments with health care provider and physical therapist, medications prescribed, activity level, and wound care

PREOPERATIVE CARE: USE IN CONJUNCTION WITH THE STANDARDIZED PREOPERATIVE CARE PLAN

PREOPERATIVE NURSING/COLLABORATIVE DIAGNOSIS

Nursing Diagnosis   **ACUTE PAIN** NDx

Definition: Unpleasant sensory and emotional experience associated with actual or potential tissue damage, or described in terms of such damage (International Association for the Study of Pain); sudden or slow onset of any intensity from mild to severe with an anticipated or predictable end, and with a duration of less than 3 months.

Related to:
- Fracture of the bone
- Tissue trauma
- Muscle spasm

CLINICAL MANIFESTATIONS

Subjective	Objective
Verbalization of pain	Grimacing; reluctance to move; clutching hip/thigh; restlessness; diaphoresis; increased BP; tachycardia, tachypnea

RISK FACTORS
- Trauma
- Dislocation
- Fractures
- Muscle spasms
- Stress and anxiety

DESIRED OUTCOMES

The client will experience diminished hip pain as evidenced by:
a. Verbalization of a reduction in pain
b. Relaxed facial expression and body positioning
c. Stable vital signs
d. Respiratory rate within normal limits

NOC OUTCOMES

Comfort level; pain control

NIC INTERVENTIONS

Analgesic administration; pain management: acute environmental management; calming technique

NURSING ASSESSMENT	RATIONALE
Assess for and report signs and symptoms of pain • Verbalization of pain • Grimacing, clutching hip, diaphoresis, increased BP, tachycardia	*Early recognition of signs and symptoms of acute hip pain allows for prompt intervention.*
Assess the client's pain using a standardized pain scale and pain location, quality, onset, duration, precipitating factors, aggravating factors, alleviating factors	*Use of a pain intensity rating scale gives the nurse a clearer understanding of the client's pain being experienced, changes in pain over time, and promotes consistency when communicating with others.*

THERAPEUTIC INTERVENTIONS	RATIONALE

Independent Actions

Implement measures to reduce pain:
- Perform actions to reduce fear and anxiety about the pain experience:
  - Assure client that the need for pain relief is understood; plan methods for achieving pain control with client. **D** ✦

Promotes relaxation and subsequently increases the client's threshold and tolerance for pain.
Collaboration provides client some method of control over care.

- Perform actions to reduce fear and anxiety: **D** ● ✦
  - Reduce environmental stimulation.
  - Provide explanation prior to procedures.
  - Maintains a calm, supportive demeanor.
- Perform actions to promote rest:
  - Minimize environmental activity and noise. **D** ● ✦
  - Limit the number of visitors and their length of stay.

Having client focus on something other than pain. Understanding what will occur will help to decrease client's anxiety,
Actions help to reduce fatigue and subsequently increase the client's threshold and tolerance for pain.
Too much activity and noise may be stressful for the client. The nurse should collaborate with the client to determine the number and frequency of visitors.

Provide or assist with additional nonpharmacological measures for pain relief.
- Relaxation exercises (e.g., guided imagery, progressive relaxation, MBSR)
- Diversional activities such as watching television, reading, listening to music or conversing **D** ● ✦

Relaxes muscle tension and decreases anxiety. Strengthens or provides for new coping mechanisms.
Distraction techniques refocus client on something other than pain.

Dependent/Collaborative Actions

Implement measures to reduce pain:
- Administer analgesics and muscle relaxants if ordered (Opioids: morphine; NSAIDS: ketorolac; muscle relaxants: cyclobenzaprine).
- Provide medication at regular intervals.
- Request a PCA administration of medications.

Administering analgesics before activities and procedures that can cause pain and before pain becomes severe improves mobility. Ketorolac is effective in treating pain with fewer side effects.
Pain medication provided at regular intervals decreases incidence of episodes of severe pain Providing PCA pain administration allows client control over pain relief.

- Perform actions to maintain effective traction on the injured extremity.
  - Ensure that weights are hanging freely.
  - Do not allow footplate or ropes to rest on end of bed.

Client is usually placed in Buck's traction preoperatively to stabilize and reduce the fracture and reduce muscle spasms and pain.
Traction is not maintained when the weights are not hanging freely, the footplates or ropes are resting on the bed, or the rope knots are on the pulley. Muscle spasms can occur when traction is not maintained.

  - Keep affected heel off bed.
  - Keep knots away from pulley device.
  - Do not remove traction unless specifically ordered.

Protect the heel from skin breakdown.

Maintenance of traction on affected side also can decrease experience of pain.

- Do not lift the weights in order to facilitate moving the client or performing other care.
- Limit head of bed elevation to 20 to 25 degrees except for meals and toileting. **D** ● ✦
- Place a trochanter roll or sandbag firmly against the lateral aspect of injured hip and upper thigh (should extend from iliac crest to mid-thigh).

This reduces traction force and can cause severe muscle spasms.

Actions help to maintain the prescribed traction force.

Trochanter rolls/sandbags help to maintain leg in proper alignment.

NDx = NANDA Diagnosis   **D** = Delegatable Action   ● = UAP   ✦ = LVN/LPN   ⊜▶ = Go to ⊜volve for animation

Continued...

THERAPEUTIC INTERVENTIONS	RATIONALE
• Consult physician if extremity appears out of alignment; do not attempt to realign extremity.	*An attempt to realign the extremity may cause further tissue trauma.*
• Move client carefully, keeping injured extremity well supported. **D ● ✦**	*Prevents further injury; decreases client pain and anxiety when moving.*
If turning is allowed, place pillow between legs before turning. **D ● ✦**	*In order to prevent adduction and further strain on the fracture site.*
Consult appropriate health care provider if above measures fail to provide adequate pain relief:	*Notifying the appropriate health care provider allows for modification of the treatment plan.*
• Physician, pharmacist.	
• Pain management specialist.	

Nursing Diagnosis   # RISK FOR PERIPHERAL NEUROVASCULAR DYSFUNCTION NDx (FRACTURED EXTREMITY)

Definition: Susceptible to disruption in the circulation, sensation, and motion of an extremity, which may compromise health.

Related to:
• Trauma to or excessive pressure on the nerves or blood vessels as a result of the injury
• Displaced bone fragments
• Blood accumulation and edema at fracture site
• Improper alignment, application of skin traction device, or traction on the injured extremity
• Fear and anxiety

CLINICAL MANIFESTATIONS (IF NEUROVASCULAR DYSFUNCTION OCCURS)

Subjective	Objective
Self-report of numbness or tingling in leg or foot; increased pain in extremity or buttock	Diminished or absent pedal pulses; capillary refill time in toes greater than 2 to 3 seconds; pallor, cyanosis, or coolness of the extremity; inability to flex or extend foot or toes

RISK FACTORS
• Immobilization
• Fracture
• Mechanical compression
• Vascular obstruction
• Chronic illness

DESIRED OUTCOMES

The client will maintain normal neurovascular function in the injured extremity as evidenced by:
a. Palpable pedal pulses
b. Capillary refill time in toes less than 2 to 3 seconds
c. Extremity warm and usual color
d. Ability to flex and extend foot and toes
e. Absence of numbness and tingling in leg and foot
f. No increase in pain in extremity or buttock

NOC OUTCOMES

Tissue perfusion: peripheral neurological status

NIC INTERVENTIONS

Circulatory care: arterial insufficiency; circulatory care: venous insufficiency; positioning; lower extremity monitoring

NURSING ASSESSMENT	RATIONALE
Assess for and report signs and symptoms of neurovascular dysfunction in the injured extremity:	*Early recognition of signs and symptoms of neurovascular dysfunction allows for prompt intervention.*
• Numbness or tingling in leg or foot	
• Increased pain in extremity or buttock	
• Diminished or absent pedal pulses	
• Capillary refill time in toes greater than 2 to 3 seconds	
• Pallor, cyanosis, or coolness of the extremity	
• Inability to flex or extend foot or toes	

THERAPEUTIC INTERVENTIONS	RATIONALE

Independent Actions

Assess affected limb, compare findings to noninjured limb, document and report changes.

Assessment of the 6 P's is appropriate for any type of fracture:

- Pain: Assess using a pain scale including severity, quality, intensity, radiation, and onset of new and different pain.

  An increase in pain or inability to control pain with medication and increased pain experienced with passive stretching may indicate compartment syndrome.

- Pulses: Monitor and document pulses distal to the injury. Use a rating scale for intensity of palpable pulses.

  Change in pulses within injured limb and differences noted between injured and noninjured limb may indicate changes in blood flow distal to the injury.

- Paresthesia: Assess sensations proximal and distal to the site injury using light touch to the skin. Ask client about changes in sensation. Report any "pins and needles" feelings.

  Decreased feeling or "pins and needles" feeling report by client may indicate nerve damage and indicate compartment syndrome.

- Pallor: Assess capillary refill, color, and warmth distal to the injury. Track findings over time and report any decline in findings.

  Irreversible damage may occur if not resolved.

  Decreasing color, capillary refill time, and warmth to the extremity indicate arterial insufficiency and should receive immediate intervention.

- Paralysis: Ask client to dorsiflex or plantar flex the foot. Note: decreases in movement or inability to perform.

  Decreased movement or no movement is indicative of compartment syndrome and requires timely intervention.

- Pressure or edema: Assess for changes in firmness or swelling of the extremity distal to the injury.

  Edema or increased tightness of the skin correlates with increased internal pressure on the muscles and tissues and indicative of compromised circulation distal to site of injury.

Implement measures to prevent neurovascular dysfunction in injured extremity:

- Place a trochanter roll or sandbag firmly against lateral aspect of injured hip and upper thigh (should extend from the iliac crest to mid-thigh). **D** ✦

  Proper positioning is required to maintain appropriate traction tension.

- Make sure skin traction device (e.g., elastic wraps, foam boot with Velcro strap) is applied properly (if necessary to reapply, obtain assistance so that one person can maintain traction on the leg during the reapplication process). **D** ✦

  Prevents further injury due to dislocation of hip trochanter and potential for pain and discomfort.

- Make sure that excessive or prolonged pressure is not exerted on Achilles tendon and medial and lateral aspects of knee and ankle. **D** ✦

  Decreases potential for further injury and increased pain.

If signs and symptoms of neurovascular dysfunction occur:

- Notify physician if the signs and symptoms persist or worsen.

  Allow for prompt treatment of client changes.

- Prepare client for surgical intervention (e.g., internal fixation, insertion of hip prosthesis).

  Compartment syndrome, if untreated for more than 6 hrs, can result in permanent injury.

The rest of the postoperative care for the client with a hip fracture with prosthesis or internal fixation is the same as a total joint replacement.

Refer to Total Joint Arthroscopy Care Plan.

TOTAL JOINT REPLACEMENT/ARTHROSCOPY—(HIP/KNEE)

A joint replacement (arthroplasty) is a surgical procedure in which the diseased, injured, or malfunctioning part of the joint is replaced with a prothesis. A total hip replacement is performed to relieve joint pain that has been resistant to conservative management and/or improve joint mobility in persons with severe arthritis. In a total hip replacement, the damaged femoral head is replaced with a metal prosthesis that is cemented or fit into the femur. On the top of this prosthesis is attached a metal or ceramic ball that replaces the femoral head. The hip socket or acetabulum is replaced with a metal socket where the new femoral head articulates with the hip bone. A spacer or liner, made of metal, plastic, or ceramic, may be placed between the new ball and socket to provide a smooth gliding surface. A partial hip replacement involves replacing the top of the femur with a prosthesis and ball that fits into the hip joint, but the hip socket or acetabulum is not replaced. The type of replacement depends on the level of damage or injury to the hip.

A total knee replacement is a surgical procedure in which the knee joint and articulating surfaces of the tibia, femur, and patella are replaced with mental and plastic prosthetic devices. These devices are held together either using cement or a porous prosthesis is used that allows for endogenous bone growth and over time will hold the joint together. A knee replacement is performed to relieve joint pain that has not been controlled by conservative management and/or to improve joint mobility in persons with severe arthritis, congenital knee deformity, hemophilic arthropathy, or severe intra-articular injury.

Joint replacement surgery may involve traditional open procedure or robotic-assisted minimally invasive surgery. Minimally invasive joint replacement has a decreased incidence of complications including less tissue trauma, blood loss, and a smaller scar. Clients also experience a decreased length of hospital stay and shorter recovery time. The determination of which approach to use for joint replacement is a decision made by the physician and client. It is based on multiple client factors including but not limited to age, level injury or disease process, and previous hip/knee surgery.

Hip and knee replacements are the most commonly performed joint replacements, but replacement surgery can be performed on other joints, as well, including the ankle, wrist, shoulder, and elbow.

This care plan focuses on the adult client hospitalized for a total hip/knee replacement. Much of the postoperative information is applicable to client care following a joint replacement and receiving care in an extended care facility or home setting.

OUTCOME/DISCHARGE CRITERIA

The client will:
1. Have evidence of normal healing of the surgical wound
2. Maintain clear, audible breath sounds throughout lungs
3. Have reduced/controlled joint pain
4. Have expected degree of mobility of replaced joint
5. Exhibit no signs and symptoms of infection or postoperative complications
6. Demonstrate correct transfer and ambulation techniques and proper use of ambulatory aids if required.
7. Demonstrate the ability to correctly perform the prescribed exercises
8. Verbalize an understanding of activity and position restrictions necessary to prevent dislocation of prosthesis
9. Identify ways to reduce the risk of loosening prosthesis
10. Identify ways to reduce the risk of falls in the home environment
11. State signs and symptoms to report to the health care provider
12. Identify community resources that can assist with home management and provide transportation
13. Develop a plan for adhering to recommended follow-up care including future appointments with health care provider and physical therapist, medications prescribed, activity level, and wound care

PREOPERATIVE: USE IN CONJUNCTION WITH THE STANDARDIZED PREOPERATIVE CARE PLAN

POSTOPERATIVE: USE IN CONJUNCTION WITH THE STANDARDIZED POSTOPERATIVE CARE PLAN

Nursing Diagnosis **ACUTE PAIN** NDx

Definition: Unpleasant sensory and emotional experience associated with actual or potential tissue damage or described in terms of such damage (International Association for the Study of Pain); sudden or slow onset of any intensity from mild to severe with an anticipated or predictable end, and with a duration of less than 3 months.

Related to: Surgical procedure—injury to bone and tissues

CLINICAL MANIFESTATIONS

Subjective	Objective
Verbalization of pain	Grimacing; reluctance to move; restlessness; diaphoresis; increased BP; tachycardia, tachypnea, grimacing with movement

RISK FACTORS
- Trauma
- Dislocation
- Fractures
- Muscle spasms
- Fear and anxiety

DESIRED OUTCOMES

The client will experience diminished hip pain as evidenced by:
a. Verbalization of a reduction in pain
b. Relaxed facial expression and body positioning
c. Stable vital signs
d. Respiratory rate within normal limits

NOC OUTCOMES	NIC INTERVENTIONS
Comfort level; pain control	Analgesic administration; pain management: acute environmental management; calming technique

NURSING ASSESSMENT	RATIONALE
Assess for and report signs and symptoms of pain • Verbalization of pain • Grimacing, diaphoresis, increased BP, tachycardia, tachypnea	*Early recognition of signs and symptoms of acute pain allows for prompt intervention.*
Assess the client's pain using a standardized pain scale and location, quality, onset, duration, precipitating factors, aggravating factors, alleviating factors	*Use of a pain intensity rating scale gives the nurse a clearer understanding of the client's pain experienced, changes in pain over time, and promotes consistency when communicating with others.*

THERAPEUTIC INTERVENTIONS	RATIONALE

Independent Actions
Implement measures to reduce pain:
• Perform actions to reduce fear and anxiety about the pain experience:
  • Assure client that the need for pain relief is understood; plan methods for achieving pain control with client.
  • Provide explanation prior to procedures.
  • Maintains a calm, supportive demeanor.
	Promotes relaxation and subsequently increases the client's threshold and tolerance for pain.

Provide or assist with additional nonpharmacological measures for pain relief. • Relaxation exercises (e.g., guided imagery, progressive relaxation, MBSR) • Diversional activities such as watching television, reading, listening to music or conversing	*Having client focus on something otherthan pain. Understanding what will occur will help to decrease client's anxiety.* *Relaxation techniques relax muscle tension and decrease anxiety. Strengthens or provides for new coping mechanisms. Distraction techniques refocus client on something other than pain.*
Maintain appropriate positioning/alignment of affected extremity.	*Decreases incidence of muscle spasms, pain, and tension on the operative site.*
Dependent/Collaborative Actions Implement measures to reduce pain:	
	Administering analgesics before activities and procedures that can cause pain and before pain becomes severe improves mobility.
Administer pain medication every 3 to 4 hrs during the first 24 hrs postoperatively and prior to physical therapy or exercises • Analgesics (opioids: morphine; etc. • NSAIDS: ketorolac IV)	*Pain medication provided at regular intervals decreases incidence of episodes of severe pain.* *Ketorolac IV is as effective in treating pain and has less side effects that opioids.*
Intermittently apply ice packs to surgical area if ordered	*Cold numbs sore tissues, decreases localized swelling, and decreases vasodilation, thus decreasing pain-producing chemical transmission.*
Consult appropriate health care provider if above measures fail to provide adequate pain relief or client reports sudden severe pain: • Physician, pharmacist; pain management specialist	*Notifying the appropriate health care provider allows for modification of the treatment regimen.*

Nursing Diagnosis **IMPAIRED PHYSICAL MOBILITY** NDx

Definition: Limitation in independent, purposeful movement of the body or of one or more extremities.

Related to:
• Pain and weakness in weight-hearing extremity associated with surgery
• Prescribed activity and weight-bearing restrictions following surgery
• Generalized weakness associated with surgery
• Depressant effect of anesthesia and some pain medications
• Fear of falling, dislodging drainage tubes if present, dislocating prosthesis and compromising surgical wound

NDx = NANDA Diagnosis   **D** = Delegatable Action   ● = UAP   ✦ = LVN/LPN   ⊖▶ = Go to ⊖volve for animation

CLINICAL MANIFESTATIONS

Subjective	**Objective**
Expression of fear about moving	Deceased reaction time, difficulty turning, limited ability to perform gross motor movements, limited range of motion, postural instability, slowed and/or uncoordinated movements

RISK FACTORS

- Malnutrition
- Musculoskeletal impairment
- Pain
- Fear and anxiety

NOC OUTCOMES

Mobility; joint movement; ambulation; bone healing

NIC INTERVENTIONS

Musculoskeletal rehabilitation participation; joint mobility; exercise therapy participation and ambulation

DESIRED OUTCOMES

The client will maintain maximum physical mobility as evidenced by:
a. Participation in prescribed exercises
b. Participation in ambulation within prescribed weight-bearing limitations

NURSING ASSESSMENT	**RATIONALE**
Assess for and report signs and symptoms of impaired physical mobility: • Assess fear/anxiety and client's concerns about increasing activity and ambulation • Assess client's gross motor skill and range of motion and determine limitations to implementing prescribed exercises and weight-bearing ambulation restrictions • Assess client's understand concerning required activity and ambulation • Assess client's postural stability	*Early recognition of causes of impaired mobility allows for prompt intervention.*

THERAPEUTIC INTERVENTIONS	**RATIONALE**
Independent Actions Allow client to express fears and concerns about exercise and activities following surgery. Encourage client to use overhead trapeze to move self. Reinforce physical therapist's instructions regarding muscle strengthening exercises, transfer and ambulation techniques, and use of ambulatory aids. Encourage client to perform prescribed exercises on affected and unaffected limb. Hip Replacement: Perform actions and instruct client in ways to prevent extreme (beyond 90 degrees) hip flexion or bending at the waist: • Instruct client not to learn forward to reach objects out of reach or at the foot of the bed • Do not elevate operative leg when client is sitting in the chair	*Decreasing anxiety and fear about postsurgical exercises and ambulation allows client to focus on correct technique.* *Engages client in self-care and strengthens self-confidence in ability.* *Actions when practiced increase muscle strength and increase confidence and skill in activities and techniques.* *Increases client's self-confidence in completing the exercises and increases muscular strength.* *Decreases incidence of pain and dislocation of hip joint. Movement precautions should be utilized for at least 6 weeks or until removed by the physician.* *The client should not bend the hip more than a 90-degree angle and should not bend from the waist. This movement may dislodge hip joint and delay healing.*

THERAPEUTIC INTERVENTIONS	RATIONALE
• Turn patient using an abduction device or pillows between the legs. The client should not be positioned on the surgical side and should maintain pillows between legs when lying on the nonoperative side. Do not allow the operative limb to cross the midline of the body. **D** ● ✦	*Prevents dislocation of the hip joint and decreases pain and discomfort.*
• Support foot with a pillow when lying on nonoperative side. **D** ● ✦	*Prevents the foot from dangling, twisting, and increasing pressure on the hip.*
• Never cross ankles or legs when sleeping in supine position. **D** ● ✦	*Increases risk for dislocation of hip joint.*
• Do not allow the client to sleep in a prone position. **D** ● ✦	*In this position there may be the tendency to turn the leg outward or flex at the hip, which increases the risk for dislocation.*
Knee Replacement:	
• Monitor and appropriately align client limbs when using a continuous passive movement (CPM) machine.	*Use of CPM device to improve range of motion, improve wound healing, and decrease the incidence of adhesions in the operative knee. However, research shows that the use of CPM minimally improves the ability to bend knee.*
• When in bed and if not in a CPM device, support the operative knee by placing a pillow under the calf.	*Supports/promotes full-leg extension.*
• Assist with and encourage client to perform weight-bearing exercises and sitting in a chair with legs dependent.	*Support ambulation with restricted weight-bearing and sitting in the chair. Legs should not be propped up but placed in a dependent position.*

Dependent/Collaborative Actions

Consult the appropriate health care provider (i.e., physical therapist, physician) if client is unable to achieve expected level of mobility	*Allows for modification of treatment regimen.*

Nursing Diagnosis ## RISK FOR PERIPHERAL NEUROVASCULAR DYSFUNCTION NDx (OPERATIVE EXTREMITY)

Definition: Susceptible to disruption in the circulation, sensation, and motion of an extremity, which may compromise health.

Related to:

Hip
- Trauma to or excessive pressure on the nerves or blood vessels during surgery
- Blood accumulation and edema in the surgical area
- Improper alignment of operative extremity
- Dislocation of the prosthesis(es)

Knee
- Trauma to or excessive pressure on the nerves or blood vessels during surgery
- Blood accumulation and edema in the surgical area
- Improper alignment of operative extremity
- Pressure exerted by the dressing, knee immobilizer, or CPM machine
- Dislocation of the prosthesis(es)

CLINICAL MANIFESTATIONS

Subjective	Objective
Self-report of increased pain in the extremity; numbness or tingling in the foot or toes (knee); pain in the foot during passive motion of toes or foot; numbness or tingling in the leg or foot (hip)	Diminished or absent pedal pulses; capillary refill time in toes greater than 2 to 3 seconds; pallor, cyanosis, or coolness of the extremity; inability to flex or extend knee, foot, or toes (knee)

RISK FACTORS

- Immobilization
- Mechanical compression (brace)
- Vascular obstruction
- Hypovolemia
- Chronic illness

DESIRED OUTCOMES

The client will maintain normal neurovascular function in the operative extremity as evidenced by:
a. Palpable pedal pulses
b. Capillary refill time in toes less than 2 to 3 seconds
c. Extremity warm and usual color
d. No increase in pain in extremity
e. Ability to flex and extend knee, foot, and toes (**hip**)
f. Absence of numbness and tingling in leg or foot (**hip**)
g. Ability to flex and extend foot and toes (**knee**)
h. Absence of numbness and tingling in foot and toes (**knee**)
i. Absence of foot pain during passive movement of toes and foot (**knee**)

NOC OUTCOMES

Tissue perfusion: peripheral; Neurological status: peripheral

NIC INTERVENTIONS

Circulatory care: arterial insufficiency; circulatory care: venous insufficiency; lower extremity monitoring; positioning; pressure management; heat/cold application

NURSING ASSESSMENT

Assess for and report signs of neurovascular dysfunction in the operative extremity:
- Increased pain in the extremity
- Numbness or tingling in the foot or toes (knee)
- Pain in the foot during passive motion of toes or foot
- Numbness or tingling in the leg or foot (hip)
- Diminished or absent pedal pulses
- Capillary refill time in toes greater than 2 to 3 seconds
- Pallor, cyanosis, or coolness of the extremity
- Inability to flex or extend knee, foot, or toes (hip, knee)

RATIONALE

Early recognition of signs and symptoms of neurovascular dysfunction allows for prompt intervention.

THERAPEUTIC INTERVENTIONS

Independent Actions
Assess affected limb, compare findings to noninjured limb, document and report changes.
Assessment of the 6 P's is appropriate for any type of joint replacement surgery:
- Pain: Assess using a pain scale including severity, quality, intensity, radiation, and onset of new and different pain.

- Pulses: Monitor and document pulses distal to the injury. Use a rating scale for intensity of palpable pulses.

- Paresthesia: Assess sensations proximal and distal to the site of surgery using light touch to the skin. Ask client about changes in sensation. Report any "pins and needles" sensations.
- Pallor: Assess capillary refill, color, and warmth distal to the injury. Monitor trends over time and report any decline in findings.
- Paralysis: Ask client to dorsiflex or plantar flex the feet, note decreases in movement or inability to perform.

RATIONALE

An increase in pain or inability to control pain with medication and increased pain experienced with passive stretching may indicate compartment syndrome.
Change in pulses within injured limb and differences noted between injured and noninjured limb may indicate changes in blood flow to distal to the injury.
Decreased feeling or "pins and needles" feeling report by client may indicate nerve damage and indicate compartmental syndrome.

Irreversible nerve damage may occur if not resolved.

Decreasing color, capillary refill time, and warmth to the extremity indicates arterial insufficiency and should receive immediate intervention.

THERAPEUTIC INTERVENTIONS	RATIONALE
• Pressure or edema: Assess for changes in firmness or swelling of the extremity distal to the injury. Measure calf size if indicated	*Decreased movement or no movement is indicative of compartmental syndrome and requires immediate intervention.* *Edema or increased tightness of the skin correlates with increased internal pressure on the muscles, nerves, and tissues and is indicative of compromised circulation distal to site of surgery.*
Maintain patency of wound drainage system, if present (e.g., prevent kinking of tubing, empty collection devices as needed, keep collection device below the level of surgical site, maintain suction as ordered).	*Helps to maintain vascular fluid volume.*
Encourage client intake of oral fluids if not contraindicated.	*Maintaining patency of a drainage system reduces the accumulation of fluid in the surgical area, decreasing pressure on the surgical site and surrounding tissues.*
Hip Arthroplasty:	*Dehydration increases the risk of deep vein thrombosis and potential for neurovascular insult.*
• Assure that straps on abductor wedge are not exerting pressure on the popliteal space, Achilles tendon, and medial aspects of the heel and ankle.	*Excessive pressure on the popliteal space compresses arteries, nerves, and veins, decreasing perfusion and increasing the risk for nerve damage. In addition, the risk for deep vein thrombosis increases because of altered perfusion.*
• Encourage client in range-of-motion exercises and ambulation.	*Promotes circulation and maintains muscle strength.*
Knee Arthroplasty:	
• Elevate operative leg when not in CPM machine by placing pillow under calf.	*Elevation of the affected limb reduces edema in surgical area. Limiting knee flexion reduces pressure on peroneal nerve.*
• If using CPM or immobilizer, assure the straps are not too tight and placing excessive pressure on the affected limb.	*Decreases circulation and pressure on skin, decreasing the incidence of skin injury.*
Dependent/Collaborative Actions	
Apply intermittent ice pack or cooling pad to operative site.	*Cold therapy facilitates vasoconstriction, thereby decreasing bleeding, swelling, and pain at the surgical site.*
Notify health care provider if signs and symptoms of neurovascular dysfunction occur.	*Allows for prompt modification of the treatment regimen.*
Prepare client for surgical intervention.	*Information about what is happening as part of the treatment plan decreases fear and anxiety concerning condition.*

Nursing Diagnosis IMPAIRED TISSUE INTEGRITY NDx/RISK FOR IMPAIRED TISSUE INTEGRITY NDx

Definition: Impaired Tissue Integrity NDx: Damage to the mucous membrane, cornea, integumentary system, muscular fascia, muscle, tendon, bone, cartilage, joint capsule, and/or ligament; **Risk for Impaired Tissue Integrity NDx:** Susceptible to damage to the mucous membranes, cornea, integumentary system, muscular fascia, muscle, tendon, bone, cartilage, joint capsule and/or ligament, which may compromise health.

Related to:
• Disruption of tissue associated with the surgical procedure
• Delayed wound healing associated with factors such as decreased nutritional status and inadequate blood supply to wound area
• Irritation of skin associated with contact with wound drainage, pressure from tubes, and use of tape
• Excessive or prolonged pressure on tissues from balanced suspension device, straps on abductor wedge, and elastic wraps or stockings
• Damage to the skin and/or subcutaneous tissue associated with prolonged pressure on tissues, friction, and shearing while mobility is decreased

CLINICAL MANIFESTATIONS

Subjective	Objective
N/A	Pallor and/or redness of skin in the following areas: skin in contact with wound drainage, tape, or tubing; back, coccyx, and buttocks; elbows and/or heels; skin in areas at edges of compression dressing or joint immobilizer; areas in contact with CPM machine; areas under elastic wraps or compression stockings

RISK FACTORS

- Imbalanced nutrition
- Immobility
- Mechanical pressure
- Surgical procedure

DESIRED OUTCOMES

The client will:
a. Experience normal healing of the surgical wound
b. Maintain tissue integrity as evidenced by absence of redness and irritation, and no skin breakdown

NOC OUTCOMES

Tissue integrity: skin and mucous membranes; wound healing: primary intention

NIC INTERVENTIONS

Incision site care; skin surveillance; positioning; pressure ulcer prevention; pressure management; skin care: topical treatments

---

NURSING ASSESSMENT

Assess for and report signs and symptoms of skin breakdown:
- Pallor and/or redness of skin in the following areas:
  - Skin in contact with wound drainage, tape, or tubing
  - Back, coccyx, and buttocks
  - Elbows and/or heels
  - Skin in areas at edges of compression dressing or joint immobilizer
  - Areas in contact with CPM machine
  - Areas under elastic wraps or compression stockings

RATIONALE

Early recognition of signs and symptoms of actual or impaired skin integrity allows for prompt intervention.

THERAPEUTIC INTERVENTIONS

RATIONALE

Independent Actions

Implement measures to prevent tissue irritation and breakdown in areas in contact with wound drainage, tape, and tubings:
- Maintain patency of drainage tubes. **D** ✦

- Apply collection device over drains and incisions that are draining continuously. **D** ✦
- Ensure client is not lying on drainage tubes. **D** ✦ ●
- Perform actions to decrease skin irritation from tape:
  - Use only the necessary amount of tape. **D** ✦
  - Use hypoallergenic tape.
  - Use Montgomery straps or tubular netting.

Implement measures to prevent tissue breakdown associated with decreased mobility:
- Position client properly; use pressure-reducing or pressure-relieving devices (e.g., pillows, alternating pressure mattress) if indicated. **D** ✦ ●
- Instruct client to use overhead trapeze to lift self and shift weight at least every 30 minutes.
- Gently massage around reddened areas at least every 2 hrs. **D** ✦
- Lift and move client carefully using a turn sheet and adequate assistance. **D** ●
- Perform actions to keep client from sliding down in bed (e.g., limit length of time client is in a semi-Fowler's position to 30-minute intervals). **D** ●
- If turning is allowed, turn client every 2 hrs, maintaining proper alignment. **D** ●

Implement measures to prevent irritation and breakdown on elbows and heels:
- Massage elbows and heels with lotion. **D** ✦ ●
- Encourage client to use overhead trapeze to move self rather than pushing up with heel and elbows.
- Provide elbow and heel protectors if indicated. **D** ●

Maintaining patency of drainage tubes helps to prevent the possibility of leakages around tubes.
Removes fluid from tissues and decreases pressure on the suture line and surrounding skin.
Prevents drainage tube blockage and backup into tissues.
Pressure on the skin may compromise circulation to that area.
Tape irritates the skin and some clients have tape allergies.
Decreases incidence of skin irritation and allergic reactions.
Decreases exposure of the skin to avoid repeated application and removal of tape.

Actions help to reduce constant pressure on skin and bony prominences, improving circulation to skin.

Actions prevent shearing injury to client's skin.

Actions stimulate circulation to the skin.

Prevents shearing forces against client's skin.

Decreases pressure on coccyx.

Turning from side to side decreases constant pressure on bony prominences.
Actions help to reduce the risk of skin surface abrasion and shearing and decrease the potential for skin injury. Also, can improve client comfort.

THERAPEUTIC INTERVENTIONS	RATIONALE
Implement measures to prevent tissue breakdown under elastic wraps or stockings:	
• Remove elastic wraps or stockings at least twice daily, bathe and thoroughly dry skin, and reapply smoothly. **D** ✦ ●	*Moisture facilitates skin breakdown.*
• Check wraps or stockings frequently and reapply if they have slipped or become wrinkled. **D** ✦	*Wrinkles under skin will increase pressure and increase risk of breakdown.*
• If areas of redness develop under wraps or stockings, consult physician before reapplying.	
Hip arthroplasty:	
Implement measures to prevent tissue breakdown associated with excessive pressure caused by balanced suspension device or abductor wedge:	
• Make sure metal parts on suspension device are not resting on any area of extremity.	*Balanced suspension devices or abductor wedges may promote tissue breakdown via increased tissue pressure. Straps and tape can be irritating to the skin and compromise circulation if they are too tight.*
• Maintain proper alignment of extremity in suspension device. **D** ✦	
• Make sure that straps holding abductor wedge in place are not too tight. **D** ✦	
Knee arthroplasty:	
Implement measures to prevent tissue breakdown in areas in contact with the compression dressing, knee immobilizer, and CPM machine:	
	Improves circulation.
	Keeping the dressing dry decreases potential for tissue maceration.
• Loosen straps on knee immobilizer if they appears to be too tight. **D** ✦	
• Keep dressing dry.	
• Position the operative extremity so the knee immobilizer and CPM machine are not causing excessive pressure on any area. **D** ✦	
• Ensure CPM machine is padded appropriately. **D** ✦	*Decreases pressure on skin and decreases incidence for skin injury.*
Dependent/Collaborative Actions	
If tissue breakdown occurs:	
• Notify appropriate health care provider (e.g., physician, wound care specialist).	*Notifying the physician allows for modification of the treatment plan.*
• Perform care of involved areas as ordered or per standard hospital procedure.	

DISCHARGE TEACHING/CONTINUED CARE

Nursing Diagnosis ## DEFICIENT KNOWLEDGE ɴᴅx; INEFFECTIVE HEALTH MANAGEMENT ɴᴅx; INEFFECTIVE FAMILY HEALTH MANAGEMENT* ɴᴅx

Definition: Deficient Knowledge NDx: Absence of cognitive information related to a specific topic, or its acquisition; **Ineffective Health Management NDx:** Pattern of regulating and integrating into daily living a therapeutic regimen for the treatment of illness and its sequelae that is unsatisfactory for meeting specific health goals; **Ineffective Family Health Management NDx:** A pattern of regulating and integrating into family processes a program for the treatment of illness and its sequelae that is unsatisfactory for meeting specific health goals of the family unit.

Related to:
• Decisional conflict
• Difficulty managing complex treatment regimen
• Family conflict
• Insufficient knowledge of therapeutic regimen
• Powerlessness

*The nurse should select the nursing diagnostic label that is most appropriate for the client's discharge teaching needs.

NDx = NANDA Diagnosis **D** = Delegatable Action ● = UAP ✦ = LVN/LPN ⊝▶ = Go to ⊝volve for animation

CLINICAL MANIFESTATIONS

Subjective	Objective
Self-report of lack of understanding	Demonstrated lack of knowledge about basic health practices; demonstrated lack of adaptive behaviors; impaired personal support systems; inaccurate follow-through of instructions

RISK FACTORS

- Cognitive limitations
- Economically disadvantaged
- Inadequate support system
- Family conflict
- Lifting objects or excessive twisting

NOC OUTCOMES	NIC INTERVENTIONS
Knowledge: fall prevention; prescribed activity; treatment regimen	Health system guidance; teaching: individual; teaching: prescribed activity/exercise

NURSING ASSESSMENT	RATIONALE
Assess client's readiness and ability to learn. Assess meaning of illness to client.	*Early recognition of readiness to learn and meaning of illness to client allows for implementation of the appropriate teaching interventions.*

THERAPEUTIC INTERVENTIONS	RATIONALE

Desired Outcome: The client will demonstrate correct transfer and ambulation techniques and proper use of ambulatory aids.

Independent Actions

Reinforce instructions about correct transfer and ambulation techniques and proper use of walker, quad cane, or crutches. Reinforce physician's instructions about amount of weight-bearing on operative extremity. Allow time for questions, clarification, and practice of transfer and ambulation techniques.	*Performing transfer techniques and using assistive devices correctly reduces the risk of injury.* *Early weight bearing may cause increased pain and discomfort.* *Allows the nurse to reinforce patient education and to evaluate the need for further instruction.*

THERAPEUTIC INTERVENTIONS	RATIONALE

Desired Outcome: The client will demonstrate the ability to correctly perform the prescribed exercises.

Independent Actions

Reinforce the physical therapist's instructions on prescribed exercises and the importance of continuing the exercises for the prescribed length of time. Allow time for questions, clarification, and return demonstration of prescribed exercises.	*Regular physical activity helps to maintain bone mass, increase lean muscle mass, and increase muscular strength, improving overall function and range of motion.* *Allows the nurse to reinforce patient education and to evaluate the need for further instruction.*

THERAPEUTIC INTERVENTIONS	RATIONALE

Desired Outcome: The client will identify ways to reduce the risk of loosening of the prosthesis(es).

THERAPEUTIC INTERVENTIONS	RATIONALE

Independent Actions

Hip arthroplasty:

Instruct client to adhere to the following activity and position restrictions (length of time the restrictions are necessary varies but ranges from 2 to 6 months):

These actions are important for the client to adhere to prevent dislocation of the prosthesis.
Anything that requires joint flexion beyond 90 degrees should be avoided.

- Turn only as directed by physician (many physicians allow client to turn to nonoperative side only).
- Instruct client to keep pillow between legs when lying on back or side and when turning.

Prevents overextension and increases comfort.

- Never cross legs.

Actions prevents dislocation.

- Do not sit on low chairs, stools, or toilets; place a cushion on low chairs, rent or purchase an elevated toilet seat for home use, and use the high toilets designated for the handicapped when in public facilities.
- Do not elevate operative leg higher than hip when sitting.
- Sit in chairs with arms and use the arms to raise self off chair.
- Support weight on nonoperative leg when raising self from a sitting position.
- Use assistive devices (e.g., long-handled shoe horn, long-handled grabber) to assist with activities that require flexing hip beyond 90 degrees (e.g., putting on shoes and socks, reaching objects on the floor or in low cupboards or drawers, pulling bed covers up from end of bed).

Assistive devices can improve patients ability to care for self.

- Keep operative leg in proper alignment and avoid extreme internal and external rotation of leg.
- Do not drive until approved by physician (usually about 6 weeks after surgery).

Prevents injury to self and potential injury to others.

- When riding in a car:
  - Sit on a firm pillow or cushion to prevent hip flexion of more than 90 degrees.

Prevents overextension and increases comfort.

  - Keep operative leg extended (a sudden impact of the knee against the dashboard can dislodge the prosthesis(es).
- When sexual activity is resumed, avoid positions that involve extreme rotation of the operative leg, flexing hip beyond 90 degrees, and moving operative leg past the midline.

Lifting objects or excessive twisting puts patient at risk for adding stress to operative site.

- Avoid lifting heavy objects, excessive twisting and turning of body, and activities that place excessive strain on hip (e.g., jogging, jumping).

Knee arthroplasty:

Inform client of the possibility of loosening of the prosthesis (usually does not occur until 2 to 3 years after surgery).

Provides information to the client that they should be aware of following surgery.

Instruct client to report increasing pain or instability of operative knee

May indicate loosening of the prosthesis.

- Adhere to weight-bearing restrictions if prescribed.

Decreases undue pressure on the prosthetic joint and prevents injury to residual limb.

- Avoid unusual twisting of knee.
- Avoid contact sports.
- Do not force knee beyond comfortable degree of flexion and avoid kneeling.
- Avoid placing undue stress on knees (e.g., do not lift and carry heavy objects, maintain ideal body weight, avoid activities such as jogging).

THERAPEUTIC INTERVENTIONS	RATIONALE

Desired Outcome: The client will identify ways to reduce the risk of falls in the home environment.

Independent Actions
Provide the following instructions on ways to reduce risk of falls at home:
*   Keep electrical cords out of pathways.
*   Remove unnecessary furniture and provide wide pathways for ambulation.
*   Remove scatter rugs.
*   Provide adequate lighting at all times.
*   Avoid unnecessary stair climbing.

Actions reduce potential causes of in-home falls and increases ease of movement.

THERAPEUTIC INTERVENTIONS	RATIONALE

Desired Outcome: The client will state signs and symptoms to report to the health care provider.

Independent Actions
Instruct client to report these additional signs and symptoms:
*   Persistent or increased pain or spasms in operative extremity
*   Loss of sensation or movement in operative extremity
*   Inability to bear expected amount of weight on operative extremity
*   Inability to maintain operative extremity in a neutral position
*   Instability of operative extremity (feeling of knee "giving out") or shortening of the operative extremity (noticed as a limp in a hip client)
*   Chills
*   Fever
*   Increase or change in wound drainage

Educating the client regarding signs and symptoms to report to the health care provider allows for implementing appropriate interventions, altering the plan of care, and reducing the risk of potential complications.

THERAPEUTIC INTERVENTIONS	RATIONALE

Desired Outcome: The client will identify community resources that can assist with home management and provide transportation.

Independent Actions
Provide information about community resources that can assist client and significant others with home management and provide transportation (e.g., home health agencies, Meals on Wheels, church groups, transportation services). Initiate a referral if indicated.

Social support can aid the client in obtaining necessary resources to adapt to physical changes and obtain the necessary long-term assistance to maintain independence.

THERAPEUTIC INTERVENTIONS	RATIONALE

Desired Outcome: The client, in collaboration with the nurse, will develop a plan for adhering to recommended follow-up care including future appointments with health care provider and physical therapist, medications prescribed, activity level, and wound care.

Independent Actions
Collaborate with clients to develop a plan to adhere to health care provider prescribed exercises, medications and side effects, and follow-up appointments.
Reinforce the importance of keeping appointments with physical therapist.

Provides client the confidence that they can adhere to treatment regimen.

Adherence to a plan of care reduces the risk of complications and improves patient outcomes.

THERAPEUTIC INTERVENTIONS	**RATIONALE**
Teach client the rationale for, side effects of, schedule for taking, and importance of taking prescribed medications.	*Helps client to understand the importance of adherence to medications and know what to expect related to side effects.*
Instruct client to inform other health care providers of history of total joint arthroplasty so prophylactic antimicrobials can be started before any dental work, invasive diagnostic procedures, or surgery is performed.	*Allows for maintenance of appropriate care and prevents potential for injury.*
Inform client that the prosthetic device may activate metal detector alarms. Recommend carrying an identification/information card verifying presence of the device.	*Decreases embarrassment and prevents unnecessary stress.*

RELATED CARE PLANS

Preoperative
Postoperative

ADDITIONAL NURSING DIAGNOSIS

RISK FOR INFECTION NDx
Related to:

- Introduction of pathogens into the wound during or after surgery
- Hematoma formation (increases the likelihood of infection by providing a good medium for growth of pathogens and compromising blood flow to the area)
- Increased susceptibility to infection associated with decreased effectiveness of immune system if client is elderly and immunosuppression if client has been taking corticosteroids to treat the joint disorder necessitating the surgery (e.g., rheumatoid arthritis)
- Hematogenous seeding of wound from distant sites (e.g., urinary tract)

ACTIVITY INTOLERANCE NDx
Related to:

- Tissue hypoxia associated with anemia (there can be significant blood loss because the hip is a very vascular area)
- Difficulty resting and sleeping associated with discomfort, position restrictions, fear, and anxiety

RISK FOR FALLS NDx
Related to:

- Weakness, fatigue, and postural hypotension associated with the effects of major surgery and physiological changes that may have occurred if client is elderly
- CNS depressant effect of some medications (e.g., narcotic [opioid] analgesics, centrally acting muscle relaxants, some antiemetics)
- Weakness and pain in weight-bearing extremity associated with surgery on the hip
- Difficulty with transfer and ambulation techniques

LAMINECTOMY/DISCECTOMY WITH OR WITHOUT FUSION

A laminectomy is the surgical removal of the lamina of a vertebra. It may be performed to allow for removal of a neoplasm or bone fragments that are putting pressure on nerve roots or the spinal cord or to enable a rhizotomy or cordotomy to be performed to treat intractable pain. Most commonly, a laminectomy is performed to gain access to a herniated nucleus pulposus (HNP, "ruptured disk") so that a discectomy (removal of the herniated portion of the disk) can be accomplished.

Disk herniation is usually the result of trauma (e.g., falls, vehicular accidents) or strain caused by factors such as improper or repeated lifting of heavy objects, twisting, sneezing, or coughing. Age-related degenerative changes in the disks, supporting ligaments, and vertebrae make the disks more prone to rupture. The most common sites of disk herniation are C5–6, C6–7, L4–5, and L5–S1. These areas of the spine are the most flexible and therefore are subjected to a greater amount of movement and strain. Signs and symptoms of lumbar disk herniation can include low back pain that radiates down the buttock, thigh, calf, and ankle on the affected side; muscle spasms in the lower back; muscle weakness, diminished knee and ankle reflexes, numbness, or tingling in the affected lower extremity; constipation; and/or urinary retention.

Clinical manifestations of cervical disk herniation can include neck pain that radiates to the shoulder, arm, and fingers on the affected side; stiff neck; muscle spasms in the neck; and/or muscle weakness, diminished biceps and triceps reflexes, numbness, or tingling in the affected upper extremity.

A discectomy is usually indicated if conservative measures such as rest, heat or cold applications, anti-inflammatory medications, analgesics, muscle relaxants, and local steroid injections fail to control pain or if neurological deficits persist or worsen. Disk removal is usually accomplished by a microdiscectomy or laminectomy and can be performed using an anterior and/or posterior approach. The surgical procedure performed depends on the location and size of the herniated disk and physician preference. If the vertebral column in the surgical area is unstable, a spinal fusion may be performed along with a laminectomy. The surgical immobilization of the unstable area is accomplished using a bone graft (autograft [usually from the iliac crest], allograft, or bone substitute) or implanted fixation devices such as cages, plates, screws, and rods.

This care plan focuses on the adult client admitted for a laminectomy that is being performed to remove an HNP. The care of a client hospitalized for a laminectomy

with spinal fusion is also discussed. Much of the post-operative information is applicable to clients receiving follow-up care in an extended care facility or home setting.

OUTCOME/DISCHARGE CRITERIA

The client will:
1. Have improved neurological function
2. Have evidence of normal healing of the surgical wound
3. Have intact skin under the stabilization device if one is present
4. Have pain controlled
5. Have no signs and symptoms of postoperative complications
6. Identify ways to prevent recurrent disk herniation
7. Demonstrate the ability to correctly apply and remove the stabilization device if one is required
8. Verbalize an understanding of ways to maintain skin integrity when wearing a stabilization device
9. State signs and symptoms to report to the health care provider
10. Develop a plan for adhering to recommended follow-up care including future appointments with health care provider, medications prescribed, activity level, and wound care

PREOPERATIVE: USE IN CONJUNCTION WITH THE STANDARDIZED PREOPERATIVE CARE PLAN

RELATED PREOPERATIVE NURSING/COLLABORATIVE DIAGNOSIS:

DEFICIENT KNOWLEDGE NDx
Definition: Absence of cognitive information related to a specific topic, or its acquisition.

Related to: The surgical procedure, routines associated with surgery, physical preparation for laminectomy and spinal fusion (if planned), sensations that normally occur after surgery and anesthesia, and postoperative care.

POSTOPERATIVE: USE IN CONJUNCTION WITH THE STANDARDIZED POSTOPERATIVE CARE PLAN

Nursing Diagnosis | RISK FOR PERIPHERAL NEUROVASCULAR DYSFUNCTION NDx

Definition: Susceptible to disruption in circulation, sensation, or motion of an extremity, which may compromise health.

Related to:
- Trauma to the nerves or blood vessels during surgery
- Blood accumulation and inflammation in the surgical area
- Dislocation of the bone graft or implanted fixation devices (if a fusion was performed)
- Excessive external pressure on the nerves or blood vessels associated with improper fit or application of the stabilization device (e.g., cervical collar, back brace, corset)

CLINICAL MANIFESTATIONS

Subjective	Objective
Verbal self-report of numbness or tingling in extremities; development of or increase in pain in extremities	Diminished or absent peripheral pulses; capillary refill time greater than 2 to 3 seconds; pallor, cyanosis, or coolness of extremities; inability to flex or extend feet, toes, hands, or fingers; diminished or absent reflexes in extremities; development of or increase in muscle weakness

RISK FACTORS
- Mechanical compression
- Vascular obstruction
- Immobilization

DESIRED OUTCOMES

The client will have usual or improved peripheral neurovascular function as evidenced by:
a. Palpable peripheral pulses
b. Capillary refill time less than 2 to 3 seconds
c. Extremities warm and usual color
d. Ability to flex and extend feet, toes, hands, and fingers
e. Usual or improved reflexes, muscle tone, and sensation in extremities
f. No new or increased pain in extremities

NOC OUTCOMES	NIC INTERVENTIONS
Neurological status: spinal sensory/motor function; tissue perfusion: peripheral	Neurological monitoring; positioning: neurological; circulatory care: arterial insufficiency; circulatory care: venous insufficiency

NURSING ASSESSMENT	RATIONALE
Assess for and report signs and symptoms of peripheral neurovascular dysfunction (check upper extremities after surgery on the cervical area and lower extremities after surgery on the lumbar area):	*Early recognition of signs and symptoms of peripheral neurovascular dysfunction allows for prompt intervention.*

- Numbness or tingling in extremities
- Development of or increase in pain in extremities
- Diminished or absent peripheral pulses
- Capillary refill time greater than 2 to 3 seconds
- Pallor, cyanosis, or coolness of extremities
- Inability to flex or extend feet, toes, hands, or fingers
- Diminished or absent reflexes in extremities
- Development of or increase in muscle weakness

THERAPEUTIC INTERVENTIONS	RATIONALE

Independent Actions

Implement measures to reduce the risk for peripheral neurovascular dysfunction:

- Perform actions to reduce strain on the surgical area: **D** ✦
  - Keep spine in proper alignment.
  - Prevent hyperextension, extreme flexion, or twisting of spine.
  - Position to maintain flattening of lumbosacral spine:
    1. Side lying with knees flexed
    2. Supine with slight knee flexion
- Maintain wound suction and patency of wound drain.

- Apply stabilization device properly; notify orthotist if it appears to create excessive pressure on any area.

Reducing strain on the surgical area helps to prevent bleeding and subsequent hematoma formation in the surgical area and to reduce the risk for dislocation of the bone graft or implanted fixation devices (if fusion was performed).

Reduces the accumulation of blood in the surgical area and subsequently prevents increased pressure on nerves and blood vessels.

Prevents injury.

Dependent/Collaborative Actions

Implement measures to reduce the risk for peripheral neurovascular dysfunction:

- Perform actions to reduce strain on the surgical area.
  - Ensure client is always positioned with spine in proper alignment.
  - Apply stabilization device.
- Administer corticosteroids if ordered.

If signs and symptoms of peripheral neurovascular dysfunction occur:

- Assess for and correct improper body alignment and external cause of excessive pressure (e.g., tight or improperly applied stabilization device).
- Notify physician if signs and symptoms persist or worsen.
- Prepare client for surgical intervention (e.g., evacuation of hematoma, repositioning of dislocated bone graft or implanted fixation devices) if planned.

Actions help to stabilize surgical area and decrease incidence of complications.

Corticosteroids help to reduce inflammation in the surgical area.

Allows for prompt intervention to reduce complications resulting in permanent nerve dysfunction (e.g., hematoma, dislocated bone graft).

| Nursing Diagnosis | **ACUTE PAIN** NDx |

Definition: Unpleasant sensory and emotional experience associated with actual or potential tissue damage, or described in terms of such damage (International Association for the Study of Pain); sudden or slow onset of any intensity from mild to severe with an anticipated or predictable end, and with a duration of less than 3 months.

Related to:
- Tissue trauma and reflex muscle spasms associated with the surgery
- Removal of bone if an autograft was used to achieve spinal fusion (the bone is usually taken from the client's iliac crest)
- Stretching and compression of sensory nerves associated with blood accumulation and inflammation in the surgical area
- Irritation from drainage tube (wound drain may be present, especially after a spinal fusion)
- Stress on surgical area associated with movement
- Release of pressure on compressed spinal nerve root after removal of the HNP (improved sensory nerve function can cause a temporary increase in pain in area[s] of previously ditminished sensation).

CLINICAL MANIFESTATIONS

Subjective	**Objective**
Verbal self-report of pain; reluctance to move	Grimacing; restlessness; diaphoresis; increased BP; tachycardia

RISK FACTORS	**DESIRED OUTCOMES**
• Altered limited mobility • Inadequate pain relief	The client will experience diminished pain.

NOC OUTCOMES	**NIC INTERVENTIONS**
Pain control; comfort level	Pain management; analgesic administration

NURSING ASSESSMENT	**RATIONALE**
Assess the patient for signs and symptoms of pain: • Verbalization of pain • Reluctance to move • Grimacing • Restlessness • Diaphoresis • Increased BP • Tachycardia	*Early recognition of signs and symptoms of pain allows for prompt intervention.*

THERAPEUTIC INTERVENTIONS	**RATIONALE**

Independent Actions

Implement additional measures to reduce pain:
- Perform actions to reduce strain on the surgical area: **D** ✦
  - Ensure that client is always positioned with spine in proper alignment. **D** ✦

  - Apply stabilization device if ordered.
  - If stabilization device loosens, reapply it or tighten straps or screws if allowed, or consult orthotist about adjustment of the device.
  - Implement measures to prevent hyperextension, extreme flexion, and/or twisting of spine (e.g., instruct and assist client to logroll when turning; put needed items within easy reach; if a cervical laminectomy was performed, place a small pillow or folded pad under client's head rather than a full-size pillow; assist with bathing and dressing as needed). **D** ✦ ●

Reducing strain on the surgical area helps to prevent bleeding and subsequent hematoma formation in the surgical area and to reduce the risk for dislocation of the bone graft or implanted fixation devices (if fusion was performed).

Stabilization helps to provide additional support to surgical area. Prevents chance for injury.

THERAPEUTIC INTERVENTIONS	**RATIONALE**
• If lumbar laminectomy was performed, assist client to maintain a position that results in flattening of the lumbosacral spine (e.g., slight knee flexion when supine, knees flexed while in side-lying position, feet elevated on footstool when sitting in chair). **D ✦ ●**	*Interventions help to reduce injury from stretching of the nerves and muscles in the lower back.*
• Instruct client to avoid sitting or standing for longer than 20- to 30-minute intervals (some physicians instruct clients to sit only during meals and ambulate only short distances when progressive activity begins).	
• Instruct client to avoid straining to have a bowel movement (especially after lumbar laminectomy) and vigorous coughing; consult physician about an order for a laxative and antitussive if indicated.	*Helps to reduce tension on incision lines.*
• If appropriate, perform actions to reduce pressure on bone graft donor site (e.g., position client so he/she is not lying on site, protect the site with padding if stabilization device is worn over it).	

Dependent/Collaborative Actions

Implement additional measures to reduce pain:
| • Administer corticosteroids if ordered. | *Steroids help to reduce inflammation in the surgical area.* |

Nursing Diagnosis **IMPAIRED SKIN INTEGRITY** NDx; **RISK FOR IMPAIRED SKIN INTEGRITY** NDx

Definition: Impaired Skin Integrity NDx: Altered epidermis and/or dermis; **Risk for Impaired Skin Integrity NDx:** Susceptible to alteration in epidermis and/or dermis, which may compromise health.

Related to:
• Disruption of tissue associated with the surgical procedure
• Irritation of skin associated with contact with wound drainage, use of tape, and pressure from tubes and/or stabilization device if present

CLINICAL MANIFESTATIONS

Subjective	**Objective**
Verbal self-report of pain	Color changes, redness, swelling, warmth (signs of infection); surgical incisions; abrasions/tears

RISK FACTORS
• Physical immobility
• Shearing forces
• Pressure over bony prominence
• Inadequate nutrition

DESIRED OUTCOMES

The client will:
a. Experience normal healing of the surgical wound
b. Maintain tissue integrity in areas in contact with wound drainage, tape, tubings, and stabilization device as evidenced by absence of redness and irritation, and no skin breakdown

NOC OUTCOMES

Wound healing: primary intention; tissue integrity: skin and mucous membranes

NIC INTERVENTIONS

Skin surveillance; positioning; wound care; pressure management

---

NDx = NANDA Diagnosis   **D** = Delegatable Action   ● = UAP   ✦ = LVN/LPN   ⊜▶ = Go to ⊜volve for animation

NURSING ASSESSMENT	RATIONALE
Assess the patient for signs and symptoms of skin irritation and breakdown: • Areas in contact with wound drainage, tape, and tubings • Area under stabilization device • Color changes, redness, swelling, warmth (signs of infection) • Surgical incisions • Abrasions/tears Assess the site of impaired tissue integrity and determine the cause	*Early recognition of signs and symptoms of actual or impaired skin integrity allows for prompt intervention.*

THERAPEUTIC INTERVENTIONS	RATIONALE
Independent Actions Implement measures to prevent skin irritation and breakdown under stabilization device: • Apply stabilization device securely enough to keep it from rubbing and irritating the skin but not too tightly. **D** ✦ • Position client so that stabilization device is not causing excessive pressure on any area. **D** ✦ • Assist client to put a cotton T-shirt on under back brace or corset and ensure that the shirt is dry and wrinkle-free. **D** ✦ ● • Apply a thin layer of a dry lubricant such as powder or cornstarch to skin under stabilization device in order to reduce friction. **D** ✦ ● • Pad areas over bony prominences before applying stabilization device. • Instruct client to refrain from inserting anything under the stabilization device. • Consult physician or orthotist if stabilization device is putting excessive pressure on the skin. If tissue breakdown occurs: • Notify appropriate health care provider (e.g., physician, wound care specialist). • Perform care of involved area(s) as ordered or per standard hospital procedure.	*Constant pressure applied to the skin reduces blood flow to the tissues.* *Actions improve comfort when wearing the stabilization device and decreases incidence for injury.* *Notifying the appropriate health care provider allows for modification of the treatment plan.*

Collaborative Diagnosis   RISK FOR RESPIRATORY DISTRESS

Definition: Severe difficulty breathing.

Related to:

• Trauma to the phrenic nerve during surgery and/or compression of the phrenic nerve after surgery associated with inflammation or accumulation of blood in the surgical area (can occur with a cervical laminectomy because the phrenic nerve arises at the C3–5 level)
• Tracheal compression associated with inflammation or accumulation of blood in the surgical area after a cervical laminectomy (particularly if the anterior approach was used)
• Closure of the glottis associated with paralysis of the vocal cords (can occur as a result of injury to the bilateral recurrent laryngeal nerves during an anterior cervical laminectomy)

CLINICAL MANIFESTATIONS

Subjective	Objective
Cervical laminectomy: statements of difficulty swallowing or choking sensation	Cervical laminectomy: increased swelling in the neck or bulging of the wound; rapid and/or labored respirations, stridor, sternocleidomastoid muscle retraction, restlessness, agitation; abnormal arterial blood gas values; decrease in pulse oximetry values

RISK FACTORS
- Coagulopathy
- Elevated blood pressure
- Third spacing of fluid

DESIRED OUTCOMES

The client will not experience respiratory distress as evidenced by:
a. Unlabored respirations at 12 to 20 breaths/min
b. Absence of stridor and sternocleidomastoid muscle retraction
c. Usual mental status
d. Oximetry results within normal range
e. Arterial blood gas values within normal range

NURSING ASSESSMENT

Assess client for signs and symptoms of respiratory distress:
- Verbalization of difficulty swallowing
- Swelling in neck; rapid, labored respiration, stridor, retractions, agitation

Monitor pulse oximetry and arterial blood gas values for abnormalities

RATIONALE

Early recognition of signs and symptoms of respiratory distress allows for prompt intervention.

THERAPEUTIC INTERVENTIONS

Independent Actions

Have tracheostomy and suction equipment readily available after cervical laminectomy.

Implement measures to prevent respiratory distress after a cervical laminectomy:
- Implement measures to reduce strain on the surgical area:
  - Keep neck in proper alignment. **D** ✦
  - Ensure that cervical collar is applied correctly.
  - Instruct and assist client to support neck when moving.
- Elevate head of bed 30 to 45 degrees unless contraindicated.
- Apply ice pack to incisional area as ordered. **D** ✦ ●

Dependent/Collaborative Actions
- Administer corticosteroids if ordered. **D** ✦
- Maintain wound suction and patency of wound drain. **D** ✦

If signs and symptoms of respiratory distress occur:
- Place client in a high-Fowler's position unless contraindicated.
- Loosen neck dressing or cervical collar if it appears tight.
- Administer oxygen as ordered.
- Assist with intubation or emergency tracheostomy if performed.
- Prepare client for surgical evacuation of hematoma or repair of the bleeding vessel(s) if planned.

RATIONALE

Provides ready access to life support equipment if required.

Actions help to reduce inflammation and/or prevent bleeding and subsequent hematoma formation in the surgical area.

Application of ice reduces postsurgical swelling along incision site. Corticosteroids help to prevent edema at the site which decrease strain on the surgical area.

Patent drains help to prevent the accumulation of blood in the surgical area.

Improves lung expansion.
Prevents increased pressure on trachea which may decrease airflow.
Provides supplemental tissue oxygenation.
Provides temporary maintenance of airway.

Collaborative Diagnosis ## RISK FOR CEREBROSPINAL FLUID LEAK

Definition: Leakage of the cerebrospinal fluid (CSF) into the tissues and out of the CNS compartment.

Related to: Inadvertent damage to and/or incomplete closure of the dura (care is taken during surgery to keep the dura intact; however, it is sometimes necessary to incise dura that extends along the involved nerve)

CLINICAL MANIFESTATIONS

Subjective	Objective
Verbal self-report of headache	Clear drainage from the incision; presence of glucose in wound drainage as shown by positive results on a glucose reagent strip (be aware, blood will test positive for glucose); yellowish ring ("halo") around bloody or serosanguineous drainage on lower back or neck dressing, sheet, or pillowcase (CSF dries in concentric circles)

NDx = NANDA Diagnosis   **D** = Delegatable Action   ● = UAP   ✦ = LVN/LPN   ⊜▶ = Go to ⊜volve for animation

RISK FACTORS
- Surgical Damage
- Injury

DESIRED OUTCOMES

The client will have resolution of CSF leak if it occurs as evidenced by:
a. Absence of CSF drainage from lower back or neck incision
b. No reports of headache

NURSING ASSESSMENT	**RATIONALE**
Assess for and report signs and symptoms of a CSF leak: • Reports of headache • Clear drainage from incision • Presence of glucose in wound drainage	*Early recognition of signs and symptoms of CSF leak allows for prompt intervention.*

THERAPEUTIC INTERVENTIONS	**RATIONALE**
Dependent/Collaborative Actions Implement measures to reduce strain on the surgical area. • Keep neck in proper alignment. • Instruct and assist client when moving. If signs and symptoms of CSF leak occur:	*Actions help to promote healing of the dura and subsequent resolution of CSF leak.*
• Maintain activity restrictions as ordered to reduce stress on the meningeal tear. **D** ✦ ●	*Prevents further damage and decreases incidence of infection.*
• Change dressing as soon as it becomes damp; maintain meticulous sterile technique when changing dressing. **D** ✦	*Keeps area clean and dry as much as possible.*
• Administer antimicrobials if ordered. **D** ✦ • Assess for and report signs and symptoms of meningitis (e.g., fever; chills; new, increasing, or persistent headache; nuchal rigidity; photophobia; positive Kernig and Brudzinski signs).	*Decreases potential for and consequences of infection.*
• Prepare client for surgical repair of the torn dura if planned (usually the torn dura heals spontaneously within a few days).	*Requires change in treatment regimen.*

Collaborative Diagnosis ▏ # RISK FOR LARYNGEAL NERVE DAMAGE

Definition: Injury to one or both of the nerves that are attached to the voice box.

Related to: Surgical trauma or pressure on the nerve(s) associated with inflammation or accumulation of blood in the surgical area (can occur with an anterior cervical laminectomy)

CLINICAL MANIFESTATIONS

Subjective	**Objective**
Reports of voice changes (hoarseness; weak, whispery voice; inability to speak)	Respiratory distress (rapid and/or labored respirations, stridor, sternocleidomastoid muscle retraction, restlessness, agitation; abnormal arterial blood gas values; decrease in pulse oximetry values)

RISK FACTORS
- Hematoma at surgical site
- Edema/swelling at surgical site

DESIRED OUTCOMES

The client will experience resolution of laryngeal nerve damage if it occurs as evidenced by:
a. Improved voice tone and quality
b. Gradual resolution of hoarseness
c. Absence of respiratory distress

NURSING ASSESSMENT	RATIONALE
Assess for the following indications of laryngeal nerve damage: • Hoarseness • Weak, whispery voice • Respiratory distress • Stridor • Retractions • Restlessness • Agitation	*Early recognition of signs and symptoms of laryngeal nerve damage allows for prompt intervention.*

THERAPEUTIC INTERVENTIONS	RATIONALE
Independent Actions	
Implement measures to reduce pressure on the laryngeal nerves (e.g., elevated head of bed, ice to surgical site, monitor for swelling).	*Maintains patent airway and decreases potential for injury.*
Assess arterial blood gases for abnormal values and pulse oximetry.	*Monitors oxygenation status.*
• Encourage client to avoid unnecessary talking. **D** ✦ ●	*Action helps to rest the vocal cords.*
• Implement measures to facilitate communication (e.g., provide pad and pencil, flash cards, or Magic Slate; ask questions that require a short answer or nod of head). **D** ✦ ●	*Allows for ongoing communication when resting the voice.*
Reinforce physician's explanation regarding the permanence of voice changes (voice tone and quality usually return to normal as inflammation subsides).	*Helps client understand need for resting the voice and may improve adherence.*
If signs and symptoms of laryngeal nerve damage occur:	
• Notify physician immediately if signs and symptoms of respiratory distress occur, client is unable to speak, or hoarseness or voice changes worsen.	*Notifying the physician allows for modification of the treatment plan.*

Collaborative Diagnosis RISK FOR PARALYTIC ILEUS

Definition: Paralysis of the intestinal musculature caused by trauma, peritonitis, electrolyte imbalance, or spasmolytic agent

Related to:
• Impaired innervation of the intestinal tract after a lumbar laminectomy associated with stimulation of sympathetic nerves and/or loss of parasympathetic nerve function in the operative area
• Depressant effect of anesthesia and some medications (e.g., centrally acting muscle relaxants, narcotic [opioid] analgesics, some antiemetics)

CLINICAL MANIFESTATIONS

Subjective Reports of persistent abdominal pain and cramping	**Objective** Firm, distended abdomen; absent bowel sounds; failure to pass flatus

RISK FACTORS
• Immobility
• Medication administration

DESIRED OUTCOMES
The client will not develop a paralytic ileus as evidenced by:
a. Absence or resolution of abdominal pain and cramping
b. Soft, nondistended abdomen
c. Gradual return of bowel sounds
d. Passage of flatus

NDx = NANDA Diagnosis   **D** = Delegatable Action   ● = UAP   ✦ = LVN/LPN   ⊖▶ = Go to ⊖volve for animation

NURSING ASSESSMENT	RATIONALE
Assess for and report signs and symptoms of paralytic ileus: • Abdominal pain • Cramping • Distended abdomen • Absent bowel sounds • Failure to pass stool Monitor results of abdominal radiographs for abnormalities (distended bowel)	*Early recognition of signs and symptoms of paralytic ileus allows for prompt intervention.*

THERAPEUTIC INTERVENTIONS	RATIONALE
Dependent/Collaborative Actions Implement measures to prevent paralytic ileus: • Increase activity as soon as allowed and tolerated. • Administer gastrointestinal (GI) stimulants.	*Ambulation helps to stimulate motility of the GI tract.* *GI stimulants increase peristalsis without adding a purgative effect.*

DISCHARGE TEACHING/CONTINUED CARE

Nursing Diagnosis   **DEFICIENT KNOWLEDGE** NDx; **INEFFECTIVE FAMILY HEALTH MANAGEMENT** NDx; **OR INEFFECTIVE HEALTH MAINTENANCE*** NDx

Definition: **Deficient Knowledge NDx:** Absence of cognitive information related to a specific topic, or its acquisition; **Ineffective Family Health Management NDx:** A pattern of regulating and integrating into family processes a program for the treatment of illness and its sequelae that is unsatisfactory for meeting specific health goals of the family unit; **Ineffective Health Maintenance NDx:** Inability to identify, manage, and/or seek out help to maintain well-being.

Related to:
• Insufficient information for self-care
• Insufficient knowledge of resources
• Difficulty navigating complex health care system
• Difficulty managing complex treatment regimen
• Family conflict

CLINICAL MANIFESTATIONS

Subjective	Objective
Verbalization of the problems and concerns with treatment regimen	Demonstrated lack of knowledge about basic health practices; demonstrated lack of adaptive behaviors; impaired personal support systems; inaccurate follow-through of instructions

RISK FACTORS
• Cognitive deficit
• Financial concerns
• Inability to care for oneself

NOC OUTCOMES	NIC INTERVENTIONS
Knowledge: treatment regimen	Health system guidance; teaching: individual; teaching: prescribed activity/exercise

*The nurse should select the nursing diagnostic label that is most appropriate for the client's discharge teaching needs.

NURSING ASSESSMENT	RATIONALE
Assess client's readiness and ability to learn. Assess meaning of illness to client.	*Early recognition of readiness to learn and meaning of illness to client allows for implementation of the appropriate teaching interventions.*

THERAPEUTIC INTERVENTIONS	RATIONALE

Desired Outcome: The client will identify ways to prevent recurrent disk herniation.

Independent Actions

Inform client about ways to reduce back and/or neck strain and subsequently reduce the risk of recurrent disk herniation:

- Lose weight if overweight.

  Maintaining a normal body weight reduces stress/strain on the back.

- Support the spine adequately (e.g., sleep on a firm mattress; sit on firm, straight-backed or contoured chairs; wear stabilization device as prescribed).

  Appropriate alignment reduces risk for injury.

- Use proper body mechanics (e.g., bend at the knees rather than waist, push rather than pull heavy objects, carry items close to body).

  Use of proper body mechanics reduces the risk of injury.

- Keep spine in good alignment (e.g., avoid excessive bending or twisting, maintain good posture).

  Reduces stress on back, reducing the risk of injury.

- Wear flat or low-heeled shoes; avoid wearing high heels.

  Helps to maintain proper posture.

- Adhere to prescribed, progressive exercise program to strengthen back, neck, shoulders, arms, legs, and abdominal muscles.

  Stronger, well-developed muscles provide better support to bony spine.

Provide a dietary consult regarding a weight reduction program if indicated.

Helps client to develop a plan including foods client likes to eat.

Refer client to an occupational therapist and/or vocational rehabilitation specialist.

Provides assistance in modifying daily routines or pursuing different job opportunities, if indicated.

Allow time for client to practice proper body alignment when sitting, standing, and walking; proper positioning when resting; and any exercises allowed in immediate postoperative period. Encourage client to think about and plan movements before doing them.

Ensuring client's understanding of proper body mechanics reduces the risk of additional injury. Allow time for questions and return demonstration to assess the need for further instruction.

THERAPEUTIC INTERVENTIONS	RATIONALE

Desired Outcome: The client will demonstrate the ability to correctly apply and remove stabilization device if one is required.

Independent Actions

Reinforce instructions on the correct way to apply and remove stabilization device (e.g., cervical collar, back brace, corset) if client needs to wear one after discharge.

Reduces the risk of injury associated with improper use of stabilization devices.

THERAPEUTIC INTERVENTIONS	RATIONALE

Desired Outcome: The client will verbalize an understanding of ways to maintain skin integrity when wearing a stabilization device.

Independent Actions

If client is to be discharged with a stabilization device, instruct client to examine skin daily when device is off (if device should not be removed, demonstrate how to examine underneath it using a mirror and flashlight).

Early, prompt recognition of potential areas of skin breakdown allows for prompt intervention.

NDx = NANDA Diagnosis   **D** = Delegatable Action   ● = UAP   ✦ = LVN/LPN   ⊝▶ = Go to ⊝volve for animation

Continued...

THERAPEUTIC INTERVENTIONS	RATIONALE

Instruct client in ways to maintain skin integrity if a stabilization device needs to be worn:
- Apply device properly and maintain spine in good alignment to avoid undue pressure in any area.
- Wear a cotton T-shirt under back brace or corset and keep shirt dry and wrinkle-free.
- Apply a thin layer of powder or cornstarch to skin under stabilization device to reduce irritation caused by friction.
- Avoid inserting anything under the device.
- Place padding between stabilization device and bony prominences.

THERAPEUTIC INTERVENTIONS	RATIONALE

Desired Outcome: The client will state signs and symptoms to report to the health care provider.

Independent Actions
Instruct client to report these additional signs and symptoms:
- Decreased movement or sensation in extremities.
- Coolness or bluish color of extremities.
- Increasing or recurrent numbness, tingling, or pain in surgical area or extremities.
- Difficulty standing up straight (after lumbar surgery) or keeping neck straight (after cervical surgery).
- Persistent and/or severe headache.
- Drainage of clear or bloody fluid from incision.
- Persistent hoarseness or difficulty swallowing (after cervical laminectomy).
- Reddened or irritated area on skin underneath stabilization device.

Educating the client regarding signs and symptoms to report to the health care provider allows for implementing appropriate interventions, altering the plan of care, and reducing the risk of potential complications.

THERAPEUTIC INTERVENTIONS	RATIONALE

Desired Outcome: The client, in collaboration with the nurse, will develop a plan for adhering to recommended follow-up care including future appointments with health care provider, medications prescribed, activity level, and wound care.

Independent Actions
Reinforce physician's instructions regarding activity (the restrictions will vary depending on extensiveness of surgery, client's condition, and physician preference):
- Avoid lifting objects weighing more than 5 to 10 lbs.
- Progress through exercise program as prescribed.
- Avoid sitting or standing for longer than 30 minutes at a time (especially after surgery on lumbar area).
- Schedule adequate rest periods.
- Avoid driving a car (causes increased flexion of the spine) and taking long car rides (the vibrations can jar the spine and long periods without significant changes in position can increase stiffness and discomfort) until allowed.
- Do not participate in contact sports.

Following activity restrictions allows for healing of surgical site and increased muscle strength and tolerance for activity.

RELATED CARE PLANS

- Preoperative
- Postoperative

The Client With Alterations in the Breast and Reproductive System

HYSTERECTOMY

Hysterectomy is the surgical removal of the uterus. It is performed to treat a variety of conditions including malignant and nonmalignant growths in the uterus and cervix, symptomatic endometriosis, uterine prolapse, intractable pelvic infection, irreparable rupture of the uterus, and dysfunctional or life-threatening uterine bleeding. Both the uterus and cervix are removed in a total hysterectomy. A panhysterectomy is the removal of the uterus, cervix, fallopian tubes, and ovaries and is often referred to as a total abdominal hysterectomy with bilateral salpingectomy and oophorectomy (TAH–BSO). A radical hysterectomy is done to treat some cancers of the cervix. It involves removal of the uterus, cervix, ligaments, and part of the vagina as well as dissection of the pelvic lymph nodes.

A vaginal or abdominal approach can be used to perform a hysterectomy. Minimally invasive robotic surgery is also used to perform a hysterectomy. Not everyone is a candidate for minimally invasive surgery. The approach used depends on factors such as the woman's pelvic anatomy and size of the uterus, whether repairs to the vaginal wall or pelvic floor are needed, the presence of other medical conditions, previous abdominal surgeries, and the diagnosis.

This care plan focuses on the adult client hospitalized for a TAH with salpingectomy and oophorectomy.

OUTCOME/DISCHARGE CRITERIA

The client will:
1. Have evidence of normal healing of surgical wound
2. Have clear, audible breath sounds throughout lungs
3. Maintain adequate urine output
4. Have surgical pain controlled
5. Have no signs and symptoms of postoperative complications
6. Verbalize an understanding of the effects of surgical menopause
7. Identify ways to achieve sexual satisfaction
8. Verbalize an understanding of medications ordered including the rationale for the prescription, food and drug interactions, side effects, schedule for taking, and importance of taking as prescribed
9. State signs and symptoms to report to the health care provider
10. Share feelings about the loss of reproductive ability
11. Develop a plan for adhering to recommended follow-up care including future appointments with health care provider, activity limitations, and wound care

POSTOPERATIVE: USE IN CONJUNCTION WITH THE STANDARDIZED POSTOPERATIVE CARE PLAN

Nursing Diagnosis **URINARY RETENTION** NDx

Definition: Inability to empty bladder completely.

Related to:
- Obstruction of the urinary catheter
- Impaired urination after removal of catheter associated with:
  - Decreased perception of bladder fullness associated with the depressant effect of anesthesia and some medications (e.g., narcotic [opioid] analgesics)

- Increased tone of the urinary sphincters associated with sympathetic nervous system stimulation resulting from pain, fear, and anxiety
- Relaxation of the bladder muscle associated with nerve trauma and/or edema in the bladder area resulting from surgical manipulation; the depressant effect of anesthesia and some medications (e.g., narcotic [opioid] analgesics); stimulation of the sympathetic nervous system (can result from pain, fear, and anxiety)

CLINICAL MANIFESTATIONS

Subjective	Objective
Self-report of bladder fullness or suprapubic discomfort; inability to empty bladder	Bladder distention, absence of fluid in urinary drainage tubing, output that continues to be less than intake 48 hrs after surgery; frequent voiding of small amounts (25 to 60 mL) of urine

RISK FACTORS

- Surgery
- Medication regimen
- Age

DESIRED OUTCOMES

The client will not experience urinary retention as evidenced by:
a. No reports of bladder fullness and suprapubic discomfort
b. Absence of bladder distention
c. Balanced intake and output (I&O) within 48 hrs after surgery
d. Voiding adequate amounts at expected intervals after removal of the catheter

NOC OUTCOMES

Urinary elimination

NIC INTERVENTIONS

Urinary retention care; Urinary elimination management; Urinary catheterization; Urinary retention care

NURSING ASSESSMENT

Assess for and report signs and symptoms of urinary retention:
- Normal voiding pattern
- Verbal reports of bladder fullness or suprapubic discomfort
- Palpable bladder distention
- Absence of fluid in urinary drainage tubing
- Output that continues to be less than intake 48 hrs after surgery
- Frequent voiding of small amounts (20–60 mL) of urine
- Bladder scan of residual > 100 mL urine after voiding

RATIONALE

Early recognition of signs and symptoms of urinary retention allows for prompt intervention.

THERAPEUTIC INTERVENTIONS

Independent Actions
Implement measures to prevent urinary retention if client has a catheter:
- Keep drainage tubing free of kinks. **D** ● ✦

- Keep collection container below level of bladder. **D** ● ✦
- Anchor catheter tubing securely to prevent inadvertent removal. **D** ● ✦

RATIONALE

Actions help prevent urinary retention by maintaining patency of urinary catheter.
Promotes catheter drainage.
Prevents injury and in-and-out movement which decreases introduction of microbes.

THERAPEUTIC INTERVENTIONS	RATIONALE
After removal of catheter:	
• Instruct client to urinate when the urge is first felt.	*Actions help prevent urinary retention after removal of urinary catheter.*
• Promote actions that facilitate relaxation during voiding attempts.	*Relaxation of perineal muscles supports voiding efforts.*
• Provide privacy. **D** ● ✦	
• Hold a warm blanket against abdomen. **D** ● ✦	
• Run water in sink. **D** ● ✦	
• Pour warm water over perineum. **D** ● ✦	
• Allow client to assume a normal position for voiding if allowed. **D** ● ✦	
Consult physician if urinary retention persists or if actions fail to alleviate urinary retention.	*Notifying the physician allows for modification of the treatment plan.*

Nursing Diagnosis | RISK FOR INEFFECTIVE PERIPHERAL TISSUE PERFUSION NDx

Definition: Susceptible to a decrease in blood circulation to the periphery, which may compromise health.

Related to:
• Trauma to pelvic veins during surgery
• Venous stasis associated with:
  • Decreased activity
  • Increased blood viscosity that can result from decreased fluid volume
  • Pelvic congestion resulting from inflammation in the surgical area
  • Abdominal distention (the distended intestine may put pressure on the abdominal vessels)
  • Pressure on the pelvis and calf vessels during surgery if a vaginal approach was used
• Hypercoagulability associated with increased release of tissue thromboplastin into the blood from surgical trauma and hemoconcentration and increased blood viscosity from decreased fluid volume.

CLINICAL MANIFESTATIONS

Subjective	Objective
Self-report of pain and tenderness in lower extremities; and sudden onset of chest pain	Calf swelling; unusual warmth, and/or increase in calf diameter; decreased or absent peripheral pulses; coolness in extremities; decreased level of consciousness; increased restlessness; decreasing SaO_2

RISK FACTORS
• Immobility
• Age
• Smoking
• Inadequate fluid volume
• Surgery
• Decreased venous return

DESIRED OUTCOMES

The client will not develop decreased peripheral tissue perfusion as evidenced by:
a. Absence of pain, tenderness, swelling, and numbness in extremities
b. Usual temperature and color of extremities
c. Palpable peripheral pulses
d. Usual mental status
e. Usual sensory and motor function
f. Absence of sudden chest pain and dyspnea

NOC OUTCOMES

Circulation status; risk control: thrombus

NIC INTERVENTIONS

Tissue perfusion management; Fluid management

NDx = NANDA Diagnosis   **D** = Delegatable Action   ● = UAP   ✦ = LVN/LPN   ⊝▶ = Go to ⓔvolve for animation

NURSING ASSESSMENT	RATIONALE
Assess for impaired peripheral circulation:	*Early recognition of signs and symptoms of impaired peripheral circulation allows for prompt intervention.*
• Assess peripheral pulses and compare side to side	*Changes indicate possible impaired circulation.*
• Assess for pain, tenderness, swelling, unusual warmth or positive Homan sign in extremities	*Possible development of thrombus.*
• Assess for numbness, pallor, and coolness in extremities	*Possible indication of arterial insufficiency.*
• Assess for sudden onset of chest pain, dyspnea, increasing restlessness, apprehension	*Possible indication of thromboembolism.*
• Declining SaO_2 levels	

THERAPEUTIC INTERVENTIONS	RATIONALE
Independent Actions:	
• Monitor dressings and perineal pads, documenting amount of bleeding, color, amount, and odor of drainage.	*Increased blood on dressing and perineal pads and increased drainage may indicate potential for alterations in clotting and possible hemorrhage.*
• Support and encourage client with frequent turning, coughing, deep breathing and use of incentive spirometry every 2 hrs.	*Prevents stasis of respiratory secretions and promotes oxygenation to tissues.*
• Encourage ambulation as soon as possible.	
• When client is in bed, encourage range of motion exercises and food and leg exercises.	*Improves circulation and supports venous return to the heart. Helps to prevent venous stasis complications.*
• Encourage fluid intake, if not contraindicated.	*Enhances venous return and prevents venous stasis.*
• Avoid high-Fowler's positions and crossing legs when in bed or sitting.	*Supports vascular volume.*
	Prevents venous stasis and pooling of blood in pelvis and extremities
Dependent/Collaborative Actions:	
• Maintain adequate fluid volume of at least 2500 mL/day unless contraindicated.	*Adequate hydration supports circulating volume, reducing risk for thrombus formation.*
• Apply antiembolic stockings and/or sequential compression devices if client is inactive and on bedrest. **D ● ✦**	*Supports venous return to the heart and decreases venous stasis.*
• Notify health care provider if signs and symptoms of impaired peripheral perfusion occur.	*Allows for prompt alteration in treatment regimen.*

Nursing Diagnosis **RISK FOR SITUATIONAL LOW SELF-ESTEEM** NDx

Definition: Susceptible to developing a negative perception of self-worth in response to a current situation, which may compromise health.

Related to:
• Surgical procedure that removes ability to bear children
• Age of individual at time of surgery
• Number of children or desire to have children at time of surgery
• Change in sexual identity
• Change in femininity

CLINICAL MANIFESTATIONS

Subjective	Objective
Verbal self-report of feeling less than others due to loss of childbearing capabilities	N/A

RISK FACTORS

* Age
* Marital/partner status
* Religious beliefs

DESIRED OUTCOMES

The client will not experience situational self-esteem as evidenced by:
a. Verbalization of concerns and ways to address them
b. Verbalization of changed body/self-image
c. Engagement in care and interaction with significant others
d. Verbalization of acceptance of self and new body image

NOC OUTCOMES

Self-esteem enhancement

NIC INTERVENTIONS

Self-esteem monitoring

NURSING ASSESSMENT	RATIONALE
• Assess client's emotional status and changes in interactions with others • Assess client's willingness to discuss body-image changes.	*Early recognition of decreased self-esteem allows for prompt intervention.*

THERAPEUTIC INTERVENTIONS	RATIONALE

Independent Actions:

* Provide time to listen to client's concerns about changes in lifestyle and self-image.
* Determine meaning of the loss to client and significant other.
* Identify with client's coping mechanisms that have worked in the past and identification of new ones if client is interested.
* Provide accepting and open communication allowing client to discuss concerns about physical changes.
* Refer client to community services or support groups.

Provides an accepting environment for client to express concerns, hopes, and fears.
Provides opportunity to understand client's expectations and clarify any areas of concern or misunderstanding.
Helps to strengthen client's ability to deal with change and possibly add to currently used coping mechanisms.
Allows client to discuss feelings, fears, etc. without fear of judgment.

Provides for continuation of care.

Dependent/Collaborative Actions:

Request consultation for professional counseling.

Provides for continuum of care following discharge.

DISCHARGE TEACHING/CONTINUED CARE

Nursing Diagnosis **DEFICIENT KNOWLEDGE** NDx

Definition: Absence of cognitive information related to specific topic, or its acquisition.

CLINICAL MANIFESTATIONS

Subjective	Objective
Verbal self-report of inability to manage illness and/orto follow prescribed regimen; expresses concern about physical and functional changes	Inaccurate follow-through with instructions; inappropriate behavior; refusal to participate in care

RISK FACTORS

* Cognitive deficit
* Inability to care for self

NOC OUTCOMES

Knowledge: treatment regimen; prescribed activity; prescribed medications; sexual functioning

NIC INTERVENTIONS

Health system guidance; teaching: individual; prescribed medication; prescribed exercise; prescribed medication regimen; sexuality

NDx = NANDA Diagnosis   **D** = Delegatable Action   ● = UAP   ✦ = LVN/LPN   ⊖▶ = Go to ⊖volve for animation

NURSING ASSESSMENT	RATIONALE
Assess client's readiness and ability to learn. Assess meaning of illness to client.	*Early recognition of readiness to learn and meaning of illness to client allows for implementation of the appropriate teaching interventions.*

THERAPEUTIC INTERVENTIONS	RATIONALE

Desired Outcomes: The client will verbalize an understanding of the effects of surgical menopause.

Independent Actions

Reinforce the physician's explanation of surgical menopause and its possible effects (e.g., hot flashes, facial hair growth, decrease in vaginal lubrication, insomnia, fatigue, nervousness, palpitations, depression).	*Having a greater understanding of the physiological effects of surgery will aid the client in understanding potential effects of surgery and allow for time to grieve, develop effective coping skills, and seek out the social support necessary to adjust to the effects of surgery.*
Explain the probable effects of the surgery on sexual functioning (e.g., decreased libido, vaginal dryness, painful intercourse).	*Provides information to client on how physiological changes impact sexual functioning.*
Instruct client on methods available to address physical changes specific to sexual functioning.	*Assists client in identification of resources and methods to support sexual functioning and decrease impact of menopause changes.*

THERAPEUTIC INTERVENTIONS	RATIONALE

Desired Outcomes: The client will identify ways to achieve sexual satisfaction.

Independent Actions
Instruct client in ways to promote sexual satisfaction:

• Use a water-soluble lubricant in the vagina to prevent pain during intercourse.	*The amount of vaginal lubrication decreases as a result of the effects of surgically induced menopause.*
• Take hormone replacements (e.g., estrogen) as prescribed.	*Hormone replacement is not available from all health care providers. If client is interested in hormone replacement, they should discuss this with their health care provider.*
• Try different positions for intercourse to determine whether some positions are more comfortable than others.	*Provide accepting environment to allow client to explore various methods of obtaining sexual satisfaction for self and partner.*
Reinforce physician's instructions regarding when client can resume sexual intercourse (usually 4–6 weeks).	*Waiting to resume sexual intercourse provides time for appropriate healing.*

THERAPEUTIC INTERVENTIONS	RATIONALE

Desired Outcomes: The client will verbalize an understanding of medications ordered including rationale for prescription, food and drug interactions, side effects, schedule for taking, and importance of taking as prescribed.

Independent Actions

Explain the rationale for, side effects of, schedule for taking, and importance of taking hormone replacement therapy as prescribed.	*Taking medications as prescribed is important to achieve maximum benefits of therapy and prevent adverse effects. Understanding the purpose and side effects of medications improves adherence.*
Inform client of pertinent interactions between estrogen and other medications she is taking.	
Instruct client to inform physician of any other prescription and nonprescription medications she is taking and to inform all health care providers of medications being taken.	*Decreases potential for adverse drug effects.*

THERAPEUTIC INTERVENTIONS	RATIONALE

Desired Outcomes: The client will state signs and symptoms to report to the health care provider.

THERAPEUTIC INTERVENTIONS	RATIONALE

Independent Actions

Instruct the client to report these additional signs and symptoms:

- Foul-smelling vaginal discharge (it is normal to have an increased amount of discharge about 2 weeks postoperatively when internal sutures are absorbed).
- Heavy, bright-red vaginal bleeding or the passage of clots that are thumb-size or larger.
- Excessive depression or difficulty dealing with changes in body image.
- Excessive discomfort associated with effects of surgical menopause.
- Adverse reactions to estrogen replacement therapy.

These clinical manifestations are indications of infection, trauma, and other complications. These should be reported to the health care provider for modification of the treatment plan.

May require consultation with psychologist or other trained professional.

May require increased or change in pain medications or implementation of adjuvant methods of pain control/support.

THERAPEUTIC INTERVENTIONS	RATIONALE

Desired Outcomes: The client, in collaboration with the nurse, will develop a plan for adhering to recommended follow-up care including future appointments with health care provider, activity limitations, and wound care.

Independent Actions

Collaborate with the client in developing a plan to implement physician's discharge instructions.

- Client should understand activity restrictions and importance of increasing activity over time.
- Avoid lifting objects over 10 pounds, sitting for long periods, stair climbing, and strenuous physical activity (e.g., vacuuming, aerobics) for 6 to 8 weeks postoperatively.
- Avoid driving for at least a week after surgery.

Avoid douching, using tampons, tub baths and having sexual intercourse for 4 to 6 weeks postoperatively.

- Stress importance of increasing fiber and fluid in diet.
- Stress importance of maintenance of appropriate complex carbohydrates, protein, and low fat in diet.

Reinforce importance of keeping follow-up appointments with the health care provider.

Implement measures to improve client adherence:

- Include significant others in teaching sessions if possible.
- Encourage questions and allow time for reinforcement and clarification of information.
- Provide written instructions.

Adhering to a prescribed treatment plan helps promote positive outcomes and prevents complications.

Client may become easily fatigued and should be aware that this is normal. The client should plan gradual resumption of activities.

Avoiding heavy lifting allows for appropriate physical healing.

Prevents strain on surgical area.

Decreases potential for vaginal or incisional infections.

Prevention of constipation and potential straining with a bowel movement. Straining could cause increased bleeding and delay healing time.

Nutritional intake including protein promotes healing.

Follow-up appointments are important to monitor progress.

Involving the client's significant other improves client adherence to treatment regimen.

ADDITIONAL CARE PLANS

ACUTE PAIN NDx
Related to:
- Tissue trauma and reflex muscle spasms associated with the surgical procedure

DISTURBED BODY IMAGE NDx
Related to:
- Loss of reproductive organs with subsequent inability to bear children
- Feeling of loss of femininity and sexuality

GRIEVING NDx
Related to:
- Loss of reproductive ability, early menopause, diagnosis of cancer (if present), and the possibility of premature death

RISK FOR INFECTION NDx
Related to:
- Wound contamination associated with introduction of pathogens during or following surgery
- Decreased resistance to infection associated with factors such as age and an inadequate nutritional status
- Increased growth and colonization of microorganisms associated with urinary stasis
- Introduction of pathogens associated with the presence of an indwelling catheter

MASTECTOMY

A mastectomy is the surgical removal of all or part of the breast. It is most commonly conducted to treat breast cancer. The type of mastectomy is based on factors such as the location, type, and size of the tumor; the number of tumors; breast size; axillary lymph node status; whether the client has received prior irradiation of the breast; and client preference. The two major types of surgeries performed to treat breast cancer are a modified radical mastectomy and breast-conserving surgery (e.g., lumpectomy, quadrantectomy).

A modified radical mastectomy includes removal of the breast and an axillary node dissection. The pectoral muscles and surrounding nerves are left intact. This allows the client to retain the shape of her breast and avoid the shoulder and arm limitations and skin graft requirements that accompany a radical mastectomy. Leaving the muscles and nerves intact facilitates reconstructive surgery, which may be performed at the time of the mastectomy or delayed for several months, depending on physician and client preference and additional treatment planned.

Post breast surgery, additional treatment (e.g., chemotherapy, hormone therapy, external radiation therapy) may be considered after a modified radical mastectomy. Treatment depends on factors such as the immunological and menopausal status of the client, tumor type and size, and amount of lymph node involvement.

Breast-conserving surgery is an option for many women with stage I or stage II breast cancer. It involves excision of the tumor, a surrounding margin of normal tissue, and an axillary lymph node dissection. It is often followed by a course of radiation therapy to eradicate any residual tumor and reduce the risk for tumor recurrence.

Axillary node dissection has traditionally been performed with all invasive breast cancer to stage the tumor. Sentinel node biopsy (lymphatic mapping) is used to identify axillary node involvement and avoid unnecessary lymph node dissection. This procedure can be done the day of surgery. If the sentinel node is negative for cancer cells, an axillary dissection is not necessary, which eliminates the need for axillary drains and reduces the risk for lymphedema.

This care plan focuses on the female adult client hospitalized for a modified radical mastectomy. Much of the postoperative information is applicable to clients receiving follow-up care in a home setting.

OUTCOME/DISCHARGE CRITERIA

The client will:
1. Have evidence of normal healing of surgical wounds
2. Maintain clear, audible breath sounds throughout lungs
3. Maintain adequate surgical pain relief
4. Have no signs and symptoms of postoperative complications
5. Identify ways to reduce the risk of trauma to and infection in the arm on the operative side
6. Identify ways to prevent and treat lymphedema of the arm on the operative side
7. Demonstrate the ability to care for wound drainage device if present
8. Demonstrate the ability to perform the prescribed exercises and verbalize an understanding of additional exercises to be done once the incision has healed
9. Verbalize the importance of and demonstrate the ability to perform a breast self-examination (BSE) on the remaining breast and operative site
10. State the factors to consider in selecting a breast prosthesis
11. State signs and symptoms to report to the health care provider
12. Share thoughts and feelings about the change in body image
13. Identify community resources that can assist with adjustment to the diagnosis of cancer and the loss of a breast
14. Develop a plan for adhering to recommended follow-up care including future appointments with health care provider, medications prescribed, activity level, wound care, and plans for subsequent treatment

PREOPERATIVE: USE IN CONJUNCTION WITH THE STANDARDIZED PREOPERATIVE CARE PLAN

Nursing Diagnosis **DEFICIENT KNOWLEDGE** NDx

Definition: Absence of cognitive information related to a specific topic, or its acquisition.

Related to:
- Surgical procedure
- Changes in body image
- Diagnosis that required surgical intervention
- Postoperative care

CLINICAL MANIFESTATIONS

Subjective	Objective
Verbalization of a lack of understanding of what is going to occur	Exaggerated behaviors

RISK FACTORS

- Unfamiliar environment
- Anxiety about the future
- Barriers in culture or communication
- Diagnosis

DESIRED OUTCOMES

The client will:
- Verbalize an understanding of the surgical procedure, preoperative care, and postoperative sensations and care
- Demonstrate the ability to perform activities designed to prevent postoperative complications

NOC OUTCOMES

Knowledge: disease process; treatment regimen

NIC INTERVENTIONS

Teaching: preoperative; teaching: individual; teaching: prescribed exercise

NURSING ASSESSMENT

Assess client's readiness and ability to learn.
Assess meaning of illness to client.

RATIONALE

Early recognition of readiness to learn and meaning of illness to client allows for implementation of the appropriate teaching interventions.

THERAPEUTIC INTERVENTIONS

Independent Actions

Provide the following information about sensations that may occur after a mastectomy:

- Explain to client that it is common to have sensations of pain, numbness, and tingling in the operative area (these sensations usually subside over time and may last for a year).
- Assure client that the sense that both breasts are present and phantom breast sensation is common.
- Explain to client that she may feel a change in balance at first, particularly if breasts are large.

Provide additional instructions regarding ways to prevent complications after a mastectomy:

- Inform the client that she must keep upper arm on operative side close to her body for a few days after surgery (length of time will vary according to physician preference).
- Demonstrate recommended postmastectomy exercises (e.g., squeezing a ball, flexion and extension of the fingers and wrist, wall climbing, rope pulley exercises, arm swings, rope turning); inform client that hand and wrist exercises are usually begun the day after surgery with gradual progression to full range-of-motion exercises of arm and shoulder on operative side when incision has healed.

Instruct client on ways to minimize or prevent lymphedema of the arm on operative side:

- Keep arm on operative side elevated on pillows with elbow above heart level and hand higher than elbow in the early postoperative period.
- Perform recommended postmastectomy exercises as soon as allowed.
- Avoid having BP measurements, injections, blood draws, and intravenous infusions in arm on operative side.

RATIONALE

Clients vary in physical and cognitive ability to learn. When educating clients, nurses need to determine a client's ability to read and understand written materials. If literacy barriers are present, alternative educational materials should be provided. Allow time for questions, clarification, and return demonstration of any learned actions.

Prevents tension on the suture lines and subsequent hematoma formation and seroma formation.

These are essential to facilitate and improve lymphatic and blood circulation, maintain muscle tone, and prevent contractures.

Supports lymphatic drainage.

These procedures increase the risk of infection or trauma and subsequent lymphedema.

POSTOPERATIVE: USE IN CONJUNCTION WITH THE STANDARDIZED POSTOPERATIVE CARE PLAN

Nursing Diagnosis ACUTE PAIN NDx (CHEST AND ARM ON OPERATIVE SIDE)

Definition: Unpleasant sensory and emotional experience associated with actual or potential tissue damage, or described in terms of such damage (International Association for the Study of Pain); sudden or slow onset of any intensity from mild to severe with an anticipated or predictable end, and a duration of less than 3 months.

Related to:
- Tissue trauma and reflex muscle spasms associated with surgery
- Irritation from drainage tubes
- Strain on the surgical area postoperatively

CLINICAL MANIFESTATIONS

Subjective	Objective
Verbal self-report of pain	Grimacing; reluctance to move; restlessness; diaphoresis; increased BP; tachycardia; dyspnea

RISK FACTORS
- Surgical procedure
- Fear and anxiety

DESIRED OUTCOMES

The client will experience diminished pain in the chest and arm on the operative side as evidenced by:
a. Verbalization of a decrease in or absence of pain
b. Relaxed facial expression and body positioning
c. Increased participation in activities
d. Stable vital signs

NOC OUTCOMES

Pain control; comfort level; pain: adverse psychological reaction

NIC INTERVENTIONS

Pain management; analgesic administration

NURSING ASSESSMENT	RATIONALE
Assess for and report signs and symptoms of pain: • Verbalization of pain • Grimacing • Reluctance to move • Restlessness • Diaphoresis • Increased BP • Tachycardia • Dyspnea	*Early recognition of signs and symptoms of pain allows for prompt intervention.*

THERAPEUTIC INTERVENTIONS	RATIONALE

Independent Actions

Assess pain using a standardized pain scale that includes location, duration, frequency, and intensity of pain.

Provides for a baseline of experienced pain and a standardized method for communication to the health care team.

Discuss phantom breast pain.

Assure client that sensations are occurring and discuss the physiological reasons they occur. Assure client it is not just their imagination. They will be treated accordingly.

Perform actions that will help prevent or alleviate pain:
- Place client in a semi-Fowler's position during the immediate postoperative period.

Actions help reduce pain in the chest and arm on the operative side.

- Elevate the arm on the operative side on pillows, keeping elbow above the level of the heart and hand higher than the elbow. **D** ✦

Improves vascular and lymph return and decreases extremity edema.

THERAPEUTIC INTERVENTIONS	RATIONALE
• Do not use arm on the operative side for intravenous therapy, blood draws, injections, and BP measurements. **D** ● ✦	*Actions help decrease tension on the incision, promote circulation, and prevent venous congestion in affected arm. Also prevents potential for infection and decreased lymphatic return.*
• Move the operative extremity gently. **D** ● ✦	*Movement may increase client's pain.*
• Reinforce the importance of adhering to arm and shoulder movement restrictions.	*Decreases pain, and supports venous and lymphatic return.*
• Maintain patency of wound drainage system (e.g., prevent kinking of tubing, empty collection device as needed, maintain suction as ordered, keep collection device below surgical wound). **D** ● ✦	*Actions help prevent fluid accumulation in the operative site, thereby reducing pain.*
• Securely anchor drainage tubes and collection device.	*Prevents in-and-out movement of tube that decreases potential for injury and potential for the introduction of bacteria.*
• If a sling is ordered, apply it to the client's arm before client gets out of bed.	*Action reduces pain by supporting the affected arm and reducing strain on the surgical site.*
• Instruct client to get out of bed on the unaffected side.	*Action helps reduce pain by reducing strain on the surgical site. Action promotes the use of the unaffected arm rather than the arm on the operative side.*
• Place needed items within easy reach.	*Prevents stretching/straining to reach desired object.*
Provide nonpharmacologic measures to decrease pain: guided imagery, relaxation exercises, distraction—listening to music, watching TV	*Promotes relaxation, refocuses attention, and augments clients current coping mechanisms while implementing new ones.*
Dependent/Collaborative Actions	
Administer analgesics as ordered:	*Opioid, non-opioid analgesics, and NSAIDs are used for pain relief.*
• Opioid analgesics	
• Non-opioid analgesics	
• Nonsteroidal anti-inflammatory agents (NSAIDs)	
Consult appropriate health care provider if above measures fail to provide adequate pain relief.	*Notifying the appropriate health care provider allows for modification of the treatment plan.*

Nursing Diagnosis RISK FOR PERIPHERAL NEUROVASCULAR DYSFUNCTION NDx

Definition: Susceptible to disruption in the circulation, sensation, and motion of an extremity, which may compromise health.

Related to: Chronic swelling or feeling of tightness in the arm or hand due to an accumulation of lymphatic fluid in the soft tissue of the arm
Interruption in usual lymph flow associated with surgical removal of axillary lymph nodes and channels, edema in the operative area, and infection of or trauma to operative arm

CLINICAL MANIFESTATIONS

Subjective	Objective
Self-report of numbness, tingling, pain, sensation of heaviness or tightness or weakness, or decreased movement in affected arm	Edema (measure arm on operative side at points 5 to 10 cm above and below elbow); decreased or inability to move arm on the surgical side Diminished pulses in arm; pallor or cyanosis

RISK FACTORS
- Surgical procedure
- Exposure to pathogens
- Age

DESIRED OUTCOMES

The client will not develop ineffective peripheral tissue perfusion or neurovascular changes of the arm on the operative side as evidenced by:
a. Absence or gradual resolution of numbness, tingling, and weakness of the arm
b. Absence of pain and feeling of heaviness and tightness in the arm
c. Absence of edema in the arm
d. Capillary refill < 2 to 3 seconds
e. Extremity maintains usual warmth and color
f. No decrease in movement of affected arm

NOC OUTCOMES

Tissue perfusion: peripheral

NIC INTERVENTIONS

Circulatory care: arterial insufficiency; circulatory care: venous insufficiency; positioning; upper extremity monitoring

NURSING ASSESSMENT

Assess for and report signs and symptoms of ineffective peripheral tissue perfusion of the arm on the operative side:
- Verbal reports of numbness, tingling, pain, sensation of heaviness or tightness or weakness or paralysis in affected arm
- Capillary >2 to 3 seconds
- Edema (measure arm on operative side at points 5–10 cm above and below elbow)
- Peripheral pulses

RATIONALE

Early recognition of signs and symptoms of ineffective peripheral tissue perfusion or neurovascular changes allows for prompt intervention.

THERAPEUTIC INTERVENTIONS

Independent Actions
Monitor the 6 P's of neurovascular changes:
- Pain: Assess using a pain scale including severity, quality, intensity, radiation, and onset of new and different pain.

- Pulses: Monitor and document pulses on the upper extremity on the surgical side; use a rating scale for intensity of palpable pulses.
- Paresthesia: Assess sensations on the upper extremity on the surgical side. Ask client about changes in sensation. Report any "pins and needles" feelings.
- Pallor: Assess capillary refill, color, and warmth of the upper extremity on the surgical side. Track findings over time and report any decline in findings.
- Paralysis: Ask client to squeeze nurse's hand; note decrease in movement or inability to perform.
- Pressure or edema: Assess for changes in firmness or swelling of the surgical side extremity.

Perform actions to prevent ineffective tissue perfusion:
- Place client in a semi-Fowler's position during the immediate postoperative period.
- Elevate arm on the operative side on pillows, keeping elbow above the level of the heart and hand higher than elbow. **D** ✦
- Place a sign above bed to remind personnel not to use arm on operative side for intravenous therapy, blood draws, injections, and BP measurements. **D** ● ✦

RATIONALE

An increase in pain or inability to control pain with medication and increased pain experienced with passive movement may indicate compartmental syndrome.
Change in pulses within injured limb and differences noted between injured and noninjured limb may indicate changes in blood flow to distal to the injury.
Decreased feeling or "pins and needles" feeling report by client may indicate nerve damage and/or indicate compartmental syndrome.
Irreversible damage may occur if not resolved. Decreasing color, capillary refill time, and warmth to the extremity indicates arterial insufficiency and should receive immediate intervention.
Decreased movement or no movement is indicative of compartment syndrome and requires timely intervention.
Edema or increased tightness of the skin correlates with increased internal pressure on the muscles and tissues and is indicative of compromised circulation on the upper extremity on the surgical side.

Measures help prevent lymphedema of arm on operative side.

Enhances lymph and venous return to the heart.

Actions help decrease risk of infection or trauma and subsequent lymphedema.

THERAPEUTIC INTERVENTIONS	RATIONALE

Perform actions to prevent wound infection:
- Instruct and assist client to perform postmastectomy exercises as soon as allowed.

Actions help promote lymphatic drainage.

Dependent/Collaborative Actions

If signs and symptoms of lymphedema occur:
- Notify the appropriate health care provider.
- Apply an elastic pressure gradient sleeve to the affected arm if ordered to reduce edema.
- Assist and instruct client in manual massage of the affected arm and/or use of sequential compression device on affected arm if ordered.
- Administer antimicrobial agents if ordered.

Notifying the appropriate health care provider allows for modification of the treatment plan.

Medications help prevent or treat cellulitis and lymphangitis.

Nursing Diagnosis IMPAIRED PHYSICAL MOBILITY NDx

Definition: Limitation in independent, purposeful movement of the body or of one or more extremities.

Related to: Transection of or trauma to the nerves during surgery; pressure on nerves associated with lymphedema if it occurs; nonadherence with prescribed exercise program

CLINICAL MANIFESTATIONS

Subjective	**Objective**
Reports of new or increased numbness, tingling, or weakness in arm	Inability to move joints through expected range of motion

RISK FACTORS	DESIRED OUTCOMES

RISK FACTORS
- Surgery
- Fatigue
- Edema

DESIRED OUTCOMES

The client will have expected mobility of the arm and shoulder on the operative side as evidenced by:
a. Ability to put hand, arm, and shoulder through expected range of motion
b. No reports of new or increased numbness, tingling, or weakness in arm

NOC OUTCOMES	NIC INTERVENTIONS
Mobility status	Mobility monitoring

NURSING ASSESSMENT	RATIONALE

Assess for and report signs and symptoms of motor and/or physical impairment of the arm and shoulder on operative side:
- Reports of new or increased numbness, tingling, change in sensations, or weakness in arm from surgical side
- Inability to move joints through expected range of motion
- Capillary refill <2 to 3 seconds

Early recognition of signs and symptoms of impaired physical mobility allows for prompt intervention.

THERAPEUTIC INTERVENTIONS	RATIONALE

Independent Actions

Perform actions to prevent lymphedema:
- Initiate postmastectomy exercises as soon as allowed.

Measures help prevent arm and shoulder dysfunction. Interventions aimed at prevention of lymphedema reduce pressure on surrounding nerves.

NDx = NANDA Diagnosis   **D** = Delegatable Action   ● = UAP   ✦ = LVN/LPN   ⊖▶ = Go to ⊖volve for animation

Continued...

THERAPEUTIC INTERVENTIONS	RATIONALE
• Encourage use of arm on operative side to perform activities of daily living as soon as allowed, such as feeding, combing hair, washing face • Assist with ambulation when able and range-of-motion exercises if on bed rest.	*Improves circulation, decreases edema, improves muscle strength, and enhances ability to care for self. Exercises help to strengthen muscles.*

Dependent/collaborative Actions

Administer medications as ordered:
- Analgesics
- Diuretics

If signs and symptoms of impaired arm or shoulder function occur, consult occupational therapist or physical therapist.

Rationale

Analgesics decrease pain and should be given before exercises.
Diuretics help to decrease edema.
Prompt notification of changes allows for modification of treatment regimen.

Collaborative Diagnosis **IMPAIRED TISSUE INTEGRITY** NDx

Definition: Damage to mucous membrane, cornea, integumentary system, muscular fascia, muscle, tendon, bone, cartilage, joint capsule, and/or ligament.

Related to: Delayed or impaired flap adherence associated with irregular shape of chest wall, impaired wound drainage, and excessive movement of operative area with arm and shoulder use

CLINICAL MANIFESTATIONS

Subjective	Objective
N/A	Unusual swelling around incision site, less than expected amount of drainage in collection device, continued drainage from incision

RISK FACTORS
- Ineffective therapeutic regimen
- Excessive movement of upper extremities
- Age

DESIRED OUTCOMES

The client will not develop impairment of skin integrity at the surgical site as evidenced by:
a. No unusual swelling around incision
b. Expected amount of wound drainage in collection device
c. Absence of continued drainage from incision

NOC OUTCOMES

Skin integrity; wound healing: primary intention

NIC INTERVENTIONS

Skin surveillance; wound monitoring

NURSING ASSESSMENT	RATIONALE
Assess for and report signs and symptoms of seroma formation: • Unusual swelling around incision site • Less than expected amount of drainage in collection device • Continued drainage from incision	*Early recognition of signs and symptoms of seroma formation allows for prompt intervention.*

THERAPEUTIC INTERVENTIONS	RATIONALE
Independent Actions Implement measures to promote healing: • Maintain compression dressing over operative site if one is in place. **D** ✦	*Action helps promote skin flap adherence so that fluid cannot accumulate in any dead space beneath the flap.*

THERAPEUTIC INTERVENTIONS	**RATIONALE**
• Maintain patency of wound drainage system (e.g., prevent kinking of tubing, empty collection device as needed, keep collection device below surgical wound, maintain suction as ordered). **D** ✦	*Prevents blockage and helps to promote drainage and helps to decrease edema.*
• Place needed items within easy reach to prevent excessive arm and shoulder movement. **D** ● ✦	*Decreases stretching of arms, which decreases wound healing.*
• If a sling is ordered, apply it to client's arm before client gets out of bed.	*Supports the arm and reduces strain on the surgical site.*
• Reinforce importance of adhering to arm and shoulder movement restrictions.	*Decreases strain/pulling at the surgical site.*
• Encourage appropriate diet with complex carbohydrates and quality proteins.	*Promotes wound healing.*
• Encourage ambulation and frequent position changes.	*Promotes circulation and decreases risk of immobility and potential skin breakdown.*
• Use aseptic/sterile technique with dressing changes.	*Prevents cross contamination.*
• Encourage adequate rest and sleep.	*Helps to promote healing and decreases fatigue.*

Dependent/Collaborative Actions

If tissue breakdown occurs or seroma formation occurs:

• Notify the appropriate health care provider.	*Notifying the appropriate health care provider allows for modification of the treatment plan.*
• Prepare client for needle aspiration of fluid if hematoma or seroma occurs.	
• Assist with application of compression dressing if not already present.	*Protects surgical wound and surrounding tissues.*
• Administer antimicrobials if ordered.	*Treatment of infections.*

Nursing Diagnosis **DISTURBED SELF-CONCEPT***

Definitions: Disturbed Body Image NDx: Confusion in mental picture of one's physical self; **Situational Low Self-Esteem NDx:** Development of a negative perception of self-worth in response to a current situation; **Grieving NDx:** A normal, complex process that includes emotional, physical, spiritual, social, and intellectual responses and behaviors by which individuals, families, and communities incorporate an actual, anticipated, or perceived loss into their daily lives.

Related to: Loss of a breast; temporary dependence on others for assistance with self-care associated with restricted arm movement; possible altered sexuality patterns associated with decreased libido, perceived loss of femininity, and fear of rejection by partner

CLINICAL MANIFESTATIONS

Subjective	**Objective**
Verbalization of negative feelings about self	Lack of participation in activities of daily living, refusal to look at mastectomy site, withdrawal from significant others; frequent crying

RISK FACTORS

- Surgical procedure
- Loss of image of self
- Age

DESIRED OUTCOMES

The client will demonstrate beginning adaptation to the loss of her breast and integration of the change in body image as evidenced by:
a. Verbalization of feelings of self-worth and sexual adequacy
b. Active participation in activities of daily living
c. Willingness to look at surgical site
d. Maintenance of relationships with significant others

---

*The nurse should select the diagnostic label that is most appropriate for the client.

NDx = NANDA Diagnosis   **D** = Delegatable Action   ● = UAP   ✦ = LVN/LPN   ⊝▶ = Go to ⊝volve for animation

NOC OUTCOMES	NIC INTERVENTIONS
Body image; self-esteem; psychosocial adjustment: life change; sexual functioning; sexual identity	Body-image enhancement; grief work facilitation; self-esteem enhancement; role enhancement; counseling: emotional support; support system enhancement; sexual counseling

NURSING ASSESSMENT	RATIONALE
Assess for signs and symptoms of a disturbed self-concept: • Verbalization of negative feelings about self • Lack of participation in activities of daily living • Refusal to look at mastectomy site • Withdrawal from significant others • Expression of concern about personal sexuality	*Early recognition of signs and symptoms of disturbed self-concept allows for prompt intervention.*

THERAPEUTIC INTERVENTIONS	RATIONALE

Independent Actions

Implement measures to facilitate the grieving process:

Assist the client to identify and use coping techniques that have been helpful in the past.

Discuss grieving process and assist client to accept the phases of grieving as an expected response to loss of breast tissue.

Allow client to verbalize expressions of anger and/or sadness about changes in body image and self-concept. Involve partner/significant other in discussion if client is willing.

Implement measures to facilitate client's adjustment to the effects of the loss of a breast on her sexuality:

• Facilitate communication between client and partner; focus on feelings the couple share and assist them to identify factors that may affect their sexual relationship.

• Arrange for uninterrupted privacy during hospital stay if desired by the couple.

• Assist client with usual grooming and makeup habits.

• Demonstrate acceptance of client using techniques such as touch and frequent visits.

• Encourage significant others to visit frequently and to use touch when interacting with the client.

• Stay with client during first dressing change and encourage her to express feelings about appearance of incision and change in body. If the client is reluctant to look at the surgical site, provide support and encouragement to do so before discharge.

• Encourage client's participation in activities that can assist her to integrate the physical change that has occurred (e.g., exercise, grooming, bathing, wound care).

If breast reconstruction has not been performed:

• Encourage client to discuss possibilities for future reconstruction of breast with physician if desired.

• Discuss the variety of prostheses available and ways to obtain one.

• Assist client's and significant others' adjustment by listening, facilitating communication, and providing information.

• Support behaviors suggesting positive adaptation to the loss of a breast (e.g., willingness to look at and care for wound, compliance with exercise program, maintenance of relationships with significant others).

A change in body appearance can initiate a grieving response. Resolution of grief assists the client to accept changes experienced and integrate the changes into self-concept.

Involving partner in care of the client can help facilitate partner's adjustment to the change in client's appearance and subsequently decrease the possibility of partner's rejection of client.

Allows for discussions in safe, supportive environment.

Engages client in self-care and may help improve acceptance of body changes.

Establishes trust with client.

Allows client to visualize a more "normal" future.

Provides support to client. Maintain an accepting countenance when working with client.

Enhances self-care ability, improves circulation, and increases muscle strength. Increases client's confidence in ability to care for self.

Explores options available for client following healing process.

Provides client/family support following discharge from acute care facility.

Enhances ability to work through grieving process.

THERAPEUTIC INTERVENTIONS	RATIONALE
• Reinforce the temporary nature of operative side arm movement restrictions.	*Prevents injury.*
• Encourage client contact with others so that she can test and establish a new self-image.	
• Encourage visits and support from significant others.	*Helps client to feel supported and accepted by significant others.*
• Encourage client to pursue usual roles and interests and to continue involvement in social activities.	
• Provide information about and encourage use of community agencies and support groups (e.g., Reach to Recovery; sexual, family, and individual counseling services).	*Helps client understand that life goes on and supports her ability to maintain engagement in things the client likes to do.* *Provides for continuum of care and support from individuals who have experienced a mastectomy.*

Dependent/Collaborative Actions

Consult appropriate health care provider (e.g., psychiatric nurse clinician, physician) if client seems unwilling or unable to adapt to the loss of her breast.	*Notifying the appropriate health care provider allows for modification of the treatment plan.*

DISCHARGE TEACHING/CONTINUED CARE

Nursing Diagnosis ## DEFICIENT KNOWLEDGE NDx; INEFFECTIVE HEALTH MANAGEMENT NDx*

Definition: **Deficient Knowledge NDx:** Absence or deficiency of cognitive information related to specific topic or its acquisition; **Ineffective Health Management NDx:** Pattern of regulating and integrating into daily living a therapeutic regimen for the treatment of illness and its sequelae that is unsatisfactory for meeting specific health goals.

CLINICAL MANIFESTATIONS

Subjective	**Objective**
Verbalizes inability to manage illness and inability to follow prescribed regimen	Inaccurate follow-through with instructions; inappropriate behavior; refusal to participate in care

RISK FACTORS
- Cognitive deficit
- Failure to reduce risk factors
- Inability to care for self
- Unfamiliar with resources
- Economically disadvantaged
- Lack of social support

NOC OUTCOMES	NIC INTERVENTIONS
Knowledge: disease process; treatment regimen; treatment procedure(s); health resources; sexual functioning; sexual identity	Health system guidance; teaching: individual; teaching: disease process; teaching: prescribed exercise; teaching: prescribed medication; teaching: psychomotor skill; teaching: sexuality; sexual counseling

NURSING ASSESSMENT	RATIONALE
Assess client's readiness and ability to learn. Assess meaning of illness to client.	*Early recognition of readiness to learn and meaning of illness to client allows for implementation of the appropriate teaching interventions.*

*The nurse should select the diagnostic label that is most appropriate for the client's discharge teaching needs.

NDx = NANDA Diagnosis   **D** = Delegatable Action   ● = UAP   ✦ = LVN/LPN   ℮▶ = Go to ℮volve for animation

THERAPEUTIC INTERVENTIONS	RATIONALE

Desired Outcome: The client will identify ways to reduce the risk of trauma to and infection in the arm on the operative side.

Independent Actions

Provide the following instructions:

* Avoid cuts by pushing cuticles back instead of cutting them and trimming fingernails carefully.
* Wear heavy work gloves when gardening and rubber gloves when in contact with steel wool, harsh chemicals, abrasive compounds, or water for prolonged periods.
* Wear insulated gloves when reaching into a hot oven or handling hot items.
* Use a thimble when sewing to avoid pinpricks.
* Keep pressure off the affected arm (e.g., avoid wearing tight jewelry and clothes with constricting bands, carry heavy objects such as purse or packages with the unaffected arm).
* Offer only the unaffected arm for blood pressure readings, injections, blood drawing, and intravenous therapy.
* Wash any break in the skin on the affected arm with soap and water and cover the area with a protective dressing.
* Use an electric rather than a straight-edge razor when shaving underarm area.
* Use insect repellant when in an area where stinging or biting insects may be located.
* Avoid prolonged exposure to the sun to prevent burns.

Actions help reduce the risk of trauma to and infection in the arm on operative side.

Prevents exposure to new bacteria.

Prevents injury and potential for infection.

Promotes circulation and lymph drainage.

Helps to maintains skin integrity and decreases potential for cross-contamination.
Prevention of injury and risk for bleeding.

THERAPEUTIC INTERVENTIONS	RATIONALE

Desired Outcome: The client will identify ways to prevent and treat lymphedema of the arm on the operative side.

Independent Actions

Instruct client in ways to prevent lymphedema of the arm on operative side:

* Elevate the affected arm on pillows for 30 to 45 minutes at least 3 times a day for the prescribed length of time (usually 6–12 weeks).
* Sleep on unaffected side or back with affected arm elevated for the prescribed length of time (usually 6–12 weeks).
* Avoid placing the affected extremity in a dependent position for extended periods.

Reinforce physician's instructions regarding ways to treat lymphedema if present:

* Perform manual massage of the affected arm if prescribed.
* Wear an elastic pressure gradient sleeve as recommended.

These actions help facilitate lymph drainage by gravity.

Prevents development of edema.

These actions decrease lymphedema and promotes lymph return.

THERAPEUTIC INTERVENTIONS	RATIONALE

Desired Outcomes: The client will demonstrate the ability to care for wound drainage device if present.

Independent Actions

If the client is to be discharged with wound drain(s) and a suction device, demonstrate how to empty and establish negative pressure in the collection device and provide these additional instructions:

* Keep the collection device positioned below the insertion site.

Proper wound care is necessary to prevent infection and promote optimum wound healing. Allow time for return demonstration to assess client understanding of instructions and the need for further education.
Decreases edema, stasis of fluid, and potential for infection.

THERAPEUTIC INTERVENTIONS	RATIONALE
• Keep the tubing pinned to the dressing and avoid kinks and strain on the tubing.	*Monitor changes in drainage, as this may indicate a change in condition. Increases or change in consistency or color should be reported to the health care provider.*
• Empty the collection device at least twice daily or more often if needed.	
• Keep a record of the amount of drainage (drains will typically be removed once the drainage is <20–30 mL in 24 hrs).	

THERAPEUTIC INTERVENTIONS	RATIONALE

Desired Outcomes: The client will demonstrate the ability to perform the prescribed exercises and verbalize an understanding of additional exercises to be done once the incision has healed.

Independent Actions

Reinforce teaching about postmastectomy exercises:	
• Emphasize the need to perform hand and elbow exercises regularly and begin full range-of-motion exercises of the arm and shoulder once the incision has healed.	*Postoperative exercises are necessary to prevent contraction and promote return of optimum range of motion.*
• Encourage appropriate diet with complex carbohydrates and quality proteins.	*Appropriate nutrition is required to provide energy for activities and to promote healing.*
• Encourage client to maintain adequate fluid intake.	*Supports circulatory volume*
• Encourage client to maintain adequate rest/sleep pattern.	*Provides energy to maintain exercise regimen and decreases incidence of fatigue.*

THERAPEUTIC INTERVENTIONS	RATIONALE

Desired Outcomes: The client will verbalize the importance of and demonstrate the ability to perform a BSE on the remaining breast and operative site.

Independent Actions

Explain the reasons for monthly BSE of the remaining breast and operative site.	*Performance of preventative screening measures at regular intervals can alert clients to findings that require further evaluation by a health care provider.*
• Explore with client ways to remember to carry out BSE. The examination should be done a week after conclusion of menses or on a specific date if postmenopausal.	
• Demonstrate, using a model, film, or chart, how to do a BSE.	

THERAPEUTIC INTERVENTIONS	RATIONALE

Desired Outcomes: The client will state the factors to consider in selecting a breast prosthesis.

Independent Actions

If acceptable to client, invite a Reach to Recovery volunteer or prosthetist to share information about the various prostheses available.	*Selection of a prosthetic will be a very personal choice by the client and including members of a social support network may facilitate appropriate selection.*
Suggest that client wear a soft, temporary prosthesis until complete healing of the incision has occurred.	
Encourage the client to take significant other or a close friend with her for the initial fitting of the prosthesis in order to provide emotional support.	
Emphasize that it is important to select or make a prosthesis that will balance the chest to avoid difficulties with posture and subsequent back, shoulder, and neck discomfort.	

NDx = NANDA Diagnosis　　**D** = Delegatable Action　　● = UAP　　✦ = LVN/LPN　　⊙▶ = Go to ⊖volve　for animation

THERAPEUTIC INTERVENTIONS	RATIONALE

Desired Outcomes: The client will state signs and symptoms to report to the health care provider.

Independent Actions

Instruct client to report these additional signs and symptoms:

- New or increased sensations of numbness, tingling, heaviness, or tightness in hand, arm, or shoulder on operative side.
- Increasing weakness of the affected arm.
- Decreased ability to move shoulder or arm on operative side (full range of motion should be regained within 3–6 months).
- Warmth or redness of the affected arm.
- Increase in size of arm on affected side (client may be instructed to measure arm circumference weekly at points about 2–4 inches above and below elbow and compare with unaffected arm); inform client that transient edema may occur as she increases use of the affected arm and that this should subside as collateral lymphatic circulation develops.
- Increased swelling around incision(s).
- Purulent, foul-smelling drainage from incision site(s) or wound drain insertion site.
- Dressings that become saturated with drainage more than once a day.
- Unexpected increase in or absence of drainage in collection device.

Educating the client regarding signs and symptoms requiring evaluation by a health care provider can help to reduce the occurrence of complications and improve health outcomes.

Lymphedema may not occur in the immediate postoperative period. It may occur up to 2 years following surgery. The client should be informed of what to monitor and to notify health care provider when it occurs.

May indicate infection.
May indicate infection and/or delayed wound healing.

THERAPEUTIC INTERVENTIONS	RATIONALE

Desired Outcomes: The client will identify community resources that can assist with adjustment to the diagnosis of cancer and the loss of a breast.

Independent Actions

Provide information about community resources that can assist the client and significant others with adjustment to the diagnosis of cancer and the mastectomy (e.g., American Cancer Society, Reach to Recovery, National Lymphedema Network, National Breast Cancer Coalition, home health agencies, individual and family counselors).

- Initiate a referral if appropriate.

Identification of a social support network can assist the client in selection of the appropriate type of support system to meet the adjustment needs of the individual.

THERAPEUTIC INTERVENTIONS	RATIONALE

Desired Outcomes: The client, in collaboration with the nurse will, develop a plan for adhering to recommended follow-up care including future appointments with health care provider, medications prescribed, activity limitations, exercises, wound care, and plans for subsequent treatment.

Independent Actions

Collaborate with client to develop a plan for adhering to discharge instructions.

Reinforce physician's explanations and instructions regarding future treatment (e.g., chemotherapy, radiation therapy, hormone therapy such as tamoxifen, breast reconstruction) if planned.

- Explain the importance of having follow-up breast exams and mammography as prescribed.

Helps client to have confidence in ability to care for self.

Ensuring the client understands the importance of adhering to a treatment plan may reduce the occurrence of adverse outcomes. The client should be given time to clarify and ask questions as appropriate.

THERAPEUTIC INTERVENTIONS	RATIONALE
Reinforce the physician's instructions regarding activity limitations. Instruct client to:	
• Avoid lifting heavy objects (over 5–10 pounds) until wound has healed (usually about 4–6 weeks).	*Prevents injury, develops muscle strength slowly.*
• Avoid driving until approved by physician (usually about 2 weeks).	*Prevents strain on surgical site/side and decreases risk for potential injury.*
Review physician's instructions regarding exercises (e.g., squeezing a ball, bending and flexing wrist and elbow, hand wall climbing, pulley exercises, rope turning, arm swings, elbow pull-in, scissors). Instructions should include when to start exercises, frequency, and a written description and/or pictures of how to perform them.	*Assure the client understand how and when to do exercises.* *A written plan provides a resource for client following discharge.*

ADDITIONAL CARE PLANS

BATHING SELF-CARE DEFICIT/DRESSING SELF-CARE DEFICIT NDx
Related to:
• Impaired physical mobility associated with pain, the depressant effect of anesthesia and some medications (e.g., narcotic [opioid] analgesics, some antiemetics), fear of dislodging tubes and compromising surgical wound, and prescribed arm movement restrictions on the operative side

INEFFECTIVE COPING NDx
Related to:
• Perceived loss of femininity and embarrassment associated with loss of a breast
• Fear of rejection by significant others
• Fear, anxiety, and feelings of loss of control associated with the diagnosis of cancer, subsequent treatment (e.g., external radiation therapy, chemotherapy, hormone therapy) if planned, and possibility of disease recurrence

RADICAL PROSTATECTOMY

⊖▶ A radical prostatectomy is performed to treat cancer of the prostate. The surgery includes removal of the prostate gland, prostatic capsule, seminal vesicles, and part of the vas deferens. In addition, a portion of the bladder neck is sometimes removed before the anastomosis of the remaining urethra to the bladder neck. A pelvic lymphadenectomy is usually performed concurrently if the cancer has spread into the pelvic lymph nodes. A radical prostatectomy is accomplished via several methods. The retropubic or perineal approach is used depending on the size and position of the prostate, the anticipated extensiveness of surgery, and physician preference. A laparoscopic or robotic-assisted laparoscopic approach may also be used.

Occasionally, the client will receive external radiation therapy before surgery to reduce the tumor size. If there is evidence of lymph node involvement, a course of external radiation therapy may be done after the client recovers from the surgery.

This care plan focuses on the adult client with cancer of the prostate who is admitted for a radical prostatectomy. Much of the postoperative information is applicable to clients receiving follow-up care in an extended care facility or home setting.

OUTCOME/DISCHARGE CRITERIA

The client will:
1. Maintain adequate urine output
2. Have normal healing of the surgical wound
3. Have surgical pain controlled
4. Have no signs and symptoms of infection or postoperative complications
5. Demonstrate the ability to perform care related to the urinary catheter and drainage system
6. Identify ways to manage urinary incontinence if it occurs after catheter removal
7. Identify ways to manage bowel incontinence if present
8. Share feelings and concerns about the diagnosis of cancer, the prognosis, and changes in body functioning that may occur as a result of a radical prostatectomy
9. Discuss methods of obtaining sexual gratification if permanent damage occurs.
10. State signs and symptoms to report to the health care provider
11. Develop a plan for adhering to recommended follow-up care including future appointments with health care provider, medications prescribed, activity level, wound care, and plans for subsequent treatment

---

NDx = NANDA Diagnosis   **D** = Delegatable Action   ● = UAP   ✦ = LVN/LPN   ⊖▶ = Go to ⊖volve for animation

| Nursing Diagnosis | **URINARY RETENTION** NDx |

Definition: Inability to empty bladder completely.

Related to:
- Blockage in the urinary tract
- Injury following surgery

CLINICAL MANIFESTATIONS

Subjective	Objective
Self-report of bladder fullness or suprapubic discomfort	Bladder distention, absence of urine in urinary catheter drainage tubing, output that continues to be less than intake 48 hrs after surgery

RISK FACTORS
- Surgery
- Strictures of the urethra

DESIRED OUTCOMES

The client will not experience urinary retention as evidenced by:
a. No reports of bladder fullness and suprapubic discomfort
b. Absence of bladder distention
c. Balanced I&O within 48 hrs of surgery

NOC OUTCOMES

Urinary elimination

NIC INTERVENTIONS

Tube care: urinary; bladder irrigation

NURSING ASSESSMENT	RATIONALE
Assess for and report signs and symptoms of urinary retention: • Report of bladder fullness or suprapubic discomfort • Bladder distention • Absence of urine in the urinary catheter drainage tubing • Output less than intake 48 hrs after surgery	*Early recognition of signs and symptoms of urinary retention allow for prompt intervention.*

THERAPEUTIC INTERVENTION	RATIONALE
Independent Actions: Monitor I&O. **D ● ✦**	*Indicates fluid balance. When client is receiving bladder irrigation, the intake of irrigation fluid should be subtracted from catheter output, thus equaling urine output.*
Monitor vital signs and monitor changes.	*Increased or decreased vital signs indicate fluid volume increases or dehydration.*
Note any behavioral changes including restlessness and confusion.	*May indicate increased cerebral edema from excessive solution absorbed from bladder irrigation and decreased urine output.*
Monitor bladder irrigation I&O.	*Flushes bladder of bacteria and clots from surgical procedure.*
Monitor catheter drainage, noting color, volume of clots.	*Bright red urine with clots indicated bleeding. The physician should be notified, as aggressive treatment is required.*
Assure catheter tubing is free of kinks, and maintain collection bag below bladder and off floor.	*Dark red/burgundy urine indicates venous clots and does not require intervention, as it usually subsides without additional therapy.* *Maintains patency of catheter to prevent urinary retention.*

THERAPEUTIC INTERVENTION	RATIONALE
Dependent/Collaborative Actions:	
Monitor laboratory values:	*For evaluation of ongoing bleeding or decrease in bleeding. A decrease in H/H may also indicate increased fluid volume.*
• Hct/Hgb	
• Coagulation studies	*Indicates bleeding and consumption of clotting factors.*
Anchor catheter to thigh or abdomen.	*Anchoring catheter decreases in-and-out movement, and anchoring the catheter to the abdomen places traction on arterial blood supply to the prostate, decreases bleeding, prevents introduction of microbes, and prevents inadvertent removal.*
Release traction every 4 to 6 hrs.	*Prevents tissue damage or injury from prolonged pressure.*
Administer stool softeners or laxative if ordered.	*Prevents constipation and straining associated with defecation, which may increase bleeding.*
Notify health care provider if bleeding remains bright red and there is an increase of clots.	*Notification of health care provider allows for prompt change in treatment regimen.*

Nursing Diagnosis　RISK FOR INFECTION NDx

Definition: Susceptible to invasion and multiplication of pathogenic organisms, which may compromise health.

Related to:
• Wound infection:
  • Wound contamination associated with introduction of pathogens during or after surgery (especially with a perineal approach because incision is close to the anus)
  • Delayed wound healing associated with factors such as diminished tissue perfusion of wound area (especially if client received external radiation therapy before surgery) and decreased nutritional status (if present)
• Urinary tract infection:
  • Introduction of pathogens associated with presence of indwelling catheter
  • Increased growth and colonization of microorganisms associated with urinary stasis (can occur with decreased activity and catheter obstruction)

CLINICAL MANIFESTATIONS

Subjective	Objective
Perineal wound infection: report of increased pain in wound area	**Perineal wound infection:** chills, fever, redness, heat, swelling in wound area, unusual wound drainage; foul smelling odor from wound area, persistent elevation in WBC count; change in differential count; positive wound cultures
Urinary tract infection: verbal reports of frequency, urgency and burning on urination	**Urinary tract infection:** cloudy urine; positive urine culture, abnormal urinalysis

RISK FACTORS

• Surgery
• Poor preoperative nutrition
• Catheterization

DESIRED OUTCOMES

The client will remain free of wound and urinary tract infection as evidenced by:
a. Absence of chills/fever
b. Absence of redness, heat, swelling, and increased pain in wound area
c. Usual drainage from wounds
d. Clear urine
e. White blood cell (WBC) and differential counts returning toward normal
f. Urinalysis showing fewer than 5 WBCs, negative leukocyte esterase and nitrites, and absence of bacteria
g. Negative cultures of wound drainage
h. Negative urine cultures

NOC OUTCOMES	NIC INTERVENTIONS
Immune severity; infection status; wound healing: primary intention	Infection protection; infection control; wound care; tube care: urinary

NURSING ASSESSMENT	RATIONALE
Perineal wound infection: • Increased wound pain • Chills • Fever • Redness • Heat • Swelling in wound area • Persistent elevation in WBC count • Change in differential count • Positive wound culture Urinary tract infection: Frequency; urgency; burning on urination; cloudy urine; positive urine culture; abnormal urinalysis	*Early recognition of signs and symptoms of infection allows for prompt intervention.*

THERAPEUTIC INTERVENTIONS	RATIONALE

Independent Actions:

Implement measures to prevent urinary tract infection:

- Maintain sterile technique during bladder irrigations if performed. **D**

  Actions to prevent urinary retention and subsequent stasis of urine.

- Perform catheter care as often as needed. **D ● ✦**

  Actions help prevent accumulation of mucus and blood around the meatus.

- Keep urine collection container below bladder level at all times. **D ● ✦**

  Actions help prevent reflux or stasis of urine.

- Anchor tubing securely.

  Actions help reduce the amount of in-and-out movement of the catheter (this movement can result in the introduction of pathogens into the urinary tract and can cause tissue trauma, which can result in colonization of microorganisms).

If a perineal approach was used, implement additional measures to prevent wound infection:

- Instruct and assist client to perform good perineal care immediately after bowel movements.

- Use a double-tailed T-binder, scrotal support, or jockey shorts to secure perineal dressings.

  Movement of loose dressings can cause skin irritation and subsequent breakdown.

Dependent/Collaborative Actions

Implement measures to prevent urinary tract infection:

  Actions help promote urine formation and subsequent flushing of pathogens from the bladder.

- Maintain a fluid intake of at least 2500 mL/day unless contraindicated.

  Maintenance of a closed system helps to prevent infections.

- If frequent bladder irrigations are necessary, consult physician about initiation of continuous, closed system irrigation (frequent intermittent irrigations increase the risk of introduction of pathogens).

- Increase activity as allowed.

  Improves circulation

- Administer antimicrobials as ordered.

  Antimicrobials prevent/treat infection.

- If signs and symptoms of urinary tract infection are present, notify health care provider

  Notifying the appropriate health care provider allows for modification of the treatment plan.

Nursing Diagnosis DISTURBED SELF-CONCEPT*

Definition: Disturbed Body Image* NDx: Confusion in mental picture of one's physical self; **Situational Low Self-Esteem* NDx**: Development of a negative perception of self-worth in response to a current situation; **Sexual Dysfunction* NDx**: A state in which an individual experiences a change in sexual function during the sexual response phases of desire, and or/orgasm, which is viewed as unsatisfying, unrewarding, or inadequate.

Related to: Temporary presence of urinary catheter (the catheter is usually not removed until 2–3 weeks after surgery); bowel incontinence if present and possible urinary incontinence after removal of the catheter; sterility and absence of ejaculation associated with removal of the prostate gland, seminal vesicles, and a portion of the vas deferens; possibility of impotence (especially after a perineal approach)

CLINICAL MANIFESTATIONS	RATIONALE
Subjective Verbalization of negative feelings about self and sexual function	**Objective** Lack of participation activities of daily living; refusal to perform catheter care; withdrawal from significant others and partner

RISK FACTORS

- Changes in genitourinary functioning

DESIRED OUTCOMES

The client will demonstrate beginning adaptation to changes in body functioning as evidenced by:
a. Verbalization of feelings of self-worth and sexual adequacy
b. Maintenance of relationships with significant others
c. Active participation in activities of daily living
d. Discuss with partner potential changes in sexual functioning

NOC OUTCOMES

Body image; personal autonomy; self-esteem; psychosocial adjustment: life change; sexual functioning

NIC INTERVENTIONS

Body-image enhancement; grief work facilitation; self-esteem enhancement; role enhancement; counseling; emotional support; counseling: sexuality; support system enhancement

NURSING ASSESSMENT	RATIONALE
Assess for signs and symptoms of a disturbed self-concept: • Negative feelings about self • Lack of participation in activities of daily living • Refusal to perform catheter care • Withdrawal from significant others • Changes in sexual functioning	*Early recognition of signs and symptoms of disturbed self-concept allows for prompt intervention.*

THERAPEUTIC INTERVENTIONS	RATIONALE
Independent Actions: Implement measures to facilitate the grieving process: • Discuss with client improvements in bowel, bladder, and sexual function that can realistically be expected. • Assist client to identify and use coping techniques that have been helpful in the past.	*Working through the grieving process helps the client work through their physical changes.* *Helps the client understand the healing process and functional ability over time.* *Reinforces client's normal defense mechanisms.*

*The nurse should select the nursing diagnostic label that is most appropriate for the client's discharge teaching needs.

NDx = NANDA Diagnosis   **D** = Delegatable Action   ● = UAP   ✦ = LVN/LPN   ⊜▶ = Go to ⊜volve for animation

Continued...

THERAPEUTIC INTERVENTIONS	RATIONALE
• Inform client that when he is discharged, he will be able to connect his urinary catheter to a leg bag and that this bag will allow easier mobility and will not be visible when wearing long pants.	*Helps client understand that he can care for self and no one will be aware of the leg bag.*
If client is incontinent of stool and/or if incontinence of urine is an anticipated problem after catheter removal:	
• Reinforce the importance of doing perineal exercises when allowed.	*Improves bowel and bladder control.*
• Assist him to establish a routine bowel care program.	*Reduces the risk of bowel incontinence.*
• Instruct in ways to minimize incontinence (e.g., placing disposable liners in underwear, wearing absorbent undergarments such as attends).	*Allows for social interaction without wearing a catheter.*
Because sterility is expected, discuss alternative methods of becoming a parent (e.g., adoption) if of concern to client.	*Allows client to make appropriate decisions related to family planning and potential future sexual functioning.*
Reinforce physician's explanation about the temporary or permanent nature of the impotence; if it is expected to be permanent, encourage client to discuss various treatment options (e.g., medication, vacuum erection aids, penile prosthesis) with physician if appropriate.	*Allows time and a supportive environment for client to ask questions concerning nature of changes and available actions they can take to maintain sexual functioning.*
• Suggest alternative methods of sexual gratification if appropriate.	*Assist client in exploring alternative methods of sexual gratification.*
• Discuss ways to be creative in expressing sexuality (e.g., massage, fantasies, cuddling).	
Support behaviors suggesting positive adaptation to changes that have occurred (e.g., verbalization of feelings of self-worth, compliance with treatment plan, maintenance of relationships with significant others).	
Assist client's and significant others' adjustment by listening, facilitating communication, and providing information.	*Improves communication between client and significant others related to physical changes.*
• Encourage visits and support from significant others.	
• Encourage client to pursue usual roles and interests and to continue involvement in social activities.	
• Provide information about and encourage use of community agencies and support groups (e.g., sexual, family, or individual counseling).	*Provides for continuum of care once discharged from the acute care facility.*
Dependent/Collaborative Actions:	
Consult appropriate health care provider (e.g., psychiatric nurse clinician, physician, sexual counseling) if client seems unwilling or unable to adapt to changes resulting from the radical prostatectomy.	*Notifying the appropriate health care provider allows for modification of the treatment plan.*

DISCHARGE TEACHING/CONTINUED CARE

Nursing Diagnosis **DEFICIENT KNOWLEDGE** NDx; **INEFFECTIVE HEALTH MANAGEMENT** NDx; **INEFFECTIVE FAMILY HEALTH MANAGEMENT*** NDx

Definition: Deficient Knowledge NDx: Absence of cognitive information related to a specific topic, or its acquisition; **Ineffective Health Management NDx:** Pattern of regulating and integrating into daily living a therapeutic regimen for the treatment of illness and its sequelae that is unsatisfactory for meeting health goals; **Ineffective Family Health Management NDx:** A pattern of regulating and integrating into family processes for the treatment of illness and its sequelae that is unsatisfactory for meeting specific health goals of the family unit.

*The nurse should select the diagnostic label that is most appropriate for the client's discharge teaching needs.

CLINICAL MANIFESTATIONS

Subjective	**Objective**
Self-report of inability to manage illness and inability to follow prescribed regimen	Inaccurate follow-through with instructions; inappropriate behavior; refusal to participate in care

NOC OUTCOMES

Knowledge: disease process; treatment regimen; exercise; medication regimen; sexual functioning; sexual identity

NIC INTERVENTIONS

Health system guidance; teaching: individual; teaching: disease process; teaching: prescribed exercise; teaching: psychomotor skill; pelvic muscle exercise

NURSING ASSESSMENT

- Assess client's readiness and ability to learn
- Assess meaning of illness to client

RISK FACTORS
- Cognitive deficits
- Failure to take action to reduce risk factors
- Inability to care for self

RATIONALE

Early recognition of readiness to learn and meaning of illness to client allows for implementation of the appropriate teaching interventions.

- Financial concerns
- Lack of social support

THERAPEUTIC INTERVENTIONS

Desired Outcome: The client will demonstrate the ability to perform care related to the urinary catheter and drainage system.

Independent Actions:
Instruct client regarding care related to the urinary catheter and drainage system including:
- Washing the urinary meatus with soap and water at least twice a day.
- Anchoring catheter tubing securely.
- Keep catheter and collection bag tubing free of kinks.
- Keep urine collection bag below the level of the bladder.

- Changing the leg bag to bedside collection bag when laying down for more than a few hours.
- Regular emptying the leg bag and the bedside collection bag.
- Measuring and recording the amount of urine output if prescribed.
- Monitor fluid intake as prescribed.
- Allow time for return demonstration and involve significant other in teaching if appropriate or client allows.

RATIONALE

Ensuring that the client understands proper care of the catheter and drainage system will help prevent infection.

Maintains perineal integrity and decreases incidence for infection.

Prevents in-and-out activity and decreases introduction of microbes.
Prevents stasis of urine and potential for infection.
Ensures urine flow out of the bladder and prevents backup into the kidney.
Prevents stasis of urine in the bag and decreases potential for infection.

Monitors urine output to assure that client has adequate urine production.
Prevents decreased intake and subsequent decreased urine production.

Increases client's confidence in ability to care for self and for the nurse to assess when further instruction is required. Involving the client's significant other allows them to engage in client's care and support prescription for self-care.

THERAPEUTIC INTERVENTIONS

Desired Outcome: The client will identify ways to manage urinary incontinence if it occurs after catheter removal.

Independent Actions:
Provide information about ways to reduce the risk of urinary incontinence after removal of the urinary catheter:

- Teach client to attempt to urinate every 2 to 3 hrs and when the urge is felt.

RATIONALE

Incontinence can occur as a result of trauma to urinary sphincters during surgery and/or irritation from the urinary catheter, damage to the pelvic nerves during surgery, and/or a temporary decrease in bladder function while the catheter was in place.
Bladder training to begin urinating regularly following catheter removal.

Continued...

THERAPEUTIC INTERVENTIONS	RATIONALE
• Urinate in a standing or sitting position.	*Facilitates complete bladder emptying.*
• Avoid drinking large quantities of liquid over a short period of time.	*Increases urine production and increases potential for incontinence.*
• Limit intake of alcohol and caffeine-containing beverages.	*Alcohol and caffeine have a mild diuretic effect and act as irritants to the bladder; products containing alcohol and caffeine may make urinary control more difficult.*
• Stop drinking liquids a few hours before bedtime.	*Reduces risk of nighttime incontinence.*
• Avoid activities that make it difficult to empty bladder as soon as the urge is felt (e.g., long car rides, lengthy meetings)	*May increase the incidence of incontinence.*
• Reinforce the importance of performing perineal exercises regularly when allowed (e.g., stopping and starting urine stream during voiding without holding breath or tensing muscles in buttocks, legs, or abdomen; squeeze buttocks together and then relaxing muscles; develop a Kegel exercise plan).	*These activities strengthen the pelvic floor and can decrease or eliminate the incidence of incontinence. They should be practiced daily for the rest of the client's life.*
• If incontinence occurs, the client should wash and dry perineal area after each episode.	*Decreases incidence of infection.*
• Wear disposable underwear liners or absorbent undergarments.	*Keeps perineal area clean and dry, prevents irritation and potential for infection.*

THERAPEUTIC INTERVENTIONS	RATIONALE

Desired Outcome: Discuss methods of obtaining sexual gratification if permanent damage occurs.

Independent Actions:
Provide time for client and significant other to discuss the following:

• Impact of physical changes on their lives.	
• Discussion of new methods to provide sexual gratification agreeable to both parties.	*Allows for expression of concerns, grief, and loss in a safe, protected environment.*
• Allow time for client and partner to grieve loss of function due to surgery.	
• Provide time and privacy, if interested, to explore and possibly experiment prior to discharge.	
• Consult sex therapist to work with client and partner.	*Consult with an expert that can assist client and partner to explore options for sexual gratification.*
• Refer client to community resources or groups that are dealing with post radical prostatectomy changes that impact quality of life.	*Provides for continuum of care and support from others who have experienced the same changes.*

THERAPEUTIC INTERVENTIONS	RATIONALE

Desired Outcome: The client will state signs and symptoms to report to the health care provider.

Independent Actions:
Instruct the client to report the following signs and symptoms:

• Urinary or bowel incontinence that persists longer than expected, worsens, or interferes with daily life.	*Educate the client regarding signs and symptoms requiring evaluation by a health care provider can help reduce the occurrence of complications and improve health outcomes.*
• Persistent or unexpected impotence.	
• Difficulty coping with the diagnosis of cancer and/or the effects of the radical prostatectomy on body functioning.	*Indicates possible urinary tract infection and/or system blockage.*
• Fever, chills, elevated temperature.	
• Cloudy urine.	
• Decreased urine output.	

THERAPEUTIC INTERVENTIONS	RATIONALE

Independent Actions:

The client, in collaboration with the nurse, will develop a plan for adhering to recommended follow-up care including future appointments with health care provider, medications prescribed, activity level, wound care, and plans for subsequent treatment.

- Collaborate with client to develop a daily and weekly schedule integrating all prescribed activities required to promote recovery and improved health.
- Discuss appropriate diet and exercises to implement.
- Encourage client to stop smoking, if appropriate, and provide community resources for success.
- Reinforce health care provider's instructions, prescriptions, and answer any follow-up questions.
- Explain importance of follow-up appointments with health care provider.
- Instruct client to avoid lifting heavy objects (over 5 lbs) until allowed by health care provider.
- Avoid driving until allowed by health care provider.
- Discuss importance of adhering with follow-up appointments with health care provider.

Assures that client has a written plan in place for follow-up, understands all instructions, and has a schedule for implementation of exercise plan, self-care, and follow-up appointments with health care provider. This also allows the nurse additional time to reinforce information, support, and access to community resources post discharge.

THERAPEUTIC INTERVENTIONS	RATIONALE

Desired Outcome: The client will state signs and symptoms to report to the health care provider.

Independent Actions:

Instruct the client to report the following signs and symptoms:

- Urinary or bowel incontinence that persists longer than expected, worsens, or interferes with daily life.
- Persistent or unexpected impotence.
- Difficulty coping with the diagnosis of cancer and/or the effects of the radical prostatectomy on body functioning.
- Fever, chills, elevated temperature.
- Cloudy urine.
- Changes in urine output or increase in bleeding or expelling clots.
- Continued bladder fullness after voiding.
- Unable to pass urine.

Educate the client regarding signs and symptoms requiring evaluation by a health care provider can help reduce the occurrence of complications and improve health outcomes.

Possible infection
Possible urinary tract infection and/or system blockage.

THERAPEUTIC INTERVENTIONS	RATIONALE

Desired Outcome: The client will identify ways to manage bowel incontinence if present.

Independent Actions:

If the client is experiencing bowel incontinence, instruct to:

- Adhere to a routine bowel care program.
- Perform perineal exercises regularly when allowed (e.g., stopping and starting urine stream during voiding without holding breath or tensing muscles in buttocks, legs, or abdomen; squeeze buttocks together and then relax muscles; develop a Kegel exercise plan).
- Wash and dry perineal area following each episode of incontinence.
- Wear disposable underwear liners or absorbent undergarments such as Attends if needed.

Prevent or decrease potential for uncontrolled defecation.

Improves sphincter control and decreases potential for inability to hold urine.
Prevents potential cross contamination and infection.
Prevents potential embarrassing events.

TRANSURETHRAL RESECTION OF THE PROSTATE

Transurethral resection of the prostate (TURP) is the surgical removal of a prostatic adenoma through the urethra, while leaving the true prostate and its fibrous capsule intact. It may be performed to remove a small cancerous prostatic tumor but most frequently is done to remove a benign prostatic neoplasm that has enlarged enough to block the bladder neck or urethra.

Benign prostatic hyperplasia (BPH) is common in men over 50 years of age and results from age-associated changes in androgen levels. Hyperplasia usually occurs gradually and involves the medial portion of the prostate gland, which surrounds the urethra. Treatment is indicated when signs and symptoms of prostatism (e.g., urgency, frequency, hesitancy, decreased force of urinary stream, nocturia, post-void dribbling) become problematic or when complications such as recurrent urinary tract infection, urinary retention, hematuria, renal calculi, or hydronephrosis occur.

TURP is the most common surgical method for treating BPH. If the prostate gland is very large, an open prostatectomy using a suprapubic or retropubic approach may be necessary. There are a variety of methods to treat BPH. Medical therapy includes pharmacological intervention with doxazosin, tamsulosin, terazosin, or finasteride. When medical intervention is no longer effective, surgery is indicated. There are a variety of surgical procedures to treat BPH. These include but are not limited to laser incision or removal of prostatic tissue, transurethral resection "roto rooter," placement of a stent or coil in the prostatic urethra, balloon dilation,

transurethral vaporization, and transurethral microwave thermotherapy. Factors influencing the treatment method selected include the client's age and health status, size of the enlarged prostate, presence of complications, and physician/client preference and physician expertise.

This care plan focuses on the adult client with BPH who is undergoing a TURP. The information is applicable to clients having surgery in a hospital or outpatient (e.g., surgical care center) setting.

OUTCOME/DISCHARGE CRITERIA

The client will:
1. Maintain adequate urine output
2. Have bladder spasms controlled
3. Exhibit no signs and symptoms of infection or postoperative complications
4. Identify ways to decrease or prevent bleeding in the surgical area
5. Practice exercises to regain or maintain control of bladder emptying
6. State signs and symptoms to report to the health care provider
7. Develop a plan for adhering to recommended follow-up care including future appointments with health care provider, medications prescribed, and activity level

POSTOPERATIVE: USE IN CONJUNCTION WITH THE STANDARDIZED POSTOPERATIVE CARE PLAN

Nursing Diagnosis   IMPAIRED URINARY ELIMINATION NDx

Definition: Dysfunction in urine elimination.

Related to: **Retention**:
- Obstruction of the urinary catheter
- Difficulty urinating after removal of the catheter associated with:
  - Loss of bladder muscle tone resulting from hypertrophy of the detrusor muscle as BPH developed, overdistention of the bladder preoperatively, and/or decompression of the bladder when the catheter was present
  - Relaxation of the bladder muscle resulting from stimulation of the sympathetic nervous system (can result from surgical site discomfort, fear, and anxiety) and the depressant effect of some medications (e.g., narcotic [opioid] analgesics)
  - Decreased perception of bladder fullness resulting from the depressant effect of some medications (e.g., narcotic [opioid] analgesics)
  - Obstruction of the urethra and bladder neck by blood clots, tissue debris, and/or edema (can occur as a result of surgical instrumentation, irritation from the urethral catheter, and/or pressure from the catheter balloon if traction was applied postoperatively)

Incontinence after catheter removal: Trauma to the urinary sphincter(s) associated with surgical instrumentation, irritation from the urethral catheter, and/or pressure from the catheter balloon if traction was applied postoperatively

CLINICAL MANIFESTATIONS

Subjective	**Objective**
Verbal reports of bladder fullness; increasing need to strain to empty bladder; increasing urgency; feeling of bladder fullness after voiding	Bladder distention; absence of urine in urinary drainage bag; output that continues to be less than intake 48 hrs after surgery; voiding frequent small amounts of urine (after removal of catheter)

RISK FACTORS

- Surgical procedure
- Preoperative urinary retention
- Medication regimen
- Age

DESIRED OUTCOMES

The client will:
a. Not experience impaired urinary elimination as evidenced by:
  - No reports of bladder fullness and suprapubic discomfort
  - Absence of bladder distention
  - Balanced I&O within 48 hrs after surgery
  - Voiding adequate amounts at expected intervals after catheter removal
b. Experience urinary continence

NOC OUTCOMES

Urinary continence; urinary elimination

NIC INTERVENTIONS

Urinary incontinence care; urinary retention care; bladder irrigation; catheter care: urinary; pelvic muscle exercise

NURSING ASSESSMENT

Assess for and report signs of impaired urinary elimination:
- Reports of bladder fullness
- Increasing need to strain to empty bladder
- Increasing urgency
- Bladder distention
- Absence of urine in urinary drainage bag
- Output that continues to be less than intake 48 hrs after surgery
- Voiding frequent small amounts of urine (after removal of catheter)
- Experience of incontinence

RATIONALE

Early recognition of signs and symptoms of impaired urinary elimination allows for prompt intervention.

THERAPEUTIC INTERVENTIONS

Independent Actions
Implement measures to maintain patency of the urinary catheter:
- Keep drainage tubing free of kinks. **D** ● ✦
- Keep collection container below level of bladder.
- Tape catheter securely to abdomen or thigh. **D** ✦
Monitor I&O.

Implement measures to prevent trauma to the urinary sphincter(s) while the catheter is in place to reduce the risk of urinary incontinence after removal of the catheter:
- Anchor catheter securely to client's abdomen or thigh. **D** ✦
After removal of the catheter, implement measures to reduce the risk of urinary incontinence:
- Offer urinal or assist client to bathroom every 2 to 4 hrs if indicated. **D** ● ✦
- Keep urinal within easy reach of client.

RATIONALE

Maintaining patency of urinary catheter helps prevent urinary retention.
Prevents backup of urine into the kidney.
Promotes urine drainage.
Prevents inadvertent removal of the catheter.
To assure adequate urine output particularly when client is receiving continuous bladder irrigation.

Prevents excessive movement of the catheter. In-and-out movement of the catheter may introduce microbes into the bladder.

Encourages voiding to prevent status of urine.
Prevents the bladder becoming too full and overstretching prior to voiding.

NDx = NANDA Diagnosis **D** = Delegatable Action ● = UAP ✦ = LVN/LPN ⊖▶ = Go to ⊖volve for animation

Continued...

THERAPEUTIC INTERVENTIONS	RATIONALE
• Instruct client to urinate when the urge is first felt.	*A hypotonic bladder can be easily distended and client needs to become more aware of urge to void following catheter removal.*
• Perform actions to promote relaxation during voiding attempts (e.g., provide privacy, have client sit to void, hold a warm blanket against abdomen).	*Actions promote relaxation of the bladder sphincter and promote voiding.*
• Perform actions that may help trigger the micturition reflex and promote a sense of relaxation during voiding attempts (e.g., run water, place client's hands in warm water, encourage client to urinate when in shower). **D** ● ✦	
• Allow client to assume a normal position for voiding unless contraindicated. **D** ● ✦	
• Instruct client to perform perineal exercises (e.g., stopping and starting stream during voiding; squeezing buttocks together, then relaxing the muscles) regularly.	*Actions help strengthen pelvic floor muscles and improve tone of the external urinary sphincter that leads to better bladder elimination control.*
• Limit oral fluid intake in the evening. **D** ✦	*Actions help decrease the possibility of nighttime incontinence.*
• Instruct client to limit intake of alcohol and beverages containing caffeine.	*Alcohol and caffeine have a mild diuretic effect and act as irritants to the bladder; these factors may make urinary control more difficult.*
• Instruct client to space fluids evenly throughout the day rather than drinking a large quantity at one time.	*Rapid filling of bladder can result in increased urine production and the potential for incontinence.*

Dependent/Collaborative Actions
• Perform and monitor bladder irrigations as ordered.	*Promotes excretion of clots and debris from surgical procedure.*
If signs and symptoms of urinary retention occur after removal of the catheter, consult physician about intermittent catheterization or reinsertion of an indwelling catheter.	*Notifying the appropriate health care provider allows for modification of the treatment plan.*
If continued bleeding occurs during bladder irrigation or urinary incontinence persists, consult physician regarding intermittent catheterization, reinsertion of an indwelling catheter, or use of external collection device (e.g., condom catheter).	*Allows for prompt modification of treatment plan.*

Nursing Diagnosis IMPAIRED COMFORT NDx (BLADDER SPASMS), ACUTE PAIN NDx

Definition: Impaired Comfort NDx: Perceived lack of ease, relief, and transcendence in physical, psychospiritual, environmental, cultural, and/or social dimensions; **Acute Pain NDx:** Unpleasant sensory and emotional experience associated with actual or potential tissue damage, or described in terms of such damage (International Association for the Study of Pain); sudden or slow onset of any intensity from mild to severe with an anticipated or predictable end, and with a duration of less than 3 months.

Related to: Irritation of the bladder wall associated with tissue trauma during surgery, presence of urinary catheter, rapid infusion of irrigation solution, and distention of the bladder (can occur if urine flow becomes obstructed); increased pressure on the bladder neck and prostatic fossa if traction is applied to the urethral catheter (traction may be applied to pull the catheter balloon into the prostatic fossa to put pressure on bleeding vessels)

CLINICAL MANIFESTATIONS

Subjective	Objective
Verbal self-report of suprapubic discomfort; urgent need to urinate or defecate; verbal self-report of pain	Leakage of urine around the urinary catheter; intermittent periods of increase in bloody urine/bladder irrigation

RISK FACTORS
- Surgery
- Three-way urinary catheterization
- Bladder irrigation

DESIRED OUTCOMES

The client will experience relief of impaired comfort and pain as evidenced by:
a. Verbalization of relief of suprapubic discomfort and pain
b. No reports of an urgent need to urinate or defecate
c. No leakage of urine around the urinary catheter

NOC OUTCOMES

Comfort level; symptom control; comfort status: physical

NIC INTERVENTIONS

Medication administration; catheter care

NURSING ASSESSMENT	RATIONALE
Assess for and report signs and symptoms of altered comfort: bladder spasms: • Suprapubic discomfort • Urgent need to urinate or defecate • Leakage of urine around the urinary catheter • Intermittent periods of increase in bloody urine/bladder irrigation • Assess for and report symptoms of acute pain: • Assess the client's pain using a standardized pain scale including location, quality, onset, duration, precipitating factors, aggravating factors, alleviating factors	*Early recognition of signs and symptoms of altered comfort/bladder spasms allows for prompt intervention.* *Use of a pain intensity rating scale gives the nurse a clearer understanding of the client's pain experienced, changes in pain over time, and promotes consistency when communicating with others.*

THERAPEUTIC INTERVENTIONS	RATIONALE
Independent Actions Maintain patency of the urinary catheter (e.g., irrigate as needed, keep tubing free of kinks).	*Maintains flow and prevents stasis of urine.*
Perform actions to reduce movement of the catheter: • Anchor catheter securely to client's abdomen or thigh. • Instruct client to avoid pulling on and twisting the catheter.	*Actions help decrease the impaired comfort and pain including risk of bladder spasms and prevent bladder distention.* *Decreases ongoing irritation of the urethra and bladder.*
Release traction on the catheter every 4 to 5 hrs or more frequently as ordered. **D** ✦	*Reduces pressure on the bladder neck and fossa.*
Do not increase frequency of bladder irrigations or speed up continuous irrigation unless bleeding is noted or blood clots or tissue debris are present. **D** ✦	*Excessive or rapid bladder irrigation can irritate the bladder mucosa.*
Instruct client to avoid attempting to urinate around the catheter and straining to urinate after catheter is removed.	*Attempts to forcefully contract bladder can stimulate bladder spasms.*
If bladder spasms occur: Encourage client to take deep breaths, use guided imagery, watch Tv or listen to music.	*Reduces muscle tension, refocuses client's attention, and provides relaxation that may decrease bladder spasms.*
• Encourage client to take short, frequent walks unless contraindicated. **D** ✦	*Walking seems to reduce spasms.*
• Decrease the rate of continuous bladder irrigation if urine is not red and blood clots and tissue debris are not present.	*May decrease bladder spasms and client's feeling of bladder fullness and pressure.*
Dependent/Collaborative Actions If bladder spasms occur: • Administer belladonna and opium (B&O) rectal suppositories if ordered (this is a combination of an antimuscarinic and narcotic analgesic).	*Reduces spasm of the bladder muscle and the client's perception of pain and discomfort; it is only prescribed when the urinary catheter is present because it can cause urinary retention.*
• Anticholinergics: Propantheline bromide.	*Relieves bladder spasms while client has a catheter.*
Consult physician if above measures fail to control bladder spasms.	*Notifying the appropriate health care provider allows for modification of the treatment plan.*

NDx = NANDA Diagnosis   **D** = Delegatable Action   ● = UAP   ✦ = LVN/LPN   ⊖▶ = Go to ⊖volve for animation

| Nursing Diagnosis | **RISK FOR BLEEDING NDx** |

Definition: Susceptible to a decrease in blood volume, which may compromise health.

Related to: Surgical procedure of the prostate gland, which is very vascular

CLINICAL MANIFESTATIONS

Subjective	Objective
N/A	Bright red drainage (could indicate arterial bleeding) or persistent darker drainage (venous bleeding) and blood clots in urinary catheter; persistent redness of and blood clots in urine after removal of the catheter; significant decrease in RBC, Hct, and Hgb levels; tachypnea; hypotension; tachycardia; decreased urine output; pallor; cool, clammy skin; anxiety; confusion; agitation; capillary refill > 2 to 3 seconds; declining SaO_2

RISK FACTORS
- Inadequate fluid volume replacement
- Trauma from surgery
- Age
- History of taking NSAIDS, anticoagulants

DESIRED OUTCOMES

The client will not develop excessive bleeding as evidenced by:
a. Usual mental status
b. Stable vital signs
c. Skin warm and usual color
d. Palpable peripheral pulses
e. Urine output at least 30 mL/h

NOC OUTCOMES

Blood loss severity

NIC INTERVENTIONS

Bleeding precautions; bleeding reduction; bladder irrigation

NURSING ASSESSMENT	**RATIONALE**
Assess for and report signs and symptoms of excessive bleeding:	*Early recognition of signs and symptoms of excessive bleeding allows for prompt intervention.*
• Bright red drainage (could indicate arterial bleeding) or persistent darker drainage (venous bleeding) and blood clots in urine.	
• After removal of the catheter; significant decrease in RBC, Hct, and Hgb levels.	
• Tachypnea; hypotension; tachycardia; decreased urine output; pallor; cool, clammy skin; anxiety; confusion and agitation.	
• Capillary refill >2 to 3 seconds.	
• Declining SaO_2.	
Assess serum Hgb/Hct and report any abnormalities.	*Changes indicate extent of blood loss.*

THERAPEUTIC INTERVENTIONS	**RATIONALE**
Independent Actions	
Monitor I&O, noting color, consistency, and volume of clots.	*Indicates fluid balance and if replacement is required. When client is on bladder irrigation, monitoring of the volume of clots and color and consistency of urine is an indication of bleeding. Bright red indicates arterial bleeding; dark red/burgundy with increased viscosity and clots indicate venous bleeding, which may decrease without intervention.*
Monitor vital signs: BP; heart rate, respirations, and capillary refill.	*Decreased blood pressure and increased heart rate are indications of hypovolemia. Compare these findings to I&O and extent of bleeding noted in urinary drainage. Increased capillary refill time and increased reparations may indicate excessive bleeding and decreased fluid volume.*

THERAPEUTIC INTERVENTIONS	RATIONALE
Monitor for any behavioral changes, restlessness. or confusion.	*Indicates declining fluid volume and cerebral perfusion pressure, which may be associated with increased bleeding.*
Encourage fluid intake greater than 2000 mL/day if not contraindicated once catheter is removed.	*Helps to maintain vascular fluid volume.*
Instruct client to take short rather than long walks and to avoid sitting for long periods.	*Ambulation improves circulation and venous return.*
Instruct client to avoid straining to have a bowel movement.	*Prevents stress on surgical site.*
Implement measures to prevent urinary retention.	*Actions help prevent distention of the bladder and subsequent pressure on the newly coagulated blood vessels in the operative area.*
Instruct client to return to bed and limit activity for a few hours if urine has increased redness when ambulating or sitting in chair.	*Rest decreases pressure on bladder and surgical area.*

Dependent/Collaborative Actions:

Monitor laboratory values:	
Hgb/Hct.	*Decrease in values may indicate dilutional results or based on I&O could indicate active bleeding.*
Coagulation studies and platelet count.	*Decrease in findings indicates active bleeding and consumption of clotting factors.*
Administer IV fluids and blood products as ordered.	*Replacement for vascular volume and oxygen-carrying capabilities.*
Maintain traction on the urethral catheter as ordered (provides direct pressure on the bleeding vessels).	*Measures help to prevent or control hemorrhage to prevent hypovolemic shock.*
• Anchor catheter tubing securely to client's abdomen or thigh to minimize movement of catheter.	*Actions help to prevent trauma to and/or unnecessary pressure on the prostatic area, thereby reducing the risk of hemorrhage.*
• Administer stool softeners if indicated.	*Decreases risk of constipation and potential for straining with a bowel movement, thus decreasing pressure on surgical site and risk for bleeding.*

Nursing Diagnosis **RISK FOR IMBALANCED FLUID VOLUME** NDx

Definition: Susceptible to a decrease, increase, or rapid shift from one to the other of intravascular, interstitial, and/or intracellular fluid, which may compromise health. This refers to body fluid loss, gain, or both.

Related to:
• Vigorous fluid therapy during and immediately after surgery; increased secretion of antidiuretic hormone (output of antidiuretic hormone [ADH] is stimulated by trauma, pain, and anesthetic agents); excessive absorption of irrigation solution via the prostatic veins during and after surgery. "TUR syndrome" resulting from the absorption of large volumes of bladder irrigation fluid in surgery and early postoperative period.
• Potential for bleeding during and after surgical procedure
• Increased diuresis following removal of prostate and opening of urinary tract

CLINICAL MANIFESTATIONS

Subjective	Objective
Fluid volume excess: reports of dyspnea; orthopnea, confusion	**Fluid volume excess:** elevated BP; presence of S3 heart sound; bounding pulse, change in mental status; intake greater than output; decreased BUN, Hct, serum sodium and osmolality; chest radiograph results demonstrating pulmonary congestion
Fluid volume deficit: complaints of thirst and dry mouth	**Fluid volume deficit:** decreased blood pressure, normal or high serum sodium and osmolality; increased Hct, and urine osmolality

---

NDx = NANDA Diagnosis   **D** = Delegatable Action   ● = UAP   ✦ = LVN/LPN   ⊖▶ = Go to ⊖volve for animation

RISK FACTORS

- Surgery
- Excessive bladder irrigation
- Endocrine response to trauma
- Age

DESIRED OUTCOMES

The client will not experience imbalanced fluid volume as evidenced by:
a. Stable weight
b. Stable BP
c. Absence of S_3 heart sound
d. Normal pulse volume
e. Balanced I&O within 48 hrs after surgery
f. Usual mental status
g. BUN, Hct, serum sodium, and osmolality within normal range
h. Absence of dyspnea, orthopnea, edema, and distended neck veins

NOC OUTCOMES

Fluid overload severity; fluid balance; fluid volume

NIC INTERVENTIONS

Fluid monitoring; fluid management

NURSING ASSESSMENT	RATIONALE
Assess for and report signs and symptoms of **fluid volume excess**: • Dyspnea, orthopnea • Increased blood pressure • S_1 heart sound: bounding pulse, change in mental status • Intake greater than output Assess serum electrolytes, BUN, Hct, serum sodium, and osmolality, reporting any abnormal values. Assess chest radiograph results, reporting any abnormalities. Assess for and report **fluid volume deficit**: • Decreased blood pressure, heart rate • High serum sodium and osmolality • Increased Hct and urine osmolality • Complaints of thirst and dry mouth	*Early recognition of signs and symptoms of fluid volume imbalance allows for prompt intervention.*

THERAPEUTIC INTERVENTIONS	RATIONALE
Independent Actions: Monitor I&O.	*While patient is on bladder irrigation, the potential for increased fluid volume is great and strict I&O will alert the health care team of changes.*
Monitor vital signs, documenting and analyzing trends.	*Both dehydration and fluid volume excess require prompt intervention to prevent shock.*
Monitor mental status, noting restlessness, confusion, or change in behavior.	*Changes in mental status and behavior reflect cerebral perfusion and edema from excessive bladder irrigation fluids.*
Monitor catheter drainage, noting extent and continuation of bleeding.	*Bleeding may occur with the first 24 hrs following surgery. Ongoing or excessive bleeding should be reported due to potential vascular deficit and depletion of clotting factors.*
Dependent/Collaborative Actions Monitor laboratory values: • Hct/Hgb and sodium. • Urine osmolality. • Coagulation studies. Administer IV fluids as ordered. Infuse packed red blood cells (RBCs) if ordered. Maintain traction on urinary catheter by taping to abdomen or thigh.	*Indicate fluid volume status and impact of bleeding, if occurring.* *Indicates status of clotting factors.* *Maintain vascular fluid volume status.* *May be required due to excessive bleeding.* *Traction on catheter applies pressure on the artery supply to the prostate and helps to control bleeding.*

THERAPEUTIC INTERVENTIONS	RATIONALE
Release traction every 4 to 5 hrs or per hospital policy.	Continuous traction may cause long-term or permanent nerve damage. Diuretics are given to decrease excess fluid volume.
Administer medication as ordered: • Diuretics • Stool softeners	Stool softeners are given to decrease straining with bowel movement. Straining increases pressure on the perineum and may cause increased bleeding.
Use normal saline rather than hypotonic solutions for bladder irrigations.	Decreases fluid volume shifts.
Do not increase frequency of bladder irrigations or increase speed of continuous irrigation unless indicated.	Actions help reduce absorption of fluid via the prostatic veins to further reduce the risk for excess fluid volume and/or water intoxication.
Notify physician if signs and symptoms of fluid deficit or overload develop.	Notifying the appropriate health care provider allows for modification of the treatment plan.

DISCHARGE TEACHING/CONTINUED CARE

Nursing Diagnosis **DEFICIENT KNOWLEDGE NDx, INEFFECTIVE FAMILY HEALTH MANAGEMENT, INEFFECTIVE HEALTH MANAGEMENT* NDx**

Definition: **Deficient Knowledge NDx:** Absence of cognitive information related to specific topic, or its acquisition; **Ineffective Family Health Management NDx:** A pattern of regulating and integrating into family process a program for the treatment of illness and its sequelae that is unsatisfactory for meeting specific health goals of the family unit; **Ineffective Health Management NDx:** Pattern of regulating and integrating into daily living a therapeutic regimen for treatment of illnesses and its sequelae that is unsatisfactory for meeting specific health goals.

CLINICAL MANIFESTATIONS

Subjective	Objective
Verbal self-report of inability to manage illness and inability to follow prescribed regimen	Inaccurate follow-through with instructions; inappropriate behavior; refusal to participate in care

RISK FACTORS
• Cognitive deficit
• Failure to reduce risk factors
• Inability to care for oneself
• Difficulty in modifying personal habits and integrating treatments into lifestyle
• Changes in body functioning

NOC OUTCOMES	NIC INTERVENTIONS
Knowledge: disease process; treatment regimen	Health system guidance; teaching: individual; teaching: disease process; teaching: prescribed exercise; pelvic muscle exercise; teaching: catheter care

---

*The nurse should select the nursing diagnostic label that is most appropriate for the client's discharge teaching needs.

NDx = NANDA Diagnosis   **D** = Delegatable Action   ● = UAP   ✦ = LVN/LPN   ⊖▶ = Go to ⊖volve for animation

NURSING ASSESSMENT	RATIONALE
Assess client's ability to learn and readiness to learn Assess understanding of patient teaching	*Learning is more effective when the client is motivated and under-stands the importance of what is to be learned. Readiness to learn is based on situations and physical and emotional challenges.*

THERAPEUTIC INTERVENTIONS	RATIONALE

Desired Outcomes: The client will identify ways to prevent bleeding in the surgical area.

Independent Actions
Instruct client in ways to prevent bleeding in the surgical area:

• Avoid straining during defecation (provide instructions about increasing fluid intake and intake of foods high in fiber if client tends to be constipated).	*Prevents stress on perineum and surgical site.*
• Avoid long walks, prolonged sitting, long car rides, running, climbing stairs quickly, strenuous exercise, sexual intercourse, and lifting objects over 10 pounds for as long as recommended by physician (usually for 2–6 weeks after discharge).	*Increased pressure on perineal area will increase potential for bleeding. Client should increase activity slowly over time.*
• Consult physician before resuming preoperative medications such as aspirin and other NSAIDs, warfarin, and clopidogrel (physicians often recommend waiting 1–2 weeks after surgery if possible before resuming these medications).	*These medications impact blood clotting and may increase risk for bleeding.*

THERAPEUTIC INTERVENTIONS	RATIONALE

Desired Outcome: The client will identify ways to regain or maintain control of bladder and bowel emptying.

Independent Actions
Instruct client in ways to regain or maintain control of bladder emptying:

• Try to urinate every 2 to 3 hrs and whenever the urge is felt.	*Prevents bladder from getting too full and decreases incidence of incontinence.*
• Urinate in a standing or sitting position.	*Assuming normal voiding position will help to facilitate bladder emptying.*
• Instruct client in ways to regain or maintain control of bowel emptying.	
• Attempt to have a bowel movement at routine times consistent with client's habits before surgery.	
• Attempt to have a bowel movement when the urge is first felt.	*Facilitates bowel evacuation. Will begin to train bowel of when to defecate and attempting to have frequent bowel movements will decrease incidence of bowel incontinence.*
• Begin bowel training routine if necessary. Eat a well-balanced diet full of fiber and fluids.	*Adequate fiber is necessary to maintain bowel patterns. May need to decrease volume of fiber during periods of incontinence.*
• Avoid drinking large quantities of liquids over a short period.	*Increases urine production and the need to void.*
• Limit intake of alcohol and caffeine-containing beverages.	*Alcohol and caffeine have a mild diuretic effect and act as irritants to the bladder; these factors may make urinary control more difficult.*
• Drink fluids at regular times throughout the day. Drink less in the evening a few hours before bedtime.	*Stop drinking liquids a few hours before bedtime (reduces risk of urine retention and nighttime incontinence).*
• Avoid long car rides, lengthy meetings, etc. that require holding urine for an extended period of time.	*Avoid activities that make it difficult to empty bladder as soon as the urge is felt. Prevents risk for increased retention and for incontinence. This also prevents increased bowel incontinence due to lack of an available bathroom.*

THERAPEUTIC INTERVENTIONS	**RATIONALE**
• Perform perineal exercises (e.g., stopping and starting stream during voiding; squeezing buttocks together, then relaxing the muscles) 10 to 20 times/hour while awake until urinary control is regained.	*Improves bladder and bowel control and muscle strength of perineum.*
• Begin routinely practicing Kegel exercises.	
If client is experiencing urinary incontinence, instruct to:	*Allows client to increase mobility and activity without potential embarrassment of incontinence.*
• Wear disposable underwear liners or absorbent undergarments such as Attends if necessary.	

THERAPEUTIC INTERVENTIONS	**RATIONALE**

Desired Outcome: The client will state signs and symptoms to report to the health care provider.

Independent Actions

Instruct client to report these additional signs and symptoms:

• Persistent burgundy-colored or bright red urine (inform client that some blood is expected intermittently for 2–3 weeks after surgery but that urine should become pink to amber after he rests and increases fluid intake for a couple of hours).	*Educating the client regarding signs and symptoms requiring evaluation by a health care provider can help reduce the occurrence of complications and improve health outcomes.*
• Presence of large blood clots or continued passage of smaller clots.	*Indicates bleeding.*
• Development of or increase in frequency, burning, or pain when urinating.	*Indicates possible infection.*
• Decrease in urine output or force and caliber of urinary stream.	
• Bladder distention.	*Indicates possible urinary blockage.*
• Unexpected loss of bladder control.	*Indicates changes in muscular or neurologic control.*
• Cloudy urine unrelated to orgasm.	*It is expected that urine will be cloudy after orgasm if client is experiencing retrograde ejaculation.*
• Persistent or increased bladder spasms.	
• Chills, fever.	
• Difficulty in voiding or inability to urinate.	
Consult physician if urinary incontinence persists, worsens, or interferes with daily life so that various options (e.g., biofeedback, insertion of artificial urinary sphincter) can be discussed.	*Allows for changes in therapeutic regimen.*

THERAPEUTIC INTERVENTIONS	**RATIONALE**

Desired Outcome: Discuss methods of obtaining sexual gratification if permanent damage occurs.

Independent Actions:

Provide time for client and partner to discuss concerns related to:	*Explain in terms that the client and partner can understand concerning the anatomy of an erection and ejaculation and how that has changed with the surgical procedure.*
Urinary incontinence	
Bowel incontinence	
Retrograde ejaculation	
Reinforce information provided by the physician concerning sexual performance changes.	*Reinforcement of information provided by the physician provides for consistent information and whether changes are permanent.*
Encourage client to continue with pelvic strengthening exercises and Kegels.	*Client needs to be aware that over time these exercises will reduce or eliminate urinary or bowel incontinence.*
Refer client to community resources, support groups, or counselor as indicated.	*Provides for continuum of care.*
If changes in sexual functioning occur, recommend client to discuss situation with health care provider.	*Allows for changes in treatment regimen.*

THERAPEUTIC INTERVENTIONS	RATIONALE

Desired Outcomes: The client, in collaboration with the nurse, will develop a plan for adhering to recommended follow-up care including future appointments with health care provider, medications prescribed, and activity level.

Independent Actions

Collaborate with client to develop a written plan that includes prescribed activity, exercises, self-care, and follow-up appointments.

This should include a sample of all daily activities allowed and someone to take them to the health care provider's office.

Reinforce the physician's instructions regarding the importance of lying down and increasing fluid intake for a few hours if amount of blood or number of blood clots in the urine increases.

Explain the importance of having a digital rectal examination and a blood test for prostate-specific antigen (PSA) done each year (cancer of the prostate and recurrent BPH can develop because the entire prostate gland is not removed during a TURP).

Creating a written plan provides the client with a resource to use following discharge. It forces client to think about what needs to be done and who will support them in their recovery. Creating a daily sample plan helps client to see how days will be structured and can increase confidence in their ability to care for self.

Ensuring the client understands the importance of adhering to a treatment plan may reduce the occurrence of adverse outcomes. The client should be given time to clarify and answer questions as appropriate.

Follow-up is critical to assure ongoing health and allows for treatment in therapeutic regimen as needed.

ADDITIONAL NURSING DIAGNOSES

RISK FOR INFECTION NDx: URINARY TRACT
Related to:

- Introduction of pathogens associated with instrumentation of urinary tract during surgery, presence of indwelling catheter, and frequent bladder irrigations
- Increased growth and colonization of microorganisms associated with urinary stasis resulting from decreased activity and urinary retention if it occurs

SEXUAL DYSFUNCTION NDx
Related to:

- Urinary incontinence; retrograde ejaculation; altered self-image

15

The Client Receiving Treatment for Neoplastic Disorders

CHEMOTHERAPY

⊖▶ This care plan focuses on the use of cytotoxic drugs in the treatment of cancer. Chemotherapy is used alone or in combination with radiation therapy, surgery, and/or biotherapy to achieve a cure, control tumor growth, or provide relief of symptoms associated with advanced disease (palliation). The success of the therapy depends on the size, type, and location of the tumor in addition to the client's physiologic and psychologic condition.

Cytotoxic drugs are classified according to chemical structure (e.g., antimetabolites, mitotic inhibitors [vinca alkaloids, plant alkaloids], alkylating agents), primary mode of action (e.g., some interfere with folic acid synthesis or produce cross-links of DNA strands), or effect on the cell life cycle. Some drugs are more effective during a specific phase of the cell cycle and are referred to as cell cycle phase specific or cell cycle specific (e.g., mitotic inhibitors, antimetabolites). The cytotoxic agents that interrupt the cell replication process without regard to the phase of the cell cycle are classified as cell cycle phase nonspecific or cell cycle nonspecific (e.g., alkylating agents, antitumor antibiotics).

The primary effect of cytotoxic drugs is to interrupt cell replication. It is believed that cytotoxic drugs kill a percentage of tumor cells with each dose and that tumors with a large percentage of growing cells will experience greater cell death than tumors with a smaller percentage of growing cells. Cells in the resting phase are less responsive to chemotherapeutic agents and are better able to repair themselves if damaged during treatment.

More than one anticancer drug is traditionally given for cancer treatment in order to prevent the cancer from becoming resistant to treatment. The additive and sometimes synergistic effects that occur when drugs are used together allow an increased percentage of tumor cells to be killed without a concomitant increase in drug-induced toxicities. The dose, combination, and treatment schedule for the drugs are determined by factors such as the physiologic status of the client and the drug's action on the cell cycle, the cell's metabolism, the drug's toxic effects, and the nadir. Cytotoxic agents are most frequently given intravenously, but routes such as oral, subcutaneous, topical, and direct instillation into the target area (e.g., peritoneum, bladder, cerebrospinal fluid) are used when appropriate.

Cytotoxic drugs do not discriminate between normal and the cancerous cells; as a result, the client may experience certain side effects and/or toxic effects after their administration. The drugs have the greatest effect on rapidly dividing cancerous and normal cells (e.g., bone marrow, skin, hair follicles, lining of the gastrointestinal tract). Because of this lack of selectivity between the cancerous and the normal cell, nursing care of the recipient of the drugs is indeed a challenge.

This care plan focuses on the adult client hospitalized for an initial or subsequent cycle of chemotherapy and/or management of side effects of treatment with cytotoxic agents. Much of the information is also applicable to clients receiving chemotherapy and/or follow-up care in an outpatient facility or home setting.

OUTCOME/DISCHARGE CRITERIA

The client will:
1. Have no signs and symptoms of toxic effects of cytotoxic agents
2. Have side effects of cytotoxic agents under control
3. Have fatigue at a manageable level
4. Have an adequate or improved nutritional status
5. Identify ways to prevent infection during periods of lowered immunity
6. Demonstrate appropriate oral hygiene techniques
7. Identify techniques to control nausea and vomiting
8. Verbalize ways to improve appetite and nutritional status
9. Verbalize ways to manage and cope with persistent fatigue
10. Verbalize ways to prevent bleeding when platelet counts are low
11. Verbalize ways to adjust to alterations in reproductive and sexual functioning
12. Verbalize ways to promote independence and prevent injury if neuropathies are present
13. Demonstrate the ability to care for a central venous catheter, a peritoneal catheter, or an implanted infusion device if in place
14. Demonstrate care and precautions necessary if a peripherally inserted central line is in place
15. Verbalize an understanding of an implanted infusion pump and precautions necessary if one is in place
16. State signs and symptoms to report to the health care provider
17. Share thoughts and feelings about changes in body image resulting from chemotherapy

18. Identify community resources that can assist with home management and adjustment to the diagnosis of cancer and chemotherapy and its effects

19. Develop a plan for adhering to recommended follow-up care including medications prescribed and schedule for chemotherapy, laboratory studies, and future appointments with health care provider

---

Nursing Diagnosis | **IMBALANCED NUTRITION: LESS THAN BODY REQUIREMENTS** NDx

Definition: Intake of nutrients insufficient to meet metabolic needs.

Related to:
- Decreased oral intake associated with:
- Oral, pharyngeal, and esophageal pain and difficulty swallowing resulting from mucositis if it has developed
  - Anorexia resulting from factors such as depression, fear, anxiety, fatigue, discomfort, early satiety, altered sense of taste and smell, and increased levels of certain cytokines that depress appetite (e.g., interleukin-1, tumor necrosis factor)
  - Altered mental status (can result from fluid and electrolyte imbalances, hypoxia, or tumor involvement of the brain)
- Loss of nutrients associated with vomiting and diarrhea if present
- Impaired utilization of nutrients associated with:
  - Accelerated and inefficient metabolism of proteins, carbohydrates, and/or fats resulting from factors such as increased levels of cortisol, glucagon, and certain cytokines (e.g., tumor necrosis factor, interleukin-1)
  - Decreased absorption of nutrients resulting from loss of intestinal absorptive surface if mucositis has developed
- Utilization of available nutrients by the malignant cells rather than the host

CLINICAL MANIFESTATIONS

Subjective	Objective
Verbal self-report of weakness and fatigue	Significant weight loss; abnormal blood urea nitrogen (BUN) and low serum prealbumin, albumin, and transferrin levels; sore, inflamed oral mucous membrane; pale conjunctiva, anorexia

RISK FACTORS
- Inability to ingest foods
- Inability to absorb nutrients
- Inability to digest foods
- Insufficient intake

DESIRED OUTCOMES

The client will have or attain an adequate nutritional status as evidenced by:
a. Weight within or returning toward normal range for client
b. Normal BUN and serum prealbumin, albumin, and transferrin levels
c. Usual strength and activity tolerance
d. Healthy oral mucous membrane

NOC OUTCOMES

Nutritional status

NIC INTERVENTIONS

Nutritional monitoring, nutrition therapy, nausea management

NURSING ASSESSMENT	**RATIONALE**
Assess for and report signs and symptoms of malnutrition: • Weakness • Fatigue • Significant weight loss • Sore, inflamed oral mucous membrane • Pale conjunctiva	*Early recognition of signs and symptoms of malnutrition allows for prompt intervention.*
Monitor percentage of meals and snacks client consumes. Report a pattern of inadequate intake.	*Provides ability to determine if client maintains adequate intake.*
Monitor serum BUN and serum prealbumin, albumin, and transferrin levels.	*Possible indication that client may have cachexia and provides indications of adequate intake of diet.*

THERAPEUTIC INTERVENTIONS	RATIONALE

Independent Actions

Implement measures to maintain or promote an adequate nutritional status:

- Implement measures to reduce nausea and vomiting (e.g., provide mints or sour candy for client to suck on to eliminate noxious odors).

  Vomiting results in loss of nutrients and these measures can help to maintain an intact oral mucosa.

- Implement measures to reduce oral, pharyngeal, esophageal, and abdominal pain (e.g., encourage client to suck on ice during infusion).

  Pain can decrease client's appetite and result in decreased oral intake.

- Implement measures that will help client to adjust psychologically to the diagnosis of cancer and treatment with chemotherapy (e.g., reassure client hair loss is temporary; encourage client to wear wig).

  Improves self-esteem and decreases depression, which may affect a client's desire to eat.

- Implement measures to compensate for taste alterations that might be present:

  Enhancing the taste of foods/fluids and providing nutritious alternatives to those that taste unpleasant to the client help to stimulate appetite and improve oral intake.

  - Encourage client to select mild-tasting fish, cold chicken or turkey, eggs, and cheese as protein sources if beef or pork tastes bitter or rancid.

    Action helps to stimulate salivation.
    Increases ability to maintain adequate protein intake.

  - Provide meat for breakfast if aversion to meat tends to increase as day progresses.

    May help to increase flavor of food and desire to eat.

  - Experiment with different flavorings, seasonings, and textures.

    May decrease some peculiar tastes.

  - Serve food cold or at room temperature.

    Decreases impact of metallic taste clients desire to eat.

  - Provide client with plastic rather than metal eating utensils if metallic taste is present. **D** ●

    Decreased dryness of the oral mucosa decreases difficulty in swallowing food.

If client is having difficulty swallowing:

- Implement measures to reduce the severity of stomatitis and/or relieve dryness of the oral mucous membrane (e.g., encourage client to suck on sugarless candy).

  Decreases discomfort while allowing client to maintain intake.

- Help client to select foods that require little or no chewing and are easily swallowed (e.g., custard, eggs, canned fruit, mashed potatoes).

  Sticky and dry foods increase difficulty in swallowing food.

- Avoid serving foods that are sticky (e.g., peanut butter, soft bread, honey).

  Moisture decreases dependence on saliva to moisten food.

- Moisten dry foods with gravy or sauces.
- Serve food warm if indicated. **D** ● ✦

  Warm food can stimulate sense of smell and subsequent appeal of certain foods.

- Increase activity as tolerated. **D** ● ✦

  Activity usually promotes a sense of well-being, which can improve appetite.

- Obtain a dietary consult if necessary to assist client in selecting foods/fluids that are appealing and adhere to personal and cultural preferences.

  Foods/fluids that appeal to the client's senses and are in accordance with personal and cultural preferences are most likely to stimulate appetite and promote interest in eating.

- Encourage a rest period before meals. **D** ●

  The physical activity of eating requires some expenditure of energy. Fatigue can reduce the client's desire and ability to eat.

- Maintain a clean environment and a relaxed, pleasant atmosphere. **D** ● ✦

  Noxious sights and odors can inhibit the feeding center in the hypothalamus. Maintaining a clean environment helps prevent this from occurring. In addition, maintaining a relaxed, pleasant atmosphere can help reduce the client's stress and promote a feeling of well-being, which tends to improve appetite.

- Provide oral hygiene before meals. **D** ● ✦
- Provide largest amount of calories and protein when appetite is best (usually at breakfast).

  Oral hygiene moistens the mouth, which makes it easier to chew and swallow; it also removes unpleasant tastes, which often improves the taste of foods/fluids.

- Serve frequent, small meals rather than large ones if client is weak, fatigues easily, and/or has a poor appetite.

  Small rather than large meals can enable a client who is weak or fatigues easily to finish a meal. Smaller meals also seem less overwhelming.

NDx = NANDA Diagnosis   **D** = Delegatable Action   ● = UAP   ✦ = LVN/LPN   ⊜▶ = Go to ⊜volve for animation

Continued...

THERAPEUTIC INTERVENTIONS	RATIONALE
• Encourage significant others to bring in client's favorite foods and eat with him or her.	*Favorite foods eaten along with family members help to make eating more of a familiar social experience.*
• Limit fluid intake with meals (unless the fluid has high nutritional value).	*Limiting fluids helps to reduce early satiety and subsequent decreased food intake.*
• Allow adequate time for meals; reheat foods/fluids if necessary.	*Clients who feel rushed during meals tend to become anxious, lose their appetite, and stop eating.*
• Ensure that meals are well balanced and high in essential nutrients; offer high-calorie, high-protein dietary supplements (e.g., milkshakes, puddings, or eggnog made with cream or powdered milk reconstituted with whole milk; commercially prepared dietary supplements) if indicated.	*Clients must consume a diet that is well balanced and high in essential nutrients in order to meet their nutritional needs. Dietary supplements are often needed to help accomplish this.*
• Perform actions to control diarrhea (e.g., avoid foods high in fiber, caffeine, alcohol, spices, or fats).	*Foods may irritate the bowels or cause the stool to be more liquid which can lead to fluid and electrolyte losses.*
• Encourage the use of relaxation techniques (e.g., visualization, guided imagery) and exercise.	*Relaxation may help to decrease nausea and anorexia. Exercise may stimulate appetite.*

Dependent/Collaborative Actions

Implement measures to maintain or promote an adequate nutritional status:	
• Administer appetite stimulants (e.g., megestrol acetate, dronabinol) if ordered.	*These drugs can increase appetite.*
• Administer vitamins and minerals if ordered. **D** ✦	*Vitamins and minerals are needed to maintain metabolic function.*
• Perform a calorie count if ordered. Report information to dietitian and physician.	*A calorie count provides information about the caloric intake and nutritional value of the foods/fluids the client consumes. This information helps the dietician and physician to determine whether an alternative method of nutritional support is needed.*
Evaluation laboratory values: BUN, serum prealbumin, albumin, and transferrin levels	*Helps to identify degree of biochemical change with changes in diet and to monitor the adequacy of the client's diet.*
Consult physician regarding an alternative method of providing nutrition (e.g., parenteral nutrition, tube feedings) if client does not consume enough food or fluids to meet nutritional needs.	*Notification of the appropriate health care provider allows for modification of the treatment plan.*

Nursing Diagnosis **ACUTE PAIN** NDx**/CHRONIC PAIN** NDx

Definitions: Acute Pain NDx: Unpleasant sensory and emotional experience associated with actual or potential tissue damage, or described in terms of such damage (International Association for the Study of Pain); sudden or slow onset of any intensity from mild to severe with an anticipated or predictable end, and with a duration of less than 3 months; **Chronic Pain NDx:** Unpleasant sensory and emotional experience associated with actual or potential tissue damage, or described in terms of such damage (International Association for the Study of Pain); sudden or slow onset of any intensity from mild to severe, constant or recurring without an anticipated or predictable end, and with a duration of greater than 3 months.

Related to:

- **Oral, pharyngeal, esophageal, and/or abdominal pain** related to mucositis associated with the effects of cytotoxic drugs on the rapidly dividing cells of the gastrointestinal mucosa
- **Muscle and bone pain** (the cause is not known but it sometimes occurs in persons receiving paclitaxel and high doses of vinblastine or etoposide)
- **Neuropathic pain** related to the effects of some cytotoxic drugs (e.g., paclitaxel, cisplatin, vinca alkaloids) on the peripheral nerves

CLINICAL MANIFESTATIONS

Subjective	Objective
Verbal self-report of oral, pharyngeal, esophageal, and/or abdominal pain; statements of painful swallowing; reports of gastric pain induced by spicy or acidic foods; reports of achiness (usually in lower extremities); reports of numbness, tingling, burning, or shooting pain in an extremity or extremities	Grimacing; reluctance to eat or move; clutching abdomen; restlessness

RISK FACTORS

- Chronic disability
- Injurious chemical agents

DESIRED OUTCOMES

The client will experience diminished pain as evidenced by:
a. Verbalization of a decrease in or absence of pain
b. Relaxed facial expression and body positioning
c. Increased participation in activities

NOC OUTCOMES

Pain control; comfort level

NIC INTERVENTIONS

Pain management; environmental management: comfort; analgesic administration; oral health maintenance

NURSING ASSESSMENT	RATIONALE
Assess for and report signs and symptoms of acute/chronic pain.	*Early recognition of signs and symptoms of acute/chronic pain allows for prompt intervention.*
Assess client's perception of the severity of pain using a pain intensity rating scale.	*Use of a pain scale provides for a baseline with which to measure pain and facilitates the transfer of knowledge about a client's pain experience.*
Assess the client's pain pattern (e.g., location, quality, onset, duration, precipitating factors, alleviating factors).	*Each of these affects the treatment of pain.*

THERAPEUTIC INTERVENTIONS	RATIONALE

Independent Actions
Implement measures to reduce pain:

- Perform actions to reduce fatigue (e.g., schedule frequent rest periods; minimize environmental noise). **D** ● ✦

  The reduction of fatigue helps to increase the client's threshold and tolerance for pain.

- Perform actions to reduce fear and anxiety in order to promote relaxation and subsequently increase the client's threshold and tolerance for pain (e.g., maintain calm, supportive, confident manner).

  Fear and anxiety can decrease the client's threshold for pain and thereby heighten the perception of pain.

- Provide or assist with nonpharmacologic methods for pain relief (e.g., massage; position change; progressive relaxation exercises; guided imagery; acupuncture; restful environment; diversional activities such as watching television, reading, or conversing). **D** ● ✦

  Nonpharmacologic interventions may be be effective as they stimulate closure of the gating mechanism in the spinal cord and block the transmission of pain impulses.

- If client has oral, pharyngeal, esophageal, or abdominal pain:
  - Perform actions to reduce the severity of stomatitis (e.g., encourage client to perform oral hygiene frequently using soft-bristle toothbrush or soft-tip swab).

    Actions help to reduce irritation to dry, inflamed oral mucosa.

  - Instruct client to avoid extremely hot, spicy, or acidic foods/fluids; dry or hard foods; raw vegetables.

    Decreased experience of pain may improve client's nutritional intake. Spicy, hot, and acidic foods cause further irritation to the oral and GI mucosa

  - Offer cool, soothing liquids such as nonacidic juices and ices. **D** ● ✦

    Decreases discomfort and provides moisture for the oral cavity which can help to decrease breakdown.

Continued...

THERAPEUTIC INTERVENTIONS	RATIONALE
Dependent/Collaborative Actions Implement measures to reduce pain: If client has oral, pharyngeal, esophageal, or abdominal pain,	
• Instruct client to gargle with a saline solution every 2 hrs or spray mouth with a solution containing diphenhydramine and water (1 oz diphenhydramine and 1 qt water) if ordered.	Actions help to soothe the oral mucous membrane. Protects and soothes oral mucosa which can decrease pain and helps to prevent potential infection.
• Administer topical anesthetics/analgesics and oral protective agents (e.g., mixture of diphenhydramine, antacid, and xylocaine viscous; sucralfate oral suspension) if ordered. **D** ✦	Topical anesthetics decrease pain and can help to improve oral intake.
• Administer the following medications if ordered to manage pain: **D** ✦	Pharmacologic therapy is an effective method of relieving pain.
• Nonopioid analgesics • Skeletal muscle relaxants • Antidepressants	Muscle relaxants help to reduce pain associated with muscle spasms. Antidepressants are often used to treat neuropathic pain.
• Opioid analgesics or opioid analgesics combined with N-methyl-D-aspartate receptor antagonists • Corticosteroids.	
• Apply a cooling pad or ice pack to painful extremity unless contraindicated. **D** ● ✦ `	Steroids help to reduce inflammation, which may cause gain. Action may help reduce mild neuropathic pain.
Consult appropriate health care provider (e.g., pharmacist, physician, pain management specialist) if pain persists or worsens.	Notification of the appropriate health care provider allows for modification of the treatment plan.

Nursing Diagnosis   IMPAIRED INTEGRITY OF ORAL MUCOUS MEMBRANE NDx

Definition: Injury to lips, soft tissue, buccal cavity, and/or oropharynx.

Related to:
• **Dryness** due to reduced oral intake
• **Stomatitis** due to:
  • Malnutrition and inadequate oral hygiene
  • Disruption in the renewal process of mucosal epithelial cells associated with toxic effects of cytotoxic drugs (particularly antimetabolites, antitumor antibiotics, mitotic inhibitors, and taxanes)
  • Infection, particularly gingival, during the period of myelosuppression

CLINICAL MANIFESTATIONS

Subjective	Objective
Verbal self-report of burning pain in mouth; difficulty swallowing; taste changes	Dryness of the oral mucosa; inflamed and/or ulcerated oral mucosa; viscous saliva; positive results of cultured specimens from oral lesions

RISK FACTORS
• Chemical irritants
• Decreased salivation
• Barriers to oral self-care
• Malnutrition
• Medication side effects

DESIRED OUTCOMES
The client will maintain a healthy oral cavity as evidenced by:
  a. Absence of inflammation
  b. Pink, moist, intact mucosa
  c. No reports of oral dryness and burning
  d. Ability to swallow without discomfort

NOC OUTCOMES
Oral hygiene; oral health status

NIC INTERVENTIONS
Oral health maintenance; oral health restoration

NURSING ASSESSMENT	RATIONALE
Assess client for dryness of the oral mucosa and signs and symptoms of stomatitis: • Reports of burning pain in mouth • Difficulty swallowing • Taste changes • Dryness of the oral mucosa • Inflamed and/or ulcerated oral mucosa • Viscous saliva • Positive results of cultured specimens from oral lesions	*Early recognition of signs and symptoms of impaired oral mucosa allows for prompt intervention.*

THERAPEUTIC INTERVENTIONS	RATIONALE

Independent Actions

Implement measures to prevent or reduce the severity of stomatitis and/or relieve dryness of the oral mucous membrane: • Encourage client to chew on ice during chemotherapy infusion, especially if receiving 5-fluorouracil.	*Maintaining moisture in the oral cavity helps to prevent breakdown.*
• Reinforce importance of oral hygiene and assist client with this after meals and snacks; avoid use of products that contain lemon/glycerin and mouthwashes containing alcohol.	*Lemon/glycerin or alcohol-containing products have a drying and irritating effect on the oral mucous membrane. Client should be taught to avoid commercial oral mouthwash unless ingredients do not include glycerin or alcohol.*
• Instruct and assist client to perform oral hygiene using a soft-bristle toothbrush or sponge-tipped swab and to floss teeth gently.	*Use of appropriate oral hygiene devices and techniques helps to effectively remove food particles and debris from client's mouth without causing trauma to the oral mucous membrane.*
• Have client rinse mouth frequently with warm saline solution, baking soda and warm water, chlorhexidine gluconate (Peridex), or mist oral cavity frequently, using a spray bottle. **D** ● ✦	*Increases moisture in the oral cavity and cleans mouth of debris.*
• Lubricate client's lips frequently. **D** ● ✦	*Lubricating lips helps prevent drying and cracking.*
• Encourage client to suck on sugarless candy or chew sugarless gum. **D** ● ✦	*Sucking on candy stimulates saliva secretion.*
• Encourage client not to smoke or chew tobacco.	*Smoking dries the oral mucous membrane.*
• Encourage client to use a saliva substitute (such as Salivart) if indicated.	*Exogenous saliva helps to decrease oral cavity drying.*
• Instruct client to avoid substances that might further irritate the oral mucosa (e.g., hot, spicy, or acidic foods/fluids).	*Irritation and subsequent inflammation can occur when tobacco is in contact with the oral mucosa.*
• Perform actions to promote an adequate nutritional status (e.g., serve food cold or at room temperature; experiment with different seasonings, textures).	*Actions help to compensate for taste alterations that the client may be experiencing.*
If stomatitis is not controlled: • Increase frequency of oral hygiene. **D** ● ✦	*Removes toxins and bacteria that may increase the potential for inflammation or breakdown.*
• If client has dentures, remove them and replace only for meals. **D** ●	

Dependent/Collaborative Actions

Implement measures to prevent or reduce the severity of stomatitis and/or relieve dryness of the oral mucous membrane: • Encourage a fluid intake of at least 2500 mL/day unless contraindicated.	*Adequate hydration helps keep the oral mucosa moist, which reduces the risk of cracking and breakdown.*
• Provide client with a prophylactic antifungal oral suspension or lozenge (e.g., nystatin) if ordered. **D** ✦	*Prevents development of suprainfection due to destroyed intestinal flora.*
Consult appropriate health care provider (e.g., oncology nurse specialist, physician) if signs and symptoms of dryness and stomatitis persist or worsen.	*Notification of the appropriate health care provider allows for modification of the treatment plan.*

Nursing Diagnosis **RISK FOR BLEEDING** NDx

Definition: Susceptible to a decrease in blood volume, which may compromise health.

Related to: Thrombocytopenia, associated with chemotherapy-induced bone marrow suppression

CLINICAL MANIFESTATIONS

Subjective	Objective
N/A	Petechiae, purpura, or ecchymoses; gingival bleeding; prolonged bleeding from puncture sites; epistaxis, hemoptysis; unusual joint pain; frank or occult blood in stool, urine, or vomitus; increase in abdominal girth; menorrhagia; restlessness, confusion; decreasing blood pressure (BP) and increased pulse rate; decrease in hematocrit (Hct) and hemoglobin (Hgb) levels

RISK FACTORS

- Trauma

DESIRED OUTCOMES

The client will not experience unusual bleeding, as evidenced by:
a. Skin and mucous membranes free of petechiae, purpura, ecchymoses, and active bleeding
b. Absence of unusual joint pain
c. Absence of frank and occult blood in stool, urine, and vomitus
d. No increase in abdominal girth
e. Usual menstrual flow
f. Usual mental status
g. Vital signs within normal range for client
h. Stable or improved Hct and Hgb levels

NOC OUTCOMES

Blood coagulation; blood loss severity

NIC INTERVENTIONS

Bleeding precautions, administration of blood products

NURSING ASSESSMENT

Assess client for unusual bleeding and report signs and symptoms such as:
- Petechiae
- Purpura
- Ecchymoses
- Gingival bleeding
- Prolonged bleeding from puncture sites
- Epistaxis
- Hemoptysis
- Unusual joint pain
- Frank or occult blood in stool, urine, or vomitus
- Increase in abdominal girth
- Menorrhagia
- Restlessness
- Confusion
- Decreasing BP and increased pulse rate
- Decrease in Hct and Hgb levels

Monitor platelet count and coagulation test results (e.g., bleeding time). Report significant worsening of values.

If platelet count is low, coagulation test results are abnormal, or Hct and Hgb levels decrease, test stools, urine, and vomitus for occult blood. Report positive results.

RATIONALE

Early recognition of signs and symptoms of bleeding allows for prompt intervention.

THERAPEUTIC INTERVENTIONS	**RATIONALE**
Dependent/Collaborative Actions Implement measures to prevent bleeding:	*Thrombocytopenia predisposes patients to bleeding. Actions that increase the risk for bleeding should be avoided in clients with thrombocytopenia.*
• Avoid giving injections whenever possible; consult physician about prescribing an alternative route for medications ordered to be given intramuscularly or subcutaneously.	
• When giving injections or performing venous and arterial punctures, use the smallest gauge needle possible.	*Decreases volume of bleeding with injections or blood draws.*
• Apply gentle, prolonged pressure to puncture sites after injections, venous and arterial punctures, and diagnostic tests such as bone marrow aspiration.	*Increases coagulation from breaks in the skin.*
• Take BP only when necessary and avoid overinflating the cuff.	*Decreases trauma and potential for bruising.*
• Caution client to avoid activities that increase the risk for trauma (e.g., shaving with a straight-edge razor, using stiff-bristle toothbrush or dental floss).	*Decreases incidence of trauma and subsequent bleeding.*
• Whenever possible, avoid intubations (e.g., nasogastric) and procedures that can cause injury to rectal mucosa (e.g., taking temperatures rectally, inserting a rectal suppository or tube, administering an enema).	*Injuries to these areas are painful and may increase incidence of bleeding and/or infection.*
• Pad side rails if client is confused or restless.	
• Perform actions to reduce the risk for falls (e.g., keep bed in low position with side rails up when client is in bed, avoid unnecessary clutter in room, instruct client to wear slippers/shoes with nonslip soles when ambulating).	*These measures help to ensure safety and prevent injury.*
• Instruct client to avoid blowing nose forcefully or straining to have a bowel movement; consult physician about an order for a decongestant and/or laxative if indicated.	*These measures prevent trauma and subsequent bleeding.*

• Administer the following if ordered:
  • Platelet-stimulating factor
  • Estrogen-progestin preparations to suppress menses
  • Platelets
	Exogenous factors that improve blood clotting ability and decrease bleed loss.

If bleeding occurs and does not subside spontaneously, • Apply firm, prolonged pressure to bleeding area(s) if possible.	*These actions help to decrease bleeding temporarily, support adequate oxygenation in the presence of loss of red blood cells (RBCs), and replace deficient blood components.*
• If epistaxis occurs, place client in a high-Fowler's position and apply pressure and ice pack to nasal area.	*Helps to stop bleeding with a nose bleed.*
• Maintain oxygen therapy as ordered.	*Increases oxygen provided to the tissues.*
• Administer whole blood or blood products (e.g., platelets) as ordered.	*Whole blood and blood products increase the blood's oxygen-carrying capacity as well as vascular volume.*

Collaborative Diagnosis | ## RISK FOR IMPAIRED RENAL FUNCTION

Definition: Inability of the kidney to appropriately concentrate urine and excrete waste products.

Related to:
• Toxic effects of some cytotoxic agents (e.g., cisplatin, high doses of methotrexate, streptozocin) on renal cells
• Nephropathy associated with:
  • Excessive uric acid accumulation resulting from the rapid lysis of large numbers of tumor cells
  • Precipitation of certain drugs (e.g., high doses of methotrexate) in the renal tubules and collecting ducts as a result of low urinary pH and inadequate hydration before, during, and after drug administration

CLINICAL MANIFESTATIONS

Subjective	**Objective**
N/A	Urine output less than 30 mL/h; urine specific gravity fixed at or less than 1.010; elevated BUN and serum creatinine levels; decreased creatinine clearance

RISK FACTORS

- Chemotherapeutic agents
- Impaired volume status

DESIRED OUTCOMES

The client will maintain adequate renal function, as evidenced by:
a. Urine output at least 30 mL/h
b. BUN and serum creatinine levels and creatinine clearance within normal range

NURSING ASSESSMENT	RATIONALE

Assess for and report signs and symptoms of impaired renal function:
- Urine output less than 30 mL/h
- Urine specific gravity fixed at or less than 1.010
- Elevated BUN and serum creatinine levels
- Decreased creatinine clearance

Assess for and report a urine output below 100 mL/h during and for 24 hrs after administration of nephrotoxic drugs.

Early recognition of signs and symptoms of impaired renal function allows for prompt intervention.

Monitoring of changes can alert the health care team of negative consequences of nephrotoxic drugs.

THERAPEUTIC INTERVENTIONS	RATIONALE

Dependent/Collaborative Actions

Implement measures to maintain adequate renal function:

- Hydrate client with at least 150 mL/h of fluid unless contraindicated, for 6 to 24 hrs before administering drugs known to be nephrotoxic (e.g., cisplatin, high doses of methotrexate, streptozocin).
- Administer intravenous fluids as ordered during administration of nephrotoxic drugs and for 24 hrs after. **D** ✦

Adequate hydration ensures optimum perfusion of the kidney, which is necessary for the health of the functional nephron units.

Adequate hydration helps to maintain a high rate of glomerular blood flow. Increased blood flow helps to flush the medication out of the kidneys and decreases potential damage to the kidneys.

Administer the following medications as ordered:
- Diuretics (e.g., furosemide, mannitol)

- Xanthine oxidase inhibitor (e.g., allopurinol)

- Sodium bicarbonate

- Leucovorin calcium (e.g., folic acid)

- Chemoprotectant agent (e.g., amifostine)

Diuretics help to promote more rapid plasma clearance of the cytotoxic agent.

Xanthine oxidase inhibitors help to decrease the formation of uric acid.

Sodium bicarbonate helps to alkalinize the urine and subsequently increase the solubility of uric acid in the urine, thus preventing the precipitation of methotrexate in renal tubules and collecting ducts.

Folic acid helps to diminish the toxic effects of cytotoxic agents such as methotrexate on the renal cells.

Chemoprotective agents help to protect the renal cells against toxicity from some cytotoxic agents (e.g., cisplatin).

If signs and symptoms of impaired renal function occur:
- Assess for and report signs of acute renal failure (e.g., oliguria or anuria; weight gain of 2% or greater over a short time; edema; elevated BP; lethargy and confusion; increasing BUN and serum creatinine, phosphorus, and potassium levels).
- Prepare client for dialysis if indicated.

Recognition of signs and symptoms of impaired renal function allows for prompt intervention and potential preservation of kidney function.

Collaborative Diagnosis RISK FOR HEMORRHAGIC CYSTITIS

Definition: Inflammation of the bladder resulting in bleeding.

Related to: Irritation and ulceration of the bladder mucosa by toxic metabolites of certain cytotoxic agents, particularly cyclophosphamide and ifosfamide

CLINICAL MANIFESTATIONS

Subjective	Objective
Verbal self-reports of dysuria; suprapubic pain	Frank or occult blood in urine; urinary frequency/urgency

RISK FACTORS

- Chemotherapy

DESIRED OUTCOMES

The client will not develop hemorrhagic cystitis as evidenced by absence of dysuria, urinary frequency and urgency, suprapubic pain, and hematuria.

NURSING ASSESSMENT	RATIONALE
Assess for and report signs and symptoms of hemorrhagic cystitis: • Dysuria • Suprapubic pain • Frank or occult blood in urine • Urinary frequency/urgency	*Early recognition of signs and symptoms of hemorrhagic cystitis allows for prompt intervention.*

THERAPEUTIC INTERVENTIONS	RATIONALE

Dependent/Collaborative Actions
 Implement measures to prevent hemorrhagic cystitis:
 • Ensure that client is vigorously hydrated; maintain intravenous fluids at the rate ordered (often as high as 200 mL/h during chemotherapy). **D** ✦
 • Administer cyclophosphamide early in the day and encourage client to void at least every 4 hrs, before going to bed, and at least once during the night.
 • Administer mesna (Mesnex) if ordered.
 	
 • Maintain continuous bladder irrigation before and after administration of cyclophosphamide or ifosfamide if ordered.
 If signs and symptoms of hemorrhagic cystitis occur,
 • Discontinue cytotoxic drug administration and notify physician.
 • Continue with fluid administration as ordered. **D** ✦
 • Administer diuretics as ordered. **D** ✦
 	
 • Assist with or perform bladder irrigations as ordered.
 • Maintain continuous bladder irrigation with silver nitrate or alum (potassium aluminum sulfate) solution if ordered to stop bleeding.
 • Prepare client for the following if planned:
   • Cystoscopy to cauterize bleeding vessels
   • Intravesical instillation of formalin to control persistent severe bleeding
	Adequate hydration ensures ability to reduce the concentration of toxic drug metabolites in the bladder.
	
	 Actions help to prevent stasis of toxic drug metabolites in the bladder.
	
	 Mesna helps to interact with and inactivate the toxic drug metabolites of ifosfamide.
	 Continuous bladder irrigation helps to flush metabolites from the bladder and prevent the formation of obstructive clots should bleeding occur.
	 Prevents further bladder injury.
	
	 Maintains adequate urine production to flush the bladder.
	 To increase urine output and thereby decrease the concentration of toxic drug metabolites in the urine.
	
	 Bladder irrigations help to facilitate the removal of drug metabolites and flush clots from the bladder.
	
	 Prevents further injury.

Collaborative Diagnosis   **RISK FOR DRUG EXTRAVASATION**

Definition: Infiltration of drugs into soft tissues leading to local tissue irritation and sloughing.

Related to: Extravasation of vesicant drugs (e.g., most antitumor antibiotics, teniposide, vinblastine, vincristine, paclitaxel)

CLINICAL MANIFESTATIONS

Subjective	Objective
Verbal self-report of stinging or burning pain at infusion site or along vein	Swelling, blanching, or coolness of skin around infusion site

RISK FACTORS

- Infiltration of intravenous lines
- Multiple punctures in the same vein

DESIRED OUTCOMES

The client will not experience drug extravasation as evidenced by:
a. Absence of swelling, blanching, and coolness of skin around infusion site
b. No reports of stinging or burning pain at infusion site or along the vein

NURSING ASSESSMENT	RATIONALE
Assess for signs and symptoms of drug extravasation: • Reports of stinging or burning pain at infusion site or along vein • Swelling, blanching, or coolness of skin around infusion site Ensure that infusion site and surrounding tissue are visible at all times.	*Early recognition of signs and symptoms of drug extravasation allows for prompt intervention.*

THERAPEUTIC INTERVENTIONS	RATIONALE
Dependent/Collaborative Actions Implement measures to prevent drug extravasation: • Select the best vein possible for vesicant drug administration:	*Use of a fragile vein and previous use increase the risk for extravasation.*
• Do not use a vein that has been previously used for vesicant agents.	
• Use a large vein in the forearm if possible; avoid the antecubital fossa and small veins in the hand.	*Extravasation in these areas can destroy nerves and tendons.*
• Do not use an existing peripheral intravenous catheter that is more than 24 hrs old.	*This prevents excessive damage to the vein and decreases the risk of extravasation.*
• Avoid extremities with compromised circulation.	
• Consult physician about insertion of a central venous catheter or Peripherally Inserted Central Catheter (PICC) line if large and/or frequent doses of a vesicant are planned.	*Vessels with compromised circulation are at increased risk for stasis of the medication and vessel damage.*
• Do not perform multiple punctures in the same vein.	*Prevents leakage from the vessel after infusion has begun.*
• Tape intravenous catheter securely but not too tightly.	*Prevents skin irritation.*
• Do not irrigate catheter forcefully or use a high-pressure setting on infusion device.	*Irrigating forcefully may disrupt the integrity of the vessel, resulting in infiltration.*
Perform actions to ensure that the drug is infusing into the vein: • Test patency of vein before administering a cytotoxic drug. • Stay with client while a vesicant drug is infusing; check site every 2 to 3 minutes.	*Ensuring adequate blood return prior to the administration of cytotoxic agents reduces the risk of extravasation.*
Perform actions to prevent increased irritation of the vein: • Dilute drug according to manufacturer's recommendations. • Administer drug at recommended rate of infusion.	*High concentration of the medication and rapid administration will increase trauma to blood vessels.*

THERAPEUTIC INTERVENTIONS	RATIONALE
• Stop infusion if there is any indication that the drug is not infusing properly.	*Prevents injury.*
• When the drug infusion is complete, flush intravenous catheter with a minimum of 30 mL of normal saline; apply pressure to site for at least 4 minutes after catheter removal to minimize oozing.	*Ensures medication is fully administered and prevents injury or leakage of medication onto the skin.*
If signs and symptoms of drug extravasation occur:	
• Stop infusion immediately.	*Infusion must be discontinued immediately and area treated per hospital protocol to avoid extensive tissue damage.*
• Treat area of extravasation as ordered (treatment varies depending on drug used) or per standard hospital procedure.	
• Assess the site frequently for signs of increased inflammation, blistering, and necrosis.	*Document and measure changes to monitor healing. Provides information concerning changes over time.*
• Administer analgesics as ordered (severe pain is common after extravasation).	*Decreases pain and discomfort in the area.*

Nursing Diagnosis RISK FOR CARDIAC DYSRHYTHMIAS NDx

Definition: Disturbance of the heart rhythm.

Related to: Cardiotoxic effects of certain cytotoxic drugs (e.g., cyclophosphamide, high doses of ifosfamide, doxorubicin, daunorubicin, paclitaxel)

CLINICAL MANIFESTATIONS

Subjective	Objective
Verbal self-report of light-headedness; palpitations; fainting	Irregular apical pulse; pulse rate below 60 or above 100 beats/min; apical-radial pulse deficit; syncope; palpitations; abnormal rate, rhythm, or configurations on electrocardiogram (ECG)

RISK FACTORS

• Electrolyte imbalance

DESIRED OUTCOMES

The client will experience resolution of cardiac dysrhythmias if they occur as evidenced by:
a. Regular apical pulse at 60 to 100 beats/min
b. Equal apical and radial pulse rates
c. Absence of syncope and palpitations
d. ECG reading showing normal sinus rhythm

NOC OUTCOMES

Cardiac pump effectiveness

NIC INTERVENTIONS

Dysrhythmia management

NURSING ASSESSMENT	RATIONALE
Assess for and report signs and symptoms of cardiac dysrhythmias:	*Early recognition of signs and symptoms of cardiac dysrhythmias allows for prompt intervention.*
• Reports of lightheadedness, palpitations	
• Irregular apical pulse	
• Pulse rate below 60 or above 100 beats/min	
• Apical-radial pulse deficit	
• Syncope	
• Abnormal rate, rhythm, or configurations on ECG	

Continued...

NURSING ASSESSMENT	RATIONALE
Monitor liver and kidney function studies and report abnormal results.	*Cardiotoxicity can result from delayed metabolism or excretion of cytotoxic drugs by the liver or kidneys.*

THERAPEUTIC INTERVENTIONS	RATIONALE
Dependent/Collaborative Actions Administer a cardioprotectant agent (e.g., dexrazoxane) if ordered. If cardiac dysrhythmias occur: • Initiate cardiac monitoring and prepare client for an ECG if ordered. • Administer antidysrhythmic agents (e.g., lidocaine, digoxin, diltiazem, esmolol, amiodarone, atropine) if ordered. • Monitor client manifestations of decreased cardiac output. • Restrict client's activity based on his or her tolerance and the severity of the dysrhythmia. • Maintain oxygen therapy as ordered. • Assess cardiovascular status frequently and report signs and symptoms of inadequate tissue perfusion (e.g., decrease in BP, cool skin, cyanosis, diminished peripheral pulses, declining urine output, restlessness and agitation, shortness of breath). • Have emergency cart readily available for defibrillation, cardioversion, or cardiopulmonary resuscitation.	*Cardioprotective agents help to reduce the risk of anthracycline-induced cardiac damage.* *Allows for proper identification of dysrhythmias and the implementation of the appropriate interventions.* *If cardiac output decreases, implement safety measures to decrease risk of falls.* *Decreases risk of injury.* *Enhances oxygenation.* *Allows for prompt changes in treatment regimen.* *Life-threatening dysrhythmias such as ventricular fibrillation require the use of equipment maintained on emergency carts.*

Collaborative Diagnosis RISK FOR INFLAMMATION AND FIBROSIS OF LUNG TISSUE

Related to: The effects of some cytotoxic agents on the lung (e.g., busulfan, bleomycin, carmustine, mitomycin).

CLINICAL MANIFESTATIONS

Subjective	Objective
Verbal self-report of shortness of breath	Dry, hacking, persistent cough; fever; tachypnea; dyspnea on exertion; wheezing; crackles

RISK FACTORS
• Chemotherapeutic agents
• Radiation therapy

DESIRED OUTCOMES

The client will experience decreased signs and symptoms of pulmonary inflammation and fibrosis if they occur as evidenced by:
a. Decreased coughing
b. Afebrile status
c. Decreased dyspnea
d. Improved breath sounds

NURSING ASSESSMENT	RATIONALE
Assess for and report signs and symptoms of pulmonary inflammation and fibrosis, particularly if client is reaching total allowable cumulative dose of cytotoxic agent or agents known to cause pulmonary toxicity: • Verbal reports of shortness of breath • Dry, hacking, persistent cough • Fever • Tachypnea • Dyspnea on exertion • Wheezing • Crackles	*Early recognition of signs and symptoms of pulmonary inflammation/fibrosis allows for prompt intervention.*

THERAPEUTIC INTERVENTIONS	**RATIONALE**

Dependent/Collaborative Actions

If signs and symptoms of pulmonary inflammation and fibrosis occur:

- Discontinue infusion of cytotoxic agent as ordered.   *Discontinuing use of the medication prevents further exposure to the toxic agents.*

    Maintains supplemental tissue oxygenation.

- Prepare client for diagnostic studies (e.g., chest radiograph, pulmonary function studies, computed tomography (CT) or gallium scan, fiberoptic bronchoscopy) if planned.

Maintain oxygen therapy as ordered.

Administer the following medications if ordered:

- Corticosteroids   *Corticosteroids reduce the inflammatory response.*
- Bronchodilators   *Bronchodilators dilate the bronchi and bronchioles, decrease airway resistance, and improve airflow.*

Collaborative Diagnosis   RISK FOR NEUROTOXICITY

Definition: Destructive or poisonous effects on nerve tissue.

Related to: The toxic effects of certain cytotoxic agents (e.g., vincristine, vinblastine, cisplatin, ifosfamide, etoposide, high doses of methotrexate or cytarabine) on the nerves

CLINICAL MANIFESTATIONS

Subjective	**Objective**
Verbal self-report of numbness and tingling of extremities; burning pain in extremity; unusual muscle weakness; blurred vision	Constipation; ataxia; gait disturbances; difficulty with fine motor movements; foot drop or wrist drop; hearing loss; nystagmus; memory loss; confusion; expressive aphasia; seizures

RISK FACTORS

- Administration of chemotherapeutic agents

DESIRED OUTCOMES

The client will adapt to the signs and symptoms of neurotoxicity if it occurs and not experience injury associated with those signs and symptoms.

NURSING ASSESSMENT	**RATIONALE**

Assess for and report signs and symptoms of neurotoxicity:

- Numbness and tingling of extremities
- Burning pain in extremity
- Unusual muscle weakness
- Blurred vision
- Constipation
- Ataxia, gait disturbances
- Difficulty with fine motor movements
- Foot drop or wrist drop
- Hearing loss
- Nystagmus
- Memory loss
- Confusion
- Expressive aphasia
- Seizures

Early recognition of signs and symptoms of neurotoxicity allows for prompt intervention.

THERAPEUTIC INTERVENTIONS	RATIONALE
Dependent/Collaborative Actions	
If signs and symptoms of neurotoxicity occur:	Recognition of signs and symptoms of neurotoxicity allows for implementation of the appropriate interventions and modification of the treatment plan.
• Implement measures to prevent falls:	
• Keep bed in low position. **D** ●	Neurotoxicity can result in ataxia, which may predispose the client to falls.
	Common clinical manifestations associated with neoplastic drugs include numbness in the extremities (polyneuropathy), which may interfere with a normal response to hot foods and water.
• Avoid unnecessary clutter in the room. **D** ●	Decreases potential for falls and subsequent injury.
• Implement measures to prevent burns and cuts:	
• Let hot foods/fluids cool slightly before serving.	Prevents burning of oral mucosa and skin.
• Assess temperature of bath water before bathing.	
• Institute seizure precautions if indicated.	
• Implement measures to help client adapt to the following if present:	
• Constipation	
(1) Encourage fluid intake. **D** ✦	Fluid and fiber intake are effective in reducing the incidence of constipation.
(2) Increase fiber intake.	
• Pain in extremities	Musculoskeletal effects associated with neurotoxicity include myalgia, joint stiffness, and muscle weakness.
(1) Assist with position changes. **D** ●	Decreases joint stiffness.
(2) Assist with guided imagery. **D** ● ✦	Provides alternative methods of pain control.
• Foot drop	
(1) Instruct client to perform active foot exercises every 1 to 2 hrs while awake. **D** ● ✦	Prevents muscle wasting and improves muscle strength.
• Wrist drop	
(1) Instruct client to perform active wrist exercises every 1 to 2 hrs while awake. **D** ● ✦	
• Impaired hearing	
(1) Face client when speaking.	Improves communication between patient and health care provider.
(2) Use gestures.	
(3) Provide written information	
• Memory loss	
(1) Assist to make lists. **D** ● ✦	Actions assist clients with memory loss, visual or auditory hallucinations, and the confusion that can result from neurotoxicity.
(2) Repeat information as needed.	
• Confusion	
(1) Decrease environmental stimuli. **D** ● ✦	Prevents overstimulation of client that can increase confision.
(2) Keep daily routines consistent. **D** ● ✦	Allows client a level of independence.
• Expressive aphasia	
(1) Encourage client to use short words.	Take time with client to make sure that they are heard and support their concerns related to this.
(2) Encourage client to use gestures.	
Consult physician if signs and symptoms of neurotoxicity persist or worsen.	Allows for prompt change in treatment regimen.

Nursing Diagnosis ## RISK FOR DISTURBED SELF-CONCEPT*

Definition: **Disturbed Body Image NDx:** Confusion in mental picture of one's physical self; **Situational Low Self-Esteem NDx:** Development of a negative perception of self-worth in response to a current situation.

Related to
• Changes in appearance associated with the side effects of chemotherapy (e.g., alopecia, excessive weight loss, skin and nail changes) and external drug infusion catheter if present

---

* This diagnostic label includes the nursing diagnoses of disturbed body image and situational low self-esteem.

- Possible alteration in usual sexual activities associated with weakness, fatigue, reduced levels of testosterone (can occur with chemotherapy for prostate or testicular cancer or lymphoma), psychologic factors, and vaginal discomfort (may result from mucositis and premature menopause if ovarian failure occurs)
- Possible temporary or permanent infertility associated with gonadal dysfunction resulting from extensive therapy with some cytotoxic drugs (e.g., some alkylating agents)
- Increased dependence on others to meet self-care needs
- Changes in lifestyle and roles associated with effects of the disease process and its treatment

CLINICAL MANIFESTATIONS

Subjective	**Objective**
Verbal self-report of negative feelings about self; lack of plan to adapt to necessary changes in lifestyle	Withdrawal from significant others; lack of participation in activities of daily living

RISK FACTORS

- Treatment of illness
- Altered body image

DESIRED OUTCOMES

The client will demonstrate beginning adaptation to changes in appearance, body functioning, lifestyle, and roles as evidenced by:
a. Verbalization of feelings of self-worth and sexual adequacy
b. Maintenance of relationships with significant others
c. Active participation in activities of daily living
d. Develop a beginning plan for adapting lifestyle to changes resulting from the disease process and residual effects of chemotherapy

NOC OUTCOMES

Self-esteem, body image

NIC INTERVENTIONS

Body image enhancement, self-esteem enhancement, role enhancement, emotional support, support system enhancement

NURSING ASSESSMENT

Assess for signs and symptoms of a disturbed self-concept:
- Verbalization of negative feelings about self
- Lack of planning to adapt to necessary changes in lifestyle
- Withdrawal from significant others
- Lack of participation in activities of daily living

RATIONALE

Early recognition of signs and symptoms of disturbed self-concept allows for prompt intervention.

THERAPEUTIC INTERVENTIONS

Independent Actions

Implement measures to facilitate the grieving process.
Discuss with client improvements in appearance and functioning that can realistically be expected.
Implement measures for the following changes in body functioning and appearance if appropriate:
- Alopecia
  - Inform client that hair loss can be expected approximately 2 weeks after initiation of chemotherapy; may be sudden, gradual, partial, or complete and can include scalp hair, pubic hair, beard, eyebrows, and eyelashes.

  - Reassure client that hair loss is temporary (regrowth sometimes occurs before cessation of treatment but usually occurs 2–3 months after it).
  - Inform client that hair regrowth may be a different color, texture, and consistency.

RATIONALE

Allows client to discuss specific concerns they have in relation to changes that may occur while undergoing chemotherapy.
These actions help to assist client to adapt to changes in body functioning and appearance.

Clients may exhibit a range of emotional responses at the prospect of losing hair, including anger, grief, embarrassment, and fear. Educating the client regarding hair loss may alleviate anxiety and allow the client to explore feelings associated with this side effect. Allow patient to choose wig and have control during selection process.
Helps client to realize that the change is not permanent.

Continued...

THERAPEUTIC INTERVENTIONS	RATIONALE
• Encourage client to cut hair very short. • Brushing hair gently using a soft-bristle brush. • Shampooing hair only once or twice a week and using a gentle shampoo and lukewarm water.	*Prepares client for potential changes when hair regrowth occurs. Cutting the hair very short helps to decrease the anxiety related to seeing large quantities of hair fall out.*
• Avoiding use of equipment/products that dry hair (e.g., hot rollers, hair dryers, curling iron, dyes). • Avoiding hairstyles that create tension on hair (e.g., ponytails, braids). • Encourage client to wear a wig, scarf, hat, false eyelashes, or makeup if desired to camouflage hair loss.	*Helps to prevent hair breakage and subsequent loss. These actions give the client methods to help control hair loss.*
• Inform client of community resources that can provide information and assistance with ways to facilitate adjustment to changes in appearance (e.g., American Cancer Society, Look Good–Feel Better Program).	*Provides client with choices concerning what to do when hair loss occurs. Use of these helps to improve client's self-esteem.* *Provides resource for client once discharged from the acute care facility.*
• Skin changes (e.g., redness, rashes, peeling, increased sensitivity to sun, acne, darkening along the vein used for cytotoxic drug administration).	*Educating the client about skin changes associated with chemotherapy may help alleviate anxiety and allow client to explore feelings associated with this side effect.*
• Inform client that skin and vein hyperpigmentation may occur if cytotoxic drugs such as bleomycin, busulfan, methotrexate, and fluorouracil are being administered. • Inform client that skin and vein discoloration is usually temporary.	*Informs client of what to expect when undergoing chemotherapy.*
Instruct client to avoid exposure to sunlight and to use sunscreen. • Help client to identify types of clothing that can be worn to camouflage skin changes.	*Provides client with information to determine type of clothing require to prevent an increase in photosensitivity reactions.*
• Nail changes • Inform client that nails may thicken and stop growing, develop ridges, darken, and detach from nail bed during treatment with certain cytotoxic drugs (e.g., cyclophosphamide, doxorubicin, bleomycin, fluorouracil). • Reassure client that normal nail growth will resume when chemotherapy is completed.	*Informing client about nail changes associated with chemotherapy may help to alleviate anxiety. Information received before treatment can help client identify ways to adapt to changes or how to camouflage changes.* *Helps client to understand that changes are temporary.*
• Infertility • Clarify physician's explanation that infertility is a possible permanent effect of chemotherapy.	*Educating client about infertility may help alleviate anxiety and allow client to explore alternative treatments. Or to make reproductive decisions prior to initiating treatment (i.e., sperm or egg harvesting and preserving for future use)*
• Discuss alternative methods of becoming a parent (e.g., artificial insemination, adoption) if of concern to client. • Impotence. • Encourage client to discuss this with his or her physician.	*Educating client about impotence may help alleviate anxiety and allow client to explore alternative treatments.* *Impotence usually resolves after cessation of chemotherapy. Discussing this before it occurs may help client be prepared if of does occur.*
• Suggest alternative methods of sexual gratification if appropriate. • Discuss ways to be creative in expressing sexuality (e.g., massage, fantasies, cuddling).	*Gives client time to explore other methods of obtaining sexual pleasure.*
Help client with usual grooming and makeup habits if necessary. **D** ●	*Client may need assistance in this activity and nursing staff should be able to help.*
Support behaviors suggesting positive adaptation to changes that have occurred (e.g., interest in personal appearance, maintenance of relationships with significant others).	*These actions promote positive self-esteem and client's ability to maintain supportive relationships.*
Support client's and significant others' adjustment to changes by listening, facilitating communication, and providing information.	*Demonstrates accepts of client and provides a resource for client to ask questions and explore feelings about changes.*
Encourage significant others to allow client to do what he or she is able.	*Actions help encourage client to be independent and/or develop self-esteem.*

THERAPEUTIC INTERVENTIONS	RATIONALE
Encourage client contact with others.	*Contact with others helps client to test and establish a new self-image.*
Encourage visits and support from significant others.	*Provides additional resources to help client make life changes.*
Consult appropriate health care provider (e.g., psychiatric nurse clinician, physician) if client seems unwilling or unable to adapt to changes that have occurred as a result of cancer and its treatment.	

DISCHARGE TEACHING/CONTINUED CARE

Nursing Diagnosis **KNOWLEDGE DEFICIT*NDx, INEFFECTIVE HEALTH MANAGEMENT*NDx, INEFFECTIVE FAMILY HEALTH MANAGEMENT*NDx**

Definitions: **Deficient Knowledge NDx:** Absence of cognitive information related to a specific topic, or its acquisition; **Ineffective Health Management NDx:** Pattern of regulating and integrating into daily living a therapeutic regimen for the treatment of illness and its sequelae that is unsatisfactory for meeting specific health goals; **Ineffective Family Health Management NDx:** A pattern of regulating and integrating into family processes a program for the treatment of illness and its sequelae that is unsatisfactory for meeting specific health goals of the family unit.

RISK FACTORS
- Cognitive limitations
- Lack of recall
- Diminished fine/gross motor skills
- Fear and anxiety

NOC OUTCOMES	NIC INTERVENTIONS
Knowledge: disease process; treatment regimen; energy conservation; treatment procedures	Health system guidance; teaching: disease process; teaching: prescribed medication; teaching: prescribed exercise; teaching: procedure/treatment; nutrition management

CLINICAL MANIFESTATIONS

Subjective Verbal self-report of challenges related to learning; verbal self-report of concerns about one's ability to care for self	**Objective** Exaggerated behaviors; inaccurate follow-through of instructions

NURSING ASSESSMENT	RATIONALE
• Assess client's willingness to learn and knowledge related to the disease and treatment process	*The client's willingness to learn and knowledge base provide the foundation for education.*
• Assess for indications that the client may be unable to manage the therapeutic regimen effectively	*Early recognition of inability to understand disease process or provide self-care allows for changes in the teaching plan.*

THERAPEUTIC INTERVENTIONS	RATIONALE
Desired Outcome: The client will identify ways to prevent infection during periods of lowered immunity.	
Independent Actions Explain to client that his or her resistance to infection is reduced when white blood cell (WBC) counts are low. Emphasize the need to adhere closely to recommended techniques to prevent infection.	*Information about what changes occur is important to provide to client and family to help prevent the negative sequelae of cancer treatment.*

NDx = NANDA Diagnosis   **D** = Delegatable Action   ● = UAP   ✦ = LVN/LPN   ⊖▶ = Go to ⊖volve for animation

Continued...

THERAPEUTIC INTERVENTIONS	RATIONALE
Instruct the client in ways to prevent infection:	
• Avoid crowds, persons with any sign of infection, and persons who have recently been vaccinated.	*Prevents exposure to individuals who may be carrying microbes that can have a negative impact on a client undergoing chemotherapy.*
• Use good hand hygiene (e.g., wash hands using an anti-bacterial soap, use an alcohol-base hand rub).	*Good hand hygiene is paramount in preventing infection.*
• Wear gloves to protect hands during activities such as cleaning and gardening.	*Animal feces are often present in garden soil and if ingested can lead to infection in an immunocompromised client.*
• Take axillary rather than oral temperature if stomatitis is present.	*Axillary temperature assessment is more comfortable for a client with stomatitis.*
• Lubricate skin frequently to prevent dryness and subsequent cracking.	*Prevents skin breakdown and decreases potential for infection.*
• Maintain sterile technique when caring for a central venous or peritoneal catheter, an Ommaya reservoir, or an implanted infusion device (e.g., MediPort) if in place.	*Sterile technique is paramount when dealing with indwelling catheters to prevent catheter line sepsis.*
• Avoid unnecessary rectal invasion (e.g., temperature taking, enemas, suppositories, sexual activity) to prevent rectal trauma.	*Damage or perforation of the bowel can lead to sepsis in an immunocompromised client.*
• Avoid constipation to prevent damage to the bowel mucosa from hard or impacted stool.	*Adequate hydration helps to prevent constipation.*
• Wash perianal area thoroughly with soap and water after each bowel movement and after sexual activity; instruct female client to always wipe from front to back after urination and defecation.	*Prevents cross-contamination between the vagina and the rectum. Actions prevent urinary tract contamination from fecal bacteria.*
• Drink at least 10 glasses of liquid a day unless contraindicated.	*Helps to maintain adequate hydration.*
• Cough and deep breathe or use incentive spirometer every 2 hrs until usual activity is resumed.	*Supports lung expansion and movement of secretions if present. Coughing and deep breathing keep alveoli expanded, improve gas exchange, and facilitate expectoration of secretions, preventing pneumonia.*
• Stop smoking.	*Smoking damages the mucociliary system, which helps facilitate the expectoration of secretions. Prevents chronic lung irritation and paralysis of the cilia.*
• Perform meticulous oral hygiene after meals and at bedtime, change denture care solution daily, and replace toothbrush routinely.	*Maintains oral hydration and prevents oral infections.*
• Avoid douching unless ordered.	*Douching disturbs normal vaginal flora and may cause trauma to the vaginal mucosa. Prevents loss of normal flora.*
• Maintain an optimal nutritional status (e.g., diet high in protein, calories, vitamins, and minerals).	*Maintains wellness and body's ability to fight infection.*
• Avoid sharing eating utensils.	*Prevents infection.*
• Maintain an adequate balance between activity and rest.	*Adequate rest will help decrease incidence of fatigue.*
• Cleanse respiratory equipment as instructed; change water in humidifiers daily.	*Prevents infection.*
• Decrease risk of food-borne illness:	*Prevents infection or illness from food sources.*
• Avoid intake of foods with a high microorganism content (e.g., unwashed fruits and vegetables; undercooked eggs, meat, poultry, and seafood).	
• Be sure that juices and ciders are pasteurized or processed and that milk and cheese are pasteurized.	*Prevents unnecessary exposure to microbes in unpasteurized, unclean, or inappropriately prepared foods.*
• Thoroughly wash hands, food preparation items, and surfaces (e.g., knives, cutting board, countertop) before and after cooking, especially when working with raw meat, poultry, and fish.	
• Thaw food items in the refrigerator rather than on kitchen counter.	

THERAPEUTIC INTERVENTIONS	**RATIONALE**
• Avoid picking up animal waste or cleaning animal litter boxes and bird cages.	*These products may contain agents that can be harmful to a patient undergoing chemotherapy.*
• Avoid elective surgery and dental work.	*Decreases risk for bleeding and infection.*
• Reinforce the importance of taking prescribed medications such as colony-stimulating factors and prophylactic antimicrobial agents.	*Medications provide additional support to the immune system to fight off infectious agents.*

THERAPEUTIC INTERVENTIONS	**RATIONALE**

Desired Outcome: The client will demonstrate appropriate oral hygiene techniques.

Independent Actions

Explain the rationale for and importance of frequent oral hygiene.	*Frequent oral hygiene is necessary in the neutropenic client to keep the oral cavity clean, moist, and free of bacterial infection so adequate nutritional intake can occur.*
Provide instructions regarding oral hygiene techniques:	
• Cleanse mouth after eating and at bedtime; increase frequency to every 2 hrs if stomatitis is present.	*Helps to flush debris out of the oral cavity, prevent possible gum irritation and potential infection.*
• Use a soft-bristle toothbrush.	*Prevents trauma to fragile mucous membranes.*
• Rinse mouth with the following solutions as prescribed:	
• Salt or baking soda and warm water	*These solutions help to reduce oral dryness.*
• Chlorhexidine gluconate (Peridex)	
• Avoid commercial mouthwashes that have an alcohol base.	*These agents are drying to the oral mucosa.*

THERAPEUTIC INTERVENTIONS	**RATIONALE**

Desired Outcome: The client will verbalize ways to improve appetite and nutritional status.

Independent Actions

Instruct client in ways to control nausea and vomiting:	*Nausea and vomiting commonly occur after chemotherapy and/or radiation. Prevention and control of nausea and vomiting are necessary to ensure adequate nutrition.*
• Eat foods that are cool or at room temperature (hot foods frequently have a strong aroma that stimulates nausea).	*Helps to decrease nausea and calm an irritated stomach.*
• Eat dry foods (e.g., toast, crackers) or sip cold carbonated beverages if you are feeling nauseous.	
• Eat several small meals a day instead of three large ones.	*Prevents overdistention of the stomach and potential for nausea.*
• Avoid drinking liquids with meals.	*Fluids will decrease the amount of food the client may be willing to eat as fluids increase the feeling of fullness.*
• Select bland foods (e.g., mashed potatoes, cottage cheese) rather than fatty, spicy foods.	
• Rest after eating.	*Spicy food can irritation the stomach and increase the incidence of nausea.*
	Allows for easier digestion of food. Exercising would pull blood away from the stomach and increase digestion time.
• Avoid offensive odors and sights.	
• Cleanse mouth frequently.	*Increases incidence of nausea and can decrease appetite.*
• Take deep, slow breaths when nauseated.	*Maintains oral hydration.*
• Take antiemetics on a regular basis for prescribed length of time and if nausea is persistent.	*Deep breathing helps to decrease nausea,*
	Reduce nausea when taken on a regular basis and before nausea occurs.
Teach client about ways to improve appetite and maintain an adequate nutritional status:	*Cells of the mucosal lining of the stomach are highly proliferative. Intestinal mucosa is very sensitive to radiation and chemotherapy. Nausea, vomiting, diarrhea, mucositis, and anorexia are all gastrointestinal effects that can affect a client's nutritional status. These actions help to facilitate optimum nutritional status for clients undergoing chemotherapy.*
• Try fish, cheese, chicken, and eggs as protein sources instead of beef and pork if taste distortion is a problem.	
• Increase amount of sugar or sweeteners and seasonings usually used in foods and beverages.	
• Use plastic utensils and cook food in glass or plastic containers if metallic taste is present.	
• Eat in a pleasant environment with company if possible.	*Metallic taste is off-putting and may decrease intake.*
• Perform frequent meticulous oral hygiene.	

Continued...

THERAPEUTIC INTERVENTIONS	RATIONALE
• Try recommended methods of controlling nausea.	*Helps to relax the client and can potentially increase intake.*
	Eliminates unpleasant taste in mouth that may decrease appetite.
• Eat several high-calorie, high-protein, nutritious small meals each day rather than three large ones; use nutritional supplements if needed.	*Decreased nausea can lead to increased intake and improvement in nutritional status.*
Plan ahead for low-energy days (e.g., have some prepared meals available; maintain an ample supply of nutritious, minimal preparation foods such as eggs, tuna fish, cheese, peanut butter, and yogurt; keep nutritious snacks and beverages within easy reach).	*Prevents overdistention of the stomach and increases caloric intake.* *Supplements help to maintain adequate caloric intake.* *Having food readily available makes it easier to maintain adequate nutrition when one is not feeling well or not wanting to cook.*
• Take vitamins, minerals, and appetite stimulants (e.g., megestrol acetate, dronabinol) as prescribed.	*These supplements increase appetite, support caloric intake, and improve nutritional status.*

THERAPEUTIC INTERVENTIONS	RATIONALE

The client will verbalize ways to manage and cope with persistent fatigue.

Independent Actions

Instruct client in ways to manage and cope with persistent fatigue:	*Fatigue affects most clients undergoing chemotherapy and/or radiation. Fatigue may be related to anemia or side effects of therapy.*
• View fatigue as a protective mechanism rather than a problematic limitation.	
• Determine ways in which daily patterns of activity can be modified to conserve energy and prevent excessive fatigue (e.g., spread light and heavy tasks throughout the day, take short rests during an activity whenever possible, sit during an activity whenever possible, take several short rest periods during the day instead of one long one).	*Client must identify ways to decrease fatigue and put a plan in place to get enough rest and exercise to maintain muscle strength.*
• Determine whether life demands are realistic in light of physical state and adjust short- and long-term goals accordingly.	
• Avoid situations that are particularly fatiguing, such as those that are boring, frustrating, or require prolonged or strenuous physical activity.	
• Participate in a moderate exercise program (e.g., walking or bicycling 20–30 minutes three or four times a week).	*Exercise improves muscle strength and may decrease frequency of fatigue.*
• Participate in "attention-restoring" activities (e.g., walking outdoors, gardening).	

THERAPEUTIC INTERVENTIONS	RATIONALE

Desired Outcome: The client will verbalize ways to prevent bleeding when his or her platelet counts are low.

Independent Actions

Instruct client in ways to minimize risk of bleeding:	*A client who is thrombocytopenic is at risk for increased bleeding and should be instructed on actions to prevent and/or control bleeding.*
• Avoid taking aspirin and other nonsteroidal anti-inflammatory agents (e.g., ibuprofen).	
• Consult health care provider before routinely taking herbs that can increase the risk of bleeding (e.g., ginkgo, arnica, chamomile).	
• Brush teeth gently using a soft-bristle toothbrush; do not use dental floss or put sharp objects (e.g., toothpicks) in mouth.	*Prevents oral trauma.*
• Use an electric rather than a straight-edge razor. Cut nails and cuticles carefully.	*Decreases risk for nicks with shaving.* *Prevents bleeding and potential for infection.*
• Use caution when ambulating to prevent falls or bumps and do not walk barefoot.	

THERAPEUTIC INTERVENTIONS	**RATIONALE**

- To reduce the risk of cuts, be attentive when using scissors, knives, and tools.
- Avoid contact sports and other activities that could result in injury.
- Avoid straining to have a bowel movement.
- Avoid blowing your nose forcefully.
- Avoid wearing constrictive clothing (e.g., garters, knee-high stockings).
- Use an ample amount of water-soluble lubricant before sexual intercourse and avoid anal sexual activity, douching, use of rectal suppositories, and enemas in order to prevent trauma to the vaginal and rectal mucosa.
- Avoid heavy lifting.

Instruct client to control any bleeding by applying firm, prolonged pressure to the area if possible.

Prevents personal injury and potential for increased bleeding.

THERAPEUTIC INTERVENTIONS	**RATIONALE**

Desired Outcome: The client will verbalize ways to adjust to alterations in reproductive and sexual functioning.

Independent Actions

Assure client that many of the side effects of chemotherapy (e.g., decreased libido, impotence) are temporary or can be treated.

Explain to the female client that ovarian failure during chemotherapy may result in irritability, hot flashes, and other symptoms of premature menopause.

Instruct client in the childbearing years to use contraception during chemotherapy and for at least 2 years after completion of chemotherapy.

Encourage client to rest before sexual activity if fatigue is a problem.

Instruct client in measures to decrease discomfort associated with decreased vaginal secretions and mucositis:
- Use an ample amount of water-soluble lubricant before intercourse.
- Use vaginal steroid cream if prescribed to ease dryness and inflammation if present.
- Take a sitz bath two or three times a day.
- Avoid intercourse until mucositis of the vaginal canal resolves.

Instruct client to take hormone replacements (e.g., estrogen, testosterone) as prescribed.

Reproductive and sexual dysfunction vary depending on treatment protocol. Clients should be educated as to appropriate alternatives to reproductive and sexual dysfunction.

Knowledge of what can occur during chemotherapy allows the client to plan for what he or she will do to decrease symptoms.

Client needs to know that many cytotoxic drugs cause genetic abnormalities in the developing fetus.

Prevents discomfort, potential for trauma and improve sexual satisfaction.

THERAPEUTIC INTERVENTIONS	**RATIONALE**

Desired Outcome: The client will verbalize ways to promote independence and prevent injury if neuropathies are present.

Independent Actions

Instruct client in measures to promote independence and prevent injury if neuropathies are present:
- Use adaptive devices to facilitate performance of activities of daily living (e.g., zipper pulls; buttoners; molded sock aids; elastic shoelaces or Velcro straps; special pens, pencils, or utensils that are easy to grasp).

Helps client to maintain independence as much as possible and prevent injury.

Continued...

THERAPEUTIC INTERVENTIONS	RATIONALE
• Take extra precautions to prevent falls (e.g., have handrails in hallways and tubs and showers, avoid unnecessary clutter in pathways, wear shoes/slippers with nonskid soles, secure all carpets/rugs). • Adhere to precautions to prevent burns (e.g., check temperature of bath water [should be <110°F], wear mitts when handling hot items) and cuts (e.g., shield fingers when using a sharp knife, avoid the use of motorized tools such as lawnmowers and saws, use adapted nail clippers).	

THERAPEUTIC INTERVENTIONS	RATIONALE

Desired Outcome: The client will demonstrate the ability to care for a central venous catheter, a peritoneal catheter, or an implanted infusion device if in place.

Independent Actions

Provide instructions related to care of a central venous catheter (e.g., Groshong) if appropriate:	*Client and significant other should be instructed on the proper care of indwelling catheters to avoid catheter-related sepsis.*
• Change dressing if present according to protocol using aseptic technique.	
• Observe exit site for changes in appearance, redness, swelling, and unusual drainage.	*Symptoms of a potential infection should be reported to the health care provider.*
• Flush catheter according to protocol to maintain patency.	*Prevents clotting of indwelling catheter.*
• Replace injection cap as directed.	
• Tape catheter securely to chest wall. Notify physician if unable to flush catheter, if signs and symptoms of infection occur at exit site, or if catheter appears to be leaking.	*Taping of the indwelling catheter prevents in and out movement of the catheter which causes irritation to the urinary meatus, prevents accidental dislodgement and decreases potential for infection. Notifying the health care provider allows for prompt treatment of infection.*
Provide instructions related to care of a peritoneal catheter if in place:	*Proper care of a peritoneal catheter prevents dislodgement, damage, and infection.*
• Change dressing according to protocol using aseptic technique.	
• Keep catheter capped between treatments.	
• Keep water below the level of the catheter when taking a tub bath.	
• Observe for and notify physician if any of the following occurs:	*May indicate an infection.*
• Redness, swelling, or change in appearance of insertion site.	*May indicate infection or changes in patency or skin around catheter.*
• Unusual drainage from exit site.	
• Increasing abdominal pain.	*May indicate dislodgement or movement of catheter.*
• Chills or fever.	
• Increased abdominal distention between treatments.	
• Persistent nausea or vomiting.	
• Dyspnea.	
Provide instructions related to care of an implanted infusion device (e.g., MediPort, Port-a-Cath) if in place:	*Clients should be instructed on the proper maintenance of implanted infusion devices to ensure catheter patency and prevent infection.*
• Keep appointment to have device flushed or flush as instructed.	
• Avoid trauma to insertion site.	
• Notify physician if area around infusion device becomes reddened or painful.	

THERAPEUTIC INTERVENTIONS	RATIONALE

Desired Outcome: The client will verbalize an understanding of an implanted infusion pump and precautions necessary if one is in place.

Independent Actions

Reinforce physician's explanation about the purpose of the infusion pump and how it works.

Allows for client understanding and ability to care for self while maintaining some degree of independence.

Instruct client to avoid activities that could result in abdominal trauma and dislodgment of pump.

Caution client to notify physician if:

• Air travel is planned.

The client should carry an explanatory letter since pump may trigger airport weapon security devices; flow rate of pump may also need to be adjusted if the flight time is lengthy.

• Redness, swelling, or drainage occurs at incisional or refilling site.

May indicate an infection.

Emphasize importance of keeping appointments to have pump refilled.

Permanent blockage of the catheter can occur if pump is allowed to empty completely.

THERAPEUTIC INTERVENTIONS	RATIONALE

Desired Outcome: The client will state signs and symptoms to report to the health care provider.

Independent Actions

Instruct client to observe for and report the following:

• Signs and symptoms of infection (stress that usual signs of infection are diminished in people with altered bone marrow function and/or a suppressed immune system and that it is necessary to monitor closely for the following signs and symptoms):

  • Temperature above 38°C (100.4°F)
  • Changes in odor, color, or consistency of urine or pain with urination
  • White patches in mouth
  • Crusted ulcerations around or in oral cavity
  • Swollen, reddened, coated tongue
  • Painful rectal or vaginal area
  • Unusual vaginal drainage
  • Changes in the appearance or temperature of skin, particularly around puncture sites
  • Persistent productive or nonproductive cough.

Prompt reporting of adverse signs and symptoms allows for modification of the treatment plan and may reduce the risk of complications. Client must understand the importance of notifying the health care provider at the first sign of change. This can prevent deleterious outcomes.

• Signs and symptoms of bleeding (e.g., excessive bruising, black stools, persistent nosebleeds or bleeding from gums, sudden swelling in joints, red or smoke-colored urine, blood in vomitus).

• Signs and symptoms of hemorrhagic cystitis (e.g., blood in urine, pain on urination, urinary frequency or urgency).

• Signs and symptoms of extravasation (e.g., coolness, pain, swelling, and/or skin changes at infusion site).

• Signs and symptoms of pulmonary dysfunction (e.g., shortness of breath; persistent dry hacking cough; fever).

• Signs and symptoms of dehydration (e.g., dry mouth, significant weight loss, concentrated urine, light-headedness).

• Signs and symptoms of cardiotoxicity (e.g., irregular or rapid heart rate, increased weakness and fatigue, shortness of breath, unexplained weight gain, swelling of extremities); emphasize that cardiotoxicity can occur several days to months after administration of drugs known to cause it.

Continued...

THERAPEUTIC INTERVENTIONS	RATIONALE
• New or increased signs and symptoms of neurotoxicity (e.g., numbness and tingling of extremities, change in hearing acuity, blurred vision, constipation, change in motor function and coordination, burning pain in extremity, impaired memory or ability to communicate).	
• Persistent diarrhea, nausea, vomiting, and/or decreased oral intake.	
• Significant weight loss.	
• Inability to cope with the effects of the diagnosis and treatment	
Instruct client to keep a record of signs and symptoms, activities at the time the symptoms occur, measures taken to achieve relief, and the effect of the measures taken.	*Detailed accounts of signs and symptoms can aid health care practitioners in the formulation of appropriate interventions.*
Instruct client to take the information to each appointment with the health care provider.	*Allows for ongoing evaluation of the client's condition and provides time for client to express concerns and have questions answered.*

THERAPEUTIC INTERVENTIONS	RATIONALE

Desired Outcome: The client will identify community resources that can assist with home management and adjustment to the diagnosis of cancer and chemotherapy and its effects.

Independent Actions

Provide information about and encourage use of community resources that can help client and significant others with home management and adjustment to diagnosis of cancer and chemotherapy and its effects (e.g., American Cancer Society, counselors, social service agencies, Meals on Wheels, Make Today Count, Look Good–Feel Better Program, hospice, community support groups).	*These actions can help clients to cope with the emotional issues associated with chemotherapy. They can help clients manage their illness and normalize their experience.*

THERAPEUTIC INTERVENTIONS	RATIONALE

Desired Outcome: The client, in collaboration with the nurse, will develop a plan for adhering to recommended follow-up care including medications prescribed and schedule for chemotherapy, laboratory studies, and future appointments with health care provider.

Independent Actions

Collaborate with client to develop a written plan of how to adhere to treatment regimen.	*Improves client's adherence to treatment regimen.*

Thoroughly explain rationale for medications, their side effects, and the importance of taking them as prescribed. Inform client of pertinent food and drug interactions.

Reinforce physician's explanation of planned chemotherapy schedule.

Discuss with client any difficulties with adhering to the schedule and help him or her to plan ways of overcoming these.

Reinforce importance of keeping appointments for chemotherapy and laboratory studies.

Reinforce importance of keeping follow-up appointments with health care provider.

Implement measures to improve client compliance:

• Include significant others in teaching sessions.

• Encourage questions and allow time for reinforcement and clarification of information provided.

• Provide written instructions regarding ways to maintain nutritional status, future appointments with health care provider and laboratory, medications prescribed, and signs and symptoms to report.

ADDITIONAL NURSING DIAGNOSES

FEAR/ANXIETY NDx
Related to:
- Unfamiliar environment
- Lack of knowledge about chemotherapy including administration procedure, expected side effects, and impact on usual lifestyle and roles if admitted for chemotherapy
- Need for hospitalization to manage current side effects and/or toxic effects of chemotherapy and possibility of additional untoward effects with a subsequent cycle of chemotherapy
- Financial concerns
- Diagnosis of cancer with potential for premature death

NAUSEA NDx
Related to:
Stimulation of the vomiting center associated with:
- The effect of some cytotoxic drugs (those with a high emetic potential include carboplatin, cisplatin, dacarbazine, mechlorethamine, streptozocin, and carmustine), the by-products of cellular destruction, and the foul taste created by some cytotoxic agents
- Stimulation of the visceral afferent pathways resulting from inflammation of the gastrointestinal mucosa if mucositis is present
- Stimulation of the cerebral cortex resulting from stress and a conditioned response to previous experience with nausea and vomiting after the administration of cytotoxic drugs

FATIGUE NDx
Related to:
- A buildup of cellular waste products associated with rapid lysis of cancerous and normal cells exposed to cytotoxic drugs
- Difficulty resting and sleeping associated with fear, anxiety, and discomfort
- Tissue hypoxia associated with anemia (a result of malnutrition and chemotherapy-induced bone marrow suppression)
- Overwhelming emotional demands associated with the diagnosis of cancer and treatment with chemotherapy
- Increased energy expenditure associated with an increase in the metabolic rate resulting from continuous, active tumor growth and increased levels of certain cytokines (e.g., tumor necrosis factor, interleukin-1)
- Malnutrition
- Side effects of other medications client may be receiving (e.g., narcotic [opioid] analgesics, antiemetics, antianxiety agents, biotherapy agents such as interferons and interleukins)

DIARRHEA NDx
Related to:
Increased peristalsis and disorders of intestinal secretion and absorption associated with inflammation and ulceration of the gastrointestinal mucosa resulting from effects of cytotoxic drugs (particularly many of the antimetabolites, topoisomerase-1 inhibitors, and antitumor antibiotics) on the rapidly dividing epithelial cells in the intestine

RISK FOR INFECTION NDx
Related to:
Lowered natural resistance associated with:
- Malnutrition
- Chemotherapy-induced bone marrow suppression

- Long-term treatment with corticosteroids (may be used in treatment of certain types of cancer)
- Disruption in normal, endogenous microbial flora resulting from antimicrobial therapy
- Impaired immune system functioning resulting from certain malignancies (e.g., Hodgkin's disease, lymphoma, multiple myeloma, leukemia)
- Break in mucosal surfaces
- Break in skin integrity
- Stasis of secretions in lungs

GRIEVING NDx
Related to:
- Changes in body image and usual roles and lifestyle
- Diagnosis of cancer with potential for premature death

RISK FOR IMPAIRED SKIN INTEGRITY NDx
Related to:
- Increased skin fragility associated with malnutrition and dryness (a result of the effects of cytotoxic drugs on sebaceous and sweat glands)
- Frequent contact of the skin with irritants associated with diarrhea if present
- Damage to the skin and/or subcutaneous tissue associated with prolonged pressure on tissues, friction, or shearing if mobility is decreased

RISK FOR CONSTIPATION NDx
Related to:
- Autonomic neuropathy resulting from some cytotoxic drugs (e.g., vinblastine, teniposide, vindesine, vinorelbine)
- Depressant effect of medications administered to control symptoms such as pain, nausea, and vomiting (e.g., narcotic [opioid] analgesics, some antiemetics)
- Decreased activity
- Increased sympathetic nervous system activity resulting from anxiety
- Decreased intake of fiber and fluids

DISTURBED SLEEP PATTERN NDx
Related to:
- Nausea, vomiting, and pain
- Anxiety, fear, and grief
- Frequent need to defecate associated with diarrhea if present

RISK FOR POWERLESSNESS NDx
Related to:
- The possibility of disease progression and death despite treatment
- Dependence on others to assist with basic needs as a result of fatigue, weakness, and discomfort
- Possible alterations in roles, relationships, and future plans associated with changes that occur as a result of the cancer and the side effects/toxic effects of the cytotoxic drugs

NDx = NANDA Diagnosis   **D** = Delegatable Action   ● = UAP   ✦ = LVN/LPN   ⊜▶ = Go to ⓔvolve for animation

CLIENT TEACHING

Nursing Diagnosis DEFICIENT KNOWLEDGE NDx PRE-RADIATION

Definition: Absence or deficiency of cognitive information related to a specific topic, or its acquisition.

Related to: Lack of knowledge regarding how radiation works, preradiation and postradiation routines, what to expect during actual radiation treatment, and expected side effects of radiation

CLINICAL MANIFESTATIONS

Subjective	Objective
Verbal self-report of lack of knowledge of proposed treatment regimen.	Exaggerated behaviors, inaccurate follow-through of instructions, inappropriate behaviors (e.g., hostile, hysterical, agitated, apathetic)

RISK FACTORS
- Unfamiliarity with information
- Lack of exposure
- Cognitive limitations

DESIRED OUTCOMES

The client will demonstrate understanding of prescribed procedure as evidenced by:
a. Verbalization of understanding of what will occur during radiation treatment
b. Verbalization of required treatment regimen following treatment

NOC OUTCOMES

Knowledge: treatment regimen; treatment procedure(s)

NIC INTERVENTIONS

Teaching: treatment/procedure; teaching: individual

NURSING ASSESSMENT	RATIONALE
Assess client's readiness and ability to learn. Assess meaning of illness to client.	*Early recognition of readiness to learn and meaning of illness to client allows for implementation of the appropriate teaching interventions.*

THERAPEUTIC INTERVENTIONS	RATIONALE

Desired Outcome: The client will verbalize an understanding of radiation therapy and what to expect before, during, and after radiation treatments.

Independent Actions
Provide the client with the following information about radiation therapy:
- How radiation therapy works and why the total radiation dose prescribed is fractionated.
- That the client will be alone in the room during the few minutes of therapy but will be observed continuously via a television monitor, and that communication will be possible by means of an intercommunication system.
- That the machine may click or make a whirring noise but no discomfort will be felt during the treatment.
- The possible general side effects of radiation therapy (e.g., fatigue; anorexia; itchy, dry, reddened skin; moist desquamation and increase in skin pigmentation at radiation site), anticipated side effects for the particular site being irradiated, and when the side effects can be expected to occur and resolve.

Clients vary in physical and cognitive ability. When educating clients, nurses must determine a client's ability to read and understand written materials. If literacy barriers are present, alternative educational materials should be provided. Allow time for questions, clarification, and return demonstration of any learned actions.

THERAPEUTIC INTERVENTIONS	RATIONALE
• The treatment simulation process that occurs before initiation of therapy (the simulation process is done to accurately determine the treatment field and design devices such as plastic or plaster molds or lead blocks that will be used to ensure proper positioning and/or shield vital body organs within the treatment field).	
• The treatment field will include the smallest amount of normal tissue possible, and the field may be changed or reduced as the tumor shrinks in size. The vital organs are shielded during treatment to prevent unnecessary exposure.	
• The treatment field will be identified with skin markings with an indelible dye, ink, or felt tipped markers. These markings will be replaced by pinpoint tattoos once the reproducibility of the field is ensured.	
Arrange for client and significant others to visit the radiation department and meet those individuals responsible for client's care.	*Exposing clients to unfamiliar care environment can lessen anxiety associated with unfamiliar situations.*
Prepare client for waiting room experiences with others receiving radiation therapy. Emphasize that each individual has a different treatment plan, response, and prognosis and that comparisons should be avoided.	

Nursing Diagnosis ## IMBALANCED NUTRITION: LESS THAN BODY REQUIREMENTS NDx

Definition: Intake of nutrients insufficient to meet metabolic needs.

Related to:
• Decreased oral intake associated with:
• Anorexia resulting from factors such as depression, fear, anxiety, fatigue, discomfort, early satiety, an altered sense of taste (often reported by persons with cancer; can also result from damage to the taste buds and salivary glands with radiation to the head and neck), and increased levels of certain cytokines that depress appetite (e.g., interleukin-1, tumor necrosis factor)
• Impaired swallowing resulting from pharyngitis, esophagitis, dry mouth, and/or viscous oral secretions if present as a result of radiation treatment to the head, neck, or mediastinum
• Loss or impaired utilization of nutrients associated with vomiting and diarrhea if present
• Accelerated and inefficient metabolism of proteins, carbohydrates, and/or fats resulting from factors such as increased levels of cortisol, glucagon, and certain cytokines (e.g., tumor necrosis factor, interleukin-1)
• Decreased absorption of nutrients resulting from loss of intestinal absorptive surface if mucositis has developed (can occur with radiation to the abdomen or lower back)
• Utilization of available nutrients by the malignant cells rather than the host

CLINICAL MANIFESTATIONS

Subjective	Objective
Verbal self-report of weakness and fatigue	Significant weight loss (a loss of 1–2 lb during each week of radiation therapy is often expected); abnormal BUN and low serum prealbumin, albumin, hematocrit (Hct), hemoglobin (Hgb), and transferrin levels; inflamed oral mucous membrane; pale conjunctiva

RISK FACTORS

- Inability to ingest foods
- Inability to digest foods
- Inability to absorb nutrients

DESIRED OUTCOMES

The client will have or attain an adequate nutritional status as evidenced by:
a. Weight within or returning toward normal range for client
b. Normal BUN and serum prealbumin, albumin, Hct, Hgb, and transferrin levels
c. Usual strength and activity tolerance
d. Healthy oral mucous membrane

NOC OUTCOMES

Nutritional status; appetite

NIC INTERVENTIONS

Nutritional monitoring; nutrition management; nutrition therapy; pain management; nausea management

NURSING ASSESSMENT

Assess for and report signs and symptoms of malnutrition:
- Weakness and fatigue
- Significant weight loss (a loss of 1–2 lb during each week of radiation therapy is often expected)
- Inflamed oral mucous membrane
- Pale conjunctiva
- Monitor for abnormal BUN and low serum prealbumin, albumin, Hct, Hgb, and transferrin levels.
- Monitor percentage of meals and snacks client consumes.
- Report a pattern of inadequate intake.

RATIONALE

Early recognition of signs and symptoms of malnutrition allows for implementation of the appropriate interventions.

Abnormality in listed lab values can indicate malnutrition and should be reported to the primary care provider.

THERAPEUTIC INTERVENTIONS

Independent Actions
Implement measures to maintain or promote an adequate nutritional status:
Perform actions to improve oral intake:
Implement measures to control nausea/vomiting:
- Eliminate noxious sights and odors from the environment. **D** ● ✦

Implement measures to improve client's ability to swallow (e.g., assist client to select foods that are easily swallowed, such as eggs, custard, canned fruit, and mashed potatoes).
Implement measures to compensate for taste alterations if present:
- Encourage client to select mild-tasting fish, cold turkey or chicken, eggs, and cheese as protein sources if beef or pork tastes bitter or rancid.
- Provide meat for breakfast if aversion to meat tends to increase during day.
- Marinate meats in red wine or sweet-and-sour sauce.
- Add extra sweeteners to foods if acceptable to client.
- Experiment with different flavorings, seasonings, and textures.
- Serve food cold or at room temperature (can decrease some peculiar tastes). **D** ● ✦

Encourage a rest period before meals.
Maintain a clean environment and a relaxed, pleasant atmosphere. **D** ●
Provide oral hygiene before meals. **D** ● ✦

Provide largest amount of calories and protein when appetite is best (usually at breakfast). **D** ● ✦

RATIONALE

Noxious stimuli can cause stimulation of the vomiting center.

Improves nutritional status, in particular intake of protein.

Loss of sense of taste often occurs within 2 weeks of initiation of radiation treatment to head and neck, may persist for 4 to 6 weeks after completion of therapy, and usually is not permanent.
Improves intake of protein.

Enhances flavors that may improve intake.

Rest helps to minimize fatigue and improve appetite.
Allows client to take time while eating and may improve caloric intake.
Oral hygiene moistens the mouth, which makes it easier to chew and swallow; it also removes unpleasant tastes, which often improves the taste of foods/fluids.
Assures client is able to maintain caloric intake.

THERAPEUTIC INTERVENTIONS	RATIONALE
Serve frequent, small meals rather than large ones if client is weak, fatigues easily, and/or has a poor appetite. **D** ● ✦	*Prevents gastric distention and potential for nausea, vomiting, and feeling of being full.*
Allow adequate time for meals; reheat foods/fluids if necessary. **D** ● ✦	*Provides client ability to take time while eating and not feel rushed. Reheating food may increase intake.*

Dependent/collaborative actions

Implement measures to maintain or promote an adequate nutritional status;

• Perform actions to improve oral intake.	
• Increase activity as tolerated.	*Activity usually promotes a sense of well-being, which can improve appetite.*
• Obtain a dietary consult if necessary to help client select foods/fluids that meet nutritional needs, are appealing, and adhere to personal and cultural preferences.	*Provides information over time that the dietitian or nutritionist can use to develop a client specific diet.*
• Encourage significant others to bring in client's favorite foods and eat with client.	*Favorite foods eaten along with family members help to make eating more of a familiar social experience.*
• Limit fluid intake with meals (unless the fluid has high nutritional value). **D** ✦	*Limiting fluids help to reduce early satiety and subsequent decreased food intake.*
• Administer appetite stimulants if ordered. **D** ✦	*Appetite stimulates increase hunger and enhance caloric intake.*
• Ensure that meals are well balanced and high in essential nutrients; offer high-protein, high-calorie dietary supplements (e.g., milkshakes, puddings, or eggnog made with cream or powdered milk reconstituted with whole milk; commercially prepared dietary supplements) if indicated.	*Ensures adequate nutrition.*
• Avoid foods/fluids that stimulate or irritate the bowel (e.g., coffee, alcohol, foods made with synthetic sugars).	*Foods that stimulate the colon and may cause diarrhea lead to loss of fluid and electrolytes.*
• Administer vitamins and minerals if ordered. **D** ✦	*Supplements may be required to maintain adequate intake.*
• Perform a calorie count if ordered. Report information to dietitian and physician.	*Helps to determine if client is eating adequate about of calories.*
• Consult physician about an alternative method of providing nutrition (e.g., parenteral nutrition, tube feedings) if client does not consume enough food or fluids to meet nutritional needs.	*Notification of the appropriate health care provider allows for modification of the treatment plan.*

Nursing Diagnosis   IMPAIRED SWALLOWING NDx

Definition: Abnormal functioning of the swallowing mechanism associated with deficits in oral, pharyngeal, or esophageal structure or function.

Related to:

• Oral, pharyngeal, or esophageal pain associated with inflammation and/or ulceration of the mucosa if the treatment field includes the head, neck, or mediastinum
• Dry mouth and viscous oral secretions associated with destruction of the salivary glands (particularly the parotids) if the treatment field includes the head and neck
• Decreased oral intake

CLINICAL MANIFESTATIONS

Subjective	Objective
Statements of difficulty swallowing; stasis of food in oral cavity	Coughing or choking when eating or drinking

NDx = NANDA Diagnosis   **D** = Delegatable Action   ● = UAP   ✦ = LVN/LPN   ⊖▶ = Go to ⊖volve for animation

RISK FACTORS
- Upper airway abnormalities
- Oropharyngeal abnormalities
- Esophageal defects

DESIRED OUTCOMES

The client will experience an improvement in swallowing as evidenced by
a. Verbalization of same
b. Absence of food in oral cavity after swallowing
c. Absence of coughing and chocking when eating and drinking

NOC OUTCOMES

Swallowing status

NIC INTERVENTIONS

Swallowing therapy; pain management; oral health restoration

NURSING ASSESSMENT	**RATIONALE**
Assess for signs and symptoms of impaired swallowing. • Statements of difficulty swallowing • Stasis of food in oral cavity • Coughing or choking when eating or drinking	*Early recognition of signs and symptoms of impaired swallowing allows for implementation of the appropriate interventions.*

THERAPEUTIC INTERVENTIONS	**RATIONALE**
Independent Actions Perform actions to reduce oral, pharyngeal, and esophageal pain: • Offer cool, soothing liquids.	*Measures that act to reduce oral, pharyngeal, and esophageal pain help to improve the ability to swallow. Oral and pharyngeal discomfort can interfere with the client's ability and willingness to swallow effectively.*
• Instruct client to gargle with saline solution every 2 hrs to sooth mucous membranes. • Perform frequent oral hygiene.	*Decreases irritation of the mouth and throat that may decrease pain or discomfort upon swallowing.* *A moist mouth helps to lubricate food, making it easier to chew form into a bolus, and manipulate it toward the back of the mouth. A formed, moist bolus triggers the swallowing reflex more effectively and moves more easily through the esophagus.*
• Help client to select foods that require little or no chewing and are easily swallowed (e.g., custard, eggs, canned fruit, mashed potatoes). • Avoid serving foods that are sticky (e.g., peanut butter, soft bread, honey). • Perform actions to stimulate salivation at mealtime.	*Improves client nutrition without additional irritation to the oral and throat mucosa.* *Sticky foods are difficult to move through the mouth because they adhere to various structures, especially the hard palate.* *A moist mouth helps to lubricate food, making it easier to chew and swallow.*
• Provide oral hygiene before meals. • Provide a piece of hard candy for client to suck on just before meals unless contraindicated. • Serve foods that are visually pleasing.	*Removes residue in the mouth that may decrease appetite.* *Improves salivation that decreases oral irritation and enhances swallowing of food.* *Involves more senses than taste and smell that may improve appetite.*
Dependent/Collaborative Actions Implement measures to improve client's ability to swallow. Perform actions to reduce oral, pharyngeal, and esophageal pain: • Administer oral protective agents and topical anesthetics or analgesics if ordered. • Perform actions to reduce and/or liquefy viscous oral secretions. • Encourage a fluid intake of 2500 mL/day unless contraindicated.	*Thick oral secretions interfere with movement of food in the mouth. Liquefying these secretions makes it easier for a bolus of food to be formed and moved to the back of the mouth.* *Prevents ongoing oral irritation.* *Removes excess secretions from the oral cavity.* *Enhances moisture of the oral cavity and throat.*

THERAPEUTIC INTERVENTIONS	RATIONALE
• Encourage client to avoid milk, milk products, and chocolate (when combined with saliva, they produce very thick secretions).	*Prevents thick secretions which may be difficult to swallow.*
Consult appropriate health care provider (e.g., oncology nurse specialist, physician) if swallowing difficulties persist or worsen.	*Notification of the appropriate health care provider allows for modification of the treatment plan.*

Nursing Diagnosis · IMPAIRED COMFORT NDx PRURITUS

Definition: Perceived lack of ease, relief, and transcendence in physical, psychospiritual, environmental, cultural, and/or social dimensions.

Related to: Decreased function of skin sebaceous and sweat glands within the treatment field

CLINICAL MANIFESTATIONS

Subjective	Objective
Verbal self-report of itchiness	Persistent scratching or rubbing of skin; dryness and redness or excoriation of skin within the treatment field

RISK FACTORS

• Prescribed treatment regimen

DESIRED OUTCOMES

The client will experience relief of pruritus as evidenced by:
a. Verbalization of same
b. No scratching and rubbing skin

NOC OUTCOMES	NIC INTERVENTIONS
Comfort level; symptom control	Pruritus management

NURSING ASSESSMENT	RATIONALE
Assess the client for signs and symptoms of pruritus: • Reports of itchiness • Persistent scratching or rubbing of skin; dryness and redness or excoriation of skin within the treatment field	*Early recognition of signs and symptoms of pruritus allows for implementation of the appropriate interventions.*

THERAPEUTIC INTERVENTIONS	RATIONALE
Implement measures to help relieve pruritus in the treatment area: • Apply cool, moist compresses to pruritic areas. • Maintain a cool environment. • Perform actions to reduce skin dryness. • Use tepid water and mild soaps for bathing, being careful not to remove temporary skin markings. • Apply water-based lubricant lotions (e.g., Lubriderm, Eucerin) two to three times daily and after bath. **D** ● ✦ • Limit bathing to once every other day. **D** ● ✦ • Use a room humidifier to increase moisture in the air. **D** ● ✦ • Add emollients, cornstarch, baking soda, or colloid-based bath products to bath water. **D** ● ✦	*The client experiencing pruritus is likely to scratch the affected areas, which irritates the skin and can cause excoriation.* *Implementing measures to reduce the itching sensation helps prevent scratching and reduces trauma to the skin.* *Dry skin is more prone to crack and has decreased elasticity, which makes it susceptible to damage.* *Avoid lotions that contain lanolin or petrolatum because they must be removed before treatments* *Prevents skin from becoming dry.* *Moisturizing lotions and emollients provide a source of moisture to the skin.*

NDx = NANDA Diagnosis   **D** = Delegatable Action   ● = UAP   ✦ = LVN/LPN   ⊖▶ = Go to ⊖volve for animation

Continued...

THERAPEUTIC INTERVENTIONS	RATIONALE
• Apply a light dusting of cornstarch to areas of dry desquamation (cornstarch should not be used if moist desquamation is present). **D** ● ✦	*Absorbs excessive moisture on skin and decreases itching.*
• Make an oatmeal paste, apply to pruritic areas, let dry for 3 to 5 minutes, and then rinse with cool water. **D** ● ✦	*Oatmeal binds to the skin and provides a protective barrier against irritants. It can also help to normalize skin pH.*
• Pat skin dry after bathing, making sure to dry it thoroughly. **D** ● ✦	*Rubbing of the skin after bathing can irritate the skin and stimulate itching.*
• Encourage participation in diversional activities and use of relaxation techniques (e.g., music, imagery, watching TV). **D** ● ✦	*Diversional activities, such as guided imagery, have a calming effect on the body and have been used to improve comfort.*
• Use cutaneous stimulation techniques (e.g., stroking with a soft brush, light massage, pressure) at sites of itching or acupressure points.	*Skin within the treatment field should never be rubbed or deeply massaged.*
• Encourage client to wear loose cotton garments.	*Cotton is a natural fiber that is less irritating to the skin. Loose garments allow air to circulate over the skin and decrease the sensation to itch.*

Dependent/Collaborative Actions

Implement measures to help relieve pruritus in the treatment area.
• Perform actions to reduce skin dryness:
  • Encourage a fluid intake of 2500 mL/day unless contraindicated. **D** ● ✦ — *Adequate fluid intake helps to keep the skin well hydrated.*
  • Administer antihistamines and/or apply topical anesthetic cream (e.g., Lanacane) if ordered. **D** ✦ — *Antihistamines block the release of histamine which can increase skin irritaton.*
Consult appropriate health care provider (e.g., oncology nurse specialist, physician) if above measures fail to relieve pruritus or if the skin becomes more excoriated. — *Notification of the appropriate health care provider allows for modification of the treatment plan.*

Nursing Diagnosis **RISK FOR IMPAIRED SKIN INTEGRITY NDx**

Definition: Susceptibility to alteration in epidermis and/or dermis, which may compromise health.

Related to:
• Dry desquamation of irradiated site associated with increased sensitivity of skin in certain areas (e.g., opposing skin surfaces, face, perineum) and destruction of rapidly dividing epithelial cells of the skin
• Moist desquamation of irradiated area associated with damage to the basal cells of the skin
Increased skin fragility is associated with:
• Tissue edema resulting from vascular changes in irradiated area
• Malnutrition
• Excessive scratching associated with pruritus
• Frequent contact of the skin with irritants associated with diarrhea if present

CLINICAL MANIFESTATIONS

Subjective	Objective
Verbal self-report of painful dermal areas	Pallor; redness; change in skin temperature; firm or boggy tissue; pruritus; abrasions; blisters

RISK FACTORS
• Prescribed treatment regimen
• Imbalanced nutritional state
• Impaired sensation

DESIRED OUTCOMES

The client will maintain or regain skin integrity as evidenced by:
a. Minimal redness and irritation within the treatment field.
b. Absence of redness and irritation in body areas not in treatment field.
c. No skin breakdown

NOC OUTCOMES	NIC INTERVENTIONS
Tissue integrity; skin and mucous membranes, wound healing, secondary intention	Skin surveillance, skin care, topical treatments, wound care

NURSING ASSESSMENT	RATIONALE
Assess the client for signs and symptoms of actual or impaired skin integrity: • Verbal reports of painful dermal areas • Pallor, redness, change in skin temperature • Firm or boggy tissue • Pruritus • Abrasions • Blisters • Inspect the following anatomic fields: • Treatment field and area on the body surface opposite to it (should be assessed before treatment, every week during treatment, and on every subsequent visit) • Opposing skin surfaces • Bony prominences • Dependent, pruritic, and edematous areas • Perineum	*Early recognition of signs and symptoms of impaired skin integrity allows for implementation of the appropriate interventions.*

THERAPEUTIC INTERVENTIONS	RATIONALE
Independent Actions Implement measures to maintain or regain skin integrity:	*These actions help to prevent or treat skin irritation or breakdown within the treatment field.*
• Cleanse irradiated area gently each shift with tepid water and mild soap.	*May be contraindicated initially when temporary skin markings rather than tattoos are used.*
• Pat skin dry using soft materials, paying particular attention to opposing skin surfaces within the treatment field.	*Decreases irritation and potential for scratching.*
• Expose irradiated area to the air as much as possible, avoiding extremes of temperature.	
• Avoid use of tape within irradiated area.	*Prevents skin irritation and potential breakdown.*
Instruct client to:	
• Wear loose cotton clothing.	*Cotton is a natural fabric that is less irritating to the skin.*
• Avoid use of perfumed lotions or soaps, cosmetics, and deodorants.	*Avoiding the use of perfumed soaps, cosmetics, and deodorants helps to prevent chemical irritation (many of these products contain heavy metals that will augment effects of radiation on the skin).*
• Apply a light dusting of cornstarch to areas of dry desquamation.	*Cornstarch helps to reduce friction.*
• Apply a mild, water-based lubricant lotion (e.g., Lubriderm, Eucerin). **D** ● ✦	*Lubricants help to reduce skin dryness and subsequent cracking.*
• Avoid use of hydrophobic products (e.g., Vaseline). **D** ● ✦	*Hydrophobic products are difficult to remove.*
• Use an electric rather than a straight-edge razor if it is absolutely necessary to shave in the irradiated area.	*Use of an electric razor decreases irritation and potential for skin injury.*
• Avoid applications of heat and cold to irradiated area. **D** ● ✦	*Heat and cold may be drying to the skin.*
Implement measures to prevent skin breakdown associated with scratching:	
• Perform actions to relieve pruritus (e.g., apply water-based lubricant lotion). **D** ● ✦	*Water-based lubricants decrease itching without drying the skin as do lotions with alcohol.*
• Keep nails trimmed and/or apply mittens if necessary.	*Prevents further skin irritation with scratching.*
• Instruct client to apply firm pressure to pruritic areas rather than scratching.	*Prevents further irritation and decreases stimulus to scratch area.*
• Implement measures to treat a moist desquamation reaction if it has occurred.	
• Keep involved area exposed to the air as much as possible. **D** ● ✦	

NDx = NANDA Diagnosis   **D** = Delegatable Action   ● = UAP   ✦ = LVN/LPN   ⊝▶ = Go to ⊝volve for animation

Continued...

THERAPEUTIC INTERVENTIONS	RATIONALE
Perform actions to decrease skin irritation and prevent break-down associated with diarrhea:	These actions help to reduce the risk of breaks in the integrity of skin, which increases the client's exposure to pathogens.
• Avoid extremely hot or cold foods; encourage foods high in pectin, such as bananas and apple juice).	Foods that are very hot or cold and that are high in pectin can cause diarrhea.
• Help client to thoroughly cleanse and dry perineal area with soft tissue or cloth after each bowel movement; apply a protective ointment or cream, being sure to remove it before treatments if rectal area is within treatment field. **D** ● ✦	Reduces itching and potential for infection.
• If use of absorbent products such as pads or undergarments is necessary, select those that effectively absorb moisture and keep it away from the skin. **D** ● ✦	Prevents skin irritation and potential for itching.
Perform actions to reduce fluid accumulation in dependent areas:	Fluid accumulation in dependent areas increases pressure and increases the risk of disruption in normal skin integrity.
• Instruct client in and assist with range-of-motion exercises.	Improves circulation and decrease potential for edema.
• Elevate affected extremities whenever possible. **D** ● ✦	Promotes lymph drainage of extremities.
• Handle edematous areas carefully.	Prevents skin damage.
• Perform actions to promote an adequate nutritional status.	

Dependent/Collaborative Actions

Implement measures to maintain or regain skin integrity:	
• Perform actions to prevent or treat skin irritation or break down within the treatment field.	
• Apply a skin sealant to the area to be irradiated if ordered.	Prevents skin breakdown or improves healing if breakdown has occurred.
Implement measures to treat a moist desquamation reaction if it has occurred.	
• Cleanse area well with a saline solution, water, or a dilute solution of chlorhexidine three times a day; apply an astringent soak if ordered.	Decreases itch sensation and decreases potential for scratching of the skin.
• Apply a metal-free gel (e.g., RadiaCare) to involved area if ordered.	Helps to maintain skin integrity.
• Apply a topical antimicrobial agent as ordered if signs and symptoms of a localized infection occur.	Helps to prevent infection.
If unexpected skin irritation or breakdown occurs:	
• Notify appropriate health care provider (e.g., oncology nurse specialist, wound care specialist, physician).	Notification of the appropriate health care provider allows for modification of the treatment plan.
• Perform care of involved areas as ordered or per standard hospital procedure.	

Nursing Diagnosis **RISK FOR IMPAIRED ORAL MUCOUS MEMBRANE INTEGRITY** NDx

Definition: Susceptibility to injury to the lips, soft tissues, buccal cavity, and/or oropharynx, which may compromise health.

Related to:
- Dryness associated with decreased oral intake and destruction of salivary glands if the treatment field includes the head and neck
- Stomatitis associated with malnutrition, inadequate oral hygiene, and disruption in the renewal process of mucosal epithelial cells if the oral cavity is irradiated

CLINICAL MANIFESTATIONS

Subjective	Objective
Verbal self-report of burning pain in mouth; difficulty swallowing, taste changes	Dryness of the oral mucosa; thick, ropey saliva; inflamed and/or ulcerated oral mucosa; positive results of cultured specimens from oral lesions

RISK FACTORS

- Radiation therapy
- Chemical irritants
- Ineffective oral hygiene
- Malnutrition

DESIRED OUTCOMES

The client maintains a healthy oral cavity as evidenced by
a. No reports of oral dryness and burning
b. Pink, moist, intact mucosa
c. Absence of inflammation
d. Ability to swallow without discomfort

NIC OUTCOMES

Oral hygiene

NIC INTERVENTIONS

Oral health maintenance; oral health restoration

NURSING ASSESSMENT	RATIONALE
Assess the client for signs and symptoms of impaired oral mucous membranes: - Reports of burning pain in mouth - Difficulty swallowing or taste changes - Dryness of the oral mucosa - Thick, ropey saliva - Inflamed and/or ulcerated oral mucosa - Positive results of cultured specimens from oral lesions	*Early recognition of signs and symptoms of impaired oral mucous membranes allows for implementation of the appropriate interventions.*

THERAPEUTIC INTERVENTIONS	RATIONALE
Independent Actions Implement measures to prevent or reduce the severity of stomatitis and/or relieve dryness of the oral mucous membrane:	
- Instruct and assist client to perform oral hygiene after eating and as often as needed; avoid use of products that contain lemon and glycerin and mouthwashes containing alcohol.	*Lemon/glycerin and alcohol-based products have a drying and irritating effect on the oral mucous membrane.*
- Instruct and help client to perform oral hygiene using a soft-bristle toothbrush or a sponge-tipped swab and to floss teeth gently.	*Helps to maintain health gums and removes debris.*
- Have client rinse mouth frequently with warm saline solution, baking soda and warm water, or chlorhexidene gluconate (Peridex) or mist oral cavity frequently using a spray bottle.	*Provides additional moisture to the oral cavity.*
- Lubricate client's lips frequently.	*Prevents cracking of lips.*
- Encourage client not to smoke or chew tobacco.	*Smoking dries the mucosa; tobacco acts as an irritant to the oral mucosa.*
Perform actions to stimulate salivation:	
- Encourage client to suck on sugarless candy or chew sugarless gum.	*Stimulates salivation decrease irritation of the oral mucosa and enhance appetite.*
- Instruct client to avoid substances that might further irritate the oral mucosa (e.g., hot, spicy, or acidic foods/fluids).	*Decreases irritation of the oral cavity and oral pharynx.*
- Perform actions to promote an adequate nutritional status (e.g., provide oral hygiene before meals).	*Enhance appetite and removes debris from the mouth.*
- Encourage client to use a saliva substitute such as Salivart if indicated.	*Provides additional moisture to the mouth and throat.*
If stomatitis is not controlled:	
- Increase frequency of oral hygiene.	*Helps to maintain moisture and removal debris.*
- If client has dentures, remove them and replace only for meals.	*Helps to prevent breakdown of oral mucosa.*

NDx = NANDA Diagnosis   **D** = Delegatable Action   ● = UAP   ✦ = LVN/LPN   ⊖▶ = Go to ⊖volve for animation

Continued...

THERAPEUTIC INTERVENTIONS	RATIONALE
Dependent/Collaborative Actions	
Implement measures to prevent or reduce the severity of stomatitis and/or relieve dryness of the oral mucous membrane:	
• Administer amifostine 15 to 30 minutes before radiation treatment that includes the parotid glands in client with head and neck cancer.	*Amifostine is used as a protectant agent to reduce the incidence of xerostomia.*
• Administer sialagogues (e.g., oral pilocarpine [Salagen]) if ordered.	*This drug increases the natural production of saliva.*
• Encourage a fluid intake of 2500 mL/day unless contra-indicated.	*Maintains overall hydration and provides ongoing moisture to the alimentary canal.*
• Provide client with a prophylactic antifungal oral suspension or lozenge (e.g., nystatin) if ordered.	*Helps to prevent suprainfections.*
Consult appropriate health care provider (e.g., oncology nurse specialist, physician) if oral dryness and signs and symptoms of stomatitis persist or worsen.	*Notification of the appropriate health care provider allows for modification of the treatment plan.*

Nursing Diagnosis **RISK FOR BLEEDING** NDx

Definition: Susceptible to a decrease in blood volume, which may compromise health.

Related to: Thrombocytopenia associated with bone marrow suppression if large amounts of active bone marrow are included in the treatment field

CLINICAL MANIFESTATIONS

Subjective	Objective
N/A	Petechiae, purpura, or ecchymoses; gingival bleeding; prolonged bleeding from puncture sites; epistaxis, hemoptysis; unusual joint pain; frank or occult blood in stool, urine, or vomitus; increase in abdominal girth; menorrhagia; restlessness, confusion; decreasing blood pressure (BP) and increased pulse rate; decrease in hematocrit (Hct) and hemoglobin (Hgb) levels; platelet levels

RISK FACTORS
• Treatment regimen
• Impaired liver function

DESIRED OUTCOMES

The client will not experience unusual bleeding, as evidenced by:
a. Skin and mucous membranes free of petechiae, purpura, ecchymoses, and active bleeding
b. Absence of unusual joint pain
c. Absence of frank and occult blood in stool, urine, and vomitus
d. No increase in abdominal girth
e. Usual menstrual flow
f. Usual mental status
g. Vital signs within normal range for client
h. Stable or improved Hct and Hgb levels
i. Stable or improve platelet levels

NOC OUTCOMES

Blood coagulation; blood loss severity

NIC INTERVENTIONS

Bleeding precautions; administration of blood products

NURSING ASSESSMENT	RATIONALE
Assess the client for signs and symptoms of bleeding: • Unusual joint pain • Petechiae, purpura, or ecchymoses • Gingival bleeding; prolonged bleeding from puncture sites • Epistaxis, hemoptysis • Increase in abdominal girth • Frank or occult blood in stool, urine, or vomitus; menorrhagia • Restlessness, confusion • Decreasing BP and increased pulse rate • Decrease in Hct and Hgb levels • Monitor platelet count and coagulation test results (e.g., bleeding time). Report significant worsening of values.	*Early recognition of signs and symptoms of bleeding allows for implementation of the appropriate interventions.*

THERAPEUTIC INTERVENTIONS	RATIONALE

Dependent/Collaborative Actions

If platelet count is low, coagulation test results are abnormal, or Hct and Hgb levels decrease, test all stools, urine, and vomitus for occult blood. Report positive results.

Implement measures to prevent bleeding:

• Avoid giving injections whenever possible; consult physician about prescribing an alternative route for medications ordered to be given intramuscularly or subcutaneously.

Intramuscular injections in a client that is thrombocytopenic may lead to the formation of hematomas.

• When giving injections or performing venous or arterial punctures, use the smallest gauge needle possible and apply gentle, prolonged pressure to the site after the needle is removed. **D** ●✦

Providing pressure to the site helps facilitate hemostasis.

• Take BP only when necessary and avoid overinflating the cuff. **D** ● ✦

BP cuff inflation in a client that is thrombocytopenic may lead to petechiae in the affected extremity.

• Caution client to avoid activities that increase the risk for trauma (e.g., shaving with a straight-edge razor, using stiff-bristle toothbrush or dental floss).

Potential for injury and increase bleeding.

• Whenever possible, avoid intubations (e.g., nasogastric) and procedures that can cause injury to rectal mucosa (e.g., taking temperature rectally, inserting a rectal suppository, administering an enema).

Prevents injury to mucosa and decrease the potential for bleeding.

• Pad side rails if client is confused or restless.

Precaution to prevent client injury.

Perform actions to reduce the risk for falls (e.g., keep bed in low position with side rails up when client is in bed, avoid unnecessary clutter in room, instruct client to wear slippers/shoes with nonslip soles when ambulating).

Decreases risk for potential injury.

Instruct client to avoid blowing nose forcefully or straining to have a bowel movement; consult physician regarding an order for a decongestant and/or laxative if indicated.

Administer the following if ordered:

• Platelet-stimulating factor (romiplostim)

Platelet stimulation factors help the bone marrow increase production of platelets.

• Estrogen-progestin preparations.

Estrogen-progesterone preparations help suppress menses.

• Platelets.

Administration of platelets replaces components necessary for optimum clot formation.

If bleeding occurs and does not subside spontaneously:

• Apply firm, prolonged pressure to bleeding area(s) if possible.

Application of pressure helps facilitate hemostasis.

• If epistaxis occurs, place client in a high-Fowler's position and apply pressure and ice pack to nasal area.

Application of ice helps to facilitate hemostasis through vasoconstriction of vessels.

• Maintain oxygen therapy as ordered.

Supplemental oxygen is necessary in clients with reduced hemoglobin.

• Administer whole blood or blood products (e.g., platelets) as ordered.

Actions help to replace deficit of components necessary to achieve hemostasis.

Collaborative Diagnosis **RADIATION CYSTITIS**

Definition: Inflammation of cells lining the bladder.

Related to: Irritation of the bladder mucosa if the bladder is in the treatment field

CLINICAL MANIFESTATIONS

Subjective	Objective
Verbal self-report of dysuria; urinary frequency and/or urgency; suprapubic discomfort	Frank or occult blood in the urine

RISK FACTORS

- Localized radiation therapy

DESIRED OUTCOMES

The client will experience resolution of radiation cystitis if it occurs as evidenced by:
a. Reports of decreasing dysuria, urinary frequency and urgency, and suprapubic discomfort
b. Absence of hematuria

NURSING ASSESSMENT	RATIONALE
Assess for and report signs and symptoms of radiation cystitis: • Reports of dysuria, urinary frequency and/or urgency, or suprapubic discomfort • Frank or occult blood in the urine	*Early recognition of signs and symptoms of radiation cystitis allows for implementation of the appropriate interventions.*

THERAPEUTIC INTERVENTIONS	RATIONALE
Dependent/Collaborative Actions Implement measures to reduce discomfort associated with cystitis: • Encourage a minimum fluid intake of 2500 mL/day unless contraindicated. • Instruct client to avoid substances that can cause bladder irritation (e.g., caffeinated beverages, alcohol, tobacco, spicy foods). • Administer urinary tract analgesic/anesthetic agents and bladder smooth muscle relaxants if ordered. **D** ✦ • Assist with measures to control bleeding (e.g., continuous bladder irrigation with silver nitrate, cystoscopy to cauterize bleeding vessels, instillation of formalin into the bladder) if bleeding occurs and is persistent or severe.	*Adequate fluid intake helps to keep urine dilute and thereby reduce further irritation of the bladder lining.* *Avoidance of stimulants can decrease bladder irritation.* *Analgesia can prevent pain and improve urination.* *Preparation of client for procedures decreases anxiety.*

Collaborative Diagnosis **RADIATION PNEUMONITIS**

Definition: Localized inflammation of the lung.

Related to: Inflammation of lung tissue resulting from radiation to the chest

CLINICAL MANIFESTATIONS

Subjective	Objective
Verbal reports of shortness of breath	Cough; fever; night sweats; finding of infiltrates on chest radiograph; dyspnea

RISK FACTORS
- Localized radiation therapy

DESIRED OUTCOMES

The client will have improvement of radiation pneumonitis if it occurs as evidenced by:
a. Decreased dyspnea and coughing
b. Temperature declining toward normal

NURSING ASSESSMENT

Assess for and report signs and symptoms of radiation pneumonitis:
- Dyspnea
- Cough
- Fever
- Night sweats

Assess chest radiograph and report abnormal findings.
Assess pulse oximetry and arterial blood gas values, and report abnormal findings.

RATIONALE

Early recognition of signs and symptoms of radiation pneumonitis allows for implementation of the appropriate interventions.

THERAPEUTIC INTERVENTIONS

Dependent/Collaborative Actions

Implement measures to improve respiratory function:
- Instruct and assist client to turn, cough, and breathe deeply every 1 to 2 hrs.
- Reinforce correct use of incentive spirometer every 1 to 2 hrs. **D** ✦
- Maintain oxygen therapy if ordered. **D** ✦

Administer the following medications if ordered:
- Corticosteroids.
- Bronchodilators.

Consult physician if signs and symptoms of pneumonitis worsen or signs and symptoms of impaired gas exchange (e.g., restlessness, irritability, confusion, decreased partial pressure of oxygen in arterial blood [PaO_2], and increased partial pressure of carbon dioxide in arterial blood [$PaCO_2$]) develop.

RATIONALE

These actions help to reexpand alveoli, improving oxygenation.

Improves lung expansion and increases oxygenation.

Supplemental oxygen increases the partial pressure of oxygen in the blood.

Corticosteroids help to reduce inflammation.
Bronchodilators dilate larger airways, improving ventilation.
Notifying the appropriate health care provider allows for modification of the treatment plan.

Collaborative Diagnosis   LYMPHEDEMA

Definition: Accumulation of lymph fluid in soft tissue.

Related to: Damage to and subsequent obstruction of lymphatic vessels in the area being irradiated (seen most frequently in persons having radiation for breast cancer, melanoma in an upper or lower extremity, gynecologic cancer, or prostate cancer)

CLINICAL MANIFESTATIONS

Subjective	Objective
Verbal self-report of pain or feeling of heaviness, fullness, or tightness in extremity	Increase in size of extremity; sensory or motor deficits in extremity

RISK FACTORS
- Surgical excision of lymph nodes
- Radiation of lymph nodes

DESIRED OUTCOMES

The client will have decreasing signs and symptoms of lymphedema if it occurs as evidenced by:
a. Decreased pain and feeling of heaviness and tightness in involved extremity
b. Reduction in size of involved extremity
c. Improved motor and sensory function in involved extremity

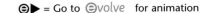

NURSING ASSESSMENT	RATIONALE
Assess extremities in or near the treatment field for signs and symptoms of lymphedema: • Verbal reports of pain or feeling of heaviness, fullness, or tightness in extremity • Increase in size of extremity • Sensory or motor deficits in extremity • Assess daily measurement of limb circumference.	*Early recognition of signs and symptoms of lymphedema allows for implementation of the appropriate interventions.*

THERAPEUTIC INTERVENTIONS	RATIONALE
Dependent/Collaborative Actions If signs and symptoms of lymphedema occur: • Elevate the involved extremity. **D** ● ✦ • Avoid use of involved extremity for BP measurements, injections, and venipunctures. **D** ● ✦ • Apply a graded-pressure or sequential compression device to involved extremity if ordered. **D** ● ✦ Administer the following medications if ordered: • Antimicrobial agents. **D** ✦ • Analgesics. **D** ✦ Consult physician if signs and symptoms of lymphedema persist or worsen or if signs and symptoms of infection (e.g., redness or unusual warmth in extremity, fever) develop.	*Elevation of an edematous extremity helps promote excess fluid drainage, promoting reabsorption.* *Clients must protect the integrity of the skin as the first barrier to the prevention of infection.* *Helps to promote drainage of lymphatic fluid.* *Agents help to prevent or treat cellulitis and lymphangitis.* *Agents help to alleviate pain associated with soft tissue swelling.* *Notification of the appropriate health care provider allows for modification of the treatment plan and reduces the risk of complications.*

Nursing Diagnosis DISTURBED SELF-CONCEPT*

Definition: **Disturbed Body Image NDx:** confusion in mental picture of one's physical self; **Risk for Situational Low Self-Esteem NDx:** Susceptibility to developing a negative perception of self-worth in response to current situation, which may compromise health.

Related to:
• Changes in appearance (e.g., temporary or permanent hair loss within the treatment field; skin changes such as erythema, uneven skin texture, or hyperpigmentation within the treatment field; excessive weight loss)
• Possible alteration in usual sexual activities associated with:
  • Fatigue, decreased levels of testosterone (if testes are in the treatment field), psychologic factors, and vaginal and/or urethral discomfort (if the lower abdomen, pelvis, or perineal area is irradiated)
  • Temporary or permanent impotence resulting from psychologic factors, decreased levels of testosterone (if testes are in the treatment field), and/or injury to pelvic nerves and blood vessels if included within the treatment field
• Altered reproductive function:
  • Sterility associated with exposure of testes or ovaries to radiation
  • Potential for genetic mutations associated with sperm or ova chromosomal damage resulting from irradiation of the gonads
• Increased dependence on others to meet self-care needs
• Changes in lifestyle and roles associated with the effects of the disease process and its treatment

CLINICAL MANIFESTATIONS

Subjective	Objective
Verbal self-report of negative feelings about self; withdrawal from significant others; lack of planning to adapt to necessary changes in lifestyle	Lack of participation in activities of daily living

*This diagnostic label includes the nursing diagnoses of Disturbed Body Image and Situational Low Self-Esteem.

RISK FACTORS

- Illness treatment
- Disturbed body image
- Social role change

DESIRED OUTCOMES

The client will demonstrate beginning adaptation to changes in appearance, body functioning, lifestyle, and roles as evidenced by:
a. Verbalization of feelings of self-worth and sexual adequacy
b. Maintenance of relationships with significant others
c. Active participation in activities of daily living
d. Verbalization of a beginning plan for adapting lifestyle to changes resulting from the disease process and the residual effects of radiation therapy

NOC OUTCOMES

Self-esteem; psychosocial adjustment: life change; personal autonomy; body image

NIC INTERVENTIONS

Body image enhancement; self-esteem enhancement; role enhancement; emotional support; support system enhancement

NURSING ASSESSMENT

Assess for signs and symptoms of a disturbed self-concept:

- Verbalization of negative feelings about self
- Withdrawal from significant others
- Lack of planning to adapt to necessary changes in lifestyle
- Lack of participation in activities of daily living

RATIONALE

Early recognition of signs and symptoms of disturbed self-concept allows for implementation of the appropriate interventions.

THERAPEUTIC INTERVENTIONS

Independent Actions
Implement measures to assist client to adapt to the following changes in appearance and body functioning if appropriate:
- Alopecia.

- Inform client that hair loss in the treatment field usually begins 2 to 3 weeks after initiation of therapy.
- Reassure client that regrowth of hair within the treatment field will occur within 2 to 3 months after cessation of therapy if the loss is temporary (temporary or patchy loss will usually occur with a radiation dose of 2000–3000 cGy; delayed hair growth or complete, permanent hair loss within the treatment field may result from a radiation exposure >4000 cGy); explain that regrowth may be a different color, texture, and thickness.
- Instruct the client in ways to minimize scalp hair loss if thinning or partial hair loss is anticipated.
- Brush and comb hair gently.
- Wash hair only when necessary and avoid harsh shampoo, cream rinse, and other hair care products.
- Do not use hair dryer, curling iron, curlers, or constrictive decorations (e.g., clips, rubber bands) on hair.
- Avoid hairstyles that create tension on hair (e.g., ponytails, braids).
- Encourage the client to wear a wig, scarf, hat, or turban if desired to conceal hair loss; contact the American Cancer Society for a wig if client is unable to obtain one but desires to do so.
- Encourage use of the wig before hair loss.

- Caution client to remove wig several times a day to allow for exposure of treatment area to the air.
- Skin changes within the treatment field.

RATIONALE

Measures that help to minimize changes in appearance reduce the impact of these changes on self-concept.
Instructing the client about hair loss associated with radiation therapy may reduce anxiety and allow for implementation of temporary measures that help improve self-esteem.

Provides client methods to help in controlling hair loss.

Provides client with choices concerning what to do when hair loss occurs. Use of these help to improve client's self-esteem.

Use of the wig before hair loss facilitates adjustment to the wig and its integration into body image.
Protects scalp from ongoing irritation.

Continued...

THERAPEUTIC INTERVENTIONS	RATIONALE
• Reinforce physician's explanation about skin changes that will occur and when they can be expected.	*Explain what skin changes may occur and help client be ready for when they occur.*
• Suggest possible clothing styles that will make changes in skin texture and pigmentation less obvious.	*Natural fabrics such as cotton are less irritation to the skin.*
• Sterility or chromosomal damage.	*Inform client of potential reproductive changes that impact one's ability to have children.*
• Clarify physician's explanation about probable effects of radiation therapy on the gonads if they are in the treatment field.	*Allows client time to ask question concerning potential changes.*
• Discuss alternative methods of becoming a parent (e.g., artificial insemination, adoption) if of concern to client.	*Allows client to prepare for changes and determine methods that may be used for reproduction prior to treatment, when possible.*
• Impotence.	*Sexual functioning is an important component of one's sense of self. Assistance may be necessary to help the client adjust to changes experienced and/or to identify alternative ways of sexual expression.*
• Reinforce physician's explanation about the temporary or permanent nature of impotence; if it will be permanent, encourage client to discuss various treatment options (e.g., vacuum erection aids, penile prosthesis) with physician.	*Allows client time to ask question concerning treatment options to maintain as much sexual functioning as possible.*
• Suggest alternative methods of sexual gratification if appropriate.	
• Discuss ways to be creative in expressing sexuality (e.g., massage, fantasies, cuddling).	*Allows client to ask questions in a supportive environment.*
• Assist client with usual grooming and makeup habits if necessary.	*Appearance is an essential component of self-esteem and one's concept of self.*
Support behaviors suggesting positive adaptation to changes that have occurred (e.g., interest in personal appearance maintenance of relationships with significant others).	*Maintaining an appearance the client is comfortable with has a positive effect on self-concept.*
Encourage significant others to allow client to do what he/she is able so that independence can be reestablished and/or self-esteem redeveloped.	*Allowing the client to do as much as he/she is able facilitates the reestablishment of independence, which enhances feelings of self-esteem.*
Assist client's and significant others' adjustment by listening, facilitating communication, and providing information.	*Listening, facilitating communication, and providing information assist the client and significant others to cope with the present situation.*
Encourage visits and support from significant others.	
Provide information about and encourage use of community agencies and support groups (e.g., vocational rehabilitation; sexual, family, individual, and/or financial counseling).	*Community agencies and support groups provide the opportunity for the client to see that he/she is not experiencing a unique problem, to share feelings and concerns, to profit from the experience of others with similar difficulties, and to learn new skills necessary to rebuild self-esteem.*
Consult appropriate health care provider (e.g., psychiatric nurse clinician, oncology nurse specialist, physician) if client seems unwilling or unable to adapt to changes resulting from cancer and radiation therapy.	*Additional counseling may be necessary to facilitate positive adaptation to the changes in appearance and/or body functioning that have occurred.*

DISHCHARGE TEACHING/CONTINUED CARE

Nursing Diagnosis   **DEFICIENT KNOWLEDGE* NDx INEFFECTIVE HEALTH MANAGEMENT* NDx INEFFECTIVE FAMILY HEALTH MANAGEMENT* NDx**

Definition: **Deficient Knowledge NDx:** Absence of cognitive information related to a specific topic, or its acquisition; **Ineffective Health Management NDx:** Pattern of regulating and integrating into daily living a therapeutic regimen for the treatment of illness and its sequelae that is unsatisfactory for meeting specific health goals; **Ineffective Family Health Management NDx:** A pattern of regulating and integrating into family processes a program for the treatment of illness and its sequelae that is unsatisfactory for meeting specific health goals of the family unit.

Related to: Lack of understand of illness and long-term impact on life and family.

*The nurse should select the nursing diagnostic label that is most appropriate for the client's discharge teaching needs.

CLINICAL MANIFESTATIONS

Subjective	Objective
Verbalization of the problem	Exaggerated behaviors; inaccurate follow-through of instructions; lack of attention to illness; lack of interest in improving health behaviors

RISK FACTORS
- Lack of exposure
- Unfamiliarity with information resources
- Economically disadvantaged patient

NOC OUTCOMES

Knowledge: disease process; treatment regimen; energy conservation; treatment procedure(s)

NIC INTERVENTIONS

Health system guidance; teaching: disease process; teaching: prescribed activity/exercise; teaching: procedure/treatment; nutrition management

THERAPEUTIC INTERVENTIONS	RATIONALE

Desired Outcome: The client will verbalize an understanding of appropriate skin care for site of irradiation.

Independent Actions

- Reinforce teaching about the expected skin reaction at the site of irradiation (e.g., redness, tanned appearance, peeling, itching, loss of hair, decreased perspiration).

  Skin contains rapidly proliferating cells that are readily damaged by radiation.
  Interventions should be directed at maintaining the integrity of the skin and preventing wound development and infection.

- Instruct the client to:
  - Clean irradiated area gently using a mild soap and tepid water, being careful not to wash off temporary skin markings.
  - Pat skin dry with a soft cotton towel.
  - Avoid rubbing, scratching, and massaging irradiated skin.

  Helps to prevent skin breakdown and potential for infection.

Relieve itching by:
- Applying a light dusting of cornstarch to area of dry desquamation.

  Moisturizing lotions and emollients provide a source of moisture to the skin.

- Adding emollients, colloidal-based bath products, corn starch, or baking soda to bath water.
- Relieve dryness by applying a water-based lubricant lotion (e.g., Lubriderm, Eucerin).

  Prevents skin drying as seen with alcohol-based products.

- Avoiding use of deodorant if treatment field includes axillae.

  Prevents skin irritation.

- Check with physician before using cosmetics or perfumed lotions or creams in treatment area.

  Chemicals contained in perfumes and lotions may exacerbate imitated skin.

- Protect irradiated skin from exposure to temperature extremes and wind.
- Avoid exposure of treated area to direct sunlight or tanning beds during treatment period and for at least 1 month after therapy is complete and always use sunscreen with sun protection factor of 15 or greater.

  Burns can occur easily because melanin production in new epidermal cells is slowed.

- Wear soft cotton garments next to treatment area; use a gentle detergent to launder clothing.

  Decreases irritation and potential for itching which can lead to breakdown.

- Avoid wearing tight or constrictive clothing over irradiated area.

  Action helps to reduce mechanical irritation.

- Avoid shaving and using tape within treatment field; use an electric razor if shaving is absolutely necessary.

  Prevents injury.

Continued...

THERAPEUTIC INTERVENTIONS	RATIONALE
• Care for a moist desquamation reaction by:	
• Performing wound care and applying sterile dressings as prescribed (stretchable netting should be used instead of tape to hold dressings in place).	*Moist desquamation produces pain and drainage, and increases the risk of infection. Actions help to maintain or prevent increased irritation to irradiated skin areas.*
• Exposing area to the air as much as possible.	*Helps to decrease skin irritation.*
• Demonstrate care of treatment site.	*Allows health care provider to correct any actions by the client or family.*
• Allow time for questions, clarification, and return demonstration of skin and wound care.	*Allows the health care provider to assess the client's understanding of information and allow reinforcement if needed.*

THERAPEUTIC INTERVENTIONS	RATIONALE
Desired Outcome: The client will identify techniques to control nausea and vomiting.	
Independent Actions	
Instruct client in the following techniques to control nausea and vomiting:	*Interventions aimed at controlling nausea and vomiting can assist with improving appetite.*
• Clean mouth frequently.	
• Avoid offensive odors and sights.	*Decrease potential nausea and vomiting and can improve appetite.*
• Eat several small meals each day instead of three large ones.	*Prevents excessive stomach expansion which can lead to nausea and vomiting.*
• Eat the largest meal 3 to 4 hrs before treatments and eat lightly for at least 3 to 4 hrs after a treatment.	*Nausea and vomiting commonly occur after chemotherapy and/or radiation.*
• Eat foods that are cool or at room temperature (hot foods frequently have a strong aroma that stimulates nausea).	*Prevention and control of nausea and vomiting are necessary to ensure adequate nutrition.*
• Eat dry foods (e.g., toast, crackers) or sip cold carbonated beverages if nausea is present.	
• Select bland foods (e.g., mashed potatoes, cottage cheese) rather than fatty, spicy foods.	*Decreases irritation to the oral mucosa and decreases potential for nausea.*
• If feasible, have someone else prepare the food.	
• Avoid drinking liquids with meals.	*Drinking at meals increases feeling of fullness.*
• Rest after eating.	
• Take deep, slow breaths when nauseated.	*Decreases sensation of nausea.*
• Follow prescribed antiemetic regimen.	

THERAPEUTIC INTERVENTIONS	RATIONALE
Desired Outcome: The client will verbalize ways to improve appetite and nutritional status	
Independent Actions	
Instruct client in ways to improve appetite and maintain an adequate nutritional status:	*The stress of illness increases the metabolic needs of clients. Caloric requirements are greatly increased during illness. Maintaining an optimal nutritional status helps support the client during hypermetabolic periods and prevents complications associated with malnutrition, which may include sepsis.*
• Try chicken, fish, cheese, and eggs as protein sources instead of beef and pork if taste distortion is a problem.	*Assures adequate intake of protein.*
• Increase the amount of sweeteners and seasonings usually used in foods or beverages.	*May improve appetite.*
• Use plastic eating utensils and cook foods in glass or plastic containers rather than metal ones.	*Decreases potential for metallic taste when eating.*
• Moisten dry foods with sauces, salad dressing, or sour cream if mouth is dry or sore.	*Improves client's ability to swallow food.*
• Eat in a pleasant environment with company if possible.	*May increase caloric intake.*
• Perform frequent oral hygiene to eliminate unpleasant tastes in mouth.	*Removes unpleasant taste in the mouth and helps maintains oral health.*
• Try recommended methods of controlling nausea.	

THERAPEUTIC INTERVENTIONS	**RATIONALE**
• Eat several high-calorie, high-protein, nutritious small meals each day rather than three large ones; use nutritional supplements if needed to maintain an adequate calorie intake.	*Prevents oral distention of the stomach while improving caloric intake.*
• Plan ahead for low-energy days (e.g., have some prepared meals available; maintain an ample supply of nutritious, minimal preparation foods such as eggs, tuna fish, cheese, peanut butter, and yogurt; keep nutritious snacks and beverages within easy reach).	*When foods are readily available, it helps client to maintain adequate nutritional intake.*
• Take vitamins and minerals as prescribed.	*Supplements may be required to maintain nutritional status.*

THERAPEUTIC INTERVENTIONS	**RATIONALE**

Desired Outcome: The client will identify ways to reduce the risk of dental caries and periodontal disease and manage stomatitis if present.

Independent Actions
Inform client that dental caries and periodontal disease can occur months to years after irradiation of the jaw, neck, or oral cavity. Emphasize that a meticulous daily oral hygiene program is essential, particularly if salivary flow is permanently reduced.

Frequent oral hygiene is necessary in the neutropenic client to keep the oral cavity clean, moist, and free of bacterial infection so adequate nutritional intake can occur.

Instruct client in ways to reduce the risk of dental caries and periodontal disease:
- Use appropriate technique for cleansing teeth.
- Brush teeth with a fluoride toothpaste several times a day, particularly after eating.
- Use a small, soft, flexible toothbrush to brush teeth.
- Rinse mouth with a fluoride solution after brushing.
- If stomatitis is present, instruct client to:
  - Rinse mouth with the following solutions as prescribed:
    - Salt or baking soda and warm water.

These techniques help to prevent oral injury and support dental health.

Removes debris from the oral cavity and is soothing to the mucus membranes.

    - Chlorhexidine gluconate (Peridex). — *Prevents gingivitis.*
    - Consult physician about use of preparations to soothe the oral mucous membrane (e.g., diphenhydramine and water mixture) if mouth is painful. — *Decrease oral pain and irritation.*
- Wear dentures only at mealtime. — *Prevents ongoing irritation.*
- Eat soft, bland foods and avoid substances that might further irritate the mouth (e.g., extremely hot, spicy, or acidic foods/fluids). — *These types of foods are irritants to the oral cavity and may cause diarrhea, which can lead to loss of fluid and electrolytes.*
- Allow time for questions, clarification, and practice of oral hygiene techniques. — *Actions allow the health care provider to assess client's understanding of information and provide reinforcement as needed.*
- Instruct client to discuss any planned dental care with the radiologist and to inform the dentist that he/she is receiving or has had radiation to the oral cavity.

THERAPEUTIC INTERVENTIONS	**RATIONALE**

Desired Outcome: The client will identify ways to prevent bleeding if platelet counts are low.

Independent Actions
Instruct client in ways to minimize the risk of bleeding:

A client who is thrombocytopenic is at risk for increased bleeding and should be instructed on actions to prevent and/or control bleeding.

- Avoid taking aspirin and other nonsteroidal antiinflammatory agents (e.g., ibuprofen). — *Aspirin and NSAIDS decrease the platelets ability to participate in the clotting process.*

NDx = NANDA Diagnosis   **D** = Delegatable Action   ● = UAP   ✦ = LVN/LPN   ⊖▶ = Go to ⊖volve for animation

Continued...

THERAPEUTIC INTERVENTIONS	RATIONALE
• Consult health care provider before routinely taking herbs that can increase the risk of bleeding (e.g., ginkgo, arnica, chamomile).	*Several herbal products may increase the risk of bleeding and should be avoided.*
• Brush teeth gently using a soft-bristle toothbrush; do not use dental floss or put sharp objects (e.g., toothpicks) in mouth.	*Decrease the risk of gingival injury.*
• Be attentive when using scissors, knives, and tools to reduce the risk of cuts.	*These actions decrease the potential for injury, bleeding, and possible infection.*
• Use an electric rather than a straight-edge razor.	
• Cut nails and cuticles carefully.	
• Use caution when ambulating to prevent falls or bumps and do not walk barefoot.	
• Avoid blowing nose forcefully.	
• Avoid contact sports and other activities that could result in injury.	
• Avoid straining to have a bowel movement.	
• Avoid wearing constrictive clothing (e.g., garters, knee high stockings).	*Decreases circulation to the extremities.*
• Use an ample amount of water-soluble lubricant before sexual intercourse and avoid anal sexual activity, douching, use of rectal suppositories, and enemas in order to prevent trauma to the vaginal and rectal mucosa.	
• Avoid heavy lifting.	
• Instruct client to control any bleeding by applying firm, prolonged pressure to the site.	*Helps to promote clotting.*

THERAPEUTIC INTERVENTIONS	RATIONALE

Desired Outcome: The client will identify ways to prevent infection if WBC counts are low.

Independent Actions

Explain to client that his/her resistance to infection is reduced when WBC counts are low. Emphasize the need to adhere closely to recommended techniques to prevent infection.

Instruct client in ways to prevent infection:

• Avoid crowds, persons with any sign of infection, and persons who have recently been vaccinated.	*Prevents exposure to infection.*
• Use good hand hygiene (e.g., wash hands using an antibacterial soap, use an alcohol-based hand rub).	*Good hand hygiene is paramount in preventing infection.*
• Wear gloves to protect hands during activities such as cleaning and gardening.	*Animal feces are often present in garden soil and if ingested, can lead to infection in an immunocompromised client.*
• Take an axillary rather than an oral temperature if stomatitis is present.	*Axillary temperature assessment is more comfortable for a client with stomatitis.*
• Lubricate the skin outside irradiated area frequently to prevent dryness and subsequent cracking.	*Dry, cracked skin provides an avenue for bacteria to enter the body.*
• Cleanse and care for skin within treatment field as recommended.	*Helps to maintain skin intetrity.*
• Avoid unnecessary rectal invasion (e.g., temperature taking, enemas, suppositories, sexual activity) to prevent trauma to the rectal mucosa.	*Decreases potential for injury and potential introduction of infectious organisms.*
• Avoid constipation to prevent trauma to the bowel mucosa from hard or impacted stool.	*Damage or perforation of the bowel can lead to sepsis in an immunocompromised client.*
• Wash perianal area thoroughly with soap and water after each bowel movement; inform female client to always wipe from front to back after defecating and urinating.	*Prevents irritation and exposure to infectious bacteria.*

THERAPEUTIC INTERVENTIONS	RATIONALE
• Avoid douching unless ordered.	*Douching disturbs normal vaginal flora and may cause trauma to the vaginal mucosa.*
• Drink at least 10 glasses of liquid per day unless contra-indicated.	*Adequate hydration prevents constipation.*
• Cough and deep breathe or use incentive spirometer every 2 hrs until usual activity level is resumed.	*Coughing and deep breathing keep alveoli expanded, improve gas exchange, and facilitate expectoration of secretions, preventing pneumonia.*
• Stop smoking.	*Smoking damages the mucociliary system, which helps facilitate the expectoration of secretions.*
• Perform meticulous oral hygiene after meals and at bedtime or more often if directed, change denture care solution daily, and replace toothbrush routinely.	*Proper oral hygiene reduces oral bacteria and helps to keep oral mucosa intact.*
• Maintain an optimal nutritional status (e.g., diet high in protein, calories, vitamins, and minerals).	*Helps body to maintain adequate immune system.*
• Avoid sharing eating utensils.	*Decreases exposure to infectious organisms.*
• Maintain an adequate balance between activity and rest.	*Prevents fatigue.*
• Cleanse respiratory equipment as instructed; change water in humidifiers daily.	*Prevents growth of and subsequent exposure to infectious organisms.*
• Decrease risk of food-borne illness.	*Inadequate preparation of foods may predispose the client with a weakened immune system to food-borne pathogens that precipitate illness.*
• Avoid intake of foods with a high microorganism content (e.g., unwashed fruits and vegetables; under-cooked eggs, meat, poultry, and seafood).	*Decreases exposure to infectious organisms.*
• Be sure that juices and ciders are pasteurized or processed and that milk and cheese are pasteurized.	*Prevents exposure to unpasteurized products which decrease potential for infection.*
• Thoroughly wash hands and food preparation items and surfaces (e.g., knives, cutting boards, countertop) before and after cooking, especially when working with raw meat, poultry, and fish.	*Handwashing and cleaning food preparation surfaces are critical in decreasing exposure to infectious organisms.*
• Thaw food items in the refrigerator rather than on kitchen counter.	*Prevents bacteria growth during food thawing.*
• Avoid picking up animal waste or cleaning animal litter boxes and bird cages.	*Animal feces contain pathogens that can be harmful in a client with a compromised immune system.*
• Avoid elective surgery and dental work.	*Prevents injury and potential exposure to infection.*
• Reinforce the importance of taking prescribed medications such as colony-stimulating factors and prophylactic anti-microbial agents.	*Improves body's ability to fight infections.*

THERAPEUTIC INTERVENTIONS	RATIONALE
Desired Outcome: The client will verbalize an understanding of and ways to manage the effects of radiation therapy on sexual and reproductive functioning.	
Independent Actions	
Clarify physician's explanation about the possible effects of irradiation on the gonads if included in the treatment field.	*Reproductive and sexual dysfunction will vary according to radiation treatment protocols. Reproductive effects may be enhanced when area is included in the radiation treatment field.*
Explain that a temporary decrease in libido may occur as a result of radiation treatment.	
Encourage client to rest before sexual activity if fatigue is a problem.	
Instruct client in measures to reduce discomfort associated with decreased vaginal secretions and mucositis.	*Radiation therapy can result in tenderness, irritation, and loss of lubrication. These actions help client minimize discomfort encountered as a result of these side effects.*
• Use an ample amount of water-soluble lubricant.	*Improves conform and decreases potential for trauma to the vaginal mucosa.*

Continued...

THERAPEUTIC INTERVENTIONS	RATIONALE
• Use a vaginal steroid cream, if prescribed.	*Decreases vaginal dryness and inflammation.*
• Avoid intercourse until mucositis of the vaginal canal and/or urethra resolves.	*Prevents injury and potential spread of infectious organisms.*
• Have male partner use a condom during intercourse to prevent contact of vaginal area with semen.	*Semen can cause a burning sensation in the early months after vaginal irradiation.*
• Emphasize the need for frequent intercourse or vaginal dilatation once mucositis has resolved to prevent stenosis of the vaginal canal.	*Stenosis may develop several weeks or months after cessation of treatment that includes the vaginal area.*
• Explain to the female client that ovarian failure during therapy may result in decreased libido, irritability, hot flashes, and other symptoms of premature menopause.	*Allows client to mentally prepare for changes and speak to health care provided about ways to decrease impact of changes.*
• Inform the female client that her usual menstrual cycle will resume within 6 months to 1 year after treatment if sterility is temporary.	*Reproductive function may be temporarily altered and as such appropriate precautions should be taken.*
• Emphasize the need for both male and female clients to practice birth control during treatment and for at least 2 years after it.	
• Encourage both male and female clients to seek genetic counseling before attempting conception to ascertain the risk of chromosomal anomalies.	*Allows for continuum of care and information sharing prior to pregnancy.*
• Instruct client to take hormone replacements (e.g., estrogen, testosterone) as prescribed.	*Hormone replacement therapy may reduce symptoms associated with ovarian failure.*

THERAPEUTIC INTERVENTIONS	RATIONALE

Desired Outcome: The client will verbalize ways to manage and cope with persistent fatigue.

Independent Actions

Instruct client in ways to manage and cope with persistent fatigue:	*Fatigue affects most all clients undergoing chemotherapy and/or radiation. Fatigue may be related to anemia or side effects from therapy.*
• View fatigue as a protective mechanism rather than a problematic limitation.	
• Determine ways that daily patterns of activity can be modified to conserve energy and prevent excessive fatigue (e.g., spread light and heavy tasks throughout the day, take short rests during an activity whenever possible, take several short rest periods during the day instead of one long one).	
• Determine whether life demands are realistic in light of physical state and adjust short- and long-term goals accordingly.	
• Avoid situations that are particularly fatiguing such as those that are boring, frustrating, or require prolonged or strenuous physical activity.	*Ignoring fatigue or participating in activities that increase stress or fatigue may exacerbate symptoms.*
• Participate in a moderate exercise program (e.g., walking or bicycling 20–30 minutes three to four times a week).	*Walking is an effective way for a client to be active without overtaxing the body.*
• Participate in "attention-restoring" activities (e.g., walking outdoors, gardening).	*Improves clients muscle tone and self-esteem.*

THERAPEUTIC INTERVENTIONS	RATIONALE

Desired Outcome: The client will verbalize an understanding of the signs and symptoms of lymphedema and ways to manage it if it occurs.

Independent Actions

Instruct the client at risk for lymphedema (e.g., person receiving radiation for breast cancer, melanoma in an extremity, gynecologic cancer, or prostate cancer) to:	*Lymphedema occurs as a result of excision or radiation of lymph nodes. Fluid accumulates in the soft tissues as lymph nodes are unable to return fluid to the circulation fluid accumulation can result in impaired motor function in the affected area.*
• Monitor for and report signs and symptoms of lymph edema (e.g., pain or a feeling of heaviness or tightness in involved extremity).	*Allows for early identification of problem and appropriate treatment to be prescribed.*

THERAPEUTIC INTERVENTIONS	**RATIONALE**

- Measure the circumference of involved arm or leg daily if the extremity appears swollen and report a sudden increase in size to the physician.
- Provide the following instructions about ways to manage and prevent complications associated with lymphedema if it occurs:
  - Keep pressure off the involved extremity (e.g., avoid wearing tight jewelry, clothes with constricting bands, and elastic stockings with constricting bands; carry bags on unaffected arm; do not cross legs).

    Clients must protect the integrity of the skin as the first barrier to the prevention of infection.
  - Keep involved extremity elevated as much as possible.

    Elevation of an edematous extremity helps promote excess fluid drainage, promoting reabsorption.
  - Perform prescribed exercises.

    This helps to promote drainage of lymphatic fluid.
  - Gently clean and apply oil or skin cream to involved extremity daily.

    Presents skin injury and helps to maintain intact skin.
  - Avoid injury to the involved extremity (e.g., do not allow finger sticks or venipunctures in involved extremity, use an electric rather than straight-edge razor when shaving involved extremity, wear gardening and cooking gloves and use a thimble for sewing if upper extremity is affected, do not walk barefoot if lower extremity is affected, avoid extreme hot or cold on affected extremity, do not cut cuticles on hand or foot of involved extremity).

    Prevents further complications from decreasing circulation and lymphatic drainage.

THERAPEUTIC INTERVENTIONS	**RATIONALE**

Desired Outcome: The client will state signs and symptoms to report to the health care provider.

Independent Actions
Instruct the client to observe for and report the following:

Prompt reporting of adverse signs and symptoms allows for modification of the treatment plan and may reduce the risk of complications.

- Signs and symptoms of infection (stress that the usual signs of infection are diminished in people with a suppressed immune system and that it is necessary to monitor closely for the following signs and symptoms).
- Temperature above 38°C (100.4°F).
- Changes in odor, color, or consistency or urine.
- Signs and symptoms of bleeding.
- Signs and symptoms of radiation cystitis.
- Signs and symptoms of radiation pneumonitis.
- Signs and symptoms of tissue fibrosis within treatment field.
- Excessive tooth decay.
- Persistent nausea, vomiting, or decreased oral intake.
- Significant weight loss (weight loss of 1–2 lb/week during radiation therapy is not unusual).
- Persistent diarrhea.
- Excessive depression or difficulty coping with the effects of the diagnosis and treatment.
- Instruct client to keep a record of signs and symptoms, activities at the time the symptoms occur, measures to achieve relief, and the effect of the measures taken. Instruct client to take the information to each appointment with the health care provider.

THERAPEUTIC INTERVENTIONS	RATIONALE

Desired Outcome: The client will identify community resources that can assist with home management and adjustment to the diagnosis of cancer and radiation therapy and its effects.

Independent Actions

Provide information about and encourage use of community resources that can assist the client and significant others with home management and adjustment to cancer and the effects of radiation therapy (e.g., local support groups, American Cancer Society, home health agencies, counselors, social service agencies, Meals on Wheels, Make Today Count, hospice).

Knowledge of community resources can aid client in identification of services that may facilitate adherence to the treatment plan and provide the social support necessary during the treatment process.

THERAPEUTIC INTERVENTIONS	RATIONALE

Desired Outcome: The client, in collaboration with the nurse, will develop a plan for adhering to recommended follow-up care including medications prescribed and future appointments with health care provider, radiation department, and laboratory.

Independent Actions

Explain the rationale for, side effects of, and importance of taking medications prescribed. Inform client of pertinent food and drug interactions:

* Reinforce physician's explanation of planned radiation therapy schedule.
* Discuss with client any difficulties he/she might have adhering to the schedule and assist in planning ways to overcome these.
* Reinforce the importance of keeping appointments for radiation treatments and follow-up laboratory studies.
* Reinforce the importance of keeping follow-up appointments with health care provider.

Implement measures to improve client compliance:

* Include significant others in teaching sessions.
* Encourage questions and allow time for reinforcement and clarification of information provided.
* Provide written instructions regarding future appointments with health care provider, radiation department, and laboratory; medications prescribed; and signs and symptoms to report.

These actions help client adhere to the prescribed treatment regimen.

Allows client to ask questions and to determine actions necessary to meet appointments.

ADDITIONAL NURSING DIAGNOSIS

FEAR NDx/ANXIETY NDx
Related to:
* Unfamiliar environment
* Lack of knowledge about radiation therapy if admitted to initiate therapy
* Need for hospitalization to manage existing side effects of radiation therapy and concern that additional untoward effects will occur with subsequent radiation treatments
* Financial concerns
* Diagnosis of cancer with potential for premature death

ACUTE PAIN NDx
Related to:
Inflammation and/or moist desquamation (if it occurs) in irradiated area

NAUSEA NDx
Related to:
Stimulation of the vomiting center associated with:
* Presence of byproducts of cellular destruction if client is receiving a large daily fraction of radiation or daily treatments over a period of several weeks

- Stimulation of the visceral afferent pathways resulting from inflammation of the gastrointestinal mucosa (occurs when areas of the chest, back, abdomen, or pelvis are irradiated)
- Stimulation of the cerebral cortex resulting from cerebral inflammation (if client is receiving whole-brain irradiation) and stress

FATIGUE NDx
Related to:
- A buildup of cellular waste products associated with rapid lysis of cancerous and normal cells exposed to radiation
- Tissue hypoxia associated with anemia (can result from malnutrition or depression of bone marrow activity if large amounts of active bone marrow are included in the treatment field)
- Difficulty resting and sleeping associated with fear, anxiety, and discomfort
- Overwhelming emotional demands associated with the diagnosis of cancer and treatment with radiation
- Increased energy expenditure associated with an increase in the metabolic rate resulting from continuous active tumor growth and increased levels of certain cytokines (e.g., tumor necrosis factor, interleukin-1)
- Malnutrition
- Side effects of medications client may be receiving (e.g., narcotic [opioid] analgesics, antiemetics, antianxiety agents)

Related to:
Increased peristalsis and disorders of intestinal secretion and absorption associated with damage to the intestinal mucosa if the treatment field includes the pelvis, abdomen, or lower back

RISK FOR INFECTION NDx
Related to:
- Break in the integrity of the skin associated with dry or moist desquamation
- Lowered natural resistance associated with
- Malnutrition
- Neutropenia resulting from bone marrow suppression if large amounts of active bone marrow are included in the treatment field
- Impaired immune system functioning resulting from certain malignancies (e.g., Hodgkin disease, lymphoma)
- Stasis of respiratory secretions and urinary stasis if mobility is decreased

GRIEVING NDx
Related to:
- Changes in body image and usual lifestyle and roles
- Diagnosis of cancer with potential for premature death

16

Nursing Care of the Elderly Client

Individuals 65 years of age and older are the fastest-growing segment of the population, making the elderly a major portion of the health care consumer population. Older persons experience many physiologic changes that occur with aging. The extent or degree of the changes that take place depends on genetic and environmental factors as well as on the client's previous attention to health maintenance. As clients reach old age, there may also be many changes in roles, relationships, and the ability to maintain their usual lifestyles. These factors create psychosocial concerns that must be addressed, particularly when the client requires health care interventions.

This care plan focuses on the elderly client requiring health care intervention. It includes the nursing diagnoses that reflect the biopsychosocial changes that commonly occur with old age and are intensified with the stressors of illness. This care plan can be used in conjunction with the care plans in this text that are appropriate to the client's specific medical diagnosis or surgery and is intended for use in an acute or extended care facility or in a home setting.

Nursing Diagnosis | **INEFFECTIVE PERIPHERAL TISSUE PERFUSION NDx/RISK FOR DECREASED CARDIAC OUTPUT NDx**

Definition: **Ineffective Peripheral Tissue Perfusion NDx:** Decreased in blood circulation to the periphery, which may compromise health; **Risk For Decreased Cardiac Output NDx:** Susceptible to inadequate blood pumped by the heart to meet the metabolic demands of the body, which may compromise health.

Related to:
Ineffective tissue perfusion NDx:
- Increased vascular resistance associated with decreased elasticity and increased rigidity of the arterial vessels, associated with changes in the proportion of elastin and collagen in the vessel walls and accumulation of substances such as calcium and lipids
- Decrease in baroreceptor sensitivity
- Peripheral pooling of blood associated with loss of muscle tone in extremities, decreased competence of venous valves, and venous dilation (resulting from loss of vascular elasticity)

Decreased cardiac output NDx Related to:
- Impaired relaxation and contractility of the heart associated with stiffening of the ventricular walls
- Increased cardiac workload resulting from an increase in vascular resistance, thickened and rigid cardiac valves, and stress of current illness

CLINICAL MANIFESTATIONS

Subjective	Objective
Verbal self-report of increased fatigue and weakness; confusion; dizziness or lightheadedness, and syncopal episodes	Variations in blood pressure (BP); irregular, rapid, or slow pulse; dyspnea; increased crackles; edema; jugular vein distention (JVD); changes in electrocardiogram (ECG); restlessness; cool, pale skin; decreased or absent peripheral pulses; capillary refill greater than 2 to 3 seconds; elevated levels of blood urea nitrogen (BUN) and serum creatinine; oliguria; claudication; angina

RISK FACTORS

- Immobility
- Inadequate fluid intake
- Cardiovascular changes
- Aging process

DESIRED OUTCOMES

The client will maintain adequate cardiac output and tissue peripheral perfusion as evidenced by:

a. BP and heart rate within normal range for client
b. Usual mental status
c. Absence of dizziness or light-headedness and syncope
d. Extremities warm with absence of pallor or cyanosis
e. Palpable peripheral pulses
f. Capillary refill time less than 2 to 3 seconds
g. Absence of edema
h. BUN and serum creatinine levels within normal limits for an elderly client
i. Urine output $\geq$ 30 mL/h
j. Absence of exercise-induced pain

NOC OUTCOMES

Tissue perfusion: peripheral circulation status, effectiveness of cardiac pump

NIC INTERVENTIONS

Circulatory care for arterial/venous insufficiency; cardiac monitoring.

NURSING ASSESSMENT	RATIONALE
Assess for and report signs and symptoms of: • Decreased cardiac output (can lead to diminished tissue perfusion)	*Early recognition of signs and symptoms of decreased cardiac output and decreased tissue perfusion allows for prompt intervention.*
• Variations in BP	*BP may be increased because of compensatory vasoconstriction and may be decreased when compensatory mechanisms and pump fail.*
• Irregular, rapid, or slow pulse	*The incidence of dysrhythmias increases with age and is of concern because of the coexisting decrease in cardiac reserve.*
• Increase in loudness of existing systolic murmurs or presence of diastolic murmur	*Soft systolic murmurs are often present in elderly clients because of sclerosed valves.*
• Development of or an increase in loudness of S_3 and/or S_4 gallop rhythm	*An S_4 can be present in healthy adult clients.*
• Development of or increase in fatigue and weakness	*Muscles do not receive adequate oxygenation.*
• Development of or increase in dyspnea	*Crackles in the morning are a common finding in an elderly adult client.*
• New finding of or increased crackles	
• Edema	*Expected age-related changes include left axis deviation and some prolongation of the PR and QT intervals.*
• JVD	
• Changes in ECG readings	
• Chest radiograph showing pleural effusion or pulmonary edema	*Pleural effusion or pulmonary edema can occur with increased afterload and decreased cardiac output.*
• Diminished peripheral tissue perfusion: • Significant decrease in BP	*Elevated systolic BP is often present in elderly clients because of the age-related stiffening of the arteries and impaired baroreceptor function.*
• Decline in systolic BP of more than 20 mm Hg when client changes from a lying to a sitting or standing position	*In an elderly client, there is often a decline in systolic BP of 12 to 20 mm Hg with this positional change because of a decrease in baroreceptor sensitivity and vasomotor responsiveness. Can indicate decreased cardiac output and decreased cerebral perfusion pressures.*
• Restlessness, confusion, or other change in mental status	
• Reports of dizziness or light-headedness or occurrence of syncopal episodes	
• Cool, pale, or cyanotic skin	*Indicates decreased peripheral tissues perfusion potentially caused by decreased cardiac output.*
• Diminished or absent peripheral pulses	
• Capillary refill time greater than 2 to 3 seconds	
• Peripheral edema	*Indicated decrease blood return to the heart.*
• Elevated BUN and serum creatinine levels	*The BUN and serum creatinine levels tend to be slightly elevated because of the age-related decline in renal function.*

THERAPEUTIC INTERVENTIONS	RATIONALE

Independent Actions

Implement measures to maintain adequate tissue perfusion:

- Perform actions to reduce cardiac workload and help maintain an adequate cardiac output:
  - Place client in a semi- to high-Fowler's position whenever possible. **D** ● ✦

    Prevents slumping and decreases pressure on abdominal organs.
  - Instruct client to avoid activities that create a Valsalva response (e.g., straining to have a bowel movement, holding breath while moving up in bed).

    These activities decrease the heart rate and subsequently cardiac output.
  - Implement measures to promote rest and conserve energy (e.g., maintain activity restrictions, minimize environmental noise, limit number of visitors and length of stay). **D** ● ✦

    Decreases stress on the heart and body's oxygenation demands.

    Implement measures to maintain an adequate respiratory status (place in high-Fowler's positions, change position every 2 hrs, instruct client in deep breathing exercises, to be done every 2 hrs). **D** ● ✦

    Promotes adequate tissue oxygenation by allowing full expansion of the lungs.
  - Discourage smoking.

    Nicotine has a cardiostimulatory effect and causes vasoconstriction which can decrease cardiac ouptut; the carbon monoxide in smoke reduces the availability of oxygen (O_2).
  - Discourage excessive intake of beverages high in caffeine, such as coffee, tea, and colas. **D** ✦

    Caffeine is a myocardial stimulant that can increase myocardial O_2 consumption and can decrease cardiac output.
  - Provide small meals rather than large ones. **D** ✦

    Large meals can increase cardiac workload because they require an increase in blood supply to the gastrointestinal tract to aid digestion.
  - Increase activity gradually as allowed and tolerated. **D** ✦

    This will improve stamina and cardiac function.
- Perform actions to reduce peripheral pooling of blood and increase venous return:
  - Instruct client in active foot and leg exercises every 1 to 2 hrs during periods of decreased activity and assist with these.

    Improve venous return to the heart through the muscle pump system.
  - Encourage and assist client with ambulation as allowed and tolerated. **D** ● ✦

    Increases muscle strength, improves the ability to extract oxygen from the blood, reducing the heart to pump more frequently and decreases stress hormones impact on the heart. It also provides the nurse a chance to assess exercise tolerance.
- Instruct and assist client to change from a supine to an upright position slowly. **D** ● ✦

  Allows time for autoregulatory mechanisms to adjust to the change in the distribution of blood associated with an upright position.
- Discourage positions that compromise blood flow in lower extremities (e.g., crossing legs, use of knee gatch, sitting for long periods, prolonged standing). **D** ● ✦

  These positions increase pooling of blood in the feet and legs, thus decreasing venous return to the heart.
- Maintain a comfortable room temperature and provide client with adequate clothing and blankets. **D** ● ✦

  Exposure to cold causes generalized vasoconstriction.

Dependent/Collaborative Actions

Implement measures to maintain adequate tissue perfusion:

- Maintain a fluid intake of 1500 to 2000 mL/day unless contraindicated; if oral intake is inadequate or contraindicated, maintain intravenous and/or enteral fluid therapy as ordered.

  There is a greater risk for fluid overload in the elderly client because of the age-related decline in the kidneys' ability to excrete a large volume of water in response to sudden volume excess.

Consult appropriate health care provider if signs and symptoms of diminished tissue perfusion persist or worsen.

Allows for prompt alterations in the treatment plan.

Nursing Diagnosis   IMPAIRED RESPIRATORY FUNCTION*

Definitions: **Ineffective Breathing Pattern NDx:** Inspiration/expiration that does not provide adequate ventilation; **Ineffective Airway Clearance NDx:** Inability to clear secretions or obstructions from the respiratory tract to maintain a clear airway; **Impaired Gas Exchange NDx:** Excess or deficit in oxygenation and/or carbon dioxide elimination at the alveolar-capillary membrane.

Related to:

Ineffective breathing pattern NDx
- Loss of alveolar elasticity (results in reduced efficiency of air expulsion)
- Decreased chest expansion associated with calcification of costal cartilage and weakened respiratory muscles
- Decreased responsiveness of chemoreceptors to hypoxia and hypercapnia

Ineffective airway clearance NDx
- Stasis of secretions associated with decreased activity during illness and an age-related decrease in ciliary activity and cough effectiveness
- Weakening of respiratory muscles

Impaired gas exchange NDx
- Loss of effective lung surface associated with a reduced number of alveoli, changes in the alveolar walls, and accumulation of secretions in the bronchioles and alveoli (can result from ineffective airway clearance)
- Reduced airflow associated with loss of alveolar elasticity, restricted chest expansion, and premature closure of small airways
- Decreased pulmonary blood flow associated with a decrease in the number of capillaries surrounding the alveoli, fibrosis of the pulmonary vessels, and a generalized decrease in tissue perfusion

CLINICAL MANIFESTATIONS

Subjective	Objective
Verbal self-report of shortness of breath; Self-report of inability to cough up secretions	Irritability, confusion, somnolence, dyspnea, orthopnea, use of accessory muscles when breathing, asymmetric chest excursion, adventitious breath sounds, diminished or absent breath sounds, abnormal breath sounds, decreased oximetry results, abnormal chest radiograph

RISK FACTORS
- Sedentary lifestyle
- Chronic illness
- Respiratory system changes

DESIRED OUTCOMES

The client will experience adequate respiratory function as evidenced by:
a. Normal rate and depth of respirations
b. Absence of dyspnea
c. Symmetrical chest excursion
d. Usual or improved breath sounds
e. Usual mental status
f. Oximetry results within normal range for an elderly client
g. Arterial blood gas values within normal range for an elderly client

NOC OUTCOMES

Respiratory status: ventilation; airway patency; gas exchange

NIC INTERVENTIONS

Respiratory monitoring; airway management; chest physiotherapy; oxygen therapy; cough enhancement

---

*This diagnostic label includes the following nursing diagnoses: ineffective breathing pattern, ineffective airway clearance, and impaired gas exchange.

NDx = NANDA Diagnosis   **D** = Delegatable Action   ● = UAP   ✦ = LVN/LPN   ⊖▶ = Go to ⊖volve for animation

NURSING ASSESSMENT	RATIONALE
Assess for and report signs and symptoms of impaired respiratory function:	*Early recognition of signs and symptoms of impaired respiratory function allows for prompt intervention.*
• Rapid, shallow, or slow respirations	*Decreased oxygenation to the tissues.*
• Dyspnea, orthopnea	*Results from alveolar collapse associated with age-related hypoventilation and decreased activity.*
• Use of accessory muscles when breathing	
• Asymmetric chest excursion	
• Adventitious breath sounds (e.g., crackles [rales], rhonchi; crackles may be heard especially on initial morning assessment)	*Diminished sounds are often present in the elderly client because of reduced airflow.*
• Diminished or absent breath sounds	
• Cough	*Will have decreased cough effort due to decreased muscle tone.*
• Restlessness, irritability	
• Confusion, somnolence	*Decreased cerebral oxygenation leads to restlessness, irritability, confusion, and somnolence.*
• Abnormal arterial blood gas values (partial pressure of O_2 in arterial blood [PaO_2] is normally lower in the elderly client)	*Changes in ABG's provide the best indication of oxygen in the blood.*
• Decrease in oximetry results	*O_2 saturation is normally lower in the elderly client.*
• Abnormal chest radiograph results	

THERAPEUTIC INTERVENTIONS	RATIONALE

Independent Actions

Implement measures to maintain an adequate respiratory status:	
• Place client in a semi- to high-Fowler's position unless contraindicated; position with pillows. **D** ● ✦	*This will prevent slumping and improve lung expansion.*
• If client must remain flat in bed, assist with position change at least every 2 hrs. **D** ● ✦	*This will improve lung expansion and decrease stasis of lung secretions.*
• Instruct client to breathe deeply or use incentive spirometer every 1 to 2 hrs.	*These actions improve lung expansion and mobilization of secretions.*
• Perform actions to decrease pain if present (e.g., splint/protect painful area during movement, administer prescribed analgesics before planned activity). **D** ● ✦	*Client will be hesitant to take deep breaths if pain is present. Splinting helps to support painful area when coughing.*
• Perform actions to decrease fear and anxiety (e.g., explain procedures, provide a calm environment). **D** ● ✦	*Fear and anxiety can cause the client to breathe in shallow and/or rapid breaths.*
• Instruct client in and assist with diaphragmatic and pursed-lip breathing techniques if indicated.	*These techniques improve oxygenation.*
• Instruct and assist client to cough or "huff" every 1 to 2 hrs. **D** ✦	*This improves lung expansion and oxygenation.*
• Discourage smoking.	*Irritants in smoke increase the production of mucus, further impair ciliary function, and can damage the bronchial and alveolar walls; the carbon monoxide also decreases O_2 availability.*
• Instruct client to avoid intake of gas-forming foods (e.g., beans, cabbage, cauliflower, onions), carbonated beverages, and large meals.	*These measures will help to reduce gastric distention and pressure on the diaphragm.*
• Maintain activity restrictions as ordered; increase activity gradually as allowed and tolerated. **D** ● ✦	*This will improve cardiac output and exercise stamina.*

Dependent/Collaborative Actions

Implement measures to thin tenacious secretions and reduce dryness of the respiratory mucous membrane:	
• Maintain a fluid intake of 1500 to 2000 mL/day unless contraindicated. **D** ● ✦	*Maintains adequate vascular fluid volume and increased hydration helps to thin secretions.*
• Humidify inspired air if ordered. **D** ✦	*Moisturizes air and helps to thin secretions.*
If client has difficulty mobilizing secretions:	
• Assist with or perform postural drainage therapy if ordered.	*Helps to mobilize and excrete secretions.*
• Consult physician about use of a mucolytic (e.g., acetylcysteine) or diluent or hydrating agent (e.g., water, saline) via nebulizer.	*These medications improve client's ability to expectorate secretions.*
• Suction as needed.	*Manually removes secretions.*

THERAPEUTIC INTERVENTIONS	RATIONALE
• Assist with positive airway pressure techniques (e.g., continuous positive airway pressure [CPAP], bilevel positive airway pressure [BiPAP], flutter/positive expiratory pressure [PEP] device) if ordered.	*Improves oxygenation by helping to expand alveoli and force air into the lungs.*
• Maintain O$_2$ therapy if ordered. **D** ✦	*Provides supplemental oxygenation to support tissue requirements.*
• Administer central nervous system depressants judiciously because of their respiratory depressant effect; hold medication and consult physician if respiratory rate is below 12 breaths/min.	*The possibility of respiratory depression is increased in the elderly because of their altered metabolism, distribution and excretion of drugs, and decreased responsiveness of chemoreceptors to hypoxia and hypercapnia.*
Consult appropriate health care provider (e.g., physician, respiratory therapist) if signs and symptoms of impaired respiratory function persist or worsen.	*Allows for prompt alteration in treatment plan.*

Nursing Diagnosis RISK FOR DEFICIENT FLUID VOLUME NDx

Definition: Susceptible to experiencing decreased intravascular, interstitial, and/or intracellular fluid volumes, which may compromise health.

Related to:
• Age-related decrease in total body water
• Decreased fluid intake associated with:
  • Restrictions imposed by current illness and/or treatment plan
  • Diminished thirst sensation
  • Desire to avoid nocturia and/or urinary incontinence
• Age-related decline in the kidney's ability to conserve water when a deficit is caused by disease or environmental factors

CLINICAL MANIFESTATIONS

Subjective	Objective
Verbal self-report of dry mouth, self-report of confusion	Decreased skin turgor; dry skin and mucous membranes; weight loss of 2% or greater over a short period; hypotension; weak, rapid pulse; capillary refill time greater than 2 to 3 seconds; flat neck veins when lying flat; elevated BUN, serum creatinine, and hematocrit (Hct) levels; oliguria; change in mental status; decreased urine output

RISK FACTORS
• Changes in regulatory systems
• Inadequate fluid intake
• Medication regimen

DESIRED OUTCOMES

The client will not experience deficient fluid volume as evidenced by:
a. Normal skin and tongue turgor for client
b. Moist mucous membranes
c. Stable weight
d. BP and pulse within normal range for client with no further increase in postural hypotension
e. Capillary refill time below 2 to 3 seconds
f. BUN and Hct levels within normal range for age
g. Usual mental status
h. Balanced intake and output

NOC OUTCOMES

Fluid balance

NIC INTERVENTIONS

Fluid monitoring; fluid management; hypovolemia management; intravenous therapy

---

NDx = NANDA Diagnosis   **D** = Delegatable Action   ● = UAP   ✦ = LVN/LPN   ⊖▶ = Go to ⊖volve for animation

NURSING ASSESSMENT	RATIONALE
Assess for and report signs and symptoms of deficient fluid volume:	*Early recognition of signs and symptoms of deficient fluid volume allows for prompt intervention.*
• Decreased skin turgor	*This is not always a reliable indicator because decreased skin turgor is a normal age-related change; turgor is best assessed over the forehead or sternum in an elderly client.*
• Decreased tongue turgor	*The tongue may be smaller than usual and have more than one longitudinal furrow.*
• Dry mucous membranes, thirst	*Thirst may not be a reliable indicator because saliva production and sensation of thirst are diminished in elderly clients.*
• Weight loss of 2% or greater over a short period	*May indicate fluid loss.*
• Low BP and/or decline in systolic BP of more than 20 mm Hg when client sits up	*A drop of 15 to 20 mm Hg is not unusual in elderly clients because of decreased baroreceptor sensitivity and vasomotor responsiveness.*
• Weak, rapid pulse	*These clinical manifestations indicate decreased vascular fluid volume.*
• Capillary refill time greater than 2 to 3 seconds	
• Neck veins flat when client is supine	
• Elevated BUN and Hct levels	
• Change in mental status (e.g., confusion)	*Indicates decreased volume below the level required to maintain cerebral perfusion pressure.*
• Decreased urine output	*Indicates an actual rather than potential fluid volume deficit.*

THERAPEUTIC INTERVENTIONS	RATIONALE
Independent Actions Implement measures to prevent deficient fluid volume:	
• Maintain a fluid intake of 1200 to 2500 mL/day and instruct client to continue this regimen after discharge unless contraindicated. **D** ● ✦	*Maintains adequate vascular volume. Adequate fluid intake is required to maintain vascular status.*
• Monitor intake and output **D** ● ✦	*Aging decreases kidney function and decreased fluid volume and further decrease output.*
Dependent/Collaborative Actions Implement measures to prevent deficient fluid volume:	
• Maintain intravenous and/or enteral fluid therapy if ordered.	*Administer intravenous fluids cautiously because the elderly client is also at risk for fluid overload.*
• Monitor laboratory values:	*These values indicate fluid volume deficit, and dehydration that can cause increased levels.*
• BUN, creatinine, Hct	

Nursing Diagnosis   **IMBALANCED NUTRITION: LESS THAN BODY REQUIREMENTS** NDx

Definition: Intake of nutrients insufficient to meet metabolic needs.

Related to:
• Decreased oral intake associated with:
  • Anorexia resulting from factors such as depression, loneliness, diminished sense of smell and/or taste, early satiety, and dyspepsia
  • Difficulty chewing and swallowing food resulting from poor dentition, a decreased amount of saliva, and weakened chewing and swallowing muscles
  • Decreased ability to purchase and/or prepare healthy foods
• Decreased utilization of nutrients associated with impaired digestion resulting from:
  • Decreased ability to chew foods thoroughly
  • Reduced secretion of digestive enzymes (e.g., salivary ptyalin, hydrochloric acid, pepsin, lipase)
• Reduced absorption of nutrients associated with hypochlorhydria, decreased intestinal blood flow, and atrophy of the absorptive surface of the intestine

CLINICAL MANIFESTATIONS

Subjective	Objective
Verbal self-report of abdominal pain and cramping; sore buccal cavity	Aversion to eating; body weight 20% or more under ideal; capillary fragility; hair loss; lack of food; lack of interest in food; pale mucous membranes; low serum albumin, prealbumin, Hct, and hemoglobin (Hgb) levels, and low lymphocyte count

RISK FACTORS

- Living on a fixed income
- Changes in taste sensation
- Medication regimen
- Mental status changes—dementia, anxiety, depression

DESIRED OUTCOMES

The client will maintain an adequate nutritional status as evidenced by:
a. Weight within normal range for client
b. Normal serum albumin, prealbumin, Hct, and Hgb levels and normal lymphocyte count for client's age
c. Usual strength and activity tolerance
d. Healthy oral mucous membrane

NOC OUTCOMES

Nutritional status

NIC INTERVENTIONS

Nutritional monitoring; appetite; nutrition management; nutrition therapy; nutritional counseling

NURSING ASSESSMENT	RATIONALE
Assess for and report signs and symptoms of malnutrition: - Weight significantly below client's usual weight or below normal for client's age, height, and body frame - Low serum albumin, prealbumin, Hct, and Hgb levels and low lymphocyte count - Weakness and fatigue - Sore, inflamed oral mucous membrane - Pale conjunctiva - Lower-than-normal anthropometric measurements such as skinfold thickness, body circumferences (e.g., hip, waist, mid- and upper arm), and bioelectric impedance analysis	*Early recognition of signs and symptoms of malnutrition allows for prompt intervention.* *Indicates that client has not maintained a proper diet. When using height and weight charts, be aware that weight is expected to decline gradually with age.* *These indicate protein depletion. Low Hct and Hgb levels and low white blood cell (WBC) counts lead to anemia and potential infections. Clinical manifestations of decreased intake and potential anemia, and weight loss.*

THERAPEUTIC INTERVENTIONS	RATIONALE

Independent Actions
Implement measures to maintain an adequate nutritional status:
- Perform actions to improve oral intake:
  - Implement measures to relieve dyspepsia, gastric fullness, and gas pain. **D** ● ✦   *Decreases pressure in the abdomen, which helps to improve appetite.*
  - Increase activity as allowed and tolerated. **D** ● ✦   *Activity usually promotes a sense of well-being, which can improve appetite; it also promotes gastric emptying, which reduces the feeling of gastric fullness.*
  - Maintain a clean environment and a relaxed, pleasant atmosphere. **D** ● ✦   *These help to improve appetite.*
  - Implement measures to decrease the sense of isolation and aloneness (e.g., use touch to demonstrate acceptance, encourage significant others to visit, schedule time to sit and speak with the client each day).   *These promote a sense of well-being, which can improve appetite.*
  - Encourage a rest period before meals if client is weak or fatigues easily. **D** ● ✦   *Fatigue can reduce the client's desire and ability to eat.*
  - Provide frequent, small meals rather than large ones if client is weak, fatigues easily, and/or has a poor appetite. **D** ● ✦   *This may help to improve intake and decrease fatigue associated with eating a large meal.*

NDx = NANDA Diagnosis   **D** = Delegatable Action   ● = UAP   ✦ = LVN/LPN   ⊖▶ = Go to ⊖volve for animation

Continued...

THERAPEUTIC INTERVENTIONS	RATIONALE
• Provide oral hygiene before eating. **D** ● ✦	*Oral hygiene moistens the mouth, which may make it easier to chew and swallow; it also removes unpleasant tastes, which often improves the taste of foods/fluids.*
• Serve foods/fluids that are appealing to the client. **D** ● ✦	*Visual appeal is especially important if client's sense of smell is diminished.*
• Encourage significant others to bring in client's favorite foods unless contraindicated and eat with client to make eating more of a familiar social experience. **D** ✦	*Clients may be more inclined to eat food they like. When family members eat with client, it helps to increase intake.*
• Provide a soft, ground, or pureed diet if client has difficulty chewing.	*Easier for client to chew and swallow.*
• Implement measures to compensate for taste alterations and/or dislike of prescribed diet.	
(1) Serve foods warm to stimulate sense of smell. **D** ● ✦	*Improves taste of foods that should be served warm and can improve intake.*
(2) Encourage client to experiment with different flavorings and seasonings. **D** ● ✦	*Adds different flavors, which may stimulate appetite.*
(3) Instruct client to use salt substitutes and salt-free herbs and spices if receiving a low-sodium diet.	*Decreases salt intake and subsequent fluid retention. Use with caution as they may increase intake of potassium.*
(4) Encourage client to add extra sweeteners to foods unless contraindicated.	*Helps improve taste of foods.*
(5) Provide alternative sources of protein if meats such as beef or pork taste bitter or rancid.	*Improves nutritional status and assure adequate protein intake.*
• Limit fluid intake with meals. **D** ✦	*Unless the fluid has high nutritional value, the fluid should be avoided as it may cause early satiety and subsequent decreased food intake.*
• Allow adequate time for meals; reheat foods/fluids if necessary. **D** ● ✦	*Improves intake of nutrients.*
• Ensure that meals are well balanced and high in essential nutrients; offer high-protein supplements if client is having difficulty maintaining an adequate caloric intake.	*Ensures adequate nutrition is maintained.*

Dependent/Collaborative Actions

Implement measures to maintain an adequate nutritional status:

• Administer vitamins and minerals if ordered. **D** ✦	*Supplements regular diet and increases importance for clients with poor or those not eating a-nutritional diet.*
• Perform a calorie count if ordered. Report this information to dietitian and physician.	*It is important to know how many calories and what type client is eating.*
• Consult physician regarding an alternative method of providing nutrition (e.g., parenteral nutrition, tube feedings) if client does not consume enough food or fluids to meet nutritional needs.	*Allows for alteration in treatment plan to provide adequate nutrition.*
• If indicated, obtain a social service consult to assist client in arranging for services such as Meals on Wheels and home health aides for feeding assistance at home.	*Provides for continuum of care and provides support for client following discharge from the health care facility.*
• Obtain a dietary consult, if necessary, to assist client in selecting foods/fluids that meet nutritional needs as well as personal and cultural preferences whenever possible.	*Provides a multidisciplinary approach to care.*
• If client has dentures, assist with putting them in before meals; if dentures do not fit properly, obtain a dental consult.	*Improves client's ability to macerate foods and decreases pain and trauma associated with loose fitting dentures.*

| Nursing Diagnosis | **RISK FOR IMPAIRED SKIN INTEGRITY** NDx |

Definition: Susceptibility to alteration in epidermis and/or dermis, which may compromise health.

Related to:
- Increased fragility of the skin associated with decreased nutritional status and age-related dryness, loss of elasticity, and thinning of skin
- Frequent contact with irritants if urinary incontinence is present
- Accumulation of waste products and decreased O_2 and nutrient supply to the skin and subcutaneous tissue associated with decreased blood flow to the skin due to:
  - An age-related decrease in dermal vascularity
  - Prolonged pressure on the tissues if mobility is decreased

NOC OUTCOMES

Tissue integrity: skin and mucous membranes

NIC INTERVENTIONS

Skin surveillance; positioning, skin care, topical, pressure ulcer prevention

RISK FACTORS
- Poor nutritional status
- Chronic illness
- Sedentary lifestyle
- Inadequate fluid intake

DESIRED OUTCOMES

The client will maintain skin integrity as evidenced by:
a. Absence of redness and irritation
b. No skin breakdown

NURSING ASSESSMENT	**RATIONALE**
Determine client's risk for skin breakdown using a risk-assessment tool (e.g., Norton Scale, Braden Scale, Gosnell Scale).	*Early recognition of signs and symptoms of skin breakdown allows for prompt intervention.*
Inspect the skin (especially bony prominences, dependent areas, perineum, and areas of decreased sensation and/or edema) for pallor, redness, and breakdown.	*Use of a scale provides for standardized assessment.*

THERAPEUTIC INTERVENTIONS	**RATIONALE**

Independent Actions
Implement measures to prevent skin breakdown:

• Assist client to turn at least every 2 hrs. **D** ● ✦	*Elderly clients may require more frequent position changes because of decreased blood flow to the skin, reduced amounts of protective subcutaneous fat, and a decreased ability to sense pressure and discomfort.*
• Position client properly; use pressure-reducing or pressure-relieving devices (e.g., pillows, gel or foam cushions, alternating pressure mattress, air-fluidized bed) if indicated. **D** ● ✦	*Decreases the amount of pressure placed on the skin.*
• Gently massage around reddened areas at least every 2 hrs. **D** ● ✦	*Improves circulation, which increases supply of O_2 and nutrients.*
• Apply a thin layer of a dry lubricant such as powder or cornstarch to bottom sheet or skin and to opposing skin surfaces (e.g., axillae, beneath breasts) if indicated. **D** ● ✦	*Reduces friction between client's skin and the bed linens.*
• Lift and move client carefully, using a turn sheet and adequate assistance. **D** ● ✦	*Prevents accidental skin tears.*
• Perform actions to keep client from sliding down in bed (e.g., gatch knees slightly when head of bed is elevated 30 degrees or higher, limit length of time client is in a semi-Fowler's positions to 30-minute intervals). **D** ● ✦	*Reduces the risk of skin surface abrasion and shearing.*
• Instruct or assist client to shift weight at least every 30 minutes. **D** ● ✦	*Changes area of pressure on the skin and decreases incidence of skin breakdown.*
• Keep client's skin clean. **D** ● ✦	*Removes surface microorganisms which, if allowed to accumulate, increase the risk of irritation and infection.*

Continued...

THERAPEUTIC INTERVENTIONS	RATIONALE
• Keep bed linens dry and wrinkle-free. **D** ● ✦	Moisture harbors microorganisms that can cause irritation and/or infection. Keeping linens wrinkle free decreases the possibility of friction.
• Thoroughly dry skin after bathing and as often as needed, paying special attention to skinfolds and opposing skin surfaces (e.g., axillae, perineum, beneath breasts); pat skin dry rather than rub. **D** ● ✦	Excessive moisture or prolonged skin exposure softens the epidermal cells and makes them less resistant to damage.
• Make sure that external devices such as braces, casts, and restraints are applied properly.	Prevents accidental skin tears and allows for adequate circulation.
• Provide elbow and heel protectors if indicated. **D** ● ✦	Reduces pressure on these areas.
• Encourage client to wear socks while in bed. **D** ● ✦	Helps reduce friction on heels and decreases incidence of skin breakdown.
• Increase activity as allowed and tolerated.	Improves circulation and improves muscle strength.
• Avoid use of harsh soaps and hot water; use a mild soap and tepid water for bathing. **D** ● ✦	Reduces dryness of the skin and potential for breakdown.
• Apply moisturizing lotion and/or emollient to skin at least once a day.	Reduces friction and helps prevent skin surface irritation and abrasion.
• Assist client with total bath or shower every other day rather than daily. **D** ● ✦	Reduces drying of the skin.
• Encourage a fluid intake of 1500 to 2000 mL/day unless contraindicated.	Ensures skin is well hydrated.
• Protect skin from wound drainage and urinary incontinence (e.g., change dressing when damp, apply drainage collection device; take client regularly to the bathroom, encourage client to urinate when urge is felt, allow client to assume normal position for voiding). **D** ✦	Prevents skin irritation resulting from exposure to wound drainage or urine.
• Assist client to thoroughly clean and dry perineal area with soft tissue or cloth after each episode of incontinence; apply a protective ointment or cream. **D** ● ✦	Excessive exposure of skin to urine increases the potential for skin breakdown.
• If use of absorbent products such as pads or undergarments is necessary, select those that effectively absorb moisture and keep it away from the skin. **D** ● ✦	Decreases skin exposure to moisture and potential for irritation and breakdown.
• Apply a protective covering such as a hydrocolloid or transparent membrane dressing to areas of the skin susceptible to breakdown (e.g., coccyx, elbows, heels).	Decreases friction between skin and bed linens or clothing and decreases incidence of tears and/or breakdown.
• Use caution with application of heat or cold to areas of decreased sensation or circulatory impairment. **D** ✦	Aging process decreases sensation and the client may not realize that skin is being affected. Prevents potential burn to the skin.
• Maintain optimal nutritional status. **D** ✦	Proper nutrition is required to maintain the appropriate amount of subcutaneous tissue and prevent skin from becoming thin and losing its elasticity.

Dependent/Collaborative Actions

If skin breakdown occurs:

• Notify appropriate health care provider (e.g., physician, wound care specialist).	Allows for alteration in treatment plan.
• Perform care of involved areas as ordered or per standard hospital procedure. **D** ✦	Provides standardized care for skin breakdown.

Nursing Diagnosis   **IMPAIRED ORAL MUCOUS MEMBRANE INTEGRITY** NDx

Definition: Injury to the lips, soft tissues, buccal cavity, and/or oropharynx.

Related to:
- Dryness due to decreased saliva production associated with a gradual decline in salivary gland activity
- Irritation and breakdown related to dryness and thinning of the oral mucosa

CLINICAL MANIFESTATIONS

Subjective	Objective
Verbal self-report of oral dryness, irritation	Breakdown of oral mucosa

RISK FACTORS
- Chronic changes
- Inadequate fluid intake
- Medication regimen

DESIRED OUTCOMES

The client will maintain a moist, intact oral mucous membrane.

NOC OUTCOMES

Oral health, tissue integrity, skin and mucous membranes

NIC INTERVENTIONS

Oral health maintenance, oral health restoration, oral health promotion.

NURSING ASSESSMENT	RATIONALE
Assess client for dryness, irritation, and breakdown of the oral mucosa.	*Early recognition of signs and symptoms of impaired mucous membranes allows for prompt intervention.*

THERAPEUTIC INTERVENTIONS	RATIONALE

Independent Actions

Implement measures to decrease dryness and irritation of the oral mucous membrane:

- Instruct and assist client in performing oral hygiene as often as needed; avoid products that contain lemon and glycerin and mouthwashes containing alcohol. **D** ✦

  These products have a drying and irritating effect on the oral mucous membrane. Commercial mouthwashes should be avoided as they contain alcohol. Teach client to read labels.

- Instruct and assist client to perform oral hygiene using a soft-bristle toothbrush or sponge-tipped swab and to floss teeth gently. **D** ✦

  A soft-bristle toothbrush or sponge-tipped swab decreases potential for mucous membrane irritation. Gentle flossing will clean between teeth while not traumatizing the gums.

- Encourage client to rinse mouth frequently with water. **D** ● ✦

  Helps to keep mucous membranes moist and remove debris from the mouth.

- Lubricate client's lips frequently. **D** ● ✦

  Helps prevents lips from chafing.

- Encourage client to breathe through nose rather than mouth.

  Breathing through the nose prevents air from drying out the oral mucous membranes.

- Encourage client not to smoke or chew tobacco. **D** ✦

  Smoking dries the mucosa; tobacco acts as an irritant to the oral mucosa.

- Encourage a fluid intake of 1500 to 2000 mL/day unless contraindicated. **D** ✦

  Maintains adequate vascular fluid volume and oral hydration.

- Encourage client to chew sugarless gum or suck on sugarless hard candy. **D** ✦

  Stimulates salivation and helps to maintain moist mucous membranes.

- Encourage client to use artificial saliva. **D** ✦

  Lubricates the mucous membranes and prevents dryness or irritation.

If mucosa is irritated or cracked,
- Assist client to select soft, bland foods.
- Instruct client to avoid foods/fluids that are extremely hot.

  Spicy foods can cause irritation to the oral mucosa. Client may not realize how hot food is due to decreased sensation in the mouth.

- If client has dentures, remove and replace only for meals. **D** ✦

  Relieves discomfort, prevents further irritation, decreases incidence of breakdown, and promotes healing.

Dependent/Collaborative Actions

Implement measures to decrease dryness and irritation of the oral mucous membrane:
- Inspect client's dentures; obtain a dental consult if dentures are rough, cracked, or ill-fitting.

  Improves client's ability to eat without discomfort.

If mucosa is irritated or cracked:
- Administer topical anesthetics, oral protective agents, and analgesics as ordered.

  These medications protect oral mucosa from further breakdown, decrease pain, and promote healing.

Consult appropriate health care provider (i.e., dentist) if dryness, irritation, breakdown, or discomfort persists.

  Allows for multidisciplinary care.

Nursing Diagnosis **RISK FOR ACTIVITY INTOLERANCE** NDx

Definition: Susceptible to experiencing insufficient physiological or psychological energy to endure or complete required or desired daily activities, which may compromise health.

Related to:
- Decreased tissue oxygenation associated with diminished functional reserve capacity of the respiratory and cardiac systems during stress/illness
- Decrease in strength and endurance associated with the loss of muscle mass that occurs with aging
- Inadequate nutritional status
- Inadequate rest and sleep associated with age-related changes in sleep pattern and effects of current illness and hospitalization on sleep pattern

CLINICAL MANIFESTATIONS

Subjective	Objective
Verbal self-report of weakness or fatigue; report of exertional chest pain and/or dizziness	Exertional dyspnea; exertional changes in heart rate and BP

RISK FACTORS
- Medication regimen
- Poor dietary intake
- Changes in the musculoskeletal system
- Sedentary lifestyle

DESIRED OUTCOMES

The client will not experience activity intolerance, as evidenced by:
a. No reports of fatigue and weakness
b. Ability to perform activities of daily living (ADLs) without exertional dyspnea, chest pain, diaphoresis, dizziness, and a significant change in vital signs

NOC OUTCOMES

Activity tolerance, energy status

NIC INTERVENTIONS

Activity therapy, energy management, nutrition management, nutrition therapy, sleep enhancement

NURSING ASSESSMENT	RATIONALE
Assess for signs and symptoms of activity intolerance: • Statements of fatigue or weakness • Exertional dyspnea, chest pain, diaphoresis, or dizziness • Abnormal heart rate response to activity (e.g., increase in rate of 20 beats/min above resting rate, rate not returning to preactivity level within 10 minutes after stopping activity, change from regular to irregular rate); be aware that the pulse rate increases only slightly with activity and returns to preactivity level slowly in an elderly client. • A significant change (15–20 mm Hg) in BP with activity	*Early recognition of activity intolerance allows for prompt intervention.*

THERAPEUTIC INTERVENTIONS	RATIONALE
Independent Actions Implement measures to maintain adequate activity tolerance: • Maintain activity restrictions as ordered. **D** ● ✦ • Minimize environmental activity and noise. **D** ● ✦ • Implement group nursing interventions. **D** ● ✦ • Limit the number of visitors and their length of stay. **D** ● ✦ • Assist client with self-care activities as needed. **D** ● ✦ • Keep supplies and personal articles within easy reach. **D** ● ✦ • Assist client in using energy-saving techniques (e.g., using shower chair when showering, sitting to brush teeth or comb hair). **D** ● ✦	*Promotes rest and/or conserves energy.* *A quiet environment supports sleep and rest.* *Allows for periods of uninterrupted rest.* *Reduces client fatigue.* *Conserves client energy.* *Prevents client from having to get up to obtain supplies and personal articles.* *Conserves energy.*

THERAPEUTIC INTERVENTIONS	RATIONALE
• Slow pace of providing care.	*Client may need extra time to complete activities. Hurrying the client may increase the risk for falls and cause anxiety related to ability to care for self.*
• Discourage smoking and excessive intake of beverages high in caffeine such as coffee, tea, and colas. **D ✦**	*Both nicotine and excessive caffeine intake can increase cardiac workload and myocardial O_2 utilization.*
• Perform actions to maintain an adequate respiratory status (e.g., encourage use of incentive spirometer; elevate head of bed; assist with turning, coughing, and deep breathing). **D ✦**	*Maintaining or improving respiratory status increases the amount of O_2 available for energy production.*
• Maintain adequate nutritional status.	*Provides energy for activities.*
• Increase client's activity gradually as allowed and tolerated; periods of activity should be short, frequent, and interspersed with rest periods.	*Improves stamina for increasing activity.*
• Instruct client to report a decreased tolerance for activity; caution client that tolerance for vigorous activity may be diminished.	*This is due to age-related changes in thermoregulatory mechanisms and sympathetic nervous system response.*
• Instruct client to stop any activity that causes chest pain, shortness of breath, dizziness, or extreme fatigue or weakness.	*These symptoms indicate that insufficient O_2 is reaching the tissues and that activity has been increased beyond a therapeutic level.*

Dependent/Collaborative Actions

Implement measures to maintain adequate activity tolerance:

• Implement measures to increase cardiac output (e.g., administer positive inotropic agents, vasodilators, or antidysrhythmics as ordered; elevate the head of the bed) if decreased cardiac output is contributing to the client's activity intolerance.	*Sufficient cardiac output is necessary to maintain an adequate blood flow and O_2 supply to the tissues. Adequate tissue oxygenation promotes more efficient energy production, which subsequently improves client's activity tolerance.*
Consult physician if signs and symptoms of activity intolerance develop and persist or worsen.	*Allows for prompt alteration in treatment plan.*

Nursing Diagnosis   # IMPAIRED PHYSICAL MOBILITY NDx

Definition: Limitation in independent, purposeful movement of the body or of one or more extremities.

Related to:
- Decreased muscle strength associated with the loss of muscle mass that occurs with aging
- Weakness and fatigue associated with decreased functional reserve capacity of the respiratory and cardiac systems during stress and illness, inadequate nutritional status, and difficulty resting and sleeping
- Joint aching and stiffness that may be present as a result of degenerative changes in the joints
- Fear of falling
- Physical limitations/activity restrictions associated with current diagnosis and/or treatment plan
- Polypharmacy

CLINICAL MANIFESTATIONS

Subjective	**Objective**
Verbal self-report of pain, discomfort, or fatigue with activities	Decreased reaction time; difficulty moving; engages in substitution for movement; supporting the affected limb; exertional dyspnea; contractures; limited ability to perform gross and fine motor skills; limited range of motion; intentional movement-induced tremor; postural instability; uncoordinated movements

RISK FACTORS

- Pain
- Chronic illness
- Decreased muscle mass
- Sedentary lifestyle

DESIRED OUTCOME

The client will maintain an optimal level of physical mobility within prescribed activity restrictions.

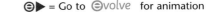

NDx = NANDA Diagnosis   **D** = Delegatable Action   ● = UAP   ✦ = LVN/LPN   ⊝▶ = Go to ⊝volve for animation

NOC OUTCOMES	NIC INTERVENTIONS
Mobility; ambulation: balance	Exercise therapy and promotion: joint mobility, ambulation, strength training, stretching, balance, muscle control

NURSING ASSESSMENT	RATIONALE
Assess client's movement ability and activity tolerance. Use a tool such as the Assessment Tool for Safe Patient Handling and Movement or the Functional Independence Measures (FIM).	*Assessment of mobility is used to best determine how to facilitate movement. Assessment of activity tolerance provides a baseline for patient strength and endurance with movement.*
Assess for cause of immobility.	*It is important to determine whether the cause of immobility is physical or psychologic and to plan interventions to improve mobility.*
Assess circulation, motion, and feeling in digits.	*Circulation may be compromised by edema of extremities, which can lead to tissue necrosis and/or contractures.*
Assess skin integrity.	*Routine examination of the skin provides for early detection and intervention of pressure sores. Pressure sores develop quickly in patients who are immobile.*
Assess need for assist devices.	*Determine client's need for assistive devices as well as proper use of wheelchairs, walkers, canes, etc., to reduce incidence of falls.*

THERAPEUTIC INTERVENTIONS	RATIONALE

Independent Actions
Encourage and implement strength training activities:
- Active and/or passive range of motion **D** ● ✦
- Ambulation **D** ● ✦
- Use of trapeze for pull-ups
- Allow client to perform as many ADLs as they are able **D** ● ✦

Inactivity contributes to muscle weakening. Contractures can develop as early as 8 hrs after a client becomes immobile. These activities maintain and increase client's strength and ability to move.
Allowing client to perform self-care increases confidence in ability to maintain ADLs.

Use assistive devices to help client with movement:
- Crutches
- Gait belt **D** ● ✦
- Walker **D** ● ✦

Use of assistive devices helps the caregivers decrease the potential for client falls and/or injuries.

Encourage patient with positive reinforcement during activities. **D** ● ✦

A positive approach to activities supports the client's accomplishment and engagement in new activities, and improves self-esteem.

If client complains of joint aching or stiffness:
- Encourage client to perform mild exercise of affected joint or joints upon awakening in the morning. **D** ✦

Reduces stiffness, improves mobility and muscle strength.

Encourage activity and participation in self-care as allowed and tolerated. **D** ● ✦

Client should be as active as possible to prevent potential loss of mobility.

Encourage client to continue a regular exercise program after discharge.

Improves strength and stamina for activities. Client must understand the importance of continuing an exercise program postdischarge to maintain mobility.

Encourage the support of significant others.

Involves significant others in client care.

Allow them to assist with range-of-motion exercises, positioning, and activity unless contraindicated. **D** ✦

Exercises improve stamina for activities and improve muscle strength. Allowing significant others to engage in care of the client helps them to understand what is required to assist the client in maintaining mobility.

Dependent/Collaborative Actions
If client complains of joint aching or stiffness:
- Consult physician regarding application of heat to affected joint or joints.

Application of heat helps to relax joints and relieve stiffness.

- Administer analgesics (e.g., nonsteroidal anti-inflammatories) if ordered.

Analgesics reduce joint pain and stiffness.

Consult appropriate health care provider if client is unable to achieve expected level of mobility or if range of motion becomes more restricted.

Allows for prompt alteration in treatment plan.

Nursing Diagnosis   **IMPAIRED URINARY ELIMINATION*** NDx

Definitions: **Risk for Urge Urinary Incontinence NDx:** Susceptible to involuntary passage of urine occurring soon after a strong sensation or urgency to void, which may compromise health; **Stress Urinary Incontinence NDx:** Sudden leakage of urine with activities that increase intra-abdominal pressure; **Reflex Urinary Incontinence NDx:** Involuntary loss of urine at somewhat predictable intervals when a specific bladder volume is reached. **Overflow Urinary Incontinence NDx:** Involuntary loss of urine associated with overdistention of the bladder. **Functional Urinary Incontinence NDx:** Inability of usually continent person to reach toilet in time to avoid unintentional loss of urine.

Related to:
Frequency and urgency:
* Incomplete bladder emptying, decrease in bladder capacity, and uninhibited bladder contractions in response to small volumes of urine (bladder detrusor muscle hyperactivity or instability)

Urinary retention:
* Decreased tone of bladder muscle
* Obstruction of the bladder outlet by an enlarged prostate or fecal impaction
* Decreased attention to the urge to urinate
* Difficulty urinating associated with anxiety about a lack of privacy and possibly having to use a bedpan or urinal
* The effect of some medications (e.g., sedatives, narcotic [opioid] analgesics, anticholinergics)

Incontinence (urge, stress, reflex, overflow, functional):
* Decreased tone of the external urinary sphincter and an incompetent bladder outlet (a result of lessening of the urethrovesical junction angle in women) associated with degenerative changes in the urethra and pelvic floor muscles and structural supports of the bladder (occurs more in women as a result of childbearing and estrogen deficiency)
* Decreased bladder capacity and an increase in uninhibited bladder contractions in response to small volumes of urine (bladder detrusor muscle hyperactivity or instability)
* Overflow of urine associated with overdistention of the bladder if urinary retention is present
* Delays in toileting associated with:
  * Inability to get to the toilet in time to urinate resulting from unfamiliar environment and impaired physical mobility
  * Difficulty removing clothing in a timely manner when needing to urinate resulting from reduced manual dexterity

CLINICAL MANIFESTATIONS

Subjective	Objective
Urge incontinence: Self-reports of involuntary loss of urine	**Urge incontinence:** Observed inability to reach commode in time to avoid urine loss
Stress incontinence: Self-reports of leakage of small amounts of urine on exertion, with coughing, sneezing, and/or laughing	**Stress incontinence:** Observe leakage of urine during exertion, coughing, sneezing, and/or laughing
Reflex incontinence: Self-reports of inability to inhibit or initiate voiding or sensation of bladder fullness	**Reflex incontinence:** N/A
Overflow urinary incontinence: Self-report of leaking urine due to overdistention of the bladder	**Overflow urinary incontinence:** Observed leakage of urine following intake of fluids.
Functional incontinence: Self-reports of loss of urine prior to getting to the commode; amount of time to reach commode exceeds length of time between sensing the urge to void and uncontrolled voiding; report of being incontinent only in the morning	**Functional incontinence:** N/A

---

* The nurse should select the appropriate nursing diagnosis that is most appropriate based on the nursing assessment.

RISK FACTORS

- Medication regimen
- Changes in urinary system functioning
- Childbearing

DESIRED OUTCOMES

The client will maintain or regain optimal urinary elimination as evidenced by:
a. Voiding at normal intervals
b. No reports of urgency, frequency, bladder fullness, and suprapubic discomfort
c. Absence of bladder distention
d. Absence of incontinence
e. Balanced intake and output

NOC OUTCOMES

Urinary continence; urinary elimination

NIC INTERVENTIONS

Urinary incontinence care; urinary retention care; urinary elimination management; urinary habit training; urinary bladder training

NURSING ASSESSMENT	RATIONALE
Assess for signs and symptoms of impaired urinary elimination: • Frequent voiding of small amounts (25–60 mL) of urine • Nocturia • Reports of urgency, frequency, bladder fullness, or suprapubic discomfort • Bladder distention • Incontinence • Output less than intake	*Early recognition of signs and symptoms of impaired urinary elimination allows for prompt intervention.*

THERAPEUTIC INTERVENTIONS	RATIONALE

Independent Actions

Monitor client's pattern of fluid intake and urination (e.g., times and amounts of fluid intake, types of fluids consumed, times and amounts of voluntary and involuntary voiding, reports of sensation of the need to void, activities preceding incontinence).

Knowledge of the client's fluid intake and urination pattern assists in the identification of factors that may be causing urinary incontinence. This information helps the nurse plan individualized interventions that promote urinary continence.

Implement measures to promote optimal urinary elimination:

- Offer bedpan or urinal or assist client to bedside commode or bathroom every 2 to 4 hrs if indicated. **D** ● ✦

Urinary incontinence occurs when the pressure in the bladder becomes greater than the pressure exerted by the urinary sphincters.

- Instruct client to urinate when the urge is first felt. **D**

Emptying the bladder before the pressure becomes too great reduces the risk of incontinence.
Improves the client's ability to completely empty the bladder.

- Implement measures to promote relaxation during voiding attempts (e.g., provide privacy, encourage client to read). **D** ● ✦

- Implement measures involving use of water and warmth to promote voiding (e.g., run water, place client's hands in warm water, pour warm water over perineum). **D** ● ✦

Triggers the micturition reflex and promotes relaxation, which improves client's ability to empty the bladder.

- Allow client to assume a normal position for voiding unless contraindicated. **D** ● ✦

A sitting or standing position uses gravity to facilitate bladder emptying. The more completely the bladder is emptied, the less risk there is of incontinence.

- Instruct client to lean upper body forward and/or gently press downward on lower abdomen during voiding attempts unless contraindicated.

This puts pressure on the bladder, which helps create a sensation of bladder fullness, which stimulates the micturition reflex.

- Maintain normal bowel function measures.

Constipation increases pressure on the bladder outlet causing increased urinary retention.

- Implement measures to reduce delays in toileting (e.g., have call signal within client's reach and respond promptly to requests for assistance; have bedpan, urinal, or bedside commode readily available to client; provide easy access to bathroom; provide client with easy-to-remove clothing such as pajamas with Velcro closures or an elastic waistband). **D** ● ✦

Delays in toileting or the distance needed to get to the bathroom increase the chance of urinary incontinence.

THERAPEUTIC INTERVENTIONS	RATIONALE
• Instruct client to perform pelvic floor muscle exercises (e.g., stopping and starting stream during voiding; squeezing buttocks together, then relaxing the muscles) several times a day if appropriate.	*Strengthens pelvic floor muscles and improves tone of the external urinary sphincter.*
• Instruct client to continue these exercises after discharge, emphasizing that it will take several weeks of exercise before improvement may be noted.	*Provides for continuum of care once discharged from the acute care facility.* *Decreases frustration in knowing that improvement will not be seen for several weeks.*
• Instruct client to space fluids evenly throughout the day rather than drinking a large quantity at one time.	*Rapid filling of the bladder can result in incontinence if client has decreased urinary sphincter control.*
• Limit oral fluid intake in the evening. **D** ● ✦	*Decreases the possibility of nighttime incontinence.*
• Instruct client to avoid drinking alcohol and beverages containing caffeine.	*Alcohol and caffeine have a mild diuretic effect and act as irritants to the bladder; both factors may make urinary control more difficult.*

Dependent/Collaborative Actions

Implement measures to promote optimal urinary elimination.

• Administer the following medications if ordered:	
• Cholinergic (parasympathomimetic) agents (e.g., bethanechol). **D** ✦	*Cholinergics stimulate bladder contractions and promote complete bladder emptying if incontinence is associated with overflow resulting from urinary retention.*
• Estrogen preparations. **D** ✦	*May be used to treat stress incontinence in postmenopausal women.*
• Anticholinergics (e.g., oxybutynin, tolterodine) **D** ✦	*Anticholinergics decrease bladder detrusor muscle hyperactivity and reduce episodes of urge incontinence.*
• Sympathomimetic agents (e.g., ephedrine) **D** ✦	*Sympathomimetics increase urethral sphincter tone.*
• Catheterize client if ordered. **D** ✦	*Determination of the amount of residual urine.*
• Assist with urodynamic studies (e.g., urethral pressure profile, uroflowmetry, cystometrogram) if ordered.	*These can help to determine the cause of altered urinary elimination.*
• If urinary incontinence persists:	
• Use biofeedback techniques if appropriate.	*Assists client in regaining control over the pelvic floor muscles and external urinary sphincter.*
• Instruct and assist client with bladder retraining program if appropriate.	*Establishes a schedule of when client should empty his or her bladder with the goal of decreasing urinary elimination problems.*
• Consult physician regarding intermittent catheterization, insertion of an indwelling catheter, or use of an external collection device (e.g., condom catheter).	*Allows for alteration in treatment plan.*

Nursing Diagnosis   **RISK FOR CONSTIPATION** NDx

Definition: Susceptible to a decrease in normal frequency of defecation accompanied by difficult or incomplete passage of stool, which may compromise health.

Related to:

- Decreased gastrointestinal motility associated with age and exacerbated by decreased activity and anxiety during illness
- Failure to respond to the urge to defecate associated with dulling of the impulses that sense the signal to defecate, inability to get to the toilet independently, and/or reluctance to use a bedpan or bedside commode
- Difficulty evacuating stool associated with weakened abdominal muscles and decreased lubrication of stools (a result of diminished intestinal production of mucus)
- Decreased intake of fiber and fluids
- Possible chronic laxative use

CLINICAL MANIFESTATIONS

Subjective	Objective
Verbal self-report of pain on defecation	Infrequent bowel movements; hard, dry stool; chronic laxative use

NDx = NANDA Diagnosis   **D** = Delegatable Action   ● = UAP   ✦ = LVN/LPN   ⊜▶ = Go to ⊜volve for animation

RISK FACTORS

- Poor muscle tone
- Inadequate fluid/fiber intake
- Medication regimen
- Sedentary lifestyle

DESIRED OUTCOMES

The client will not experience constipation, as evidenced by:
a. Usual frequency of bowel movements
b. Passage of soft, formed stool
c. Absence of abdominal distention and pain, feeling of rectal fullness or pressure, and straining during defecation

NOC OUTCOMES

Bowel elimination; status

NIC INTERVENTIONS

Bowel incontinence care; bowel management; bowel training

NURSING ASSESSMENT

Assess for signs and symptoms of constipation (e.g., decrease in frequency of bowel movements; passage of hard, formed stools; anorexia; abdominal distention and pain; feeling of fullness or pressure in rectum; straining during defecation).

Assess bowel sounds. Report a pattern of decreasing bowel sounds.

RATIONALE

Early recognition of signs and symptoms of constipation allows for prompt intervention.

THERAPEUTIC INTERVENTIONS

Independent Actions

Determine if the client regularly uses laxatives.

Implement measures to prevent constipation:
- Encourage client to defecate whenever the urge is felt. **D** ✦
- Encourage client to relax, provide privacy, and have call signal within reach during attempts to defecate. **D** ● ✦

- Encourage client to establish a regular time for defecation, preferably within an hour after a meal.
- Instruct client to increase intake of foods high in fiber (e.g., bran, whole-grain breads and cereals, fresh fruits and vegetables) unless contraindicated.
- Determine if client has irregular mealtimes.
- Instruct client to maintain a minimum fluid intake of 1500 to 2000 mL/day unless contraindicated.
- Encourage client to drink hot liquids (e.g., tea) upon arising in the morning. **D** ● ✦
- Increase activity as allowed and tolerated. **D** ● ✦

- Encourage client to perform isometric abdominal strengthening exercises unless contraindicated.
- Perform actions to reduce fear and anxiety (e.g., explain procedures, provide care in a confident manner). **D** ✦
- If client is taking analgesics for pain management, encourage the use of nonopioid rather than opioid analgesics when appropriate. **D** ✦
- Instruct client to continue with actions to promote regular bowel function after discharge (e.g., maintain a fluid intake of at least six to eight glasses per day, increase intake of foods high in fiber, participate in regular exercise program).

RATIONALE

Laxative abuse decreases the colon's musculature and decreases the urge to defecate.

Prevents stool from remaining too long in the bowel and becoming hard.

Measures that promote relaxation enable the client to relax the levator ani muscle and external anal sphincter, which facilitates evacuation of stool.

Promotes routine defecation.

Fiber adds bulk to the intestinal contents.

Changes in or irregular meal times can lead to constipation.

Adequate hydration is important in having a soft stool.

Stimulates peristalsis which promotes passage of stool through the colon.

Activity improves peristalsis and strengthens the abdominal muscles.

This type of exercise strengthens the abdominal muscles and stimulates peristalsis.

Promotes relaxation.

Analgesics decrease peristalsis and promote constipation.

Provides for continuum of care postdischarge from the acute care facility.

THERAPEUTIC INTERVENTIONS	RATIONALE

Dependent/Collaborative Actions
Implement measures to prevent constipation:
- Administer laxatives, stool softeners, and/or enemas if ordered. **D** ● ✦

- Consult physician about checking for an impaction and digitally removing stool if client has not had a bowel movement in 3 days, if client is passing liquid stool, or if other signs and symptoms of constipation are present.
- Consult appropriate health care provider if signs and symptoms of constipation persist and appear to be an ongoing problem.

These medications promote evacuation of the bowel.
Stool softeners decrease hardness of the stool that allows for easier passage.
Minimizes risk for bowel obstruction.

Allows for prompt alterations in treatment plan.

Nursing Diagnosis	**DISTURBED SLEEP PATTERN** NDx

Definition: Time-limited awakenings due to external factors.

Related to:
- Fear, anxiety, change in environment if in hospital or extended care facility, and discomfort associated with present illness
- Age-related nocturia
- Age-related changes in the stages of sleep resulting in frequent awakenings and less deep restorative sleep

CLINICAL MANIFESTATIONS

Subjective	**Objective**
Verbal self-report of difficulty falling asleep; statements of not feeling well rested	Frequent awakenings

RISK FACTORS
- Sedentary lifestyle
- Chronic illness
- Medication regimen
- Daytime napping
- Decrease in exercise

DESIRED OUTCOMES

The client will attain optimal amount of sleep as evidenced by statements of feeling well rested.

NOC OUTCOMES	NIC INTERVENTIONS
Sleep; status	Sleep enhancement

NURSING ASSESSMENT	RATIONALE

Assess for signs and symptoms of a disturbed sleep pattern (e.g., statements of difficulty falling asleep, frequent awakenings, or not feeling well rested).
Assess client's regular sleep patterns (e.g., hour of bedtime, frequency and length of naps).

Early recognition of signs and symptoms of disrupted sleep patterns allows for prompt intervention.

THERAPEUTIC INTERVENTIONS	RATIONALE

Independent Actions
Implement measures to promote sleep:
- Discourage excessive napping during the day unless signs and symptoms of sleep deprivation exist. **D** ✦

- Perform actions to reduce fear and anxiety (e.g., explain procedures, provide care in a confident manner). **D** ● ✦

Clients will have more hours of sleep if they do not nap during the day. Elderly clients may have short naps during the day because of shorter sleep time at night.
Promotes relaxation and rest.

NDx = NANDA Diagnosis   **D** = Delegatable Action   ● = UAP   ✦ = LVN/LPN   ⊙▶ = Go to ⊖volve for animation

Continued...

THERAPEUTIC INTERVENTIONS	RATIONALE
• Perform actions to reduce dyspepsia, gastric fullness, and gas pain if present (tell client not to eat foods that promote gas and to avoid sodas) and discomfort associated with client's diagnosis and treatment.	*Causes discomfort and interferes with sleep.*
• Inform client of normal changes in sleep pattern that occur with aging.	*Reduces concerns about quality and amount of sleep necessary to maintain health.*
• Encourage participation in relaxing diversional activities during the evening. **D** ● ✦	*Decreases stress and promotes relaxation.*
• Discourage intake of foods and fluids high in caffeine (e.g., chocolate, coffee, tea, colas) in the evening. **D** ● ✦	*Caffeine is a stimulant and will make it difficult for the client to rest.*
• Offer client an evening snack that includes milk unless contraindicated. **D** ● ✦	*Milk contains L-tryptophan, which is believed to help induce and maintain sleep.*
• Allow client to continue usual sleep practices (e.g., position; time; presleep routines such as reading, watching television, and listening to music) whenever possible. **D** ● ✦	*Allowing client normal sleep practices will decrease disruption of sleep patterns while in the acute care facility.*
• Satisfy basic needs such as comfort and warmth before sleep. **D** ● ✦	*Promotes relaxation.*
• Encourage client to limit intake of fluids in the evening and urinate just before bedtime. **D** ✦	*Reduces nocturia.*
• Encourage client to avoid drinking alcohol in the evening.	*Alcohol interferes with rapid eye movement (REM) sleep.*
• Encourage client to avoid smoking before bedtime. **D** ● ✦	*Nicotine is a stimulant.*
• Reduce environmental distractions (e.g., close door to client's room; use night-light rather than overhead light whenever possible; lower volume of paging system; keep staff conversations at a low level and away from client's room; close curtains between clients in a semiprivate room or ward; keep beepers and alarms on low volume; have earplugs available for client if needed). **D** ✦	*Most individuals sleep in a dark, quiet environment.*
• Perform actions to reduce interruptions during sleep (70–100 minutes of uninterrupted sleep is usually needed to complete one sleep cycle).	*Interruptions decrease REM sleep, causing disruption of sleep patterns.*
• Restrict visitors.	
• Group care (e.g., medications, treatments, physical care, assessments) whenever possible.	
• Encourage client to use relaxation techniques.	*These measures help to promote relaxation and increase potential for adequate sleep.*

Dependent/Collaborative Actions

Implement measures to promote sleep:

• Review medications that client takes with pharmacist or physician and identify those that can interfere with sleep (e.g., nicotine transdermal systems, theophylline, corticosteroids, diuretics, diphenhydramine or other over-the-counter sleep aids, some antidepressants); if possible, administer medications such as corticosteroids and diuretics early in the day rather than late afternoon or evening and encourage client to continue this schedule for these medications at home.	*Medications that may interfere with sleep should be given as early in the day as possible.*
Administer a prescribed sedative-hypnotic only if indicated; administer these agents cautiously; inform client that over-the-counter sleep aids (e.g., diphenhydramine) can interfere with the quality of sleep and daytime functioning and should not be taken on a regular basis. **D** ✦	*The metabolism, distribution, and excretion of drugs are often altered in the elderly client.*
Consult appropriate health care provider if signs and symptoms of sleep deprivation (e.g., irritability, lethargy, agitation, inability to concentrate) occur and persist or worsen.	*Allows for prompt alterations in treatment plan.*

Nursing Diagnosis **RISK FOR INFECTION** NDx

Definition: Susceptible to invasion and multiplication of pathogenic organisms, which may compromise health.

Related to:
- Stasis of respiratory secretions associated with decreased activity during illness and age-related decrease in ciliary activity and cough effectiveness
- Decrease in immunity associated with:
  - An age-related decline in T-cell and B-cell function and the number of functional macrophages in the skin and alveoli
  - An inadequate nutritional status if present
- Decrease in effectiveness of the body's physical barriers associated with changes in the skin and mucous membranes
- Urinary stasis associated with decreased activity during illness and the urinary retention that can result from a decrease in bladder muscle tone, the effect of certain medications, an enlarged prostate, and difficulty urinating in a new environment
- Favorable environment for growth of pathogens in vagina associated with an increase in the pH of vaginal secretions

CLINICAL MANIFESTATIONS

Subjective	Objective
Verbal self-report of fatigue and lack of appetite Reports of frequency, urgency, or burning when urinating	Elevated temperature; chills; increased pulse rate; malaise, lethargy, acute confusion; abnormal breath sounds; productive cough of purulent, green, or rust-colored sputum; cloudy urine; urinalysis showing a WBC count greater than 5, positive leukocyte esterase or nitrites, or presence of bacteria; heat, pain, redness, swelling, or unusual drainage in any area; elevated WBC count and/or significant change in differential

RISK FACTORS

- Chronic illness
- Injury
- Inadequate immune system response
- Increased susceptibility to pathogens
- Decrease in exercise

DESIRED OUTCOMES

The client will remain free of infection, as evidenced by:
a. Absence of fever and chills
b. Pulse rate within normal limits
c. Normal breath sounds
d. Cough productive of clear mucus only
e. Voiding clear urine without reports of burning and increased frequency and urgency
f. Absence of heat, pain, redness, swelling, and unusual drainage in any area
g. Usual mental status
h. WBC and differential counts within normal range for elderly client
i. Negative results of cultured specimens

NOC OUTCOMES

Immune status

NIC INTERVENTIONS

Infection control; infection protection; immunization/vaccination management

NURSING ASSESSMENT

Assess for and report signs and symptoms of infection.

- Increase in temperature above client's usual level (be aware that normal temperature in the elderly client may be <37°C)

RATIONALE

Early recognition of signs and symptoms of infection allows for prompt intervention.
Be aware that some signs and symptoms vary because of an age-related decline in thermoregulatory, immune, and sympathetic nervous system responses.

Continued...

NURSING ASSESSMENT	RATIONALE
• Chills • Increased pulse rate • Abnormal breath sounds • Cough productive of purulent, green, or rust-colored sputum • Loss of appetite • Cloudy urine • Reports of burning when urinating • Reports of increased urinary frequency or urgency • Urinalysis showing a WBC count >5 per high-power field, positive leukocyte esterase or nitrites, or the presence of bacteria • Heat, pain, redness, swelling, or unusual drainage in any area • Malaise, lethargy, acute confusion • Increase in WBC count and/or significant change in differential • Positive results of cultured specimens (e.g., urine, vaginal drainage, wound drainage, sputum, blood)	*The elderly individual may have a diminished shivering reflex.* *The elderly client may not demonstrate the classic elevation in pulse rate that occurs with infection because of a decreased sympathetic nervous system response.*

THERAPEUTIC INTERVENTIONS	RATIONALE

Independent Actions
Implement measures to prevent infection:

• Maintain a fluid intake of ≥1500 to 2000 mL/day unless contraindicated.	*Maintains adequate hydration and vascular fluid volume.*
• Use good hand hygiene and encourage client to do the same. **D** ● ✦	*Hand hygiene removes transient flora, which reduces the risk of transmission of pathogens.*
• Adhere to the appropriate precautions established to prevent transmission of infection to the client (standard precautions, transmission-based precautions on other clients, neutropenic precautions). **D** ● ✦	*Helps prevent the transmission of microorganisms and reduces the client's risk of infection.*
• Use sterile technique during invasive procedures (e.g., urinary catheterizations, venous and arterial punctures, injections, wound care) and dressing changes. **D** ✦	*Reduces the possibility of introducing pathogens into the body*
• Anchor catheters/tubings (e.g., urinary, intravenous, wound drainage) securely. **D** ● ✦	*Reduces the risk for trauma to the tissues and the risk for introduction of pathogens associated with in-and-out movement of the tubing.*
• Change equipment, tubings, and solutions used for treatments such as intravenous infusions, respiratory care, irrigations, and enteral feedings according to hospital policy.	*The longer that equipment, tubings, and solutions are in use, the greater the chance of colonization of microorganisms, which can then be introduced into the body.*
• Change peripheral intravenous line sites according to hospital policy.	*Peripheral intravenous line sites are changed routinely to reduce persistent irritation of one area of a vein wall and the resultant colonization of microorganisms at that site.*
• Maintain a closed system for drains (e.g., wound, chest tube, urinary catheter) and intravenous infusions whenever possible.	*Prevents introduction of pathogens into the body.*
• Protect client from others with infections and instruct client to continue this after discharge. **D** ● ✦	*Protecting the client from others with infections reduces the client's risk of exposure to pathogens.*
• Maintain adequate nutritional status. **D** ✦	*Adequate nutrition is needed to maintain normal function of the immune system.*
• Perform actions to prevent and treat irritation and breakdown of the oral mucous membrane (e.g., maintain oral hydration, use a soft-bristle toothbrush, do not use glycerin swabs for mouth care). **D** ● ✦	*Frequent oral hygiene helps prevent infection by removing most of the food, debris, and many of the microorganisms that are present in the mouth. It also helps maintain the integrity of the oral mucosa, which provides a physical and chemical barrier to pathogens.*
• Instruct and assist client to perform good perineal care routinely and after each bowel movement. **D** ● ✦	*The perineal area contains a large number of organisms. Routine cleaning of the area reduces the risk of colonization of organisms and subsequent perineal, urinary tract, and/or vaginal infection.*

THERAPEUTIC INTERVENTIONS	RATIONALE
• Perform actions to maintain an adequate respiratory status (e.g., use incentive spirometry every 2 hrs, change position every 2 hrs, ambulating as able).	*Reduces stasis of respiratory secretions and the risk of a respiratory tract infection.*
• Perform actions to prevent or treat urinary retention (e.g., encourage clients to void when they experience the urge, maintain adequate fluid volume). **D ● ✦**	*Prevents urine accumulation in the bladder, which creates an environment conducive to the growth and colonization of microorganisms, and reduces the risk of urinary tract infection.*
• Perform actions to prevent skin breakdown (promote ambulation, change positions of bedridden clients every 2 hrs, maintain adequate hydration). **D ● ✦**	*Skin breakdown removes one of the physical barriers to the body.*
• If client has a wound, provide appropriate wound care (e.g., use dressing materials that maintain a moist wound surface, assist with debridement of necrotic tissue, use dressing materials that absorb excess exudate, maintain patency of wound drains). **D ✦**	*Facilitates wound healing and reduces the number of pathogens that enter or are present in the wound.*
• Perform actions to reduce stress (e.g., reduce fear, anxiety, and pain; help client identify and use effective coping mechanisms). **D ● ✦**	*Prevents an increase in cortisol secretion, which is important because cortisol interferes with some immune responses.*

Dependent/Collaborative Actions

Implement measures to prevent infection.

• Instruct client to receive immunizations and vaccinations (e.g., pneumococcal pneumonia, tetanus, influenza) at recommended intervals if appropriate.	*Immunizations are often recommended to reduce the possibility of some infections in high-risk clients (e.g., those clients who are immunosuppressed, elderly, or have a chronic disease).*
• Consult appropriate health care provider regarding the following:	
• Initiation of antimicrobial therapy if indicated. **D ✦**	*Prevents and/or treats infection.*
• Antimicrobial orders that do not seem appropriate (e.g., prolonged use of antimicrobials, excessively high doses of an antimicrobial, unnecessary use of broad-spectrum or multiple antimicrobials). **D ✦**	*Reduces the risk of elimination of the client's natural flora and/or the development of drug-resistant microorganisms.*

Nursing Diagnosis **RISK FOR FALLS** NDx

Definition: Susceptible to increased susceptibility to falling, which may cause physical harm and compromise health.

Related to:

- Dizziness or syncope associated with decreased cerebral tissue perfusion that can result from certain medications (e.g., antihypertensive agents) and from age-related vascular changes, decrease in cardiac output, and postural hypotension
- Loss of balance associated with the effect of certain medications (e.g., sedatives, narcotic [opioid] analgesics) and the changes in posture, reduced coordination, delayed reaction time, and impaired proprioception that can occur with aging
- Tripping associated with age-related gait abnormalities (e.g., decreased step height and length) and impaired vision
- Weakness associated with an age-related decrease in muscle strength and the general deconditioning that can occur with reduced physical activity

CLINICAL MANIFESTATIONS

Subjective	Objective
Self-expressed concern for safety during ambulation; stated history of previous falls	Unsteadiness when ambulating, use of ambulation aids, visual field deficits, confusion, orthostatic hypotension, medication therapy (e.g., antihypertensives, diuretics, hypnotics, antianxiety agents, narcotics, tranquilizers, antidepressants), anemias, arthritis

RISK FACTORS

- Medication
- Sedentary lifestyle
- Safety hazards in the home
- Weakness

DESIRED OUTCOMES

The client will not experience falls.

NOC OUTCOMES

Fall Prevention Behavior; Falls Occurrence

NIC INTERVENTIONS

Fall Prevention; Environmental Management

NURSING ASSESSMENT	RATIONALE
Assess client's risk for falls using standardized assessment tool (e.g., Fall Risk Assessment).	*A client's risk for falls increases with the number of risk factors. Determining the client's risk for falls allows implementation of the appropriate preventive measures.*
Assess client's balance and mobility skills.	*Determining the client's baseline status allows for the implementation of the appropriate preventive measures.*
Evaluate client's medications to determine whether they place the client at increased risk for falls.	*Some medications may cause excessive drowsiness, altered mental states, or physiologic changes such as orthostatic hypotension that can increase the risk of falls in clients. Early identification of such medications allows for implementation of appropriate preventive measures.*

THERAPEUTIC INTERVENTIONS	RATIONALE

Independent Actions
Implement measures to reduce the risk for falls:

- Keep bed in low position with side rails up when client is in bed. **D** ● ✦
  Prevents client from falling when getting out of bed.
- Keep needed items within easy reach and help client to identify their location. **D** ● ✦
  Prevents client from stretching to obtain items, losing balance, and falling.
- Encourage client to request assistance whenever needed; have call signal within easy reach. **D** ● ✦
  Provides assurance to client that someone will assist him or her as needed and that he or she can remain in bed until assistance arrives.
- Use lap belt when client is in chair if indicated. **D** ● ✦
  Prevents client from sliding out of a chair.
- Instruct client to wear well-fitting slippers/shoes with nonslip soles and low heels when ambulating.
  Decreases potential for falls and improves ambulation.
- Keep floor free of clutter and wipe up spills promptly. **D** ● ✦
  Prevents client from tripping over clutter or slipping on wet floors.
- Instruct and assist client to get out of bed slowly.
  Reduces dizziness associated with postural hypotension.
- Carefully position tubings and equipment. **D** ● ✦
  Prevents client from tripping over equipment.
- Accompany client during ambulation and use a transfer safety belt if client is weak or dizzy. **D** ● ✦
  Provides stability when ambulating and helps prevent falls.
- Provide ambulatory aids (e.g., walker, cane) if client is weak or unsteady on feet. **D** ● ✦
  Provides stability when ambulating.
- Reinforce instructions from physical therapist on correct ambulation and transfer techniques.
  Improves client adherence and improves safety.
- If vision is impaired, orient client to surroundings, room, and arrangement of furniture and identify obstacles during ambulation.
  Ensures that client will be able to see obstacles in his or her path when ambulating.
- Instruct client to move slowly, use wider stance when ambulating, and avoid turning head or body rapidly.
  Prevents loss of balance when ambulating.
- Instruct client to ambulate in well-lit areas and to use handrails if needed.
  Allows client to see obstacles that may be in his or her path when ambulating.
- Do not rush client; allow adequate time for ambulation to the bathroom and in hallway. **D** ● ✦
  Elderly clients may move more slowly; allowing them adequate time for ambulation decreases their frustration and risk for falls.
- Make sure that shower has a nonslip bottom surface and that shower chair; make sure that bath mat, call signal, grab bars, and adequate lighting are present.
  Decreases risk for slipping and falling while on wet surfaces.

THERAPEUTIC INTERVENTIONS	RATIONALE
• Maintain adequate strength and activity tolerance and an optimal level of physical mobility.	*Provides for client stamina while performing ADLs.*
• If client is at high risk for falls and gets up without assistance despite reminders to request assistance,	*Institute facility's fall protocol.*
• Attach an alarm device to bed or chair. **D** ● ✦	*Notifies health care personnel if client leaves the chair or bed.*
Include client and significant others in planning and implementing measures to prevent falls. **D** ● ✦	*Helps family understand what they can do to assist client and reduce risk for falls.*
Discuss with client and significant other:	
• The need to evaluate living environment for hazards (e.g., thick or loose carpets, inadequate or loose railings, insufficient lighting) and make necessary modifications.	*Improves safety.*
• The importance of participating in a regular exercise program for conditioning and muscle strengthening and continuing with therapy for gait and balance training if needed.	*Provides conditioning and muscle strengthening and improves balance.*
• Stress the importance of continuing appropriate safety precautions after discharge.	*Prevents falls.*
If falls occur, initiate appropriate first aid and notify physician.	*Allows for prompt intervention.*

Dependent/Collaborative Actions

Implement measures to reduce the risk for falls:	
• If client is at high risk for falls and gets up without assistance despite reminders to request assistance:	
• Consult physician about the temporary use of jacket or wrist restraints.	*Helps prevent falls of clients who won't remain in the bed or chair to protect them from falling.*
• Administer central nervous system depressants judiciously. **D** ✦	*Central nervous system depressants decrease client's level of consciousness and increase risk for falls.*

Nursing Diagnosis # RISK FOR ASPIRATION NDx

Definition: Susceptible to entry of gastrointestinal secretions, oropharyngeal secretions, solids, or fluids to the tracheobronchial passages, which may compromise health.

Related to: Diminished gag reflex and the gastroesophageal reflux that can occur as a result of decreased tone of the lower esophageal sphincter

CLINICAL MANIFESTATIONS

Subjective	Objective
Verbal self-report of difficulty swallowing and choking on food or liquids	Choking on food or liquids. Cough presence of tube feeding in tracheal aspirate, chest radiograph showing pulmonary infiltrate

RISK FACTORS
- Changes in esophageal sphincter tone
- Medication regimen

DESIRED OUTCOMES

The client will not aspirate secretions or foods/fluids as evidenced by:
a. Clear breath sounds
b. Resonant percussion note over lungs
c. Absence of cough, tachypnea, and dyspnea

NOC OUTCOMES

Aspiration prevention

NIC INTERVENTIONS

Aspiration precautions

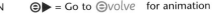

NDx = NANDA Diagnosis   **D** = Delegatable Action   ● = UAP   ✦ = LVN/LPN   ⓔ▶ = Go to ⓔvolve for animation

NURSING ASSESSMENT	RATIONALE
Assess for and report signs and symptoms of aspiration of secretions or foods/fluids (e.g., rhonchi, dull percussion note over affected lung area, cough, tachypnea, dyspnea, tachycardia, presence of tube feeding in tracheal aspirate, chest radiograph showing pulmonary infiltrate).	*Early recognition of signs and symptoms of aspiration of secretions or foods/fluids allows for prompt intervention.*
Assess client's gag reflex.	*Aging individuals have a decreased rate of swallowing. Silent aspirations may occur in an elderly client.*

THERAPEUTIC INTERVENTIONS	RATIONALE

Independent Actions

Implement measures to reduce the risk for aspiration:

- Perform actions to reduce gastroesophageal reflux (e.g., provide small frequent meals rather than three large ones; instruct client to ingest food slowly; maintain client in high Fowler's positions during ingestion of foods and fluids and for ≥30 minutes thereafter). **D** ● ✦

- Instruct client to avoid laughing and talking while eating and drinking.

- Encourage client to concentrate on eating and drinking and allow ample time for meals and snack. **D** ● ✦

- Instruct and assist client to perform oral hygiene after meals. **D** ● ✦

- If client is receiving tube feedings, check tube placement before each feeding or on a routine basis if tube feeding is continuous, and do not administer tube feeding if the residual exceeds a specified amount (usually 75–100 mL). **D** ✦

Prevents stomach from becoming too full and incidence gastric fluid reflux into the oropharynx. Reflux is decreased when the head of the bed is elevated at least a 35- to 45-degree angle.

Maintaining a sitting position after eating decreases the incidence of aspiration in the elderly.

Prevents food/fluids from moving into the trachea rather than the esophagus.

Allows client to fully chew foods, which makes them easier to swallow and reduces the risk of aspiration. Eating slowly assures the client does not feel rushed and tries to swallow food too quickly which may lead to aspiration.

Ensures that food particles do not remain in the mouth.

Prevents overdistention of the stomach and subsequent increased pressure, which can force gastric contents into the oropharynx and increase the risk for aspiration.

Dependent/Collaborative Actions

If signs and symptoms of aspiration occur:

- Perform tracheal suctioning.
- Withhold oral intake.
- Prepare client for chest radiograph.

Manually removes contents from the trachea.
Prevents further aspiration.
Helps to determine degree of aspiration and treatment required.

Nursing Diagnosis **RISK FOR INJURY** NDx

Definition: Susceptible to physical damage due to environmental conditions interacting with the individual's adaptive and defensive resources, which may compromise health.

Related to:

Visual: The lens becoming more opaque, losing elasticity, and yellowing; loss of ciliary muscle tone; decreased pupil size; and changes in the cornea, retina, macula, and vitreous humor

Gustatory: A diminished sense of smell and atrophy of the taste buds (there usually only a modest, quality-specific loss of taste in elderly clients)

Kinesthetic: A decrease in vestibular sensitivity and ability to perceive movement

Tactile: A decreased number of sensory receptors in the skin

Age-related: Decrease in tactile sensation; changes in vision and incidence of cataracts; hearing loss

RISK FACTORS
- Changes in sensations
- Visual disturbances
- Polypharmacy

CLINICAL MANIFESTATIONS

Subjective	Objective
Verbal self-report of difficulty with vision, hearing, taste, and difficulty moving.	Visible injury on client's body

DESIRED OUTCOMES

The client will not experience an injury related to declines in his or her senses.

NOC OUTCOMES

Knowledge personal safety and medication

NIC INTERVENTIONS

Environmental management, safety, medication management

NURSING ASSESSMENT

Assess client for the following:
- Vision changes (e.g., statements of decreased visual acuity, altered depth perception, inability to adjust to changes in lighting, increased sensitivity to glare, or altered color perception; overreaching or underreaching for objects which may lead to injury)
- Diminished kinesthetic sense (e.g., unsteadiness on feet, swaying, lack of coordination which may lead to falls
- Diminished tactile sensation (e.g., statements of diminished feeling in extremities, holding or touching very hot objects, use of heating pad at higher-than-expected temperatures; increases potential for burns)

RATIONALE

Early recognition of changes in sensory functioning allows for prompt intervention.

THERAPEUTIC INTERVENTIONS

Independent Actions
If client's vision is impaired:
- Ensure that lighting is adequate but not too bright. **D** ● ✦
- Avoid sudden changes in light intensity. **D** ● ✦
- Reduce the glare from windows by partially closing blinds or curtains. **D** ● ✦
- Provide a night-light. **D** ● ✦

- Provide large-print reading material if available. **D** ● ✦

- Keep frequently used items within the visual range. **D** ● ✦
- Encourage client to wear his/her glasses; make sure glasses are clean. **D** ● ✦
- Provide auditory rather than visual diversionary activities if indicated. **D** ● ✦
- Inform client of resources available if additional information about visual aids is desired (e.g., American Foundation for the Blind).
- Assist with activities such as filling out menus and reading mail and legal documents as needed.

Implement measures to prevent burns if client has decreased tactile sensation:
- Let hot foods and fluids cool slightly before serving. **D** ● ✦
- Supervise client while smoking if indicated. **D** ● ✦
- Assess temperature of bath water and direct heat application (e.g., heating pad, warm compress) before and during use. **D** ● ✦

RATIONALE

Elderly individuals have increased sensitivity to glare.
Elderly clients often adjust more slowly to changes in lighting.
Increased sensitivity to glare makes it more difficult to see.

Facilitates adaptation to a darkened environment and improves night vision. Decreases potential for falls.
Easier for client to read with reading glasses. Decreases potential for medication errors.
The visual field narrows with aging and keeping things within the visual range decreases risk of falls.
Improves visual acuity and ability to see through lenses.

Relieves boredom.

Provides for continuum of care once discharged from the acute care facility.

Assists the client in making decisions and decreases potential for being abused.
These safety measures help prevent injury from burns.

NDx = NANDA Diagnosis   **D** = Delegatable Action   ● = UAP   ✦ = LVN/LPN   ⊖▶ = Go to ⊖volve for animation

Continued...

THERAPEUTIC INTERVENTIONS	RATIONALE
Implement measures to reduce the risk for falls if client's vision and/or sense of position or balance seems impaired:	
• Keep bed in low position. **D** ● ✦	*Prevents potential for client falling when getting out of bed.*
• Keep needed items within easy reach and assist client to identify their location. **D** ● ✦	*Prevents stretching to reach objects and possible loss of balance or falling out of bed.*
• Encourage client to request assistance whenever needed; have call signal within easy reach. **D** ● ✦	*Assures client that someone is available to help them.*
• Use lap belt when client is in chair if indicated. **D** ● ✦	*Prevents client from sliding out of the chair.*
• Keep floor free of clutter and wipe up spills. **D** ● ✦	*Improves client safety.*
• Instruct and assist client to get out of bed slowly and change position slowly.	*Reduces dizziness associated with postural hypotension.*
• Provide ambulatory aids (e.g., walker, cane) if appropriate. **D** ● ✦	*Improves balance when walking.*
Instruct client and significant others in above methods of adapting to disturbed sensory perceptions.	*Provides for continuum of care.*
Dependent/Collaborative Actions	
Consult appropriate health care provider if disturbed sensory perceptions worsen.	*Allows prompt alteration in intervention.*

Nursing Diagnosis ## RISK FOR INJURY NDx (PATHOLOGIC FRACTURES)

Definition: Susceptible to physical damage due to environmental conditions interacting with the individual's adaptive and defensive resources, which may compromise health.

Related to:
• Pathologic fractures osteoporosis associated with an imbalance between bone resorption and bone formation resulting from decreased estrogen levels in women
• Calcium deficiency (results from decreased dietary intake and decreased absorption due to vitamin D deficiency), and
• Decreased activity

CLINICAL MANIFESTATIONS

Subjective	**Objective**
Verbal self-report of pain in joints and/or bones	Decrease in mobility and range of motion of extremities, abnormal joint positioning; swelling over skeletal structures, radiographs showing pathologic fractures

RISK FACTORS
• Decreased calcium absorption
• Sedentary lifestyle
• Medication regimen
• Chronic illness
• Poor diet

DESIRED OUTCOMES

The client will not experience pathologic fractures, as evidenced by:
a. Usual mobility and range of motion
b. Absence of unusual motion, abnormal joint position, and obvious deformity of any body part
c. Absence of pain and swelling over skeletal structures
d. Radiographs showing absence of fractures

NOC OUTCOMES

Knowledge of personal safety and medication

NIC INTERVENTIONS

Environmental management, safety, medication management

NURSING ASSESSMENT	RATIONALE
Assess for and report signs and symptoms of pathologic fractures (e.g., decrease in mobility or range of motion, motion at site where motion does not usually occur, abnormal joint position or obvious deformity, pain or swelling over skeletal structures, radiographs showing pathologic fracture).	*Early recognition of signs and symptoms of fractures allows for prompt interventions.*

THERAPEUTIC INTERVENTIONS	RATIONALE

Independent Actions
Implement measures to prevent pathologic fractures:

• Move client carefully; obtain adequate assistance as needed. **D ● ✦**	*Prevents falls and fractures.*
• When turning client, logroll and support all extremities. **D ● ✦**	*Prevents dangling of extremities during turning and decreases the potential for injury.*
• Use smooth movements when moving client; avoid pulling or pushing on body parts. **D ● ✦**	*Prevents sharp, jerking movements, which may cause fractures.*
• Initiate and follow facility safety protocol. **D ● ✦**	*Provides standardized care to prevent accidental falls and bone injury.*
• Help client to maintain maximum mobility. **D ● ✦**	*Weight-bearing exercises reduce bone breakdown.*
• Discourage smoking and excessive caffeine and alcohol intake. **D ✦**	*Nicotine and caffeine increase cardiac workload and may increase shortness of breath. Alcohol will increase diuresis requirement and increase activity and the potential for falls.*
• Encourage client to consume a diet that includes adequate amounts of protein, vitamins, and calcium.	*Ensures an adequate amount of nutrients required for healthy bones.*
• Emphasize need for client to follow a regular exercise program after discharge.	*Provides for continuum of care once client is discharged from the acute care facility.*

Dependent/Collaborative Actions
Implement measures to prevent pathologic fractures:

• Consult physician about use of a tilt table if client is immobile.	*Facilitates weight bearing.*
• Administer calcium preparations, vitamin D, and medications that inhibit bone resorption (e.g., calcitonin, alendronate) if ordered. **D ● ✦**	*These preparations improve potential for bone health and decrease in pathologic fractures.*

If fractures occur:

• Maintain activity restrictions if ordered. **D ● ✦**	*Prevents further bone injury.*
• Apply external stabilization device (e.g., cervical collar, brace, splint, sling) if ordered.	*Stabilizes bone for healing.*
• Prepare client for surgery (e.g., internal fixation) if planned.	*Decreases client's fear and anxiety.*
• Administer analgesics and/or muscle relaxants if ordered. **D ✦**	*Controls pain associated with pathologic fractures.*

Collaborative Diagnosis | DRUG TOXICITY

Definition: An accumulation drug or drugs in the bloodstream that may lead to severe side effects.

Related to:
- An increase in cell receptor sensitivity to some drugs
- Changes in the usual distribution of drugs associated with factors such as a decrease in total body water, a decrease in lean body mass, an increase in total body fat, and a decrease in serum albumin
- Impaired metabolism and excretion of drugs associated with diminished liver and kidney function
- Synergistic effect that occurs with some combinations of medications (elderly clients are often taking a number of medications)

CLINICAL MANIFESTATIONS

Subjective	Objective
Verbal self-report of confusion, blurred vision, anorexia, nausea, dizziness, itchy skin	Ataxia; vomiting; diarrhea; dysrhythmias; postural hypotension; stridor; rash; urticaria; agitation; elevated BUN, serum creatinine, and serum transaminase levels

---

RISK FACTORS

- Polypharmacy
- Changes in distribution
- Inadequate fluid intake
- Poor diet
- Changes in mental status: dementia, anxiety, depression

DESIRED OUTCOMES

The client will not develop drug toxicity as evidenced by absence of signs and symptoms commonly associated with drug toxicity, such as:
a. Ataxia, agitation, confusion, and blurred vision
b. Anorexia, nausea, vomiting, and diarrhea
c. Dizziness, dysrhythmias, and postural hypotension
d. Dyspnea and stridor
e. Rash and urticaria
f. Elevated BUN, serum creatinine, and serum transaminase levels

NURSING ASSESSMENT	RATIONALE
Assess client for signs and symptoms that might be indicative of drug toxicity (e.g., ataxia, agitation, confusion, blurred vision, anorexia, nausea, vomiting, diarrhea, dizziness, dysrhythmias, postural hypotension, dyspnea, stridor, rash, urticaria, elevated BUN, serum creatinine, and serum transaminase levels).	*Early recognition of signs and symptoms of drug toxicity allows for prompt intervention.* *Signs and symptoms will vary depending on drugs being taken.*

THERAPEUTIC INTERVENTIONS	RATIONALE

Independent Actions

Implement measures to prevent drug toxicity:

- Educate client about common adverse effects of drugs being taken and ways to avoid toxicity; encourage client to report adverse effects or any other unusual symptoms immediately.

  Informs client of what to observe for and what to do should adverse effects occur. Also improves adherence to medication regimen.

- Obtain baseline vital signs and results of laboratory studies indicative of renal and hepatic function.

  Facilitates assessment of the effects of medications on these systems.

- Monitor blood levels (e.g., peak, trough) of drugs as ordered and report results to physician; be aware that the elderly client may experience toxic effects when drug levels are within the "normal" therapeutic range.

  Helps to appropriately determine amount of medication client should receive and prevents drug toxicity.

- Before discharge:
  - Provide client and family members with clear, simple, written instructions for taking medications prescribed; include drug name, dose, schedule, route of administration, special precautions such as incompatible foods or drugs, and adverse reactions to observe for.

    Provides an ongoing source of information about client's medications.

- Assist client to set up a system for remembering to take medications as prescribed (e.g., divided pill container, use of timer).

  Facilitates appropriate administration of client's medications.

- Emphasize the importance of taking only those medications that are prescribed, following the directions carefully, and keeping the physician informed of adverse effects experienced.

  Prevents interaction between medications that may decrease or increase the potency of the client's medications.

- Provide client with a written schedule for any laboratory tests that are to be done to monitor the therapeutic effect or side effects of medications being taken.

  Facilitates client taking medications at the appropriate times and what should be monitored.

- Encourage client to get all of medications from one pharmacy and to provide that pharmacy with a complete medical history and list of medications being taken.

  Prevents potential drug interactions if client received multiple prescriptions from multiple pharmacies.

If signs and symptoms of drug toxicity occur, withhold dose and notify appropriate health care provider (e.g., physician, practitioner, pharmacist).

Prevents further buildup of drug toxicity and allows for prompt intervention.

THERAPEUTIC INTERVENTIONS	RATIONALE

Dependent/Collaborative Actions

Implement measures to prevent drug toxicity:

- Consult appropriate resource (e.g., pharmacist, physician, drug book, geriatrician) for the following:

  Provides multidisciplinary approach to medication administration.

  - Information about possible drug interactions of the medications client is taking

    Facilitates monitoring of drug toxicity effects.

  - Appropriate dosages of medications for elderly clients

    The smallest effective dose of a medication should be ordered for elderly persons to reduce the risk of adverse effects.

  - Schedule for and order of administration of medications

    The absorption, distribution, metabolism, and excretion of many medications may be altered by other medications as well as the age-related changes in body function and the client's current illness.

Administer central nervous system depressants judiciously.

Central nervous system depressants decrease client's level of consciousness so that drug toxicity may be difficult to recognize.

Nursing Diagnosis ## INEFFECTIVE SEXUALITY PATTERN NDx

Definition: Expressions of concern regarding own sexuality.

Related to:

- Fear of rejection associated with feelings of loss of physical attractiveness
- Inadequate opportunities for sexual expression associated with lack of available partner
- Misconceptions about sexual functioning in old age
- Fear of urinary incontinence
- Dyspareunia associated with vaginal changes (e.g., decreased vaginal lubrication, thinning and loss of elasticity of the vaginal wall, shortening and narrowing of the vagina) resulting from decreased estrogen levels
- Embarrassment associated with possible impotence (erections are usually less intense and slower in the elderly male; may be further affected by certain disease processes [e.g., diabetes, vascular disorders, chronic renal failure] and medications [e.g., thiazide diuretics, tricyclic antidepressants, certain antihypertensive agents])

CLINICAL MANIFESTATIONS

Subjective	**Objective**
Verbal self-report of sexual concerns; report of difficulties in performing sexual activities	N/A

RISK FACTORS

- Lack of interest and/or partner
- Medication regimen
- Chronic illness
- Changes in sexual response
- Absence of significant other

DESIRED OUTCOMES

The client will demonstrate beginning adaptation to changes in sexuality patterns as evidenced by:
a. Verbalization of a perception of self as sexually acceptable and adequate
b. Statements reflecting ways to adjust to effects of aging on sexual functioning

NOC OUTCOMES

Sexual identity

NIC INTERVENTIONS

Body image enhancement, sexual counseling

NDx = NANDA Diagnosis   **D** = Delegatable Action   ● = UAP   ✦ = LVN/LPN   ⊖▶ = Go to ⊖volve for animation

NURSING ASSESSMENT	RATIONALE
Assess for symptoms of altered sexuality patterns (e.g., verbalization of sexual concerns, limitations, or difficulties; reports of changes in sexual activities or behaviors).	*Early recognition of signs and symptoms of altered sexuality patterns allows for prompt intervention.*
Determine client's perception of desired sexuality, usual pattern of sexual expression, recent changes in sexuality patterns, and knowledge of age-related changes in sexual functioning.	*Be aware that the client may be reluctant to express concerns because of the common stereotype that the elderly are not sexually active.*

THERAPEUTIC INTERVENTIONS	RATIONALE

Independent Actions

Implement measures to promote an optimal sexuality pattern:

- Educate client on the age-related changes in sexual functioning (e.g., sexual responses are slower and less intense, vaginal secretions are diminished, erections take longer to achieve, seminal fluid volume is reduced, erection is rapidly lost after orgasm, refractory time between orgasms is longer); encourage questions and clarify misconceptions.

  Gives client factual information about changes in sexual performance that client may not have known.

- Facilitate communication between client and partner; focus on feelings shared by the couple and assist them to identify changes that may affect their sexual relationship.

  Allows client and significant other to discuss and make changes in a safe environment.

- Discuss ways to be creative in expressing sexuality (e.g., massage, fantasies, cuddling).

  Client may not be aware of alternative methods of expressing sexuality.

- Arrange for uninterrupted privacy if desired by couple.

  Allows client and significant other to explore identified changes.

- Perform actions to improve client's self-concept (e.g., limit negative self-reflection, assist client in identification of effective coping mechanisms).

  Positive self-esteem should have a positive effect on client's sexuality.

- If dyspareunia is a problem:
  - Encourage female client to use a water-soluble lubricant before sexual intercourse.

    Reduces vaginal dryness.

  - Suggest experimentation with different positions during intercourse.

    Reduces the depth of penetration.

- If impotence is a problem:
  - Encourage client to discuss it with physician.

    Impotence may be due to reversible factors such as medication therapy, alcohol, and poorly controlled chronic disease conditions.

  - Assure client that occasional episodes of impotence are normal.

    Assures client of normalcy.

  - Suggest alternative methods of sexual gratification if appropriate.

    May improve sexual gratification.

  - Encourage client to discuss various treatment options (e.g., penile prosthesis, sildenafil, vardenafil, intraurethral alprostadil pellet placement, external vacuum device) with physician if appropriate.

    Allows client to know there are options available to treat impotence and the appropriateness of discussing this with his physician.

- Reinforce the importance of rest before sexual activity.

  Improves ability to perform sexually.

- If incontinence of urine is a problem, encourage client to void just before intercourse and other sexual activity.

  Decreases incidence of incontinence during sexual activity.

- Include partner in above discussions and encourage continued support of the client.

  Demonstrates support for client and partner and allows them to receive factual information.

Dependent/Collaborative Actions

Implement measures to promote an optimal sexuality pattern:

- If dyspareunia is a problem:
  - Administer estrogen if ordered or provide client with information about estrogen therapy.

    Reduces vaginal dryness and thinning of vaginal epithelium.

Consult appropriate health care provider (counselor, sex therapist, physician) if counseling appears indicated.

Allows for a multidisciplinary treatment plan.

Nursing Diagnosis **RISK FOR FRAIL ELDERLY SYNDROME** NDx

Definition: Susceptible to a dynamic state of unstable equilibrium that affects the older individual experiencing deterioration in one or more domains of health (physical, functional, psychological, or social) and leads to increased susceptibility to adverse health effects, in particular disability.

Related to:
- Reduced opportunities for socialization associated with inadequate financial resources, death or disability of friends and family members, reluctance of others to include the elderly in activities, reluctance to establish new relationships and try new activities, and/or a move to a different location (e.g., family member's home, foster home, extended care facility)
- Decreased desire to communicate with others associated with an imbalance between the effort required to interact with others and the anticipated rewards of the interaction
- Decreased participation in usual activities associated with changes in sensory and motor function and fear of falls
- Withdrawal from others associated with fear of embarrassment resulting from functional changes such as incontinence or hearing loss

CLINICAL MANIFESTATIONS

Subjective	Objective
Expression of feelings of rejection; being different from others or being lonely	Sad, dull affect; hostility; uncommunicative and withdrawn; absence of supportive significant others

RISK FACTORS
- Chronic illness
- Sedentary lifestyle
- Loss of friends and/or family
- Lack of interest in interacting with others

DESIRED OUTCOMES

The client will not experience a sense of isolation and loneliness, as evidenced by:
a. Maintenance of relationships with significant others
b. No expression of feelings of isolation and loneliness

NOC OUTCOMES

Social support, quality of life

NIC INTERVENTIONS

Enhancement of socialization, facilitation of visits

NURSING ASSESSMENT

Assess for indications of isolation and loneliness (e.g., absence of supportive significant others; uncommunicative and withdrawn; expressing feelings of rejection, being different from others, or being lonely; hostility; sadness; dull affect).

RATIONALE

Early recognition of signs and symptoms of loneliness allows for prompt intervention.

THERAPEUTIC INTERVENTIONS

RATIONALE

Independent Actions
Implement measures to decrease isolation and reduce the risk for loneliness:
- Help client to identify reasons for feeling isolated and alone; aid client in developing a plan of action to reduce these feelings.
- Use touch to demonstrate acceptance of client. **D** ● ✦
- Encourage significant others to visit. **D** ● ✦
- Encourage client to maintain telephone contact with others. **D** ● ✦
- Schedule time each day to sit and talk with client. **D** ● ✦

- Help client to identify a few persons they she feels comfortable with and encourage interactions with them.
- Make objects such as telephone, television, radio, newspapers, and greeting cards accessible to client. **D** ● ✦

Helps clients to realize they have to be actively involved in changing feelings of loneliness.

Decreases loneliness and connects client with others.
Helps client to understand that he or she is not alone.
Helps client become actively engaged in decreasing feelings of loneliness.
Demonstrates acceptance of client and shows client that having positive interactions with others is possible.
Help client role play with interactions to provide self-esteem in ability to relate others in social interactions.
Allows client to interact with others, and electronics may provide distractions.

NDx = NANDA Diagnosis **D** = Delegatable Action ● = UAP ✦ = LVN/LPN ⊝▶ = Go to ⊝volve for animation

Continued...

THERAPEUTIC INTERVENTIONS	RATIONALE
• Have significant others bring client's favorite objects from home and place in room. **D** ● ✦	*Makes client feel more at home in the health care environment.*
• Change room assignments if necessary.	*Provide the client with a roommate with similar interests.*
• Encourage interaction between client and roommate.	*Demonstrates to client that others find client interesting and are willing to spend time with him or her.*
• Emphasize the importance of maintaining active friendships and seeking out new relationships; encourage participation in support groups if appropriate.	*Encourages client to engage in interactions with others.*
• Encourage client to participate in structured activity programs after discharge; provide information about community senior centers and the programs they offer.	*Provides for continuum of care after discharge from the acute care facility.*

Nursing Diagnosis   DEFICIENT KNOWLEDGE NDx

Definition: Absence of cognitive information related to a specific topic, or its acquisition.

Related to:
• Lack of motivation, inadequate support and supervision, and insufficient financial resources
• Confusion about appropriate health care practices and a decreased level of trust associated with conflicting advice from multiple health care providers
• Conflicting values between client and health care providers
• Knowledge deficit regarding current diagnosis, medications and treatments prescribed, and consequences of failure to comply with treatment plan

CLINICAL MANIFESTATIONS

Subjective	Objective
Verbal self-report of inability to care for self at home; statements reflecting lack of understanding of self-care; statements reflect understanding of disease progression with or without treatment; statements of unwillingness to engage in required treatment regimen	Nonadherence to diet; refusal to be involved in treatment regimen.

RISK FACTORS
• Chronic illness
• Medication regimen
• Lack of resources both social and financial

DESIRED OUTCOMES

The client will demonstrate the probability of effective management of therapeutic regimen as evidenced by:
a. Willingness to learn about and participate in treatments and care
b. Statements reflecting ways to modify personal habits and integrate treatments into lifestyle
c. Statements reflecting an understanding of the implications of not following the prescribed treatment plan

NOC OUTCOMES

Knowledge: treatment regimen; disease process; participation in health care decisions; compliance behavior; health beliefs.

NIC INTERVENTIONS

Discharge planning; health system guidance; teaching: disease process; teaching: treatment; financial resource assistance

NURSING ASSESSMENT	RATIONALE
Assess for indications that the client may be unable to effectively manage the therapeutic regimen: • Statements reflecting inability to manage care at home. • Failure to adhere to treatment plan (e.g., not adhering to dietary modifications, refusing medications, refusing to ambulate). • Statements reflecting a lack of understanding of the factors that will cause further progression of current illness and/or accelerate aging process. • Statements reflecting an unwillingness or inability to modify personal habits and integrate necessary treatments into lifestyle. • Statements reflecting view that situation is hopeless and that efforts to comply are useless.	*Early recognition of signs and symptoms of ineffective therapeutic management allows for prompt intervention.*

THERAPEUTIC INTERVENTIONS	RATIONALE
Independent Actions Implement measures to promote effective management of the therapeutic regimen:	
• Discuss with client the specific factors that may interfere with management of care (e.g., inadequate financial resources, religious or cultural conflicts, lack of support systems).	*Helps client identify underlying cause of ineffective treatment management.*
• Explain the aging process and current diagnosis in terms the client can understand; stress the fact that adherence to the treatment plan is necessary in order to delay and/or prevent complications associated with the diagnosis and minimize some of the changes that occur with aging.	*Helps client understand that some physiologic changes are part of the aging process, but others require adherence to a treatment regimen.*
• Help client to clarify values and identify ways to incorporate the therapeutic goals and priorities into his or her value system.	*Values clarification and lifestyle changes.*
• Encourage questions and clarify misconceptions the client may have about aging and his or her diagnosis and effects of each.	*Ensures client's understanding of physiologic changes and impact on his or her ability to maintain earlier lifestyle.*
• Perform actions to promote trust in caregivers (e.g., validate conflicting advice, explain reasons for treatment plan).	*Helps improve adherence.*
• Encourage client to participate in treatment plan (e.g., take medications as prescribed, perform recommended exercises).	*Helps to improve client's self-confidence in ability to care for self.*
• Provide instruction regarding medications and treatments prescribed; allow time for return demonstration of procedures; determine areas of difficulty and misunderstanding and reinforce teaching as necessary.	*Knowledge of medications and how they impact the system improves client adherence to treatment regimen and understanding of the importance of adhering to the prescribed medication regimen. The client must be able to recognize alterations in functioning related to medication administration and what clinical manifestations that should be reported to the health care provider.*
• Provide client with written instructions about medications and treatments.	*Provides a reference once discharged from the acute care facility.*
• Help client to identify ways to incorporate treatments into his or her lifestyle; focus on modifications of lifestyle rather than complete change, if possible.	*Clients will adhere more closely to lifestyle modifications that they identify.*
• Encourage client to discuss his or her financial concerns; obtain a social service consult to help client with financial planning and to obtain financial aid if indicated.	*Provides for ongoing support post discharge from the acute care facility.*
• Provide information about and encourage use of community resources that can assist client to make necessary lifestyle changes if appropriate.	*Provides ongoing support and continuum of care post discharge from the acute care facility.*

Continued...

THERAPEUTIC INTERVENTIONS	RATIONALE
• Encourage client to attend follow-up educational classes if appropriate.	*Increases client's understanding of disease process and ongoing self-care.*
• Reinforce behaviors suggesting future compliance with the therapeutic regimen (e.g., statements reflecting plans for integrating treatments into lifestyle, active participation in exercise program, changes in personal habits).	*Improves client's self-confidence in abilities to adhere to treatment regimen and to care for self.*
• Include significant others in explanations and teaching sessions and encourage their support; reinforce the need for client to assume responsibility for managing as much of his or her care as possible.	*Provides ongoing support once the client is discharged from the acute care facility.*

Dependent/Collaborative Actions

Consult appropriate health care provider about referrals to community health agencies if continued instruction, support, or supervision is needed.	*Allows for multidisciplinary client care and for continuum of care once in the community.*

Nursing Diagnosis INTERRUPTED FAMILY PROCESSES NDx

Definition: Break in the continuity of family functioning which fails to support the well-being of its members.

Related to:
• Financial, physical, and psychologic stresses associated with family member's illness and/or progressive disability
• Inadequate knowledge about the normal aging process, client's current diagnosis, and necessary care
• Inadequate support services
• Decreased ability of client to fulfill usual family roles
• Guilt associated with the need to change client's living situation, resulting from family's inability to provide necessary care

CLINICAL MANIFESTATIONS

Subjective	Objective
Verbal self-reports of increased stress related to financial, physical, and/or psychologic associated with disability	Change in financial situations; change in psychologic stress; change in communication patterns; changes in intimacy; changes in participation in problem solving; changes in rituals; changes in satisfaction with family; changes in somatic behavior; changes in stress-reduction behavior

RISK FACTORS
• Chronic illness
• Sedentary lifestyle
• Changes in roles and responsibilities
• Poor self-esteem
• Poor social support system
• Loss of family members
• Changes in mental status: dementia, anxiety, depression

DESIRED OUTCOMES

Client's significant others will demonstrate beginning adjustment to changes in functioning of family member and family roles and structure as evidenced by:
a. Meeting client's needs
b. Verbalization of ways to adapt to required role and lifestyle changes
c. Active participation in decision making and client's rehabilitation
d. Positive interactions among one another

NOC OUTCOMES

Family integrity; family support

NIC INTERVENTIONS

Promotion of family integrity; maintenance of family process; family support

NURSING ASSESSMENT	RATIONALE
Assess for signs and symptoms of interrupted family processes (e.g., inability to meet client's needs, statements of not being able to accept client's disabilities or make necessary role and lifestyle changes, inability to make decisions, inability or refusal to participate in client's care and/or rehabilitation, negative family interactions). Identify components of the family and their patterns of communication and role expectations.	*Early recognition of signs and symptoms of interrupted family processes allows for prompt intervention.*

THERAPEUTIC INTERVENTIONS	RATIONALE

Independent Actions

Implement measures to facilitate family members' adjustment to age- or diagnosis-related changes in client and resultant changes in family roles and structure:

- Encourage family members to verbalize feelings about changes in client and the effect of these changes on family structure; actively listen to each family member and maintain a nonjudgmental attitude about feelings shared.

Helps them work through their issues and concern related to changes in the family structure. Family members must be open and honest and focused on working through changes in family structure and support.

- Instruct client and family about normal aging processes (e.g., sensory deficits, decreased muscle strength, reduced coordination).

Provides client and family with factual information related to changes being experienced.

- Reinforce physician's explanation of the effects of the current diagnosis and planned treatment and rehabilitation.

Reinforcing important information allows the nurse to both summarize key concepts and further assess client's understanding of instructions.

- Help family members to gain a realistic perspective of client's situation, conveying as much hope as appropriate.

Improves family members' support and understanding of client's situation and the importance of their support.

- Provide privacy so that family members and client can share their feelings; stress the importance of good communication techniques and facilitate their use.

Allows for open communication between family members and client.

- Help family members to progress through their grieving processes; explain that they may encounter times when they must focus on meeting their own rather than the client's needs.

Helps family members understand that a significant change has occurred and it is OK to grieve about the changes.

- Emphasize the need for family members to obtain adequate rest and nutrition and to identify and use stress management techniques.

Helps them to deal emotionally and physically with the changes experienced.

- Encourage and assist family members to identify coping strategies for dealing with client's age-related changes and changes in health status and their effect on the family.

Helps them learn what mechanisms work best for them in dealing with client and family changes.

- Help family members to identify realistic goals and ways of reaching these goals.

Helps to decrease disappointment when unrealistic goals are not met.

- Include family members in decision making about client's care; convey appreciation for their input and continued support of the client.

Helps family have some sense of control over the situation.

- Encourage and allow family members to participate in client's care and rehabilitation; instruct family in any special procedures and allow them to practice with supervision before discharge of the client.

Improves family's understanding of treatment regimen and their ability to support client.

- Help family members to identify resources that could assist them in coping with their feelings and meeting their immediate and long-term needs (e.g., counseling and social services; pastoral care; service, church, and support groups); initiate a referral if indicated.

Provides for continuum of care once client is discharged from the acute care facility.

Dependent/Collaborative Actions

Consult appropriate health care provider if family members continue to demonstrate difficulty adapting to changes in client's functioning, roles, and family structure.

Allows for multidisciplinary input into continuum of care.

NDx = NANDA Diagnosis **D** = Delegatable Action ● = UAP ✦ = LVN/LPN ⊖▶ = Go to ⊖volve for animation

ADDITIONAL NURSING DIAGNOSES

DISTURBED BODY IMAGE NDx
Related to:
- Changes in appearance and body functioning (e.g., graying and thinning of hair; sagginess of eyelids, earlobes, and breasts; dry, wrinkled skin; reduced height; increase in and change in distribution of body fat; reduction in lean body mass; decreased bladder control; diminished visual acuity and hearing)
- Increased dependence on others to meet basic needs
- Feelings of powerlessness
- Change in usual lifestyle and roles associated with decreased strength and endurance and disturbed sensory perception

RISK FOR POWERLESSNESS NDx
Related to:
- Increased dependence on others to meet basic needs
- Inability to pursue usual life activities and roles associated with age-related changes in body functioning, current diagnosis and its treatment, and inadequate financial resources
- Inability to control many of the changes that occur with aging

End-of-Life Nursing Care

This care plan focuses on care of the adult client who is expected to die soon. The information included is appropriate for clients in acute or extended care settings or in the home. The major goals of nursing care are to prevent or control physiological problems that could reduce the quality of the client's remaining life; facilitate the client's psychological adjustment to his/her imminent death; and assist the client to experience a peaceful, dignified death. The nurse also assists the significant others (SO) to understand the dying process, support the dying person, meet their own physical and emotional needs, and adjust to their loss of the client.

This care plan does not deal with any specific medical diagnosis. The nursing diagnoses included are those that are common to all persons facing death. Care plans that pertain to the client's specific medical diagnosis will provide additional guidelines for nursing care during the terminal stages of that illness.

Use in conjunction with the Care Plan on Immobility and care plans that pertain to the client's medical diagnosis.

Nursing Diagnosis **RISK FOR ASPIRATION** NDx

Definition: Susceptible to entry of gastrointestinal secretions, oropharynx secretions, solids, or fluids to the tracheobronchial passages, which may compromise health.

Related to:

- Decreased level of consciousness
- Absent or diminished gag reflex associated with the underlying disease process and/or the depressant effect of some medications (e.g., narcotic [opioid] analgesics, some antiemetics and antianxiety agents)
- Supine positioning
- Increased risk for gastroesophageal reflux associated with increased gastric pressure resulting from decreased GI motility
- Impaired swallowing associated with dry mouth and absent or diminished swallowing reflex (can occur as a result of the underlying disease process)

CLINICAL MANIFESTATIONS

Subjective	Objective
Not applicable	Rhonchi; dull percussion note over affected lung area; cough; tachypnea; tachycardia; development of or increase in dyspnea; presence of tube feeding in tracheal aspirate; chest radiograph showing pulmonary infiltrate

RISK FACTORS

- Delayed gastric emptying
- Impaired swallowing
- Decreased level of consciousness
- Tube feeding
- Immobility and positioning

DESIRED OUTCOMES

The client will not aspirate secretions or foods/fluids as evidenced by:

a. Clear or usual breath sounds
b. Resonant percussion note over lungs
c. Absence of cough and tachypnea
d. Absence of or no increase in dyspnea

NOC OUTCOMES	NIC INTERVENTIONS
Aspiration prevention; respiratory status: gas exchange	Respiratory monitoring; aspiration precautions; airway precautions

NURSING ASSESSMENT	RATIONALE
Assess for and report signs and symptoms of aspiration of secretions, vomitus, or foods/fluids: • Rhonchi • Dull percussion note over affected lung area • Cough, tachypnea, tachycardia • Development of or increase in dyspnea • Presence of tube feeding in tracheal aspirate Assess chest radiograph for evidence of pulmonary infiltrates.	*Early recognition of signs and symptoms of aspiration allows for prompt intervention.*

THERAPEUTIC INTERVENTIONS	RATIONALE

Independent Actions

Implement measures to reduce the risk for aspiration:
- Position client in side-lying or semi- to high-Fowler's positions at all times. **D** ● ✦

  These positions decrease the incidence of aspiration by decreasing the direct access to the trachea of fluids and/or food.

- Perform actions to prevent nausea and vomiting:
  - Eliminate noxious sights/odors.

    Noxious sights/odors can cause nausea and vomiting. Eliminating these reduces the risk for aspiration.

- Perform actions to reduce the accumulation of GI gas and fluid (e.g., expel flatus, eructate).

  Reducing gastric distention and gastroesophageal reflux reduces the movement of fluids/foods into the upper esophagus.

- Withhold oral food/fluids if gag reflex is depressed or absent, client is not alert, or client is experiencing severe dysphagia.

  Risk for aspiration is high when mechanisms to protect the client's airway (e.g., gag reflex) are impaired.

- If client is taking foods/fluids orally:
  - Offer foods/fluids that promote an effective swallow (e.g., thick rather than thin fluids, moist rather than dry foods). **D**

    Thin fluids rapidly pass through the mouth and can pour over the back of the tongue without triggering an effective swallow, increasing the risk for aspiration.

Maintain client in a high-Fowler's position during and for at least 30 minutes after client eats unless contraindicated. **D** ● ✦

Head-of-bed elevation facilitates movement of foods and fluid through the pharynx into the esophagus, where the risk for aspiration is greatly reduced.

- Encourage client to concentrate on eating and drinking and allow ample time for meals. **D** ✦

  If a client becomes distracted during meals or is rushed, swallowing and breathing attempts can become uncoordinated, increasing the risk for aspiration.

- Instruct client to avoid talking or laughing when swallowing.

  Laughing or talking results in the larynx remaining open during eating and increases the risk of aspiration.

  A high-Fowler's position uses gravity to aid in the flow of fluids/foods through the esophagus.

- Assist client with oral hygiene after eating. **D** ● ✦

  Good oral hygiene after meals results in the removal of remaining food particles that could enter the larynx and be aspirated into the lungs.

If signs and symptoms of aspiration occur:
- Perform tracheal suctioning.
- Withhold oral intake.
- Prepare client for chest radiograph if ordered.

Dependent/Collaborative Actions

Implement measures to reduce the risk for aspiration:
- Perform oropharyngeal suctioning and oral hygiene as often as needed.

  Oropharyngeal suctioning helps to remove excess secretions, vomitus, and food particles.

- If client is receiving tube feedings:
  - Check tube placement before each feeding or on a routine basis if continuous feeding. **D** ✦

    Validation of appropriate location of feeding tube ensures that tube feeding solution goes into the alimentary tract and not the lungs.

Do not increase rate of continuous tube feeding unless allowed and tolerated; administer intermittent tube feedings slowly.

High residual volumes can lead to upward pressure placed on the lower esophagus, increasing the risk for regurgitation.

Stop tube feeding and notify physician if residuals exceed established parameters.

Allows for prompt changes in treatment regimen.

Nursing Diagnosis **ACUTE/CHRONIC PAIN** NDx

Definition: **Acute pain NDx:** Unpleasant sensory and emotional experience associated with actual or potential tissue damage, or described in terms of such damage (International Association for the Study of Pain); sudden or slow onset of any intensity from mild to severe with anticipated or predictable end, and with a duration of less than 3 months; **Chronic Pain NDx:** Unpleasant sensory and emotional experience associated with actual or potential tissue damage, or described in terms of such damage (International Association for the Study of Pain); sudden or slow onset of any intensity from mild to severe, constant or recurring without an anticipated or predictable end, and with a duration of greater than 3 months.

Related to:
- The underlying disease process
- Muscle spasms or stiff joints associated with decreased mobility
- Reluctance to take pain medication associated with fear of loss of control and/or oversedation, feeling that taking medication is a sign of weakness, or that pain has redemptive qualities and/or need to be stoic

CLINICAL MANIFESTATIONS

Subjective	Objective
Verbal self-report of pain	Grimacing; reluctance to move; restlessness; diaphoresis; increased blood pressure; tachycardia

RISK FACTORS

- Injury agents
- Immobility/positioning
- Chronic disability

DESIRED OUTCOMES

The client will experience diminished pain as evidenced by:
a. Verbalization of decrease in or absence of pain
b. Relaxed facial expression and body positioning
c. Stable vital signs

NOC OUTCOMES	NIC INTERVENTIONS
Comfort level; pain control	Analgesic administration; pain management; patient-controlled analgesia (PCA) assistance; environmental management: comfort; dying care

NURSING ASSESSMENT	RATIONALE
Assess for signs and symptoms of pain: • Grimacing • Reluctance to move • Restlessness • Diaphoresis • Increased BP • Tachycardia • Verbalization of pain	*Early recognition of signs and symptoms of pain allows for prompt intervention.*
Assess client's perception of the severity of pain using a pain intensity rating scale. Assess the client's pain pattern (e.g., location, quality, onset, duration, precipitating factors, aggravating factors, alleviating factors).	*Use of a pain intensity rating scale gives the nurse a clearer understanding of the client's pain being experienced, changes in pain over time, and promotes consistency when communicating with others.*
Ask the client to describe previous pain experiences and methods used to manage pain effectively.	*Provides comparison to determine if pain and associated factors are changing.*

THERAPEUTIC INTERVENTIONS	RATIONALE

Independent Actions

Implement measures to reduce pain:

- Perform actions to reduce fear and anxiety about the pain experience (e.g., assure client that the need for pain relief is understood; plan methods for achieving pain control with client).

Actions help promote relaxation and subsequently increase the client's threshold and tolerance for pain.

- Perform actions to promote rest:
  - Cluster nursing care. **D** ● ✦
- Plan methods for achieving pain control with client.

Actions help reduce fatigue and subsequently increase the client's threshold and tolerance for pain.

Actions help assist client to maintain a sense of control over the pain experience.

- Provide or assist with nonpharmacological methods for pain relief (e.g., massage; position change; progressive relaxation exercise; restful environment; diversional activities such as watching television, reading, or conversing). **D** ✦

Nonpharmacological pain management includes a variety of interventions. These interventions are believed to be effective because they stimulate closure of the gating mechanism in the spinal cord.

Dependent/Collaborative Actions

Implement measures to reduce pain:

- If client has a PCA device, encourage client to use it as instructed.

Maintain integrity of analgesia delivery system (e.g., epidural, intravenous, subcutaneous, transdermal).

Provides the client a sense of control over care and experience of pain.

- Administer analgesics before activities and procedures that can cause pain and before pain becomes severe.

Prevents or decreases the experience of pain and allows the client to engage in activities as able.

- Administer the following medications as ordered to provide maximum pain relief with minimal side effects: **D** ✦
  - Opioid analgesics
  - Nonopioid analgesics
  - Local anesthetics
  - Muscle relaxants

Medications help to decrease pain experience. Client may need medications on a regular schedule to remain pain free. Be sure to address issues such as constipation when client is regularly taking opioids.

Consult appropriate health care provider (e.g., hospice nurse, palliative care nurse, pharmacist, physician, pain management specialist) if above measures fail to provide adequate pain relief.

Consulting the appropriate health care provider allows for modification of the treatment plan.

Nursing Diagnosis **RISK FOR IMPAIRED SKIN INTEGRITY** NDx

Definition: Susceptible to alteration in epidermis and/or dermis, which may compromise health.

Related to:

- Accumulation of waste products and decreased oxygen and nutrient supply to the skin and subcutaneous tissue associated with reduced blood flow from prolonged pressure on the tissues resulting from decreased mobility
- Damage to the skin and/or subcutaneous tissue associated with friction or shearing
- Frequent contact with irritants associated with incontinence of urine or stool
- Increased fragility of skin associated with inadequate nutritional status, dryness, and dependent edema

CLINICAL MANIFESTATIONS

Subjective	Objective
Verbalization of problem	Pallor; redness; obvious areas of skin breakdown

RISK FACTORS

- Immobility
- Shearing/pressure forces
- Impaired circulation
- Changes in fluid status

DESIRED OUTCOMES

The client will maintain tissue integrity as evidenced by:
a. Absence of redness and irritation
b. No skin breakdown

NOC OUTCOMES	NIC INTERVENTIONS
Tissue integrity: skin and mucous membrane	Skin surveillance; skin care: topical treatments; pressure ulcer prevention; positioning

NURSING ASSESSMENT	RATIONALE
Determine client's risk for skin breakdown using a risk assessment tool (e.g., Norton Scale, Braden Scale, Gosnell Scale).	*Early recognition of signs and symptoms of skin breakdown allows for prompt intervention.*
Inspect the skin (especially bony prominences; dependent, edematous, and pruritic areas; and perianal area) for pallor, redness, and breakdown.	

THERAPEUTIC INTERVENTIONS	RATIONALE

Independent Actions

Implement measures to prevent skin irritation resulting from incontinence of urine or stool in order to help prevent tissue breakdown:

- Perform actions to reduce the episodes of urinary and bowel incontinence:
  - Offer assistance to defecate at regular intervals during the day. **D** ●
- Assist client to thoroughly cleanse and dry perineal area with soft tissue or cloth after each episode of incontinence; apply a protective ointment or cream. **D** ● ✦
- Apply a fecal incontinence pouch if bowel incontinence is a persistent problem. **D** ✦
- If use of absorbent products such as pads or undergarments is necessary, select those that effectively absorb moisture and keep it away from the skin.

Helps to avoid skin irritation from exposure to fecal material and urine.
Helps to prevent incontinence and subsequent exposure to fecal material and urine
Keeping skin dry and protected prevents breakdown.

Protects skin from exposure to irritating substances.

Constant exposure to moisture will increase the potential for skin breakdown.

Dependent/Collaborative Actions

If tissue breakdown occurs:

- Notify appropriate health care provider (e.g., wound care specialist, physician).
- Perform pressure ulcer care as ordered or per standard hospital procedure (extensiveness of treatment is usually limited to that necessary to maintain comfort).

Consulting the appropriate health care provider allows for modification of the treatment plan.

Nursing Diagnosis **FUNCTIONAL URINARY INCONTINENCE/BOWEL INCONTINENCE** NDx

Definition: Functional Urinary Incontinence NDx: Inability of a usually continent person to reach toilet in time to avoid unintentional loss of urine. **Bowel Incontinence NDx:** Involuntary passage of stool.

Functional urinary incontinence NDx

Related to:

- Decreased ability to respond to the urge to urinate associated with decreased level of consciousness and impaired physical mobility
- Decreased awareness of full bladder and poor urinary sphincter control associated with decreased level of consciousness and/or the underlying disease process

Bowel incontinence NDx

Related to:

- Decreased ability to respond to the urge to defecate associated with decreased level of consciousness and impaired physical mobility.
- Decreased awareness of urge to defecate and poor anal sphincter control associated with decreased level of consciousness
- Fecal impaction if present (continuous stimulation of the defecation reflex by the fecal mass that inhibits the internal anal sphincter and results in loss of ability to retain the mucus and fluid that collects proximal to and leaks around the fecal mass)

CLINICAL MANIFESTATIONS

Subjective	Objective
Verbal report of urgency	Leakage of urine during body movements Leakage of fecal material

RISK FACTORS
- Immobility
- Impaired cognition
- Toileting self-care deficit

DESIRED OUTCOME
The client will not experience functional urinary and bowel incontinence

NOC OUTCOMES

Urinary continence; bowel continence

NIC INTERVENTIONS

Urinary incontinence care; self-care assistance: toileting; urinary catheterization
Bowel incontinence care

NURSING ASSESSMENT	RATIONALE
Assess for urinary incontinence: - Leakage of urine during body movements - Verbal report of urgency with post-void residuals - Assess for bowel incontinence: - Leakage of fecal material from the body - Assess the number of incontinence events.	*Early recognition of signs and symptoms of urinary and bowel incontinence allows for prompt intervention.*

THERAPEUTIC INTERVENTIONS	RATIONALE

Independent Actions

Implement measures to maintain or regain urinary and bowel continence:
- Offer bedpan or urinal or assist client to bedside commode or bathroom every 2 to 4 hrs if indicated. **D** ● ✦

  Bladder and bowel training programs help to reduce the incidence of incontinence.

- Allow client to assume a normal position for voiding and a bowel movement unless contraindicated.

  Promotes evacuation of the bladder and bowel.

- Perform actions to reduce delays in toileting (e.g., have call signal within client's reach and respond promptly to requests for assistance; have bedpan, urinal, or bedside commode readily available to client; provide client with easy-to-remove clothing such as pajamas with Velcro closures or an elastic waistband). **D** ● ✦

  Actions help to promote complete bladder emptying.

- If client has a good fluid intake, encourage him/her to space fluids evenly throughout the day rather than drinking a large quantity at one time.

  Rapid filling of bladder can result in incontinence if client has decreased urinary sphincter control.

- Encourage client to avoid drinking alcohol and beverages containing caffeine.

  Alcohol and caffeine have a mild diuretic effect and act as irritants; these factors may make urinary control more difficult.

If urinary and/or bowel incontinence persists:
- Provide client with or apply disposable undergarments (e.g., Depends, Attends) if indicated. **D** ● ✦

  Helps prevent exposure of skin to urine, preventing skin breakdown. Be sure to check client regularly to prevent the skin being exposed for a long period of time to urine or fecal material.

Dependent/Collaborative Actions

If urinary and/or bowel incontinence persists:
- For urinary incontinence:
  - Consult appropriate health care provider about intermittent catheterization, insertion of indwelling catheter, or use of external collection device (e.g., condom catheter).

  Consulting the appropriate health care provider allows for modification of the treatment plan.

THERAPEUTIC INTERVENTIONS	RATIONALE

- For bowel incontinence:
  - Consult appropriate health care provider (e.g., Hospice nurse, palliative care nurse, physician) about the use of a fecal incontinence pouch.

Nursing Diagnosis ## DEATH ANXIETY NDx

Definition: Vague, uneasy feeling of discomfort or dread generated by perceptions of a real or imagined threat to one's existence.

Related to:
- Concern about the well-being of caregivers and the impact of death on SO
- Fear of loss of physical and mental capabilities during dying process
- Anticipated discomfort (e.g., pain, nausea, difficulty breathing) during dying process
- Feeling of powerlessness over issues related to death
- Feeling of doubt about existence of a God or higher being
- Unfinished business and unresolved conflicts
- Fear of abandonment and dying alone

CLINICAL MANIFESTATIONS

Subjective	Objective
Verbal self-report of concerns about death and dying	Acting out with anger or aggression; mood swings

RISK FACTORS
- Uncertainty about a higher power
- Pain/suffering
- Terminal illness
- Loss of control

DESIRED OUTCOMES

The client will experience a reduction in death anxiety as evidenced by:
a. Verbalization of feeling less anxious
b. Usual sleep pattern
c. Relaxed facial expression and body movements
d. Stable vital signs
e. Statements reflecting resolution of unfinished business, conflicts, and concerns

NOC OUTCOMES

Anxiety self-control; fear self-control; dignified life closure; spiritual health

NIC INTERVENTIONS

Anxiety reduction; presence; emotional support; spiritual support; decision-making support; self-esteem enhancement

NURSING ASSESSMENT	RATIONALE
Assess client for concerns related to death and the dying process: • Increased anxiety • Acting out with anger and aggression • Mood swings	*Early recognition of signs and symptoms of death anxiety allows for prompt intervention.*

THERAPEUTIC INTERVENTIONS	RATIONALE
Independent Actions Implement additional measures to reduce fear and anxiety about death and dying: Establish a trusting relationship with the client and SO. Spend quality time with client and SO.	*Establishing a trusting relationship is the first step in the process of supporting the patient and SO through this difficult time. Spend time with the patient and make sure that they don't feel rushed or unimportant due to other responsibilities.*

NDx = NANDA Diagnosis   **D** = Delegatable Action   ● = UAP   ✦ = LVN/LPN   ⊖▶ = Go to ⊖volve for animation

Continued...

THERAPEUTIC INTERVENTIONS	RATIONALE
Provide a supportive environment in which the client and SO can explore concerns about death: • Advance directives, living will, and durable power of attorney. • Planning funeral/burial arrangements. • Organ/tissue donation. • How to spend remaining time. • Spend quality time with client.	*Allow client and SO time to determine what they would like to happen and how they can maintain control of what happens to them if they are unable to communicate their wishes for care.*
• Assist client to formulate plans for completing unfinished business and providing for care of SO if appropriate.	*Provides an opportunity for client and SO to consider these things and what needs to be put in place to care for others if the client was a part of the support system.*
• If appropriate, encourage and assist client to record (e.g., write, audiotape, videotape) information he/she would like others to know at the present time and after his/her death.	*Gives client and family lasting memories and a way for the SO to retain memories and ability to introduce the client to new members of the family after his/her death.*
• Encourage SO to stay with client and participate in care if their presence seems to relieve the client's fear and anxiety.	*This provides a time for the client to spend time with his/her family members and for the family to feel involved in their SO's care. It also helps the client not to feel alone in this journey and can decrease fear and anxiety.* *Gives the client a sense of control over their belongings, ability to support their family and pets, and to provide for them once they are deceased.*
Consult appropriate individuals (e.g., attorneys, social services, Hospice nursing) to help meets client's need to put systems in place for remaining friends, family, and pets. • Consult with patient regarding potential spiritual or religious needs.	*Provides for interprofessional client focused care.*

Nursing Diagnosis GRIEVING NDx

Definition: A normal, complex process that includes emotional, physical, spiritual, social, and intellectual responses and behaviors by which individuals, families, and communities incorporate an actual, anticipated, or perceived loss into their daily lives.

Related to: Loss of control over life and body functioning, changes in body image, loss of SO, and imminent death

CLINICAL MANIFESTATIONS

Subjective	Objective
Expression of distress about terminal illness and dying; denial of impending death	Change in eating habits; inability to concentrate; insomnia; anger; sadness; withdrawal from SO

RISK FACTOR

• Anticipatory loss of body processes

DESIRED OUTCOMES

The client will demonstrate progression through the grieving process as evidenced by:
a. Verbalization of feelings about dying
b. Usual sleep pattern
c. Use of available support systems

NOC OUTCOMES

Grief resolution

NIC INTERVENTIONS

Grief work facilitation; emotional support; presence; support system enhancement; dying care

NURSING ASSESSMENT	RATIONALE
Assess for signs and symptoms of grieving: • Expression of distress about terminal illness and dying • Denial of impending death • Change in eating habits • Inability to concentrate • Insomnia • Anger • Sadness • Withdrawal from SO	*Early recognition of signs and symptoms of grieving allows for prompt intervention.*

THERAPEUTIC INTERVENTIONS	RATIONALE

Independent Actions

Implement measures to facilitate the grieving process:

- Assist client to acknowledge that death is imminent. *Acknowledgment of imminent death allows grief work to progress.*
- Assess for factors that may hinder and facilitate acknowledgment.
- Discuss the grieving process and assist client to accept the phases of grieving as an expected response to anticipated losses and impending death. *Phases of grieving vary among theorists, but progress from shock and alarm to acceptance.*
- Allow time for client to progress through the phases of grieving. Be aware that not every phase is expressed by all individuals, that phases do not necessarily occur in sequential order, and that recurrence of phases is common during the course of an illness and the dying process.
- Provide an atmosphere of care and concern (e.g., provide privacy, be available and nonjudgmental, display empathy and respect). *Action helps client to feel free to express feelings.*
- Perform actions to promote trust (e.g., answer questions honestly, provide requested information).
- Encourage the verbal expression of anger and sadness about anticipated losses; recognize displacement of anger and assist client to see the actual cause of angry feelings and resentment; establish limits on abusive behavior if demonstrated. *Allows client time to express concerns and fears and feel that they are heard. Helps client work through issues associated with imminent death.*
- Encourage client to express feelings in whatever ways are comfortable (e.g., writing, drawing, conversation).
- Assist client to identify and use techniques that have helped him/her cope in previous situations of loss.
- If desired by client, assist with after-death arrangements (e.g., funeral, religious service, who should be called). *Allows client a measure of control over future events when they are no longer here.*
- Perform actions to assist the client to maintain a positive self-concept and feel good about the life he/she has experienced: *Use of personal clothing helps client to maintain his/her identity.*
  - Visit frequently and encourage verbalization about past events, life accomplishments, interests, and feelings.
  - Help client to focus on positive rather than negative aspects of his/her life experience. *Provides closure for client in relation to their life and life experiences. The more involved the client is in self-care, the more they feel they have control of care.*
  - Maintain a nonjudgmental attitude about the kind of life client has led and his/her beliefs.
  - Encourage participation in decisions about care.
  - Encourage and assist client with good physical hygiene and grooming; suggest use of personal rather than hospital clothing.
- Support behaviors suggesting successful grief work (e.g., verbalizing feelings about dying, statements reflecting that dying is difficult but a part of life, comfortable and realistic remembrances about significant relationships, use of available support systems). *The nurse should be available to spend time with client and encourage family and friends to be involved in celebrating client's life with them.*
- Explain the phases of the grieving process to SO; encourage their support and understanding.

NDx = NANDA Diagnosis   **D** = Delegatable Action   ● = UAP   ✦ = LVN/LPN   ⊜▶ = Go to ⊜volve for animation

Continued...

THERAPEUTIC INTERVENTIONS	RATIONALE
• Facilitate communication between the client and SO; be aware that they may be in different phases of the grieving process.	*Helps family and others to understand what the client is going through and what their role can be in the process.*
• Provide information about counseling services and support groups that might assist client and SO in working through grief.	*The client and family members may require counseling to work through the grief and loss processes.*
Consult spiritual advisor or pastor.	*Allows client to obtain spiritual support and work to get "right" with God if they are interested in this aspect of life.*
Dependent/Collaborative Actions	
Consult appropriate health care provider (e.g., hospice nurse, palliative care nurse, psychiatric nurse clinician, physician) regarding a referral for counseling if signs of dysfunctional grieving (e.g., persistent denial of terminal state, excessive anger or sadness, emotional lability) occur.	*Consulting the appropriate health care provider allows for modification of the treatment plan.*

Nursing Diagnosis RISK FOR SPIRITUAL DISTRESS NDx

Definition: Susceptible to an impaired ability to experience and integrate meaning and purpose in life through connectedness with self, literature, nature, and/or a power greater than oneself, which may compromise health.

Related to:
• Challenged belief and value system as a result of intense or prolonged suffering and imminent death
• Separation from religious/cultural ties
• Overwhelming grief and sense of hopelessness

CLINICAL MANIFESTATIONS

Subjective	Objective
Verbalization of conflict about beliefs and relationship with deity; reports of anger toward God; questioning the purpose for suffering; verbalizing that illness and imminent death are a punishment	Refusal to participate in usual religious practices or to have visits from clergy; apathy; hostility; withdrawal

RISK FACTORS	DESIRED OUTCOMES
• Active dying • Chronic illness • Pain • Social alienation	The client will not experience spiritual distress as evidenced by: a. Expression of a sense of spiritual well-being b. Participation in usual religious/spiritual practices when possible c. Maintaining connectedness with SO

NOC OUTCOMES	NIC INTERVENTIONS
Hope; spiritual health	Hope; inspiration; spiritual support; grief work facilitation; coping enhancement; dying care

NURSING ASSESSMENT	RATIONALE
Assess client's religious/spiritual beliefs and practices: • Verbalization of conflict about beliefs and relationship with deity • Reports of anger toward God • Questioning the purpose for suffering • Verbalizing that illness and imminent death are a punishment • Refusal to participate in usual religious practices or to have visits from clergy • Apathy, hostility, withdrawal	*Provides baseline understanding of client's beliefs.*

NURSING ASSESSMENT	RATIONALE
Assess for signs and symptoms of spiritual distress.	*Early recognition of signs and symptoms of spiritual distress allows for prompt intervention.*

THERAPEUTIC INTERVENTIONS	RATIONALE

Independent Actions

Implement measures to promote a sense of spiritual well-being:

- Give client permission to express feelings and concerns about his/her religious/spiritual beliefs.
- Maintain a nonjudgmental attitude about client's beliefs and any inner conflicts client is experiencing.
- Encourage client to use available spiritual resources (e.g., clergy, prayer, religious rituals) for support.
- Perform actions to facilitate the grieving process. Encourage verbalization of anger (e.g., allow time for client to progress through phases of grief).
- Perform actions to reduce feelings of hopelessness (e.g., allow client to exert control over activities as much as possible).

Dependent/Collaborative Actions

Consult appropriate resource (e.g., clergy, psychiatric nurse clinician, physician, palliative care nurse, hospice nurse) if signs and symptoms of spiritual distress occur and client's response is inappropriate and/or destructive.

Spirituality, whether it is religion or other beliefs, has been associated with decreased despair in patients at the end of life.

Provide support based on client's specific beliefs

This gives the client time to work through the grieving process and may reduce experience of anxiety.

Consulting the appropriate health care provider allows for modification of the treatment plan.

Nursing Diagnosis **HOPELESSNESS** NDx

Definition: Subjective state in which an individual sees limited or no alternatives or personal choices available and is unable to mobilize energy on own behalf.

Related to: Deteriorating physical condition, feelings of abandonment, loss of belief in religious/cultural values, and inability to reach self-fulfillment associated with terminal state

CLINICAL MANIFESTATIONS

Subjective	Objective
Statements of feeling hopeless	Decreased response to SO; decreased participation in self-care and decision-making; decreased verbalization; flat affect

RISK FACTORS

- Long-term stress
- Deteriorating physical condition
- Terminal illness

DESIRED OUTCOMES

The client will maintain hope as evidenced by:
a. Verbal expression of same
b. Maintenance of satisfying relationships with others
c. Participation in self-care and decision-making as able
d. Identification of realistic goals

NOC OUTCOMES

Hope; decision-making; quality of life; spiritual well-being

NIC INTERVENTIONS

Decision-making support; presence; grief work facilitation; hope instillation

---

NDx = NANDA Diagnosis   **D** = Delegatable Action   ● = UAP   ✦ = LVN/LPN   ⊖▶ = Go to ℮volve for animation

NURSING ASSESSMENT	RATIONALE
Assess client for signs and symptoms of hopelessness: • Decreased response to SO • Decreased participation in self-care and decision-making • Decreased verbalization • Flat affect • Statements of feeling hopeless	*Early recognition of signs and symptoms of hopelessness allows for prompt intervention.*

THERAPEUTIC INTERVENTIONS	RATIONALE
Independent Actions Implement measures to assist client to reduce feelings of hopelessness: • Perform actions to facilitate the grieving process: • Provide an atmosphere of care and concern.	*Grieving occurs in phases or stages over time.* *Stages must be allowed to occur in order to reduce the risk for dysfunctional grieving.*
• Perform actions to promote a sense of spiritual well-being (e.g., encourage client to use available spiritual resources). • Allow client to retain as much control as possible over activities of daily living; involve client in as much self-care and decision-making as feasible.	*Spiritual support can be a great source of strength and solace to the client and can facilitate resolution of grief.* *Provides client a sense of control over life and care.*
• Assist client to identify goals that are achievable in the time that client has left, ways to continue working toward goals previously set even if not possible to achieve them totally, and the purpose remaining in client's life such as role model or advisor to SO.	*Helps client to see purpose in their end-of-life journey and ability to impact others.*
Dependent/Collaborative Actions Consult appropriate health care provider (e.g., palliative care nurse, hospice nurse, psychiatric nurse clinician, physician) if client demonstrates increased feelings of hopelessness.	*Consulting the appropriate health care provider allows for modification of the treatment plan.*

Nursing Diagnosis   INTERRUPTED FAMILY PROCESSES NDx

Definition: Break in the continuity of family functioning which fails to support the well-being of its members.

Related to: Excessive anxiety, grief, disorganization, and current and future role changes within the family unit, inadequate support systems, and fatigue

CLINICAL MANIFESTATIONS

Subjective	Objective
Statements of not being able to accept client's imminent death or to make necessary role and lifestyle changes, verbalization of guilt	Inability to make decisions; infrequent visits; inappropriate response to client's situation; preoccupation with other aspects of life; negative family interactions

RISK FACTORS
• Situational crisis
• Shift in health status of family member
• Terminal illness

DESIRED OUTCOMES
The family members will demonstrate beginning adjustment to loss of client and changes in family roles and structure as evidenced by:
a. Verbalization of ways to adapt to required role and lifestyle changes
b. Active participation in decision-making and client's care
c. Positive interactions with one another

NOC OUTCOMES

Family coping; family functioning; family resiliency; family normalization

NIC INTERVENTIONS

Family involvement promotion; family process maintenance; family support; caregiver support; support system enhancement

NURSING ASSESSMENT

Assess for signs and symptoms of interrupted family processes:
- Statements of not being able to accept client's imminent death or to make necessary role and lifestyle changes
- Verbalization of guilt
- Inability to make decisions
- Infrequent visits
- Inappropriate response to client's situation
- Preoccupation with other aspects of life
- Negative family interactions

Identify components of the family and their patterns of communication and role expectations.

RATIONALE

Early recognition of signs and symptoms of interrupted family processes allows for prompt intervention.

THERAPEUTIC INTERVENTIONS

Independent Actions

Implement measures to facilitate family members' adjustment to imminent loss of client and altered family roles and structure:
- Encourage and assist family members to verbalize feelings about the death of the client and the effect of it on their lifestyle and family structure; actively listen to each family member and maintain a nonjudgmental attitude about feelings shared.
- Assist family members to confront the reality of the client's imminent death when they are ready; encourage them to imagine life after death of the client and to set some personal goals if appropriate.
- Provide privacy so that family members can share their feelings and grief with one another; stress the importance of and facilitate the use of good communication techniques.
- Explain the phases of grieving and assist family members to progress through their own grieving process; explain that they may encounter times when they need to focus on meeting their own rather than the client's needs.
- Emphasize the need for family members to obtain adequate rest and nutrition and to identify and use stress management techniques so that they are better able to emotionally and physically deal with the death of the client; assure them that the client will be well cared for in their absence.
- Encourage and assist family members to identify coping strategies for dealing with the client's death and its effect on those left behind.
- Include family members in decision-making about client and his/her care; convey appreciation of their input and continued support of the client.
- Encourage and allow family members to participate in client's care if desired by both client and family members.
- Assist family members to make necessary postmortem arrangements for or with the client (e.g., funeral home, burial place, clergy visitation).

RATIONALE

Client and family member must be given time to openly and honestly express feelings to facilitate the grieving process.

Discussion of feelings helps the client and family work through the grieving process.

Assistance with funeral planning may be needed, based on the coping abilities of the family.

Work with family to assure that they are able to deal with the stress of loss and ability to support client until that time.

Helps the family members determine what works best for them and to implement those processes.

Allows family and client to be involved in client care.

NDx = NANDA Diagnosis   **D** = Delegatable Action   ● = UAP   ✦ = LVN/LPN   ⊖▶ = Go to ⊖volve for animation

Continued...

THERAPEUTIC INTERVENTIONS	RATIONALE

• Provide information to family members about:
  • The current status of client.
  • Behaviors to expect as the client progresses through terminal stages of disease and his/her own grieving.
  • Physical signs and symptoms of approaching death (e.g., decrease in appetite and thirst; lack of interest in environment; withdrawal from relationships; disorientation; restlessness; agitation; vision-like experiences; "out-of-character" statements or requests; increased sleeping; incontinence; decreased level of consciousness; reduced urine output; cool, mottled extremities; respiratory sounds such as gurgling or rattling, labored breathing, or periods of no breathing).
  • Ways they can best assist in meeting client's needs.
	Keeps family members informed on client's condition and what they can expect in the dying process.

• When appropriate, help and encourage family members to "let go" of client and say goodbye.	*Family members must be given time to acknowledge sadness, forgive one another, and say goodbye.*
• Assist family members to identify resources that can assist them in coping with their feelings and in meeting their immediate and long-term needs (e.g., counseling and social services; pastoral care; service, bereavement, and church groups; hospice); initiate a referral if indicated.	*Provides for continuum of care for family members.*
• Assist family members to contact appropriate persons (e.g., funeral home director, clergy) when death occurs.	
Dependent/Collaborative Actions Consult appropriate health care provider (e.g., hospice nurse, palliative care nurse, physician) if family members continue to demonstrate difficulty adjusting to the loss of the client and role changes within the family unit.	*Consulting the appropriate health care provider allows for modification of the treatment plan.*

ADDITIONAL NURSING DIAGNOSES

NAUSEA NDx/IMPAIRED COMFORT NDx
Related to:
• An accumulation of gas and fluid in the gastrointestinal GI tract associated with decreased gastrointestinal GI motility resulting from depressant effect of some medications (e.g., narcotic [opioid] analgesics) and decreased activity and nausea

RISK FOR DEFICIENT FLUID VOLUME NDx
Related to:
• Decreased oral intake and increased fluid loss associated with vomiting and/or diaphoresis if client has a fever

IMPAIRED PHYSICAL MOBILITY NDx
Related to:
• Weakness and fatigue
• Dyspnea and/or sensory and motor deficits (can occur as a result of the underlying disease process)
• Reluctance to move associated with pain and nausea if present
• Decreased level of consciousness

IMPAIRED ORAL MUCOUS MEMBRANE NDx (DRYNESS AND IRRITATION) START
Related to:
• Decreased salivation associated with decreased oral intake and some medications (e.g., tricyclic antidepressants, anticholinergics, narcotic [opioid] analgesics, phenothiazines)
• Deficient fluid volume associated with decreased fluid intake and increased fluid loss
• Prolonged oxygen therapy (especially if administered by mask)
• Mouth breathing
• Inadequate nutritional status

SELF-CARE DEFICIT (BATHING, DRESSING FEEDING AND TOILETING) NDx
Related to:
• Weakness and fatigue
• Activity limitations associated with the underlying disease process
• Pain, nausea, dyspnea, and/or disturbed thought processes if present
• Decreased level of consciousness

DISTURBED SLEEP PATTERN **NDx**
Related to:
* Decreased physical activity, fear, anxiety, unfamiliar environment, discomfort, and inability to assume usual sleep position associated with orthopnea if present

RISK FOR FALLS **NDx**
Related to:
* Weakness, fatigue, and attempting activity unassisted because of agitation or confusion

RISK FOR CONSTIPATION **NDx**
Related to:
* Diminished defecation reflex associated with decreased nervous system responses in terminal state, suppression of the urge to defecate because of reluctance to use bedpan, and decreased gravity filling of lower rectum resulting from horizontal positioning
* Decreased ability to respond to the urge to defecate associated with weakened abdominal muscles, impaired physical mobility, and decreased level of consciousness
* Decreased GI motility associated with decreased activity, increased sympathetic nervous system activity that occurs with anxiety, and use of some medications (e.g., narcotic [opioid] analgesics, antacids containing aluminum or calcium)
* Decreased intake of fluids and foods high in fiber

Bibliography

GENERAL BIBLIOGRAPHY

Ackley B, Ladwig G, Makic, M. *Nursing Diagnosis Handbook: An Evidence-based Guide to Planning Care.* 11th ed. St Louis: Mosby-Elsevier; 2017.

Berman A, Snyder S, Jackson C. *Skills in Clinical Nursing.* 8th ed. Upper Saddle River, NJ: Pearson Prentice Hall; 2016.

Berman AJ, Snyder S, Kosier B, et al. *Fundamentals of Nursing: Concepts, Process, and Process.* 10th ed. Upper Saddle River, NJ: Prentice Hall; 2015.

Butcher HK, Bulechek GM, eds. *Nursing Interventions Classification (NIC).* 7th ed. St Louis: Mosby-Elsevier; 2018.

Frandsen G, Pennington S. *Abrams' Clinical Drug Therapy: Rationales for Nursing Practice.* 11th ed. Philadelphia: Lippincott Williams & Wilkins; 2017.

Gulanick M, Myers J. *Nursing Care Plans: Nursing Diagnosis and Intervention.* 9th ed. St Louis: Mosby-Elsevier; 2017.

Hartjes, T. ed. 7th ed. AACN Core Curriculum for High Acuity, Progressive, and Critical Care Nursing. St. Louis: Elsevier (2018).

Herdma H Kamitsuru S, eds. *NANDA International Nursing Diagnosis: Definitions & classification 2018–2020.* 11th ed. New York: Thieme; 2018.

Huether S, McCance K. Understanding Pathophysiology. 6th ed. St Louis: Mosby-Elsevier; 2016.

Ignatavicius D, Workman M, Rebar, C. *Medical-Surgical Nursing: Concepts for Interprofessional Collaborative Care.* 9th ed. Philadelphia: Saunders; 2018.

Jarvis C. *Physical Examination & Health Assessment.* 7th ed. St Louis: Saunders-Elsevier; 2016.

Lewis S, Bucher L, Heitkemper M, et al. *Medical-Surgical Nursing: Assessment and Management of Clinical Problems.* 10th ed. St. Louis: Mosby-Elsevier; 2017.

McCance K, Huether S. *Pathophysiology: The Biologic Basis for Disease in Adults and Children.* 8th ed. St Louis: Mosby-Elsevier; 2019.

Moorhead S, Johnson M, Maas M, et al. *Nursing Outcomes Classification (NOC).* 6th ed. St Louis: Mosby-Elsevier; 2018.

Pagana K, Pagana T. *Mosby's Diagnostic and Laboratory Test References.* 13th ed. St Louis: Mosby-Elsevier; 2017.

Perry A, Potter P. *Clinical Nursing Skills & Techniques.* 9th ed. St Louis: Mosby-Elsevier; 2018.

Potter A, Perry P. *Fundamentals of Nursing.* 9th ed. St Louis: Mosby-Elsevier; 2017.

Sartorius-Mergenthaler S. Complementary and alternative care initiatives. In: Hoffman J, Sullivan N, eds. *Medical-Surgical Nursing: Making Connections to Practice.* Philadelphia: F. A. Davis; 2017:202-212.

Sole M, Klein D, Moseley M. *Introduction to Critical Care Nursing.* 7th ed. St Louis: Saunders; 2017.

Swearingen P, Wright J. *All-In-One Care Planning Resource.* 5th ed. St Louis: Mosby-Elsevier; 2019.

Urden, JD, Stacy, KM, Lough, ME. Critical Care Nursing: Diagnosis and Management. 8th ed. St. Louis: Mosby. 2018.

Van Leeuwen A, Bladh M. *Davis's Comprehensive Handbook of Laboratory and Diagnostic Tests with Nursing Implications.* 7th ed. Philadelphia: F. A. Davis; 2017.

CHAPTER-BY-CHAPTER BIBLIOGRAPHY

1 PRIORITIZATION, DELEGATION, AND CRITICAL THINKING IN CLIENT MANAGEMENT

Alfaro-Lefevre R. *Critical Thinking and Clinical Judgment: A Practical Approach to Outcome-Focused Thinking.* 6th ed. St Louis: Elsevier; 2017.

ANA and NCSBN. Joint Statement on Delegation American Nurses Association (ANA) and the National Council of State Boards of Nursing (NCSBN). 2018. Available at: www.ncsbn.org/Joint_statement.pdf.

Hansten R, Jackson M. *Clinical Delegation Skills: A Handbook for Clinical Practice.* 4th ed. Sudbury, Mass: Jones and Bartlett; 2009.

LaCharity L, Kumagai C, Bartz B. *Prioritization, Delegation & Assignment: Practice Exercises for Medical-Surgical Nursing.* 5th ed. St Louis: Mosby-Elsevier; 2019.

National Council of State Boards of Nursing. National guidelines for nursing delegation. *J Nurs Regulation.* 2016;7(1):5-14.

Silvestri L. *Saunders Comprehensive Review for the NCLEX-RN® Examination.* 7th ed. St. Louis: Saunders; 2017.

2 NURSE-SENSITIVE INDICATORS

Agency for Healthcare Research and Quality. Preventing pressure ulcers in hospitals: are we ready for this change? 2014. Available at: https://www.ahrq.gov/professionals/systems/hospital/pressureulcertoolkit/putool1.html.

Agency for Healthcare Research and Quality. Understanding quality measurement. 2017. Available at: https://www.ahrq.gov/professionals/quality-patient-safety/quality-resources/tools/chtoolbx/understand/index.html.

American Nurses Association. The national database of nursing quality indicators (NDNQI). 2017. Available at: http://ojin.nursingworld.org/MainMenuCategories/ANAMarketplace/ANAPeriodicals/OJIN/TableofContents/Volume122007/No3Sept07/NursingQualityIndicators.html.

Centers for Disease Control. Strategies to prevent ventilated—associated pneumonia in acute care hospitals: 2014 update. 2014. Available at: http://www.jstor.org/stable/10.1086/677144.

Centers for Disease Control. Strategies to prevention central line—associated blood stream infections in acute care hospitals: 2014 update. 2014. Available at: http://www.jstor.org/stable/10.1086/676533.

Centers for Disease Control. Guideline for the prevention of catheter—associated urinary tract infections 2009. 2017. Available at: https://www.cdc.gov/infectioncontrol/pdf/guidelines/cauti-guidelines.pdf.

Centers for Disease Control. HAI data and statistics. 2018. Available at: https://www.cdc.gov/hai/surveillance/index.html.

Heslop L, Lu S. Nursing—sensitive indicators: a concept analysis. *J Adv Nurs.* 2014;70(11):2469-2482.

Institute of Medicine. Crossing the quality chasm: The IOM healthcare quality initiative. 2006. Available at: http://www.nationalacademies.org/hmd/Global/News%20Announcements/Crossing-the-Quality-Chasm-The-IOM-Health-Care-Quality-Initiative.aspx.

Klompas M, Branson R, Eichenwald E. Strategies to prevent ventilator—associated pneumonia in acute care hospitals: 2014 update. 2014.

Available at: http://www.jstor.org/stable/10.1086/677144

Lo E, Nicolle N, Coffin S, et al. SHEA/IDSA practice recommendation: Strategies to prevent catheter—associated urinary tract infections in acute care hospitals: 2014 update. 2014. Available at: http://www.jstor.org/stable/10.1086/675718.

Marschall J, Mermel L, Fakih M, et al. Strategies to prevent central-line associated blood stream infections in acute care hospitals: 2014 update. 2015. Available at: http://www.jstor.org/stable/10.1086/676533

National Pressure Ulcer Advisory Panel, European Pressure Ulcer Advisory Panel and Pan Pacific Pressure Injury Alliance. *Prevention and Treatment of Pressure Ulcers: Quick Reference Guide.* In: Emily Haesler, ed. *Osborne Park.* Western Australia: Cambridge Media; 2014.

National Pressure Ulcer Advisory Panel. Pressure injury prevention points. n.d. Available at: http://www.npuap.org/wp-content/uploads/2016/04/Pressure-Injury-Prevention-Points-2016.pdf.

National Pressure Ulcer Advisory Panel. New 2014 prevention and treatment of pressure ulcers: Clinical practice guideline. 2014. Available at: http://www.npuap.org/resources/educational-and-clinical-resources/prevention-and-treatment-of-pressure-ulcers-clinical-practice-guideline/.

National Pressure Ulcer Advisory Panel. NPUAP pressure injury stages. 2016. Available at: http://www.npuap.org/resources/educational-and-clinical-resources/npuap-pressure-injury-stages/.

Rechtoris, M. Becker's healthcare: Hospital review: 7 facts on patient falls. 2017. Available at: https://www.beckersasc.com/asc-quality-infection-control/7-facts-on-patient-falls.html.

Staggs V, Davidson J, Dunton N, et al. Challenges in defining and categorizing falls on diverse unit types: lessons from expansion of the NDNQI falls indicator. *J Nurs Care Qual.* 2015;30(2):106-112.

The Joint Commission. Preventing Pressure Injuries. 2016. Available at: https://www.jointcommission.org/assets/1/23/Quick_Safety_Issue_25_July_20161.PDF.

4 NURSING CARE OF THE CLIENT HAVING SURGERY

American Society of Anesthesiologists. Continuum of depth of sedation: definition of general anesthesia and levels of sedation/analgesia. 2014.

Available at: http://www.asahq.org/~/media/Sites/ASAHQ/Files/Public/Resources/standards-guidelines/continuum-of-depth-of-sedation-definition-of-general-anesthesia-and-levels-of-sedation-analgesia.pdf. Accessed January 1, 2018.

American Association of Nurse Anesthetists. Non-anesthesia provider procedural sedation and analgesia: policy considerations. 2016. Available at: https://www.aana.com/docs/default-source/practice-aana-com-web-documents-(all)/non-anesthesia-provider-procedural-sedation-and-analgesia.pdf?sfvrsn=670049b1_2. Accessed January 1, 2018.

American Society of PeriAnesthesia Nurses. 2019-2020 *Perianesthesia Nursing Standards, Practice Recommendations and Interpretive Statements.* New Jersey: ASPAN; 2018.

Heuer, A., & Kossick, M. A. (2017). Update on Guidelines for Perioperative Antibiotic Selection and Administration From the Surgical Care Improvement Project (SCIP) and American Society of Health-System Pharmacists. AANA Journal, 85(4), 293–299. Retrieved from https://search-ebscohost-com.ezproxy.net.ucf.edu/login.aspx?direct=true&db=rzh&AN=124667338&site=eds-live&scope=site

Odom-Forren J, Watson, DS. *Practical Guide to Moderate Sedation/Analgesia.* 2nd ed. St. Louis, MO: Mosby; 2005.

Paser, C., McCaffery, M. Pain assessment and pharmacological management. 1st ed. St. Louis: Mosby Elsevier.

Schick, L., Windle P eds. Peranesthesisa Nursing Core Curriculum: Preprocedure, Phase I, and Phase II PACU Nursing. 3rd ed. St. Louis: Elsevier; 2016.

The Joint Commission on Accreditation of Healthcare Organizations. Speak-up: the universal protocol for preventing wrong site, wrong procedure, and wrong person surgery. n.d. Available at: https://www.jointcommission.org/assets/1/18/UP_Poster1.PDF. Accessed January 15, 2018.

The Joint Commission (2010). Specifications manual for Joint Commission national quality core measures: Surgical care improvement project (SCIP). Available from https://manual.jointcommission.org/releases/archive/TJC2010B/SurgicalCareImprovementProject.html

5 THE CLIENT WITH ALTERATIONS IN RESPIRATORY FUNCTION

Agency for Healthcare Research and Quality (AHRQ). Preventing hospital - associated venous thromboembolism: A guide for effective quality improvement. (2016). Available from https://www.ahrq.gov/sites/default/files/wysiwyg/professionals/quality-patient-safety/patient-safety-resources/resources/vtguide/vteguide.pdf

American Society of Hematology Clinical Practice Guidelines on Venous Thromboembolism 2018. Available from https://www.hematology.org/VTE/

Gao, S., Zhang, Z., Aragon, J., Brunelli, A., Cassivi, S......& Zhou, Q. The society for translational medicine: clinical practice guidelines for the postoperative mangaement of chest tube for patients undergoing lobectomy. Journal of Thoracic Disease, 9(9), 3255-3264 (2017).

Global Initiative for Chronic Obstructive Lung Disease (2019). Global initiative for chronic obstructive lung disease. Retrieved from https://goldcopd.org/wp-content/uploads/2018/11/GOLD-2019-v1.7-FINAL-14Nov2018-WMS.pdf

Hsu, J., Sircar, K., Herman, E., & Garbe, P. EXHALE: A technical package to control asthma. Asthma and Community Health Branch Division Centers for Disease Control and Prevention. Available from https://www.cdc.gov/asthma/pdfs/EXHALE_technical_package-508.pdf

International Council of Nurses. TB Guidelines for Nurses in the Care and Control of Tuberculosis and Multi-drug Resistant TB. 3rd ed. International Council of Nurses (2015). Available from https://www.icn.ch/sites/default/files/inline-files/tb_mdrtb_guideline.pdf

Kalil et al. (2016). Management of Adults With Hospital-acquired and Ventilator-associated Pneumonia: 2016 Clinical Practice Guidelines by the Infectious Diseases Society of America and the American Thoracic Society. Available from https://watermark.silverchair.com/ciw353.pdf?token=AQECAHi208BE49Ooan9kkhW_Ercy7Dm3ZL_9Cf3qfKAc485ysgAAAjgwggI0BgkqhkiG9w0BBwagggIlMIICIQIBADCCAhoGCSqGSIb3DQEHAT AeBglghkgBZQMEAS4wEQQQMw4_kcsoCvBTHSVa7AgEQgIIB633vq CUkqZ6Fc7C2-7HCp8fWORFG WttlXYwTW0nCpqMeYafwdcCTPiG2j oT2UrgFA3u8kPMOFjeu0qCo_-iQvpu W_mcRvyfPXjiBtK8FkLp1PnPBIf_

zc_doFNJfwdaskUOdE_q5ynay
FGbwwFcziUHZraH3WmqEpn
Mm9Gn4bvN8csB2Tp3DuflEO5
dsPvSinapRq5p5PN2lGUtyTTqQY
qt-4XTYQSTh6-97XzdUFe00_Aiq75
A3DyU6ycVAkzEfgkW9_kijNKWg
ZITOT5KXx0ug0_qBt4jodQr9
D-qT39QPTvQYTxPJKIVQbPGTT
ThqfwuZ_Icspd5BCpfe5k0XN
MeukzO5wqAbX0OCvb8d_VDK4
Ao542d5ASK7F3O5laqhT7w76vyv
R3yHSn-cX0B9cYHsh5mQ-7sMz
UsEj191BOuC6WjbdbRgrqaeUhdcj
IYRF24DexhpqvNPB0rufJmHcd
AEk5Ye1JlQUToZvCa_FNg6o3s
CLjzTY5yFk75QTBwxY-1dNuUAJVa
EfIijyjBsxUFtZayVz3oMKTDXhs
3mboE6CxT5oBWyaORdn

Mandell et al. (2007). Infectious Diseases Society of America/American Thoracic Society Consensus Guidelines on the Management of Community-Acquired Pneumonia in Adults. Available from https://www.cdc.gov/pneumonia/management-prevention-guidelines.html

Nici, L., ZuWallack, R. An official american thoracic society workshop report: The integrated care of the COPD patient. Retrieved from https://www.atsjournals.org/doi/pdf/10.1513/pats.201201-014ST

Ouellette D. Pulmonary embolism guidelines. 2017. Available at: https://emedicine.medscape.com/article/300901-guidelines#showall.

World Health Organization (2017). Update: Guidelines for treatment of drug-susceptible tuberculosis and patient care. World Health Organization. Available from: https://apps.who.int/iris/bitstream/handle/10665/255052/9789241550000-eng.pdf

World Health Organization (2010). Guidelines for the treatment of tuberculosis. World Health Organization. Available from https://www.who.int/tb/publications/2010/9789241547833/en/

6 THE CLIENT WITH ALTERATIONS IN CARDIOVASCULAR FUNCTION

American Heart Association. Heart failure guidelines go-to-guide. 2017. Available at: http://hfguidelines.ksw-gtg.com/publication/?i=451480#{"issue_id":451480,"page":16}.

American Heart Association. Angina pectoris. 2018. Available at: http://www.heart.org/HEARTORG/Conditions/HeartAttack/DiagnosingaHeartAttack/Angina-Pectoris-Stable-Angina_UCM_437515_Article.jsp#.Wpsv-kxFzOb.

Coven D, Shirani J, Kalyanasundaram A. Acute coronary guidelines. 2016. Available at: https://emedicine.medscape.com/article/1910735-guidelines.

Ellenbogen, K, Wilkoff, B., Kay, N., Lau, C.P. Auricchio. Clinical Cardiac Pacing, Defibrillation, and Resynchronization Therapy. 5th ed. St. Louis: Elsevier.

Hickey, JV. The Clinical Practice of Neurological and Neurosurgical Nursing 8th ed. Solters Kluwer; 2020

Society for Vascular Surgery. Surgical bypass. n.d. Available at: https://vascular.org/patient-resources/vascular-treatments/surgical-bypass.

Society for Vascular Surgery. Vascular conditions. n.d. Available at: https://vascular.org/patient-resources/vascular-conditions/abdominal-aortic-aneurysm.

Topol EJ. *Textbook of Interventional Cardiology*. 4th ed. Philadelphia: Saunders; 2003.

Whelton et al. (2018). 2017 ACC/AHA/AAPA/ABC/ACPM/AGS/APhA/ASH/ASPC/NMA/PCNA Guideline for the Prevention, Detection, Evaluation, and Management of High Blood Pressure in Adults: A Report of the American College of Cardiology/American Heart Association Task Force on Clinical Practice Guidelines. Hypertension, 71(6), e13-e115

Yancy CW, Jessup M., Bozkurt B, et al. ACC/AHA/HDFSA focused update of the 2013 ACFF/AHA guideline for the management of heart failure: a report of the American College of Cardiology/American Heart Association Task Force on clinical practice guidelines and the heart failure society of America. *J Card Fail.* 2017;23(8):628-651.

7 THE CLIENT WITH ALTERATIONS IN NEUROLOGICAL FUNCTION

Alzheimer's Assocation. 2017 Alzheimer's disease facts and figures. 2017. Available at: https://www.alz.org/documents_custom/2017-facts-and-figures.pdf. Accessed January 19, 2017.

Alzheimer's Association. Wandering and getting lost. 2017. Available at: https://m.alz.org/wandering.asp. Accessed February 6, 2018.

Carney N, Totten, AM, O'Reilly C, et al. Guidelines for the Management of Severe Traumatic Brain Injury. 2016. Available at: https://www.braintrauma.org/uploads/13/06/Guidelines_for_Management_of_Severe_TBI_4th_Edition.pdf. Accessed February 9, 2017.

Friedland DP. Improving the classification of traumatic brain injury: the Mayo classification system for traumatic brain injury severity. *J Spine*. 2013;S4:005. doi:10.4172/2165-7939.S4-005.

Geeraerts, T., Velly, L., Abdennour, L., Asehnoune, K., Audibert, G., Bouzat, P., ... Payen, J.-F. (2018). Management of severe traumatic brain injury (first 24hours). Anaesthesia, Critical Care & Pain Medicine, 37(2), 171–186. https://doi-org.ezproxy.net.ucf.edu/10.1016/j.accpm.2017.12.001

Hadley, M.N., & Walters, B.C. (2013). Introduction to the guidelines for the management of acute cervical spine and spinal cord injuries. Neurosurgery, 72(3), 5-16.

Hemphill 3rd, J. C., Greenberg, S. M., Anderson, C. S., Becker, K., Bendok, B. R., Cushman, M., ... Hemphill, J. C., 3rd. (2015). Guidelines for the Management of Spontaneous Intracerebral Hemorrhage: A Guideline for Healthcare Professionals From the American Heart Association/American Stroke Association. Stroke (00392499), 46(7), 2032–2060. https://doi-org.ezproxy.net.ucf.edu/10.1161/STR.0000000000000069

Kirshblum SC, Burns SP, Biering-Sorensen F, et al. International standards for neurological classification of spinal cord injury. *J Spinal Cord Med.* 2011;34(6):535-546. doi:10.1179/2045 7711X13207446293695.

National Institute for Health and Care Excellence. Parkinson's disease in adults. NICE Guideline [NG71]. July 2017. www.nice.org.uk/guidance/ng71 (accessed April 2018).

Parkinson's Foundation. Statistics. 2018. Available at: http://parkinson.org/Understanding-Parkinsons/Causes-and-Statistics/Statistics.

Powers, W. J., Rabinstein, A. A., Ackerson, T., Adeoye, O. M., Bambakidis, N. C., Becker, K., & Biller, J. (2018). 2018 Guidelines for the Early Management of Patients With Acute Ischemic Stroke: A Guideline for Healthcare Professionals From the American Heart Association/American Stroke Association. Stroke, (3), 46. https://doi.org/10.1161/STR.0000000000000158

Ramesh, V. J., & Chakrabarti, D. (2018). Guidelines for the Management of Severe Traumatic Brain Injury, Fourth Edition. Neurosurgery, 82(5), E143. Retrieved from https://search.ebscohost.com/login.aspx?direct=true&db=edo&AN=129172994&site=eds-live&scope=site

Sacco R, Kasner S, Broderick J, et al. An updated definition of stroke for the 21st century. 2013. Available at: http://stroke. ahajournals.org/content/44/7/2064. Accessed February 6, 2018.

8   THE CLIENT WITH ALTERATIONS IN HEMATOLOGIC AND IMMUNE FUNCTION

Al-Khafaji A, Sharma S, Eschun G, et al. Multiple Organ Dysfunction Syndrome in Sepsis. *Medscape.* https://emedicine.medscape.com/ January 2018. Accessed April 27, 2018.

Bonsall L. Management of Sepsis and Septic Shock, Lippincott Nursing Center. 2018. Available at: https:// www.nursingcenter.com/clinical-resources/guideline-summaries/ management-of-sepsis-and-septic-shock.

Brotfain E, Koyfman L, Toledano R, et al. Positive fluid balance as a major predictor of clinical outcome of patients with sepsis/septic shock after ICU discharge. *Am J Emerg Med.* 2016;34(11):2122-2126.

Centers for Disease Control and Prevention. HIV/AIDS Guidelines and Recommendations. December, 2018. Available at: https://www.cdc.gov/hiv/ guidelines/.

Fagan B. Sepsis 3: definitions, identification and management. *Can J Crit Care Nurs.* 2018;29(2): 36-37.

Guberski T. Coordinating care for patients with HIV. In: Hoffman J, Sullivan N, eds. *Medical-Surgical Nursing: Making connections to practice.* Philadelphia: F. A. Davis; 2017: 408-420.

Kalil, A & Bailey, K. Septic Shock Treatment & Management. *Medscape.* Available at: https://emedicine. medscape.com/article/168402-treatment. Accessed January, 2018.

Lester D, Haties T, Bennett A. A review of the revised sepsis care bundles: the rationale behind the new definitions, screening tools, and treatment guidelines. *Am J Nurs.* 2018;18(8): 40-45.

Levi M. Disseminated Intravascular Coagulation Treatment & Management. *Medscape.* https:// emedicine.medscape.com/ article/199627-treatment. Accessed October 07, 2018.

Levi M, Scully M. How I Treat In Brief: Managing Disseminated Intravascular Coagulation; Available at: https:// www.ashclinicalnews.org/training-education/managing-disseminated-intravascular-coagulation/. Accessed September 1, 2018.

Moyle S. What is sepsis? Guidelines for clinical nursing. Available at: https:// www.ausmed.com/articles/what-is-sepsis/. Accessed May, 2017.

National Institute of General Medication Sciences. Sepsis. Available at: https:// www.nigms.nih.gov/education/ Documents/Sepsis.pdf. Accessed January, 2018.

Reyes B, Chang J, Vaynberg L, et al. Early identification and management of sepsis in nursing facilities: challenges and opportunities. *J Am Med Directors Assoc.* 2018;19(6): 465-471.

Schorr C. Surviving sepsis campaign hour-1 bundle. *Am Nurse Today.* 2018;13(9):16-19.

Sepsis Alliance. Sepsis and DIC. 2017. Available at: https://www.sepsis.org/ sepsis-and-sepsisdisseminated-intravascular-coagulation-dic/.

Sevillano-Barbero M. Sepsis in adults: recognition and treatment in clinical guidelines. *Pract Nurs.* 2018;29(11): 544-548.

Sullivan N. Overview of shock and sepsis. In: Hoffman J, Sullivan N, eds. *Medical-Surgical Nursing: Making Connections to Practice.* Philadelphia: F. A. Davis; 2017:246-272.

Sirvent J, Ferri C, Baro A, et al. Fluid balance in sepsis and septic shock as a determining factor of mortality. *Am J Emerg Med.* 2015;33(2):186-189. doi:10.1016/j.ajem.2014.11.016.

US Department of Health and Human Services. AIDS Info Fact Sheets. December, 2018. Available at: https:// aidsinfo.nih.gov/understanding-hiv-aids/fact-sheets.

Vincent J, Abraham E, Kochanek P, et al. *Textbook of Critical Care.* 7th ed. Philadelphia: Elsevier; 2017.

World Health Organization. Guidelines for managing advanced HIV disease and rapid initiation of antiretroviral therapy. *World Health Organization;* 2017. Available at: https://www.who.int/hiv/pub/ guidelines/advanced-HIV-disease/en/.

9   THE CLIENT WITH ALTERATIONS IN METABOLIC FUNCTION

American Diabetes Association. Diabetes care in the hospital. Sec. 14 in Standards of Medical Care in Diabetes—2017. *Diabetes Care.* 2017;40(suppl 1):S120-S127.

American Diabetes Association. Glycemic targets. Sec. 6 in Standards of Medical Care in Diabetes—2017. *Diabetes Care.* 2017;40(suppl 1):S48-S56.

American Diabetes Association. Standards of medical care in diabetes—2017. *Diabetes Care.* 2017;40(suppl 1):S1-S135.

Beck et al. (2017). 2017 National Standards for Diabetes Self-Management Education and Support. Available from https://www. diabeteseducator.org/docs/default-source/practice/deap/standards/ nationalstandards_2017.pdf?sfvrsn=2

Dhatariya, K. K., & Vellanki, P. (2017). Treatment of Diabetic Ketoacidosis (DKA)/Hyperglycemic Hyperosmolar State (HHS): Novel Advances in the Management of Hyperglycemic Crises (UK Versus USA). Current Diabetes Reports, (5), 1. https://doi. org/10.1007/s11892-017-0857-4

Gosmanov AR, Gosmanova EO, Kitabchi AE. Hyperglycemic Crises: Diabetic Ketoacidosis (DKA), And Hyperglycemic Hyperosmolar State (HHS) [Updated 2015 May 19]. In: De Groot LJ, Chrousos G, Dungan K, et al., editors. Endotext [Internet]. South Dartmouth (MA): MDText.com, Inc.; 2000. Available at: https://www.ncbi. nlm.nih.gov/books/NBK279052/.

Liamis G, Liberopoulos E, Barkas F, et al. Diabetes mellitus and electrolyte disorders. *World J Clin Cases.* 2014;2(10):488-496.

Moghissi E, Korytkowski M, DiNardo M, et al. American Association of Clinical Endocrinologists and American Diabetes Association consensus statement on inpatient glycemic control. *Endocr Pract.* 2012; 15(4):1-17.

Ross et al. (2016). 2016 American Thyroid Association Guidelines for Diagnosis and Management of Hyperthyroidism and Other Causes of Thyrotoxicosis. Thyroid, 26(10), 1343-1421

10   THE CLIENT WITH ALTERATIONS IN THE GASTROINTESTINAL TRACT

Alison A. Taylor, Oliver C. Redfern, & Marinos Pericleous. (2014). The Management of Acute Upper Gastrointestinal Bleeding: A Comparison of Current Clinical Guidelines and Best Practice. European Medical Journal Gastroenterology, (1), 73. Retrieved from https://search.ebscohost.com/ login.aspx?direct=true&db=edsdoj&A N=edsdoj.90b4eb97f7e140f0ac47b160 e1227452&site=eds-live&scope=site

American Association of Critical Care Nurses. AACN practice alert: initial and ongoing verification of feeding tube placement in adults. *Crit Care Nurse.* 2016;36(2):e8-e13.

American Society for Metabolic and Bariatric Surgery. Bariatric surgery procedures. 2018. Available at:

https://asmbs.org/patients/bariatric-surgery-procedures.

Association of Stoma Nurses UK. ASCN Stoma Care: National Clinical Guidelines. 2016. Available at: http://ascnuk.com/wp-content/uploads/2016/03/ASCN-Clinical-Guidelines-Final-25-April-compressed-11-10-38.pdf.

Boullata, J. I., Carrera, A. L., Harvey, L., Escuro, A. A., Hudson, L., Mays, A., ... Guenter, P. (2017). ASPEN Safe Practices for Enteral Nutrition Therapy [Formula: see text]. JPEN. Journal Of Parenteral And Enteral Nutrition, 41(1), 15–103. https://doi.org/10.1177/0148607116673053

Clinical Practice Guidelines for the Perioperative Nutritional, Metabolic, and Nonsurgical Support of the Bariatric Surgery Patient—2013 Update: Cosponsored by American Association of Clinical Endocrinologists, The Obesity Society, and American Society for Metabolic & Bariatric Surgery. (2013). Surgery for Obesity and Related Diseases, (2), 159. https://doi.org/10.1016/j.soard.2012.12.010

Kim BSM, Li B, Engel A, et al. Diagnosis of gastrointestinal bleeding: a practical guide for clinicians. 2014. Available at: https://www.ncbi.nlm.nih.gov/pmc/articles/PMC4231512/.

Legome E, Geibel J. Blunt abdominal trauma. 2017. Available at: https://emedicine.medscape.com/article/1980980-overview.

Lichtenstein, G. R., Loftus, E. V., Jr, Isaacs, K. L., Regueiro, M. D., Gerson, L. B., & Sands, B. E. (2018). Correction: ACG Clinical Guideline: Management of Crohn's Disease in Adults. The American Journal Of Gastroenterology, 113(7), 1101. https://doi.org/10.1038/s41395-018-0120-x

McClave S, Taylor B, Martindale R, et al. Guidelines for the provision and assessment of nutrition support therapy in the adult critically ill patient: Society of critical care medicine (SCCN) and American society for parenteral and enteral nutrition (ASPEN). 2016. Available at: http://journals.sagepub.com/doi/pdf/10.1177/0148607115621863.

Rubin, D. T., Ananthakrishnan, A. N., Siegel, C. A., Sauer, B. G., & Long, M. D. (2019). ACG Clinical Guideline: Ulcerative Colitis in Adults. The American Journal Of Gastroenterology, 114(3), 384–413. https://doi.org/10.14309/ajg.0000000000000152

Satoh, K., Yoshino, J., Akamatsu, T., Itoh, T., Kato, M., Kamada, T., ... Shimosegawa, T. (2016). Evidence-based clinical practice guidelines for peptic ulcer disease 2015. Journal of Gastroenterology, (3), 177. https://doi.org/10.1007/s00535-016-1166-4

WOCN Society Clinical Guideline: Management of the Adult Patient With a Fecal or Urinary Ostomy—An Executive Summary. (2018). Journal of Wound, Ostomy & Continence Nursing, 45(1), 50–58. https://doi-org.ezproxy.net.ucf.edu/10.1097/WON.0000000000000396

11 NURSING CARE OF THE CLIENT WITH DISTURBANCES OF THE LIVER, BILIARY TRACT, AND PANCREAS

Bager P. The assessment and care of patients with hepatic encephalopathy. Br J Nurs. 2017;26(13):724-729.

Branstetter-Hall J, Felicilda-Reynaldo D. Antiviral medications, part 3: evidence-based treatment of Hepatitis B. MEDSURG Nurs. 2017;26(6):393-398.

Brenner P, Kautz D. Postoperative care of patients undergoing same-day laparoscopic cholecystectomy. AORN J. 2015;102(1):16-29.

Chawla L, Eggers P, Star R, et al. Acute kidney injury and chronic kidney disease as interconnected syndromes. N Eng J Med. 2014;371(1):58-66.

Ferri F. Pancreatitis, chronic. In Ferri FF, ed. 2018 Ferri's Clinical Advisor: 5 Books in 1 2018. Philadelphia, PA: Elsevier; 2018.

Fullwood D, Purushothaman A. Managing ascites in patients with chronic liver disease. Nurs Stand. 2014;28(23):51-58.

Garber A, Frakes C, Arora Z, et al. Mechanisms and management of acute pancreatitis. Gastroenterol Res Pract. 2018;1-8. doi:10.1155/2018/6218798.

Greenslade L. Providing high-quality care for patients with liver disease. Br J Nurs. 2017;26(13):739.

Henriques J, Correia M. Are postoperative intravenous fluids in patients undergoing elective laparoscopic cholecystectomy a necessity? A randomized clinical trial. Surgery. 2018;63(4):721-725.

Jack K, Cooper J, Ryder S. Hepatitis B virus part 1: risk factors, blood results and nursing care. Gastrointest Nurs. 2013;11(3):37-41.

Jack K, Barnett J, Holiday A, et al. Hepatitis C therapy at home: a hospital and home care partnership. Br J Nurs. 2013;22(9):518-523.

Kornusky J, Caple C. Quick Lesson: Acute Pancreatitis, CINAHL Nursing Guide. July 20, 2018.

Leaper J, Hamlim S. Dispelling dietary myths of liver disease. Gastrointest. Nurs. 2013;12(2):45-49.

Lin E, Chertow G, Yan B, et al. Cost-effectiveness of multi-disciplinary care in mild to moderate chronic kidney disease in the United States: a modeling study. PLOS Med. 2018;15(3):1-29.

Majumder S, Chari S. Chronic pancreatitis. Lancet. 2016;387(10031):1957-1966.

Nicoll R, Robertson L, Gemmel E, et al. Models of care for chronic kidney disease: a systematic review. Nephrology. 2018;23:389-396.

Nordqvist C. What to know about cholecystitis? Medical News Today. Available at: https://www.medicalnewstoday.com/articles/172067.php. Accessed January, 2018

Oshodi T, Bench C. Ventilator-associated pneumonia, liver disease and oral chlorhexidine. Br J Nurs. 2013;22(13):751-758.

Pak M, Lindseth G. Risk factors for cholelithiasis. Gastroenterol. Nurs. 2016;39(4):297-309.

Pilger E, Costanzo C. Screening and management of hepatitis C: use education to dispel the myths about the disease and increase screening and treatments. Am Nurse Today. 2018;13(9):70-72.

Roberts G. Pancreatitis. Contin Educ Top Issues. 2018;4-10.

Staubli SM, Oertli D, Nebiker CA. Laboratory markers predicting severity of acute pancreatitis. Crit Rev Clin Laborat Sci. 2015;52(6):273-283.

Swoboda S. Coordinating care for patients with biliary and pancreatic disorders. In: Hoffman J, Sullivan N, eds. Medical-Surgical Nursing: Making Connections to Practice. Philadelphia: F.A. Davis; 2017:1321-1339.

Swoboda S. Coordinating care for patients with hepatic disorders. In: Hoffman J, Sullivan N, eds. Medical-Surgical Nursing: Making Connections to Practice. Philadelphia: F.A. Davis; 2017:1300-1320.

Tang F, Markus T. Acute pancreatitis. Medscape. February 13, 2017. Available at: https://emedicine.medscape.com/article/181364-overview.

Tenner S, Baillie J, DeWitt J, et al. American college of gastroenterology guideline: management of acute pancreatitis. Am J Gastroenterol. 2013;1-16. Available at: www.amjgastro.com.

The National Pancreas Foundation. Acute pancreatitis risks and treatment. Available at: https://pancreasfoundation.org/patient-information/acute-pancreatitis/acute-pancreatitis-risks-and-treatment/.

Valizadeh L, Zamanzadeh V, Bayani M, et al. The social stigma experience in patients with Hepatitis B infection: a qualitative study. *Gastroenterol Nurs.* 2017;40(2):143-150.

Verhaegh B, Reijven P, Prins M, et al. Nutritional status in patients with chronic pancreatitis. *Eur J Clin Nutr.* 2013;67:1271-1276.

Webster A, Nagler E, Morton R, et al. Chronic kidney disease. *The Lancet.* 2017;389(10075):1238-1252.

Williams S. Nursing Interventions on medication adherence during hepatitis C treatment: application of self-regulation model. *Gastroenterol Nurs.* 2018;41(6):525-531.

Xiaolan W, Cuiqing L, Yulan Z, et al. The effect of nursing intervention of postoperative thirst in patients after laparoscopic cholecystectomy. *Am J Nurs Sci.* 2018;7(3):106-108.

Zou L, Ke L, Li W, et al. Enteral nutrition within 72 h after onset of acute pancreatitis vs delayed initiation. *Eur J Clin Nutr.* 2014;68:1288-1293.

12 THE CLIENT WITH ALTERATIONS IN THE KIDNEY AND URINARY TRACT

Abdelmowla RAA, Hussein AH, Shahat AA, et al. Impact of nursing interventions and patients education on quality of life regarding renal stones treated by percutaneous nephrolithotomy. *J Nurs Educ Pract.* 2017;7(12):52-63.

American Nephrology Nurses' Association. *Nephrology Nursing Scope and Standards of Practice.* 8th ed. Pittman, NJ: American Nephrology Nurses' Association; 2017.

American Nephrology Nurses' Association. *Core Curriculum for Nephrology Nurses.* 6th ed. Pittman, NJ: ANNA; 2016.

Anderson B. Bladder cancer: overview and disease management. part 1: non-muscle-invasive bladder cancer. *Br J Nurs* (Urology Supplement). 2018;27(9):S27-S37.

Brick N; Cochrane Nursing Care Field. Nutritional support for acute kidney injury. *Renal Soc Australas J.* 2011;7(2):94-95.

Bonfield B. Acute kidney injury: what is it and how can it be prevented? *Pract Nurs.* 2018;29(1):I10-115.

Dirkes S. Acute kidney injury: causes, phases, and early detection. *Am Nurse Today.* 2015;10(7):20-24.

Farling K, Walker J. Coordinating care for patients with urinary disorders. In: Hoffman J, Sullivan N, eds. *Medical-Surgical Nursing: Making Connections to Practice.* Philadelphia: F.A. Davis; 2017:1401-1415.

Godin M, Bouchard J, Mehta R. Fluid balance in patients with acute kidney injury: emerging concepts. *Neph Clin Pract.* 2013;123(3-4):238-245.

Goetz LL, Klausner AP, Cardenas DD. Bladder dysfunction. In: Cifu DX, ed. *Braddom's Physical Medicine and Rehabilitation.* 5th ed. Philadelphia: Elsevier; 2016.

Gomez, N. *Nephrology Nursing Scope and Standards from Practice.* Pitman, NJ: American Nephrology Nurses Association; 2017.

Harty J. Prevention and management of acute kidney injury. Ulster Med J. 2014;83(3):149-157.

Hain D, Paixao R. The perfect storm: older adults and acute kidney injury. *Crit Care Nurs Q.* 2015;38(3):271-279.

Hess C, Linnebur S, Rhyne D, et al. Over-the-counter drugs to avoid in older adults with kidney impairment. *Nephrol Nurs J.* 2016;43(5):389-400.

Lang J. Taking action against acute kidney injury in primary care. *Clin Adv.* 2014;17(11):41-48.

Lang J, Zaber Davis J. Acute kidney injury. *J Am Acad Phys Assist.* 2016;29(4):5-54.

Lewis R. An overview of chronic kidney disease in older people. *Nurs Older People.* 2014;25(10):31-38.

Moore P, Hsu R, Liu K. Management of acute kidney injury: core curriculum 2018. *Am J Kidney Dis.* 2018;72(1):136-148.

Newman D, Burgio K. Conservative management of urinary incontinence: behavioral and pelvic floor therapy and urethral and pelvic devices. In: Wein A, Kavoussi L, Partin A, et al., eds. *Campbell-Walsh Urology.* 11th ed. Philadelphia, PA: Elsevier; 2016.

Pfau A, Knauf F. Update on nephrolithiasis: core curriculum 2016. *Am J Kidney Dis.* 2016;68(6):973-985.

Pinnington S, Ingleby S, Hanumapura P, et al. Assessing and documenting fluid balance. *Nursing Stand.* 2016;31(15):46-54.

Thomas-Hawkins C, Zazworsky D. Self-management of chronic kidney disease. *Am J Nurs.* 2005;105(10):40-48.

Thornburg B, Gray-Vickrey P. Acute kidney injury: limiting the damage. *Nursing.* 2016;46(6):24-34.

Weber J, Purvis S, VanDenBergh S, et al. Standardizing practice for intermittent irrigation of indwelling urinary catheters. *J Nurs Care Qual.* 2017; 32(3):202-206.

Williams J, Baptiste D, Sullivan N. Coordinating care for patients with renal disorders. In: Hoffman J, Sullivan N, eds. *Medical-Surgical Nursing: Making Connections to Practice.* Philadelphia: F.A. Davis; 2017:1367-1400.

13 THE CLIENT WITH ALTERATIONS IN MUSCULOSKELETAL FUNCTION

A'Court J, Lees D, Harrison W, et al. Pain and analgesia requirements with hip fracture surgery. *Orthopaed Nurs.* 2017;36(3):224-228.

Alviar M, Hale T, Lim-Dungca M. Pharmacologic interventions for treating phantom limb pain. *Cochrane Database Systemat Rev.* 2016;(10):CD006380. Available at: https://www.cochranelibrary.com/cdsr/doi/10.1002/14651858.CD006380.pub3/epdf/full.

Andrews L. Different types of intermittent pneumatic compression devices for preventing venous thromboembolism in patients after total hip replacement. *Orthop Nurs.* 2016;35(6):424-425.

Biz C, Fantoni I, Crepaldi N, et al. Clinical practice and nursing management of pre-operative skin or skeletal traction for hip fractures in elderly patients: a cross-sectional three-institution study. *Int J Orthop Trauma Nurs.* 2018; S1878–1241(18)30048-0.

Bonner L, Johnson J. Deep vein thrombosis: diagnosis and treatment. *Nurs Stand.* 2014;28(21):51-58.

Corbett M, South E, Harden M, et al. Brain and spinal stimulation therapies for phantom limb pain: a systematic review. *Health Technol Assess.* 2018;22(62):1-94.

D'Alesandro M. Focusing on lower extremity DVT. *Nursing.* 2016;46(4):28-35.

Dykes P. Preventing falls in hospitalized patients. *Am Nurse Today.* 2018;13(9):8-13.

Esoga P, Seidl K. Best practices in orthopaedic inpatient care. *Orthop Nurs.* 2012;31(4):236-240.

Finn DM, Agarwal RR, Ilfeld BM, et al. Fall risk associated with continuous peripheral nerve blocks following knee and hip arthroplasty. *MEDSURG Nurs.* 2016;25(1):25-49.

Forsh D. Deep Venous Thrombosis Prophylaxis in *Orthopedic Surgery.* *MedScape.* Available at: https://emedicine.medscape.com/article/1268573-overview. Accessed August 30, 2018.

Grigoryan K Javedan H, Rudolph J. Ortho-Geriatric care models and outcomes in hip fracture patients: a systematic review and meta-analysis. *J Orthop Trauma.* 2014;28(3):e49-e55. doi:10.1097/BOT.0b013e3182a5a045.

Gwynne-Jones D, Martin G, Crane C. Enhanced recovery after surgery for hip and knee replacements. *Orthop Nurs.* 2017;35(3):203-210.

Haertel S. Postoperative knee bracing. *Orthop Nurs.* 2018;37(5):325-327.

Lee M, Moorhead S. Nursing care patterns for patients receiving total hip replacements. *Orthop. Nurs.* 2014;33(3):149-158.

Majid N, Plummer V. The effectiveness of orthopedic patient education in improving patient outcomes: a systematic review protocol. *JBI Database System Rev Implement Rep.* 2015;13(1):122-133. doi:10.11124/jbisrir-2015-1950.

McNichol L, Lund C, Rosen T, et al. Medical adhesives and patient safety: consensus statements for the assessment, prevention, and treatment of adhesive-related skin injuries. *Orthop Nurs.* 2013;32(5):267-281.

Nonpharmacologic Management of Pain in Adults and Children. University of Florida College of Medicine-Jacksonville, Department of Emergency Medicine. Pain Assessment and Management Initiative (PAMI): A Patient Safety Project. Available at: http://pami.emergency.med.jax.ufl.edu/. Accessed October 17, 2018.

Ouellette D. Pulmonary Embolism. *MedScape.* Available at: https://emedicine.medscape.com/article/300901-overview. Accessed June 21, 2018.

Richardson C, Kulkarni J. A review of the management of phantom limb pain: challenges and solutions. *J Pain Res.* 2017;10:1861-1870.

Twig R, Kulik S. Coordinating care for patients with musculoskeletal disorders. In: Hoffman J, Sullivan N, eds. *Medical-Surgical Nursing: Making Connections to Practice.* Philadelphia: F. A. Davis; 2017:1142-1172.

Virani A, Green T, Turin TC. Phantom limb pain: a nursing perspective. *Nurs Stand.* 2014;29(1):44-50.

White D, Kulik S. Coordinating care for patients with musculoskeletal trauma. In: Hoffman J, Sullivan N, eds. Medical-Surgical Nursing: *Making Connections to Practice.* Philadelphia: F. A. Davis; 2017:1173-1194.

Wilson K, Devito D, Zavotsky K, et al. Keep it moving and remember to P.A.C. (pharmacology, ambulation, and compression) for venous thromboembolism prevention. *Orthop Nurs.* 2018;37(6):339-345.

Yager M, Stichler J. The effect of early ambulation on patient outcomes for total joint replacement. *Orthop. Nurs.* 2014;34(4):197-200.

14 THE CLIENT WITH ALTERATIONS IN THE BREAST AND REPRODUCTIVE SYSTEM

Ahern T, Gardner A, Courtney M. A survey of the breast care nurse role in the provision of information and supportive care to Australian women diagnosed with breast cancer. *Nurs Open.* 2015;2(2):62-71.

American Cancer Society. Surgery for breast cancer. 2016. Available at: https://www.cancer.org/cancer/breast-cancer/treatment/surgery-for-breast-cancer.html. Accessed November 27, 2018.

Bernier F. Kegel Exercises for Men for Pelvic Floor Strengthening. Available at: https://simonfoundation.org/kegel-exercises-for-men/. Accessed October 2018.

Cancer Information Network. Available at: www.cancerlinksusa.com.

Caple C, Schub T. Breast cancer in women: the effect on the family. *CINAHL Nursing Guide;* May 18, 2018; (Evidence-Based Care Sheet) AN: T700924.

Chun C. What you need to know about breast cancer. *Medical News Today.* Available at: https://www.medicalnewstoday.com/articles/37136.php. Accessed November, 2018.

Collins M. Transurethral resection of the prostate. *MedScape.* Available at: https://emedicine.medscape.com/article/449781-overviewMedscape. Accessed November 27, 2016.

DePolo J. Regular Exercise During Treatment After Breast Cancer Surgery Offers Benefits. 2018. Breastcancer.org. Available at: https://www.breastcancer.org/research-news/exercise-during-tx-after-sx-offers-benefits.

DeVita V, Hellman JR. Rosenberg S, eds. *Cancer: Principles and Practice of Oncology.* 11th ed. Philadelphia: Lippincott Williams & Wilkins; 2018.

Ferrari C. Nursing care orientations for women under treatment for breast cancer. *J Nurs UFPE.* 2018;12(3):676-683.

Freire M, Hagen BM, de Lima CF, et al. Breast cancer and its treatments: repercussions in Sexuality lived by women. *J Nurs UFPE.* 2017;11(11):4511-4514.

Gilmore F, Williams A. Support with nutrition for women receiving chemotherapy for breast cancer. *Br J Nurs.* 2018;27(4):S4-S9.

Guthrie C. Finding strength after fighting breast cancer. *Health.com;*88-89.

Isardas G, Holle M. Breast cancer: psychological adjustment. *CINAHL Nursing Guide.* December 01, 2017.

(Evidence-Based Care Sheet) AN: T700965.

Javid S, Lawrence S, Lavallee D. Prioritizing patient-reported outcomes in breast cancer surgery quality improvement. *Breast J.* 2017;23(2):127-137.

Kim N, Shin BC, Shin JS, et al. Dietary pattern and health-related quality of life among breast cancer survivors. *BMC Women's Health.* 2018;18:65. doi:10.1186/s12905-018-0555-7.

Kruger, N. Improving patient outcomes: decorative tattoos, breast cancer and lymphedema. *Wounds UK.* 2018;14(2):12-16.

Lambadiari M, Aikaterini,L, Ioannis I, et al. General health condition of young women with breast cancer depending on surgical and adjuvant treatment. *Int J Caring Sci.* 2017;10(3):1201-1207.

Lee A. Coordinating care for female patients with reproductive and breast disorders. In: Hoffman J, Sullivan N, eds. *Medical-Surgical Nursing: Making connections to practice.* Philadelphia: F. A. Davis; 2017:1434.

Lesiuk T. The effect of mindfulness-based music therapy on attention and mood in women receiving adjuvant chemotherapy for breast cancer: a pilot study. *Oncol Nurs Forum.* 2015;42(3):276-282.

Leysen L, Beckwée D, Nijs J, et al. Risk factors of pain in breast cancer survivors: a systematic review and meta-analysis. *Support Care Cancer.* 2017;25:3607-3643.

Lynn S. Coordinating care for male patients with reproductive and breast disorders. In: Hoffman J, Sullivan N, eds. *Medical-Surgical Nursing: Making connections to practice.* Philadelphia: F.A. Davis; 2017:1459-1478.

Montpetit C, Singh-Carlson S. Engaging patients with radiation related skin discomfort in self-care. *Can Oncol Nurs J.* 2018;28(3):191-211.

Pilgrim J, Morgan H. Breast cancer: treatment with surgery. *CINAHL Nursing Guide.* January 26, 2018. (Evidence-Based Care Sheet) AN: T700811.

Reis D, Jones T. Aromatherapy: using essential oils as a supportive therapy. *Clin J Oncol Nurs.* 2017;21(1):16-21.

Reis A, Gradim C. Alopecia in breast cancer. *J Nurs UFPE.* 2018;12(2):447-455.

Schub T, Holle M. Breast cancer in older women. *CINAHL Nursing Guide.* June 08, 2018; (Evidence-Based Care Sheet) AN: T700983.

Schreiber M. Postoperative nursing considerations: transurethral resection of the prostate. *MEDSURG Nurs.* 2017;26(6):419-422.

Schub, T, Holle M. Breast cancer: treatment with systemic therapy. *CINAHL Nursing Guide.* November 17, 2017. (Evidence-Based Care Sheet - CEU) AN: T700839.

Schub E, Kornusky J. Breast cancer: treatment and disease-related fatigue. *CINAHL Nursing Guide.* July 27, 2018. (Evidence-Based Care Sheet) AN: T700993.

Uribe L, DeVesty G. Breast cancer: management of treatment-induced hot flashes. *CINAHL Nursing Guide.* December 29, 2017. (Evidence-Based Care Sheet) AN: T700884.

Ward-Sullivan C, Leutwyler H, Dunn LB, et al. Differences in symptom clusters identified using symptom occurrence rates versus severity ratings in patients with breast cancer undergoing chemotherapy. *Eur J Oncol Nurs.* 2017;122-132.

Ward-Sullivan C. Stability of symptom clusters in patients with breast cancer receiving chemotherapy. *J Pain Symptom Manag.* 2018;55(1):39-54.

Ward-Sullivan C, Leutwyler H, Dunn LB, et al. A review of the literature on symptom clusters in studies that included oncology patients receiving primary or adjuvant chemotherapy. *J Clin Nurs.* 2017;1-30.

Waterkemper R. Nursing consultation for patients with continuous cancer description of the diagnosis, interventions and results. *J Nurs UFPE.* 2017;11(12):4838-4844.

Whisenant M, Wong B, Mitchell SA, et al. Distinct trajectories of fatigue and sleep disturbance in women receiving chemotherapy for breast cancer. *Oncol Nurs Forum.* 2017;44(6):739-750.

Yang S, Park DH, Ahn SH, et al. Prevalence and risk factors of adhesive capsulitis of the shoulder after breast cancer treatment. *Support Care Cancer.* 2017;25:1317-1322.

15 THE CLIENT RECEIVING TREATMENT FOR NEOPLASTIC DISORDERS

Abbott L, Hooke C. Energy Through Motion© An activity intervention for cancer-related fatigue in an ambulatory infusion center. *Clin J Oncol Nurs.* 2017;21(5):618-626.

American Cancer Society. Available at: www.cancer.org.

Bakker R, Mens JMW, de Groot HE, et al. A nurse-led sexual rehabilitation intervention after radiotherapy for gynecological cancer. *Support Care Cancer.* 2017;25:729-737.

Bauer C, Laszewski P, Magnan M. Promoting adherence to skin care practices among patients receiving radiation therapy. *Clin J Oncol Nurs.* 2015;19(20):196-203.

Bostock S, Bryan J. Radiotherapy-induced skin reactions: assessment and management. *Br J Nurs.* 2016;25(4):S18-S24.

Brachytherapy. Mayoclinic.com. Available at: https://www.mayoclinic.org/tests-procedures/brachytherapy/about/pac-20385159.

Brant JM, Eaton LH, Irwin MM. Cancer-related pain: assessment and management with putting evidence into practice interventions. *Clin J Oncol Nurs.* 2017;21(suppl 3):4-6.

Bratton S, Iannotta J. Nutritional interventions for managing adverse effect. *Oncol Nurse Adv.* 2017;22-26. Available at: www.OncologyNurseAdvisor.com.

Brigle K. Myelosuppression, bone disease, and acute renal failure. *Clin J Oncol Nurs.* 2017;21(suppl 5):60-76.

Chino F, Peppercorn JM, Rushing C, et al. Out-of-pocket costs, financial distress, and underinsurance in cancer care. *AMA Oncol.* 2018. [E-pub ahead of print], doi:10.1001/jamaoncol.2017.2148.

Coolbrandt A, Wildiers H, Aertgeerts B, et al. Systematic development of CHEMOSUPPORT, a nursing intervention to support adult patients with cancer in dealing with chemotherapy-related symptoms at home. *BMC Nurs.* 2018;17:28. doi:10.1186/s12912-018-0297-8.

Cuba F, Salum G. Cherubini K, et al. Cannabidiol: an alternative therapeutic agent for oral mucositis? *J Clin Pharm Therap.* 2017;42(3):245-250.

Danhauer S, Addington E, Sohl S, et al. Review of yoga therapy during cancer treatment. *Support Care Cancer.* 2017;25:1357-1372.

de Oliveira M, de Oliveira G, de Souza-Talarico J, et al. Surgical oncology: evolution of postoperative fatigue and factors related to its severity. Clin J Oncol Nurs. 2016;20(1):E3-E8.

de Oliveira T, de Jesus C. Uncertainties experiences by post-surgical patients diagnosed with neoplasms. *J Nurs UFPE.* 2018;12(10):2873-2882.

DeVita VT Jr, Hellman S, Rosenberg SA, eds. *Cancer: Principles and Practice of Oncology.* 11th ed. Philadelphia: Lippincott Williams & Wilkins; 2018.

Eaton L, Brant J, McLeod K, et al. Nonpharmacologic pain interventions: a review of evidence-based practices for reducing chronic cancer pain. *Clin J Oncol Nurs.* 2017;21(suppl 3):54-70, A1-A9.

Gallagher E, Rogers B, Brant J. Cancer-related pain assessment: monitoring the effectiveness of interventions. *Clin J Oncol Nurs.* 2017;21(suppl 2):8-12.

Hartnett E. Integrating oral health throughout cancer care. *Clin J Oncol Nurs.* 2017;19(5):615-619.

Haryani H, Fetzer J, Wu C, et al. Chemotherapy-induced peripheral neuropathy assessment tools: a systematic review. *Oncol Nurs Forum.* 2017;44(3):E111-E123.

Hitchcock J, Savine L. Medical adhesive-related skin injuries associated with vascular access. *Br J Nurs* (IV Therapy Supplement). 2017;26(8):S4-S12.

Johns S, Brown LF, Beck-Coon K, et al. Randomized controlled pilot trial of mindfulness-based stress reduction compared to psychoeducational support for persistently fatigued breast and colorectal cancer survivors. *Support Care Cancer.* 2016;24:4085-4096.

Jordan K, Feyer P, Höller U, et al. Supportive treatments for patients with cancer. *Dtsch Arztebl Int.* 2017;11:481-487.

Kim S, Kim K, Meyer D. Self-management intervention for adult cancer survivors after treatment: a systematic review and meta-analysis. *Oncol Nurs Forum.* 2017;44(6):719-728.

Kwekkeboom K. Cancer symptom cluster management. *Semin Oncol Nurs.* 2016;32(4):373-382. Available at: https://www.ncbi.nlm.nih.gov/pmc/articles/PMC5143160/pdf/nihms-781147.pdf.

McCoy C, Paredes M, Allen S, et al. Catheter-associated urinary tract infections: implementing a protocol to decrease incidence in oncology populations. *Clin J Oncol Nurs.* 2017;21(4):460-465.

Milligan F, Martinez F, Aal SHMA, et al. Assessing anxiety and depression in cancer patients. *Br J Nurs.* 2018;27(10):S18-S23.

Mitra S, Dash R. Natural products for the management and prevention of breast cancer. *Evidence-Based Complementary Alternative Med.* 2018;23.

Muzumder S, Nirmala S, Avinash H, et al. Analgesic and opioid use in pain associated with head-and-neck radiation therapy. *Ind J Palliat Care.* 2018;24(2):176-178.

National Cancer Institute. Available at: www.nci.nih.gov.

Pai R, Ongole, R. Nurses' knowledge and education about oral care of cancer patients undergoing chemotherapy and radiation therapy. *Ind J Palliative Care.* 2015;21(2):225-230.

Pessi R, Feuercgutte KK, da Rosa LM, et al. Prevention of vaginal stenosis after brachytherapy: nursing intervention. *J Nurs UFPE.* 2016;10(9):3495-3502.

Riley E. Understanding oral mucositis: causes and treatments. *JCN.* 2017;31(5):69-72.

Samantarath P, Pongthavornkamol K, Olson K, et al. Multiple symptoms and their influences on health-related quality of life in adolescents with hematologic malignancies undergoing chemotherapy. *Pacific Rim Int J Nurs Res.* 2018;22(4):319-331.

Scot A. Non-sting barrier cream in radiotherapy-induced skin reactions. *Br J Nurs.* 2015;24(10):S32-S37.

Shelton B. Overview of cancer care. In: Hoffman J, Sullivan N, eds. *Medical-Surgical Nursing: Making Connections to Practice.* Philadelphia: F. A. Davis; 2017:213-245.

Sundaramurthi T, Gallagher N, Sterling B. Cancer-related acute pain: a systematic review of evidence-based interventions for putting evidence into practice. *Clin J Oncol.* 2017;21(suppl 3):13-30, A1-A6.

Wodzinski A. Potential benefits of oral cryotherapy for chemotherapy-induced mucositis. *Clin J Oncol Nurs.* 2016;20(5):462-465.

Yarbro CH, Wujcik D, Holmes-Gobel B, eds. *Cancer Nursing: Principles and Practice.* 8th ed. Burlington, Mass: Jones & Bartlett; 2018.

16 NURSING CARE OF THE ELDERLY CLIENT

Boltz M, Capezuti E, Fulmer T, Zeicker D. *Evidence-based Geriatric Nursing Protocols for Best Practice.* 5th ed. New York: Springer.

Brook S. Nutritional considerations in older adults. *Br J Commun Nurs.* 2018;23(9):449-452.

Brown L. Untangling polypharmacy in older adults. *MEDSURG Nurs.* 2016;25(5):408-411.

Cost D. Geriatric implications for Medical-Surgical Nursing. In: Hoffman J, Sullivan N, eds. *Medical-Surgical Nursing: Making Connections to Practice.* Philadelphia: F. A. Davis; 2017:55-72.

de Lima P. Educational activities on cardiovascular health for the elderly people at home. *J Nurs UFPE.* 2017;11(11):4498-4504.

Geriatric Nursing. Psychological care of the Elderly. Available at: https://geriatricnursing.org/psychological-care-of-the-elderly/.

Gothe N, Kramer A, McAuley E. Hatha yoga practice Improves Attention and processing speed in older adults: results from an 8-week randomized control trial. *J Alternat Complement Med.* 2017;23(1):35-40.

Gray M. Case Studies in geriatric urology: focus on continence in the older adult. *Urol Nurs.* 2017;37(3):143-170.

Lee P. Effect of exercise on depressive symptoms and body balance in the elderly. *Educ Gerontol.* 2017;43(1):33-44.

Moreira M, Bilton T, Dias C, et al. What are the main physical functioning factors associated with falls among older people with different perceived fall risk? *Physiother Res Int.* 2017;22:1-11.

Ojo O. Meeting the nutritional needs of older patients in the hospital setting. *Br J Nurs.* 2018;27(8):426-428.

Sampoornam W, Soorya C, Ranjana G, et al. Efficiency of walking exercise on sleep pattern among geriatrics-A dose response analysis. *Int J Nurs Educ.* 2016;8(3):138-142.

Stuart E. Importance of good nutrition for the older community. *JCN.* 2018;32(3):16.

Suzuki K, Miyamoto M, Hirata K. Sleep disorders in the elderly: diagnosis and management. *J Gen Fam Med.* 2017;18:61-71.

Touhy T, Jett K. *Ebersole and Hess' Gerontological Nursing & Healthy Aging.* 5th ed. St. Louis: Mosby-Elsevier, Inc; 2018.

Touhy T, Jett K. *Ebersole & Hess' Toward Healthy Aging: Human Needs and Nursing Response.* 9th ed. St. Louis: Mosby-Elsevier, Inc; 2016.

Vieira C. Risk factors associated with falls in elderly. *J Nurs UFPE.* 2016;10(11):4028-4035.

Williams P. *Basic Geriatric Nursing.* 6th ed. St. Louis: Mosby-Elsevier, Inc; 2016.

Wood C. Ensuring good nutrition for older patients in the community. *JCN.* 2017;31(3):49-51.

Yates A. Urinary continence care for older people in the acute setting. *Br J Nurs* (Urology Supplement). 2017;26(9):S28-S30.

17 END-OF-LIFE NURSING CARE

Albert R. End-of-life care: managing common symptoms. *Am Fam Phys.* 2017;95(6):356-361.

American Nephrology Nurses Association. Position statement: nephrology nurse's role in palliative and end-of-life care. *Nephrol Nurs J.* 2018;45(6):549-551.

American Nurses Association. Nurses' roles and responsibilities in providing care and support at the end of life. Available at: https://www.nursingworld.org/~4af078/globalassets/docs/ana/ethics/endoflife-positionstatement.pdf.

Bükki J, Unterpaul T, Nübling G, et al. Decision making at the end of life—cancer patients' and their caregivers' views on artificial nutrition and hydration. *Support Care Cancer.* 2014;22:3287-3299.

Campbell M. Ensuring breathing comfort at the end of life: the integral role of the critical care nurse. *Am J Critical Care.* 2018;27(4):264-269.

Coelho A, Parola V, Cardoso D, et al. Use of non-pharmacological interventions for comforting patients in palliative care: a scoping review. *JBI Database Systemat Rev Implement Rep.* 2017;15(7):1867-1904.

Cook L. Fluid and electrolyte management. In: Hoffman J, Sullivan N, eds. *Medical-Surgical Nursing: Making Connections to Practice.* Philadelphia: F. A. Davis; 2017:103-132.

Coyne P, Mulvenon C, Paice J. American society for pain management nursing and hospice and palliative nurses association position statement: pain management at the end of life. *Pain Manag Nurs.* 2018;19(1):3-7.

Farrington N, Fader M, Richardson A. Managing urinary incontinence at the end of life: an examination of the evidence that informs practice. *Int J Palliative Nurs.* 2013;19(9):449-456.

Grewe F. The soul's legacy: a program designed to help prepare senior adults cope with end-of-life existential distress. *J Health Care Chaplaincy.* 2017;23:1-14.

Lessans S. Pain management. In: Hoffman J, Sullivan N, eds. Medical-Surgical Nursing: *Making connections to practice.* Philadelphia: F. A. Davis; 2017:164-201.

Matzo M, Sherman D, eds. *Palliative Care Nursing: Quality Care to the End of Life.* 4th ed. New York: Springer; 2015.

Muecke R. Complementary and alternative medicine in palliative care: a comparison of data from surveys among patients and professionals. *Integr Cancer Ther.* 2016;15(1):10-16.

Nunn C. It's not just about pain: symptom management in palliative care. *Nurse Prescrib.* 2014;12(7):338-344.

Owens D. Oxygen therapy management. In: Hoffman J, Sullivan N, eds. *Medical-Surgical Nursing: Making Connections to Practice.* Philadelphia: F. A. Davis; 2017:73-102.

Phillips C, McNab C, Loewen L. Advance care planning and chronic kidney disease: what do patients know and what do they want? *Nephrol Nurs J.* 2018;45(6):513-523.

Pickstock S. Breathlessness at end of life: what community nurses should know. *JCN.* 2017;31(5):74-77.

Prichard D, Bharucha A. Management of opioid-induced constipation for people in palliative care. *Int J Palliat Nurs.* 2015; 21(6):272-280.

Sartorius-Mergenthaler S. Complementary and alternative care initiatives. In: Hoffman J, Sullivan N, eds. *Medical-Surgical Nursing: Making connections to practice.* Philadelphia: F. A. Davis; 2017:202-212.

Silva R, Caldeira S, Coelho A, et al. Forgiveness facilitation in palliative care: a scoping review protocol. *JBI Database Systemat Rev Implement Rep.* 2017;15(10):2469-2479.

Zeng Y, Wang C, Ward K, et al. Complementary and alternative medicine in hospice and palliative care: a systematic review. *J Pain Symptom Manag.* 2018;56(5): 781-794.

Index